NEURAL MECHANISMS
OF LEARNING
AND MEMORY

The nervous system of a representative invertebrate, the gastropod mollusc *Pleurobranchaea californica*, which is the subject of experiments on the cellular basis of choice and learning (see Chapter 29). A, dorsal view of an intact specimen. The anterior feeding proboscis is extended from beneath the oral veil at the top of the photograph. This specimen was 15 cm in length. B, a view of the nervous system, exposed by a dorsal longitudinal incision in the anterior third of the animal. The anterior brain (top) is 1 cm wide and connected to the buccal ganglion by two nerves, the cerebrobuccal connectives. Note the many cell bodies, some of which reach 1 mm in diameter and are plainly visible with the unaided eye. C, a living, unstained brain (dorsal view), showing the numerous, brightly pigmented nerve-cell bodies as they appear through the dissecting microscope. D, a brain following back-injection of the left cerebrobuccal connective with cobalt chloride and subsequent precipitation of cobalt sulfide in the filled neurons. This technique has been used in this instance to identify anatomically and map the positions of interneurons that turn on the feeding behavior (Davis et al., 1974), in preparation for electrophysiological studies. These interneurons may be the loci of physiological changes that underlie learning in this preparation. E, a living, unstained buccal ganglion (dorsal view). Most of the cell bodies that are visible belong to motoneurons that supply feeding musculature (Siegler, Mpitsos, and Davis, 1974). F, a buccal ganglion following back-injection of the third buccal root, a nerve that supplies feeding musculature active during withdrawal of the feeding proboscis. Most of the filled cell bodies belong to identified feeding motoneurons. G, a brain following back-injection of the right cerebrovisceral connective. H, an isolated nervous system showing the brain (top), buccal ganglion (bottom), and lateral pedal ganglia. Neurophysiological experiments on associative learning are being conducted on this relatively simple preparation. (See Chapter 29 for references.)

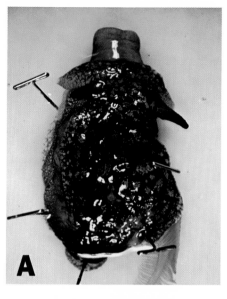

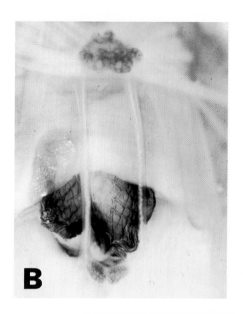

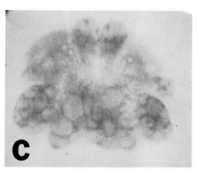

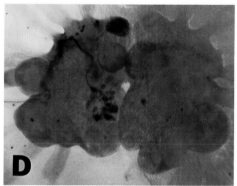

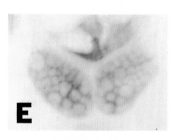

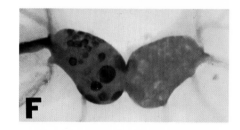

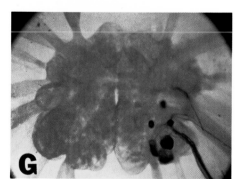

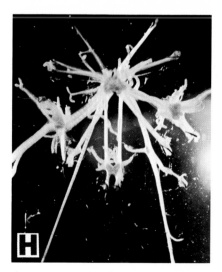

NEURAL MECHANISMS OF LEARNING AND MEMORY

Mark R. Rosenzweig and Edward L. Bennett
EDITORS

PREPARED WITH THE SUPPORT OF
THE NATIONAL INSTITUTE OF EDUCATION

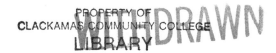

The MIT Press
Cambridge, Massachusetts, and
London, England

This work was developed under a contract with (or grant from)
Department of Health, Education, and Welfare, National
Institute of Education. However, the opinions and other con-
tent do not necessarily reflect the position or policy of the
Agency, and no official endorsement should be inferred.

This book was printed and bound
by The Colonial Press Inc.
in the United States of America

Library of Congress Cataloging in Publication Data
Main entry under title:

Neural mechanisms of learning and memory.

    Papers presented at a conference held at Asilomar,
Calif., June 24–28, 1974.
      Bibliography: p.
      Includes indexes.
      1. Memory—Congresses. 2. Information theory in
biology—Congresses. 3. Neuropsychology—Congresses.
I. Rosenzweig, Mark R. II. Bennett, Edward L.
III. National Institute of Education. [DNLM: 1. Learn-
ing—Congresses. 2. Memory—Congresses. 3. Neuro-
physiology—Congresses. WL102 N4933 1974]
QP406.N48   612′.82   75–35780
ISBN 0–262–18076–6

Contents

41430

Preface

This volume presents papers given during a five-day conference dealing with current research approaches being used to find out how learning and memory occur in terms of neural processes. The conference, sponsored by the National Institute of Education, took place on 24–28 June 1974 at Asilomar, California. It included about seventy participants, who came from England, France, and the U.S.S.R., as well as from all parts of the United States. Most of the papers had been circulated in draft form in advance of the meeting, and they have been revised for publication on the basis of extensive discussions at Asilomar and continued work after the conference.

The product of the conference was intended to be helpful to a number of groups: (1) researchers and students working on these problems; (2) members of government agencies and private foundations who need to be informed about the state of research in this area; and (3) members of the public who want to keep in touch with this active and challenging field.

Since the goal of understanding the neural bases of learning and memory involves workers in many disciplines, the two conveners of the conference were fortunate in recruiting a well-informed and creative Planning Committee. Many of the main decisions about format and participants in the conference were made at the meeting of the Planning Committee in July 1973. The committee included Richard Atkinson, Murray E. Jarvik, Arnold L. Leiman, James L. McGaugh, Robert Y. Moore, Burton Rosner, and Felix Strumwasser, as well as the two editors.

In some cases participants who were nominated originally proved not to be available or had to withdraw for various reasons, but excellent replacements were enlisted, some on rather short notice. Participants agreed to prepare their contributions well in advance, and most of the drafts were circulated before the meeting. Each participant also agreed to arrive the day before the opening session and to remain throughout the week in order to maximize exchanges. The conference was meant to be not simply a set of formal presentations, but also an opportunity for researchers to get to know each other and to talk to each other. Since progress in the field will depend upon young scientists, each participant was invited to nominate a junior participant (an advanced student or young postdoctoral researcher), and twenty junior participants attended and took part in the discussions.

Since the desirability of informal discussion was a major consideration, it was decided to keep the number of presentations relatively small. The Planning Committee also decided not to try to cover all current research approaches, but to limit the program to certain main ones. The final scope of the conference was determined partly by judgments of the committee and partly by the availability of participants to represent various approaches.

In order to provide for journalistic coverage without having this influence the form of presentations or discussions, we invited Dr. Irving Bengelsdorf to attend and to prepare a report for science writers and for the public. We requested participants to cooperate with him before, during, and after the meeting, and he has worked closely with us in preparing the report that was circulated by NIE.

Each major topic was the subject of one or two review papers. In addition, each review paper was taken up from a different point of view by one or two designated discussants, as well as being the subject of free discussion from the floor. Needless to say, no difference in competence was implied by inviting certain investigators to be reviewers and others to be discussants; the roles could just as well have been reversed. Furthermore, as it turned out, some of the discussion papers are fuller and broader than some of the reviews. The reviewers and discussants were asked to keep certain basic goals and objectives in mind when preparing their papers. It was emphasized that we wanted, not simply a report of each participant's own research, but, rather, reviews of main fields. The aims set forth for the reviewers and discussants were these:

1. To produce critical evaluations of the progress and potentialities of several of the main current research approaches.

2. To acquaint participants with a variety of approaches other than their own, and to encourage a consideration of the use of other methods.

3. Through the wide interdisciplinary participation, to try to note and bring to the attention of the group developments and techniques of other sciences that might be brought to bear on problems of learning and memory.

4. To suggest areas that may be ready or nearing readiness for application, or where applied research should be undertaken.

5. To bring the results of the conference to a wide audience through publication of the proceedings.

It was our intention that each chapter should be understandable by scientists not in the particular specialized field, and also by students in advanced college courses and in graduate courses. These broad aims were realized to a greater or lesser extent in the various chapters, depending in part upon the state of the subfield and in part upon the interests and inclinations of the writers. Each of the papers gives a current view of a facet of the field by a highly qualified investigator, and, taken together, these chapters present a broad, varied, and comprehensive portrayal of the field.

Finally, we are happy to render a number of sincere acknowledgments. First, to the National Institute of Education, which sponsored the conference, and to Dr. John Mays, science advisor to the National Institute of Education, who worked closely with us through all of the planning stages, who participated in the conference at Asilomar, and with whom we have been in close contact during the preparation of this volume. Next, we would like to thank the committee with whom we met in July 1973 to plan the details of the conference. During the week of the conference, Hillary Katz and Bogdan Roman helped in many ways with the physical arrangements and with the operation of the projectors.

Our very special thanks go to Mrs. Jessie Langford, who has worked with us from the very first ideas about this conference through the final editing of this volume. She helped to prepare the initial plans and then corresponded with all the participants; she set up all of the formal matters necessary for the smooth running of the conference and was on the spot to solve any problems that arose. Later she handled the voluminous correspondence with the authors, and she participated in the detailed editing of all the chapters. We are deeply indebted to Mrs. Langford for her effective, accurate, and tireless work from the conception of the conference to the appearance of this volume.

Introduction: Prospects for Application of Research on Neural Mechanisms of Learning and Memory

MARK R. ROSENZWEIG AND
EDWARD L. BENNETT

The chapters of this volume offer a rich and varied panorama of research largely directed toward understanding the biological processes involved in learning and memory. Such basic research is undertaken with the hope, often implicit but amply justified by history, that it will eventually lead to applications that become socially beneficial. As such basic research is pursued, it may supply concepts and techniques that can be applied to problems such as improving classroom teaching, alleviating the difficulties of the retarded, the aphasic, and the senile, and fostering the fullest development of human intellectual potential. To a large degree, of course, responsibility for application is incumbent on those individuals and groups who are keenly aware of specific social problems upon which scientific knowledge needs to be focused. Becoming aware of current scientific resources, they may be able to select concepts and techniques that will provide a solution. Or, finding the absence of suitable knowledge, they can call attention to the need. The recognition of a need has been a prime factor in achieving outstanding applied advances, according to a recent study, "Interactions of Science and Technology in the Innovative Process: Some Case Studies" (NSF, 1973). We hope, therefore, that this volume will not only aid and encourage basic researchers, but will also serve as a survey of the state of the art that can be drawn upon for applications and used to find areas where fresh efforts are needed. We already have evidence that the conference will aid researchers, since some of the participants have told us that their experiences at the meeting have led them to make changes in their research programs. We hope in the longer run to see evidence that the conference and this volume have led to applications.

What are some specific applications to practical problems of learning and of teaching that may come, sooner or later, from the lines of basic research described in the chapters of this volume? For an overview of the many and varied directions of research, we can describe seven levels (see also Table 40.1, p. 599):

A. Behavioral descriptions of learning and memory
B. Formal systems approaches

C. Molar or general neural processes
D. Regional localization of neural processes involved in learning and memory
E. Changes in synapses and neural circuits as bases of learning and memory
F. Use of simpler systems for detailed study of neural processes in learning and memory
G. Study of learning, memory, and neural changes in developing subjects.

We shall now note some possible applications that may emerge as research is pursued at each of these levels, although in many cases, of course, applications will come from joint results at more than one level. Occasionally, the application of a research advance will be rather prompt and direct, but the study of major advances shows that they usually involve combinations of specific discoveries made over a span of many years.

POSSIBLE APPLICATIONS OF RESEARCH AT VARIOUS LEVELS

A. Behavioral descriptions of learning and memory

Behavioral studies have shown that learning takes place over a much wider range of circumstances than earlier observers and theorists had supposed. Knowledge of this range can broaden the perspective of researchers and can suggest a greater variety of measures and experimental strategies that may prove useful. For example, in searching for neural correlates and bases of learning and memory (C–F below), it may be better to use simpler behavioral paradigms than the rather complex instrumental learning which has often been employed for this purpose. Our recognition of the diversity of learning situations may enable a closer understanding of the specific rules governing particular forms of information acquisition and storage.

B. Formal systems approaches

Where in the human learner are the main limitations or constraints in the amount of information that can be stored or retrieved? This has become a meaningful question and one on which fruitful research has been done since the 1950s when the learner was first conceptualized as an information-processing system—one that has identifiable, sequentially arranged components for the initial detection, temporary storage, permanent storage, retrieval, and use of information. Given the limited channel capacity that has been found, how can information be "packaged" better for efficient learning and retrieval? (Research utilizing the information-processing approach has demonstrated that much more information can be acquired when it is grouped in "chunks" rather than being presented in small units.) How can a person's time be allocated most efficiently for learning? Since channel capacity is limited and since repetition and depth of analysis favor long-term storage, a major factor in assuring storage may be to motivate the learner to spend sufficient time and effort on the material. Thus the formal systems approach may lead to renewed stress upon motivational factors in learning and memory.

C. Molar or general neural processes
What conditions (e.g., diet, health, diseases) favor or impair the general processes that mediate learning and memory? What kinds of intervention (e.g., diet, drugs, general health measures) can improve learning, retention, and retrieval?

Since various antibiotics and other drugs are found to impair formation of long-term memory in animals, clinicians should be alerted to the possibility of such effects in the therapeutic use of these drugs.

Senile decline of memory and mental retardation that is not caused by disease or birth trauma represent major problems for which no biological correlate has yet been established. A few reports suggest that retardates may be characterized by abnormal dendritic spines or by decreased concentrations of synaptic vesicles. If such neural abnormalities could be established, this would be a first step toward prevention and treatment of retardation and senility. In the case of hyperkinetic children, a variety of drugs have been employed on an empirical basis in the attempt to improve learning. Again, the establishment of the cellular bases of learning and memory could lead to a more rational selection of therapeutic agents.

D. Regional localization of neural processes involved in learning and memory
Can relations be clearly established between damage to certain parts of the brain and certain disorders of learning and memory? If so, then tests of learning and memory can aid in diagnosis of brain damage.

Can certain brain regions important in learning and memory be shown to be susceptible to certain deleterious agents? This appears to be true in a few cases (e.g., Korsakoff's syndrome resulting from damage to mamillary bodies due to a lack of vitamin B in alcoholism; impairment of formation of long-term memory in cases of hippocampal lesions caused by herpes encephalitis). Designation of such specific regional effects can help to focus research on prevention and therapy for such damage.

E. Changes in synapses and neural circuits as bases of learning and memory
Research done at the molar level could be made sharper and more productive if we could establish the detailed processes underlying learning and memory. Just as research and application in the area of public health was greatly advanced when the germ theory of infection was established, so we can expect major advances in research on learning and memory when we have discovered the detailed cellular bases of these phenomena.

F. Use of simpler systems for detailed study of neural processes in learning and memory
In relation to the statement in the paragraph above, it may well be true that the cellular processes underlying learning and memory can be identified and studied more exhaustively in simpler organisms, in parts of organisms, or in tissue preparations, rather than in intact complex mammals. Just as work with the bacterium *E. coli* is the basis for modern understanding of hereditary mechanisms in all living beings, so some researchers in this area hope to make fundamental contributions to the understanding of learning and memory through their studies of simpler systems.

G. Study of learning, memory, and neural changes in developing subjects
Research with developing subjects may help to solve questions about the neural processes involved in learning and memory, and the answers found may in turn help to aid in the education of children. For example, there have been many hypotheses that have attempted to account for the paucity of memories of early childhood—"infantile amnesia" for a period during which the child is clearly learning a great deal. Now research with animals has demonstrated that the immature brain learns quickly but also forgets quickly; retention requires repetition even more at an early age than later. It remains to determine what aspects of neural immaturity are related to poor retention, and animal studies can furnish this knowledge. At least it is already clear that neural immaturity is responsible for infantile amnesia, rather than other hypothesized factors such as a lack of verbal

facility or a repression of the infantile personality trauma. Therefore, it should be possible to apply this knowledge to the scheduling of learning tasks in relation to age and also to the planning of training for the early childhood years.

THE RELEVANCE OF RESEARCH WITH ANIMAL SUBJECTS

Since social concerns with learning and memory are related to problems of human learners, it may be asked why many researchers work with animal subjects and how this may be relevant to human questions. A glance at the history of research on learning and memory shows not only that almost from the beginning there has been an interpenetration of research with human and animal subjects, but also that many of the most influential concepts about human learning and many of the most useful experimental techniques have come from the animal laboratory. Thus the classical conditioning of Pavlov, which was based on animal research, has been widely applied in studies and theories of human behavior. It provided some of the main support for the influential school of behaviorism, founded by Watson in 1913. Subsequently, the work of Skinner and others on operant conditioning of animals (beginning in 1938) led to a reinterpretation of many aspects of human behavior, and also to effective techniques of behavior modification. The persistent efforts of experimental psychologists to study the perceptions of nonverbal animals has led to the elaboration of powerful techniques that have been employed in the last decade to study the perception of the preverbal child. By use of these techniques, the infant has been discovered to be a more active and keener perceiver than his limited motor capacities had led us to suppose.

The attempts to teach systems of communication to chimpanzees have led to revised concepts about language and to unexpected aid for aphasic patients. Since chimps do not have the vocal structures necessary for speech, experimenters in the last decade have taught them manual sign language (the Gardners) or the use of arbitrary colored shapes as symbols (Premack). The success of the animals and their growing levels of competence and abstraction have met many of the criteria established for language behavior. Those who wish to maintain distinctions between human and animal ability are being forced to look more closely at language and to establish new criteria. As an unexpected by-product of this research, the artificial language devised by Premack for the chimp has been found useful to permit several aphasic patients to reestablish communica-

tion (see Glass, Gazzaniga, and Premack, *Neuropsychologia* 11 (1973) : 95–103).

Techniques developed to study human behavior have also been usefully applied to animal subjects. Thus the principle of the Békésy audiometer has been applied by Blough and others to the study of sensory thresholds of animals. Riley showed at this conference how experimental designs worked out for human experimentation are being employed to test the occurrence of selective attention in animal subjects.

Undoubtedly, the interpenetration of human and animal research will continue, to the enrichment of both. This is one of the implications of the Darwinian revolution that began over a century ago and whose fruits we are still reaping.

Biology of Human Memory

1

The Psychobiological Approach to Human Memory

PAUL ROZIN

ABSTRACT This paper considers human memory within a broad biological perspective. It deals with the evolution and development of memory, as well as the relationship between nervous-system organization and the properties of memory as determined by psychologists.

Because there is some degree of localization of function in the brain, specific brain damage may result in memory deficits. Surprisingly, rather specific memory deficits also occur after general brain trauma, such as concussion, or general brain deterioration, as in senility. The most common disorders of memory, called the amnesic syndromes, are characterized by failure to recall events of the recent past (e.g., more than 30 seconds from the present), with memory for the immediate present and general intelligence undisturbed. The syndromes can be divided into two subcomponents, involving failure to recall verbal items or failure to recall visuospatial (nonverbal) materials. The neurological and psychological bases of the syndromes are discussed. Particular attention is devoted to analysis of the memory defects as a failure to store recent experiences or as an inability to retrieve them.

Other topics discussed include disorders of immediate memory, the relationship between perception and memory, the role of the frontal areas and "intelligence" in memory, and the problem of ascribing a particular physical location to "permanent" memory "traces."

1.1 INTRODUCTION

The accomplishments of human memory are staggering. We carry around the meanings of some tens of thousands of words, the ability to recognize countless visual scenes or configurations, probably thousands of faces, the sounds of many voices, melodies, and the like, and the abilities to drive cars, hit baseballs, play pianos, and so on. We may recognize within a fraction of a second a person whom we may have met only once some months ago.

The task at hand is to attempt to account for the biological basis of such phenomena: the registration, storage, and retrieval of acquired information. In order to begin to understand this system of enormous capacity and flexibility, we have to deal with matters that are not, strictly speaking, part of the area of memory (e.g., perception, attention, intelligence, skill organization, and language). The relevant literature, dealing with the

PAUL ROZIN, Department of Psychology, University of Pennsylvania, Philadelphia, PA

necessarily intertwined biological and psychological bases of these phenomena, is itself staggering in size—indeed, it challenges the capacity of human memory itself. The problem is exacerbated by the fragmentary nature of our knowledge in all of these areas, a fragmentation which resists memory's powerful encompassing tool, the chunking of a subject into meaningful organized units. The organism can only do so much organizing and chunking—some must be provided by an inherent organization of the information.

I find myself wishing that I were writing this paper a little less than a hundred years ago, in 1890, at the close of a decade that I would consider the golden age of memory (hopefully we are entering another). During this decade Ribot composed his classic work, *Diseases of Memory* (1882), which outlined and lucidly described not only the pathology of memory, but also some fundamental aspects of the memory process, such as registration and recollection. He emphasized memory as an active process. For example, he viewed recollection as a localization in time, accomplished by construction from a series of temporal reference points. He emphasized the value of pathological material in understanding memory. Following up on this, in 1889, Korsakoff published a magnificent paper describing one form of the amnesic syndrome that now bears his name. His fine clinical observations and interpretations led to a description of the syndrome as primarily a failure in recollection, an inability to recall an experienced event as an event from the past, as a segment from a continuous temporal stream. He believed the disorder to be consequent upon a deficit in memory formation, and to be a defect in the organization or associational structure of memories. As we shall see later, this description and analysis still seems remarkably apt after 85 years.

The decade closes with the monumental *Principles of Psychology* by William James (1890). The chapter on memory here is frighteningly modern. It shows how little we have advanced today from what a little knowledge, common sense, and an extraordinary mind could put together 85 years ago. James has already outlined memory into a sequence of processes, beginning with a stage akin to a positive afterimage, followed by entry into *primary memory,* the current stream of consciousness (now called short-term memory),[1] and then *secondary memory,* a large and more permanent store outside of immediate consciousness (now called long-term memory).

Memory proper, or secondary memory as it might be styled, is the knowledge of a former state of mind after it has already once dropped from consciousness; or rather it is the knowledge of an event, or fact, of which meantime we have not been thinking, with the additional consciousness that we have thought or experienced it before. (James, 1890, p. 648)

Again, as with Ribot and Korsakoff, we see clearly the notion of temporal integration and awareness of the past. James also emphasized the organized nature of secondary memory: the associations between elements and the weaving of an organizing matrix among the "traces" in the long-term store. The search of the long-term store for a particular memory (a topic of great recent interest in psychology, but largely ignored by those with biological interests) is described as making a "search in our memory for a forgotten idea, just as we rummage our house for a lost object. In both cases we visit what seems to us to be the probable *neighborhood* of that which we miss" (James, 1890, p. 654). James spoke of two factors controlling the quality or strength of memories: physiological retentiveness, a fundamental feature of the nervous system which differs across subjects, and the richness of the organizational-associative network within which the memories are embedded. Add to these conceptions the notion of selective attention and the role of repetition in establishing memories, both dealt with by James, and we have the basic problems for a biology of human memory clearly laid out in the last century.

In 1885 Ebbinghaus began the scientific study of memory with the first experiments on memorization, using nonsense materials. These experiments showed that orderly data could be obtained and suggested that the appropriate way to study memory was, in the good tradition of the biological sciences, to simplify. Simplification was accomplished by removing the trappings of past learning and attitudes through the use of meaningless material. The contrast with the broad cognitive views of Ribot, Korsakoff, and William James is striking. Within psychology, and much of the study of the biology of memory, the Ebbinghausian view has prevailed until quite recently.

There was one other critical contribution from this golden decade that to me has profound implications for the study of memory, though it did not directly deal with memory. This is the notion of a vertical hierarchical organization in the nervous system, and hence in behavior, put forth by John Hughlings Jackson (1884). The idea of conceiving the structure of the nervous system and of behavior as a hierarchy is powerful, and it leads naturally into the idea of levels of function in memory, with classical conditioning, for example, under lower control than memory for stories. Modern work suggests that the organization of the memory store itself is almost certainly hierarchical (e.g., Bower, 1970). The notion of vertical hierarchy, in Jackson's hands, becomes powerful when coupled with the observation that the higher levels of the hierarchy are more sensitive or fragile. As a result, they are more likely to be knocked out in disease, whether of a degenerative sort or produced by general trauma. Jackson's basic notion that the stages of evolution and development of the nervous system are reversed in disease has wide application.

Alas, this paper cannot stop now. A great deal has been done since 1890, though neither the problems nor the solutions have changed substantially. Much of the progress made since 1890 has occurred in the last decade, with a rather widespread application of the information-processing approach to the study of the neuropathology of memory. This recent activity in the biological aspects of memory is most obvious in the appearance, over the last decade or so, of three journals, *Cortex, Neuropsychologia,* and *Brain and Language,* all focusing on neurological aspects of higher mental processes. Furthermore, two readable general books on biological aspects of human memory have been written in the last decade by Talland (1968) and Barbizet (1970) as well as a number of more detailed volumes (e.g., Talland and Waugh, 1969; Whitty and Zangwill, 1966).

Taking into account the recent burst in activity, it would be a difficult task for both me and the reader to attempt an exhaustive review of the area. What I propose, instead, is the dual strategy of providing, on the one hand, a general overview of the problems and types of psychobiological approaches to memory, and on the other, a consideration in detail of one particular aspect of the neurobiology of memory: the amnesic syndromes. I have selected this particular set of syndromes because it has been extensively studied, it is of particular interest to both psychologists and neurologists, and it can be utilized to illustrate many of the general points I wish to make about the psychobiological approach to memory. The general organization of the paper will thus be as follows: First, I shall present in outline the basic charac-

---

[1] James's primary memory can also be construed to include the earliest stages of registration or positive afterimages, or even to be more akin to these stages than to what is presently called short-term memory.

teristics of the amnesic syndromes. With this as an illustrative base, I shall then discuss some basic issues in psychobiological approaches to memory, including the virtues of a neuropathological approach and the ontogenetic and evolutionary aspects of human memory (more information on the amnesic syndromes will be introduced here as it becomes relevant). Then I shall return to a more detailed consideration of the amnesic syndromes. Finally, I shall briefly discuss some general issues relating to the neuropathology of memory.

The approach used in this paper will be psychobiological. Psychobiological explanation involves the description of a reference phenomenon along what might be called two orthogonal axes. One of these, a mechanistic or reductionistic axis, involves restating or describing the reference phenomenon in terms of smaller units, which might be units of behavior (e.g., a description of walking in terms of reflexes) or of the nervous system (e.g., an analysis of a system such as the speech processor into more fundamental neural circuit components). It is this enterprise that justifiably occupies most people who claim the biology of memory as their interest. It includes the description of the physiological basis of the engram, the study of the role of different anatomical areas in memory processes, and the construction of patterns of connection among known biological components to synthesize the phenomena under study. Whether viewed as a psychological, physiological, or anatomical problem, the reductionistic view requires a breaking into small units, or lower levels (Jackson, 1884; Teitelbaum, 1967), and the reassembling or synthesizing of these units into a functioning system (Teitelbaum, 1967). The enterprise is laudable, and it is progressing. I shall later deal in detail with the contribution that brain lesions can make to describing the components of the memory system within this analytic-synthetic framework.

A second "axis" of explanation, less frequently considered, has to do with the temporal dimension: explanation of the past history of a phenomenon and the consequences of the phenomenon, over both the short run and the lifetime of the organism and species. Temporal explanation moves from evolutionary origins, through ontogenetic factors, to the present time, and onwards to immediate consequences and adaptive or survival value. Questions, especially about evolutionary origins and adaptive value, are inherently important aspects of biological explanation, and they also often raise issues of fundamental importance for the analysis and synthesis of behavior. I shall try to illustrate the heuristic value of such conceptions in the course of this paper.

1.2 AN INTRODUCTION TO THE AMNESIC SYNDROMES

The amnesic syndromes comprise a variety of disease entities with multiple causes. They may be transient or permanent. Because of the variety of forms and causes, I have carefully added the "s" to the word syndrome. All amnesic syndromes are characterized by two salient symptoms, which were initially described by Korsakoff (1889): (1) the failure to recall events of the recent past, despite a more or less "normal" immediate or short-term memory; (2) the loss of a feeling of familiarity or self reference with respect to recent experiences that are either re-presented or happen to be recalled (as they occasionally are). These symptoms concern memories coming from the postmorbid period, and are hence described as anterograde amnesia.

Two relatively "pure" case histories (bilateral hippocampal damage) and one more common type (Korsakoff syndrome) follow.

The most studied and celebrated case is that of H.M., a motor winder, who was subjected to bilateral removal of mesiotemporal tissue by Scoville for the control of epileptic seizures (Scoville and Milner, 1957). This operation had been performed successfully many times before, but in this instance, possibly because it invaded somewhat more hippocampal tissue than on previous occasions, a severe memory loss resulted. H.M. had a relatively uneventful early history. Seizures began at age 7 and became worse over the years, until at age 27 he was unable to work. His memory appeared normal prior to the operation. He had passed his high-school examinations without difficulty. His Wechsler IQ was 112 (these and further facts in this description come from Scoville and Milner, 1957; Milner, 1966; Milner, Corkin, and Teuber, 1968; Milner, 1970, 1972). The operation was performed on September 1, 1953. On the return of consciousness, H.M. could no longer recognize the hospital staff, apart from Dr. Scoville, whom he had known for many years. He could not remember or learn his way around the hospital. He showed a patchy but extensive premorbid amnesia for about three years. For example, he did not remember the death of his uncle, three years prior to the operation, but did retain a few other trivial and more recent memories. His early memories seemed clear and vivid; his short-term memory (e.g., digit span), his speech, and other behaviors were quite normal and appropriate. His main problem was his inability to recall any events that occurred postoperatively once they departed from his immediate attention (consciousness). For example, six months after the operation his family moved to another house on the same street, but he could not remember the new address and continued to go to the old house. A second move, a few years later, also produced great problems, although there was dim awareness of having moved. H.M. could perform all sorts of tasks that he had learned prior to surgery. For example, he could mow the lawn, but would never remember where he left the lawnmower. He did the same puzzles day after day and reread the same newspapers and magazines. He did not recognize neighbors and friends unless they had known him for many years prior to the operation. Each time he learned of the death of his uncle, he became very moved, treating it as a new occurrence.

H.M. has remained in a stable state over the years since his operation. His epileptic seizures are under good control, and his memory deficit, when last fully evaluated in 1968 (Milner, Corkin, and Teuber, 1968), was almost as dense and complete as in the postoperative period. Remarkably, intelligence, as measured by the Wechsler (WAIS), remains above normal, with an IQ of 118 obtained in 1962. Thirteen years after the operation, H.M. remains virtually unable to recall or learn any new verbal or visual material. The premorbid amnesia may have shrunk a bit, while early memories remain intact, including memories from his twenties (he was 27 at the time of operation). He is dimly aware of his father's death, which occurred some years after the operation, and he also knows that President John F. Kennedy was assassinated (but doesn't know who succeeded him). He works at a job assembling cigarette lighters on cardboard frames, but he is unaware of this job when not at it and cannot describe it. On the other hand, he can draw the floor plan for the bungalow he has lived in for the last eight years and seems to have learned something about the neighborhood.

H.M. is of particular interest because of the purity of the case and his high intelligence. The concurrence of an IQ of 118 and a Wechsler Memory Quotient of 64 is remarkable. Careful tests of verbal and visual memory indicate no recall (see Milner, 1966, 1972). His ability to use intelligence factors as memory aids is significant: thus, when asked who became president after Kennedy's assassination, he replied that it "must have been the vice-president, because that is the law." His own descriptions of this strange state of isolation from one's own past are quite poignant:

"Every day is alone in itself, whatever enjoyment I've had, and whatever sorrow I've had. . . . Right now, I'm wondering, have I done or said anything amiss? You see, at this moment everything looks clear to me, but what happened just before? That's what worries me. It's like waking from a dream. I just don't remember" (Milner, 1970).

H.M. obviously has some awareness of his memory deficit.

Another "pure" case was described by Starr and Phillips (1970). This patient, M.K., a high-school math and science instructor, was stricken with herpes simplex encephalitis at age 43. He now shows a stable, thoroughly dense amnesia for recent events, with a normal short-term memory. As with H.M., he shows a premorbid amnesia that is patchy but extends back some years, so that he is unaware of the birth of his last two children less than five years before his illness. M.K. has learned almost nothing in the way of verbal information since the illness. His performance on tests of verbal memory that require "long-term storage" is dismal. He has learned a few names over the years, a few major events, and can get around the hospital. In spite of these severe memory defects, he tests with an IQ of 125 (WAIS). This is undoubtedly an underestimate, in the sense that his limited storage capacity for new information could compromise his effectiveness. In fact, his performance was below normal on two WAIS subtests, digit symbol and picture arrangement. The former requires, for optimum performance, learning of ten digit-figure pairs, and the latter involves consideration and rejection of various hypotheses about the logical sequence in a series of pictures. Like H.M., M.K. shows an awareness of his memory deficit, and he writes things on paper to remind himself.

Starr and Phillips report one remarkable instance of new learning. M.K. was able to play the piano, and he worked with the band in the hospital. On one occasion he was taught a new song ("South American Way") which he had never heard before. He learned it in one afternoon. (According to the band director, he is able to learn new music by heart.) On the next day he had no recall for the experience of having learned the song, nor did he show any recognition for the name of the song. However, when the beginning of the melody was hummed for him, he said, "Oh, that piece," and proceeded to play it correctly.

These two patients share most characteristic symptoms in common: above-average intelligence; normal immediate or short-term memory; a virtually complete inability to recall recent events, but some residual capacity for some types of learning (e.g., getting around the hospital, the melody for M.K.); some awareness of the memory disorder, but no sense of familiarity or continuity with the past. Incidentally, both seem to have lost the ability to name odors—itself a specific memory deficit.

A third case, less "pure" but typical of the Korsakoff syndrome, is cited by Zangwill:

A publican, aged 60, was admitted with a history of excessive alcoholic consumption for many years. Three months previously, he had had two major epileptic fits in one day, and in the past few weeks had become progressively more unsteady on his feet. His wife had noted some slurring of speech. One month previously he developed diplopia, which had, however, cleared by the time of his admission. His memory had deteriorated progressively, and there had been episodes of confusion, disorientation, and confabulation.

On admission, the patient was amnesic, disorientated, and confabulatory. There was marked peripheral neuropathy and ataxia.

The patient was seen repeatedly in the Psychological Department, over a period of seven weeks. On the Wechsler-Bellevue Full Scale, he achieved an IQ of 105, without undue scatter or other evidence of appreciable recent deterioration. Weigl's Sorting Test, which calls for some measure of conceptual grasp and flexibility, was executed satisfactorily. On the other hand, the patient failed to learn the Babcock sentence or sequences of nine or ten digits in spite of innumerable trials. He was also unable to reproduce the gist of the "Cowboy" story from immediate memory, but with the aid of prompts recalled one or two points, which he linked in a confabulatory way. When the story was repeated five minutes later, the patient denied that he had heard this particular story before, but thought he had heard a similar one. He gave a similar response on recognition tests with objects or pictures, thus exhibiting well-marked reduplicative paramnesia.

At first, the patient was completely disoriented, believing himself to be in a hospital in the vicinity of his own home. He gave the month (July) as January, the year (1963) as 1956, and his own age (60) as 52. He gave his present home address as one which he had in fact moved five years previously, and when asked about his recent doings, described activities appropriate to a newsagent, though he had in fact sold his newspaper business at about the time he moved to his present address. He betrayed no knowledge of his life as a licensed victualler, and completely denied his second marriage, which had taken place two years earlier. (Nonetheless, he recognized his present wife and accepted her as such when she visited him in hospital.) Although aware that he was in hospital (which he rationalized in a facile manner), the patient blandly denied that he was ill or that his memory was in any way affected.

There was little change in this patient's psychological state during the ensuing weeks. He continued to show dense retrograde amnesia for the four to five years prior to the onset of his illness, and appeared to retain practically nothing of his current experiences, whether tested by recall or recognition. Nonetheless, some degree of retention, at a quasi-automatic level, could be demonstrated. For example, while claiming not to recognize his examiners from day to day, the patient did not appear to react to them as total strangers. Again, although he denied that he knew the name of the hospital, he could

select it correctly from a list containing the names of several hospitals, justifying his choice in an ad hoc manner. At this time, too, he showed a tendency to reduplication, stating that he had previously been in a hospital similar to the present one, though smaller and in the vicinity of his own home. Appreciation of his memory loss remained virtually nonexistent. (Zangwill, 1966)

Based on clinical case studies and some experimental work to be discussed later, the salient features of the amnesic syndromes are as follows:

A. Anterograde amnesia, characterized by:

1. *Failure to recall or recognize recent events.*

In its densest form this can amount to complete failure to recall any events occurring more than 15–30 seconds ago if the patient has been distracted in the interval.

2. *Loss of a sense of familiarity and personal reference.*

This feature was noted by Korsakoff (1889) and emphasized as a central characteristic of the syndrome by Claparède (1911), who said that the continuity with the past was destroyed, and hence the sense of familiarity, the "I've seen that before." He pointed out that though events may be associated with each other in an amnesic, they do not form a part of a temporally integrated stream, a part of the self (translated as "me-ness"). Thus, for example, Talland (1965) describes an amnesic patient who had a few recent memories, including the fact that his brother had gotten married. When asked how he knew this, he responded by saying he must just have been told. It is a common observation that in memory testing, amnesic patients, even when they give a correct answer, have no feeling that it is correct or awareness that they have just been presented with the material under study.

3. *At least some storage of recent events.*

As initially noted by Korsakoff, some recent, apparently lost memories may reappear. Recent work (see Warrington and Weiskrantz, 1973, and Section 1.6.5) has confirmed this, and indicated that recent memories can be effectively recalled with the use of partial information cues.

4. *Particular difficulty with remembering completely new material*

(e.g., names of people met for the first time after the onset of pathology).

5. *Retained capacity for learning and perceptuomotor skills* (see Section 1.5, on ontogeny).

B. Some disorders of premorbid memory (see Section 1.5, on ontogeny).

C. Intact short-term memory and intelligence.

Other symptoms *may* accompany the syndromes, including lack of awareness of the memory disorder, confabulation, and disorientation (as in the third case history). There are also some indications that amnesics do not show the normal improvement in memory when testing is through recognition rather than recall (Warrington and Weiskrantz, 1970).

1.3. THE PSYCHOBIOLOGICAL ANALYSIS OF HUMAN MEMORY

1.3.1 The relationship between psychological and biological approaches to memory

In order to deal with memory within a reductionistic framework, we must start out with a conception of the phenomenon at some level. The most appropriate level seems to be the type of "mental" analysis offered by modern cognitive psychologists. Beginning with a conception of what the major psychological features of memory are, and of their relationship to one another, we can attempt to look into the nervous system for corresponding functions. The folly of entering the nervous system *without* a sensible notion of the structure of the phenomenon under study is well illustrated by the history of phrenology.

I would like to emphasize this point here because it is all too easy to assume that the natural direction of information flow in scientific understanding is from biology to psychology. It is certainly true that biologists have a surer data base and a more sophisticated understanding of the phenomena they study. However, with complex phenomena, where the level of understanding is low at all levels, it appears to me that the major direction of information flow is from psychology to biology. A notable example of this comes from Sherrington's (1906) discovery of the laws of the reflex, inferred from observations of behavior rather than from direct measurements of the nervous system. The relationships he described for reflexes, such as summation and inhibition, he inferred as properties of the synapse, and he was proved right. Other basic characteristics of synaptic interactions were also seen first in whole behavior. Similarly, in color vision, the notion of an opponent-process coding system (Hering, 1878; Hurvich and Jameson, 1957) came out of psychology, in particular phenomenology and psychophysics. The physiological realization of neural systems behaving in accordance with opponent-process principles occurred over 75 years after they were first suggested, and only after neurophysiologists had begun to take the opponent-process model seriously and thus to look for units with both excitatory and inhibitory responses to different wavelengths (Hurvich and Jameson, 1969). It is very easy to miss an inhibitory response if one is not looking for it. Even much of Jackson's work involved inferences about the structure of the nervous system from the normal development and dissolution of *behavior*, as well as from

pathological cases. It seems to me that over the last century, the ledger sheet favors beginning with analysis of the behavioral or mental structure of the phenomenon to be studied (see Gallistel, 1974, for further discussion and examples of this point). On the other hand, the narrow paradigmatic description of learning processes by psychologists has been a disservice to neurobiologists (see Manning, this volume, and Rozin and Kalat, 1971, 1972).

In the area of memory, the interchange of information and ideas between neurological and psychological approaches has been more reciprocal than in most other areas, as illustrated by the unusual neurosurgical-psychological collaboration at the Montreal Neurological Institute. In the case of the amnesic syndromes, modern neurologically oriented work has been heavily influenced by the information-processing approach (see Simon, this volume), while, on the other hand, modern psychological notions such as the "two-stage" (or three or four or more) memory system, gain great support from the apparent dissociation of stages in the amnesic syndromes. Similarly, the contrast between verbal and nonverbal processing mechanisms in psychology has influenced and been influenced by work in neuropsychology indicating specialization in hemispheric functions.

Figure 1.1 displays one of the all-too-familiar "box" information-processing diagrams of memory function. It represents my conception of memory processes, and though it purports to be a description of the mental processes involved in memory, it is substantially influenced by data from neuropsychology. I hesitate to add another box model to a literature already burgeoning with boxes. It is a frightening thought that with 10 billion neurons to work with, one might indeed come up with

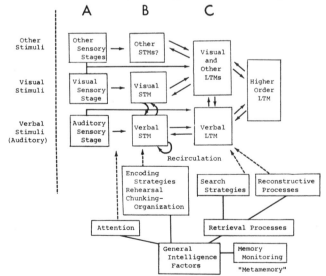

FIGURE 1.1 Hypothetical schematic diagram of processing stages in human memory.

quite a few boxes in a detailed model. Though no model I know of approaches that number, I have a feeling that the total number of boxes in all information-flow models of memory may be nearing that figure. Be that as it may, the model of memory presented here is like most others in positing three stages of processing in the formation of memories: (1) a sensory stage, (2) a limited-capacity, short-term memory stage (STM), probably synonymous with presence in consciousness, and (3) a high-capacity, long-term memory stage (LTM). It assumes a number of different channels of entry into memory (Posner, 1969; Simon, this volume), and a group of intelligence factors operating at various stages in memory processing. Data on memory pathology suggest compromise of various components of this array, and hence provide evidence for their existence. For example, the existence of parallel channels for verbal and nonverbal information is supported by neuropathological data indicating specific deficits in verbal or nonverbal memory, both at the STM level and at the level of access to LTM. Furthermore, the possibility that there is a recirculation mechanism for retaining materials in verbal STM but not in visual STM is suggested by data from H.M. and other amnesics (see Section 1.6.4).

The question now arises, how does such a model map onto the nervous system? It should be clear that given the kind of units into which we aspire to break human memory, study at the level of single cells and synapses will not have a direct mapping. Though memory must in principle be describable in terms of the activity of single neurons, this microphysiological unit is below the level of the phenomena we describe; that is to say, the basic and unique features of the human memory system do not seem to inhere in individual neurons. In the same sense, it is not necessary to understand how a carburetor is constructed to be able to fit it into a meaningful conception of the operation of an automobile engine. When we enter the nervous system, we should be looking for physiological or anatomical systems that *correspond to* inferred psychological systems.

In the ideal neurological model, each processing stage, box, store, or whatever name one prefers, would correspond to a part in the brain. A conception of the brain in terms of centers connected by tracts has certain obvious parallels to the psychological stage model, and is a viable view of brain organization (Geschwind, 1965a, b). Geschwind conceives of syndromes, when well-defined, as consisting of either obliteration of a processing center or, more commonly (for neuroanatomical reasons), severance of the connections between processing centers. For example, he explains "pure alexia" (Geschwind, 1962), the sudden loss of the ability to read while visual perception, language, and writing remain

intact, as a disconnection of the visual analyzers from the linguistic system. The brain damage accompanying this syndrome supports his interpretation. Similarly, modality-specific anomias, the loss of the ability to name objects in a particular modality, are described by Geschwind as a disruption of connections between the lexical system and various perceptual input channels (Geschwind, 1967). Although the Geschwindian view can lead to oversimplification, in many cases it seems to describe neuropsychological deficits concisely.

An alternative mapping view is associated with the eminent Russian neuropsychologist A. R. Luria (1966, 1973). Luria views both psychological functioning and brain organization in a dynamic, complex, and developmentally fluid framework. He has particular concern for the psychological analysis of phenomena preceding neuropsychology, and he is especially sensitive to the multiple systems involved in any complex function (as in the memory box diagram) and to the multiple routes to pathological functioning. The brain does not divide as neatly for him as it does for Geschwind. Luria sees three basic systems, organized both vertically and horizontally, contributing to higher mental functions. The first, axial and midline, is involved with alerting, wakefulness, and activation. The second, with substantial cortical components, is involved with the reception, analysis, and storage of information. It would correspond to all of the processing stage boxes under A, B, and C in Figure 1.1. Anatomically, it encompasses the posterior portions of the cerebral cortex, including the temporal lobes. The third system, localized in the frontal regions, is involved with programming, regulation, and verification. Many of the general intelligence factors indicated in Figure 1.1 are associated with this last system.

In Luria's view, the activating system is thought to be necessary for the operation of the other systems, and since the lesions in the amnesic syndrome concentrate in this system, Luria conceives of the defect as one of low activation or tone. The memory system is conceived as a series of processes involving increasing elaboration of the incoming signal, from the early modality-specific stages that take place in the projection areas of the senses, through an intermediate stage in the association areas bordering on each projection area, and finally to a tertiary stage of processing where modality specificity in stimulus encoding and elaboration disappears. Interestingly, this tertiary area, which Luria locates in the inferior parietal lobe, is also the area that Geschwind (1964) has pinpointed as being critical in the integration of inputs from different modalities, and hence in the formation and naming of concepts. Luria's conception of the memory system does not lend itself very easily to the box information-processing analogue. It seems to me to be more compatible with psychological models that refer to depth of processing (e.g., Craik and Lockhart, 1972), and that conceive of permanence of memory in terms of how deeply (on a scale from simple sensory registration to semantic analysis) an input is processed.

1.3.2 The extent to which pathology produces a meaningful breakdown of psychological function

One might be surprised that breakdown of function in an organized and interesting way occurs so often in cases of damage to the nervous system. There is, of course, some localization of function in the brain, so that spatially contiguous brain areas tend to mediate similar functions. In the visual projection areas of the cortex, the topological mapping is quite precise, so that small lesions produce meaningful symptoms, describable as blind spots or scotomas.

Localization is apparently precise enough so that strokes, tumors, or surgery, which by their nature produce spatially contiguous lesions, occasionally result in a clear-cut symptomatology that is pure enough to be of interest to psychologists. The possibility of specific damage is enhanced because axons mediating similar functions are formed into compact nerve tracts that can be destroyed by small lesions (Geschwind, 1965a,b). These tracts are much more likely to be completely obliterated than are more diffusely located "processing centers," if such exist. One major source of specificity or pure syndromes comes, surprisingly, from apparently general insults to the nervous system. That is, a variety of harmful physical or chemical stresses, which may appear to act equally on the whole brain, in fact act quite specifically.

Possibly more significant than the gross spatial localization of function in the brain are both visible and biochemical differences in the individual brain cells themselves. Not surprisingly, cells performing similar functions seem to look alike (allowing description of different parts of the cortex by the cell patterns and layers) and to be biochemically alike. Thus some cells seem more sensitive to anoxia or physical trauma. As a result, in senility or head trauma, certain systems tend to drop out first. As it happens, memory functions are implicated early in the response to many stressors. In fact, a particularly rich source of interesting patients arises from cases of exposure to toxins or microorganisms that have specific proclivities for particular types of brain cells. I first learned of the exquisite specificity of these lesions from a course in neurology for psychologists taught by Dr. Oscar Marin. Thus the Korsakoff syndrome, involving rather specific mammillary-body destruction, is produced by a vitamin deficiency, and amnesic syndromes

(as in M.K. above) are produced by herpes simplex viruses, which have a predilection for hippocampal cells. The biochemical specificity of the nervous system is common knowledge to neurologists, since many diseases are characterized by specific destruction of particular types of cells. For example, in amyotrophic lateral sclerosis, it appears that some toxin, deficiency, or biological agent specifically attacks motor neurons, and does so eventually throughout the nervous system, while leaving other cells, and thus other systems, intact. Similarly, carbon monoxide poisoning can produce selective damage to the globus pallidus and a parkinsonian syndrome. In a way, the purest lesions of the nervous system, which should have clear functional significance, are those based on the nature of the individual cells. Strangely, the technique of producing biochemically specific lesions has not been used much in the study of animals, though it has recently become more common with the emergence of modern neurochemistry and pharmacology. Here is a case where students of animal physiological psychology have had much to learn from neurology.

The dissolution of the nervous system in senility also provides an orderly, nonrandom sequence of neurological preparations, which will be discussed below. The basic notion (Jackson, 1884) is that higher systems tend to deteriorate first, hence reversing the order of development. Furthermore, in recovery of function, functions or systems tend to come back in the order in which they developed, allowing an analysis of fundamental stages and systems. Such an analysis, comparing development and recovery, has been made in rats for the control of feeding and drinking (Teitelbaum, Cheng, and Rozin, 1969). The parallel is almost exact. Since one observes a great deal of recovery of function in neurology, there is a natural opportunity to investigate the organization of brain and behavior. Damage to higher centers releases lower ones, allowing the study of simpler components of the total system. Similar observations can be made in the process of development.

The neuropathological approach is not without its pitfalls. Most obvious is the impossibility of obtaining a set of cases with truly comparable neurological damage. Thus inferences have to be made, if one is interested in what tissue really serves what function, from sets of different lesions with differing degrees of overlap, in conjunction with the corresponding psychological deficits. By looking at the common overlap in tissue destruction in all cases in which a particular symptom appears (the method of intersecting sums), one can tentatively assign particular areas to particular components of various mental functions (e.g., Pribram, 1969; Milner, 1972). Convincing localization of specific functions can also be accomplished by Teuber's method of double dissociation, through which complementary deficits are produced by two different lesions. For example, specific right-hemisphere lesions produce defects in visual memory, with verbal memory unaffected, and other left-hemisphere lesions produce the opposite pattern.

As Luria (1966, 1973) has pointed out, making a hole in a complex system will often disrupt its normal mode of operation without providing much insight into this mode (e.g., studying a radio by banging it with a hammer). Conversely, a critical center might be damaged with little resulting symptomatology if there exist compensating systems or alternative routes of processing (Goldstein, 1939). In short, great care is needed in the interpretation of neuropathological data. However, as I hope the reader will realize, in the discussion of the amnesic and other syndromes, with appropriate care much can be learned about basic memory and basic brain processes.

1.3.3. Component analysis of psychological systems

I would like now to address the specific advantages of a neuropathological approach for those interested in the *psychological* explanation of human memory. Neuropathological cases permit the testing and development of psychological models of higher mental functions. In particular, appropriate patients provide the opportunity to do *component analyses*. If a psychological theory, for example, claims that process A is necessary for process B, then it should not be possible to see process B in the absence of A. (The logic here is not tight, since it is conceivable that while process A may be cut off from or inaccessible to behavior, it is still present as an intermediate stage in other processes. One would certainly not want to claim there is no language function in cases of anarthria.) Thus, for example, a theory of speech perception which assumes that the speech-generation machinery in the brain is employed in the perception process is a bit embarrassed by the preservation of good speech comprehension in the face of a high-level cortical disturbance of speech production (Brain, 1965).

Psychological arguments as to whether there is a single (verbal) memory-encoding mechanism or multiple mechanisms are enlightened by neuropathological work. Here the question, in terms of neurological components, is whether the verbal-analysis machinery is deeply involved in the encoding of all memories. The answer appears to be no. The dissociation by Brenda Milner and her colleagues of memory functions into two categories, roughly verbal and nonverbal, each associated with one of the temporal lobes, suggests separate

processing mechanisms (Milner, 1972, 1974; Milner and Taylor, 1972). (In fact, the general development, within neuropsychology, of notions of differentiation of the two hemispheres, one for verbal, possibly analytic functions, and the other for nonverbal, possibly gestalt-type functions, has enormous implications for psychology; see Levy, 1969; Levy, Trevarthen, and Sperry, 1972; Sperry, Gazzaniga, and Bogen, 1969; Milner, 1973; Gazzaniga, 1970, and in this volume.) For example, there has been some debate as to whether the great enhancement of memory for word pairs produced by instructions to make interacting images in the head can be attributed to some type of conversion from a verbal to a spatial, visual, or related type of representation. Pathology helps here in a number of ways. The notion that imagery instructions lead to superiority *because* they produce a visual representation that is more cohesive or stable is probably wrong, since congenitally blind people show roughly the same enhancement after imagery instructions as do normals (Jonides, Kahn, and Rozin, 1975). On the other hand, the amazingly popular view in psychology that the effect is fundamentally verbally mediated seems quite unlikely, since patients with severe linguistic disorders and accompanying poor verbal memory show marked improvement in recall when introduced to imagery instructions (Patten, 1972). Furthermore, patients with no speech impairments at all, but with lesions in the left temporal lobe that result in relatively poor verbal, as opposed to visuospatial, memory, show major gains from the use of imagery instructions. These gains are larger than those of people with right temporal

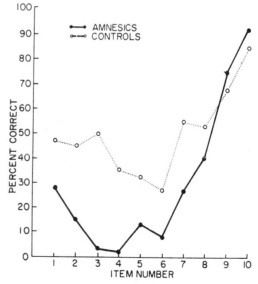

FIGURE 1.2 Mean percentage correct recall as a function of order of presentation for amnesic and control subjects with immediate recall. From Baddeley and Warrington (1970). Reproduced with permission from *Journal of Verbal Learning and Verbal Behavior* 9: 179.

damage, who would be expected to have visuospatial-memory problems (Jones, 1974).

A most instructive instance of neurological component analysis concerns the explanation of the free-recall function for word lists. If normal subjects are given one presentation of a list of about ten words and immediately after list presentation are asked to recall as many words as possible, they typically perform best on the last few words (recency effect) and also show enhanced performance on the first few words (primacy effect), as illustrated in Figure 1.2. This U-shaped function has been accounted for as the joint output of the two storage systems involved in STM and LTM (Glanzer and Cunitz, 1966). The primacy effect is attributed to readout from LTM, since these items can be transferred to LTM before STM becomes overloaded with new items. Items from the middle of the list may be squeezed out of STM by more recently presented items before they can enter LTM. On the other hand, the most recently presented items are readily available since they have just entered STM.

This dual-component theory of free recall can be tested with amnesics, who presumably have sharply curtailed access to material recently transferred to LTM, but normal STM. As might be expected, the recency component, representing STM function, is quite normal, while performance on middle and beginning items, where LTM makes the substantial contribution, is markedly depressed (Figure 1.2; Baddeley and Warrington, 1970; Miller, 1971). If recall is delayed by 30 seconds and the subject is given an intervening task that presumably fully occupies STM, normals show a loss of the recency component, as would be predicted by the theory. Moreover, the recency component also drops out or is greatly attenuated in amnesics attempting delayed recall, resulting in an almost uniformly poor performance. In contrast to these data, studies of patients with severely limited *auditory* STM yield complementary results in tests of immediate recall (see Section 1.7): there is a marked contraction of the recency component (Shallice and Warrington, 1970; Saffran and Marin, 1974). On the whole, then, data from neuropathology, by allowing component analysis, permit confirmation of a psychological theory.

1.3.4 Study of isolated or released subsystems
As a consequence of the disappearance or disconnection of some subsystems in a higher mental function, a particular subsystem may end up isolated from the systems with which it usually interacts. In some cases it may still have input and output connections, so that the hopefully uncontaminated behavior of the system can be observed.

Thus previously inferred properties of the subsystem can be verified, or new ones discovered.

A most striking example comes again from the work of Geschwind, and involves a patient who had suffered extensive cerebral damage, resulting in essential isolation of the fundamental language areas of the major hemisphere from the rest of the cerebrum (Geschwind, Quadfasel, and Segarra, 1968). The result was a "talking machine," which repeated everything uttered to it and thus retained the capability of decoding, at least briefly retaining, and encoding speech, without any contact with the rest of the brain and hence isolated from other cognitive functions.

Split-brain patients provide another excellent example of isolated systems, where what appear to be two different modes of processing, "verbal-analytic" in the dominant hemisphere and nonverbal or "wholistic-gestalt" in the minor hemisphere, are exposed for separate study by callosal section (Levy, 1969; Sperry, Gazzaniga, and Bogen, 1969). Although relatively little work has been done on memory in split brains, we know of considerable differences in the area of perception and information processing which almost certainly have memorial consequences.

The best example of study of an isolated system again concerns the amnesic syndromes. It appears that short-term memory is really quite intact in many patients suffering dense amnesia for recent events. Hence the operating characteristics of the short-term memory system can be explored quantitatively, uncontaminated from materials in long-term memory (see Section 1.6.3).

1.3.5 Interactions between human pathological and animal research
There are two ways in which human work would be of direct interest to those primarily interested in studying a system in animals. First, insofar as common systems exist, the human system has the advantage of ease in measurement and report, largely due to the mediation of language. This is of incalculable value in the study of higher mental functions. Thus, for example, in the battles that have raged over the years, in the literature on animal electroconvulsive shock (ECS), about whether the shock really has a retroactive amnesic effect, relatively little consideration has been given to the fact that experiments on ECS with humans quite clearly show memory loss for at least a brief period prior to shock (Williams, 1950a; Cronholm, 1969). It stands to reason that something similar happens in rats.

Second, there is a great contrast in methodology between human pathological and animal learning research. Psychologists studying animal learning and memory tend to be laboratory experimenters, whereas neurologists and neuropsychologists approach memory disorders in the manner of ethologists. Thus the knowledge a neurologist has of the subtle features of motor skills, affects, etc., far outstrips what very clever psychologists with their technical virtuosity can extract from animals. The knowledge of the baseline is just greater in humans: language is available as a communication tool, and the neurologist or neuropsychologist is trained to look for all sorts of subtle details and indicators of processes gone awry. The richness of human material leads to the extensive study of individual cases—the ability to pick out clear-cut instances for detailed study. Just consider what has been learned about memory from H.M. alone.

1.3.6 Other advantages of the neuropathological approach

Neuropathology also provides the psychologist with interesting patterns of disorder which may be useful, not because of their fundamental nature, but as convenient ways to study other problems. Thus split-brain patients can often be used to determine the dominant mode of processing in a particular cognitive process. If, for example, one conceives of familiar-word recognition as a visual-gestalt problem, as opposed to an analysis into visual or phonemic segments, one would be inclined to predict good word recognition by the minor hemisphere. Dense and relatively pure amnesics such as H.M. provide an excellent opportunity to obtain repeated measurements from one subject without having to worry about interactions of past experience with present performance. H.M. allows experiments that are usually run across subjects to be run within one subject, thus factoring out individual-difference variables. Indeed, it would be possible to generate free-association norms using H.M. alone, instead of asking many subjects one time each to give their first association to a particular word.

1.4 THE EVOLUTION OF HUMAN MEMORY

Three basic trends in brain evolution, moving through the primates and apes to man, can be described (Luria, 1973):

1. diminished specificity of cortical areas, with the primary sensory-projection areas occupying a smaller portion of the cortex;

2. lateralization of function, leading to a linguistically dominant hemisphere;

3. particular enlargement of two areas of the cortex: the anterior frontal areas and the inferior parietal areas.

The development of language has undoubtedly been a major factor in the evolution of the brain. Concordant with this notion, Geschwind and Levitsky (1968) have recently pointed out that a portion of the upper surface of the human temporal lobes, which appears to serve linguistic functions, is larger in the left, "linguistic" hemisphere.

Although there is no full-blown model of the evolution of memory or intelligence, it is instructive to discuss some of the issues involved. The human memory system must be built upon prior developments in "lower" primates. One cannot evolve a complex system from the ground up without building stable subsystems. Simon (1962), in an eloquent article, has pointed to the almost absolute need for a hierarchical subsystem structure in complex systems, since errors or mistakes in evolution or development could otherwise bring down the whole system. Building out of self-contained subsystems assures that a failure in one part of the mechanism results, at worst, only in loss of that particular subsystem.

In fact, in a variety of infrahuman creatures, one sees components that probably form part of the human memory system. In addition to a variety of outstanding memorial accomplishments, such as memory for food location and sun position in bees (von Frisch, 1967) or for the location and relationship of particular tidepools in gobiid fish (Aronson, 1951; see Rozin, 1976, for a general discussion of such adaptations), a variety of other abilities are seen in infrahumans which resemble human "intelligent" abilities, and which undoubtedly depend upon similar types of circuitries or programs. Considerations of this sort have led me to suggest that much of the evolution of intelligence and memory consists of the initial development of sophisticated systems to handle specific situations, and the subsequent liberation of these tightly wired systems from their original restricted context (see Rozin, 1976). In other words, particular circuitry, evolved to handle particular problems (such as size constancy in perception, or compensation for sun movement in bees), is initially only accessible to the input and output systems that it has been designed to serve. With evolution, some of these systems are connected into other systems, and become components in a hierarchy wherein they can be used more widely. It is hard to believe that such basic memory-intelligence components as scanning mechanisms or memory-storage systems evolved independently for each situation in which they turned out to be useful. Rather, these mechanisms became tied into new subsystems, and thus became more accessible, in the course of evolution.

I would like to make one other observation about the evolution of memory systems before addressing some specific issues. Much of the research on memory in animals and humans focuses on the problem of plasticity: How does new information get coded and stored in the nervous system? This emphasis is understandable. However, it is also important to realize that much of the machinery involved in human memory has little to do with plasticity per se. Thus, for example, hierarchical storage mechanisms, mechanisms for scanning over a set of stored materials for a given target, mechanisms that might well be involved in judgments of familiarity and a score of other processes, can easily be conceived as "hardware." These wired-in systems might possibly be analogous to complex motor systems or, for that matter, some aspects of the navigation systems of bees. Hence, in discussing the evolution of memory, one should look for precursors in many areas of function.

The basic question in the evolution of memory, especially as between chimpanzees and man, is, of course, the extent to which the fundamental difference is a consequence of language. Put another way, how different is the memory functioning of the human right hemisphere, or, more appropriately, the human brain with language functions excised, from that of chimpanzees? In order to explore this issue we must compare the maximal memorial achievements of apes with the achievements of humans with impoverished linguistic function.

Recently the techniques and approaches of modern cognitive psychology have penetrated into infrahuman primate research. Only beginnings have been made here, which means that we do not yet have an adequate idea of the memory capabilities of apes and monkeys. Indications are that short-term memory (obviously for nonverbal material) shows similar decay functions, as measured by the delayed matching-to-sample paradigm, in monkeys and men (Drachman and Ommaya, 1964; Jarrard and Moise, 1971; Medin, 1972). Direct comparison is difficult because monkey researchers at the moment are limited to recognition procedures, in contrast to the more informative recall procedures used with humans. Furthermore, monkeys presumably do not have a verbal-rehearsal program, which permits humans to maintain a certain amount of information in active memory over long periods, in the absence of interference. Given all these facts, the decay of memory for dot locations and the like to chance levels well within one minute (in delayed matching-to-sample procedures) does not seem out of line.

The future looks very bright for the exploration of memory function in apes, due in large part to the remarkable progress made by Premack (1971) in teaching the chimpanzee Sarah a written language. The ease with which such concepts as "color of," negation, and ques-

tion have been taught has been most striking. Surely similar techniques can be used to produce apes literate enough to be used in recall experiments and to be queried, for example, about the order of successive stimuli. Even in the absence of a convenient communication vehicle such as Premack has provided, it is in fact possible to ask infrahumans important questions about such matters as temporal sequence. Gleitman (1974) has recently described a training procedure that could be used to extract sophisticated information of this type from animals.

Approaching the evolutionary problem from the human side is very difficult. The principal problem would appear to be separating out the hopelessly entangled functions of memory and intelligence. As indicated in the memory model in Figure 1.1, there are many aspects of memory function that are tightly linked to intelligence functions. In fact, intelligence tests such as the Wechsler (WAIS) include specific memory tests. On the WAIS, three of the eleven subtests are explicitly involved with memory (vocabulary, information, and digit span), and two others (digit symbol and picture arrangement) make extensive demands on short- or medium-term storage abilities. Even the digit span, which would seem to be a pretty raw and low-level measure of short-term memory capacity, correlates about +.67 with the total verbal and performance IQ score (Wechsler, 1955). However, it must be pointed out that (1) digit-span scores include digit sequences that are repeated backwards, and (2) this is the lowest correlation of any subtest with the total score. Presumably, the increase of digit span with intelligence is related to some organizational, grouping, or chunking tendency. Though digit span and total intelligence correlate rather well in normals, they are quite dissociable. Senile dementia is often characterized by normal or near-normal digit span, despite severe loss of recent memory and severe deterioration of intelligence (see, for example, Delay and Brion, 1962, cited in Barbizet, 1970; Diamond and Rozin, unpublished data). The digit-span task apparently taps rather low-level systems or, at the least, retains access to intelligence functions that have become disconnected from most other mental functions.

A natural way to approach the ape/man interface, once we have thought about the smartest apes around, would be to look at humans with severe mental handicaps. One might hope to see, in mental retardation for example, a dropping out of the highest memorial accomplishments, leaving others intact. Unfortunately, the picture is not so simple. Though the memory performance of retardates has been described as primarily a deficit in organization, retrieval, and planning (Spitz,

1973), educable retardates have digit spans in the 3–4 range, compared to 6 $\pm$ 1 for normal agemates (Spitz, 1973).

Another approach to the ape/man comparison would be to place language in center stage, and ask about the extent to which the memories of chimps and men are similar once language is factored out. A way to get at this would be to examine the functioning of memory in congenitally deaf children, especially those with little exposure to alternative language systems. There is precious little data on this point. Surprisingly, severe language deprivation does not have the enormous effect one might expect it to have on general cognitive functioning (Furth, 1966). However, linguistic deprivation must certainly leave a mark on memory functioning. A recent study indicates a clear tendency for congenitally deaf subjects to organize a series of syllables or faces spatially rather than sequentially, though sequencing *can* be performed (O'Connor and Hermelin, 1973). The relation of temporal sequencing itself, and of language in general, to memory could certainly be further explored in deaf subjects, and also in the right hemispheres of split brains and in subjects with severe, acquired verbal deficits.

Another line of investigation that might shed light on the role of language in memory would be to examine the remarkable performances of idiot savants (e.g., Roberts, 1945; Anastasi and Levee, 1959), who seem able to memorize vast amounts of pictorial or verbal information through some sort of "visualization" process often called eidetic imagery. For example, the individual studied by Roberts (1945) could, following $2\frac{1}{2}$ hours study of a full-year calendar, give the day of the week of any date and, more impressively, indicate which of three randomly varied colors each date was written in. Most impressive is the performance of the mnemonist described in fascinating detail by Luria (1968), who seemed again to code experience in a multimodal but nonverbal manner.

The fundamental question is, what are the distinguishing features of human memory? There is no reason to believe that the speed of either learning or the incorporation of information, per se, is especially high in man. Memory-scanning "hardware" may be more elaborate in man, though on ecological-evolutionary grounds it is not obvious that man, the hunter, had much greater memory or scanning demands made on him than are made on present-day baboons or chimps. Given the enlargement of the human frontal area, it is reasonable to suspect a significant advance in the area of general memorizing strategies, plans, and the like, especially since such functions are deficient after some types of frontal lesions in man (Luria, 1966; see Section 1.8.1).

The most likely sources for differences, other than in frontal-lobe function, have to do with language and lateralization on the one hand, and the concept of "self" on the other.

The possible influence of language on the operation and organization of memory is enormous. At the least, it provides a powerful new system for coding and organizing information, as well as a way of formulating strategies for retrieving it. Verbal rehearsal, a strategy frequently used by humans and almost certainly a uniquely human process, offers the advantage of allowing material to be retained for relatively long periods in short-term memory. This facilitates both immediate access to the information and the storage of the information in permanent form. The brain lateralization that accompanied language development may well have also involved special developments in the linguistic hemisphere to facilitate the processing and memorization of temporal sequences of events (Carmon and Nachshon, 1971). In other words, it is possible that hemispheric specialization has provided alternative schemes for encoding over and above the addition of a language function (Levy, 1969).

Human memory has the characteristic of forming a temporally coherent stream. This was part of the definition of memory offered by William James. Events occur in particular spatiotemporal contexts, and they are stored in memory with respect to these contexts, so that the past has order, reality, and coherence. Aristotle pointed out that "many animals have memory and are capable of instruction, but no other animal except man can recall the past at will." Claparède (1911) strongly emphasized the temporal coherence of human memories and the associated concept of "me-ness." He rightly distinguished between recognition and the localization of an event in one's own past. He pointed out that this temporal tagging and personal association of memories, in conjunction with conscious processes, allows for voluntary memory searches. Thus, when we encounter someone who looks familiar, we may consciously and voluntarily initiate a search through our memories to locate this present event within our past experience. This powerful tool may be available only to humans.

Human/infrahuman differences in language, self-reference, and intelligence factors may help to explain the failure to obtain amnesic syndromes in animals with lesions corresponding to the effective lesions in humans (Weiskrantz, 1971; Isaacson, this volume). The animal experiments typically focus on perceptual or motor learning and involve repeated trials and primary reinforcement. On the whole, this type of learning or memory can be described as "lower-level," and it is characteristically preserved in the human amnesic syndromes.

The more complex conceptual and linguistic experiences are the ones that tend to be lost in humans, along with the ability to place experiences in a personal context. Since these capacities may exist in only rudimentary forms in animals, one should probably not expect them to reproduce the human types of amnesic syndromes.

1.5 ASPECTS OF THE ONTOGENY OF HUMAN MEMORY

1.5.1 Introduction

The basic questions in the ontogeny of human memory concern the order in which various memory functions or capacities are acquired, the relation of this order to features of the development of the nervous system, and the way in which the developmental sequence is revealed or paralleled in the dissolution of the nervous system during disease and in recovery following disease. I shall emphasize development-disease-recovery parallels, since this issue is germane to both the neuropathological aspects of memory and the amnesic syndromes.

The outline of the relationship between development, disease, and recovery was clearly laid down between 1880 and 1890, principally in the work of Jackson (1884) and Ribot (1882). Ribot described the order of decay of memory functions in progressive amnesia as follows:

1. failure of memory for recent events, with old memories preserved relatively intact;

2. loss of intellectual acquisitions, such as foreign languages, with earlier acquisitions remaining;

3. loss of memory for emotional states or highly emotional experiences;

4. finally, loss of habits and automated routines (such as dressing).

This sequence resembles that described by Delay and Brion (1962, cited in Barbizet, 1970) for the decay of cognitive functioning in senile dementia: first a loss in the ability to deal with new situations; then difficulty in chronological ordering of remembered events; then loss of powers of narration, with patchy memory; then loss of personal skills and abilities (e.g., knitting) and social habits; and eventually loss of even the awareness of deficit. The recovery-development parallel is also documented by Ribot (1882). He describes the case of a 24 year old who, following a period of two months of torpor, appeared very childlike, with no recognition of relatives. Recovery proceeded, with extension of vocabulary from few to many words, and with notions such as "opposite" coming in gradually. "Relearning" of relatives as new acquaintances occurred, as did relearning to read through regained mastery of the alphabet. The patient did not remember these experiences, according to Ribot, but relearned them.

A particularly fertile area for the study of either the reacquisition or sequential remembering of both memories and cognitive skills should be the detailed examination of trauma in children of elementary-school age, since a regression of even a few years in such children would push them into a period clearly different, both in memory and cognitive functioning, from that of their chronological age. In other words, a three-year retrograde amnesia in a seven year old would take him back to a period in which his whole cognitive structure was different, and fundamental reading and arithmetic skills had not yet been acquired. There are abundant reports in the literature (e.g., Blau, 1936; Brink et al., 1970) describing severe regressions in children following trauma, with relearning of both speech and motor abilities. Blau described a case of a fifth grader who regressed to the first-grade level and then showed complete and gradual recovery. However, none of these studies has been documented in any detail, so that precise questions about the order of return of memories, or the relative speed of recovery of different types of functions, cannot be answered.

The only significant parallel, in detail, between development and dissolution of cognitive function comes from the order of disappearance of Piagetian capacities in senility (Ajuriaguerra, Rey-Bellet-Muller, and Tissot, 1964; H. Feldman, R. Gelman, and P. Rozin, unpublished data). On the whole, the capacities last acquired in development drop out first in senility.

1.5.2 Levels of function in memory

I believe that the Jacksonian view, translated into Ribot's formulation for the study of memory, is basically correct. That is, I believe that those aspects of memory that appear first in evolution also develop first and usually disappear last in disease, and that such memories can be generally characterized as being organized at lower levels of the nervous system. The basic argument for this view is that it makes sense out of much of the data, although there is not much direct evidence relating type of memory to level of organization in the nervous system.

The best argument for Jacksonian explanations of memory dissolution concerns the different types of memory encoding or processing employed by adults. Adults seem to have at least three modes of processing or encoding: motor (enactive), ideational (e.g., iconic in vision), and symbolic or verbal (Bruner, Olver, and Greenfield, 1966). In evolution, it is almost certain that the schemes developed in the order motor, ideational, verbal. Bruner, Olver, and Greenfield have specifically suggested this sequence for human development. Certainly motor and visual memory appear in human children before the acquisition of significant verbal or symbolic capacities.

Possibly last to develop are strategies for tackling memory problems, such as organization or chunking schemes, consciously applied. These are seldom employed spontaneously by young children (Flavell, Griedricks, and Hoyt, 1970). Neuroanatomically, this might be related to the late development of the frontal areas, which seem to mediate memory monitoring and strategies (see Section 1.8.1).

The proposed evolutionary and developmental sequence (motor to ideational to symbolic encoding, followed by memorization strategies) suggests progressively higher levels of neural organization. Certainly verbal processes are carried on at the cortical level, and memory strategies are at least partly involved with the anterior frontal area, the most recently developed part of the brain.

To what extent does this sequence describe the dissolution of memory? It appears that motor skills or perceptuomotor abilities often remain intact in the amnesic syndromes. Talland (1965) noted evidence for learning by Korsakoff patients in "proprioceptive" tasks. In particular, he reported improvement in a motor-skill task involving picking up small beads with a small tool. He also cited Stern (1935) as having shown that a "total amnesic" learned to write shorthand and retained the skill. Both H.M. and M.K., though almost completely unable to remember names or faces, showed some ability to get around in their hospital or new home environments (Milner, 1966; Starr and Phillips, 1970). It is not clear how to characterize this learning, since it may well have a representational, visuospatial aspect. The most striking case of the sparing of perceptuomotor skills is M.K.'s demonstrated ability to learn a new piece of music on the piano in the face of a very dense general amnesia and no awareness of the experience of having learned the new piece (see Section 1.2).

The McGill group (see Milner, 1972, for a review) has carried out a number of investigations with H.M. in order to improve the definition of his residual memory capacities. H.M. performs normally on a mirror drawing task (Milner, 1962). The ability to draw a line between the double borders of a star, as seen through a mirror, was acquired rapidly and retained over two subsequent days (Figure 1.3). As usual, H.M., while demonstrating improved performance on days 2 and 3, had no awareness of having experienced the task before. Similarly, Corkin (1968) demonstrated improvement in performance by H.M. on rotary-pursuit, bimanual-tracking, and tapping tasks. Learning of these skills was below normal in all cases, but it was nonetheless significant. Retesting on the rotary pursuit task after a few days yielded complete retention.

The area of residual memory is further defined by studies on maze learning. Milner (1965) found H.M. completely unable to master a 28-choice-point visual stylus maze (see Figure 1.4). There was no learning in 215 trials spread over three days, in contrast to normals who usually reach a criterion of three consecutive errorless performances in about twenty trials. Similarly, Corkin (1965) found H.M. unable to make any progress, in terms of error reduction, on a 10-choice-point tactual maze. This latter study is of particular interest since, despite the fact that errors were not reduced, total time to complete the maze dropped significantly, from about 90 seconds on the first 10 trials to about 40 seconds on trials 71 to 80. Thus, although H.M. was unable to remember the turn sequence, he did develop increased skill in

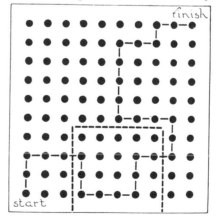

FIGURE 1.4 Plan of a visually guided stylus maze. The black circles represent metal boltheads on a wooden base. The patient must discover and remember the correct route, indicated here by a black line. The area enclosed by the dotted line is the shortened form of the maze. When this is used, the remainder of the maze is shielded from the patient's view. H. M. showed no improvement on the large maze, but substantial learning on the small maze. Modified from Milner (1962). Reproduced with permission from *Physiologie de l'Hippocampe* (Paris: Centre National de la Recherche Scientifique).

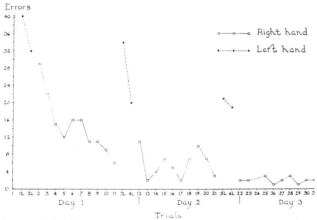

FIGURE 1.3 Mirror drawing performance of H.M., showing normal learning over a three-day period. From Milner (1962). Reproduced with permission from *Physiologie de l'Hippocampe* (Paris: Centre National de la Recherche Scientifique).

moving about through the maze (reversing at dead ends, etc.).

It is not clear why the visual maze was beyond H.M.'s capacity, given his ability to learn a little about spatial aspects of his surroundings. However, it is conceivable that the task demands of the 28-choice-point maze were too great, given the memory deficit. With considerations such as these in mind, Milner, Corkin, and Teuber (1968) studied H.M.'s performance on a small, 8-choice-point subsection of the original visual stylus maze (the dotted section of Figure 1.4). On this smaller maze H.M. reached criterion within 155 trials, and he showed significant savings as much as two *years* later, when he learned the same maze to criterion in 39 trials (Milner, 1970). This level of savings is below normal but well above chance. It is possible that there is success with 8 choice points because this number lies within the capacity of short-term memory. There is some evidence sugggesting that amnesics can show learning for tasks fully "comprehendible" within the span of STM (Drachman and Ommaya, 1964). It is also possible that 8 choices is just sufficiently easier than 28 that it can be learned with severely limited memory function.

The studies of amnesics do not clearly indicate relative superiority on visual as opposed to verbal memory, as one might expect from the ontogenetic literature. However, comparisons of the relative quality of two ill-defined types of memory are extremely difficult, and there is no simple way to equate or compare performance on visual- and verbal-recognition tests. There are a few studies suggesting relatively greater deficits in verbal encoding in amnesics (e.g., Cermak, Butters, and Gerrein, 1973). Parallel support for this view comes from the suggestion that verbal-recognition memory is more impaired than visual-recognition memory in normal subjects under partial anesthesia (Adam, 1973).

However, although it makes some neuroanatomical sense to conceive of motor skills as being organized at lower levels in the nervous system, available evidence (see Section 1.6.3) suggests that visuospatial-verbal differences are likely to be mediated by somewhat parallel structures in opposite hemispheres. Memorization strategies and the like tend to drop out in senility and are associated with the highest levels of neurological organization. They may, however, be spared in the amnesic syndromes (e.g., H.M.).

Ribot suggested that "emotional" memories and habitual acts were resistant to dissolution. I am not sure what defines emotional memories, and I therefore find it difficult to discuss their level of organization in the nervous system. That they tend to be preserved is indicated by many clinical examples, such as the classical case of Claparède (1911). He concealed a pin in his hand, and offered his hand to an amnesic patient. The patient grasped it, then withdrew her hand in pain. A few minutes later he offered his hand again, and the patient resisted shaking it. When asked why, the patient replied, "Doesn't one have the right to withdraw her hand?" Then the doctor insisted on a further explanation, and the patient said, "Is there perhaps a pin hidden in your hand?" However, the patient could not give any idea of why she had this suspicion. The clinical evidence on emotional memories is not completely clear-cut. For example, there is H.M.'s failure to remember his uncle's death prior to his (H.M.'s) surgery.

The argument with respect to habitual acts is also based primarily on their preservation in disease, especially senility. In addition, Williams (1966) reports that following electroconvulsive shock, memory for common words (e.g., the ability to name a comb from its picture) returns more rapidly than that for uncommon ones (e.g., teeth of the comb). However, it is not clear whether habitual or highly practiced memories are better described as resistant to dissolution because they are organized at lower levels and thus may be performed without conscious attention, or resistant because they are overdetermined by being reduplicated in the brain.

In summary, the relationship of level of organization in the nervous system to order of appearance in development and evolution and order of disappearance in disease is empirically weak, but it is suggestive and it seems intuitively to be correct. The case is clearest with respect to conditioning—which is at least partly intact in amnesics (Talland, 1960, 1965)—and perceptuomotor acquisitions on the one hand, and verbal or visuospatial memories and memory-strategy functions on the other.

1.5.3 The temporal organization of premorbid amnesias

Ribot asserted that the *age* of memories, that is time per se, was an important dimension in understanding diseases of memory. We now turn to this problem, and ask whether recent memories are more susceptible than older memories to destruction or loss of access. Most of the relevant data come from the amnesic syndromes and senility.

Amnesic syndromes are almost invariably accompanied by a failure in recall of at least some memories *antedating* the onset of pathology. These are often called *retrograde amnesias*. I will not use this term because it implies that the memory loss dates back continuously from the time of onset of the disease. I prefer the more neutral term *premorbid memory loss*. The distinction between premorbid and anterograde amnesias can often be made precisely, since the onset of "pathology" is often sudden, as in cranial trauma. This premorbid amnesia is one of the most puzzling aspects of the amnesic syndromes, and also one of the most controversial. It is puzzling because it involves failure to recall memories that have already been established as long-term memories. It is controversial because the basic retrograde aspect of the amnesia is in question. That is, can this memory "loss" be described as dating back more or less continuously in time from onset of pathology to some other time further in the past? Before plunging into a discussion of the temporal organization of premorbid memory "loss," it might be worthwhile to outline a few general features of the premorbid amnesias which are generally accepted.

Almost all instances of amnesic syndromes with sudden onset include a dense amnesia for the period of seconds or minutes prior to trauma (e.g., Whitty and Zangwill, 1966a). This amnesia tends to be permanent. This brief period of retrograde amnesia corresponds roughly with intervals reported in some of the literature on electroconvulsive shock in animals. It may reflect a transient disturbance of a consolidation mechanism, disturbance of rehearsal strategies (Williams, 1969), or some other disturbance of a highly sensitive just-registered memory. It does not raise the massive problems of the longer premorbid amnesias, which obviously involve previously consolidated memories.

A second point of general agreement is that there is often a defect in premorbid memories, extending well past the immediate pretrauma period. Discussion and disagreement hinges only on whether this disruption has a temporally organized basis, i.e., whether it is really retrograde.

A third area of general agreement is that the often massive disturbance of past memories almost invariably shows substantial recovery, apparently spontaneously. In many cases of extensive amnesias, after a period of recovery the only remaining amnesia is for a period of seconds to minutes prior to trauma, the same period referred to above (Whitty and Zangwill, 1966a; Russell, 1959).

A final point on which there is some consensus is that, *in general*, the more severe the damage to the memory "system," as gauged by the length of the period of anterograde amnesia (amnesia dating from the onset of injury), the more premorbid amnesia is observed (see Table 1.1, which indicates the lengths of periods of retrograde amnesia for fifty consecutive patients from four groups of anterograde amnesics). This relationship is of considerable interest, since it suggests a linkage in mechanism between the anterograde and premorbid amnesias. In some cases there is a striking relationship between termination of anterograde amnesia and shrinkage of premorbid amnesia (Benson and Geschwind, 1967;

TABLE 1.1

Relationship between anterograde amnesia and retrograde amnesia (200 subjects)

Duration of R.A.	Duration of A.A.				
	<1 hr	1–24 hr	1–7 days	>7 days	Total
Nil	9	1	1		11
< 1 min	34	35	15	12	96
1–30 min	6	13	21	18	58
0.5–12 hr	1	1	9	6	17
0.5–2 days			3	7	10
2–10 days			1	6	7
Over 10 days				1	1
Total	50	50	50	50	200

Source: Table 3 from W. R. Russell, *Brain, Memory, Learning: A Neurologist's View*, © Oxford University Press, 1969, by permission of the Oxford University Press, Oxford.

see also Figure 1.5). It is also important to realize that premorbid amnesia, whatever its cause, has a tendency to shrink spontaneously over time, whereas the experiences occurring during the period of anterograde amnesia tend not to be remembered subsequently (Whitty and Zangwill, 1966a; Russell, 1959). This makes some sense, of course, since the premorbid memories are obviously laid down prior to trauma, whereas there might be a registration or consolidation defect during the period of anterograde amnesia. At this time there is insufficient evidence to permit the assumption of a direct linkage between anterograde and premorbid amnesias. There is certainly a clear dissociation in H.M. between dense anterograde amnesia and fairly good recall of premorbid events. This has been clearly demonstrated for memories of faces of public figures in a recent study (Marslen-Wilson, 1974; see Section 1.6.6).

The interpretation of these amnesias for past events is inherently difficult. Since many past memories are recovered, and hence were not "lost," one could argue

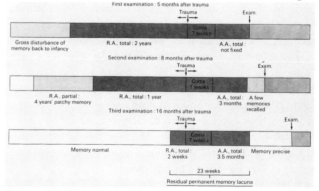

FIGURE 1.5 Amnesic symptoms at three different times following cranial trauma in a 40-year-old patient. No surgery. R.A., retrograde amnesia (premorbid amnesia). A.A., anterograde amnesia. From *Human Memory and Its Pathology* by Jacques Barbizet. Copyright 1970 by W.H. Freeman and Company.

that the last few seconds or minutes are subject to the same pathology as more distant memories, and thus could also be recovered. Indeed they sometimes are (Whitty and Zangwill, 1966a; Russell, 1959). Thus we are not logically justified in claiming that the period just prior to trauma is literally lost, or nonconsolidated, in most cases, even though there tends to be a permanent amnesia for these events. Hence both two-process and single-process theories of premorbid amnesia are tenable. As it turns out, the issue of major controversy is not the brief period of dense, permanent amnesia, but the larger disturbances of past memories.

THE ARGUMENT FOR THE EXISTENCE OF TEMPORALLY CONTIGUOUS AND TEMPORALLY ORGANIZED PREMORBID AMNESIAS. Ribot (1882) clearly stated what, in modern accounting terms, might be called the last-in/first-out principle: the more recent a memory, the more vulnerable it is. This fits, in general, with clinical and anecdotal impressions of preservation of childhood memories in old age and senility, and with the presenting characteristics of amnesic patients. Severely afflicted patients, for example, when asked who is president of the United States, frequently name a president of a few to many years back, and appear to be unaware of major events over the recent past.

This type of amnesia may even occur in mild cases. For example, Fisher (1966) describes a case of sudden onset of transient amnesic symptoms in a 41-year-old patient, without any loss of consciousness. A "retrograde" amnesia of a few years appeared suddenly, so that the patient claimed that John F. Kennedy was president, even though it was one year after the assassination, and gave her age as 39 or 40. Within five hours after the trauma, she knew that Lyndon B. Johnson was president. Clinical impressions of loss of memories for the relatively recent past prior to trauma are accompanied by impressions of clear memories of earlier days. For example, doctor D.G., densely amnesic following temporal-lobe surgery, was described as remembering minute details of his early life and medical training (Scoville and Milner, 1957). The clinically described retrograde amnesias of a few years in H.M. and M.K. (see Section 1.2) further confirm the Ribot position.

Ribot cites extensive anecdotal evidence for the general last-in/first-out principle. One of his most striking examples of temporally organized dissolution comes from a case of Dr. Rush, in Philadelphia:

Dr. Scandella, an ingenious Italian who visited this country a few years ago, was master of the Italian, French, and English languages. In the beginning of the yellow fever, which terminated his life . . . he spoke English only; in the middle of the disease, he spoke French only; but, on the day of his death he spoke only in the language of his native country. (Ribot, 1882, p. 182)

Studies of large numbers of cases of trauma suggest that most premorbid amnesias are retrograde, and extend back minutes or hours, but that amnesic intervals of days, weeks, or years occur fairly often. Russell (1959; see also Russell and Nathan, 1946) concludes that in general, "there is a vulnerability of memories which depends directly on their nearness to the injury." An instance cited by Russell demonstrates this point nicely:

A case previously described was that of P.A.S., a green-keeper, aged 22, who was thrown from his motorcycle in August 1933. There was a bruise in the left frontal region and slight bleeding from the left ear, but no fracture was seen on X-ray examination. A week after the accident he was able to converse sensibly, and the nursing staff considered that he had fully recovered consciousness. When questioned, however, he said that the date was February 1922, and that he was a schoolboy. He had no recollection of five years spent in Australia, and two years in this country working on a golf course. Two weeks after the injury he remembered the five years spent in Australia, and remembered returning to this country; the past two years were, however, a complete blank as far as his memory was concerned. Three weeks after the injury he returned to the village where he had been working for two years. Everything looked strange, and he had no recollection of ever having been there before. He lost his way on more than one occasion. Still feeling a stranger to the district he returned to work; he was able to do his work satisfactorily, but had difficulty in remembering what he had actually done during the day. About ten weeks after the accident the events of the past two years were gradually recollected and finally he was able to remember everything up to within a few minutes of the accident. (Russell, 1959, pp. 69–70)

Recovery from amnesia is characterized, according to Russell, by gradual, temporally organized shrinkage. The process is illustrated by a case in Figure 1.5. During recovery islands of memories, temporally isolated from both the present and the well-recalled past, frequently appear (Russell, 1959). These islands often form bases from which further extensions of memory occur, with "bridges" eventually occurring between the islands as a coherent past is recreated. Others also report formation and enlargement of islands, but are less sanguine about the basic temporally organized nature of the recovery (Whitty and Zangwill, 1966a; Williams and Zangwill, 1952; Williams, 1969).

Two other lines of evidence support the general notion

of temporally organized premorbid amnesia. One has to do with the general observation that the more severe the anterograde amnesia, the further back the retrograde amnesia goes, as shown by the data in Table 1.1. Under different circumstances Bickford and his colleagues (1958) produced retrograde amnesias for past periods of from a few minutes to several days by stimulating the midtemporal gyrus, 1.5–2.0 cm below the surface. The extent of the reported retrograde amnesia was related to the duration of the stimulation, suggesting again the further invasion of past events by the more severe disturbances. Extent of retrograde amnesia was measured by the patient's estimate of date, day of week, time of day, name of president, etc.

All of the studies cited up to this point have employed reasonable general techniques of assessing past memories, but have not involved detailed exploration of the extent and precision of memories from different time periods. This is probably because the clinical impression of retrograde, temporally organized amnesia is so striking. There is one precisely measured experimental case, but it unfortunately involves very brief periods of amnesia and hence may fall within the "disturbance-of-consolidation" interval described above: Cronholm (1969), studying memory for materials shown to a patient just prior to electroconvulsive-shock therapy, found that material presented 60 seconds prior to shock was remembered better than material presented just 15 seconds prior to shock.

THE CASE AGAINST TEMPORALLY ORGANIZED PREMORBID AMNESIA. It will be noted that the basic case for the Ribot position depends on a large number of instances, very few of which are described with enough precision to be compelling. Since the alternative view holds that memories. in general are disturbed during amnesias, the patchiness or poor quality of recent pretrauma memories per se is not at issue, but rather whether these memories are *relatively* severely disturbed. In fact, a number of investigators who have spent much time studying amnesic patients are not convinced of the truth of Ribot's law. The existence of islands of memories during recovery (Russell, 1959; Whitty and Zangwill, 1966a) is itself a violation of the law, though in all fairness, the law should be interpreted only to indicate a general temporal direction of memory loss or recovery. However, the islands themselves do not appear in anything like a strictly chronological sequence (Whitty and Zangwill, 1966a). Furthermore, occasionally an island of events dating from the recent pretrauma past is intact, though extensive periods before it seem inaccessible (Williams and Zangwill, 1952).

In general, Williams (1969) and Whitty and Zangwill (1966a) do *not* describe memory loss and recovery as fundamentally chronological, though they do not deny that there may be some relationship between time and the vulnerability of memories. They also question the clinical impression that memory for remote events remains intact (as does Barbizet, 1970). This doubt is supported by data from the animal literature which indicates, in most cases, an increased vulnerability of *older* memories to forgetting (Campbell and Spear, 1972).

Furthermore, any Ribot-type view must deal with the special case of amnesia for the experiences of early childhood. The period prior to about age six is only dimly remembered by most humans. This can be explained in psychodynamic terms, or as a consequence of the fundamental changes in cognition that occur around this age, which probably alter drastically the memory encoding and retrieving processes. The Ribot law, if true at all, probably applies only from about six years on in the human case.

RECENT ATTEMPTS TO RESOLVE THE ISSUE. Over the last five years there has been a sudden spurt of experiments that have attempted to measure the relationship between age of memory and resistance to forgetting in normals and amnesics. All of these attempts, by necessity, have resorted to the questionnaire technique, in which subjects are queried for their recall or recognition of faces or public events associated with different time periods. This represents a marked improvement over clinical impression, but it has problems of its own. It is hard to assure equal difficulty of items from different time periods, and it is not possible to be certain that subjects were exposed to a particular face or event at the time when it reached public prominence, rather than at some later date (as, for example, in a historical movie or history class).

The questionnaire technique was first introduced to the problem of premorbid amnesias by Warrington and her colleagues. Their work, measuring recall or recognition for events or faces (Warrington and Silberstein, 1970; Warrington and Sanders, 1971), and other work on event memory (Squire and Slater, 1975), showed a gradual decline in memory for material from the period extending back about five to ten years prior to testing, with rather stable memory performance for materials older than this. This recency effect did *not* appear in another recent questionnaire study (Seltzer and Benson, 1974).

The Squire and Slater (1975) study used a particularly well designed questionnaire, constructed of multiple-choice questions about television shows that were aired for only one season at different times in the past. With some equalization for popularity as well as exposure, these items form about as fair a test of past memories as can be imagined. The reliability of the technique is attested to by the failure of subjects who were very young, or not alive, or out of the country during a particular period, to identify the programs from this period.

Given that adults do not show a "primacy" effect, but do possibly show a "recency" effect, do diseases of memory preferentially attack more recent memories? The oldest subjects (70 years and above) in one of the questionnaire studies showed the poorest total memory performance, and showed it across a 25-year time period (Warrington and Sanders, 1971). This anti-Ribot result was confirmed in persons with specific amnesic syndromes, who showed a more or less uniform depression on face or event memory (Sanders and Warrington, 1971). However, performance of amnesics for material from all time periods was essentially random, so that a floor effect might be hiding a true retrograde memory loss. A recent study by Seltzer and Benson (1974), using event questionnaires, clearly shows the retrograde relationships: normals and Korsakoffs showed about equal recognition memory for events that occurred 35 or more years ago, while the Korsakoffs' performances became progressively poorer, with respect to normals, the more recent the events.

The weight of evidence presently seems to support a general retrograde direction in premorbid amnesias. However, more detailed day-to-day study of the process of loss and recovery of past memories is needed. In order to do this one needs a situation of sudden onset, as in cranial trauma or electroconvulsive shock. Recent work has shown that following a series of electroconvulsive shocks, there is a loss of event memories dating back at least twenty years (Squire, 1974). ECS is a scheduled event, so that adequate pretests can be performed. Coupled with the improved Squire-Slater television-program questionnaire, a definitive study could be arranged.

Another situation with special promise for clarifying this issue could be the study of football players suffering concussion injuries. Morris Moscovitch and I have, for some years, been planning such a study. These injuries occur quite frequently, and recovery is ordinarily complete. They go by the name "ding" amnesias (Yarnell and Lynch, 1973) and are associated with periods of disorientation and anterograde amnesia. Many references are made to such injuries in popular books about football (e.g., *Instant Replay: The Green Bay Diary of Jerry Kramer*). The important advantage of football players is that they carry in their heads a complex assortment of plays that change from year to year and, to some extent,

from game to game. They also have experienced a set of games and practices at particular well-defined times, which have been recorded by the coaching staff and sometimes are on videotape or film. Thus a fine-grain record of events is available, so that recovery could be mapped in detail. I am encouraged to think that this approach is viable by what I gather is a true anecdote about a professional quarterback, who, following some sort of concussion, returned to his team's huddle and began calling plays from a different team that he had been on two years before.

Having considered the evidence, we must end where we began, with certainty only that there *is* a brief period of dense retrograde amnesia for events just prior to trauma, that more global disturbances of past memories occur, and that these latter tend to recover. The data from clinical cases and some of the recent experimental data support Ribot, and hence I am inclined to believe that there is a true retrograde amnesia, i.e., a last-in/first-out principle. Why old memories should be more resistant to disease is a fascinating question. It is possible that, by virtue of age, they are more "practiced," and hence resemble habitual acts. But, then, why are habitual acts disease-resistant?

1.6. THE AMNESIC SYNDROMES

1.6.1 Neuropathology of the amnesic syndromes

Amnesic syndromes result from a wide variety of apparently different causes (Whitty and Lishman, 1966). Transient syndromes may result from transient vascular occlusions, epileptic fits, trauma (especially concussion), nutritional deficiencies, and a variety of acute toxemias. Syndromes that often have a permanent or relatively permanent character result from toxemias, anoxia, vitamin deficiencies (including those induced by chronic alcoholism), focal brain wounds (Teuber, Milner, and Vaughan, 1968), intracranial infections (e.g., herpes simplex encephalitis), vascular lesions, tumors (Kahn and Crosby, 1972), surgical procedures, senility (Kral, 1969), and presenility (Alzheimer variety: Miller, 1971).

From the point of view of the study of memory dysfunction, the majority of the patients studied probably fall into the categories of Korsakoff's psychosis (usually due to chronic alcoholism), senility, or relatively acute forms of concussion trauma. A smaller number of cases, but of special significance due to the purity of the syndrome, suffer specific brain damage consequent upon encephalitis (e.g., M.K.; see Starr and Phillips, 1970) or surgery of the temporal lobes (e.g., H.M.; see Penfield and Milner, 1958). And then there are the "psychogenic" syndromes, which share properties of the amnesic syndromes. These can sometimes be differentiated by their tendency to clear up suddenly (Stengel, 1966).

Patients carrying the diagnosis of alcoholic Korsakoff syndrome probably constitute the largest group of amnesics with relative sparing of most other functions. Characteristically, these patients develop severe neurological symptoms called Wernicke's encephalopathy, quite suddenly (Adams, 1969; Victor, Adams, and Collins, 1971). These symptoms include a variety of relatively peripheral signs such as ataxias and palsies, accompanied by global confusion. Embedded within the global confusion, but hardly salient at the onset, is an amnesic syndrome. The Wernicke syndrome seems to be due primarily to vitamin B$_1$ (thiamine) deficiency, resulting from a diet in which alcohol forms the main source of calories. Not only does alcohol contain no vitamin B$_1$, but since it is high in carbohydrates, it increases the need for this vitamin. Treatment of Wernicke patients with thiamine often causes a dramatic reversal of most of the symptoms. The amnesic disorder is most resistant to recovery, and hence the Wernicke syndrome often clears into the more focalized Korsakoff psychosis. Victor, Adams, and Collins (1971), in a large-scale study, found that the Korsakoff syndrome was not preceded by the Wernicke global syndrome in only 9 of 245 cases. The classical Korsakoff psychosis, consisting of an amnesic syndrome with confabulation and some disorientation, results at least transiently following 84 percent of Wernicke syndromes. Twenty-one percent of these Korsakoffs show complete recovery, and 26 percent show none. The bulk of patients studied as amnesics are rather severe cases of the Korsakoff syndrome. They have both a history of chronic alcoholism and, most likely, some residues from acute stages of widespread brain dysfunction.

Given the bewildering array of causes of the amnesic syndromes, it is really quite surprising, and pleasing, to discover that there are some anatomical common denominators. Focusing on cases where there is frank neuropathology (as opposed to general and usually temporary depression of brain function, as in cranial trauma; or more permanent and widespread damage, as in senility), the great majority of what seem to be critical lesions lie in what is called the circuit of Papez (Papez, 1937). This sequence of interconnected structures, arranged in a connecting "circle," is a part of the limbic system. The system has long been implicated, primarily in the animal literature, in the mediation of emotional behavior. The Papez circuit, as indicated in Figure 1.6, consists of the following principal components: from the mammillary bodies via the mamillothalamic tract to the anterior nuclear group of the dorsal thalamus; then via thalamocortical radiations to the cingulate gyrus; then to the

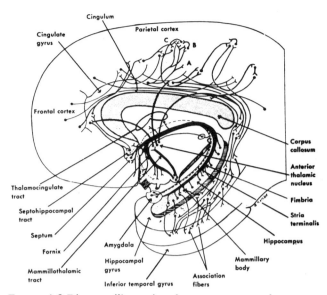

FIGURE 1.6 Diagram illustrating the components and connections of the Papez circuit. From Kahn and Crosby (1972). Reproduced with permission from *Neurology* 22: 121. Copyright 1972 by The New York Times Media Company, Inc.

hippocampal gyrus via short association bundles to the hippocampus and amygdala; and from the hippocampus, via the fimbria-fornix system, to the septum and mammillary bodies. Connections between amygdala and hypothalamus may also be considered part of the system (Kahn and Crosby, 1972).

Bilateral damage to this circuit, at any of a number of points, seems a sufficient condition for the generation of an amnesic syndrome. A number of studies and reviews of the neuropathology of the Korsakoff syndrome have converged on the conclusion that bilateral damage to the mammillary bodies is the primary neurological correlate (Brierly, 1966; Angelergues, 1969; Marin, 1955; Brion, 1969). Presumably they are especially sensitive to thiamine deficiency. The one study that expresses considerable skepticism on this point (Victor, Adams, and Collins, 1971) provides much evidence for the *sufficiency* of mammillary-body damage to produce the syndrome, since 75 percent of the Korsakoff brains analyzed by these authors showed mammillary-body damage. However, these authors were impressed by the finding of four Korsakoff cases without mammillary damage but with clear damage of the mediodorsal nucleus of the thalamus, a structure not intimately connected with the Papez circuit. Whatever the pathological causes of the syndrome in these few cases, the sufficiency of mammillary-body damage is not in serious question. Supporting evidence comes from amnesic syndromes produced by tumors in the area of the mammillary bodies (Kahn and Crosby, 1972; Angelergues, 1969). Such tumors often produce symptoms by exerting pressure on the critical tissue; this is strongly indicated by the fact that removal of some craniopharyngiomas pressing against the mammillary areas leads to a reversal of symptoms.

Bilateral damage to the anterior nucleus of the thalamus or the fornix can produce amnesic syndromes (Angelergues, 1969; Sweet, Talland, and Ervin, 1959), although the findings on fornix lesions or section are mixed (Brierly, 1966). Stimulation of the fornix (Ojemann, 1971, one clinical case) leads to disturbances of memory.

As with the mammillary bodies, evidence for critical involvement of the hippocampus is quite compelling. Some types of encephalitis (e.g., herpes simplex) seem both to attack the hippocampus specifically and to produce amnesic syndromes. Vascular lesions or tumors in the hippocampus have been associated with memory disorders (Whitty and Lishman, 1966; Brierly, 1966). In senility and presenility (Alzheimer's disease), where memory functions are especially compromised, there are reports of plaques in the hippocampal area (Brierly, 1966; Whitty and Lishman, 1966). An acute amnesic syndrome was produced in an epileptic patient by stimulation with electrodes implanted in the hippocampus (Chapman et al., 1967).

The most compelling evidence for hippocampal involvement in the amnesic syndromes comes from analysis of the brains of patients who have undergone surgery of the temporal lobes for relief of the symptoms of epilepsy. This long-term study, done by the McGill group, uniquely combines the highest levels of neuroanatomical and psychological assessment (Scoville and Milner, 1957; Penfield and Milner, 1958; Milner, 1967, 1970, 1972). Patients are carefully evaluated for a variety of memory and other cognitive functions, and these evaluations are compared with brain maps showing the location of the tissue removed during surgery. Careful analysis of the tissue necessary and sufficient to produce failures in recent memory has led Milner and her colleagues to conclude that the critical structure is the hippocampus. The extent of the midtemporal lesions that have produced syndromes like that of H.M. is shown in Figure 1.7.

Bilateral destruction of other portions of the Papez circuit has been reported to produce amnesic syndromes (Brion, 1969; Whitty and Lishman, 1966; Angelergues, 1969). There are also scattered reports of lesions in other areas, such as frontal lobes (Angelergues, 1969; Whitty and Lishman, 1966), that produce similar symptoms.

In face of the neuroanatomical data, two difficult questions arise. First, why does this particular system, which is partly subcortical and not very cognitive in neuroanatomical flavor, seem to play such a critical role in memory function? And second, why is this system

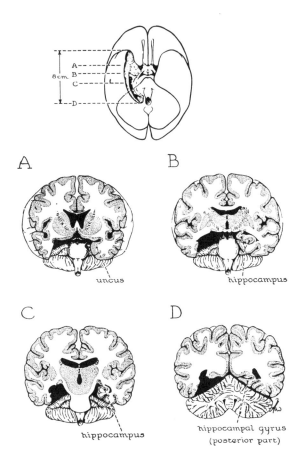

FIGURE 1.7 Diagrammatic cross sections of the human brain, showing the estimated extent of removal in Dr. Scoville's medial-temporal-lobe ablation. All operations were bilateral, single-stage procedures, but here, for illustrative purposes, one side has been left intact. From Milner (1972). Reproduced with permission from *Clinical Neurosurgery* 19: 422.

so easily compromised, so that amnesic syndromes are caused by such diverse mechanisms as general head trauma, senility, and thiamine deficiency?

There is no clear-cut answer to either of these questions. The specific involvement of the limbic system may be an important clue to the *psychological* nature of the amnesic syndrome (an example of information flow from neurology to psychology), since the limbic system is part of the general subcortical activation and arousal system described by Luria (1966, 1973). Part of the role of this system is to maintain cortical tone—presumably in order to keep the cognitive motors running. If we hold to this view, then we must assume that the interesting cognitive stuff goes on somewhere else, and that the Papez circuit is like the fuel line to the engine of the car: cutting it will stop the engine, but studying it won't give much insight into the basic *neurological* mechanisms of memory. But to hold such a view, to assume that defects in activation cause the amnesic syndrome, raises a serious problem. Why does the memory system fail while other cognitive functions, which would appear on the surface to involve at least as much activation, remain untouched? Either memory function for some reason requires an awful lot of gas, or there are somewhat separate or specialized arousal or modulation systems for different functions. Possibly the strong connections between the Papez circuit and the frontal and temporal lobes mediate such specificity.

Alternatively, one could look to more specific functions performed by the Papez circuit. Its role in the mediation of emotions and its special relationship to the olfactory system come to mind. The problem is that emotional memories and other types of memories that one would be inclined to place in the limbic system are just those that seem to be preserved when this system is damaged in humans. There is an indication of olfactory-memory deficit in H.M. and M.K. (Could they also be deficient in the stimulation of memories, à la Proust, from olfactory experiences?) But even if true, it would be difficult to get from such specific characteristics to the full amnesic syndrome. Limbic-system involvement with response selection and inhibition mechanisms (see Isaacson, this volume), a form of selective activation, could be related to memory-retrieval disorders (see Section 1.6.5 and Warrington and Weiskrantz, 1973).

As to the second question, the high frequency of occurrence of amnesic syndromes, one is forced to the conclusion that this is a highly sensitive neurological system. Data on trauma and senility suggest that it is particularly susceptible to general depression of the nervous system. This is supported by the fact that partially anesthetized humans show a transient amnesic syndrome (Adam, 1973). This is a bit puzzling, since in the Jacksonian scheme the limbic system would not ordinarily be accorded early-drop-out status, as it is not at the highest and most complex level of organization in the nervous system. However, one could claim that the memory-formation system resides somewhere else, and is simply highly sensitive to damage to systems that contribute to its function, the limbic system being one. After all, there is no direct evidence that cranial trauma, for example, acts through the limbic system (as opposed to acting upon a common neurological link further along in the processing sequence).

A parallel explanation for the frequency and diversity of causes of amnesic syndromes focuses on the critical importance of *bilateral* damage to the Papez circuit. This circuit is quite extensive, with some parts located rather close to the midline. This means that a single pathological locus could possibly induce a bilateral lesion or depression of function; this would be highly unlikely for corresponding cortical structures. Thus, for example, it is possible for tumors of the base of the brain or adjoining tissue to interfere with the function of both mammillary bodies (Kahn and Crosby, 1972). In other words, if the circuit is seen as a pair of rather long wires, often running close and parallel to each other, the chances for bilateral interruption would be much greater than in a system composed of two rather diffusely defined masses of brain tissue. These anatomical facts, plus apparent biochemical specificities in parts of the circuit (e.g., manifested as an affinity for herpes simplex in the hippocampus or a sensitivity to thiamine deficiency in the mammillary bodies), could account for much of the symptomatology. However, the explanation of the frequency of the syndrome in senility, cranial trauma, or partial anesthesia is still obscure.

This brief review has raised more questions than it has answered. It also illustrates how far one can be from a meaningful answer even with good neurological localization of function.

1.6.2. The amnesic syndromes—one or many?

I have carefully referred to the amnesic syndrome*s*. Given the multiple etiology and neuropathology, it is worthwhile to look for relationships between type of pathology and type of syndrome. This quest does not have simply neuropathological interest. The many psychological studies now in the literature on amnesic syndromes use diverse patient populations, so that interpretation of the literature requires some sensitivity to the type of subjects studied.

The irreducible core of the amnesic syndromes seems to be (1) loss of access, in recall and recognition, to at least many postmorbid memories, and (2) a lost sense of familiarity upon exposure to instances of these memories. These characteristics exist side by side with apparently normal short-term memory. In the Korsakoff syndrome these symptoms are typically associated with lack of awareness of the deficit, disorientation, and confabulation (Talland, 1965; Lhermitte and Signoret, 1972). A number of investigators have remarked on the fact that in the typical hippocampal syndromes, such as those resulting from encephalitis or bilateral midtemporal lobectomy, confabulation, disorientation, and lack of awareness of the deficit are absent (Zangwill, 1966; Lhermitte and Signoret, 1972). Careful and broadly based examination of psychological function in Korsakoff patients reveals a variety of other cognitive defects. Poor performance in divided-attention tasks, disjunctive-reaction-time tasks, and cancellation problems (e.g., crossing out all the small letters bordering on empty spaces in a written passage) (Talland, 1965), perseveration on inappropriate hypotheses in problems or identification tasks (Talland, 1965; Oscar-Berman, 1973), and deficits in attention shifting, perseveration, and set inflexibility

(Milner, 1964) are all clear signs of frontal-lobe dysfunction (Luria, 1966; P. Milner, 1970). This suggests either direct frontal damage or frontal depression via depression of the limbic system as an activator. The Papez circuit has many linkages with the frontal area.

An experiment by Lhermitte and Signoret (1972) provides a particularly clear separation between the hippocampal-encephalitic and the Korsakoff syndromes (see also Lhermitte and Signoret, this volume). In a task that involved learning the identity and location of each of nine pictures in a 3 × 3 matrix, both Korsakoffs and encephalitics performed very poorly on free recall. That is, they were unable, after numerous exposures, to name which picture belonged in each location. However, given the pictures, the Korsakoffs were able to do rather well in placing them in their appropriate locations, and the encephalitics were not. This contrasts with the superiority of the encephalitics in repeating sequences of items and in remembering over brief time intervals a display in the 3 × 3 matrix in which there was a logical plan to the arrangement (e.g., size and color varying systematically across the two axes). This pattern of results suggests a more severe deficit of "memory formation" or "consolidation" in the encephalitics and a more severe deficit of memory planning or organization in the Korsakoffs. The specific deficit in the Korsakoffs suggests frontal involvement, since patients with frontal-lobe damage are deficient both at discovery procedures (for detecting and using a plan) and at remembering the temporal order of sequences (Milner, 1971).

Given this diversity of symptomatologies, any study of the psychological or biological aspects of the amnesic syndrome faces a difficult problem in selecting subjects. The problem is exacerbated by a second factor. In general, it is desirable to use individuals with intelligence in the normal range. Since it is likely that either side effects or, possibly, direct effects of the amnesia-producing pathology compromise intelligence a bit, the range of subjects is significantly reduced. Most investigators, in order to keep intelligence in the normal range, have studied individuals with marked but often not terribly severe amnesic symptoms. The severity can be measured crudely by scores on the Wechsler Memory Scale, which includes evaluation of both short- and long-term memories and uses both verbal and nonverbal materials. The amnesics studied vary in their scores from one standard deviation below the mean to almost three below the mean. This issue is critical because most amnesics studied are not like H.M.—they show some significant recall on word lists or paired associates, and hence cannot, even at first blush, be described as lacking the ability to form long-term memories.

1.6.3 The amnesic syndrome as an instance of pure short-term memory

According to James (1890), an object in primary (short-term) memory "never was lost; its date was never cut off in consciousness from that of the immediately present moment. In fact it comes to us as belonging to the rearward portion of the present space of time, and not to the genuine past." This seems a perfect description of the clinical impression of what is spared in the amnesic. Things stay in this immediate consciousness as long as they can, and then drop off into the unknown, or the inaccessible, or the unrecallable. Even when items are recalled, they lack the feeling of having been experienced before. I know of no better description of the short-term memory space than James's version, and I am inclined to use it as the standard against which to validate the amnesic. If one does this, one can then use the other properties of the intelligent amnesic's short-term memory to help define the characteristics of this memory compartment, or memory stage.

The critical fact about amnesics' recent memory is the disappearance of an item from memorial awareness following a brief distraction. This virtually universal feature of amnesics is particularly well illustrated by H.M. (20 months after surgery):

He was able to retain the number 584 for at least 15 minutes, by continuously working out elaborate mnemonic schemes. When asked how he had been able to retain the number for so long, he replied: "It's easy. You just remember 8. You see, 5, 8, and 4 add to 17. You remember 8; subtract it from 17 and it leaves 9. Divide 9 in half and you get 5 and 4, and there you are: 584. Easy." A minute or so later, H.M. was unable to recall either the number "584" or any of the associated complex train of thought; in fact he did not know that he had been given a number to remember, because in the meantime the examiner had introduced a new topic. (Milner, 1970)

The concept of compartmentalized memory, and specifically of a distinction between short- and long-term memory, has received much attention in cognitive psychology. The distinction is based on differences in capacity (small in STM), forgetting (rapid in STM), and coding mechanisms (acoustic rather than semantic in verbal STM), along with the neurological data (see Simon, this volume). Depending on one's theoretical persuasion, particular phenomena of memory belong to the short-term or long-term compartments, or to the netherworld between. The performance of amnesics would be helpful as a means of assigning phenomena to their appropriate boxes.

Baddeley and Warrington (1970) carried out a number of experiments in which traditional measures of short-term memory were used with amnesic patients (four of whom were alcoholic Korsakoffs). These patients had intelligence that was in the normal range, showed very little recall from recently established long-term memory, and were disoriented as to date and place. Their performance on digit span was quite normal except that it deteriorated rapidly at eight digits, a point where one might expect long-term factors to play a most significant role. In the free recall of a series of ten words, as mentioned above (Section 1.3.3; see Figure 1.2), the performance of amnesics is what one would expect with the absence of an LTM component (Baddeley and Warrington, 1970; Miller, 1971).

Hebb (1961) noted that in successive digit-span experiments, if one particular group of digits longer than the subject's span was repeated at frequent intervals (unknown to the subject), the subject's performance would gradually improve on that particular span. Since this presumably results from long-term storage of these sequences, it should not occur in amnesics. Drachman and Arbit (1966) tried this with a number of amnesics, including H.M. They found little evidence for learning of supraspan digit strings. Baddeley and Warrington (1970) obtained clear evidence for improvement, though not at the same rate as in normals. This in itself is not strong evidence against the picture I have been painting since these amnesics showed some ability to recall events of the recent past.

Most of the detailed studies of the STM characteristics of amnesics are based on the Peterson-Peterson paradigm (1959) or the related Konorski paradigm (1959). In either procedure subjects are presented with some information to remember and are then tested after a brief interval (up to about one minute). In the Konorski paradigm stimulus A is presented and removed. Some seconds later another stimulus is presented, and the subject must indicate whether it is the same as or different from the previous one. In the related delayed matching-to-sample procedure the subject is offered a series of stimuli on the second presentation, and must choose the one that matches the original. In the Peterson-Peterson procedure free recall is characteristically used: the subject is asked to produce the stimuli after a fixed interval of time. In all these procedures, during the time between the standard and test stimuli, the subject can be either left alone to rehearse or busied with a distracting task.

In the initial study of this type, Prisko (1963) used the Konorski technique to compare normal subjects with patients who had undergone bilateral temporal surgery. The bitemporally lesioned patients (including H.M.) showed severe amnesic syndromes, with significant hippocampal damage bilaterally. In the same-different paradigm Prisko used five different types of stimuli: clicks of various frequencies, patterns of light flashes, tones, colors, and nonsense figures. Though performance was good when the test stimulus followed the standard immediately, it deteriorated quite rapidly in the amnesics over the one-minute period, even in the absence of interfering tasks. Introduction of such a task produced no further deterioration. (The interfering task was performance of a motor task in response to verbal instructions. In other words, it was not in the same mode as the stimuli to be remembered.) Performance was deficient on all five types of stimuli.

These data, along with H.M.'s fine performance on "584," suggest that in normals there is a rehearsal or recirculation mechanism only for verbalizable material, since without distraction H.M. could hold on to numbers but not visual or auditory "patterns" (see Figure 1.1). This difference in the handling of different materials was clearly confirmed in H.M. by Sidman, Stoddard, and Mohr (1968). On a delayed matching-to-sample procedure, without distraction, H.M. showed no deterioration at all in his memory of verbal materials for up to 40 seconds, the longest interval tested. On the other hand, when H.M. had to remember the shape of a circle or ellipse and to match it to one of a set shown to him at testing, his performance deteriorated rapidly over time. Although he performed normally with an immediate match, he was clearly below normal by 8 seconds, and he dropped to chance in the range 24–32 seconds. Normals retain the stimuli of Prisko or Sidman, Stoddard, and Mohr over periods of one minute without difficulty. Since the difference between normals and amnesics appears to lie in the ability to place or gain access to recent events in LTM, the interesting possibility arises that this ability is needed to retain nonverbal materials in STM, while verbal rehearsal or recirculation strategies suffice to hold verbalizable materials in STM.

In a design similar to Prisko's, Wickelgren (1968) studied in H.M. the decay in short-term memory for single digits, three-digit sequences, and the pitches of tones. In this case the Konorski procedure resulted in the normal type of exponential curve decaying in the normal time range. From the point of view of Wickelgren's model of short-term memory processes, H.M. is normal.

A number of investigators have used the Peterson-Peterson recall task, giving subjects consonants or words to remember, following it with verbal interference, and then testing recall at specified intervals. In general, consistent with the notion that STM is normal in amnesics, both a mixed amnesic population (Baddeley and Warrington, 1970) and M.K. (Starr and Phillips, 1970)

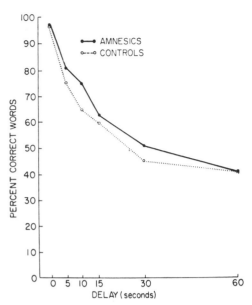

FIGURE 1.8 Retention of three words after varying intervals during which rehearsal was prevented. From Baddeley and Warrington (1970). Reproduced with permission from *Journal of Verbal Learning and Verbal Behavior* 9: 181.

showed a normal decay function (see Figure 1.8). Here again, as with the decay of nonverbal memory in H.M., we have a finding that sheds light on conceptions of short-term memory. As can be seen in Figure 1.8, the item decay function for both normals and amnesics asymptotes at about 60 seconds at a level well above chance (about 40 percent correct on a recall task). This residual memory had been attributed, by most psychologists, to storage in long-term memory. However, if storage in or retrieval from long-term memory is seriously deficient in amnesics, it is hard to imagine how the curves could overlap so well.

Three qualifications must be placed on the idea of considering amnesics as exhibiting relatively pure and isolated STM. First, some experiments on amnesics indicate deficient STM function. This work suggests a variety of encoding or retrieval deficits, especially at the semantic level, as measured by the Peterson-Peterson paradigm (Cermak and Butters, 1972; Cermak, Butters, and Gerrein, 1973).

Second, the interactions between putatively separate short- and long-term stores must occur at two levels. At one level, familiar items in STM must interact with already existing representations of themselves in LTM. In some sense this is how the meaning of a word such as "house" in a Peterson-Peterson experiment may be present in consciousness, i.e., represented in STM. Amnesics like H.M. seem to have normal access to existing LTM in this sense, as otherwise their performance on IQ tests would be dismal. Because of this

access, it would be reasonable to expect them to show semantic confusions, which are ordinarily associated with LTM. At another level, new items, or particular instances of familiar items, are normally entered into LTM and can then be retrieved into STM. It is this second LTM-STM interaction that is lost in amnesics, and that accounts for the frequent lack of an LTM component in psychological functions.

Third, there are puzzling features in the memory performance of amnesics which suggest a larger capacity in STM than is normally expected. For example, amnesics tend to be able to preserve an instructional set in a task that is challenging the capacity of their STM. Thus, in a task where they are supposed to make same-different judgments, or recall words on presentation of a specified signal, they often retain these instructions over a series of trials, even though their STM is ostensibly filled with task materials (see Talland, 1965, for examples). This finding leads to such notions as "intermediate-term" or "working" memories (see Simon, this volume).

1.6.4 Fractionation of the amnesic syndromes

The amnesic syndrome fractionates, both anatomically and psychologically, into two rather satisfying sub-deficits. These correspond roughly to a deficit in a verbal-memory system in the dominant hemisphere and a deficit in a nonverbal-memory system in the minor hemisphere (see Milner, 1972, 1973, for reviews).

DOMINANT (USUALLY LEFT)-TEMPORAL-LOBE DAMAGE AND VERBAL-MEMORY DEFICITS. Lesions of the left temporal lobe lead to specific deficits in verbal long-term memory, with visual and other forms of nonverbal memory intact. Patients who were able to learn definitions for five unfamiliar words after one exposure preoperatively, required eight exposures following dominant-temporal-lobe surgery. This same patient population, which before surgery had earned an average score of three correct responses on three trials of six arbitrary paired associates (Wechsler Memory Scale), was unable to learn any such associates after surgery (Meyer and Yates, 1955). Other types of paired associates, employing nonverbal visual or tactual materials, were readily learned postoperatively (Meyer, 1959). This specific verbal-memory deficit was stable for years (Blakemore and Falconer, 1967). A similar specific verbal deficit is seen with memory for prose materials (Wechsler Memory Scale), with a clear deficit in dominant-temporal-lobe epileptics *before* surgery, presumably as a consequence of tissue damage. The verbal deficit was increased by dominant-temporal-lobe resection (Milner, 1958). In a verbal recognition task (a series of words was presented, and subjects had to indicate which words were occurring for a second time), left temporals showed a clear deficit, but there was no corresponding deficit on a similar task for recurrence of visual figures (delays of 3–18 sec) (Figure 1.9). Finally, using a Peterson-Peterson paradigm, Corsi observed clear deficits in left temporals on memory for a consonant trigram (Corsi, 1969; Milner, 1972). (This deficit specific to the dominant side is a bit puzzling, since data from bilateral patients do not appear so abnormal on the Peterson-Peterson task. Furthermore, this task is usually associated with STM rather than LTM functions.) Right-temporal patients were normal (see Figure 1.10).

There is a small worry in this work that general verbal deficits, possibly at the perceptual level, are at least partly accounting for the specific deficit. While it is true that dysphasia is often apparent following surgery, it is characteristically transient. Verbal-memory testing carried out years after surgery still shows the deficit, even in subjects within the normal IQ range (Blakemore and Falconer, 1967). Maintenance of normal intelligence speaks strongly against an across-the-board verbal deficit. There does tend to be a decrease in verbal IQ (Meyer and Yates, 1955), which seems much more minor than the memory deficit. Verbal IQ usually returns to the premorbid range within one year of surgery, while the verbal-memory deficit persists.

The evidence is quite clear that the critical dominant-temporal-lobe structure is the hippocampus: the more hippocampus removed, the more severe the memory deficit (Figure 1.10; Corsi, 1969, 1972).

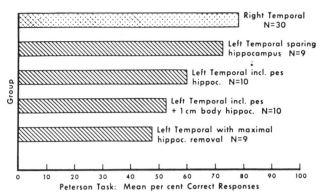

FIGURE 1.10 Verbal-memory deficit after left-temporal lobectomy as related to medial extent of temporal-lobe resection. These data for the Peterson-Peterson task show a progressive reduction in the mean number of consonant trigrams correctly recalled with increasing destruction of the left hippocampus. No impairment is seen after right-temporal lobectomy, regardless of whether or not the hippocampus has been excised. From Corsi (1969) as reproduced in Milner (1970).

MINOR(RIGHT)-TEMPORAL-LOBE DAMAGE AND DEFICITS IN NONVERBAL MEMORY. The picture of memory functions following minor-temporal-lobe surgery is almost perfectly complementary to the syndrome just described. These patients show some minimal perceptual deficits (e.g., in dealing with complex visual figures), severely compromised nonverbal long-term memory, and normal verbal memory. They perform poorly on visual or tactual stylus mazes, on which left temporals are quite normal (Corkin, 1965; Milner, 1965), with indications that the defect is not perceptual. They are poor at recurring-nonsense-figure tasks, but normal on recurring-word tasks (Kimura, 1963; Teuber, Milner, and Vaughan, 1968; see Figure 1.9). This is the inverse of the performance of left temporals. Finally, they are poor at recognition of recently presented faces (Milner, 1968), while left temporals are normal.

Right temporals also show deficiencies on Konorski or Peterson-Peterson tasks, which suggests involvement of STM. In a Konorski-type task, with flashes, clicks, tones, colors, or nonsense figures as stimuli, right temporals do more poorly than left temporals only on the nonsense figures (Figure 1.11). The nonsense figures are the only stimuli used in this experiment that would be very difficult to verbalize. Right temporals are also clearly deficient in imitating a pattern of tapping on an array of blocks (Corsi, 1972, cited in Milner, 1971). Finally, within the Peterson-Peterson paradigm, memory for location of a dot on a line is poor in right temporals, in contrast to good performance on a trigram (Corsi, 1972; Milner, 1973). Deficits in tactual memory in the dominant hemisphere of split brains (Milner and Taylor, 1972) and in memory for tonal sequence in right tem-

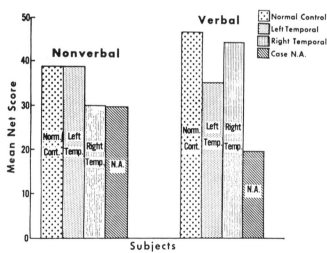

FIGURE 1.9 Performance of the patient N.A. (bilateral temporal-lobe removal), normal controls, and groups of patients with removals from right or left temporal lobes, on two visual recognition tasks. The nonverbal task involved recurring nonsense figures; the verbal task involved recurring words, nonsense syllables, and numbers. From Teuber, Milner, and Vaughan (1968). Reproduced with permission from *Neuropsychologia* 6: 277. Copyright 1968 by Pergamon Press.

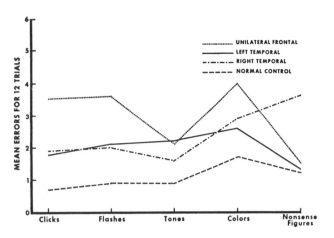

Figure 1.11 Effects of three different types of cerebral excisions on performance in a Konorski-type test with five different types of stimuli. Values indicated are for trials on which there was a 60-second interval between presentation of standard and test stimuli, with a distracting task in the interval. A score of six represents chance performance. From Prisko (1963). Reproduced with permission.

porals (Milner, 1958) further extend the scope of the specific deficit.

The specific role of the minor temporal lobe in nonverbal memories is also supported by the observation that stimulation of the right mammillothalamic tract in one patient seemed to interfere with performance on a visual, but not a verbal, memory task (Ojemann, 1971).

As with the left temporals, there are some worrisome problems about perceptual deficits being partly responsible for the memory deficit. Right temporals have difficulties in perception of tachistoscopically presented nonsense figures (Kimura, 1963) and deficits in the McGill picture-anomaly test (Milner, 1958). These deficits are small compared to the memory deficits, but slightly defective perception could be amplified in the memory process. However, there is good reason to believe that the nonverbal-memory deficits are not primarily perceptual. Right-temporal patients can do quite well on perceptual tests: one group with severe memory deficit was normal on a picture-completion task (WAIS; Meyer and Yates, 1955). Furthermore, Milner (1968) found that her right temporals were about as good as normals on face recognition with zero delay, with a deficit developing over the following seconds.

Evidence for critical involvement of the right hippocampus is quite strong. Hippocampal involvement has been related to memory deficits for tactual mazes (Corkin, 1965), faces (Milner, 1968), and dot locations (Corsi, 1972).

CONSEQUENCES AND IMPLICATIONS OF FRACTIONATION. The clear double dissociation of verbal and nonverbal memo-

ries raises many important questions. The definition of precisely what type of memories are dealt with selectively by each hemisphere would provide great insight into cognitive function, and memory in particular. It is possible that the critical dimensions might not be verbal vs. nonverbal, but rather analytic vs. "gestalt" (Levy, 1969). There are also suggestions that modality of input (e.g., visually or auditorily presented words) differentiates left from right temporals (Samuels, Butters, and Fedio, 1972). Whatever the precise description of the lateralized deficits, it is clear that there are two very different memory systems in the brain. The extent to which each system (hemisphere) can operate in the other's mode is unknown. Recovery of function following unilateral temporal lobectomy may occur most rapidly more than three years after surgery (Blakemore and Falconer, 1967). Is this recovery due to a resumption of verbal- or nonverbal-memory functions, or is it due to a compensation mechanism in which the patient improves his ability to code materials with his remaining "coding" system (Goldstein, 1934)?

The dissociation between right- and left-temporal-lobe functions is remarkably clear-cut. This, of course, suggests little contribution of each hemisphere to the memory for materials that clearly fit into the other hemisphere's coding system. Note for example, in Figure 1.9, that the performances of patients on tasks related to their nondeficient hemisphere are at about the level of normals. Similarly, in Figure 1.10, the right temporals' performances in the Peterson-Peterson trigram are at the level of normals.

If the dissociation were complete, one would expect that with "pure" verbal or nonverbal stimuli the performance of unilateral temporals with the relevant side damaged would be no better than that of bilateral temporals. On the whole, this does not appear to be so: Prisko (1963), using various "nonverbal" patterns (e.g., flashes, click patterns, nonsense figures), found bilateral temporals (including H.M.) to be slightly more deficient than right temporals. Teuber, Milner, and Vaughan (1968) show data on recurring figures or words indicating an inferiority of bilateral temporals on both tasks (see Figure 1.9, but note that N.A., the only bilateral temporal, performs considerably better than the other bilateral temporals studied). Corsi (1972) has data supporting this. These somewhat discrepant data are hard to interpret, since the availability of one memory channel must have some value even for an inappropriate type of stimulus.

A worrisome feature about the more recent work on material-specific deficits is the confounding of measures of LTM and STM. Since STM is ostensibly normal in amnesics, it is somewhat disturbing to see marked defects on Peterson-Peterson or Konorski tasks in unilateral temporals. The reader should at least be aware that the interesting results of Prisko and Corsi possibly tap into STM rather than LTM.

It is hard to explain the specific effects in terms of perceptual deficit, even though mild deficits are often present, as indicated in the review above. The perceptual-deficit explanation becomes all the more unlikely when patients with bilateral temporal lesions are considered. Some of these are remarkably normal in perceptual function and even show superiority on such visual tasks as hidden figures or figure-completion tests (Milner, Corkin, and Teuber, 1968; Starr and Phillips, 1970). It is hard to imagine, given the severe memory deficit, how H.M. or M.K. could do so well on intelligence tests if they had significant perceptual deficits; and in fact, few significant defects have been noted.

There is one very puzzling finding in the fractionation data. In reading case histories of the unilateral temporal population, who almost all have a sudden-onset semi-amnesic syndrome, I have not found mention of any specific premorbid amnesias. Naively, one might have expected a premorbid, material-specific amnesia for faces or scenes from the past in right temporals. If this does not occur, it suggests a clear distinction between lateralized encoding processes and more generalized storage and retrieval processes. Also, if true, the lack of premorbid amnesias makes the explanation of the deficit as perceptual in nature quite unlikely, since perceptual factors are critical in the recognition of familiar events.

The neat fractionation of the amnesic syndrome has important implications for the psychological issue of the coding mechanisms in memory. The notion that virtually all information is encoded verbally (Glanzer and Clark, 1963), and that STM is thus only a verbal memory, seems untenable. The normal performance of left temporals on nonverbal tasks is very striking, as is the facilitation of verbal memory in left temporals through an imagery-mnemonic technique (Patten, 1972; Jones, 1974). Here is a case where data from the neurological literature has significant influence on psychological theory.

1.6.5 Theories about the nature of the psychological defect in the amnesic syndrome
A number of theories have been proposed to account for the amnesic syndromes. As with most theories, they tend to be simplifying, that is, they try to explain the basic memory disorder as a defect in a *single* mechanism. This usually leads to an emphasis on certain particular features of the syndromes. I shall review the basic theories briefly. In the course of review I shall present some additional features of the syndromes that I have not yet mentioned; these will be most important in the discussion of retrieval-disorder theories.

CONSOLIDATION BLOCK. The most straightforward view of the amnesic syndromes is that there is a consolidation failure, or impaired transition from short-term memory to long-term memory, or failure to store information beyond the immediate present. These three alternative ways of stating the same basic view represent the basic position of Brenda Milner and her colleagues (Milner, 1970, 1972). This theory fits very well with the basic data on the syndrome, as reported so far, and with the phenomenology. It also fits extremely well with physiological conceptions of the memory process, which postulate a brief labile phase, a consolidation phase, and a more permanent, structural phase. All the data pointing to LTM-STM dissociations support this view, as does the normality of STM and intelligence. It must make the additional assumption that some types of "simpler" (e.g., motor) memories can still be consolidated. The fact that some recent materials do get recalled by dense amnesics (e.g., H.M.'s recall of the assassination of President Kennedy) can be accounted for as an almost complete, but not absolute, consolidation block.

Two arguments can be brought against a consolidation-block view as the sole explanation (see Table 1.2, below). First, premorbid amnesia, which almost invariably accompanies the syndrome, must by its very nature be a retrieval rather than a consolidation or storage disorder. Second, sensitive methods of testing show that a great many postmorbid experiences appear to be stored, even by amnesics. I shall consider these data along with retrieval theories, since they form the basis for such theories.

ENCODING DEFECTS. This view, put forward by Cermak, Butters, and their colleagues holds that quality and quantity of recall is determined by the extent or depth of encoding. The more highly processed an input is, the better it will be remembered (a levels-of-processing approach; see Craik and Lockhart, 1972). Within this scheme, defects in verbal-semantic-symbolic coding, one of the highest forms of processing, would lead to memory loss. Experiments on a population of Korsakoff patients with moderately severe memory loss support the notion of a semantic-encoding deficit. In a free-recall test of eight words, Korsakoffs were not aided by semantic-encoding cues (Cermak and Butters, 1972). In other free-recall experiments, Korsakoffs were aided by semantic category cues at the time of recall, but when they were not given explicit retrieval cues, they did not spontaneously use verbal (as opposed to acoustic or associative) means of encoding or organization (Cermak, Butters, and Gerrein, 1973). In another study, using the Peterson-Peterson paradigm, they demonstrated a deficiency in verbal memory (for three-consonant clusters), whether materials were presented in a visual, auditory, or tactual mode, in contrast to rather normal performance with nonverbal stimuli (e.g., visual forms or tone sequences) in the same modalities (Butters et al., 1973). These results have led to the postulation of a verbal-encoding deficit, which in the view of the experimenters is equivalent to a verbal-processing deficit. Such a theory can account for the failure to recall recent experiences (especially verbal ones) and the sparing of sensorimotor (nonverbal) memories. It can also explain why prompts facilitate recall (they would make up for the encoding deficit).

One problem with the semantic-encoding-deficit view is that the empirical results on which it is based are in some conflict with other results, using similar patient populations and paradigms. These patients show extensive ability to use semantic-encoding cues provided by the experimenter, and to organize materials in free-recall lists spontaneously along semantic lines (Warrington and Weiskrantz, 1971; Baddeley and Warrington, 1973).

A second problem concerns the assumption by Cermak, Butters, and their colleagues that they are dealing with what amounts to a defect in coding that affects short- as well as long-term memory (indeed, in the levels-of-processing view there is no clear distinction). If we are to assume a genuine defect in verbal processing in these subjects, how is it possible to explain normal performance on measures of verbal intelligence? The striking fact about many of the Korsakoff patients, and most especially H.M. and M.K., is that they are quite facile verbally, have large vocabularies, solve verbal problems, respond to complex instructions, and even invent elaborate verbal mnemonics (e.g., H.M.'s "584" memory trick). Furthermore, the enormous deficit in memory for nonverbal materials is hard to explain as a semantic deficit, as is the fractionation of the amnesic syndromes into verbal and nonverbal components.

The general notion of an encoding deficit has much to recommend it, if it is not restricted to semantic encoding and is not applied to STM as well as the material transferred to LTM. A more general encoding deficit is suggested by the fractionation experiments, which indicate that the amnesic syndromes are composed of a combination of subdeficits in verbal and nonverbal memory (Talland's (1965) notion of "premature closure of activation" may fit into this framework). In order to account for high intelligence, extensive semantic *processing* must be granted. We do not have to assume that semantic processing in STM (obviously with the aid of materials in LTM) is necessarily related to permanence of memory.

If certain types of *processing* are not preserved in LTM in amnesics, a more robust encoding-deficit theory would result (see Section 1.6.7).

RETRIEVAL DISORDER. We have already encountered a few characteristics of the amnesic syndromes that are difficult to handle within consolidation-block frameworks and suggest that retrieval rather than storage of information is critically involved. First is the existence of premorbid amnesias, which are, of logical necessity, a retrieval problem. It is striking that the major shrinkage in premorbid amnesias correlates in time with disappearance of the general amnesic state (see Section 1.5.4; Figure 1.5; Table 1.1; Russell, 1959; Benson and Geschwind, 1967). If this indicates a common mechanism for the two sets of symptoms, it implies a retrieval explanation of anterograde amnesias.

The conception of the amnesic syndromes as retrieval disorders can emphasize either of two types of deficit: (1) disorders in encoding or labeling of memories, so that they cannot be later retrieved, or (2) disorders in the retrieval process itself. Warrington and Weiskrantz (1973), the principal proponents of the retrieval disorder position, lean to the second possibility. In particular, they believe that amnesia occurs because of an unusual amount of interference at the time of recall: many competing memories or traces are vying for access to the output mechanism, and normal mechanisms of inhibition or selection are inoperative (Warrington and Weiskrantz, 1970, 1973). This type of defect would clearly lead to frequent "false positive" responses.

A retrieval-defect view can account for many of the salient features of amnesia (see Table 1.2, below): normal STM and defective recall of recent experiences would result from the "loss" of stored information, since it cannot be effectively retrieved. According to Warrington and Weiskrantz, the sparing of perceptuomotor skills results from their greater resistance to (or lower amounts of) interference, and hence from lack of competition at recall.

The most compelling argument for retrieval defects comes from evidence I have not presented up to this point. First of all, in the free recall of word lists, there is in the performance of amnesics a very high level of intrusions from prior lists. In one study, 50 percent of the intrusion errors were from previous lists (Warrington and Weiskrantz, 1968b). High prior-list intrusion rates, comparable to or greater than those normally seen, have been reported on a number of occasions (Baddeley and Warrington, 1970; Starr and Phillips, 1970). Clearly, one would not expect high intrusion levels from prior lists if these items had not been stored.

Another line strongly suggesting a retrieval defect is

the marked improvement in memory of amnesics when they are given prompts at the time of recall. Williams (1950a, b) demonstrated that memory for visual stimuli seen just prior to electroconvulsive shock could be improved by showing the subjects ink blots with some resemblance to the stimulus items. She later showed that the memory of amnesics could be facilitated by gradual prompting with ambiguous pictures (Williams, 1953). Warrington and Weiskrantz (1968a) have confirmed these results using fragmented pictures or words as prompts (Figure 1.12). Although normal or amnesic subjects could not guess the target word or picture from the maximally degraded stimuli prior to training, these same fragmented stimuli strongly facilitated recall after subjects had been exposed to the set of target words or pictures (Warrington and Weiskrantz, 1968a, 1970). Prompts clearly have their effect at the time of recall, since in some of these experiments subjects never saw the fragmented stimuli in the acquisition phase. The cuing effect cannot be explained in terms of "perceptual" learning, since "linguistic" cues, such as "met" for the target word "metal," are also quite effective (Weiskrantz and Warrington, 1970).

The "disinhibition" of memory traces at the time of retrieval, postulated by Warrington and Weiskrantz (1970, 1973), clearly handles these data. It also establishes contact with the hitherto puzzling lack of amnesic symptoms in animals with bilateral temporal lesions (Weiskrantz, 1971; Warrington and Weiskrantz, 1973). There are some conditions under which deficient memory is observed in such animals. These include a slowness to extinguish and poor performance on discrimination reversals. These and related symptoms have been characterized as a deficit in the stopping of ongoing behavior and as a problem of abnormal interference. These

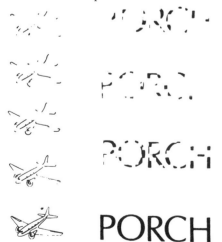

FIGURE 1.12 Examples of fragmented pictures and words used by Warrington and Weiskrantz (1968a). Reproduced with permission from *Nature* 217: 972–974.

defects clearly resemble the defect postulated in humans by Warrington and Weiskrantz.

The explanatory power of this retrieval theory is impressive, but there are a number of salient phenomena that it does not account for. The lack of a sense of familiarity once a memory *is* recalled, a constant feature of the amnesic syndrome, is not explained. Furthermore, normal intelligence and normal abilities to retrieve a variety of long-term memories, such as vocabulary items, are hard to explain within the framework of grossly disturbed retrieval. Since a global retrieval disorder is postulated, the theory must maintain that depression of access to premorbid memories is fairly uniform over time. The theory cannot easily explain true retrograde amnesia, if it exists, or the special difficulty of new learning (see next section).

1.6.6 Some recent attempts to resolve conflicts and discriminate among the theories

ACTIVATION OF EXISTING MEMORY TRACES VS. NEW LEARNING. In the examination of amnesic patients, the denial of remembrance for events that have just transpired is striking. If one discusses a subject, such as dog breeds for example, over a period of minutes with a dense amnesic, followed by a brief interruption of about 15 seconds, the patient will often claim to have no memory of the previous discussion and no idea of what it was about. However, if at this point one urges the patient to say any word that comes into his head, one is likely to hear a word relevant to the previous conversation (e.g., collie). It is as if there were no awareness of the conversation, but still some continued activation of the "memory traces" that were recently in use. This can be explained by an activation notion: recently activated traces remain especially accessible for some period of time after use (Diamond and Rozin, unpublished data). A number of cognitive psychologists have suggested processes of this sort to account for data from normal subjects (e.g., Morton, 1968), and terms such as "intermediate-term" or "working" memory have been suggested. (This may also be related to the preservation of information about task instructions in amnesics.)

Other evidence for such a process comes from patients with anomias. Weigl (1968) has shown that a patient who fails to name a picture can be aided by being exposed, during an interim period, to the spoken name in question, along with other irrelevant words. Exposure to the critical word, or to semantic associates of the word, or to the reading of the word, facilitates the subject's ability to use the word to name the picture the next time it is shown, if the test is done within a moderate time after priming. This procedure, which Weigl calls "deblocking," appears to operate by a trace-activation procedure. This normal memory process could be called a "hot-tubes" effect (Diamond and Rozin, unpublished data)—after you turn off a vacuum-tube radio, the tubes stay hot for a while.

It should be obvious that it is only possible to activate traces that already exist in memory. The phenomenon of trace activation is important for understanding the amnesic syndrome because the great majority of data on prior-list intrusions and prompts involve relatively short time periods between training and testing, which an activation process may well bridge. Furthermore, the stimuli in such experiments are almost always items already in the subject's premorbid long-term memory, (usually pictures of common objects or words). The issue is, then, the extent to which activation processes, along with some consolidation block or encoding deficit, can explain the Warrington and Weiskrantz data. To what extent do amnesics really store new memories, and to what extent have they simply preserved the ability to activate old ones? A most striking deficit in the amnesic syndrome, even in mild cases, is an inability to learn new things, such as names of people. The dismal performance of amnesics on paired-associate paradigms, where the pairs are randomly rather than meaningfully associated (so that they would not have been in memory prior to presentation), strikingly indicates new-learning inability (Diamond and Rozin, unpublished data; Scoville and Milner, 1957; Sweet, Talland, and Ervin, 1959; Meyer and Yates, 1955). Most dense amnesic subjects score zero correct on the three trials of six arbitrarily paired associates on the Wechsler Memory Scale (Meyer and Yates, 1955) or similar tasks (Figure 1.13A). Similarly, M.K. performed particularly poorly in a recognition test for new, as opposed to previously familiar, stimuli (Starr and Phillips, 1970).

If it is true that prompting effects work largely by cuing the subject as to which of his recently activated memories should be selected, and that new learning is completely or almost completely blocked, then one should not be able to demonstrate prompting effects for *new* material. Diamond and Rozin tested this hypothesis in a study using six very dense amnesics of considerably below average intelligence, but with digit spans in the normal range. In a free-recall situation subjects were presented with lists of either common English two-syllable words (e.g., candy) already in LTM, or nonsense two-syllable words (e.g., numdy) presumably not already in LTM. Over six learning trials, in each of which both the subject and the experimenter repeated each word, amnesics, unlike controls, showed almost no free recall of these items (Figure 1.13 B, C). The critical issue is the effect of prompts, which in this case were the first

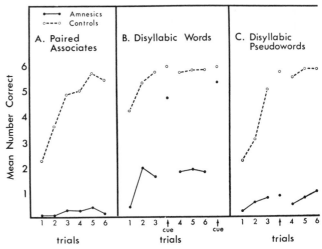

FIGURE 1.13 Combined data from six amnesic and six control subjects for three experiments. In experiment A subjects had six trials of exposure and testing for six unrelated word pairs. A perfect score on any trial would be six. In experiments B and C the six stimuli to be learned were disyllabic words (e.g., can-dy) or disyllabic pseudowords (e.g., num-dy). In addition to six free-recall tests, cued recall, prompted by the first syllable in each disyllable, was carried out after trials three and six. Unpublished data by R. J. Diamond and P. Rozin, 1974.

syllable of each word (e.g., "can" for candy, "num" for numdy). If new learning is blocked, and prompts work primarily to select from among recently activated memories, then prompts should produce significant improvement in amnesics for familiar words but not for new ones. As indicated in Figure 1.13, this is exactly what happened. There was no advantage to prompts with nonsense disyllables, with appropriate controls for guessing. Further experiments estimated the decay characteristics of the activation process, and indicated that prompting effects, under the conditions used in this experiment, disappear after about two hours. If this process is operating normally in amnesics, then they are ideal subjects in which to study it, since the decay-of-activation curve cannot be measured directly in normals, who have an alternate and more powerful way of remembering the stimulus (i.e., LTM).

There are two problems with the "hot-tubes" notion as a way of accounting for the Warrington and Weiskrantz effects. First, there is some evidence for ability to learn new things in amnesics. Warrington and Weiskrantz (1973) report some data showing that prompts aid with new materials. The problem here, of course, is that only in very dense amnesics would one expect a total block in new memory formation. Insofar as new memories can be formed, prompts would be expected to work. Warrington and Weiskrantz's subject population had both higher (normal) intelligence and better memory than Diamond and Rozin's population, so this may account for the discrepancy. A more serious problem with "hot tubes" as a pervasive explanation is that prompting or cuing effects can be demonstrated over a period of days (see, for example, Milner, Corkin, and Teuber, 1968). Even H. M. showed some improvement on incomplete figures four months after training. Clearly, traces are not activated for such periods. For the moment, then, intact-trace activation, like other postulated features, can only be used, in conjunction with other postulated deficits (e.g., consolidation block), to explain some of the phenomena of the amnesic syndromes.

AN INGENIOUS ATTEMPT TO DISCRIMINATE AMONG THE MAIN THEORIES. Marslen-Wilson (1974) has reported an excellent experiment designed to test encoding vs. consolidation-block vs. retrieval theories. It should already be clear to the reader that no one experiment can do this, since each theory is incapable of explaining some of the key phenomena, but this experiment represents nonetheless one of the finest attempts to clarify the issues.

Marslen-Wilson tested recall (identification) memory for a set of faces of public figures associated with particular decades in the range 1920 to the present. He was interested in the question of whether identification would be selectively impaired for faces associated with time periods subsequent to the onset of memory pathology. He used a population of Korsakoff amnesics, H.M., and normal controls. Clearly, retrieval theories predict uniformly poor face recall over time, whereas both encoding and consolidation-block theories predict severe drops in memory for the more recent faces. The data supported the latter contention. H.M.'s data were particularly clear: his face recall was in the normal range for faces "prior" to the 1950s, and then dropped off sharply.

Marslen-Wilson retested his subjects on those items that they had failed, this time providing additional cues. Cues were either circumstantial (e.g., for Wendell Wilkie: he was a Republican presidential nominee in 1940; he ran against FDR and lost) or "phonological" (e.g., W.W., Wend. W., and so on, providing progressively more information). For this situation a retrieval view predicts major facilitation of memory on both pre- and postmorbid items, while a consolidation-block view predicts no major facilitation in the postmorbid period. An encoding view might well predict across-the-board facilitation, but especially with postmorbid faces where the cues might counteract the initial encoding deficits. The results clearly indicate that prompts produce major improvements in memory (most noticeable, of course, in the postmorbid-memory results due to the low baseline). This holds for both the Korsakoff population and for H.M., who improved from 7.5 percent to 80 percent correct for faces of the 1960s. These last data are partic-

ularly difficult for a consolidation-block view since H.M. did quite well with postmorbid memories. Activation processes do not help much here since the faces of the last two decades are new memories.

Note, then, that retrieval theories fail to predict the preservation of old memories on the recall task, while consolidation theories fail to predict the facilitation of recent memory on the prompt task. Only the encoding view comes through both hurdles unscathed, though one has to make assumptions about the nature of the encoding deficit to explain these data.

1.6.7 A synthesis: Explanation of the amnesic syndromes

Perhaps the reader can now appreciate the wish I expressed at the beginning of this paper, that I could be writing this in 1890. The basic phenomena of the amnesic syndromes were known, and a framework was available for interpretation. We now have a number of theories, a lot more fine-grain information as to the disorder itself, and a literature on the subject which expands significantly on a monthly basis. In an attempt to create some order, I have constructed Table 1.2, which lists the basic phenomena of the amnesic syndromes on one axis and the basic theories on the other. I have indicated on the table which theories, in my opinion, can handle which phenomena. I have also created some hybrid theories which I shall describe shortly. I believe that the basic phenomena to be explained are—

1. the preserved functions: STM, intelligence, motor-skill acquisition;
2. defective recall of recent events from LTM;
3. evidence of storage of recent memories, via intrusion errors and prompted recall;
4. the lack of a feeling of familiarity about correctly recalled memories;
5. the particular difficulty with learning new things;
6. the whole problem of deficits in premorbid memories;
7. the Marslen-Wilson experiment;
8. the mismatch between animal and human data; and
9. the fractionation into two material-specific components.

I have tried to list only phenomena that have been reported a number of times and are not controversial in themselves, and I have treated the premorbid-amnesia phenomena as just an unspecified deficit in premorbid memories. The first three columns contain the three basic theories in their unelaborated form: Milner's pure consolidation block, the defect in encoding in short-term memory (Cermak, Butters, et al.), and Warrington and Weiskrantz's disinhibition at the time of retrieval.

The first point to note is that none of the basic theories

Phenomena to be explained	Theory				
	Consolidation block	Semantic encoding	Retrieval	Modified c.b.[2]	Modified retrieval[3]
Preserved functions:					
intelligence	+	−	−	+	+
short-term memory	+	−	+	+	+
perceptuomotor memories	+	+	+	+	+
LTM: memory for recent experiences:					
poor recall	+	+	+	+	+
good cued recall	−	+	+	+	+
prior-list intrusions	−	+	+	+	+
lack of a sense of familiarity	+	0	−	+	+
special difficulties with memories for new items	+	0	0	+	+
Premorbid-memory defects	−	−	+	−	+
Marslen-Wilson data	−	0	−	0	0
Absence of amnesic syndromes in animals	0	+	+	0	0
Fractionation into material-specific deficits	+	−	0	+	0

1. A plus indicates that the theory can produce a reasonable explanation for the phenomenon. A zero indicates that the phenomenon is consistent with the theory but that assumptions must be added. A minus indicates that the phenomenon is inconsistent with the theory. A number of arbitrary decisions had to be made in awarding symbols, especially as between zeros and pluses and especially on the last four phenomena. Many of the designations are thus arguable. The premorbid-memory defect simply represents the idea that something is wrong with premorbid memory, without any assumptions about true retrograde amnesia.
2. The modified consolidation-block theory assumes severe deficits in storing new information, leading to a disturbance in episodic memory, with normal memory-activation processes.
3. The modified retrieval view holds that personal references and other weakly stored memories are harder to retrieve.

can handle all of the major features of the syndrome. Specifically, consolidation block cannot explain the substantial storage of recent memories (intrusions, cued recall, Marslen-Wilson) or any of the indications of disturbances in premorbid memory. Encoding deficit in STM cannot explain the apparent normality of STM or intelligence, or any of the deficits in premorbid memories. The retrieval view has trouble with intact intelligence (which involves access to old memories, such as vocabulary), the lack of a sense of familiarity (which should appear once the item is retrieved), the special difficulty of new learning, and certain aspects of premorbid amnesia, though it is the only theory that can explain *any* of the premorbid deficit. Surprisingly, the only phenomena all three can explain are the loss of LTM recall and the sparing of motor skills—though special assumptions are needed for the latter. None of these theories is inconsistent with any of the others. Therefore, combinations of them, or combinations with modification, offer possible solutions.

I propose that the most central feature of the syndrome, and one of the few that are truly uncontroversial, is the loss of a feeling of familiarity upon either exposure to or recall of previously experienced events. The memories that really seem gone are the references to personal experience and their temporospatial relations, what Tulving (1972) calls episodic memories as opposed to semantic memories or knowledge. Most normal forgetting seems to involve episodic memories, which appear to be quite fragile.

When one sees a friend, the perceptual representation of the friend must make contact with some memorial representation in LTM. No new information need be entered in memory. However, after the meeting, the existence of the meeting as a personal experience would be lost if no new information could be stored or retrieved, because the time, place, and context of the meeting, which are unique and new, would then not be preserved. Episodic memories by their nature involve time and context tags which are experienced once (I saw my friend Bill *yesterday* at *school*), as opposed to known memory items (my friend Bill, who is experienced frequently). Thus the difference between episodic and "factual" memories is largely one of the number of exposures.

I propose that a central defect in the amnesic syndromes is a severe (but not complete) consolidation block, which results in a selective loss of recently occurring new experiences. This amounts to a personal-reference (episodic) encoding deficit, since the time-context cues are unique and new experiences. Note that this type of encoding deficit differs from that of Cermak and Butters in that it is posited at the gateway between STM and

LTM, and not as an STM deficit, and also in that it is not verbal-specific. By keeping an encoding deficit out of STM, one avoids the problem of explaining the normality of intelligence and STM. If we add the presumably normal memory-activation processes (Diamond and Rozin, unpublished data), we can explain almost all of the major features of the amnesic syndromes (see the heading "modified consolidation block" in Table 1.2).

The episodic-memory deficit directly explains the failure to recall recent items, as it is through time-context tags that it is possible to identify what was presented some seconds or minutes ago. The lack of a feeling of familiarity follows directly from the proposed deficit, as does, of course, the failure to form new memories (which is, indeed, the proposed deficit itself). Prompting works because it allows selection among activated memories or facilitates retrieval of items that are inaccessible because their time context was not well consolidated. This modified consolidation defect, with its consequent episodic encoding deficit, cannot explain any type of premorbid deficit, but it can account for the Marslen-Wilson data since the amnesics have been exposed to the faces of the public figures repeatedly, allowing some minimal learning during the postmorbid period. The failure to obtain amnesic syndromes in animals could result from the fact that most of the tasks used with animals are of the sort that human amnesics *can* perform. The fractionation data are explainable with the reasonable assumption, given hemispheric specialization, of separate mechanisms for new memory formation. The major problem for this modified consolidation-block theory is the premorbid amnesias, which *must* be viewed as retrieval failures.

This leads to a reconsideration of retrieval models. Suppose that retrieval of personal referents (time tags, contexts, etc.) were more difficult for normals than "fact" retrieval. This process might then be selectively impaired in the amnesic syndrome if the retrieval system were damaged. This would result in many of the faulty-memory phenomena we have discussed, and would also easily explain both the normal intelligence (which deals with "semantic" or "factual" memory) and the clear loss of a feeling of familiarity (see the heading "modified retrieval" in Table 1.2). Familiarity is, after all, generated by these very personal reference tags. There is still some problem accounting for both the great difficulty in learning new items and the data of Marslen-Wilson and others indicating rather intact old memories. In addition to difficulties with the possibility of selective loss of recent premorbid memories, retrieval views of any sort face great difficulty in explaining transient amnesias. In these it is often the case that when memory clears, the premorbid amnesia shrinks to almost zero

while the period of anterograde amnesia tends to remain permanent, suggesting a clear dissociation in mechanisms (Russell, 1959).

The idea that retrieval may be relatively impaired for "personal references" is reinforced by data from post-hypnotic amnesia. After a suggestion of amnesia during hypnosis, "deeply hypnotized" subjects show significant amnesia for the events transpiring while they were under hypnosis. They also show "source amnesia," that is, they may remember some facts imparted to them during hypnosis, but they have no memory of how they obtained these facts (Evans and Thorn, 1966). Furthermore, when asked to *recall* events that transpired during the hypnotic episode, deeply hypnotized subjects, unlike "controls," tend not to list the events in their actual temporal order (Evans and Kihlstrom, 1973). Since all these amnesic effects are reversed when the amnesia instructions are countermanded, this must be a retrieval disorder. It appears relatively selective to episodic information (temporal order and context).

Examination of Table 1.2 indicates that the best bets are the assumptions of just a severe consolidation block, compromising new materials especially, or of a general depression of memory which specifically affects the handling of weakly consolidated items at times of both encoding and retrieval.

Historically, it is of interest that the criticality of the episodic view was postulated at the beginning of the century, by Claparède (1911). Furthermore, while recent theoretical explanations of the sort discussed in this paper have come up short, partly because they have attempted to employ single simple deficits, the original theory of Korsakoff (1889) was appropriately more complex. He posited a dual disorder: a defect of physiological retentiveness or trace strength, which might be called consolidation block today, and a weakened associative network, which might be considered either an encoding or a retrieval disorder. (These two components, associative network and retentiveness, are the two parameters of the quality of memory described by James in the *Principles*, published the year after Korsakoff's paper.) We have not advanced very far.

It is not clear, at this point, whether there is something special about personal reference tags (time-place-context) over and above the fact that they are unique. If the construction of a continuous "stream" of personal references is specifically affected, with some sparing of new information per se, it might be possible to explain the absence of amnesic syndromes in infrahumans. It is likely that they do not have a personal reference system in the first place.

This issue aside, the selective susceptibility of unique,

episodic information fits neatly into a levels-of-function approach (Jackson, 1884). The neurological damage in the amnesic syndrome seems to be to a selective activation or regulation mechanism. The resultant loss in tone or activation should affect the most sensitive memory processes. A defect of storage or encoding for unique events, along with a retrieval failure for these same poorly encoded events, would result.

1.7 SELECTIVE IMPAIRMENT OF SHORT-TERM MEMORY: THE CONVERSE OF THE AMNESIC SYNDROMES

On the whole, the picture presented by the amnesic syndrome lends support to the basic Jamesian view of primary (short-term) and secondary (long-term) memory compartments. Further evidence of the independent existence of these theoretical entities comes from severe disturbances in STM, with LTM intact. The reference case here is K.F., a patient suffering damage to the left parietal area (Warrington and Shallice, 1969). There are some associated verbal deficits (WAIS verbal IQ is 79; performance IQ is 113). K.F. has an auditory digit span of one or at most two items, but he seems able to learn new materials rather easily. His score on the paired-associates memory portion of the Wechsler Memory Scale was less than one standard deviation below normal. A few other patients with similar patterns of disturbances have been described (Warrington, Valentine, and Pratt, 1971; Saffran and Marin, 1975).

Detailed examination of the memory capacities of these patients leads to a very satisfying dissociation, which supports many hypothesized features of short- and long-term memory. The greatly abbreviated digit spans, in the range of one to three for auditorily presented items, are significantly higher for visually presented verbal items (Warrington and Shallice, 1969; Warrington and Shallice, 1972; Saffran and Marin, 1975). The free-recall data for word lists show effects converse to those seen in amnesics: there is an abbreviated recency effect, of one or even zero items, and a reduced primacy effect, presumably due to a limited processing capacity in STM and limited rehearsal capability (Shallice and Warrington, 1970; Saffran and Marin, 1975). The digit span is improved by a slower presentation rate, as would be predicted if the LTM component were critical. (This procedure does not improve the performance of amnesics.) The memory for three items in the Peterson-Peterson paradigm is significantly reduced (Shallice and Warrington, 1970). In fact, the Peterson-Peterson decay curve for three items is flat: the subjects seem able to encompass only one or two of the items and to hold these

over the test interval. The auditory-memory span can also be extended by using familiar, meaningful, or meaningfully related items, all effects that would be expected if the LTM component, which is generally regarded as more sensitive to semantic dimensions, were largely responsible for the performance (Saffran and Marin, 1975).

Patients with this type of reduced auditory-memory span are often described as conduction aphasics. They show a marked deficit in ability to repeat verbal materials, such as sentences, which is easily traceable to their limited span of apprehension. The most fascinating feature of these patients with what amounts to limited auditory-verbal windows on the world is the way they handle complex verbal inputs. Saffran and Marin (1975) have recorded the attempts of one patient to repeat accurately auditorily presented sentences. A few examples follow:

Standard: The soldiers knew that pleasing women can be fun.
Patient: The soldiers knew that going with charming women can be fun.

Standard: The residence was located in a peaceful neighborhood.
Patient: The residence was situated in a quiet district.

What appears in both of these cases, and in many others described by the authors, is a preservation of the sense of the sentences, but a loss of much of the "surface structure." Of course, the accurate rendition of the first word or two is a primacy effect. What is remarkable is that the meanings of the sentences are extracted, even at normal speaking rates. Furthermore, in a number of cases, ambiguity in the meaning of the standard sentence is preserved in the paraphrase (e.g., the first example above). Whatever one's interpretation of this fascinating result, it is clear that at some levels a lot of material can enter LTM in these patients. Compromise of STM seems to compromise selectively preservation of the precise form of the verbal stimulus.

Just as there is a double dissociation between the amnesic syndromes and this converse of it, there is a double dissociation within each of the syndromes. In the amnesic syndrome it concerns verbal vs. nonverbal material-specific deficits. In the abbreviated STM syndrome there seem to be relatively specific auditory and visual deficits. The auditory-verbal memory deficit has just been described. There is some evidence that with lesions closer to the occipital area, there can be a selective reduction in the visual-memory span (Warrington and Rabin, 1970). For example, Luria (1966) reports a patient who was only able to comprehend one object at a time in the visual field. This would appear to be an instance of a double double dissociation.

Taken together, the amnesic syndromes and the abbreviated STM syndromes give added support to the idea of two rather independent memory systems.

1.8 SOME GENERAL QUESTIONS ABOUT MEMORY AND THE BRAIN

1.8.1 Intelligence functions in memory and the frontal lobes

From a perusal of Figure 1.1, it is clear that there are a seemingly limitless number of ways in which the functioning of the total memory system can be compromised. In addition to direct interference with any of the hypothetical stages or with the "connections" between them (should one take the model literally), there is the possibility of damage to the general cognitive or intelligence factors that in many subtle ways affect memory. These include processes such as selective attention, chunking, organization, and strategies for remembering or scanning through memory. Pathology producing significant drops in intelligence would be likely to affect many of these processes. However, there might be some dissociation between general intelligence, measured as IQ, and intelligence factors in memory. For example, many effects of organization and clustering in memory occur without the subject's conscious awareness. After all, mnemonic techniques almost certainly include procedures already in use below the level of consciousness in memory. Thus the fact that a subject may not be able explicitly and consciously to use a cognitive process or skill in an arbitrary IQ-type task does not guarantee that he does not have access to it for other purposes.

One would expect damage to various parts of the frontal lobes to have specific effects on memory, since these areas are generally associated with the operations of planning, selection among alternatives, and verification (Luria, 1966, 1973). Perseveration, an inability to turn off or inhibit an ongoing behavior or process, is characteristic of frontal patients. This may appear at the level of motor or conceptual function, depending on the individual case. Perseverative disorders, manifested as difficulties in alternation tasks or a general inability to inhibit behaviors, characterize animals with frontal damage (P. Milner, 1970). This is accompanied by a difficulty in discriminating which of two events occurred more recently (Iversen, 1973). Parallel disorders are seen in frontal humans: dorsolateral frontal damage leads to perseverative defects in card-sorting performance when subjects are required to shift from one sorting principle

to another (Milner, 1963). While short-term memory may be more or less normal in frontal patients (Samuels, Goodglass, and Brody, 1970), they have considerable difficulty in reporting which of two events occurred more recently (Milner, 1971, 1973). This makes them highly subject to proactive inhibition (Prisko, 1963).

Consistent with the general planning and overseeing functions attributed to at least parts of the frontal area, a number of characteristic memory deficits occur in these patients (Luria, 1966). Memory-monitoring functions are especially deficient: frontals are poor at estimating their own progress in a memory task (Luria, 1966). They are relatively unresponsive to mnemonic aids (Barbizet, 1970; Luria, 1966), and in learning a list of items, they do not adopt the normal strategy of "concentrating" on the items not yet learned (Milner, 1969). They therefore plateau early on such tasks. They tend to persevere on scanning tasks (Luria, 1966). In general, motivational factors seem to have a disproportionate role in controlling their memorial performance. They do better on interesting tasks (Milner, 1969). This, plus the perseverative tendency, may account for failures in proper control of selective attention (Luria, 1966). There is reason to believe that at least some of these defects can be more precisely localized in the frontal areas, and that some type of fractionation of these symptoms may occur (Milner, 1973).

1.8.2 Memory and perception

I have had occasion to refer above to the interactions of perception and memory. Defective perception must almost certainly have effects on the formation of new memories, since the deterioration of the information content of the stimulus restricts the materials upon which memory can operate. Conversely, since much of perceptual ability depends on past experience, one might expect severe memory disorders to affect perception. In keeping with these ideas, there tends to be an involvement of one of these functions in cases where the other is involved. I have referred to this issue in the case of fractionation of the amnesic syndromes, where memory deficits associated with a given temporal lobe are usually coupled with some perceptual disorders for corresponding materials (Milner, 1972). Logically, however, one might expect that perceptual abilities would remain intact, in spite of a severe amnesic syndrome, as long as the perceptual system has access to certain relevant past experiences. This does appear to be the case. First, older experiences *seem* to be available to the subject. Second, even if they are not recallable, as such, to the patient, they may be accessible to the perceptual system. This may be a "lower-level" and hence intact system, in the same sense that the system compensating for the visual displacement produced by prisms is almost certainly lower-level (Harris, 1965). The important point is that we cannot make strong inferences from a subject's performance about the presence or absence of a capacity. The disconnection syndromes (Geschwind, 1965a,b) clearly make this point. Nonetheless, it is striking how independent perception seems to be from overtly measured memory. H.M. (Milner, Corkin, and Teuber, 1968) and N.A. (Teuber, Milner, and Vaughan, 1968) perform above normal on tests of visual perception, such as hidden-figure tests, in the face of almost total loss of recall of similar materials. Poor correlations, in patients with various types of lesions, between visual-perception and visual-memory tasks have been reported (Warrington and Rabin, 1970).

On the other hand, it is at least interesting that the cognitive functions that characterize each of the hemispheres in the perceptual area extend into their memory functions. Thus the dominant hemisphere, which incorporates most speech processing and production, is also specifically involved with verbal memories, and the opposite is true for the minor hemisphere (Milner, 1972, 1973). Even if memory functions are divided in part from perceptual functions, they are at least located in the same half of the brain. I would like to discuss this interaction briefly, with face recognition as an example.

There is quite a bit of evidence indicating that right (minor)-hemisphere lesions are much more likely to interfere with face recognition or perception than are left-hemisphere lesions (see, for example, De Renzi and Spinnler, 1966). There are even some suggestions that there may be a specific visual system for recognition of faces (Yin, 1970), though it is also possible to conceive of faces as just especially difficult and subtle stimuli (De Renzi and Spinnler, 1966). At what level in the processing of faces do different neurological mechanisms become involved? Moscovitch, Scullion, and Christie (1976) have done a revealing experiment that explores the early stages. Consistent with the generally reported role of the right hemisphere in face perception, it has been found that reaction times to recognize or match faces are faster when the comparison is done in the minor visual field, i.e., the field directly connected to the minor hemisphere (Geffen, Bradshaw, and Wallace, 1971). Moscovitch, Scullion, and Christie used this type of paradigm to study the time course of appearance of minor-field and minor-hemisphere superiority. Subjects had to indicate as quickly as possible whether a target face was the same as, or different from, a test face. When the test face was presented immediately after the target, there was no clear advantage to the minor (left) over the dominant (right) visual field. However, with delays of 100 msec or more between

target and test, a clear minor-field advantage appeared. This suggests that at the level of sensory storage or "iconic" representation, the hemispheres are equivalent, but that as the stimuli are further processed, the encoding system or some other feature of the minor hemisphere establishes a superiority. This view is confirmed by the fact that a minor-hemisphere superiority can be obtained with a delay of only a few milliseconds if the target face is followed by a visual mask, which would have the effect of erasing the "sensory store." These data suggest that material-specific, hemispheric perceptuomemory abilities begin to be manifested at the point of "read-in" to short-term memory.

These early-stage minor-hemisphere advantages, as mentioned above, carry over into longer-term facial-memory performance. Most interestingly, it is possible, provisionally, to fractionate minor-hemisphere function in face memory. Right parietal lesions, which produce a variety of higher-order visual disorders, leave specific deficits in ability to do an immediate match of unfamiliar faces, without affecting memory for premorbidly familiar faces (Warrington and James, 1967). Conversely, right temporal lesions interfere with memory for the familiar faces, but not the immediate-recognition task. This suggests a perception-memory dissociation.

There is one final, rather deep issue in perception and memory that is relevant to neuropathological approaches. Some modern views of memory and perception assume that they are active processes in which full-blown percepts or memories are in some way constructed from fragments. That is, some psychologists would claim that the apparently clear memory one has of a college classmate's face, for example, is actually constructed from fragmentary memories of features of it, plus some rules for making faces from features. It would seem reasonable to assume that the machinery that does this reconstruction would be the very same machinery that is involved in face perception, since the same processes probably occur in perception. If that is so, then the recall of faces from the past should be severely compromised by disorders in face perception. The fact that the recognition of familiar faces can be intact in the face of perceptual deficit (Warrington and James, 1967) is interesting, but it is not necessarily germane to this issue since recognition may not involve these same reconstructive acts. The critical question to ask is an introspective one: Can patients with severe face-perception deficits call up a good image of a face from the past? Can the left (dominant) hemisphere of a split brain, which has defective face perception, recall faces as well as the total brain used to? I do not know the answer to these questions, and I am not sure they can be convincingly answered. It should be obvious, however, that the same question can be asked about perception and memory for any type of material, and that it has deep psychological interest and implications.

1.8.3 A final puzzle: Still in search of the engram

Up to this point there has been little reference to the trace or engram, that is, the *physical* realization of long-term memories. The amnesic syndromes deal with lack of access to long-term memories and/or failure to form them. But *where* are they when they are formed? In the classical paper in this area, "In Search of the Engram," Karl Lashley (1950), after a long series of experimental attempts at excising engrams in animals, admitted that he had not been able to locate them. The story for humans is remarkably similar. Even massive lesions to the brain do not result in what can clearly be defined as a *loss* of long-term memories, as opposed to a loss of access to such memories. Though it is logically impossible to prove that loss is not loss of access, the actual phenomena do not even suggest significant true losses. Most losses of past memories are impermanent. The agnosias, as a group of disorders, represent memory losses in the sense of failures of recognition. However, they can easily be conceived, especially when they are modality-specific (e.g., the inability to recognize visually presented objects), as loss of access by disconnection or weakening of a system (Geschwind, 1965a,b).

Even the memory disruption produced by dense amnesia of a bilateral temporal syndrome does not reliably and convincingly produce a true premorbid-memory loss of any extent. At the absolute minimum, one would like to believe that, given hemispheric specialization, verbal memories would tend to be found somewhere in the dominant side and nonverbal memories in the minor side. In face of the clear disorders in material-specific memories resulting from unilateral hippocampal damage, there is no clear evidence of any loss of *premorbid* long-term memories in these patients, of the appropriate type or otherwise. Even more striking is the lack of evidence that either hemisphere of split-brain patients, in spite of the differences in cognitive capacity between them, shows any loss in old memories, material-specific or otherwise. This problem has not yet been examined carefully. If both hemispheres are equally good on old visual and verbal memories, the omnipresence of the engram would indeed be a likely hypothesis.

The only suggestion of localization of long-term memories comes from the literature on epilepsy and brain stimulation. Jackson (1888) noted that epileptic attacks are sometimes preceded by an aura with psychic qualities. These might involve hallucinations, memories, or peculiar feelings of familiarity (déjà vu), strangeness, or dissociation. This psychic aura presumably represents discharge in a diseased portion of the brain. The nature of these psychic phenomena has been extensively studied and has been related to results coming from stimulation of the brains of epileptics during surgery, by Penfield and his collaborators (Penfield and Jasper, 1954; Penfield and Roberts, 1959; Mullan and Penfield, 1959; Penfield and Perot, 1963). They have accumulated many case studies of epileptic patients. Prior to the removal of diseased tissue at operation, they stimulate the brain of the patient electrically in the region of the suspected pathology. This aids in locating the area responsible for the onset of seizures in that they attempt, by brain stimulation, to elicit the same experiences or phenomena that precede the epileptic seizures. In general, they have found that psychically interesting responses are produced only from stimulation of the temporal lobes or their neighboring structures, including hippocampus and amygdala (see also Chapman et al., 1967). Stimulation of the temporal lobes outside the speech area occasionally gives rise to experiences related to memory. Hallucinations, which are highly organized sensations, or cruder sensations such as flashes, can be produced by stimulation closer to primary receptive areas.

Penfield and his colleagues divide the temporal-lobe responses into two categories: experiential (memories) and interpretive (feelings related to memory about ongoing experience). Experiential responses to stimulation are almost always similar to the arousal of visual or auditory memories. For example, one patient, on stimulation, reports: "Oh, a familiar memory—in an office somewhere. I could see the desk. I was there and someone was calling to me—a man leaning on a desk with a pencil in his hand" (Penfield and Roberts, 1959). Patients report that these experiences are very vivid—like living through the experiences again—and they often have double awareness. Typical experiences involve hearing or observing the action or speech of others or hearing music. The subject's own behavior is not usually a part of the experience (Penfield and Perot, 1963). The scenarios aroused from old memories move forward in time in a consistent manner (Penfield and Roberts, 1959; Chapman et al., 1967). Interpretive responses are ordinarily feelings about ongoing experiences, such as feelings of familiarity, even without referents, or strange or distant feelings (Mullan and Penfield, 1959).

Experiential or interpretive responses come almost exclusively from stimulation of the temporal lobes. A great many of the experiential responses come from the lateral superior portion of the temporal lobes. There is a tendency for more psychic responses (experiential or interpretive) to occur upon right-temporal-lobe stimulation. Normal lateralization expectations are not realized: voices and sounds both occur more commonly with right-temporal stimulation (Penfield and Perot, 1963). There may be some sort of vague topographic organization, since it is reported that neighboring areas tend to elicit related memories (Penfield and Perot, 1963). There is reported to be a rather high stability in the results produced by repeated stimulation at the same site. For example, right-temporal stimulation in one case led to a fragment of a song that the subject could not identify. Repeated stimulation apparently rearoused the same memory, so that the subject could eventually identify the song (Penfield and Jasper, 1954). In another instance four successive stimulations at the same site led to, first, a report of the search for the name of a song; second, the sound of talking; third, the song "O Marie, O Marie"; and fourth, this song again (Penfield and Jasper, 1954). It is quite possible that arousal of a particular memory facilitates its rearousal a short time later by an activation process (Penfield and Roberts, 1959).

It is critical to realize that these stimulation-elicited memories are all coming from the brains of epileptic patients in the general area of the brain pathology (Penfield and Jasper, 1954). Such responses may not be elicitable, with this type of straightforward stimulation, in normal brain tissue. There is a relationship between the psychic phenomena involved in the epileptic aura and the psychic events resulting from stimulation. For example, in ten seizure cases where interpretive feelings of familiarity were part of the aura, brain stimulation led to similar feelings in six (Mullan and Penfield, 1959).

The correspondence between fits and brain stimulation can be quite striking. Penfield and Jasper (1954) have reported a patient whose epileptic fits were preceded by an aura involving the psychic experience of someone grabbing a stick out of the mouth of a dog. They also reported two instances in which a fit was triggered in this patient by the real experiences of seeing a rifle grabbed out of a cadet's hands and a hat grabbed from a hat-check girl. During surgery, stimulation of the patient's temporal lobe at a particular site led to the experience of someone grabbing something from someone.

The linkage between stimulation and psychic experience is tight: "As long as the electrode is held in place, the experience of a former day goes forward. There is no holding it still, no turning back, no crossing with other periods. When the electrode is withdrawn, it stops as suddenly as it began" (Penfield and Roberts, 1959).

Even allowing for possible contamination of these fascinating reports by the patient's expectations of what or how he should respond, there seems to be a genuine phenomenon here. The limitation of interesting results to areas near epileptic foci is troubling but does not negate the interest of this material. The ability of the brain to inhibit what must be a variety of effects of the

stimulation, so as to result in a single coherent experience, is certainly noteworthy.

What is of course most exciting is the possibility that Penfield and his colleagues are tapping into the long-elusive engram. It is sad to report that excision of the whole area around these psychically active sites does not seem to erase any memories. Pribram (1969), in summarizing the literature on impaired memory consequent upon experimentally produced local brain damage in animals, concludes that "the impairment apparently is not so much a removal of localizable engrams as an interference with the mechanisms that code neural events so as to allow facile storage and retrieval." This holds as well for humans. We are still in search of the engram.

1.9 CONCLUSIONS

At the beginning of this paper I expressed the wish that I could have written it in the 1890s. It is indeed remarkable how close to the mark the basic schemes of Jackson and James were, and how accurately Korsakoff described the amnesic syndrome and how well he theorized about its cause. The great length of this paper results largely from the relative increase of details about memory disorders over the ensuing years, without a compensating increase in theoretical approaches in memory to accommodate the new information. I hope that if another such review is written in 1990, the intervening advances in the psychological understanding of human memory will permit someone to organize materials on the amnesic syndromes so that they can be covered in a few pages.

ACKNOWLEDGMENT

The auther would like to thank Drs. Henry Gleitman, Oscar Marin, Elisabeth Rozin, and Eleanor Saffran for their helpful comments.

REFERENCES

ADAM, N. 1973. Effects of general anesthetics on memory functions in man. *Journal of Comparative and Physiological Psychology* 83: 294–305.

ADAMS, R. D. 1969. The anatomy of memory mechanisms in the human brain. In Talland and Waugh (1969), pp. 91–106.

AJURIAGUERRA, J. DE, REY-BELLET-MULLER, M., and TISSOT, R. 1964. A propos de quelques problèmes posés par le déficit opératoire des vieillards atteints de démence dégénérative en début d'évolution. *Cortex* 1: 103–132, 232–256.

ANASTASI, A., and LEVEE, R. F. 1959. Intellectual defect and musical talent: A case report. *American Journal of Mental Deficiency* 64: 695–703.

ANGELERGUES, R. 1969. Memory disorders in neurological disease. In P. J. Vinken and G. W. Bruyn, eds., *Handbook of Clinical Neurology: Disorders of Higher Nervous Activity*, Vol. 3. New York: American Elsevier.

Aronson, L. 1951. Orientation and jumping in the gobiid fish *Bathygobius soporator*. *American Museum Novitates* 1486: 1–22.

Baddeley, A. D., and Warrington, E. K. 1970. Amnesia and the distinction between long- and short-term memory. *Journal of Verbal Learning and Verbal Behavior* 9: 176–189.

Baddeley, A. D., and Warrington, E. K. 1973. Memory coding and amnesia. *Neuropsychologia* 11: 159–166.

Barbizet, J. 1970. *Human Memory and Its Pathology*. Translated by D. K. Jardine. San Francisco: W. H. Freeman.

Benson, D. F., and Geschwind, N. 1967. Shrinking retrograde amnesia. *Journal of Neurology, Neurosurgery and Psychiatry* 30: 539–544.

Bickford, R., Mulder, D. W., Dodge, H. W., Svien, H. J., and Rome, H. P. 1958. Change in memory function produced by electrical stimulation of the temporal lobe in man. *Research Publications of the Association for Research in Nervous and Mental Diseases* 36: 227–243.

Blakemore, C. B., and Falconer, M. A. 1967. Long-term effects of anterior temporal lobectomy on certain cognitive functions. *Journal of Neurology, Neurosurgery and Psychiatry* 30: 364–367.

Blau, A. 1936. Mental changes following head trauma in children. *Archives of Neurology and Psychiatry* 35: 723–769.

Bower, G. H. 1970. Organizational factors in memory. *Cognitive Psychology* 1: 18–46.

Brain, L. 1965. *Speech Disorders*. 2nd ed. London: Butterworths.

Brierly, J. B. 1966. The neuropathology of amnesic states. In Whitty and Zangwill (1966), pp. 150–180.

Brink, J. D., Garrett, A. L., Hale, W. R., Woo-Sam, J., and Nickel, V. L. 1970. Recovery of motor and intellectual function in children sustaining severe head injuries. *Developmental Medicine and Child Neurology* 12: 565–571.

Brion, S. 1969. Korsakoff's syndrome: Clinico-anatomical and physiopathological considerations. In Talland and Waugh (1969).

Bruner, J. S., Olver, R., and Greenfield, P. M. 1966. *Studies in Cognitive Growth*. New York: John Wiley & Sons.

Butters, N., Lewis, R., Cermak, L. S., and Goodglass, H. 1973. Material-specific memory deficits in alcoholic Korsakoff patients. *Neuropsychologia* 11: 291–299.

Campbell, B. A., and Spear, N. E. 1972. Ontogeny of memory. *Psychological Review* 79: 215–236.

Carmon, A., and Nachsohn, I. 1971. Effect of unilateral brain damage on perception of temporal order. *Cortex* 7: 410–419.

Cermak, L., and Butters, N. 1972. The role of interference and enoding in the short-term memory deficits of Korsakoff patients. *Neuropsychologia* 10: 89–95.

Cermak, L. S., Butters, N., and Gerrein, J. 1973. The extent of the verbal encoding ability of Korsakoff patients. *Neuropsychologia* 11: 85–94.

Chapman, L. F., Walter, R. D., Markham, C. H., Rand, R. W., and Crandall, P. H. 1967. Memory changes induced by stimulation of hippocampus or amygdala in epilepsy patients with implanted electrodes. *Transactions of the American Neurological Association* 92: 50–56.

Claparède, E. 1911. Recognition et moiité. *Archives de Psychologie* 11: 79–90. (Recognition and "me-ness." In D. Rapaport, ed., *Organization and Pathology of Thought*. New York: Columbia University Press, 1951).

Corkin, S. 1965. Tactually-guided maze learning in man: Effects of unilateral cortical excisions and bilateral hippocampal lesions. *Neuropsychologia* 3: 339–351.

Corkin, S. 1968. Acquisition of motor skill after bilateral medial temporal-lobe excision. *Neuropsychologia* 6: 255–265.

Corsi, P. M. 1969. Verbal memory impairment after unilateral hippocampal excisions. Paper read at 4th Annual Meeting of the Eastern Psychological Association, April, 1969.

Corsi, P. M. 1972. Human memory and the medial temporal region of the brain. Unpublished Ph.D. dissertation, McGill University.

Craik, F. I. M., and Lockhart, R. S. 1972. Levels of processing: A framework for memory research. *Journal of Verbal Learning and Verbal Behavior* 11: 671–684.

Cronholm, B. 1969. Post-ECT amnesias. In Talland and Waugh (1969), pp. 81–90.

Delay, J., and Brion, S. 1962. *Les Démences Tardives*. Paris: Masson.

Delay, J., and Brion, S. 1969. *Le Syndrome de Korsakoff*. Paris: Masson.

De Renzi, E., and Spinnler, H. 1966. Facial recognition in brain-damaged patients—An experimental approach. *Neurology* 16: 145–152.

Drachman, D. A., and Arbit, J. 1966. Memory and the hippocampal complex. II. Is memory a multiple process? *Archives of Neurology* 15: 52–61.

Drachman, D. A., and Ommaya, A. K. 1964. Memory and the hippocampal complex. *Archives of Neurology* 10: 411–425.

Ebbinghaus, H. 1885. *Über das Gedachtnis*. Leipzig: Duncker. (*Memory*, trans. H. Ruyer and C. E. Bussenius. New York: Teachers College, Columbia University, 1913.)

Ellis, N. R. 1963. The stimulus trace and behavioral inadequacy. In N. R. Ellis, ed., *Handbook of Mental Deficiency*. New York: McGraw-Hill, pp. 134–158.

Evans, F. J., and Kihlstrom, J. F. 1973. Posthypnotic amnesia as disrupted retrieval. *Journal of Abnormal Psychology* 82: 317–323.

Evans, F. J., and Thorn, W. A. F. 1966. Two types of posthypnotic amnesia: Recall amnesia and source amnesia. *International Journal of Clinical and Experimental Hypnosis* 14: 162–179.

Fisher, C. M. 1966. Concussion amnesia. *Neurology* 16: 826–830.

Flavell, J. H., Griedricks, A. G., and Hoyt, J. D. 1970. Developmental changes in memorization processes. *Cognitive Psychology* 1: 324–340.

Furth, H. G. 1966. *Thinking without Language. Psychological Implications of Deafness*. New York: The Free Press.

Gallistel, C. R. 1974. Motivation as central organizing process: The psychophysical approach to its functional and neurophysiological analysis. In J. Cole and T. Sonderegger, eds., *Nebraska Symposium on Motivation*, vol. 22 (in press).

Gazzaniga, M. 1970. *The Bisected Brain*. New York: Appleton-Century-Crofts.

Geffen, G., Bradshaw, J. L., and Wallace, G. 1971. Interhemispheric effects on reaction time to verbal and nonverbal visual stimuli. *Journal of Experimental Psychology* 87: 415–422.

Geschwind, N. 1962. The anatomy of acquired disorders of reading. In J. Money, ed., *Reading Disability*. Baltimore: The Johns Hopkins Press.

Geschwind, N. 1964. The development of the brain and the evolution of language. In C. I. J. M. Stuart, ed., Monograph Series on Languages & Linguistics, no. 17. Report of the 15th Annual R.T.M. on Linguistic and Language Studies, April 1964.

GESCHWIND, N. 1965a. Disconnexion syndromes in animals and man. Part I. *Brain* 88: 237–294.

GESCHWIND, N. 1965b. Disconnexion syndromes in animals and man. Part II. *Brain* 88: 585–644.

GESCHWIND, N. 1967. The varieties of naming errors. *Cortex* 3: 97–112.

GESCHWIND, N., and LEVITSKY, W. 1968. Human brain: Left-right asymmetries in temporal speech region. *Science* 161: 186–187.

GESCHWIND, N. QUADFASEL, F. A., and SEGARRA, J. M. 1968. Isolation of the speech area. *Neuropsychologia* 6: 327–340.

GLANZER, M., and CLARK, W. H. 1963. Accuracy of perceptual recall: An analysis of organization. *Journal of Verbal Learning and Verbal Behavior* 1: 289–299.

GLANZER, M., and CUNITZ, A. R. 1966. Two storage mechanisms in free recall. *Journal of Verbal Learning and Verbal Behavior* 5: 351–360.

GLEITMAN, H. 1974. Getting animals to understand the experimenter's instructions. *Animal Learning and Behavior* 2: 1–5.

GOLDSTEIN, K. 1934. *Der Aufbau des Organismus. Einführung in die Biologie unter besonderer Berücksichtigung der Erfahrungen am kranken Menschen.* The Hague: Martinus Nijhoff. (*The Organism. A Holistic Approach to Biology Derived from Pathological Data in Man.* New York: American Book Co., 1939.)

HARRIS, C. S. 1965. Perceptual adaptation to inverted, reversed, and displaced vision. *Psychological Review* 72: 419–444.

HEBB, D. O. 1961. Distinctive features of learning in the higher animal. In J. F. Delafresnaye, ed., *Brain Mechanisms and Learning.* New York: Oxford University Press, pp. 37–46.

HERING, E. 1878. *Zur Lehre vom Lichtsinne.* Vienna.

HURVICH, L. M., and JAMESON, D. 1957. An opponent-process theory of color vision. *Psychological Review* 64: 384–404.

HURVICH, L. M., and JAMESON, D. 1969. Human color perception. *American Scientist* 57(1): 143–166.

IVERSEN, S. D. 1973. Brain lesions and memory in animals. In J. A. Deutsch, ed., *The Physiological Basis of Memory.* New York: Academic Press, pp. 305–364.

JACKSON, J. H. 1884. Croonian lectures on evolution and dissolution of the nervous system. *British Medical Journal* 1: 591. (Reprinted in J. Taylor, ed., *Selected Writings of John Hughlings Jackson,* Vol. 2. London: Staples Press, 1958, pp. 44–75.)

JACKSON, J. H. 1888. On a particular variety of epilepsy (intellectual aura), one case with symptoms of organic brain disease. *Brain* 11: 179–207. (Reprinted in J. Taylor, ed., *Selected Writings of John Hughlings Jackson,* Vol. 1. London: Staples Press, 1958, pp. 385–405.)

JAMES, W. 1890. *The Principles of Psychology.* New York: Henry Holt & Co.

JARRARD, L. E., and MOISE, S. L. 1971. Short-term memory in the monkey. In L. E. Jarrard, ed., *Cognitive Processes in Non-human Primates.* New York: Academic Press, pp. 3–24.

JONES, M. K. 1974. Imagery as a mnemonic aid after temporal lobectomy. *Neuropsychologia* 12: 21–30.

JONIDES, J., KAHN, R., and ROZIN, P. 1975. Imagery instructions improve memory in blind subjects. *The Bulletin of the Psychonomic Society* 5: 424–426.

KAHN, E. A., and CROSBY, E. C. 1972. Korsakoff's syndrome associated with surgical lesions involving the mammillary bodies. *Neurology* 22: 117–125.

KIMURA, D. 1963. Right temporal-lobe damage. *Archives of Neurology* 8: 264–271.

KONORSKI, J. 1959. A new method of physiological investigation of recent memory in animals. *Bulletin de l'Academie Polonaise des Sciences: Serie des Sciences Biologiques* 7: 115–117.

KORSAKOFF, S. S. 1889. Étude médico-psychologique sur une forme des maladies de la mémoire. *Revue Philosophique* 5: 501–530.

KRAL, V. A. 1969. Memory disorders in old age and senility. In Talland and Waugh (1969), pp. 41–48.

LASHLEY, K. S. 1950. In search of the engram. *Symposia of the Society for Experimental Biology* 4: 454–482.

LEVY, J. 1969. Possible basis for the evolution of lateral specialization of the human brain. *Nature* 224: 614–615.

LEVY, J., TREVARTHEN, C., and SPERRY, R. W. 1972. Perception of bilateral chimeric figures following hemispheric deconnexion. *Brain* 95: 61–78.

LHERMITTE, F., and SIGNORET, J.-L. 1972. Analyse neuropsychologique et différenciation des syndromes amnésiques. *Revue Neurologique (Paris)* 126: 161–178.

LURIA, A. R. 1966. *Higher Cortical Functions in Man.* Translated by B. Haigh. New York: Basic Books.

LURIA, A. R. 1968. *The Mind of a Mnemonist.* Translated by L. Solotaroff. New York: Basic Books.

LURIA, A. R. 1973. *The Working Brain. An Introduction to Neuropsychology.* Translated by B. Haigh. New York: Basic Books.

MARIN, O. S. M. 1955. Étude critique de l'Anatomie pathologique du Syndrome de Korsakoff. Unpublished thesis, Faculté de Médecine de Paris.

MARSLEN-WILSON, W. 1974. The implications of anterograde amnesia for the structure of human memory. Paper read at the Eastern Psychological Association Meeting, Philadelphia, April 1974.

MEDIN, D. L. 1972. Evidence for short- and long-term memory in monkeys. *American Journal of Psychology* 85: 117–120.

MEYER, V. 1959. Cognitive changes following temporal lobectomy for relief of temporal lobe epilepsy. *Archives of Neurology and Psychiatry* 81: 299–309.

MEYER, V., and YATES, A. J. 1955. Intellectual changes following temporal lobectomy for psychomotor epilepsy. *Journal of Neurology, Neurosurgery and Psychiatry* 18: 44–52.

MILLER, E. 1971. On the nature of the memory disorder in presenile dementia. *Neuropsychologia* 9: 75–81.

MILNER, B. 1958. Psychological defects produced by temporal lobe excision. In *Proceedings of the Association for Research in Nervous and Mental Disease.* Vol. 36: *The Brain and Human Behavior.* Baltimore: Williams & Wilkins, pp. 244–257.

MILNER, B. 1962. Les troubles de la memoire accompagnant des lesions hippocampiques bilaterales. In *Physiologie de l'Hippocampe.* Paris: Centre National de la Recherche Scientifique, pp. 257–272. (English translation in P. M. Milner and S. Glickman, eds., *Cognitive Processes and the Brain.* Princeton: Van Nostrand Co., 1965, pp. 97–111.)

MILNER, B. 1963. Effects of different brain lesions on card sorting. The role of the frontal lobes. *Archives of Neurology* 9: 90–100.

MILNER, B. 1964. Some effects of frontal lobectomy in man. In J. M. Warren and K. Akert, eds., *The Frontal Granular Cortex and Behavior.* New York: McGraw-Hill, pp. 313–334.

MILNER, B. 1965. Visually-guided maze learning in man: Effects of bilateral hippocampal, bilateral frontal, and unilateral cerebral lesions. *Neuropsychologia* 3: 317–338.

MILNER, B. 1966. Amnesia following operation on the temporal lobes. In Whitty and Zangwill (1966), pp. 109–133.

MILNER, B. 1967. Brain mechanisms suggested by studies of temporal lobes. In F. L. Darley and C. H. Millikan, eds.,

Brain Mechanisms Underlying Speech and Language. New York: Grune & Stratton, pp. 122–145.

MILNER, B. 1968. Visual recognition and recall after right temporal-lobe excision in man. *Neuropsychologia* 6: 191–209.

MILNER, B. 1970. Memory and the medial temporal regions of the brain. In K. H. Pribram and D. E. Broadbent, eds , *Biology of Memory.* New York: Academic Press. pp. 29–50.

MILNER, B. 1971. Interhemispheric differences in the localization of psychological processes in man. *British Medical Bulletin* 27: 272–277.

MILNER, B. 1972. Disorders of learning and memory after temporal lobe lesions in man. *Clinical Neurosurgery* 19: 421–446.

MILNER, B. 1974. Hemispheric specialization: Scope and limits. In F. O. Schmitt and F. G. Worden, eds., *The Neurosciences: Third Study Program.* Cambridge, Mass.: MIT Press, pp. 75–89.

MILNER, B., CORKIN, S., and TEUBER, H.-L. 1968. Further analysis of the hippocampal amnesic syndrome: 14 year follow-up study of H. M. *Neuropsychologia* 6: 215–234.

MILNER, B., and TAYLOR, L. 1972. Right-hemisphere superiority in tactile pattern-recognition after cerebral commissurotomy: Evidence for non-verbal memory. *Neuropsychologia* 10: 1–15.

MILNER, P. 1970. *Physiological Psychology.* New York: Holt, Rinehart and Winston.

MORTON, J. 1968. Repeated items and decay in memory. *Psychonomic Science* 10: 219–220.

MOSCOVITCH, M., SCULLION, D., and CHRISTIE, D. 1976. Early versus late stages of processing and their relation to functional hemisphere asymmetry for face recognition. *Journal of Experimental Psychology* (in press).

MULLAN, J., and PENFIELD, W. 1959. Illusions of comparative interpretation and emotions produced by epileptic discharge and by electrical stimulation of the temporal cortex, *Archives of Neurology and Psychiatry* 81: 269–284.

NEISSER, U. 1967. *Cognitive Psychology.* New York: Appleton-Century-Crofts.

O'CONNOR, N., and HERMELIN, B. 1973. Short-term memory for the order of pictures and syllables by deaf and hearing children. *Neuropsychologia* 11: 437–442.

OJEMANN, G. A. 1971. Alteration in nonverbal STM with stimulation in the region of the mammillothalamic tract in man. *Neuropsychologia* 9: 195–201.

OSCAR-BERMAN, M. 1973. Hypothesis testing and focusing behavior during concept formation by amnesic Korsakoff patients. *Neuropsychologia* 11: 191–198.

PAPEZ, J. W. 1937. A proposed mechanism of emotion. *Archives of Neurology and Psychiatry* 38: 725–743.

PATTEN, B. M. 1972. The ancient art of memory. *Archives of Neurology* 26: 25–31.

PENFIELD, W., and JASPER, H. 1954. *Epilepsy and the Functional Anatomy of the Human Brain.* Boston: Little, Brown.

PENFIELD, W., and MILNER, B. 1958. Memory deficits produced by bilateral lesions in the hippocampal zone. *Archives of Neurology and Psychiatry* 79: 475–497.

PENFIELD, W., and PEROT, P. 1963. The brain's record of auditory and visual experience. A final summary and discussion. *Brain* 86: 595–696.

PENFIELD, W., and ROBERTS, L. 1959. *Speech and Brain-Mechanisms.* Princeton, N.J.: Princeton University Press.

PETERSON, L. R., and PETERSON, M. J. 1959. Short-term retention of individual items. *Journal of Experimental Psychology* 58: 193–198.

POSNER, M. I. 1969. Representational systems for storing information in memory. In Talland and Waugh (1969), pp. 173–194.

PREMACK, D. 1971. Language in chimpanzee? *Science* 172: 808–822.

PRIBRAM, K. H. 1969. The amnestic syndromes: Disturbances in coding. In Talland and Waugh (1969), pp. 127–160.

PRISKO, L. 1963. Short-term memory in focal cerebral damage. Unpublished Ph. D. dissertation, McGill University.

RIBOT, T. A. 1882. *The Diseases of Memory.* New York: Appleton & Co.

ROBERTS, A. D. 1945. Case history of a so-called idiot savant. *Journal of Genetic Psychology* 66: 259–265.

ROZIN, P. 1976. The evolution of intelligence and access to the cognitive unconscious. In J. M. Sprague and A. N. Epstein, eds., *Progress in Psychobiology and Physiological Psychology.* VI. New York: Academic Press (in press).

ROZIN, P. and KALAT, J. 1972. Learning as a situation-specific adaptation. In M. E. P. Seligman and J. Hager, eds., *Biological Boundaries of Learning.* New York: Appleton-Century-Crofts, pp. 66–96.

RUSSELL, W. R. 1959. *Brain, Memory, Learning. A Neurologist's View.* Oxford: Oxford University Press.

RUSSELL, W. R., and NATHAN, P. W. 1946. Traumatic amnesia. *Brain* 69: 280–300.

SAFFRAN, E. M., and MARIN, O. S. M. 1975. Immediate memory for word lists and sentences in a patient with deficient auditory short term memory. *Brain and Language* 2 (in press).

SAMUELS, I., BUTTERS, N., and FEDIO, P. 1972. Short-term memory disorders following temporal lobe removals in humans. *Cortex* 8: 283–298.

SAMUELS, I., GOODGLASS, H., and BRODY, B. 1970. Short-term visual and auditory memory disorders after parietal and frontal damage. *Cortex* 6: 440–459.

SANDERS, H. I., and WARRINGTON, E. K. 1971. Memory for remote events in amnesic patients. *Brain* 94: 661–668.

SCOVILLE, W. B., and MILNER, B. 1957. Loss of recent memory after bilateral hippocampal lesions. *Journal of Neurology, Neurosurgery and Psychiatry* 20: 11–21.

SELTZER, B., and BENSON, D. F. 1974. The temporal pattern of retrograde amnesia in Korsakoff's disease. *Neurology* 24: 527–530.

SHALLICE, T., and WARRINGTON, E. K. 1970. Independent functioning of verbal memory stores: A neuropsychological study. *Quarterly Journal of Experimental Psychology* 22: 261–273.

SHERRINGTON, C. S. 1906. *The Integrative Action of the Nervous System.* New Haven: Yale University Press.

SIDMAN, M., STODDARD, L. T., and MOHR, J. P. 1968. Some additional quantitative observations of immediate memory in a patient with bilateral hippocampal lesions. *Neuropsychologia* 6: 245–254.

SIMON, H. A. 1962. The architecture of complexity. *Proceedings of the American Philosophical Society* 106: 467–482.

SPERRY, R. W., GAZZANIGA, M. S., and BOGEN, J. E. 1969. Interhemispheric relationships: The neocortical commissures; syndromes of hemisphere disconnection. In P. J. Vinken and G. W. Bruyn, eds., *Handbook of Clinical Neurology*, Vol. 4. Amsterdam: North Holland Publishing Co., pp. 273–290.

SPITZ, H. H. 1973. Consolidating facts into the schematized learning and memory system of educable retardates. In N. R.

Ellis, ed., *International Review of Research in Mental Retardation*. New York: Academic Press.

Squire, L. R. 1974. Amnesia for remote events following electroconvulsive therapy. *Behavioral Biology* 12: 119–125.

Squire, L. R., and Slater, P. C. 1975. Forgetting in very long-term memory as assessed by an improved questionnaire technique. *Journal of Experimental Psychology*, 104: 50–54.

Starr, A., and Phillips, L. 1970. Verbal and motor memory in the amnestic syndrome. *Neuropsychologia* 8: 75–88.

Stengel, E. 1966. Psychogenic loss of memory. In Whitty and Zangwill (1966), pp. 181–191.

Stern, W. 1935. *Allgemeine Psychologie*. The Hague: Martinus Nijhoff. (*General Psychology from the Personalistic Standpoint*. New York: Macmillan, 1938).

Sweet, W. H., Talland, G. A., and Ervin, F. R. 1959. Loss of recent memory following section of the fornix. *Transactions of the American Neurological Association* 84: 76–82.

Talland, G. A. 1960. Psychological studies of Korsakoff's psychosis: Memory and learning. *Journal of Nervous and Mental Diseases* 130: 366–385.

Talland, G. A. 1965. *Deranged Memory*. New York: Academic Press.

Talland, G. A. 1968. *Disorders of Memory and Learning*. Baltimore: Penguin Books.

Talland, G. A., and Waugh, N. C., eds., 1969. *The Pathology of Memory*. New York: Academic Press.

Teitelbaum, P. 1967. *Physiological Psychology*. Englewood Cliffs, N. J.: Prentice-Hall.

Teitelbaum, P., Cheng, M.-F., and Rozin, P. 1969. Stages of recovery and development of lateral hypothalamic control of food and water intake. *Annals of the New York Academy of Sciences* 157: 849–860.

Teuber, H.-L., Milner, B., and Vaughan, H. G. 1968. Persistent anterograde amnesia after stab wound of the basal brain. *Neuropsychologia* 6: 267–282.

Tinbergen, N. 1951. *The Study of Instinct*. Oxford: Clarendon Press.

Tulving, E. 1972. Episodic and semantic memory. In E. Tulving, ed., *Organization of Memory*. New York: Academic Press, pp. 382–403.

Victor, M., Adams, R. D., and Collins, G. H. 1971. *The Wernicke Korsakoff Syndrome. A Clinical and Pathological Study of 245 patients, 82 with Post-mortem Examinations*. Philadelphia: F. A. Davis.

von Frisch, K. 1967. *The Dance Language and Orientation of Bees*. Cambridge, Mass.: Harvard University Press.

Warrington, E. K., and James, M. 1967. An experimental investigation of facial recognition in patients with unilateral cerebral lesions. *Cortex* 3: 317–326.

Warrington, E. K., and Rabin, P. 1970. A preliminary investigation of the relation between visual perception and visual memory. *Cortex* 6: 87–96.

Warrington, E. K., and Sanders, H. I. 1971. The fate of old memories. *Quarterly Journal of Experimental Psychology* 23: 432–442.

Warrington, E. K., and Shallice, T. 1969. The selective impairment of auditory verbal short term memory. *Brain* 92: 885–896.

Warrington, E. K., and Shallice, T. 1972. Neuropsychological evidence of visual storage in short-term memory tasks. *Quarterly Journal of Experimental Psychology* 24: 30–40.

Warrington, E. K., and Silberstein, M. 1970. A questionnaire technique for investigating very long-term memory. *Quarterly Journal of Experimental Psychology* 22: 508–512.

Warrington, E. K., Valentine, L., and Pratt, R. T. C. 1971. The anatomical localization of selective impairment of auditory verbal short-term memory. *Neuropsychologia* 9: 377–388.

Warrington, E. K., and Weiskrantz, L. 1968a. A new method of testing long-term retention with special reference to amnesic patients. *Nature* 217: 972–974.

Warrington, E. K., and Weiskrantz, L. 1968b. A study of learning and retention in amnesic patients. *Neuropsychologia* 6: 283–291.

Warrington, E. K., and Weiskrantz, L. 1970. Amnesic syndrome: Consolidation or retrieval? *Nature* 228: 628–630.

Warrington, E. K., and Weiskrantz, L. 1971. Organizational aspects of memory in amnesic patients. *Neuropsychologia* 9: 67–73.

Warrington, E. K., and Weiskrantz, L. 1973. An analysis of short-term and long-term memory defects in man. In J. A. Deutsch, ed., *The Physiological Basis of Memory*. New York: Academic Press, pp. 365–396.

Wechsler, D. 1945. A standardized memory scale for clinical use. *Journal of Psychology* 19: 87–95.

Wechsler, D. 1955. *Wechsler Adult Intelligence Scale* (Manual). New York: The Psychological Corporation.

Weigl, E. 1968. On the problem of cortical syndromes: Experimental studies. In M. L. Simmel, ed., *The Reach of Mind*. New York: Springer, pp. 143–160.

Weiskrantz, L. 1971. Comparison of amnesic states in monkey and man. In L. E. Jarrard, ed., *Cognitive Processes of Nonhuman Primates*. New York: Academic Press, pp. 25–46.

Whitty, C. W. M., and Lishman, W. A. 1966. Amnesia in cerebral disease. In Whitty and Zangwill (1966), pp. 36–76.

Whitty, C. W. M., and Zangwill, O. L., eds. 1966. *Amnesia*. London: Butterworth & Co.

Whitty, C. W. M., and Zangwill, O. L. 1966a. Traumatic Amnesia. In Whitty and Zangwill (1966).

Wickelgren, W. A. 1968. Sparing of short-term memory in an amnesic patient: Implications for strength theory of memory. *Neuropsychologia* 6: 235–244.

Williams, M. 1950a. Memory studies in E.C.T. *Journal of Neurology, Neurosurgery and Psychiatry* 13: 30–35.

Williams, M. 1950b. Memory studies in E.C.T. II. The persistence of verbal response patterns. *Journal of Neurology, Neurosurgery and Psychiatry* 13: 314–319.

Williams, M. 1953. Investigation of amnesic defects by progressive prompting. *Journal of Neurology, Neurosurgery and Psychiatry* 16: 14–18.

Williams. M. 1969. Traumatic retrograde amnesia and normal forgetting. In Talland and Waugh (1969), pp. 75–80.

Williams, M. 1973. Errors in picture recognition after E.C.T. *Neuropsychologia* 11: 429–436.

Williams, M., and Zangwill, O. L. 1952. Memory defects after head injury. *Journal of Neurology, Neurosurgery and Psychiatry* 15: 54–58.

Yarnell, P. R., and Lynch, S. 1973. The "ding": Amnestic states in football trauma. *Neurology* 23:196–197.

Yin, R. K. 1970. Face recognition by brain-injured patients: A dissociable ability. *Neuropsychologia* 8: 395–402.

Zangwill, O. L. 1966. The amnesic syndrome. In Whitty and Zangwill (1966), pp. 77–91.

POSTSCRIPT: THE LITTLE MAN IN THE HEAD

Workers in memory are frustrated at the elusiveness of the engram. If we turn for advice and guidance to others who have been frustrated in their attempts to understand the mind, we might note that, from time immemorial, resort has been made to one explanatory mechanism. This is the little man (or should one say the little person?) in the head, or homunculus. This presumably mythical creature has been credited with operation of the will, action, perception, and decision, among other things. Why could he/she not be also made the keeper of the engram?

Hardheaded scientists will claim that is utter nonsense, and represents neither progress nor science. But, as scientists, I propose that we consider the little person as a serious hypothesis. When we do so, we discover, surprisingly, that there is little evidence against the idea.

What, then, is the evidence against the little person in the head? As I understand it, from briefly reviewing the literature, there are two basic arguments, one logical and one empirical.

Logical argument: Positing a little person who can perform the operations under study does not solve anything. It just puts the problem off.

Response: This is true, but it is not necessarily wrong to put a problem off by referring it to another entity or part of a system. After all, what would one do with the claim that one cannot explain visual perception by just studying the retina, since much that is important in perception (e.g., the phenomena mediated by cortical simple or complex cells) is put off for the brain to handle. That is, after all, true. Or, to take a more compelling example, consider a father and son from another planet visiting Earth and perched in their spaceship over one of our great cities. The son might say: "Dad, what are those really fast metal things with four wheels that go whipping around corners, stop at red lights, squeeze into narrow openings, and do all that without hitting each other or other things (very often)? How do you think they work?" Father: "Gee, they are pretty impressive and lively creatures. I really can't tell how they work." Son: "Maybe there is a little man inside each one who knows to stop at red lights, and knows how to turn, and even knows where he is going. Maybe that explains it." Father: "Nonsense. That doesn't explain anything. That's just putting off the problem."

I think the "logical" case against the little man has its own logical problems.

The second, more serious objection to the little-person idea is the *empirical argument*. It is really very simple: no one has ever seen or found a little man. And indeed this is true. In the many thousands of brain operations, the thousands of human brains that have been sectioned after death, there has not been a single report of a little man.

[Skeptics could also argue that the existence of split-brain humans disproves the little man, since both hemispheres seem to retain basic perceptual, conative, engrammatic, and decision-making properties. However, this minor argument can be dismissed simply with the assumption that the little man is also split in two by the operation (after all, one would expect to find him on the midline). This simple expedient also explains the reported differences between the two hemispheres of the split brain, since, of course, the left and right hemispheres of the little man show the very same differences as the full hemispheres. Of course, one would have to assume that the little man was facing frontwards at the time of brain section, so his hemispheres would sort themselves out appropriately.]

I suggest that this search may have been a misguided enterprise. We have all been fooled, I believe, by the popular use of the homunculus in the scientific literature. He appears in textbooks typically as a large and grotesque creature draped over the cerebral cortex (see Figure 1.14) and representing the topographical distribution

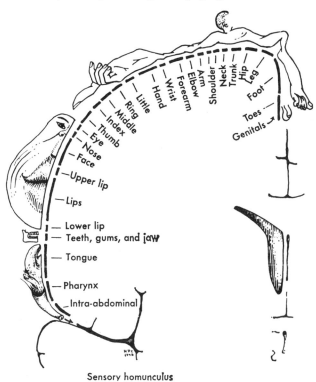

Sensory homunculus

FIGURE 1.14 Standard rendition of the sensory homunculus. From W. Penfield and T. Rasmussen, *The Cerebral Cortex of Man* (New York: Macmillan). Copyright 1950 by Macmillan Publishing Company, Inc.

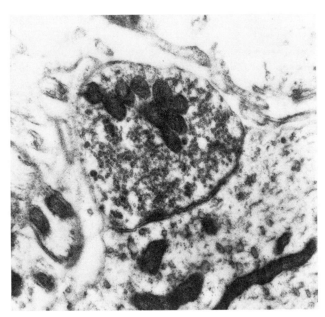

FIGURE 1.15 Electron micrograph ($\times$ 57000) of a section of the facial colliculus (unfortunately, of the rat). Preparation by S. Palay. From A. W. Ham, *Histology* (Philadelphia: Lippincott). Copyright 1957 by J. B. Lippincott Company.

of somatic sensory or motor function. I believe we have inadvertently used this ugly horror as our model. Having liberated myself from this misconception, I am now prepared to announce the first positive evidence for the little-man theory. It is shown in Figure 1.15, which is an electron micrograph of a synapse from the brain. The large central body on the picture is a presynaptic ending, abutting, on its lower right-hand side, on the surface of the postsynaptic neuron. Note within the presynaptic ending two clusters of round structures, one of five circles, the other of four. A moment's perusal will make it obvious that these are footprints.

There is a little man in the head. He just moves around a lot and is very, very small.

2

The Amnesic Syndromes and the Hippocampal-Mammillary System

F. LHERMITTE AND J.-L SIGNORET

ABSTRACT The existence of amnesic syndromes—in which recent memories are lost while premorbid events remote in time can be well recalled—following local cerebral lesions makes it possible to offer some interpretations of the functioning of memory.

Behavioral studies of patients lead to a distinction of three memory processes that can be impaired: (1) activation-consolidation, enabling storage of information beyond the immediate present; (2) information processing, enabling current information to be linked together to reduce its size; and (3) selective retrieval, making information available.

Neuropsychological analysis, that is to say, the study of disturbances of memory caused by lesions, makes it possible to differentiate certain amnesic syndromes:

1. Bilateral hippocampal lesions are responsible for a defect of the activation-consolidation process.

2. Mammillary lesions are responsible for a defect of the activation-consolidation process but are also associated with defects of selective retrieval and information processing.

3. Cingulate lesions are responsible for an isolated disorder of selective retrieval. These anatomical structures all belong to the circuit of Papez.

Psychophysiological interpretations are proposed in which the mammillary bodies would appear to constitute the nub of a system in which the hippocampus and the frontal lobes play major roles.

Human memory is of necessity the result of a structural modification in the brain. This tautology must not, however, be allowed to disguise the large gap that separates our clinical knowledge and often sophisticated psychological analyses from the biological foundations corresponding to memory traces (engrams). The clinical study of patients cannot yield any information about the nature of engrams. But the existence of amnesic syndromes following local cerebral lesions does make it possible to offer some interpretations of the functioning of memory. To do this we have to refer on the one hand to the psychological analysis of memory, and on the other to the physiology of the nervous system. The problem, then, is to join psychology and physiology together. Our discussion will fall under three main headings:

1. data supplied by behavioral studies of the amnesic syndromes;

2. neuropsychological analysis, that is to say, the studies of disturbances of memory caused by lesions; and

3. possible psychophysiological interpretations.

2.1 THE STUDY OF AMNESIC SYNDROMES

In amnesic syndromes there is a loss of recent memory, meaning that recent happenings are forgotten, whereas premorbid events remote in time can be well recalled. We shall consider the "generalized memory disorders," and we shall exclude memory loss resulting from disorders of vigilance, general intellectual impairment, or disorders of perception (see Milner and Teuber, 1968). Without any doubt the most satisfying functional definition of the amnesic syndromes is a disturbance of long-term memory (LTM) that leaves short-term memory (STM) unaffected (Drachman and Arbit, 1968; Wickelgren, 1968; Baddeley and Warrington, 1970). However, three questions arise in response to this definition:

1. Are all amnesic syndromes of an identical nature?

2. Does the observed deficiency involve a disturbance of memory only?

3. Can the amnesic syndromes be measured?

Only after these three questions have been answered will we be able to determine which memory process is impaired in the amnesic syndromes.

1. The "ideal" amnesic syndrome, such as that of H.M. (Milner, 1970; see also Rozin, this volume) consists simply of a loss of memory; the patient is conscious of the disorder, and if there is no interference, may try to counter the loss by verbal rehearsal. At the other end of the scale are some amnesic syndromes in which the patient remains unconscious of his disability and therefore denies its existence; these are generally accompanied by confabulation. It is interesting to note that confabulation is in fact an anarchical reconstruction of remote memories, often with recent memories added. Thus, in the case of one patient, the death of an Arab roommate was recounted two days later as the death of

F. LHERMITTE and J.-L. SIGNORET, Neurologie et Neuropsychologie, I.N.S.E.R.M. U84, Hôpital de la Salpêtrière, Paris, France

an Arab grocer in a district of Paris where the patient had lived twenty years before. Such confabulation is not a means of compensation. It is simply that there no longer exists any selective control over the recollection of autobiographical memories. The suggestions of the examiner and the situation may induce, rectify, or modify the "invented" reply. Similarly, faces of the present may bring about false recognition of persons familiar in the past. And finally, there is also a difficulty in reconstructing the chronology of past events. This distinction of two types of amnesic syndromes comes back to that of Zangwill (1966). The contrast is no doubt an oversimplification, since all possible intermediate stages are observed. What must be emphasized is the possibility of observing the evolution of an amnesic syndrome with confabulation toward a pure form, for in this case the disorder is clearly one of retrieval, that is to say, of the use rather than the storage of information.

2. A number of investigations, in particular those of Talland (1965) and more recently of Oscar-Berman (1973), have demonstrated the existence of a cognitive defect in the amnesic syndromes, marked by a deficiency in the information filing process, difficulty in focusing attention, bad formulation and use of hypotheses and strategies for resolving problems, and perseveration. It is remarkable that these difficulties, which are described in the frontal syndrome (Luria, 1966; Lhermitte, Derouesne, and Signoret, 1972), are observed principally in amnesic syndromes of alcoholic origin (Korsakoff's psychosis). More sophisticated research also shows that there exist disturbances involving verbal or visual encoding in these patients (Baddeley and Warrington, 1973; Cermak, Butters, and Gerrein, 1973).

3. Behavioral analysis leads to a description of the amnesic syndromes which may be summarized as follows. The core of every amnesic syndrome is a failure to retain information beyond the immediate moment, that is, an impaired transition from STM to LTM. With this core there may also be associated a retrieval disturbance and difficulties in processing information. We shall discuss the possible connections between these three functional levels below. It would make our task easier if work on the amnesic syndromes was restricted to homogeneous groups of subjects, but this is not always possible (although it does appear that, with the exception of rare cases, such as H.M., in which anterograde amnesia is almost total, patients can generally preserve a few fragments of new information). It would also be desirable to have some means of quantifying the magnitude of amnesia through the use of a genuine memory scale employing a variety of modalities (visual and verbal, for example) and different means of retrieval (free recall, cued recall, recognition). The memory scale devised by

Wechsler (1945) may still render some service, but only three of its seven subtests make use of the possibility of memorizing new material (memorization of a story; visual reproduction of three designs; and the learning of ten paired-associate words). We turn now to the description of a useful learning test.

All memory rests first upon the intake of information through some sort of sensory register, and then upon the processing of this information, according to its nature and complexity, through a strategy that has been consciously or unconsciously chosen by the subject. This processed information is then passed along to the long-term memory. The limited capacity of the short-term memory necessitates a grouping or chunking of information to produce a diminution in its size (Miller, 1956). This grouping can be carried out because the subject is able to construct links between different pieces of information, links which, in turn, rest upon data from long-term memory. This process of consolidation, based on information processing (Atkinson and Shiffrin, 1968), may vary in its level, a factor which is sometimes hard to analyze (see Craik and Lockhart, 1973). Retrieval will depend, of course, upon the manner of information processing, but it will depend also upon the means of selective search used (Luria et al., 1967; Gardner et al., 1973). Three memory processes may thus be impaired: (1) activation-consolidation, enabling the passage of information from STM to LTM; (2) information processing, enabling current information to be linked together as well as to information drawn from LTM; and (3) selective retrieval, making information available.

An easy test of learning has enabled us to analyze these three processes (Lhermitte and Signoret, 1972; Signoret, 1972). The test consists of learning the arrangement of nine pictures of familiar objects placed in a 3 × 3 grid (Figure 2.1). After an initial presentation in which the

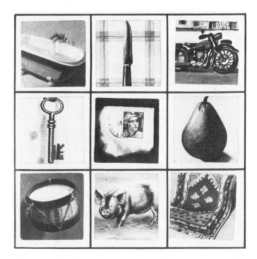

Figure 2.1 An arrangement of nine pictures into a 3 × 3 grid.

pictures are placed in their squares one at a time and in no obvious spatial order, they are presented to the subject in succession in a new order. As each picture is presented, the subject is asked to point with his finger to the corresponding square. If the answer is correct, we acknowledge it; if it is wrong, we correct it by placing the picture briefly in the proper square and then removing it. A trial consists of the presentation of all nine pictures, and the test continues until the subject succeeds in three consecutive trials. If the standard has not been met after ten trials, each figure is then left in its place, so that at the end of each trial the subject can see the arrangement of the whole grid. After warning the subject that he is supposed to remember the arrangement he has just learned, we proceed to study recall after intervals of 3 minutes, 1 hour, 24 hours, and 4 days. With the frame before the subject, we first test free recall: the subject attempts to specify orally the pictures and their corresponding squares. Then we test with cues; each figure is presented and the subject must point to the correct square.

In the case of one patient—H.R. (see Table 2.1)—learning of the arrangement was possible but difficult; after an interval of three minutes, though, it was completely forgotten. In the case of another patient—M.F.—learning was also difficult, but it was retained even after a four-day interval provided cues were supplied. In yet another patient—M.B.—learning was normal, but recall required the use of cues. Thus the disorder was one of activation-consolidation in H.R.; of activation-consolidation, information processing and selective retrieval in M.F.; and of selective retrieval only in M.B.

2.2. THE NEUROPSYCHOLOGY OF THE AMNESIC SYNDROMES

Bekhterev (1900) was the first to postulate that the medial regions of the temporal lobes might play a role in human memory processes. The truth of the postulate has been shown in cases where tissue has been removed bilaterally along the inner borders of the temporal lobes (Scoville, 1954; Scoville and Milner, 1957). The role of the hippocampus and the hippocampal gyrus in the origin of an amnesic syndrome has been confirmed by the existence of lesions following vascular diseases or encephalitis (Van Buren and Borke, 1972; Victor et al., 1961; Rose and Symonds, 1960). Some curable forms of herpes simplex encephalitis are distinguished by a necrosis affecting only the inner borders of the temporal lobes (Drachman and Adams, 1962; Hugues, 1969). Neuropathological studies have been rare, but Isaacson (1972) has made a critical review of cases following bilateral or unilateral temporal-lobe removal.

Gamper (1928) noted that the mammillary bodies seemed to be involved in all alcoholic psychoses. This was confirmed by Delay and Brion (1954). Victor, Adams, and Collins (1971) reported frequent lesions in the area of the thalamus. They emphasized the presence of lesions in the medial dorsal nucleus, but it must be noted that all their patients also presented lesions of the mammillary bodies. In support of their argument that the mammillary bodies are not necessarily involved, these authors cited the case of a patient with a bilateral lesion of the mammillary bodies who nevertheless showed no amnesic syndrome.

The hippocampus and the mammillary bodies are part of the circuit of Papez (1937). Bilateral damage to this circuit, at any of a number of points, seems to be a sufficient condition for the generation of an amnesic syndrome (Barbizet, 1963). Lesions of the fornix (Sweet, Talland, and Ervin, 1959; Brion et al., 1969), of the mammillothalamic tract (Ojemann, 1971), of the thalamus (Spiegel et al., 1956), of the thalamocingulate tract (Mabille and Pitres, 1913), of the cingulate gyrus

TABLE 2.1
Learning of the arrangement of nine pictures

Subjects	Age	I. Q.	M. Q.	Trials	Errors	Free recall	Cued recall	Disorders
Controls				1	0	9, 9, 9, 9	9, 9, 9, 9	
				4	6	7, 7, 6, 6	7, 7, 7, 7	
H. R. (hippocampus)	35	99	89	16	53	0, 0, 0, 0	0, 1, 1, 0	activation-consolidation
M. F. (mammillary)	67	107	84	12	31	0, 0, 0, 0	7, 9, 8, 8	activation-consolidation information processing selective retrieval
M. B. (cingulate)	50	107	91	1	0	1, 1, 2, 1	9, 9, 9, 9	selective retrieval

Subjects: the upper line of controls gives the best performance, the lower line gives the worst; H. R. is a patient with bilateral hippocampal lesions; M. F., a patient with mammillary lesions; and M. B., a patient with cingulate lesions. I. Q.: score on W.A.I.S. M.Q.: score on Wechsler memory scale. Trials and errors: number of trials and errors for acquisition of the arrangement. Free recall and cued recall: number of exact responses after delays of 3 min, 1 hr, 1 day, and 4 days. Disorders: disorders of the memory-processing mechanism.

(Whitty and Lewin, 1960; Brion et al., 1968), and probably of the cingulum (Dide and Botcazo, 1902), all confirm this conclusion.

The problem of amnesic syndromes following unitemporal lobectomy has not been fully cleared up. The hypothesis that amnesia involves a temporal lesion contralateral to the lobectomy is possible but not altogether proven (Stepien and Sierpinski, 1964; Dimsdale, Logue, and Piercy, 1964).

We have been able to show that the amnesic syndromes can be differentiated according to the sites of the precipitating lesions, as follows (see also Lhermitte and Signoret, 1972).

1. Bilateral hippocampal lesions—introduced during surgery or encephalitis—are responsible for pure amnesia, which can be interpreted as a defect in the activation-consolidation process. Such a defect would cause subjects to fail our nine-picture learning task since they would be unable to form "memory traces." Such patients can, however, succeed in tests where information has to be manipulated, classed, and organized in a sequential manner (see Table 2.2). For example, a subject can discover the elementary logical structure in an array of nine geometric figures presented successively in an arbitrary order (Figure 2.2); and he can also determine the code governing the successive presentation of colored counters (Figure 2.3). Success in these tests requires only brief memory work, but it does demand information processing and selective retrieval. The results obtained by such patients are equivalent to those of controls.

2. Mammillary lesions (alcoholic psychosis) are certainly responsible for a defect in the activation process since subjects with such lesions required more trials than did normals to learn the nine-picture task. But the memory traces do exist, judging by recall performances when cues are used. This recall disturbance is thus as-

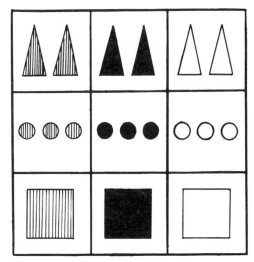

FIGURE 2.2 A logical arrangement of nine geometric figures (stripes: blue; black: red; white: yellow).

sociated with a defect of information processing; even with a short memorization period, logical and sequential learning is impossible.

3. We have also been able to observe a patient who had a double cingulate lesion after surgical treatment of an aneurism of the anterior communication artery. Confabulation was intense, but the possibility of learning was normal as long as free recall was not required. Even the recall of a simple story induced confabulated discourse in which, bit by bit, the patient associated pieces of the story with items from her own life. Results on the nine-picture and logical tests confirmed the existence of an isolated disorder of selective retrieval.

Before considering possible interpretations, it would seem to us important to consider the connections in the Papez circuit. These connections are complex, and our approach will have to be schematic. The principal extrinsic afferent tract of the hippocampus is the cingulum (Raisman, Powell, and Cowan, 1965), which arrives at the hippocampal gyrus and then attains the hippocampus via the temporoammonic tract. The principal extrinsic efferent fibers of the hippocampus make up the fornix (Raisman, Cowan, and Powell, 1966), which is composed of axons from the large pyramidal cells of the

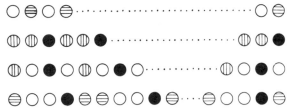

FIGURE 2.3 A code governing the successive presentation of colored counters (white: yellow; horizontal stripes: green; vertical stripes: blue; black: red).

TABLE 2.2
Learning on sequential-organization tasks

Subjects	Logical arrangement		Color code			
	T	E	YG	BBR	BYRY	GYYRG
Controls	1	0	2	2	2	2
	6	15	6	5	6	12
H.R.	4	14	2	3	3	3
M.F.	NA	67	NA	NA	NA	NA
M.B.	2	1	3	2	6	4

Subjects: see Table 2.1. Logical arrangement: arrangement of nine geometric figures. T, E: number of trials and errors for acquisition of the arrangement (NA = not acquired). Color code: code governing the successive presentation of colored counters (Y = yellow; G = green; B = blue; R = red); for each code the number of trials for acquisition is given.

hippocampus; it runs under the corpus callosum, traverses the hypothalamus, and ends in the mammillary body. Some fibers connect directly with the thalamus and the midbrain tegmentum (Guillery, 1956; Valenstein and Nauta, 1959), but in man, in contrast to animals, many fibers enter the nuclei of the mammillary body. The ratio between the number of hippocampal-mammillary fibers and the number of cells in the medial nucleus of the mammillary body ranges from 1:2 in the rat to 1:1 in the cat and monkey, to 2:1 in man (Powell, Guillery, and Cowan, 1957). Thus the number of fibers leaving the human hippocampus for cells in the mammillary body is double the number of cells in the mammillary body itself. This indicates that the human hippocampus possesses a more powerful apparatus to act upon the mammillary body than does the hippocampus in animals (Blinkov and Glezer, 1968).

The mammillary body is connected to the reticular formation by both efferent connections—the mammillotegmental tract—and afferent connections—the mammillary peduncle. It is from cells of the mammillary body especially that fibers constituting the Vicq d'Azyr or mammillothalamic tract emanate to rejoin the anterior group of nuclei of the thalamus.

The medial nucleus of the human mammillary body contains about 400,000 cells, which is 6–7 times more than in the monkey. Thus the number of cells in the human mammillary body has increased considerably during evolution, much more so than, for example, the number of cells in the parieto-occipital region. The number of fibers in the mammillothalamic tract and the number of cells in the anterior group of nuclei of the thalamus have shown proportional increases; all these structures have developed to a much greater degree than have other highly differentiated and phylogenetically new structures.

Finally, the cingulate gyrus, which receives the fibers from the anterior nucleus of the thalamus, has numerous connections with other cortical areas, principally with the frontal area and—probably through its association bundle, the cingulum—with the parieto-occipital cortex (Crosby, Humphrey, and Lauer, 1962).

2.3 PSYCHOPHYSIOLOGICAL INTERPRETATIONS

It has become habitual for those proposing memory models to design a set of boxes with information in them. But it is possible to forget the arrows linking the various boxes. The structures we have described do not by any means constitute the boxes. The role of the hippocampal-mammillary system is to be found in the arrows; the amnesic syndromes inform us only about the formation and use of memory traces, not about their nature or whereabouts. They do, however, make it possible to "situate" the three functional processes that all memory activity demands.

1. The activation-consolidation process enables information to pass from short-term memory into long-term memory. It is the impairment of this process which produces bihippocampal amnesia (Symonds, 1966; Lhermitte, 1968). It is likely that this activation first takes place at the hippocampal level, but its action is probably through the reticular formation and the thalamus. The observations made by Teuber, Milner, and Vaughan (1968) have adequately demonstrated that an amnesic syndrome can result from a lesion in the brainstem (rostral midbrain) that most likely breaks the connections between the hippocampus and the reticular formation. This role of the hippocampus in the regulation of the reticular activating influences upon the cerebral cortex was underlined by Green (1964), and the connections between the two formations were well studied by Nauta (1958). It is impossible to state exactly how long this activation-consolidation process lasts, but it probably continues beyond the time of intake of information, as is shown by some forms of posttraumatic retrograde amnesia.

It must of course be asked why certain sensorimotor activities can be preserved in amnesia (see Warrington and Weiskrantz, 1968; Corkin, 1968; Milner, Corkin, and Teuber, 1968; Sidman, Stoddard, and Mohr, 1968; Starr and Phillips, 1970). In all the reported cases it has been simply a question of elementary tasks that do not demand any information processing. It is also possible that repetition in itself brings about activation and thus allows the formation of memory traces.

The connections between the mammillary bodies and the reticular formation account for an activation defect in cases of Korsakoff's psychosis, while the persistence of certain links between the hippocampus and the reticular formation enables us to explain the possibility of learning, however limited this may be.

2. The processing of information is difficult to study. It depends on the complexity of the task to be memorized, and it is not a question of a simple encoding of information. The subject has to manipulate the information according to some strategy, which may be variable, but the result of which must be the establishment of links and associations within the information to make possible a reduction in its quantity, and the attachment of present information to information already existing in LTM (and perhaps also the constitution of a semantic system). This handling of information according to a strategy is one of the recognized functions of the frontal lobes (Luria, 1966, 1973). It is thus quite clear that cer-

tain amnesic syndromes can be interpreted as the result of a frontal disturbance. These syndromes are generally alcoholic psychoses involving lesions of the mammillary bodies, which, by means of the mammillothalamic tract and the thalamocingulate fibers, exercise control over the frontal lobes. A lesion of this system can explain the impairment observed. It must be emphasized that when information is learned by such a patient, it is never incorporated into an ensemble. In man, this ensemble is organized chronologically; the subject cannot, then, build chronological references for a bit of information that has been recorded.

3. Selective retrieval makes possible the use of information. A typical disorder in this function is demonstrated by the inability of patients to recall remote memories (Sanders and Warrington, 1971). Chronological disorganization of personal and social events may lead to a confabulated reconstruction. It must be underlined that the disorder is most clear-cut for events concerning the few years preceding the onset of the syndrome. It is also possible that posttraumatic, extensively retrograde amnesia also depends on this mechanism; the waning of this amnesia would seem to be an argument in favor of such a view. It is noteworthy that this sort of disturbance can be isolated, that is to say, it can be observed without the presence of any major difficulty in memorization. In such cases the lesion would appear to concern the cingulate gyrus and probably the cingulum. Of course, the connections between the cingulum and the hippocampal gyrus may provoke discussion as to the role of the latter formation in selective retrieval, while the mammillary bodies also exercise control over the cingulate gyrus. Recall can sometimes be facilitated in a rather spectacular way when cues are given to patients (Warrington and Weiskrantz, 1971); such was the case in the recall of our spatial arrangement of pictures.

This distinction of three different processes may appear somewhat oversimplified, for their functioning is necessarily closely linked. For example, to process information implies a certain level of activation and also the possibility of selective retrieval. Recall depends upon selective retrieval, but also upon the level of activation and the degree of processing the information has received. And finally, activation is more efficient the more treatment the information has been given.

Pathology has thus allowed us to make a hierarchical functional dissection (see also Lhermitte and Signoret, 1974). The mammillary bodies would certainly appear to constitute the nub of a system in which the hippocampus and the frontal lobes play a major role. But it is only the complete system that permits the constitution of memory traces.

REFERENCES

ATKINSON, R. C., and SHIFFRIN, R. M. 1968. Human memory: A proposed system and its control processes. In K. W. Spence and J. T. Spence, eds., *The Psychology of Learning and Motivation*, Vol. 2. New York: Academic Press.

BADDELEY, A. D., and WARRINGTON, E. 1970. Amnesia and the distinction between long- and short-term memory. *Journal of Verbal Learning and Verbal Behavior* 9: 176–189.

BADDELEY, A. D., and WARRINGTON, E. 1973. Memory coding and amnesia. *Neuropsychologia* 11: 159–165.

BARBIZET, J. 1963. Defects of memorizing of hippocampal mammillary origin: A review. *Journal of Neurology, Neurosurgery and Psychiatry* 26: 127–135.

BEKHTEREV, V. M. 1900. Demonstration eines Gehirns mit Zerstörung der vorderen und inneren Theile der Hirnrinde beider Schläfenlappen. *Neurologie Zentralblatt* 19: 990–991.

BLINKOV, S. M., and GLEZER, I. I. 1968. *The Human Brain in Figures and Tables.* New York: Plenum Press.

BRION, S., DEROME, P., GUIOT, G., and TEITGEN, M. 1968. Syndrome de Korsakoff par anévrysme de l'artère communicante antérieure: Le problème des syndromes de Korsakoff par hémorragie méningée. *Revue Neurologique (Paris)* 118: 293–299.

BRION, S., PRAGIER, G., GUERIN, R., and TEITGEN, M. 1969. Syndrome de Korsakoff par ramollissement bilatéral du fornix. Le problème des syndromes amnésiques par lésion vasculaire unilatérale. *Revue Neurologique (Paris)* 120: 255-262.

CERMAK, L. S., BUTTERS, N., and GERREIN, J. 1973. The extent of the verbal encoding ability of Korsakoff patients. *Neuropsychologia* 11: 85–94.

CORKIN, S. 1968. Acquisition of motor-skill after bilateral medial temporal lobe excision. *Neuropsychologia* 6: 255–265.

CRAIK, F. I. M., and LOCKHART, R. S. 1972. Levels of processing: A framework for memory research. *Journal of Verbal Learning and Verbal Behavior* 11: 671–684.

CROSBY, E., HUMPHREY, T., and LAUER, E. W. 1962. *Correlative Anatomy of the Nervous System.* New York: Macmillan.

DELAY, J., and BRION, S. 1954. Syndrome de Korsakoff et corps mamillaires. *Encéphale* 43: 193–200.

DIDE, M., and BOTCAZO. 1902. Amnésie continue, cécité verbale pure, perte du sens topographique; ramollissement double du lobe lingual. *Revue Neurologique (Paris)* 10: 676–680.

DIMSDALE, H., LOGUE, V., and PIERCY, M. 1964. A case of persisting impairment of recent memory following right temporal lobectomy. *Neuropsychologia* 1: 287–298.

DRACHMAN, D. A., and ADAMS, R. D. 1962. Herpes simplex and acute-inclusion body encephalitis. *Archives of Neurology* 7: 45–63.

DRACHMAN, D. A., and ARBIT, J. 1966. Memory and the hippocampal complex: Is memory a multiple process? *Archives of Neurology* 15: 52–61.

GAMPER, R. 1928. Zur Frage der Polioencephalitis haemorrhagica der chronischen Alkoholiker. Anatomische Befunde beim Alkoholischen Korsakoff und ihre Beziehungen zum Klinischen Bild. *Deutsche Zeitschrift für Nervenheilkunde* 102: 122–129.

GARDNER, H., BOLLER, F., MOREINES, J., and BUTTERS, N. 1973. Retrieving information from Korsakoff patients: Effects of categorical cues and reference to the task. *Cortex* 9: 165–175.

GREEN, J. D. 1964. The hippocampus. *Physiological Review* 44: 561–608.

GUILLERY, R. W. 1956. Degeneration in the posterior commissural fornix and the mammillary peduncle of the rat. *Journal of Anatomy* 90: 350–370.

HUGUES, J. T. 1969. Pathology of herpes simplex encephalitis. In C. W. M. Whitty, J. T. Hugues, and F. D. Mac-Callum, eds., *Virus Diseases and the Nervous System*. Oxford: Blackwell Scientific Publications.

ISAACSON, R. L. 1972. Hippocampal destruction in man and other animals. *Neuropsychologia* 10: 47–64.

LHERMITTE, F. 1968. Bases physiologiques de la mémoire. *L'Evolution Psychiatrique* 33: 579–603.

LHERMITTE, F., DEROUESNE, J., and SIGNORET, J.-L. 1972. Analyse neuropsychologique du syndrome frontal. *Revue Neurologique (Paris)* 127: 415–440.

LHERMITTE, F., and SIGNORET, J.-L. 1972. Analyse neuropsychologique et différenciation des syndromes amnésiques. *Revue Neurologique (Paris)* 126: 161–178.

LHERMITTE, F., and SIGNORET, J.-L. 1974. Analyse psychophysiologique des syndromes amnésiques. *L'Evolution Psychiatrique* 39: 203–214.

LURIA, A. R. 1966. *Higher Cortical Functions in Man*. Translated by Basil Haigh. New York: Basic Books.

LURIA, A.R. 1973. *The Working Brain*. Translated by Basil Haigh. New York: Basic Books.

LURIA, A. R., HOMSKAYA, E. D., BLINKOV, S. M., and CRITCHLEY, McD. 1967. Impaired selectivity of mental processes in association with a lesion of the frontal lobe. *Neuropsychologia* 5: 105–117.

MABILLE, H., and PITRES, A. 1913. Sur un cas d'amnésie de fixations post-apoplectiques ayant persisté pendant vingt trois ans. *Revue de Médecine* 33: 257–279.

MILLER, G. A. 1956. The magical number seven plus or minus two: Some limits of our capacity for processing information. *Psychological Review* 63: 81–97.

MILNER, B. 1970. Pathologie de la mémoire. In *La Mémoire* (Symposium de l'association de psychologie scientifique de langue française). Paris: Presses Universitaires de France.

MILNER, B., CORKIN, S., and TEUBER, H.-L. 1968. Further analysis of the hippocampal amnesic syndrome: 14 year follow-up study of H. M. *Neuropsychologia* 6: 215–234.

MILNER, B., and TEUBER, H.-L. 1968. Alteration of perception and memory in man: Reflections on methods. In L. Weiskrantz, ed., *Analysis of Behavioral Change*. New York: Harper & Row.

NAUTA, W. J. H. 1958. Hippocampal projections and related neural pathways to the midbrain in the cat. *Brain* 81: 319–340.

OJEMANN, G. A. 1971. Alteration in nonverbal STM with stimulation in the region of the mammillothalamic tract in man. *Neuropsychologia* 9: 195–201.

OSCAR-BERMAN, M. 1973. Hypothesis testing and focusing behavior during concept formation by amnesic Korsakoff patients. *Neuropsychologia* 11: 191–198.

PAPEZ, J. W. 1937. A proposed mechanism of emotion. *Archives of Neurology and Psychiatry* 38: 725–743.

POWELL, T. P. S., GUILLERY, R. W., and COWAN, W. M. 1957. A quantitative study of the fornix mammillothalamic system. *Journal of Anatomy* 91: 419–432.

RAISMAN, G., COWAN, W. M., and POWELL, T. P. S. 1965. The extrinsic afferent commissural and association fibres of the hippocampus. *Brain* 88: 963–996.

RAISMAN, G., COWAN, W. M., and POWELL, T. P. S. 1966. An experimental analysis of the efferent projections of the hippocampus. *Brain* 89: 83–108.

ROSE, F. C., and SYMONDS, C. P. 1960. Persistent memory defect following encephalitis. *Brain* 83: 195–212.

SANDERS, H. I., and WARRINGTON, E. K. 1971. Memory for remote events in amnesic patients. *Brain* 94: 661–668.

SCOVILLE, W. B. 1954. The limbic lobe in man. *Journal of Neurosurgery* 11: 64–66.

SCOVILLE, W. B., and MILNER, B. 1957. Loss of recent memory after bilateral hippocampal lesions. *Journal of Neurology, Neurosurgery and Psychiatry* 20: 11–29.

SIDMAN, M., STODDARD, L. T., and MOHR, J. P. 1968. Some additional quantitative observations of immediate memory in a patient with bilateral hippocampal lesions. *Neuropsychologia* 6: 245–264.

SIGNORET, J.-L. 1972. Memory and Korsakoff's syndrome. Persistence or extinction of memory traces. *International Journal of Mental Health* 1: 103–108.

SPIEGEL, E. A., WYCIS, H. T., ORCHINIK, C., and FREED, H. 1956. Thalamic chronotaraxis. *American Journal of Psychiatry* 113: 97–105.

STARR, A., and PHILLIPS, L. 1970. Verbal and motor memory in the amnesic syndrome. *Neuropsychologia* 8: 75–88.

STEPIEN, L., and SIERPINSKI, S. Impairment of recent memory after temporal lesions in man. *Neuropsychologia* 2: 291–303.

SWEET, W. H., TALLAND, G. A., and ERVIN, F. R. 1959. Loss of recent memory following section of the fornix. *Transactions of the American Neurological Association* 84: 76–82.

SYMONDS, C. 1966. Disorders of memory. *Brain* 89: 625–644.

TALLAND, G. A. 1965. *Deranged Memory*. London: Academic Press.

TEUBER, H.-L., MILNER, B., and VAUGHAN, JR., H. G. 1968. Persistent anterograde amnesia after stab wound of the basal brain. *Neuropsychologia* 6: 267–282.

VALENSTEIN, E. S., and NAUTA, W. J. 1959. A comparison of the distribution of the fornix system in the rat, guinea pig, cat and monkey. *Journal of Comparative Neurology* 113: 337–361.

VAN BUREN, J. M., and BORKE, R. C. 1972. The mesial temporal substratum of memory. Anatomical studies in three individuals. *Brain* 95: 599–632.

VICTOR, M., ADAMS, R. D., and COLLINS, G. H. 1971. *The Wernicke-Korsakoff Syndrome*. Oxford: Blackwell Scientific Publications.

VICTOR, M., ANGEVINE, J. B., MANCALL, E. L., and FISHER, C. M. 1961. Memory loss with lesions of hippocampal formation. Report of a case with some remarks on the anatomical basis of memory. *Archives of Neurology* 5: 244–257.

WARRINGTON, E. K., and WEISKRANTZ, L. 1970. Amnesic syndrome: Consolidation or retrieval? *Nature* 228: 628–630.

WARRINGTON, E. K., and WEISKRANTZ, L. 1971. Organizational aspects of memory in amnesic patients. *Neuropsychologia* 9: 67–73.

WECHSLER, D. 1945. A standardized memory scale for clinical use. *Journal of Psychology* 19: 87–95.

WHITTY, C. W. M., and LEWIN, W. 1960. A Korsakoff syndrome in the post-cingulectomy confusional state. *Brain* 83: 648–653.

WICKELGREN, W. A. 1968. Sparing of short-term memory in

an amnesic patient: Implications for strength theory of memory. *Neuropsychologia* 6: 235–244.

ZANGWILL, O. L. 1966. The amnesic syndrome. In C. W. M. Whitty and O. L. Zangwill, eds. *Amnesia*. London: Butterworth & Co., pp. 77–91.

3

The Biology of Memory

MICHAEL S. GAZZANIGA

ABSTRACT Recent split-brain and other clinical and animal data are reviewed with special reference to the issues of mass action, equipotentiality, and the role of motivation in memory. The picture that emerges is one in which the brain stores information about past experience in multiple ways and in multiple sites throughout the brain. With this view, the task becomes not to find the engram, but to find the network that interconnects a variety of disparate processing systems that each contribute information to the reconstruction of past experience.

3.1 INTRODUCTION

A primary objective in neuroscience is to establish how and through what processes information is stored in the central nervous system. Memory is rarely both the necessary and sufficient condition for behavioral processes (or, put differently, conscious experience), but it is invariably a necessary and key condition. Yet the long-standing questions of how and where information is stored, and by what brain mechanisms it is accessed, are as elusive today as ever before, at the molecular level as much as at the psychological level.

To begin with, most of us vault over the initial problem that must be solved by any viable model of memory —namely, how does the organism recognize either internally or externally generated stimuli and put them into a form that can be used in a relevant memory search? The trend is to bypass such questions, to proceed by accepting the notion that there is an inherent organization to information storage systems and then studying differences in organizational properties through reaction time and recognition and recall tasks at the experimental psychological level, and through brain lesions, electrical stimulation, pharmacological manipulations, and the like at the physiological level. While these studies are usually intriguing, they rarely leave us with any feeling for how the memory storage and retrieval system actually works.

In this chapter the aim will be to focus on how a variety of split-brain and other animal and clinical studies have contributed to present understanding of the physical basis of information storage. While some problems and data from animal work will be reviewed which

will highlight what I consider to be facts on the subject of memory, it is my guess that real insight into the biology of memory can be best obtained at this time by considering clinical and human experimental data. Here a case can be made that place and process are both very important in memory and that processing activities take place at identifiable regions in the brain. Moreover, evidence will be described which suggests that the brain has a variety of ways to encode and store information, and that a given information storage system in the brain is not necessarily accessible to every other network of stored information.

3.2 GENERAL BACKGROUND

A good point of departure for seeing where we stand in the 1970s is to see how far we have come from Lashley's classic and spellbinding 1950 paper "In Search of the Engram." While he made a variety of points, let me address the research that has in recent years directly challenged his main conclusions. Particularly at stake, of course, are his principles of mass action and the equipotentiality of cortical areas.

3.2.1 Mass action

The principle of mass action, defined as it was in a very general way, seems to make little sense in the light of split-brain phenomena in animals, where it has been shown time and again that little, if any, impairment is seen in *performance* when one hemisphere alone controls behavior (as opposed to the normal situation where the interaction of the two half-brains is possible via the corpus callosum) (Nakamura and Gazzaniga, 1974). Clearly a more radical deviation from normal learning and performance is caused by discrete lesions within one hemisphere, as in the inferior-temporal-lobe syndrome where 5–10 percent of the cortex is removed, than can be found in the split brain, where 100 percent of the cortical contribution of the one hemisphere is disconnected from the processing system of the opposite half-brain.

There have been, of course, a series of recent reports that split-brain cats are, in fact, impaired in learning (Sechzer, 1970). These are not ultimately convincing, however, because it is hard to determine how much of the decrement is due to the callosum surgery and how

MICHAEL S. GAZZANIGA, Department of Psychology, State University of New York at Stony Brook much to the deleterious effect of the chiasma section alone. Indeed, we have recently produced huge learning deficits in adult cats merely by making retinal lesions. In addition, Berlucchi (1974), in a recent exhaustive analysis of cat pattern-discrimination data, contends that there is no basis for the claim of a learning deficit in the single hemisphere. However, we have recently found evidence that if interproblem, rather than intraproblem, learning is examined, split-brain monkeys take more than twice as long to acquire a discrimination as do normal animals (LeDoux and Gazzaniga, unpublished observation). Thus, the issue concerning the learning capacity of the single hemisphere remains unsettled, but may be related to whether one is considering perceptual (intraproblem) or conceptual (interproblem) learning capacity.

Hebb (1942) argued for the importance of treating acquisition and performance separately. A widely used measure of performance is memory capacity. Milner (1974) has observed that split-brain humans have a spatial-memory impairment. Furthermore, Zaidel and Sperry (1974), solely on the basis of postoperative testing, claimed that split-brain humans showed deficits in short-term memory (STM) when compared to control subjects matched for IQ. We have recently had an opportunity to examine the STM issue in a callosum-sectioned patient with the appropriate control—preoperative testing. Using a variety of tasks, we were unable to find STM or other information-processing deficits (Le Doux, Risse, Wilson, and Gazzaniga, in preparation). This finding supports a series of experiments carried out by Richard Nakamura on the monkey using a nested match-to-sample task (Nakamura and Gazzaniga, 1975). This task requires that the monkey put "on hold" one piece of information (color) when another piece (pattern) comes in, and the second piece must be processed before the original information can be used. That is, first a color stimulus and then a pattern is presented to the animal. Next, two patterns are presented, one of which must be matched to the original pattern. Finally, two colors come on, one of which matches the original color. Thus, the color-matching problem starts before and finishes after the pattern-matching problem. As Figure 3.1 shows, the split-brain animals were less efficient processors. However, control experiments have demonstrated that if both hemispheres are allowed to view the problem, the split-brain animal performs at the normal level. Also, hemispherectomized animals do as well as normals on this task. These data indicate that the performance deficits seen in split-brain animals are more attributable to behavioral interference from the nonseeing hemisphere than to the direct neuro-

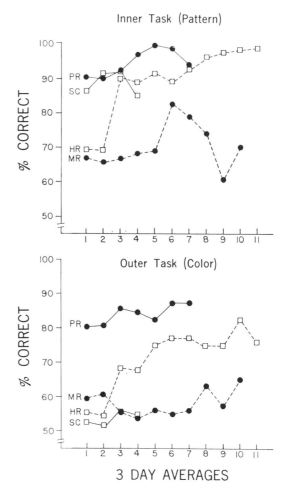

FIGURE 3.1 These graphs give a breakdown of individual performances of monkeys on nested matching tasks using one eye (one hemisphere in the split-brain animals). PR is the normal control; MR, HR, and SC are the experimental splits. The upper graph shows that the normal and two of the splits can do the inside or pattern task to above 90% level of performance. MR does worse but is clearly above the 50% chance level. The lower graph shows that no animal can attain the 90% performance level on the outer or color task. However, PR, the normal animal, is clearly superior to all splits, although one split, HR, shows signs of catching up after 33 days.

logical consequences of brain bisection (Nakamura, 1975).

This leaves us, on the whole, doubting whether there are significant costs to commissurotomy, a conclusion that markedly contrasts with Lashley's notion of mass action. However, should our recent observation on interproblem learning be confirmed, then perhaps the picture emerging from brain bisection work is that when the information-processing system is pushed, discrete impairments may be forthcoming following commissurotomy, but that these impairments tend to reveal themselves more during the learning or assimilation stage of processing, rather than during the performance of a well-learned behavior.

3.2.2 Equipotentially

The idea of cortical equipotentiality makes little sense when considered in light of the continuing studies on partial commissurotomy in both monkey and man (Gazzaniga and Freedman, 1973; Gazzaniga and Wilson, 1975; Gazzaniga, 1973b). Just as there are certainly specific deficits associated with particular cortical lesions in man, so the section of specific commissural sites produces dramatic effects in the interhemispheric exchange of information—a fact which makes little sense if cortical areas are indeed equipotential (Gazzaniga, 1973b; see Figure 3.2). As a result of these new developments, one can come to the problem of the physical basis of memory with no strings attached, and what I would like to do first is to build a case that might be best described as that of a neolocalizationist by considering in more detail some of the split-brain work as well as other clinical material. Before proceeding, however, and at the risk of sounding like I want it both ways, let me backtrack and set forth some animal work of ours on motiva-

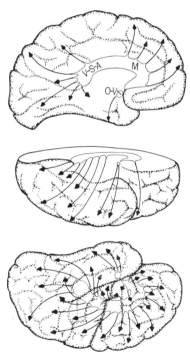

FIGURE 3.2 Major callosal projections in man and their functional specificities. Visual (V), somatosensory (S), and auditory (A) information course through the posterior third of the callosum, whereas motor (M) and, possibly, motivational information course through the more anterior regions. The anterior commissure may connect visual and olfactory (O) information.

tion that is totally consistent with many of Lashley's conclusions.

3.3 THE ROLE OF MOTIVATION IN MEMORY

Lashley warned us of how important it is to keep in mind the motivational state of an animal when testing for behavior deficits following lesions. We held this admonition in mind when we started using the split-brain monkey to study the necessary conditions for discriminative learning (Johnson and Gazzaniga, 1970, 1971). Prior to this series of studies, split-brain reports offered little insight into the underlying brain mechanisms involved in learning and memory. After the dramatic breakdown in interhemispheric transfer of discrimination learning on visual and tactile problems had been shown, which underlined the importance of the cortical commissural system in the intercortical exchange of information, little else was forthcoming from the animal literature on what the technique teaches about learning and memory per se. Indeed, it has yet to be shown that the corpus callosum can transmit "a memory" from one half-brain to the other. Experiments to date only indicate that if the corpus callosum is intact during training, sometimes there is evidence that a bilateral engram is found and sometimes there is not. While there are good indications that complex codes are transmitted in animals (Berlucchi, 1972) and especially in man (Gazzaniga, 1974), there is still little evidence for transfer of an engram per se.

Nonetheless, it has been my contention that the split-brain preparation is one of the most exciting preparations that can be used to get at questions of more general interest in the understanding of learning and memory. For example, David Johnson and I did a series of studies in which we taught a visual-pattern discrimination to one separated hemisphere. The animal was overtrained and consequently performed perfectly on the task. We then exposed the eye of the untrained hemisphere and let it observe the errorless performance of the trained half-brain for forty trials (Figure 3.3). What we discovered when we probed for knowledge of the problem by giving trials to the naive hemisphere alone was that it had learned the problem.

With errors not a necessary condition for learning, we then asked whether the organism needs a "reward." Thus, in another set of animals, we trained a discrimination to one hemisphere while the other, through the use of polaroid filters (see Trevarthen, 1962), saw a blank field. We then advanced the reward schedule so that the animal was rewarded only on every other trial. At this

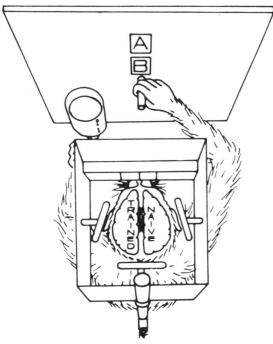

FIGURE 3.3 A split-brain monkey observing a visual discrimination through a specially designed training apparatus that allows for the separate or combined projection of visual information to each eye. Here, a naive hemisphere is free to observe the errorless performance of a trained hemisphere.

stage, this did not prove disruptive in any way. Then, on the nonrewarded trial, the naive hemisphere was allowed to see the visual discrimination. The question was, could it learn by observing the trained hemisphere perform the task perfectly in the absence of reward? What we found was that the normal response pattern was totally disrupted, and no learning took place after two experimental sessions. In a subsequent experiment (Gazzaniga, 1974), however, when we extended the number of days on which the nonrewarded observational trials were presented, learning did occur. This leaves us with one more—or, more accurately, one less—essential condition needed for discrimination learning to occur—namely, the presence of a primary reward.

These data raised in our minds the whole question of the role reward plays in learning and memory. One interpretation is that its importance lies in engaging the organism to attend to a particular task and that it plays little or no role in the brain mechanisms involved in information storage. Put differently, reward merely signals the organism that a particular event is to be stored, but the storage process itself is not dependent on the brain mechanism underlying reward. What is critical for information storage is pure, simple contiguity.

This, of course, is not to undercut the importance of reward mechanisms in learning performance. In studies done with Alan Gibson (Gibson and Gazzaniga, 1971; Gibson, 1972) on the effects of unilateral hypothalamic lesions (and others as well) on feeding behavior in monkeys, striking differences in eating rates were frequently seen between the two hemispheres in a split (Figure 3.4). We have often wondered whether the difference in learning abilities one commonly sees between hemispheres in splits (Nakamura and Gazzaniga, 1975) reflects differences in motivation—possibly brought about by hypothalamic or other brain damage incurred during split-brain surgery. The implication here for variations in normative data on cognitive tasks is, alas, that it may largely reflect motivational variables.

The role of reward needs to be considered in more detail. We subscribe to the view that reinforcement is relative and is a function of response probabilities (Premack, 1966). Thus stimulus A can reinforce stimulus B only if the organism has a higher probability of responding to A than to B. With this view, one can escape from Skinner's tautological approach in which a reinforcer is what is discovered to be reinforcing. Now, before saying A is rewarding, we separately and independently

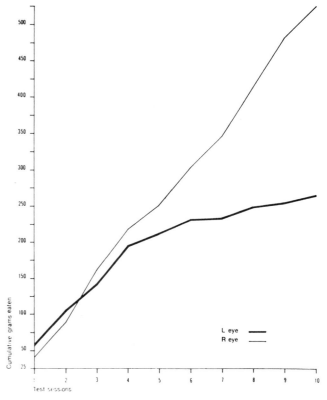

FIGURE 3.4 Unilateral lesions can differentially affect the motivational state of the separated hemispheres. The right cerebrum has a discrete hypothalamic lesion but also a considerable amount of other brain damage, which disallows conclusions on the contribution of the hypothalamus alone. The main point here is that, following cerebral commissure alone, the split-brain animal shows a striking difference in eating behavior as a function of eye use. From Gibson (1972).

measure the probability that an animal will choose A over B. If it is greater than 0.5, we can accurately predict that receiving A contingent on doing B will increase the probability of doing B.

The importance of viewing these processes in relative terms is, it seems to me, especially critical when one is trying to understand the underlying physiology. The Skinnerian view, that the organism has a repertoire of responses and that a particular one comes to the fore only as a result of external contingencies, strikes me as static and passive. The Premack view is more organic in that it sees the organism as actively and continuously assigning values to all stimuli, and in that what governs behavioral activity is response probability, which is generated by the organism.

Yet, curiously, it is the static Skinnerian view that has dominated physiological thinking. How many times have we heard about reward centers that interact with cognitive cortical centers? The view has been that it is reward which freezes or etches into the brain the particular information an organism is processing. All we have to do is locate the reward center and trace its connections to the higher centers, and we shall then know the primary neural circuits of behavior—of learning and memory. Experiments that contradict this paradigm go unnoticed. For example, it has been shown that a rat with an elec-

trode in a reward center will increase its rate of self-stimulation in order to gain the opportunity to run. In other words, running is rewarding the reward center.

In recent work, we have applied this basic insight in a more physiological setting (Gazzaniga et al., 1974). Lesions in the lateral hypothalamus predictably render rats adipsic. They show, postoperatively, essentially no probability of drinking, but will run for approximately 150 sec in 30 min. When the two events are made contingent, so that in order to run the rats have to drink, drinking commences immediately (Figure 3.5).

These data taken together serve as a fair warning not to take too literally the idea that memory and mental processing systems can be located in the brain in a simple sense. If one changes the external contingencies of training prior to or after a brain lesion, seemingly obvious and reliable neurobehavioral symptoms indicating specificity of function tend to disappear. This leaves the problem of localization of function as mercurial as ever (Gazzaniga, 1973a). On the positive side, however, these data suggest that as the motivational state changes, access to innate or learned behavioral patterns, which I think are multiply represented in the brains of both animals and men, are allowed expression. This brings us to what I mean by the multiple representation of the engram.

3.4 THE MULTIDIMENSIONALITY OF EXPERIENCE AND INFORMATION STORAGE

For years the organization of the brain was thought to be as simple as the psychological conceptions of what the organization of memory might be and entail. Thus, when it was thought that there was little more to life and memory than the relations between stimulus and response, brain scientists felt that there was little more to the brain mechanisms underlying these processes than the presence of discrete brain areas processing incoming and outgoing information (see Rozin, this volume). In this light it quickly became the dominant view in clinical neurology that most, if not all, of the processes involved in language and cognition were largely localized in the left (dominant) hemisphere. That guess, which was not a bad one given the dramatic and deleterious effects of a left lateral lesion, allowed people to conclude that little of importance went on in the right hemisphere of man. This rather pure, simple view of the neurological organization underlying behavior began to fall apart when clinical studies showed that deficits of a dramatic nature were produced by right-sided lesions, and that these were different in kind and magnitude from similarly occurring lesions on the left (see Milner, 1971).

A long series of experiments aiming at a neuropsychological analysis of fully commissurotomized patients,

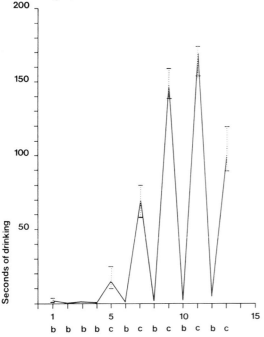

Consecutive days

FIGURE 3.5 Rats with lateral hypothalamic lesions will not drink on baseline (b) days when free access to drinking and running is allowed. They will run, however, and when the two behaviors are made contingent (c), drinking immediately commences. When the contingency is removed, drinking behavior again returns to a low level. From Gazzaniga et al. (1974).

begun some 13 years ago by Roger Sperry and myself on the Bogen (1969) series of patients, has shown that the right hemisphere in man is a nearly equal partner in most of the cognitive activities of everyday experience (Gazzaniga, Bogen, and Sperry, 1962, 1963, 1965; Gazzaniga and Sperry, 1967; Gazzaniga, 1970, 1972). In addition, there have been hints that it is specifically organized to do particular kinds of cognitive tests. Many of the insights gained here have now been brought into the experimental psychologist's laboratory; experiments have been designed to test their validity on the normal population using lateralized projection techniques and reaction time. There has been an explosion of activity in this area—so much so that one can only hope to keep straight the activities of his own lab. I should like, therefore, to report on a recent experiment that John Seamon and I have performed.

Seamon had discovered that when a subject is given an instruction to encode information in terms of an image (as opposed to a verbal-rehearsal instruction), the well-known Sternberg (1966) effect, in which the reaction time to a probe stimulus increases as a function of the number of items in the memory set, is eliminated (Seamon, 1972). For example, if a subject is instructed to rehearse one word verbally, it takes a certain amount of time to respond to a subsequent probe stimulus (a query as to whether the "probe" is a member of the memory set). If two words are given to the subject to rehearse verbally, it takes a bit longer to respond to the probe, and with three, still longer, and so on. If, on the other hand, the instructions are to take the one, two, or three words and put them into an image, Seamon found that the time required to find out whether the probe was a member of the memory set did not vary with the number of words in the set. When this test was applied in a hemisphere-specialization design, it was discovered that the right hemisphere is the system of choice and appears to be the brain site responsible for processing images (Figure 3.6).

These data would suggest that a callosum-sectioned patient might have problems making images in the manner just described. In some preliminary studies Sally Springer and I tested this possibility, using a modification of a test of Gordon Bower (1970) in which simple word pairs are presented. While a partially sectioned patient had no problems in making images to assist him in overall recall, a completely sectioned patient complained about his striking inability to make such images when requested to do so. Interestingly, though, when given the words "cat" and "car," the patient shot back with "jaguar." At the same time this patient was unable to form a picture of say, a cat in or on a car. It would seem that one can make clever inferences or associations

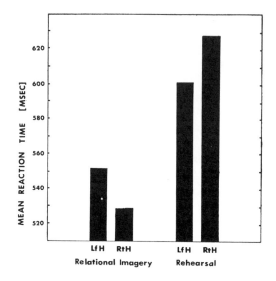

FIGURE 3.6 The brain area that is active in the encoding and retrieval of information is easily manipulated as a function of encoding instructions. When verbal rehearsal is the set, the left hemisphere is superior, whereas instructions to the subject to "remember" by forming images of the words in the memory set finds the right hemisphere superior. From Seamon and Gazzaniga (1973).

from words and yet not have them relate to imagery mechanism.

Encouraged by these results, I find myself more willing to interpret some anecdotal stories based on my observations of many of Bogen's and Wilson's patients. For instance, remembering what to buy at the store caused problems for N.G. This sort of problem makes sense when viewed in this light, because if there is one obvious use for imagery mechanism, it is to aid a person in remembering what to buy at the market. Also, it would seem likely that imagery is a powerful component of sexual arousal. There are in this regard reports that split-brain patients masturbate more frequently postoperatively. It is as if the right hemisphere, now no longer checked by the verbal self-control mechanisms of the left, feels free to initiate sexual activity more frequently. It is still too soon to say for sure whether these are real phenomena. If they do prove to be real, it would be fascinating to see whether there is a progressive change in attitudes about sex as a consequence of the left half-brain having to come to grips with overt behavior precipitated from the free-wheeling right. In other words, in order to reduce dissonance about the overt sexual behavior initiated by the right half-brain, will the left hemisphere change its values about the behavior in question? (See Festinger, 1957.)

These kinds of observations, along with others which have shown, surprisingly, that it is the right hemisphere that recognizes whether a group of letters is a word or not

(Gibson, Dimond, and Gazzaniga, 1972), leads one to the quick conclusion that there are mechanisms all over the cerebrum involved in the normal processing of our cognitive activities with respect to language, thought, and action. The question is, what does this augur for memory processes? Let me make my point, which is that aspects of one experience are differentially located in the brain, by describing a recent clinical case that had a truly dramatic course.

The patient was a 62-year-old male surgeon with no known neurological disorders prior to a transitory stroke. He was right-handed with left-hemisphere dominance for speech and language. He was intelligent, curious, and extremely positive about every aspect of the human condition. Accordingly, through all stages of the stroke he was making every effort, using every faculty available to him, in trying to engage the environment.

On a Thursday evening following dinner, the patient complained of an excruciating headache followed by dizziness and vomiting. The following morning he was taken to the hospital, where it was immediately diagnosed that a stroke had occurred. During the subsequent 72 hours his speech and language facilities were disturbed, but there were no gross signs of paralysis or somatic sensory loss. There was a right homonymous hemianopsia. On Sunday morning his condition had deteriorated considerably and edema had set in. Steroids were administered and maintained for 48 hours. On the following Monday the situation looked better, and during the following two weeks a truly remarkable recovery occurred. Thus, within a 14-day period a patient went from normal cognitive functioning into a state that totally disrupted these processes and back again to normal functioning. The observations that I would like to report here have to do with the course of recovery commencing five days after the onset of the stroke. It is the reconstruction of his cognitive and memory mechanisms that is of interest.

The main observations to be reported here suggest that memory or engrams for things or events are multiply represented in the brain because the experiences themselves have multiple aspects. Thus, for example, when a red carnation was held up in full view and the patient was asked what it was, he said, "flower." When asked what color, he said "red." But when the patient was asked what kind of flower, he was unable to say "carnation." Indeed, even when a list of names of familiar flowers was read aloud, he was still unable to make the match. This was true despite the fact that the patient's most active hobby was gardening. When the examiner finally said it was a carnation, the patient said the word aloud and accepted the assertion with equanimity. Then, spontaneously, the patient reached for the carnation, put

it in his lapel, and smiled his satisfaction. On the following day, when the edema had subsided even more, thus making active more extensive brain areas, the patient was able to name all the flowers in the room (there was quite an assortment) with little or no difficulty.

At the same time in the recovery period, the patient asked about some flowers he and his daughter had planted "down by the road at the bottom of the hill." "What was that?" he asked. When the answer was given as Gazania, a plant commonly known to him normally, he said, "Oh, Gazania." Again, it seems that the category of names given to plants or flowers was not yet available for recall or recognition.

In general these observations are consistent with the view that memory is multiply represented in the brain, not in the sense that a particular engram associated with a particular experience is multiply represented, but that a particular experience has multiple aspects to it and these are stored at a variety of sites in the cerebrum. The prediction from such a model would be that when recall of an experience takes place in the presence of new brain damage, there may be a breakdown in recalling all aspects of the experience. In the present case, because of the transitory "turning off," as it were, of local neural processes, specific aspects of the past experience were not available to the subject. Clearly, normal experience has a "what" and "where" aspect to it. Something happens at a certain place and time. In the flower case above, the patient could remember "where" on the lot a plant had been planted but could not tell you "what" until the part of the brain that stored "what" information had returned to normal functioning.

It is worth recalling in this regard the earlier work of Penfield (as summarized, for example, in Penfield and Roberts, 1959). The dramatic, though highly infrequent, responses produced by cortical stimulation of conscious patients, in which whole experiences were reported, must, of course, reflect the fact that the surgeon has successfully tapped into a neural network linking together the entire ensemble of events.

It is also worth noting the considerable mass of psychological data revealing that, within a given class or "memory network," there are distinct differences in retrieval time for "calling up" related elements (Collins and Quillian, 1969). This suggests to me that such information is located in spatially separate points in the brain.

3.5 MULTIPLE NEURAL CODING

Another frequent assumption in the study of memory is that information is stored in only one fashion. There is *a* brain mechanism for the storage of information, and this same mechanism is used in all storage processes.

We have been for some time now running a variation of the traditional carotid amytal test in an effort to understand some of the cerebral aspects of memory storage (Figure 3.7). In brief, what we do is test how the brain stores information when the language and speech system has been put to sleep through the unilateral injection of sodium amytal in the left carotid artery. These tests are only carried out when angiography is prescribed and in left-brain-damaged patients who suffer no language or speech disturbance.

Prior to the injection of the amytal, an object is placed in the left hand without the person seeing it, and he is required to name it. A correct response here shows that the stereognostic information from the left hand is taking its normal course up to the right hemisphere and then over to the left language and speech center via the corpus callosum. Subsequently, when amytal is injected, the entire right half of the body becomes flaccid, and the left hemisphere becomes unconscious and stops functioning. In this state the patient is given another object to be palpated with the left hand. After a 30-second exploration of the object, it is removed and the patient is allowed to wake up; this occurs one to two minutes later. The patient is then asked what was placed in the left hand, and the typical response is that he does not know. The patient continues to reject all knowledge of the object when pressed by the examiner. However, if a board with a variety of objects pinned to it is held up, it is discovered that the patient can easily point to the appropriate object.

What we think is occurring here is that information stored in the absence of the language and speech system is not necessarily available to that system when it returns to normal functioning. It is as if the information is stored in neural code X whereas the normal neural code of language and speech is Y, the two being mutually exclusive.

It is precisely this kind of result that leads us to speculate that in normal man there may well exist a variety of separate memory banks, each inherently coherent, organized, logical and with its own set of values. Yet these memory banks do not communicate with one another inside the brain. The only way to discover the total resources of the organism is to ask the organism to watch itself as it behaves. For example, if memory bank A takes control of the motor apparatus and produces a behavior, it is only subsequent to the event that the other memory-bank systems become aware that such impulses, so to speak, have been stored in the brain.

What is suggested here, then, is that we are beginning to see data indicating that the normal brain is indeed

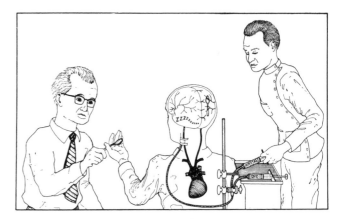

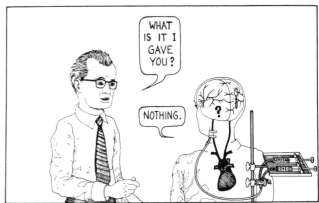

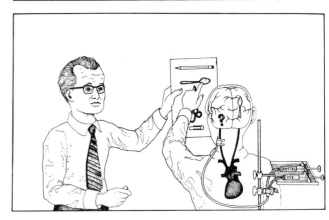

FIGURE 3.7 A picture sequence depicting methods used in amytal testing. First, amytal is administered, subsequent to angiography, into the left hemisphere, thereby anesthetizing the language and speech systems. A spoon is then placed in the left hand, and the right hemisphere takes note. When the left hemisphere regains consciousness, the subject, asked what was placed in his left hand, says "nothing." Finally, it is seen that the right hemisphere can direct the left hand to make the appropriate response in a matching-to-sample task.

split into many domains. What can be done surgically is only an exaggerated instance of a more general phenomenon, a phenomenon that may prove to be a key to a viable model of mind. For present purposes, however, suffice it to say that there is good reason to believe that there is no unitary mechanism responsible for the encoding of information in the brain and that all the information in the brain is not mutually accessible. If this is true, of course, the task of the neuroscientist is slightly more complex than has been supposed, if that is possible. We may be faced with the fact that memory storage, encoding, and decoding is a multifaceted process carried out in different ways in different areas of the brain.

3.6 SUMMARY

In the foregoing I have tried to bring together some of the split-brain and clinical data that bear on the problem of the cerebral basis of information storage. My interpretation of the general imperatives from this field is that we must be very concerned with specificity in the neural system—with the idea that the system is discrete rather than probabilistic, and that it is terribly sensitive to destruction, disconnection, or damage. The arguments against this view, coming from classical data such as Lashley's, stem largely from a failure to appreciate fully that experience is multifaceted and, as such, is multiply evoked in many ways and places in the brain.

REFERENCES

BERLUCCHI, G. 1972. Anatomical and physiological aspects of visual functions of corpus callosum. *Brain Research* 37: 371–392.

BOGEN, J. 1969. The other side of the brain. *Bulletin of the Los Angeles Neurological Society* 34: 73–105, 135–162.

BOWER, G. H. 1970. Imagery as a relational organizer in associative learning. *Journal of Verbal Learning and Verbal Behavior* 9: 529–533.

COLLINS, A., and QUILLIAN, R. 1969. Retrieval time from semantic memory. *Journal of Verbal Learning and Verbal Behavior* 8: 240.

FESTINGER, L. 1957. *A Theory of Cognitive Dissonance*. Stanford, Calif.: Stanford University Press.

GAZZANIGA, M. S. 1970. *The Bisected Brain*. New York: Appleton-Century-Crofts.

GAZZANIGA, M. S. 1972. One brain—two minds? *American Scientist* 60: 311–317.

GAZZANIGA, M. S. 1973a. Discrimination learning without reward. *Physiology and Behavior* 11: 121–123.

GAZZANIGA, M. S. 1973b. Brain theory and minimal brain dysfunction. *Annals of the New York Academy of Sciences* 205: 89–92.

GAZZANIGA, M. S. 1974. Partial commissurotomy and cerebral localization. In K. Zulch, ed., *Cerebral Localization*. New York: Springer-Verlag.

GAZZANIGA, M. S., BOGEN, J. E., and SPERRY, R. W. 1962. Some functional effects of sectioning the cerebral commissures in man. *Proceedings of the National Academy of Sciences* 48: 1765–1769.

GAZZANIGA, M. S., BOGEN, J. E., and SPERRY, R. W. 1963. Laterality effects in somesthesis following cerebral commissurotomy in man. *Neuropsychologia* 1: 209–215.

GAZZANIGA, M. S., BOGEN, J. E., and SPERRY, R. W. 1965. Observations on visual perception after disconnection of the cerebral hemisphere in man. *Brain* 88: 221.

GAZZANIGA, M. S., and FREEDMAN, H. 1973. Observations on visual processes after posterior callosal section. *Neurology* 23: 1126–1130.

GAZZANIGA, M. S., RISSE, G. L., SPRINGER, S. P., CLARK, E., and WILSON, D. H. 1975. Psychological and neurological consequences of partial and complete cerebral commissurotomy. *Neurology* 25: 10–15.

GAZZANIGA, M. S., and SPERRY, R. W. 1967. Language after section of the cerebral commissures. *Brain* 90: 131–148.

GAZZANIGA, M. S., and WILSON, D. H. 1975. Neuropsychological observations following complete and partial commissurotomy. *Neurology* (in press).

GAZZANIGA, M. S., and YOUNG, E. D. 1967. Effects of commissurotomy on the processing of increasing visual information. *Experimental Brain Research* 3: 368–371.

GIBSON, A. R. 1972. Independence of cortico-hypothalamic feeding mechanisms in brain bisected monkeys. Unpublished Ph.D. dissertation, New York University.

GIBSON, A. R., DIMOND, S. J., and GAZZANIGA, M. S. 1972. Left field superiority for word matching. *Neuropsychologia* 10: 463–466.

GIBSON, A. R., and GAZZANIGA, M. S. 1971. Hemisphere differences in eating behavior in split-brain monkeys. *The Physiologist* 14: 150.

HEBB, D. O. 1942. The effect of early and late brain injury on test scores and the nature of normal adult intelligence. *Proceedings of the American Philosophical Society* 85: 275–292.

JOHNSON, J. D., and GAZZANIGA, M.S. 1970. Interhemispheric imitation in split brain monkeys. *Experimental Neurology* 27: 206–212.

JOHNSON, J. D., and GAZZANIGA, M. S. 1971. Some effects of nonreinforcement in split-brain monkeys. *Physiological Behavior* 6: 703–706.

LASHLEY, K. 1950. In search of the engram. *Symposia of the Society for Experimental Biology* 4: 454–482.

MILNER, B. 1971. Interhemispheric differences in the localization of psychological processes in man. *British Medical Bulletin* 27: 272–277.

MILNER, B. 1974. Double écoute et fonctions mnésiques chez les sujects à cerveau dédoublé. Paper read at the Lyon Symposium, "Les Syndromes de Disconnexion Calleuse Chez L'Homme."

MILNER, B., and TAYLOR, L. 1972. Right hemisphere superiority in tactile pattern recognition after cerebral commissurotomy: Evidence for non-verbal memory. *Neuropsychologia* 10: 1–17.

MYERS, R. E., and SPERRY, R. W. 1953. Interocular transfer of a visual form discrimination habit in cats after section of the optic chiasm and corpus callosum. *Anatomical Record* 175: 351–352.

NAKAMURA, R. K. 1975. Cerebral information processing in

split-brain monkeys: One vs. two hemispheres. Unpublished Ph.D. thesis, State University of New York at Story Book.

NAKAMURA, R. K., and GAZZANIGA, M. S. 1974. Reduced information processing capabilities following commissurotomy in the monkey. *The Physiologist* 17: 294–295.

NAKAMURA, R. K., and GAZZANIGA, M. S. 1975. Comparative aspects of short-term memory mechanisms. In J. A. Deutsch and D. Deutsch, eds., *Short-Term Memory*. New York: Academic Press.

PENFIELD, W., and ROBERTS, L. 1959. *Speech and Brain-Mechanisms*. Princeton, N. J.: Princeton University Press.

PREMACK, D. 1966. Reinforcement theory. *Nebraska Symposium on Motivation* 13: 129–148.

SEAMON, J. G. 1972. Imagery codes and human information retrieval. *Journal of Experimental Psychology* 96: 468–470.

SEAMON, J. G., and GAZZANIGA, M. S. 1973. Coding strategies and cerebral lateralizing effects. *Cognitive Psychology* 5: 249–256.

SECHZER, J. A. 1970. Prolonged learning in split-brain cats. *Science* 169: 889–892.

STERNBERG, S. 1966. High-speed scanning in human memory. *Science* 153: 652–654.

TREVARTHEN, C. B. 1962. Double visual learning in split-brain monkeys. *Science* 136: 258–259.

ZAIDEL, D., and SPERRY, R. W. 1974. Memory impairment after commissurotomy in man. *Brain* 97: 263–272.

4

The Amnesic Syndromes and the Encoding Process

J.-L. SIGNORET AND F. LHERMITTE

ABSTRACT An event may produce different kinds of memory traces or engrams; its translation into an internal memory representation defines the encoding process. This process is the result of a strategy by which one selects the salient components of the item to be remembered and thus transforms the item into traces which can be stored. Frontal lesions in man prevent him from taking the initiative in choosing the correct strategy for a given situation. The encoding process involves distinct cerebral areas, depending upon the type of stimulus: thus left temporal lobectomy impairs the learning and retention of verbal material; right temporal lobectomy impairs the memorization of visual or auditory patterns. The roles of the neocortex and the hippocampus are discussed, and the disturbance of verbal learning in split-brain patients is considered.

There are two main encoding processes, verbal and visual, and of these verbal encoding is more disturbed in amnesic syndromes. The functional prevalence of verbal encoding in human memory leads us to ask if each hippocampus is equipotential. The troubles of memory after infarction in the territory of the left posterior cerebral artery, which supplies mesial temporal structures, confirm the functional importance of the left hippocampus. This importance lies in the links existing between the left hippocampus and the neocortex areas on which language is dependent. Unilateral convulsive therapy in man seems to yield evidence in favor of this interpretation.

Any event contains many different aspects. For example, a photograph of a man and a woman in a restaurant is a simple visual image, yet it may be "translated" into a verbal message, or evoke smells, or even bring about a feeling of desire. This multidimensionality of events causes them to produce different kinds of memory traces (engrams) which will be located at a variety of sites in the brain (this is a necessary consequence of the specificity of the cerebral cortex).

This argument, even if oversimplified, leads us to consider two problems in the light of pathology:

1. The analysis and memorization of the different aspects of an event depends upon the subject. It is also a question of information processing, which rests in turn upon an encoding system (which may, for example, be verbal or visual). What are the roles of the various cerebral regions in the encoding process?

2. In particular, does there exist a functional specificity in the role of the hippocampal-mammillary system?

J.-L. SIGNORET and F. LHERMITTE, Neurologie et Neuropsychologie, I.N.S.E.R.M. U84, Hôpital de la Salpêtrière, Paris, France

4.1 THE ENCODING PROCESS

Information processing is a necessity. The problem before us now is to examine the nature of the memory traces produced by events. "How events in the external world are to be translated into the internal memory representation" is indeed the problem we have to consider, and this is how Anderson and Bower (1973) have defined the encoding process.

All information has physical properties, that is to say, is engendered by particular kinds of material stimuli (visual, verbal, tactile, etc.). Of the four uses of the encoding concept noted by Bower (1972), we shall, to simplify matters, bear two in mind: (1) selection by the subject of components of a complex stimulus pattern; and (2) elaboration by the subject, after stimulation, of "associated operators" that qualitatively transform the item to be remembered. Moreover, of these associated operators, we shall consider only those that are visual (mental imagery) or verbal. Present evidence suggests the following characteristics for the encoding process:

1. It is the result of a strategy that is under the control of the subject. This strategy selects the components of the stimulus and chooses associated operators.

2. It involves specific functional cerebral areas, depending on the nature of the stimulus material.

It may now be asked if cerebral lesions in man are capable of interfering with the encoding process, thereby causing a deficiency in memory traces.

4.1.1. The encoding process as a strategy

The role of the frontal lobes in the choice and initiation of strategies is well established (Luria, 1973). We raised the question in our preceding discussion (Lhermitte and Signoret, this volume) when talking about information processing, but it is of course arbitrary to distinguish between information processing and the encoding process. We shall here take "encoding" to mean simply the recording and translation of material stimuli and "information processing" to mean operations that the subject is able to perform upon these recorded or translated elements. A subject who finds it impossible to initiate a strategy of encoding has undergone a memory disturbance.

We have been able to show such a disturbance in two patients with frontal vascular lesions. These patients did not show any major intellectual deficiency; they complained about their memories, but it was not a question of an amnesic syndrome since everyday events were retained. However, the subjects were unable to learn verbal paired associates, that is, to learn six concrete word pairs. In this test each list of six pairs was read at a rate of one pair every ten seconds, and presentation of a list was always followed immediately by a cued recall (i.e., the first word of each pair was read to the subject and he was required to respond with the second word of the pair). The response on the cued recall was not corrected if it was wrong. There were five presentations and five recalls, and a different order was used on each trial and each recall. This task was easy for control subjects (26 correct responses out of 30).

Taking our inspiration from the research of Bower and Winzenz (1970) and of Jones (1974), we then made use of "associative mediators," which may be considered factors in an encoding process. At first, a new list of six pairs of concrete words was read, but for each pair a sentence connecting the two words together was also given by the examiner (e.g., with the pair "beggar-cupboard": "the beggar carries the cupboard"). With the help of associative mediators, performance was much improved, and retesting after a ten-minute delay showed that the verbal associations had been maintained. Then, with a new list, each subject was asked to create his own sentences connecting the word pairs. Improvement was also apparent under this condition.

At a second stage we used two new lists. First, the patient was shown a picture containing the two items of each word pair in interaction (e.g., for the pair "umbrella-bottle" we had an umbrella in a bottle, as in Figure 4.1). Then, for the second list we asked the subject to imagine his own picture connecting the word pairs. As with the sentences, performance was improved;

FIGURE 4.1 A visual mediator used for the verbal pair "umbrella-bottle." (The images are shown as interacting.)

in fact, the number of correct responses was close to that obtained by control subjects in a standard situation (Figure 4.2). The patients were thus capable of creating an adequate encoding strategy if the examiner supplied the model. In contrast to these frontal patients, though, associative mediators had no practical effect on the performance of one amnesic subject with hippocampal lesions.

The data clearly show that the patients with frontal lesions retain the ability to construct and constitute memory traces; their lesions, which are probably bilateral and exist chiefly on the internal face (due to surgical treatment of a rupture of an aneurism in the anterior communicating artery), somehow prevent them from taking the initiative in choosing the right strategy. However, their performances when a verbal or visual model has been given indicate that their encoding processes may, in fact, be unimpaired. We shall see that certain focal lesions produce differing results. In this regard, pathology confirms the observations of Bower and Winzenz (1970) with normal subjects: facility is found to be greater with imagery than with sentences.

4.1.2 The encoding process and the particular kind of stimulus material: Material-specific memory changes

The encoding process involves distinct cerebral areas depending upon the nature of the stimulus. Much research over the last twenty years has been devoted to the study of material-specific memory loss in man (for a review see Beauvois, 1973). We can summarize this research as follows: (1) Left temporal lobectomy in the dominant hemisphere for speech impairs the learning and retention of verbal material (Meyer and Yates, 1955; Milner, 1958; Blakemore and Falconer, 1967). This impairment is selective: memory for visual patterns, faces, and melodies is not affected. (2) Conversely, right temporal lobectomy impairs the memory of visual patterns (Kimura, 1963; Warrington and James, 1967; Milner, 1968) and auditory patterns (Shankweiler, 1966), and it retards the learning of a stylus maze, whether visually or proprioceptively guided (Corkin, 1965; Milner, 1965), whereas left temporal lobectomy does not. Thus there is a double dissociation between the effects of these two lesions. These data confirm the interhemispheric functional difference that is clearly demonstrated in the split brain. Nevertheless, the interpretation of the data poses a certain number of problems.

The recording of an event (Penfield and Milner, 1958) and the retention of recent memory traces (Stepien and Sierpinski, 1960) would both appear to depend on cortical areas situated in the immediate proximity of the sensory-projection zones. Recording and retention both

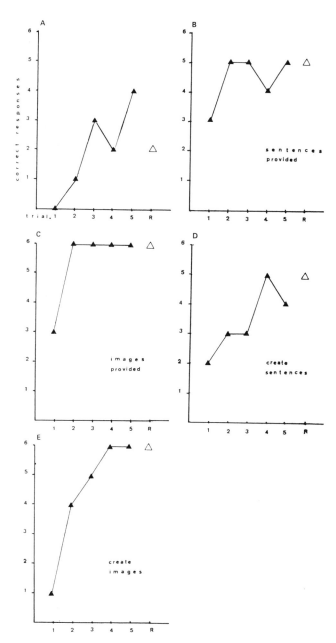

FIGURE 4.2 Curves of verbal paired-associate learning for a patient with frontal lesions. Delayed-recall score is shown by a triangle above R in each graph. A: control condition, no aids. B: sentences provided by the experimenter. C: images provided by the experimenter. D: sentences created by the subject. E: images created by the subject.

involve the encoding process, as the following five points demonstrate.

1. The encoding process is linked to the activity of perception. In tests of visual memory in particular, one might suspect a perceptual disorder to be at the origin of the memory deficiency. Unfortunately, if such a perceptual disorder exists in patients with lesions of the right hemisphere, we shall not be able to make a clear distinction between its effects and those of the memory deficiency. Warrington and Rabin (1970) have reported, however, that right parietal lesions are the cause of the perceptual disorder, and right temporal lesions the cause of the memory disorder.

Dee and Fontenot (1973) have shown that the dominance of the right hemisphere for the perception of complex figures of low verbal association appears to arise from hemispheric differences in memory rather than from purely perceptual processes. Complex figures were presented in either the left or right visual field; after a variable delay (0, 5, 10, 20 sec) the subject was required to indicate whether or not a new figure was the same as the initial figure. The analysis of the results indicates that the right hemispheric superiority was obtained only at the longer retention intervals.

2. The encoding process may enable the subject to call upon "associated operators" to accomplish contradictory performances. Failure of visual memorization tasks in subjects with left hemispheric lesions is no doubt explained by the fact that the subject cannot make a verbal code out of the visual stimuli (Boller and de Renzi, 1967; de Renzi, 1968; Brewer, 1969).

3. The encoding process may thus be affected in a selective manner by a localized lesion. Indeed, the very good work of Jones (1974) shows that in tasks requiring the learning of paired-associate words, patients with left temporal lobectomy fail, whereas patients with right temporal lobectomy succeed. The breakdown of the encoding process is selective for the verbal operators; in fact, recourse to a picture in which the images evoked by the words are shown as interacting partially compensates for the verbal-memory defect. Compensation also exists if later, with a new list, the subject is asked to create visual images. This fact demonstrates that the encoding process involving visual operators is preserved. On the other hand, patients with an amnesic syndrome following bilateral mesial temporal-lobe lesions derive no benefit from attempting to employ visual images.

4. The effects of the encoding process go beyond short-term memory. For example, the immediate recognition of unfamiliar photographed faces is normal in cases of right temporal lobectomy, but results are poor for recognition after a two-minute period (Milner, 1968).

More peculiar would appear to be the selective impairment of auditory verbal short-term memory described by Warrington, Logue, and Pratt (1971) in the case of lesions in the area of the supramarginal and angular gyri of the left hemisphere—peculiar and selective because auditory verbal long-term memory remained intact. In fact, the verbal encoding process is mainly phonèmic in short-term memory and mainly semantic in long-term memory (Baddeley, 1966). Besides this, and as opposed to patients who have undergone left temporal lobectomy, the subjects were aphasic. The comparison in aphasic patients between immediate repetition on the one hand, and the learning of a series of words on the other, confirms that there are two types of verbal encoding (Beauvois and Lhermitte, 1975).

5. The possibility of normal performance for short-term memory, contrasted with difficulties of retention for a specific kind of material, leads us to consider the role of the hippocampus in the consolidation and preservation of the encoding process. Milner (1965, 1968) has shown that deficiency in maze learning and in the recognition of photographed faces after right temporal lobectomy is proportional to the extent of the hippocampal excision. Corsi (quoted by Milner, 1971) was able to confirm this fact for right and left temporal lobectomy. Similar verbal and nonverbal tasks were employed. Simple tasks were the recall of a group of three consonants and the reproduction of a cross on a line after a short interval occupied with interpolated activity. Subjects were also tested with recurrent sequences made up of digits in the verbal modality and block-tapping in the visuospatial modality. These data must not cause us to neglect the role of the excision of the neocortex in the origin of disturbances in the encoding process. But they must lead us to reconsider the role of the hippocampus, and possibly its functional specificity. Stepien and Sierpinski (1974), studying five cases of recent-memory impairment following unilateral temporal lesions, found only one patient showing selective impairment of verbal recent memory; the lesion in this case concerned only the left hippocampal zone.

4.1.3 The encoding process and the split brain
Professor Milner has been kind enough to allow us to mention here a very recent study whose preliminary results were made known at a 1974 Lyon Symposium on the corpus callosum. Eight patients who had undergone a midline section of the interhemispheric commissures went through the learning task described by Jones (1974), that is, the learning of ten paired associates. The markedly impaired performance of the callosal patients in this straightforward verbal learning task was quite unexpected because these patients could use visual imagery as a mnemonic aid. It is clear then that inter-

hemispheric connections are necessary for efficient learning of a purely verbal task. It would seem to us impossible to attribute this defect to a specific material memory change; it is also difficult to say whether it is a question of a strategy defect that may be due to a disconnection of the two frontal lobes. What is important to note is the necessary functioning of both hemispheres together to effect verbal learning.

4.2 FUNCTIONAL SPECIFICITY AND THE HIPPOCAMPAL-MAMMILLARY SYSTEM

In man, it is impossible to analyze memory activity without, at some time or other, considering the relationship that exists between memory and language. The psychological interpretations that have led to the concept of semantic memory (Kintsch, 1972; Tulving, 1972) give us the most complete model to date. At the same time the importance of imagery in cognitive activities (Segal, 1971) has led to an emphasis upon the role of such imagery in the course of certain types of memory activity (Paivio, 1969). These two encoding processes, verbal and visual, thus complement rather than oppose each other. It would appear to us remarkable that psychological research should find a dichotomy which must be closely linked to the knowledge that the split brain has given us about the functional specificity of the hemispheres.

One may now wonder if, in amnesic syndromes, one of the two encoding processes is more disturbed than the other. After considering this problem, we shall take up the question of whether there is a dominance in the left hippocampal-mammillary system, and this will lead to a study of the data arising from unilateral electroconvulsive therapy.

4.2.1 The encoding process and amnesic syndromes
Baddeley and Warrington (1973) studied "memory coding" in amnesic syndromes by comparing the free recall of lists of unrelated control words with the recall of lists of words grouped together on the basis of phonemic similarity, taxonomic-category membership, or a composite visual image. There was no advantage from visual-imagery coding (see also Jones, 1974), but there was an advantage from both phonemic similarity and taxonomic-category grouping. Conversely, Cermak and Butters (1972) have found that, as opposed to control subjects, in whom memory performance was improved when encoding cues were provided, amnesic patients showed a decline in retention upon the use of such cues in the recall of eight words (two words from each of four different categories). These results suggest a failure to encode new

information verbally. In a later paper Cermak, Butters, and Gerrein (1973) gave reasons for this failure: amnesic patients spontaneously prefer to rely upon acoustic rote encoding, and they show an inability to employ semantic encoding strategies. In particular, there is a severe memory deficiency when verbal materials are used, and there is no deficiency for nonverbal memory tasks employing the visual, auditory, and tactile modalities of short-term memory (Butters et al., 1973). It must also be noted that in persistent anterograde amnesia after a stab wound in the basal brain, verbal material was more affected than nonverbal (Teuber, Milner, and Vaughan, 1968). Failure to use verbal encoding was fully studied in the patient H.M. (Sidman, Stoddard, and Mohr, 1968); with verbal material the delayed matching-to-sample performance of the patient was unimpaired up to 40 seconds; with nonverbal material there was failure after periods of 24 to 32 seconds. Sidman, Stoddard, and Mohr relate this to the fact that the patient cannot "devise his own verbal encoding," which normally plays an important role in extending the immediate-memory span.

This failure to use verbal encoding cannot by itself explain forgetfulness. It is, moreover, possible that this disorder, which appears to be selective, is only the result of the functional prevalence of verbal encoding in normal memory activity. In a task of delayed matching of tactile patterns, patients with cerebral commissurotomy demonstrate left-hand performances superior to right. As Milner and Taylor (1972) noted, "The fact that the non-speaking right hemisphere could bridge intratrial intervals of at least two minutes, whereas the left hemisphere could not, shows that verbal coding is neither necessary nor sufficient for the retention of complex perceptual material." Similarly, we may remark that the selected motor skills (rotary pursuit, bimanual tracking, tapping) whose acquisition was found intact in the patient H.M. (Corkin, 1965), are tasks which do not necessitate verbal encoding.

4.2.2 Is there a "dominance" in the hippocampal-mammillary system?

The functional prevalence of verbal encoding, the consequence of the many types of links (phonemic, syntactic, semantic) that language makes possible, leads us to ask if each hippocampal-mammillary system in man is equipotential. The existence of an amnesic syndrome after unilateral temporal lobectomy is now generally interpreted as involving damage to the opposite temporal lobe (Penfield and Milner, 1958). It is agreed that an amnesic syndrome may come about after right temporal lobectomy (Serafetinides and Falconer, 1962: Dimsdale, Logue, and Piercy, 1964) just as after left temporal lobectomy

(Baldwin, 1956; Walker, 1957), but the risk appears to be much greater after the left-side operation (Milner, 1966).

At the same time, troubles of memory appear frequently in the case of infarction in the territory of the left posterior cerebral artery (Mohr et al., 1971; Benson, Marsden, and Meadows, 1974; Signoret and Lhermitte, 1975). The posterior cerebral artery supplies mesial temporal structures (including the hippocampus and hippocampal gyrus) and the temporo-occipital area. During the first weeks after the infarction, there often exists a temporal disorientation regarding remote facts, not just recent ones. This disorder probably reflects a rupture in the functional equilibrium of the right and left hippocampal-mammillary systems, an equilibrium which probably rests upon rich interhippocampal connections. More often than not this disorientation disappears and patients complain of a memory disorder; it is never a question of an amnesic syndrome but, rather, of a difficulty in retaining information. Inner consciousness of the disorder is well established, and rote learning of a text is possible, which is never the case in amnesic syndromes. But this rote learning is difficult. It must be pointed out that a visual-field defect (right hemianopia) is habitually present, and sometimes there is pure alexia too.

We have studied memory performances in six patients with infarction in the territory of the left posterior cerebral artery (Table 4.1). The memory quotient (Wechsler Scale) was always deficient, whereas the intelligence quotient was satisfactory. The learning of paired associate words was particularly deficient, but this deficiency also concerned visual performances, since reproduction of the Rey figure, after the patient had copied it, showed poor memorization. All these patients failed in the following learning task: Six pairs of objects were shown consecutively (e.g., scissors-baby, tree-watch). After this presentation the first object of each pair—the cue—was shown to the subject, and he was required to indicate the right response from among the six response objects, which were now placed before him. If the response was wrong, it was corrected. This procedure made it possible to lessen any difficulty in evocation, as the subject had before him the response repertory. Five trials were made with the same six pairs. Out of these thirty responses, control subjects made a maximum of three mistakes; the average number of mistakes for the six patients was eighteen. Failure in this sort of test, often greater than that of subjects with an amnesic syndrome, has left us puzzled, but a functional hippocampal suppression could account for such a defect in the activation-consolidation process, which normally makes possible the recording of each pair in memory. Difficulty in learning the arrangement of nine pictures (see Lher-

TABLE 4.1
Results of learning tests for patients with infarction of the left cerebral posterior artery

Subjects	Age	I.Q.	M.Q.	Paired objects Errors	Arrangement of nine pictures			
					Trials	Errors	Free recall (24 hr)	Cued recall (24 hr)
Controls				0	1	0	9	9
				3	4	6	6	7
1 Bo	27	113	93	18	20	79	4	6
2 Ja	56	104	96	17	12	44	5	7
3 Le	67	100	77	14	20	58	6	7
4 Fi	68	97	77	19	12	49	5	9
5 Ca	66	120	99	20	13	36	4	6
6 Ba	43	106	74	20	14	53	4	9

Subjects: upper line of Controls gives the best performance, lower line the worst; 1–6 are the patients. I.Q.: score on W.A.I.S. M.Q.: score on Wechsler memory scale. Trials, errors: number of trials and errors for the acquisition. Free (cued) recall: number of exact responses after a 24-hr delay.

mitte and Signoret, this volume) was close to the difficulty observed in amnesic subjects, and this also supports our point of view. Even so, information can be conserved, as is shown in performances of free recall after a delay of 24 hours; this confirms the possibility of learning by rote. But the success in the same tasks obtained by two patients with right mesiotemporal lesions negates this interpretation, unless one accepts a "quantitative" difference between the two hippocampi. A possible disturbance with verbal material only, as described after left temporal lobectomies, would not seem to take account of any memory deficiency with visual material—the Rey figure and the learning of paired objects. One may indeed ask if success in these two tasks does not necessarily involve a verbal encoding process.

Very recently, two new patients with memory disorders following infarction in the territory of the posterior cerebral artery underwent our learning task of six concrete words pairs, with the mediation of sentences and then of pictures. The failure in the initial task was largely reversed when images were provided by the examiner, and moderately reduced when they were created by the subject (these results confirm those of Jones, 1974). By way of contrast, the sentences given by the examiner led to no improvement whatsoever (see Figure 4.3). Thus, in contradiction to data afforded by the two "frontal" patients which led us to conclude that there was a strategy disorder, there would now seem in these "posterior" patients to be a selective disorder in the verbal encoding process. Failure to reproduce from memory the Rey figure, and also to learn the six paired objects, could be explained by the fact that the difficult standard of the tasks compels the subjects to have recourse to a verbal encoding process.

We thus come to the problem of a functional specificity in the hippocampal-mammillary system. It does not appear that lesions in the neocortex have to be linked with lesions of the hippocampus; Ojemann (1971) reports a disorder in nonverbal short-term memory upon stimulation in the region of the right mammillothalamic tract in man. The functional importance of the verbal encoding process in memory activity could, then, take account of the difference in memory capacity observed between right and left hippocampal lesions. But it is certain that this functional difference lies in the links existing between the left hippocampus and the neocortical areas on which language depends.

4.2.3 Unilateral convulsive therapy

Unilateral convulsive therapy in man seems to us to yield evidence in favor of the interpretation just stated. Since the work of Lancaster, Steinert, and Frost (1958), numerous data have confirmed that a series of generalized seizures produced by unilateral electrical stimulation of the nondominant hemisphere does not produce any adverse effect on current-memory performance, while bilateral frontotemporal stimulation impairs both immediate reproduction and delayed reproduction (Martin et al., 1965; Canicott and Waggoner, 1967; d'Elia, 1970). A disturbance concerned uniquely with verbal memory after dominant-side electrode placement (Fleminger et al., 1970) confirms hemispheric functional specificity, but raises as well the problem that the verbal encoding process has to take account of certain anterograde memory disorders observed after bilateral electroconvulsive therapy (Williams, 1973). In the same way, verbal learning carried out 24 hours before treatment is started is more easily forgotten after either bilateral electroconvulsive therapy or dominant unilateral convulsive therapy than after nondominant unilateral convulsive therapy. It is true, of course, that precise neurophysiological repercussions from electroconvulsive

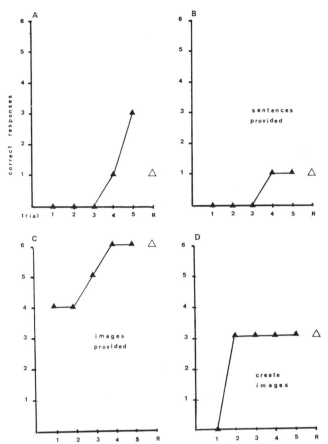

FIGURE 4.3 Curves of verbal paired-associate learning for a patient with infarction of the left cerebral artery (occipitotemporal and hippocampal lesions). Delayed-recall score is shown by a triangle above R in each graph. A: control condition. B: sentences provided by the experimenter. C: images provided by the experimenter. D: images created by the subject.

therapy are not well known. The disturbance cannot be limited to the hippocampal system, since the presence of dysphasia, which is possible after right unilateral electro-convulsive therapy in left-handers (Warrington and Pratt, 1973), implicates the neocortical repercussion of the method. But these facts appear to us to confirm the functional preponderance of the dominant "hippocampus-neocortex couple," because the verbal encoding process is fundamental to memory activity in man.

We are indeed conscious of the fact that our interpretations do not rest upon data from animal experimentation. We know what difficulties there are in trying to produce in animals memory disorders similar to those of human pathology by lesions of the hippocampal-mammillary system (Delacour, 1966). It is possible that neuropsychologists studying man are interested in memory activities which are too elaborate; it may also be that animal experimenters are interested in memory activities which are too elementary. Nevertheless it is the

biological knowledge of the latter activities which will eventually allow us to understand memory in man, even if the cerebral functional organization is somewhat different.

REFERENCES

ABRAMS, R., and TAYLOR, M. A. 1973. Anterior bifrontal ECT: A clinical trial. *British Journal of Psychiatry* 122: 587–590.

ANDERSON, J. R., and BOWER, G. H. 1973. *Human Associative Memory*. Washington, D.C.: V. H. Winston & Sons.

BADDELEY, A. D. 1966. The influence of acoustic and semantic similarity on long term memory for word sequences. *Quarterly Journal of Experimental Psychology* 18: 302–309.

BADDELEY, A. D., and WARRINGTON, E. K. 1973. Memory coding and amnesia. *Neuropsychologia* 11: 159–165.

BALDWIN, M. 1956. Modifications psychiques survenant après lobectomie temporale subtotale. *Neurochirurgie* 2: 152–167.

BEAUVOIS, M. F. 1973. Rôle des lésions corticales restreintes dans les déficits mnésiques partiels. *L'Année Psychologique* 73: 273–309.

BEAUVOIS, M. F., and LHERMITTE, F. 1975. Répétition immédiate et apprentissage d'une série de mots chez 30 sujets aphasiques. *Neuropsychologia* 13: 247–251.

BENSON, D. F., MARSDEN, C. D., and MEADOWS, J. C. 1974. The amnesic syndrome of posterior cerebral artery occlusion. *Acta Neurologica Scandinavica* 50: 133–145.

BLAKEMORE, C. B., and FALCONER, M. A. 1967. Long term effects of anterior temporal lobectomy on certain cognitive functions. *Journal of Neurology, Neurosurgery and Psychiatry* 30: 364–367.

BOLLER, F., and DE RENZI, E. 1967. Relationship between visual memory defects and hemispheric locus of lesion. *Neurology* 17: 1052–1058.

BOWER, G. H. 1970. Imagery as a relational organizer in associative learning. *Journal of Verbal Learning and Verbal Behavior* 9: 529–533.

BOWER, G. H. 1972. Stimulus-sampling theory of encoding variability. In A. W. Melton and E. Martin, eds., *Coding Processes in Human Memory*. Washington, D.C.: V. H. Winston & Sons.

BOWER, G. H. and WINZENZ, D. 1970. Comparison of associative learning strategies. *Psychonomic Science* 20: 119–120.

BREWER, W. F. 1969. Visual memory, verbal encoding and hemispheric localisations. *Cortex* 5: 145–151.

BUTTERS, N., LEWIS, R., CERMAK, L. S., and GOODGLASS, H. 1973. Material specific memory deficits in alcoholic Korsakoff patients. *Neuropsychologia* 11: 291–299.

CANICOTT, S. M., and WAGGONER, R. W. 1967. Unilateral and bilateral electroconvulsive therapy. *Archives of General Psychiatry* 16: 229–232.

CERMAK, L. S., and BUTTERS, N. 1972. The role of interference and encoding in the short-term memory deficits of Korsakoff patients. *Neuropsychologia* 10: 89–95.

CERMAK, L. S., BUTTERS, N., and GERREIN, J. 1973. The extent of the verbal encoding ability of Korsakoff patients. *Neuropsychologia* 11: 85–94.

CORKIN, S. 1965. Tactually-guided maze learning in man: Effects of unilateral cortical excisions and bilateral hippocampal lesions. *Neuropsychologia* 3: 339–351.

CORKIN, S. 1968. Acquisition of motor skill after bilateral medial temporal-lobe excision. *Neuropsychologia* 6: 255–265.

DEE, H. L., and FONTENOT, D. J. 1973. Cerebral dominance and lateral differences in perception and memory. *Neuropsychologia* 11: 167–173.

DELACOUR, J. 1966. Rôle de quelques structures cérébrales dans les processus de conditionnement. II. Cortex frontal, noyau caudé, amygdalum. *L'Année Psychologique* 66: 511–534.

D'ELIA, G. 1970. Unilateral electroconvulsive therapy. *Acta Psychiatrica Scandinavica* supp. 215: 5–98.

DE RENZI, E. 1968. Nonverbal memory and hemispheric side of lesion. *Neuropsychologia* 6: 181–189.

DIMSDALE, H., LOGUE, V., and PIERCY, M. 1964. A case of persisting impairment of recent memory following right temporal lobectomy. *Neuropsychologia* 1: 287–298.

DORNBUSH, R., ABRAMS, R., and FINK, M. 1971. Memory changes after unilateral and bilateral convulsive therapy. *British Journal of Psychiatry* 119: 75–78.

FLEMINGER, J. J., HORNE, D. J., HORNE, L., and NOTT, P. N. 1970. Unilateral electroconvulsive therapy and cerebral dominance: Effect of right and left sided electrode placement on verbal memory. *Journal of Neurology, Neurosurgery and Psychiatry* 33: 408–411.

JONES, M. K. 1974. Imagery as a mnemonic aid after left temporal lobectomy: Contrast between material specific and generalized memory disorders. *Neuropsychologia* 12: 21–30.

KIMURA, D. 1963. Right temporal lobe damage. *Archives of Neurology* 8: 264–271.

KINTSCH, W. 1972. Notes on the structure of semantic memory. In E. Tulving and W. Donaldson, eds., *Organization of Memory*. New York: Academic Press.

LANCASTER, N. P., STEINERT, R. R., and FROST, I. 1958. Unilateral electroconvulsive therapy. *Journal of Mental Science* 104: 221–227.

LURIA, A. R. 1973. *The Working Brain*. Translated by Basil Haigh. New York: Basic Books.

MARTIN, W. L., FORD, H. F., MACDONALD, E. C., and TOWLER, M. L. 1965. Clinical evaluation of unilateral EST. *American Journal of Psychiatry* 121: 1087–1090.

MEYER, V., and YATES, A. J. 1955. Intellectual changes following temporal lobectomy for psychomotor epilepsy. *Journal of Neurology, Neurosurgery and Psychiatry* 18: 44–55.

MILNER, B. 1958. Psychological defects produced by temporal lobe excision. *Research Publications of the Association for Research in Nervous and Mental Diseases* 36: 244–257.

MILNER, B. 1965. Visually-guided maze learning in man: Effects of bilateral hippocampal, bilateral frontal, and unilateral cerebral lesions. *Neuropsychologia* 3: 317–338.

MILNER, B. 1966. Amnesia following operation on the temporal lobes. In C. W. N. Whitty and O. L. Zangwill, eds., *Amnesia*. London: Butterworth & Co.

MILNER, B. 1968. Visual recognition and recall after right temporal lobe excision in man. *Neuropsychologia* 6: 191–209.

MILNER, B. 1971. Interhemispheric differences in the localization of psychological processes in man. *British Medical Bulletin* 27: 272–277.

MILNER, B. 1974. Verbal paired associate learning after cerebral commissurotomy. Paper read at the Lyon Symposium, "Le Corps Calleux."

MILNER, B., and TAYLOR, L. 1972. Right-hemisphere superiority in tactile pattern recognition after cerebral commissurotomy: Evidence for non-verbal memory. *Neuropsychologia* 10: 1–15.

MOHR, J. P., LEICESTER, J., STODDARD, L. T., and SIDMAN, M. 1971. Right hemianopia with memory and color deficits in circumscribed left posterior cerebral artery territory infarction. *Neurology* 21: 1104–1113.

OJEMANN, G. A. 1971. Alteration in non-verbal STM with stimulation in the region of the mammillo-thalamic tract in man. *Neuropsychologia* 9: 195–201.

PAIVIO, A. 1969. Mental imagery in associative learning and memory. *Psychological Review* 76: 241–263.

PENFIELD, W., and MILNER, B. 1958. Memory deficit produced by bilateral lesions in the hippocampal zone. *Archives of Neurology and Psychiatry* 79: 475–497.

PERRET, E., KOHENOF, M., and SIEGRIED, J. 1969. Influence des lésions thalamiques unilatérales sur les fonctions intellectuelles, mnésiques et d'apprentissage des malades parkinsoniens. *Neuropsychologia* 7: 79–88.

REY, A. 1959. *Test de Copie d'une Figure Complexe*. Paris: Editions du Centre de Psychologie Appliquée.

SEGAL, S. J. 1971. *Imagery. Current Cognitive Approaches*. New York: Academic Press.

SERAFETINIDES, E. A., and FALCONER, M. 1962 Some observations of memory impairment after temporal lobectomy for epilepsy. *Journal of Neurology, Neurosurgery and Psychiatry* 25: 251–255.

SHANKWEILER, D. 1966. Effects of temporal lobe damage on perception of dichotically presented melodies. *Journal of Comparative and Physiological Psychology* 62: 115–119.

SIDMAN, M., STODDARD, L. T., and MOHR, J. P. 1968. Some additional quantitative observations of immediate memory in a patient with bilateral hippocampal lesions. *Neuropsychologia* 6: 245–264.

SIGNORET, J.-L., and LHERMITTE, F. 1975. Mémoire et dominance hippocampique. A propos des troubles mnésiques observés au cours des accidents ischémiques dans le territoire de l'artère cérébrale postérieure gauche. *Revue Neurologique (Paris)* 132 (in press).

STEPIEN, L., and SIERPINSKI, S. 1960. The effect of focal lesions of the brain upon auditory and visual recent memory in man. *Journal of Neurology, Neurosurgery and Psychiatry* 23: 334–340.

STEPIEN, L., and SIERPINSKI, S. 1964. Impairment of recent memory after temporal lesions in man. *Neuropsychologia* 2: 291–303.

STONES, M. J. 1973. Electroconvulsive treatment and short-term memory. *British Journal of Psychiatry* 122: 591–594.

SUTHERLAND, E. M., OLIVER, J. E., and KNIGHT, D. R. 1969. EEG, memory and confusion in dominant, non-dominant and bitemporal ECT. *British Journal of Psychiatry* 115: 1059–1064.

TEUBER, H.-L., MILNER, B., and VAUGHAN, Jr., H. G. 1968. Persistent anterograde amnesia after stab wound of the basal brain. *Neuropsychologia* 6: 267–282.

TULVING, E. 1972. Episodic and semantic memory. In E. Tulving and W. Donaldson, eds., *Organization of Memory*. New York: Academic Press.

WALKER, A. E. 1957. Recent memory impairment in unilateral temporal lesions. *Archives of Neurology and Psychiatry* 78: 543–552.

WARRINGTON, E. K., and JAMES, M. 1967. An experimental investigation of facial recognition in patients with unilateral cerebral lesions. *Cortex* 3: 317–326.

WARRINGTON, E. K., LOGUE, V., and PRATT, R. T. C. 1971. The anatomical localisation of selective impairment of auditory verbal short-term memory. *Neuropsychologia* 9: 377–387.

WARRINGTON, E. K., and PRATT, R. T. C. 1973. Language

laterality in left-handers assessed by unilateral ECT. *Neuropsychologia* 11: 423–428.

WARRINGTON, E. K., and RABIN, P. 1970. A preliminary investigation of the relation between visual perception and visual memory. *Cortex* 1: 87–96.

WILLIAMS, M. 1973. Errors in picture recognition after ECT. *Neuropsychologia* 11: 429–436.

ZAMORA, E. M., and KAELBLING, M. D. 1965. Memory and electroconvulsive therapy. *American Journal of Psychiatry* 122: 546–554.

Information Processing
and Memory

5

The Information-Storage System Called "Human Memory"

HERBERT A. SIMON

ABSTRACT The paper undertakes to describe human memory as it looks today to psychologists who approach it from an information-processing point of view. It also undertakes to examine the relation between information processing and physiological accounts of memory.

Memories are characterized by the organization of information stored in them, the times required to store and access information, the durations over which information is retained, the conditions under which it is lost, and the nature of the cues needed to access it. Evidence from standard experimental paradigms supports the existence of two principal memories: one, a short-term memory of very limited capacity but rapid access; the other, a long-term memory requiring five to ten seconds for fixation of each new "chunk." In addition, small, short-duration memories are associated with the various sensory input channels. The long-term memory, in turn, appears to be specialized into one subsystem that is responsible for the organism's capability to recognize familiar patterns, and another that stores semantic information in an associative net.

Various properties of these memories can be inferred from recall experiments and chronometric experiments that measure processing speeds. The ways in which such inferences are drawn are illustrated by discussion of several current experimental and theoretical issues.

The first purpose of this paper is to describe human memory as it looks today to that growing group of psychologists who approach it from an information-processing point of view. A second purpose is to examine the relation between an information-processing account of human memory and a physiological account, and the implications of that relation for the division of labor between information-processing psychologists and physiological psychologists.

In the past five years there has been a great spate of books and articles that review our present knowledge about human memory and propose more or less comprehensive theories of memory organization (e.g., Anderson and Bower, 1973; Hunt, 1971, 1973; Kintsch, 1970; and Rumelhart, Lindsay, and Norman, 1972). No important purpose would be served by going over that ground again, and I shall not undertake to do so. Instead, I shall look at matters primarily from a methodological standpoint and undertake to analyze the

HERBERT A. SIMON, Department of Psychology, Carnegie-Mellon University, Pittsburgh, PA

nature of the inferences that connect theories of memory with data from experiments on memory.

5.1 INFORMATION-PROCESSING AND PHYSIOLOGICAL APPROACHES

There are numerous examples in modern science of the need for multiple explanations of complex phenomena at different levels of fineness of detail. Perhaps the classical example of this kind is found in chemistry. For many purposes, chemical reactions can be described and explained in terms of regroupings of basic units called atoms connected by ionic or covalent bonds, the reactions being accompanied by absorption or release of certain quantities of energy. With each type of atom is associated a number, its valence; and the admissibility of molecular structures is governed by rules on the valences. A body of theory erected on this basis served chemistry through the nineteenth century and well into the twentieth, and still provides the first approximation to the description of chemical processes.

By 1916 G. N. Lewis and a number of his predecessors had found a bridge, the modern electronic theory of valence, between the empirically postulated valence numbers of the chemist and the emerging physical theory of the atom. That bridge was based on the idea of stable electron shells (for ionic bonds) and the sharing of electrons between atoms (for covalent bonds). Almost immediately after the invention of quantum mechanics in 1926, the reduction of the theory of the chemical bond to the underlying physical level was carried very much farther by Condon, Heitler, London, Pauling, and many others. In principle at least, there no longer existed any boundary between physics and chemistry. Any chemical reaction could be explained in terms of an underlying atomic structure and the accompanying quantum-mechanical laws.

In practice, of course, the discovery of the quantum-mechanical explanation of the chemical bond has not made the classical chemical explanations of reactions superfluous. In the first place, the actual quantum-mechanical reduction of chemical phenomena has been carried out for only the simplest cases, and then only on the basis of ingenious approximations. Many of the largest computers in the nation today are laboring to carry out approximate quantum-mechanical analyses of molecules of quite modest size. We believe, of course, that the great mass of chemical systems that have not been analyzed in this way could be—given computers of unlimited power—but that belief is an article of our scientific faith in the uniformity of nature, not an inference from tested facts. Our reductionism remains in-principle reductionism.

In the second place, even if we could actual carry out the quantum-mechanical reduction of all chemical phenomena, we still would not want to dispense with the chemical level of theory. Research in problem solving has shown that the efficiency of problem-solving efforts can often be greatly increased by carrying out the search for a solution, not in the original problem space with all of its cluttering detail, but in an abstracted space, from which much of the detail has been removed, leaving the essential skeleton of the problem more clearly visible. The so-called planning method in problem solving involves just such a process of abstraction. In the same way, a chemist seeking to solve a typical problem of chemical synthesis would be ill-advised to immerse himself in the quantum-mechanical detail of the system before using classical chemical theory to discover one or more promising reaction paths. Thus theory at the chemical level, rather than the more "basic" theory at the physical level, remains the principal conceptual apparatus for most working chemists.

There are physicists who take the doctrine of reductionism so literally that they believe there are no "fundamental" scientific questions except the questions of elementary-particle theory. Most of us, I think, have a quite different picture of the scientific enterprise. We see the natural world as an immensely complex hierarchical system, understandable only by being represented alternatively at many levels of detail, and understood by constructing bodies of theory at each of these levels, in combination with reduction theories that show how the unanalyzed elementary structures at each level can themselves be explained in terms of the constructs available at the next level below. In this world there is need for chemistry as well as physics, biology as well as chemistry, and information-processing psychology as well as physiological psychology. Nor should the necessity for this plurality of levels of theory construction carry any implications for vitalism or mentalism, or bring any aid or comfort to antireductionists.

Information-processing psychology has sometimes been referred to as "the new mental chemistry." The atoms of this mental chemistry are symbols, which are combinable into larger and more complex associational structures called lists and list structures. The fundamental "reactions" of the mental chemistry employ elementary information processes that operate upon symbols and symbol structures: copying symbols, storing symbols, retrieving symbols, inputting and outputting symbols, and comparing symbols. Symbol structures are stored in memories, often classified as short-term and long-term memories, whose properties will be a major topic of this paper.

Symbol structures and elementary information processes are abstract entities in exactly the same sense that the molecules and reactions of classical chemistry are abstract entities. Symbol structures "exist" in exactly the same sense that molecules exist; their presence is postulated in order to explain parsimoniously a whole host of observable phenomena. Thus, the evidence for them is indirect in the same way that the evidence for molecules—at least prior to the invention of the electron microscope—was indirect. We know them by their actions, by the macroscopic phenomena that they produce.

At the same time, all of us, I believe, are committed to the proposition that thinking and other cognitive processes are performed by a biological organ called the brain, in conjunction with the peripheral nervous system and sensory and motor organs. The symbol structures and elementary information processes of information-processing psychology must therefore have their physiological counterparts in subsystems within the central nervous system that function as memory units, and subsystems that are capable of processing these physiologically stored structures. The term "system" is used here rather than "unit" to avoid commitment to any assumption of localism—any notion that each symbol structure that is stored must have its specific storage location in the brain. Nothing in contemporary information-processing theories of memory requires that memories be specifically localized; and nothing in those theories is incompatible with a distributed or even holographic theory of the physiological basis for memory.

There is no reason to suppose that the "mental chemistry" of symbols is any less complex than the chemistry of atoms and molecules. On the contrary, the best information-processing explanations we possess of problem solving and other complex cognitive performances employ intricate organizations, or programs, of information processes to account for the long sequences of events that occur (Newell and Simon, 1972), Hence it is likely that, when we come to have a bridge theory that provides an explanation of information processing in physiological terms, that bridge theory will deal explicitly and in detail only with relatively simple phenomena, handling more complex phenomena only in an "in-principle" sense. Moreover, however adequate the physiological theory turns out to be, we will still need a more aggregative and abstract theory at the information-process level to guide our thinking about the more complex phenomena.

For these reasons, the relation between physiological psychology and information-processing psychology is a complementary relation, not a competitive one. To achieve the kind of explanation of human cognition that we want to and need to have, we shall have to construct an information-processing theory to handle the complex phenomena, a bridge theory to show how the primitive structures and processes of the theory are realized physiologically, and a physiological theory to show what the basic biological and biochemical mechanisms are that implement the physiological functions.

In this scheme of things, there is plenty of work for all, and a very natural, if rough, division of labor between information-processing psychologists and physiological psychologists. Returning again to our physico-chemical analogue, we note that it was the job of the chemist to reduce the phenomena of the test tube and the beaker to rearrangements of molecular structures. It was the job of the physicist to provide physical mechanisms that could explicate "atom" and "chemical bond." Without denying the importance of the bridging theorist—the physical chemist or chemical physicist—it should be apparent that, for the most part, the physicist did not need to concern himself with complex chemical reactions, while the chemist could ignore many of the physical details of the atom. The two disciplines, while contributing in vital ways to each other's work, could specialize with respect both to the phenomena studied and the techniques for studying them.

In psychology today the subdisciplines already exist for implementing an analogous specialization, but in this specialization, it is important that the bridging function not be lost from sight. I welcome a meeting like this as an opportunity to make contact with physiological data and theories that can explain the elementary information structures and processes that theorists on my side of the boundary have postulated in order to explain complex behavior. I hope that this paper may provide to some physiological psychologists a corresponding opportunity to ascertain for what kinds of structures and processes physiological explanations are needed.

Points of contact between information-processing psychology and physiological psychology are becoming increasingly visible. One of these, reviewed at this conference by Pettigrew (see Chapter 18, this volume), concerns the extraction of features from visual stimuli

and their subsequent encoding in the central nervous system. Another, closer to the topic of the present chapter, is the relation between physiological and behavioral approaches to the phenomena of amnesia and aphasia in brain-damaged subjects. This topic, too, is reviewed elsewhere in this volume. As comparison of the relevant chapters reveals, quite similar views of the architecture of human memory are emerging from these complementary approaches.

The point of view I have taken here in my excursion into the philosophy of science is quite orthodox, and it is unlikely to evoke much disagreement or controversy. I have taken the time to present it because I think it is necessary in an interdisciplinary conversation like this one to make our frames of reference and underlying methodological assumptions fully explicit.

For the same reason, it is necessary to make some preliminary remarks about one of the main research tools of information-processing psychology—the digital computer. These remarks are the subject of the next section, at the end of which we can turn to matters of substance.

5.2 THE COMPUTER IN INFORMATION-PROCESSING PSYCHOLOGY

Over the past twenty years the electronic digital computer has played a central role as a research tool in information-processing approaches to cognitive psychology. It has, in fact, had two roles. On the one hand, computer languages have proved to be the most powerful and appropriate languages for stating psychological theories formally. Computer languages have vocabularies and syntaxes specifically designed to describe symbols and symbol structures, elementary information processes and the organizations of those processes called programs. At the same time, whenever a theory is stated in a computer language, the computer becomes available as a powerful tool for predicting the behavior of the system described by the theory, and thereby permitting a comparison of theoretical predictions with empirical data. Most of the theories of memory I shall be discussing either have been, or could rather easily be, expressed formally as computer programs.

In our book *Human Problem Solving* (1972), Allen Newell and I have discussed at some length the methods and problems of stating and testing theories expressed as computer programs. I will not repeat that discussion here, but refer the interested reader to our book. In fact, such differences as exist in the methodology for handling theories expressed in computer languages and theories not so expressed are tactical rather than fundamental.

The issues are the familiar ones of stating the theories in a form that makes them operationally testable, and devising experiments and other forms of observation that permit the predictions of theory to be confronted with empirical facts.

I shall have little to say explicitly in this paper about the computer programs that have been constructed to simulate human memory (e.g., Feigenbaum, 1961; Simon and Feigenbaum, 1964; Gregg and Simon, 1967; Anderson and Bower, 1973). These programs have played an important (and increasing) role in exploring the mechanisms required to account for memory phenomena and in searching out the indirect consequences of hypotheses about memory organization.

5.3 THE STATICS OF MEMORY: THE STORAGE SYSTEM

It is common in psychology today to use the term "memory" in the plural—to speak of "long-term memory," "short-term memory," "iconic memory," "echoic memory," and others. What is the phenomenological basis on which one makes such distinctions? How does one tell that different sets of information are held in different memories, or in the same memory?

Phenomenologically, a memory is characterized and identified by (1) the kinds of inputs that can be stored in it, (2) the time required to store new information in it, (3) the time required to access information previously stored in it, (4) the durations over which information, once stored, is retained, (5) conditions that cause loss of information over a period during which it could otherwise be retained, (6) the qualitative nature of the deterioration of stored information, (7) the nature of the cues needed for accessing stored information, and (8) the form of organization of the stored information.

5.3.1 Some standard experimental paradigms
A brief and simplified description of some standard paradigms for memory experiments will illustrate how the parameters of memory listed above can be used to infer the existence of distinct memories from experimental data. The term "distinct" here does not imply distinct spatial localization but functional specialization.

The stimulus for all of the experiments to be described is a rectangular array of English letters, selected at random and displayed in three rows of four letters each. The stimulus is displayed for 50 msec, and is of such size and intensity that there is no question of visual confusion. In the first experimental paradigm (Immediate-Recall Experiment), the subject is instructed to repeat back the sequence of stimulus letters as soon as he has seen them. Typically, a subject will recall an average of about four to six letters correctly (Simon, 1974).

In the second paradigm (Sperling paradigm), an aural cue is presented shortly after the stimulus, the subject being instructed to repeat back either the upper line of letters, the middle line, or the lower line, depending on whether the cue is a tone of high pitch, intermediate pitch, or low pitch. Performance on this task varies with the interval between exposure of the stimulus and presentation of the cue. If that interval is brief (50 msec, say), performance is nearly perfect; as the interval lengthens to one second or more, performance gradually drops to its level in the immediate-recall experiment— that is, an average of 50 percent or less correct (Sperling, 1960).

The third experimental paradigm (Delayed-Recall Experiment) is like the first, except that a delay is introduced between presentation of the stimulus and the subject's response, and during this delay the subject is instructed to perform some other task (e.g., counting backwards by threes or naming colors). Typically, the delay is some 30 seconds. Performance now depends upon the nature of the intervening task, but many tasks cause the subject's performance to fall to a level of one or two letters correct per trial (Peterson and Peterson, 1959).

In the fourth experimental paradigm (Rote-Verbal-Learning Experiment), the stimulus is exposed for a longer time, or for a number of successive trials—say, for a total exposure of several minutes. After the lapse of some time, during which there may or may not be an explicit intervening task, the subject is instructed to recall the letters. In this experiment, with sufficient redundancy, performance may be nearly perfect for delays up to several hours. Performance varies with a number of variables, including (1) total stimulus exposure time, (2) response delay, and (3) nature of intervening activity (Underwood, 1969). The strategy the subject adopts in attending to different parts of the stimulus, and the priority he assigns to fixation relative to other task activities, also affect the rate of learning (Gregg and Simon, 1967).

5.3.2 Inferences to memory structure
Many more variants can, of course, be built upon these four experimental paradigms, which have been the basis for innumerable studies published in the literature. Instead of looking in detail at these variants on the basic four themes, let us ask what the paradigms tell us about the structure of human memory. All of the inferences are based on a fundamental principle: if a subject is able to recall a stimulus that is no longer present, information about that stimulus must be stored in some memory, and if the subject is later unable to recall the stimulus, some of the stored information must have been lost or altered.

The Sperling paradigm tells us that all twelve letters can be stored for some fraction of a second—at least until the delayed cue is received that permits the perfect response. The experiment also tells us that considerable information is lost from this memory store before a second has elapsed. The immediate-recall experiment tells us that some amount of briefly presented information—but nothing like twelve letters—can be retained for an indefinite number of seconds, but that most of it is lost rapidly if certain kinds of tasks are interposed.

If we put these pieces of evidence together, we are led to one of two conclusions: either there is a single memory with a capacity of at least twelve letters, a very rapid initial forgetting rate, and then a much slower forgetting rate; or there are two memories, the first of which has the larger capacity but the faster forgetting rate. Examination of the nature of the errors of commission that subjects typically make in the immediate-recall and Sperling paradigms, respectively, suggests that the second alternative is more plausible than the first. In the immediate-recall experiment, erroneous responses are likely to be auditorily similar to the corresponding correct responses (Conrad, 1959). In the Sperling paradigm, visual similarity plays a larger role relative to aural similarity, while confusion errors tend to be relatively much less frequent than errors of omission (Sperling, 1960). The error data suggest that the memory involved in the Sperling paradigm contains information about the visual features of the stimulus elements, while the memory involved in the immediate-recall paradigm most often contains information about phoneme features of the corresponding aural letters. Under these circumstances, a recoding process occurs in transferring information from the former to the latter memory, and the two memories must be regarded as distinct.

If we turn now to a comparison of the immediate- or delayed-recall experiments with the rote-verbal-learning experiments, we obtain evidence for the existence of a memory with properties quite different from the other two. The memory produced by a stimulus of relatively long duration is capable of surviving over intervening times and tasks that would cause the loss of storage observed in the delayed-response experiments. Moreover, while there appears to be a rather definite upper limit on the amount of information that can be retained from a brief stimulus exposure, an amount which is not sensitive to the precise duration of the exposure, the amount that can be stored on longer exposure seems to be essentially unlimited—the total varying more or less proportionately with the total exposure time.

Again, the most parsimonious explanation for these phenomena is to postulate two memories: one that can acquire a specified small amount of information quite rapidly but cannot increase that amount or retain it over interrupting activities; and one that can acquire an indefinite amount of information and retain it for an indefinite length of time, even over intervening tasks, but that requires a substantial length of time for the acquisition process to take place.

This brief account sketches the logic and the non-physiological evidence on which are based current widely held beliefs about the main kinds of human memory. If one looks at the recent literature, one discerns, amidst the mass of variant detail, a fair degree of agreement that the human memory system includes distinguishable iconic (sensory), short-term, "intermediate-term," and long-term memories, and even some agreement about the characteristics those memories possess.

5.4. THE PARAMETERS OF MEMORY

Let us look a little more closely at the parameters that define the storage speeds, access speeds, and capacities of the memories we have identified, particularly the short-term and long-term memories. In the case of short-term memory, storage capacity is the parameter of primary interest because storage and retrieval times are very short—a few hundred msec to fill the entire STM, and a second or so to produce its entire contents. Before we can measure its capacity, however, we must have some units of measurement. George Miller (1956) has proposed that the amount of information that can be stored in STM depends upon the familiarity of the information and thus, specifically, upon the number of symbols into which it must be encoded. For example, in an immediate-recall experiment with sequences of random letters, each letter would be encoded as a symbol, or "chunk," since it can be assumed that the subjects are highly familiar with individual letters of the alphabet, but not with random pairs of them. But if the stimuli in the immediate-recall experiment are random sequences of simple words, each word, being familiar to the subject, would constitute a single chunk.

5.4.1 Capacity of short-term memory
Experimental data show that the capacity of STM is reasonably constant—at least to a first approximation—when the amount of information held is measured in chunks (but not at all if it is measured in bits). To test this proposition, of course, one must have some means for determining what the chunks are, and in another paper I have shown how that can be done (Simon, 1974). Short-term memory capacity measured in chunks is probably closer to four, however, than to the number seven originally proposed by Miller.

To find a plausible interpretation of the chunking hypothesis in terms of memory structures, one cannot view the STM in isolation, but must consider its relation to long-term memory. To say that a particular symbol string, say the word "cat," is a familiar chunk is to say that there is already information available in LTM that permits that string to be recognized as a word and its meaning to be retrieved from LTM. Because this information is already stored in LTM, the lexicographical information identifying the string of letters "cat" does not need to be retained in STM; instead, one need retain only a single symbol that serves as a pointer to the relevant information in LTM. Hence what is stored in STM, under the chunking hypothesis, is the set of these pointers, each one assumed to consume just as much STM capacity as each of the others. The chunk, or symbol, stored in STM is the internal representation, in memory, of the recognized familiar stimulus.

This interpretation of the chunking hypothesis carries with it the implication that the familiar stimuli corresponding to chunks are recognized before being stored in STM. As we have just seen, the recognition mechanism is a component of LTM, not STM. Thus STM is not a buffer between the senses and LTM, but is a temporary storage for pointers to LTM that have been produced by the recognition mechanisms of LTM. If the recognition process takes place before information is stored in STM, does it occur before or after the information (if presented visually) has passed through the iconic memory? I do not know of any experiments that cast much light on this question, so I will not speculate upon the answer.

The chunking hypothesis carries no particular implications for the sensory modality of the information to which the STM symbol points. When the visual stimulus "cat" is presented to a subject who reads English, the visual string may be recognized directly, or the letters may be "sounded out," i.e., recognized, and replaced by a phoneme string, which is then recognized as a familiar sound sequence. Either process is consistent with the memory-structure hypothesis, and examples of both processes can be observed in the behavior of beginning readers.

The recognition process may also take place in several stages. For example, recognition of the visual stimulus "cat" can lead to the retrieval of a chunk that points to information in LTM about the aural word "cat." Upon retrieval of this information, its passage through the recognition mechanism again would leave in STM a pointer to the stored semantic information about "cat." The experimental fact (Conrad, 1959) that phonetic similarity of stimuli is more likely to cause confusion errors in STM than visual similarity suggests that the

two-stage recognition process is the more common one for verbal material. Notice that the two-stage process does not imply that the visual stimulus is "sounded out." Rather, visual recognition of the entire word retrieves the cue that points to the phonemic information. The two-stage recognition process might be expected to be the normal one for persons to whom the aural word and its meaning are already familiar at the time they acquire familiarity with its visual counterpart.

5.4.2 Long-term memory fixation and retrieval

Turning now to the parameters of long-term memory, our interest shifts from measures of capacity to measures of storage and retrieval time. Storage capacity is uninteresting because it appears to be unlimited. To be sure, one common symptom of senility is inability or difficulty in storing new information in LTM, but this does not necessarily mean that storage capacity has been exhausted. A simpler and more plausible explanation would attribute this memory deficit to failure of the acquisition mechanism.

In order to talk about the time required to store information in LTM, or to retrieve it, we must again settle upon an appropriate unit of measurement. One candidate is the chunk—the same unit used to measure the capacity of short-term memory. Again, I have recently discussed the empirical basis for this choice in the article referred to earlier (Simon, 1974), and will therefore only sketch the argument very briefly. First, there is now a reasonably convincing body of evidence that the time required to store a given number of nonsense syllables in LTM is proportionate to that number; while, if total exposure time is held constant, the number of exposures of the stimulus is irrelevant. If the time per trial is doubled, the number of trials needed for fixation is roughly halved; while if the time per trial is halved, the number of trials is doubled. Moreover, when the fixation time for familiar words is compared with the fixation time for nonsense syllables, the time per chunk remains nearly constant, while the time per letter or phoneme varies widely. The learning time required to link together two familiar chunks into a new chunk is of the order of five to ten seconds.

Fixation of new information in LTM is a complex process because it involves not only storing the new information in semantic memory, but also elaborating the recognition memory so that the new chunks can be recognized and accessed. Very little is known about the relative amount of time or effort required for these two parts of the fixation process, but there are some slight indications, which will be discussed in the next section, that growing the recognition net is a more time-consuming process than adding chunks to the semantic store.

Probably at least two parameters are involved in defining the time it takes to retrieve information from LTM. On the one hand, a well-learned list (e.g., the alphabet) can be recovered and produced at rates not much slower than 150 msec per item. On the other hand, Dansereau (1969), in studies of mental arithmetic, found that when a subject recovered a partial product in a mental-multiplication task, he might take about two seconds to retrieve the first digit of the number and then some 300 msec for each succeeding digit. Likewise, a number of investigators (e.g., McLean and Gregg, 1967) have found that when a newly fixated list (e.g., the alphabet permuted) is recited, letters are grouped by threes and fours with substantially longer latencies between groups than within groups. All of these data suggest that chunks are stored in LTM in highly structured form, and that while a relatively long time may be required to retrieve the first item in a structure, succeeding items are retrieved more rapidly.

5.4.3 Summary

Chronometric studies of information-processing tasks that have important memory components have been flourishing in recent years. Most such studies involve much more than retrieval from memory. For example, they often involve comparison processes to determine whether two symbols are identical or different, or syntactical processes to transform language strings. In this account I have limited myself as nearly as possible to the "pure memory" components of processing time. Leaving aside the iconic memory and other sense-related stores, four parameters of memory show up prominently in experimental studies: (1) the four-chunk capacity limit of STM; (2) the fixation time of five to ten seconds per chunk for LTM; (3) the initial access time to LTM of about two seconds; and (4) the access time of several hundred msec for chunks beyond the first, These parameters provide a possible point of linkage, so far relatively little explored, with psychological studies that would seek to identify physiological constants matching in relevant ways the parameters measured behaviorally. The attempt to identify the parameters of STM and LTM leads to a number of hypotheses about the structure of the various memories, and it is to those hypotheses that we turn next.

5.5 STORAGE AND ACCESS

The first responsibility of anyone writing about human memory is to avoid the homunculus fallacy—to avoid postulating pictures within the head which must then be viewed and interpreted by a little man who sits within. The invention of the digital computer has made the avoidance of that fallacy easier than it was in the past. Computers patently have memories, and just as patently do not have little men inside to read those memories. Moreover, computers can be described in highly abstract ways that do not depend at all upon the particular hardware they employ. Vacuum tubes, transistors, relays, and solid-state circuits can all be used to realize the same abstract memory organization. Thus, when one speaks of an "associational" memory, or a "content-addressed" memory, one is describing an abstract organization of structures and processes for storing and retrieving symbols, and not a particular hardware realization of that organization.

The terms "symbol" and "pattern" used in an information-processing context are similarly abstract. A pattern is some kind of arrangement of a substrate associated with processes for creating and copying such arrangements, and for discriminating among them. The substrate may be mechanical, electrical, magnetic, or biochemical. And a symbol is simply a pattern that can be discriminated by an information-processing system (Newell and Simon, 1972, pp. 23–26).

Because of their abstract character, the terms used to describe memory structures and processes in computers are available for the description of human memory. In using this terminology, one makes only a few basic commitments to the nature of the memory being described. The most important of these commitments is that the contents of memory can be characterized as symbols and relations among symbols, and that the memory processes are symbol-manipulating processes. The advantage of a neutral and abstract terminology of this kind will become most apparent when we come, presently, to discuss mental imagery, for it is in such a discussion that the homunculus fallacy is most to be feared. If we allow nothing in memory but abstract patterns and their relations, and if we define visual imagery in terms of such patterns and the processes operating on them, then there will be no need for the homunculus, and no role for him if he tries to intrude himself. But I am getting ahead of my story, for I intend in this section to discuss general questions of memory organization, and will turn to imagery only in the next section.

5.5.1 Recognition and semantic memories

Reasons have already been presented for supposing that there are at least two different components in long-term memory possessing quite different characteristics. In general, the memory models that have been proposed in recent years have been models of one or the other of these components, but not of both. Or if both components have been included, one has been treated much more fully than the other.

The first of these components of LTM is the recognition memory, which carries out the processes of discriminating among and recognizing familiar stimulus patterns or pattern components, and retrieving for STM the chunks that point to the information about those patterns stored in LTM. The second component of LTM is the information storage itself—often called nowadays the "semantic memory." Although both components of the LTM are, in a certain sense, semantic, I will follow the current terminology and refer to recognition memory and semantic memory, respectively.

Information-processing models of recognition memory in the form of computer programs date back to the late 1950s, the earliest being the EPAM system (Feigenbaum, 1961; Simon and Feigenbaum, 1964; Gregg and Simon, 1967). A later system dealing with some of the same mechanisms and phenomena is SAL (Hintzman, 1968), while MAPP (Simon and Gilmartin, 1973) employs an EPAM-like memory to simulate some aspects of chess memory. Most other models of LTM are mainly concerned with semantic memory and have little to say about recognition memory. Among these are the systems of Lindsay (1963), Reitman, Grove, and Shoup (1964), Quillian (1968), Rumelhart, Lindsay, and Norman (1972), Schank (1972), and Winograd (1972). The Anderson and Bower (1973) HAM model, while not completely specified or programmed, contains both recognition and semantic components and is the closest approximation that exists to a theory dealing in some detail with both aspects of the memory system.

In addition to cognitive models like those just mentioned, in which memory plays the central role, there are of course a considerable number of formal theories of problem solving, concept attainment, and pattern induction that incorporate theories of memory ranging from the rudimentary to the elaborate. A problem-solving theory applied to tasks in the domains of cryptarithmetic, chess, and logic is discussed in Newell and Simon (1972).

The degree of consensus among all of these theories about the basic mechanisms of human memory is striking. In fact, all of the mechanisms postulated are variants of two basic species: (1) discrimination nets to perform the functions of recognition memory, and (2) node-link or property-list memories to perform the functions of semantic memory. A complete theory of memory would have to include components of both kinds, linked in an effective way. Whether the logic of the experimental data has forced all of these theories into the same mold, or whether their resemblances are testimony to the limitations of human imagination, is a question that must be left to the verdict of future research.

5.5.2 Organization of recognition memory

A discrimination net consists of a set of test nodes connected by branches, the aggregate of nodes and branches forming a treelike structure. At each node is stored one or more perceptual tests that can be applied to a stimulus or to a chunk in STM. The outcome of the test selects a particular one of the branches emanating from the test node and transfers the stimulus to the node at the end of that branch. After a succession of tests has been performed, and the corresponding path of branches followed, a terminal node is reached, which can be identified with the chunk that has just been recognized. Different stimuli will produce different test results at some nodes and will hence be channelled down different paths in the discrimination net to different terminal nodes. (See Newell and Simon, 1972, pp. 34–36.)

5.5.3 Organization of semantic memory

A node-link or property-list memory also consists of a set of nodes connected by relations. The whole structure takes on the form of a net, however, rather than a tree, for it may contain cycles and multiple paths that reach the same node. A particular node may, for example, correspond to a particular class of stimuli—e.g., "cat." Then the relations radiating from that node and connecting it with other nodes can be interpreted as referring to properties or descriptors of that class of stimuli. Thus the relation "class" might lead from "cat" to "mammal," or "animal," the relation "food" to "carnivore," and so on. No fixed set of descriptors is postulated, but an arbitrary number of arbitrary relations is posited for each node. A general description of such a memory can be found in Anderson and Bower (1973), Chapter 4; and in Newell and Simon (1972), pp. 26–28.

5.5.4 Relation of the memories

The relation of the discrimination net to the semantic memory is analogous to the relation of an index to a textbook. Items of information in the semantic memory may be retrieved in two ways. First, recognition of a stimulus by sorting it through the recognition net gives access to its terminal node, which is a node in semantic memory. Thus, for example, recognition of the portrait on a penny gives access to the node referencing Abraham Lincoln (i.e., his physical appearance). Second, once a node in semantic memory has been accessed, other nodes may be reached by processing the relational links that connect them. That is, once Lincoln's portrait is recognized, other information about him may be retrieved, just as it could be if his name, rather than his picture, were recognized. The first process may be called retrieval by recognition, the second, retrieval by (directed) association. (The term "directed" is included here to remind the reader that a property-list memory is organized much more like the directed associations of the Wurzburg School than the simple associations of stimulus-response behaviorism.)

Experimental evidence for the existence of these two components in LTM, and for their relation, comes from a variety of sources. (I will limit my comments to experiments with normal subjects. There is also evidence from amnesic subjects—see Rozin, this volume—of failure of access to information retained in memory.) One source of evidence is the set of paradigms in which the subjects' ability to recognize information is compared with their ability to recall information. It is easy to show that much information is stored in LTM that permits successful performance of recognition tasks, but not of recall tasks. The EPAM theory explains this phenomenon. Total learning time for an item is the sum of the time for elaborating the discrimination net, so that the item can be recognized and distinguished from others, and the time for storing a description of the item in semantic memory, so that the item, once accessed, can be reproduced. In the recall task, the information about the item stored in semantic memory must be complete, else the item cannot be reconstructed. Successful recognition can take place, however, with little or no information in semantic memory as long as the item can be discriminated from others.

A second source of data on the relations between recognition and semantic memory comes from rote-memory experiments that make use of certain mnemonic devices. (For a survey of the evidence see Norman, 1969, Chapter 6.) The subject first practices a list of words—usually concrete nouns—until they are highly over-learned. He is then given a second list of words to learn, with the instruction to associate each word on the second list with the corresponding word on the first list. Finally, he is tested on his ability to recite the second list. Whereas, as we have seen, learning a list of items in the standard rote-learning paradigms requires five to ten seconds of exposure per item, in the paradigm just described most subjects can learn the second list in a single trial at a presentation rate of about two seconds per item, a savings of more than half. The EPAM theory (Feigenbaum, 1961) would explain this phenomenon provided that, in the standard rote-learning paradigm, more than half of the total learning time is required for elaborating the discrimination net—building the recognition memory—and less than half for storing in semantic memory the information needed to reconstruct the item. When the mnemonic aid is employed, access to the second list is gained by the associational links with the first, hence learning the second list requires no augmentation of recognition memory, with a consequent time savings.

A theory of forgetting adequate to handle the empirical evidence at even the grossest level would also appear to require a distinction between recognition memory and semantic memory. We know that much forgetting consists in an inability to retrieve information that can be shown to be in LTM. If a subject is unable to retrieve information using the cues provided when he stored it, but can retrieve the same information on other cues, then what has been lost is not the text but the index. To explain this within the framework of an EPAM-like theory, we postulate that when a new stimulus is encountered that resembles closely one encountered some time previously, the discrimination net may not be altered except by a change in the "pointer" at the terminal node, so that reaching this terminal now accesses the semantic information about the new stimulus, instead of the old. Thus, if one meets and becomes acquainted with a new John Smith, access to information about another John Smith one had known previously may be lost, or at least become more difficult to recover. The oral or written stimulus "John Smith" now retrieves information about the new John Smith instead of the old one. Of course, recognition may also fail simply because the cues presented by the stimulus are different from those incorporated in the discrimination net when the discrimination was originally learned—e.g., the stimulus is now presented from another viewpoint, or in a different context.

There are strong phenomenological reasons, therefore, for postulating these two components of LTM. Experiments in the literature say very little as yet, beyond what has been suggested in the preceding paragraphs, about the relative contributions of the separate components to the aggregate LTM parameters.

5.6. VISUAL IMAGERY

Visual imagery is currently a very popular topic. Whether it means the same thing in all contexts or different things in different contexts is a debatable matter (Simon, 1972). Here are some examples of recent experiments that deal, or purport to deal, with imagery:

Cooper and Shepard (1973) title a recent paper "Chronometric Studies of the Rotation of Mental Images." Subjects are presented with two successive stimuli. The first is, say, the letter "R" in its normal orientation; the second is either a normal or a backward "R," presented either in its normal orientation or rotated some number of degrees from the horizontal. The subject's task is to decide if the second stimulus can or cannot be matched to the first.

In another study, based on geographical knowledge, Shepard and Chipman (1970) show that subjects can judge which pair in a triad of states are most similar in shape, and that these judgments can be scaled. Moreover, judgments of similarity of shape when a map is in view resemble closely the judgments made when the shapes must be imagined.

Baylor (1971) instructs a subject to imagine a three-inch cube, to paint certain sides of the cube with specified colors, to slice the cube into one-inch cubes, and then to count the number of these one-inch cubes that have specified numbers of sides of specified colors.

Bower (1972) and Paivio (1971) give subjects paired-associate verbal learning tasks. Some subjects receive standard verbal learning instructions; others are instructed to form an image associating response with stimulus. In general, subjects in the imaging condition learn faster to criterion than subjects in the standard (nonimaging) condition.

Brooks (1968) has varied simultaneously the sensory modality of stimulus and response, and has shown that reaction times are longer when stimulus and response are in the same modality than when they are in a different modality. Thus an oral response to a question about a visual stimulus is faster than a pointing response, while a pointing response to a question about an aural stimulus is faster than an oral response.

5.6.1 Internal representation

In order to discuss these experiments, we need some vocabulary and concepts for talking about how information is represented internally, in LTM, and possibly also in STM. If semantic memory is, as we have argued, a node-link structure whose components denote objects and relations among them, then it has no special affinity, so far as this basic, abstract structure is concerned, for any particular one of the sensory modalities. LTM, in this view, is no more "visual" than it is "auditory" or "tactual." What can we mean, then, by associating any of those modalities to a memory and speaking of "visual memory" or "auditory memory"? There is a twofold answer to this question.

In the first place, when the raw information from a particular sensory source is encoded, the encoding describes features of the stimulus. But the features that discriminate among visual stimuli are completely different from those that discriminate among auditory stimuli. Hence, by the time the encoding for storage in LTM has been carried out, information coming from different sensory sources will be represented by different nodes and different relational links. We will refer to this by saying that information from different senses has different content.

In the second place, informational structures derived from different sources may have different topologies. Stimuli such as auditorily received language strings might, after syntactical parsing, have a treelike topology, while visually received geometrical figures might retain the topology of the original stimulus in the encoding. A square, for example, might be encoded into a set of nodes denoting its corners, edges, and surface, together with links denoting incidence and directional relations that connect various of the nodes. We will refer to this by saying that information from different senses may have different topologies.

Unfortunately, matters are more complicated than this account would suggest. Suppose we try to use the content and topology of the stored information to distinguish among the modalities of memory. Then we must take account of the fact that the modality in which information is stored in LTM may not be the same as the sensory modality through which the information was initially received. In the Baylor task, for instance, the subject is given an oral or written description in natural language of a visualizable shape. There is every reason to suppose, however, that the information is held in LTM not as a parsed language string but as an "image"—i.e., in the visual modality. At least that is what the subject reports. Conversely, a subject can produce a verbal description of a geometric figure that he is viewing, thus translating information from the visual to the verbal modality. The metaphors of the "mind's eye" and the "mind's ear" are locutions for referring to these complications. Notice that the metaphors do not imply that there are actual physiological structures corresponding to this "eye" and "ear." All that is actually asserted is that information is encoded in LTM in a variety of forms, some of which have affinities, with respect to content or topology, with particular sensory modalities.

5.6.2 Interpretation of the experiments

Let us return now to the list of imagery experiments. The success of the paradigms used by Bower and by Paivio depends on the internal representation of the stimulus material being affected by the "imaging" instructions given to the subjects. In general, subjects receiving imaging instructions learn sets of paired associates about twice as fast as subjects not receiving such instructions. This tells us nothing very specific about either the content or the topology of the representations the subjects use (Simon, 1972).

The experiments of Shepard, on the other hand, argue rather strongly for at least a partial isomorphism between the topology (and perhaps part of the metric description) of the stimulus on the one hand, and the internal representation on the other. In the rotation tasks, the time required for performance is roughly proportional to the angle through which the figures must be rotated. In the task involving the shapes of states, there is a large correlation between judgments of similarity made when the subject has a map before him and judgments made in the mind's eye.

Baylor found that he could simulate a subject's behavior in the cube-manipulating task by postulating as the internal representation a link-node structure topologically isomorphic with a cube, and by postulating processes for operating on that structure—i.e., dividing it into smaller cubes, similarly represented. The information stored and the processes for operating upon it were substantially weaker, however, than the information-extracting processes that would have been available to the subject if he had held an actual cube before his eyes. The internal representation was in no way confusable with a "photograph" of the external scene.

5.6.3 Stimulus modality and internal modality

Mention has been made of the possibility that information received through one sensory modality may be translated, for purposes of internal storage and processing, into another. The nature of this translation depends on the subject's strategy, determined, in turn, by previous learning and by the task demands. An experiment by Chase and Clark (1972) illustrates why such translation must be postulated. Subjects see a simple picture (e.g., a star above a cross) and then hear a sentence (e.g., "The star is below the cross"). Their task is to pronounce the sentence true or false. The aim of the experiment is to discover what processing takes place in this task by measuring the latencies of the answers. But the mere possibility of conducting this experiment implies that subjects can match or compare sentences with pictures in some way. Either the information extracted from the pictures must be translated into a language modality, or the information extracted from the sentences must be translated into a pictorial modality or both must be translated into some common, neutral modality. Since the pictures and sentences used in experiments like these are usually very simple, once abstracted, they do not represent highly dissimilar topologies; hence the evidence does not foreclose any of the three possibilities. But the evidence does show that there is at least one common internal representation that permits the comparison of meanings. (The experiment of Baylor suggests that when the situation described—whether by word or picture—has a more complex structure, processing requirements may force the internal representation into a pictorial modality.)

Another line of research that has been very active in recent years casts some light on the mode of internal representation of information received in the form of natural language (oral or written). Bransford and Franks (1971) read a list of sentences, each with one to four clauses, to subjects. Then a new list of sentences was read, each made up of clauses from the original sentences. The subjects, when asked to judge whether they had heard the sentences before, were unable to discriminate accurately between sentences actually heard before, and sentences that had not been heard but were made up of components that had been heard.

Bransford and Franks inferred from their results that subjects, while encoding the meanings of sentences, discard much of the syntactical information, including information about sentence boundaries. Rosenberg (1973) carried the story several steps farther. After replicating the Bransford-Franks result, he showed that much the same results could be obtained even when some of the sentences were in French and others in English, Subjects were frequently unable to distinguish between a sentence that had been presented in one language and a translation of that sentence. That is, they frequently could not remember which they had seen. Rosenberg then ran an analogous experiment in which some of the sentences were presented in English, as before, while others were translated into simple pictures. Subjects were frequently unable to remember whether or not they had previously seen a picture when they had in fact seen the sentence describing that picture.

Rosenberg constructed a computer simulation of semantic memory that predicted in considerable detail the findings of his experiments as well as those of the earlier experiments of Bransford and Franks. The key postulate in the simulation was that individual sentences are not stored separately in semantic memory, but that the information from the sentences is stored in a relational form attached to the nodes corresponding to the sentence themes. Thus, if several sentences have the same theme, all of the information from those sentences will be stored as a single relational structure linked to the node representing that theme. Since, under these circumstances, the sentence boundaries are nowhere represented in the semantic store, the subject cannot, of course, remember whether several clauses have originated in a single sentence or in several.

Rosenberg and Parkman (1972) had earlier demonstrated a similar point with information, verbally presented, about the members of a family—their family relationships and physical characteristics. On the basis of tests of how well the information was learned in a given time, together with response latencies for various kinds of questions about the relationships, they were able to demonstrate convincingly that the stored semantic information had a close topological similarity with the genealogical chart of the family.

5.6.4 Summary

From our discussion, and the experiments that have been cited, it can be seen how the topic of visual imagery in particular, and the internal representation in semantic memory in general, can be discussed in information-processing terms. Different storage modalities can be distinguished in terms of their information content (the sorts of stimulus features they record) and topology (the sorts of relational structures they employ). We tend to associate a storage modality with a sensory modality when they resemble each other in content and topology. Processes are available to the memory system for translating information from one storage modality to another. In particular, information need not be stored in the same modality in which it is received through the senses: for example, verbal information can be stored in the same modality, whether received visually or aurally, while verbal information describing a visual scene can also be stored, after translation, in a pictorial modality. This does not mean that all information will be preserved by the translation: translation between memory modalities may be at least as difficult as translation between natural languages.

5.7 ARE THREE MEMORIES ENOUGH?

In an earlier section of this paper, the structure of the evidence and the inferences for postulating distinct memory systems was examined. The distinction that is made between STM and LTM, and the distinction between these two memories and the iconic memory, derive principally from the data obtained from four experimental paradigms. We now return to the question of the architecture of the memory system, and in particular to some recent experiments using the delayed-recall paradigm which suggest that the three memories listed above may not be enough to account for the phenomena.

It should be mentioned, before proceeding, that we have been ignoring all of the iconic or sensory memories other than the visual. For example, there is another sensory memory whose existence is quite firmly established: the "echo box," or echoic memory, which permits us to retain, for a second or two, an incoming sound stream to which we have not been attending, and to bring it into STM if our attention is called to it before it disappears. The echoic memory may be thought of as the aural analogue to the visual iconic memory, although information survives substantially longer in the former

than in the latter—several seconds as against a few hundred milliseconds. In this section we will group together all the sensory memories—visual, auditory, tactile, and so on—as though they formed a single memory, and we will ask whether there is evidence for the existence of memories in the central nervous system in addition to the three kinds we have been considering.

5.7.1 The delayed-recall paradigm revisited

Early experiments using the delayed-recall paradigm showed that when a 30-second task was interposed between presentation of stimulus and response, the number of chunks that could be retained in STM was reduced from four or more to one or two. This finding has usually been explained by the hypothesis that the intervening tasks require the use of some short-term memory, and that because of the limited capacity of STM, this additional information can be stored only by displacing a portion of the information already in STM.

Subsequent experiments have shown this interpretation to be untenable. First, the subject is able to recall almost perfectly on the first trial of the experiment: it is only after three or four trials that a sizeable decrement in recall appears (Kincaid and Wickens, 1970). Second, if a time interval of ten seconds or more is inserted between trials, recall improves, and with an interval of a minute or more, it is nearly perfect again (Kincaid and Wickens, 1970). Third, when successive stimuli are highly dissimilar, recall is nearly perfect, even after three or four trials (Wickens, 1970). This "recovery" phenomenon has been called "release from proactive inhibition." This is a label for the phenomenon, not an explanation. It smacks a little of a phlogiston theory: we invent an entity—interference—to explain why something is missing, then postulate the suppression of that entity when the something reappears. Perhaps we could arrive at a simpler explanation if we simply dispensed with the hypothesized inhibition from the beginning.

Let us examine the logic of the situation. If information can be retrieved after an intervening task under some conditions, then only the access to the information, rather than the information itself, must have been lost from memory. In terms of the metaphor used earlier, what appears to have been lost is not the text but the index. But where was the information stored during the intervening period? If it was held in the limited-capacity STM, then why could not the same information be held there when there was no interval between successive trials? And how can the similarity of successive stimuli make a difference?

5.7.2 Recall of chess positions

Recent experiments by Charness (1974) provide some

clues for the explanation of these phenomena. Charness employed the delayed-recall paradigm with visual stimuli—in particular, positions from chess games with 22 pieces standing on the board. The subjects were chess players of moderate playing strength. There were six different recall conditions. In the first two recall conditions, the delay interval imposed no new burden on STM; in the third and fourth conditions, there were easy and hard oral tasks, respectively; and in the fifth and sixth conditions, there were easy and hard visual tasks.

Charness found that the intervening tasks, whether easy or hard, oral or visual, caused only a slight decrement in memory (10 or 15 percent), in contrast with earlier experiments using the delayed-recall paradigm.

Charness did find one significant effect of the intervening tasks, however. In most of the previous experiments using this paradigm, the subjects had been required to respond within five seconds; responses after that time were counted as wrong. Charness did not place an upper limit on the response time. In the immediate-recall condition and recall after rehearsal, average latencies were under five seconds. When recall took place after an intervening task had been performed, the latency measured to the time when the first piece was replaced on the board was increased by an average of nearly four seconds over the average latency in the no-task conditions. Thus, when subjects performed no tasks during the delay interval, they were able to begin to reconstruct the chess position almost immediately upon being given the signal to do so; when they performed a task during this interval, they needed considerable additional time to begin to recall the position. This increase in latency can be interpreted as meaning either that the subjects were not recovering the information from the same memory in the two cases, or that some initial process was required after interruption to "get back into context." The latter phrase, of course, is no more an explanation than is "proactive inhibition"; it is merely a label for the phenomenon.

Charness next used the delayed-recall paradigm with consonant trigrams, presented aurally at a rate of 0.6 sec per trigram, as the stimulus material, with the same interference tasks as in the previous experiment but allowing an unlimited time for response. Only one of the intervening tasks—computing the running sum of random digits —produced a recall deficit of more than 10 or 15 percent. In all the other five conditions, recall averaged 80 percent correct or better. Thus a relatively difficult aural task interferes with recall, a simple aural task or a visual task, simple or complex, does not. The only clear difference between the conditions of this experiment and those of earlier experiments that showed large decrements in re-

call for a variety of intervening tasks was the unlimited time allowed subjects for responding.

5.7.3 A possible explanation

Many more experiments are in prospect before a definitive explanation can be provided for this whole range of phenomena. Let us see whether there are any hints as to the direction that explanation might take, starting from the earlier remark that what seems to be lost in these experiments is not the stimulus information—which reappears intact under a variety of conditions—but access to it. This notion is supported by Charness's findings of long access times for recovery after another task has intervened. The lengthening of the average response latency by four seconds is suggestive of retrieval from long-term memory rather than short-term memory.

In Section 5.5, reasons were given for supposing that LTM has two components: recognition memory and semantic memory. The speeding up of fixation when mnemonic devices are used suggests that ability to store new information in LTM is limited more by the time required to modify and elaborate the recognition memory than by the time required to add the information to the semantic memory. We now hypothesize the following sequence of events:

1. a stimulus is presented, and its familiar components are discriminated by the recognition memory;

2. the internal symbols representing these components are stored in STM;

3. a new node-link structure relating these symbols is stored in semantic memory;

4. the recognition memory is modified to incorporate a new terminal node denoting or "pointing to" the new node-link structure in semantic memory.

The first three steps in the sequence are assumed to proceed very rapidly and to be completed in a second or less. The fourth step, elaboration of the recognition memory, is assumed to require the familiar ten seconds per chunk—or about thirty seconds for a consonant trigram. The information required to carry out this fourth step is already available, however, in semantic memory as a result of Step 3. Interference occurs, with consequent loss of information, if a new stimulus, similar to the previous one, is presented and processed before the processing of the previous one has been completed. In this case, the alteration of the recognition memory is interfered with since both stimuli require modification of the same portion of the net. When the successive stimuli are dissimilar, alteration of each of the two distinct portions of the recognition memory can proceed independently.

This explanation is highly speculative, but perhaps not implausible. It has the virtue that it does not invoke any memory structures or processes whose existence has not already been postulated for other reasons and on the basis of evidence from other kinds of experiments. Even the hypothesized latencies are consistent with our other knowledge. It does not call for an inhibitory process or substance, nor for the superposition of still another process to secure release from that hypothesized inhibition. In short, it can lay claim to some measure of parsimony.

Perhaps the safest conclusion for us to carry away from the experiments with the delayed-recall paradigm is that the data do not yet provide us with a convincing reason for abandoning the main outlines of the three-memory model. They do give us additional reasons, however, to look more closely at the structure and properties of long-term memory, and particulary at the special properties of the recognition and semantic components of that memory. They add further plausibility to the notion that storage of new information in semantic memory may be quite rapid, the relatively lengthy fixation time of five or ten seconds per chunk being due mainly to the requirements for modifying the recognition memory.

5.8 THE STRUCTURE OF SHORT-TERM MEMORY

As we have seen, short-term memory is defined phenomenologically by the immediate-recall experiment. That experiment shows that STM has a small fixed capacity, measured in chunks—that is, familiar recognizable units. The study of confusion errors in STM tasks shows that, at least for verbal stimuli, the symbols designated by the contents of STM are usually encoded in terms of auditory features. These two facts neatly sum up the description of the generally-agreed-upon characteristics of STM. On most other points there is either lack of information or controversy.

Our ignorance of the structure of STM is a serious impediment to reaching a better general understanding of cognitive processes. The STM stands at the crossroads of almost everything that happens in the central nervous system. It is generally believed that any active cognitive process—certainly any conscious process—must find its inputs in STM, and must place its outputs in the same memory. When 2 is added to 2 to make 4, the 2's must reside, at the outset of the process, in STM, and the 4 must reside there when the process is complete. Thus the capacity limit of STM places a strict upper limit on the complexity (in terms of numbers of inputs and outputs) of the elementary information processes that can be executed by the system, and on the ability of the system to execute processes in parallel instead of serially. The narrowness of the span of attention and the general

seriality of the processing (except possibly for recognition processes) stems, therefore, from the structure of STM.

An information-processing system needs a memory with very fast storage and retrieval times—what is usually called "working memory"—for two important purposes. One of these, described in the last paragraph, is to hold the inputs and outputs of elementary processes. The speed at which the inputs can be loaded into working memory determines how rapidly the elementary processes can be executed, and the capacity of working memory limits the complexity of those processes. But the system has a second essential reason for needing a working memory: if its behavior is to have any organization, any shape, it must have some orderly basis for determining what to do next. The information that controls the sequence of processing is called control information, and the structure that exercises this control, the control structure.

The component of an information-processing system that stores the inputs and outputs of the elementary processes may be identical to or separate from the component that stores the control information. The specific question for psychology is whether STM harbors both kinds of information, or whether there is a working memory, separate from STM, that holds the control information.

5.8.1 Hierarchic control systems

In the computer field, the traditional answer to the problem of control is to organize programs hierarchically. Each routine may contain within it one or more subroutines. When the routine is executed and reaches the subroutine, it executes the subroutine in turn. When the subroutine has completed its processing (which may involve calling its own subroutines, and so on, to arbitrary numbers of recursions of the process), it returns control to the routine that called it.

In order for such a hierarchic structure to operate properly, information must be kept in working memory of which routine called the subroutine now active, and which superroutine called that routine, and so on, all the way back up to the top of the hierarchy. This information is needed in order for control to be returned to the right place in the program when each subroutine completes its work. The usual way of mechanizing this information requirement is to provide a so-called pushdown stack, which contains the list of ascending program locations in their proper order. Thus the current program location is at the top of the list, the location in its calling routine is immediately below it, and so on. When a subroutine is finished, the stack is "popped," leaving the proper return location at the top of the stack. When a new subroutine is entered, the stack is "pushed," and the subroutine location is placed at its top. Each time a process is executed, therefore, the pushdown stack is changed in at least one respect, and these changes must be as rapid as changes in STM if the stack is not to be the limiting factor in the speed of operation of the system.

In the usual design of hierarchic programming systems, the total working memory consists of three components: a small memory equally accessible to all routines, which has much the same central position as human STM and which is used to pass information between routines; the pushdown stack for program control; and an indefinite amount of working memory to hold intermediate inputs and outputs of the separate routines. The presence of the latter storage gives such a system an essentially unlimited total amount of working memory of kinds that are almost certainly not available to the human information processor. Hence, unless additional restrictions are placed on it, such a system does not provide a good model of the limits on human STM. Let us assume, therefore, that individual routines do not have "private" working storage available to them, but must use the common and limited STM for all outputs and inputs.

Even with the latter limitation, the existence of the unlimited pushdown stack for program control would give the system an ability to keep track of its goals and subgoals which seems greatly to exceed the ability of the human information-processing system. One is led to the conclusion that the human control system must have a different architecture from that usually found in hierarchically organized programming systems. It has been proposed (Newell and Simon, 1972) that production systems offer an appropriate model for the control system.

5.8.2 Control by production systems

In two recent papers (Newell, 1972, 1973), Allen Newell has carried forward a considerable distance the proposal just mentioned, to model the human control system upon a production system. I will describe the idea briefly here and indicate its main implications for the structure of STM. The reader who is interested in a fuller account will find it in the references that have been cited.

A production system consists of a set of productions. Each production, in turn, has two parts: a condition and an action. The basic principle on which the system operates is that whenever the condition of a production is satisfied, the action of that production is executed. In implementations of such a system, the productions are generally listed in some order, and if the conditions of more than one production are satisfied at the same time, the action of the production that occurs first in the list is executed.

The principle of control in a production system is, therefore, to have no control—at least no centralized or hierarchical control. Each production "does its thing" whenever the situation is appropriate, that is, whenever its condition is satisfied. It remains to be shown, of course, that such a system can ever behave in an organized, goal-directed fashion, as it surely must if it is to simulate certain kinds of human behavior.

Nothing has yet been said about the nature of the conditions that determine when a production will become active. The crucial assumption here is that the conditions are tests on the contents of STM. That is, if one or more of the symbols in STM match the conditions of a production, the action of that production will be executed. Let us see how such an arrangement can lead to coherent action.

The actions of productions may be of several kinds. One kind of production may take encoded sensory information and place it in STM (perception). Another kind of production may produce a symbol that designates a goal or subgoal and place it in STM (goal creation). Another kind of production may retrieve symbols from LTM and place them in STM (recall). Another kind of production may rearrange the symbols in STM, bringing one of them up to the front (rehearsal). Still another may initiate motor actions, which may themselves be controlled by one or more such systems. There will be many kinds of productions besides these five, but the ones that have been listed are the most important for the operation of the control system.

Because the symbols in STM determine which productions will be activated, the source of these symbols has much to do with the character of the system's operation. If most of these symbols are placed in STM by acts of perception, the system will behave as though it were stimulus-bound. If most of the symbols originate in goal-creating actions, the system will behave in a goal-oriented and inner-directed way. If many symbols are placed in STM by recall, the course of the system's behavior will be strongly influenced by the contents of LTM—that is, by its previous learning. If the rehearsal production is activated infrequently, information may be lost from STM. (The scheme is rather more compatible with an interference theory of forgetting from STM than with a decay theory.)

Space does not permit me to elaborate further on the nature of production systems, or the precise way in which they are applied to model psychological processes. Persons accustomed to thinking in S-R terms may find it helpful to view the C→A connection between a condition and its action as analogous to the S→R connection with which they are familiar. There are important differences between the two relations, but the comparison is a tolerable first approximation. With the production-system organization of control, the single STM serves both of the working-memory functions mentioned earlier. It holds the inputs and outputs of the information processes, and it holds the control information that determines which process will be executed next. This parsimony is one of the attractive features of the production-system hypothesis, and it also has strong implications for short-term memory that should be testable in laboratory experiments.

5.8.3 Subject strategies

It appears that a very few complex human responses are "wired in." Most are modifiable both by learning and by change in strategy—the latter being at least partially under the voluntary control of the subject. The modification of behavior by change of strategy (often induced by task instructions) is well attested in the literature (e.g., Gregg and Simon, 1967; Dansereau, 1969).

The dependence of behavior on strategy creates problems of great subtlety for experimentation. If we wish to get at the underlying invariants of memory, particularly those invariants most directly related to physiology, we must be able to control, or at least detect, the strategy the subject is using. This argues for the direct inducement of specific strategies by problem instructions or other means; it argues against the pooling of data from several subjects, who may arrive in the laboratory with quite different strategies as the result of differences in their previous experiences and training.

Training subjects in specific task strategies can push them against the limits of their information-processing capabilities. It appears to be a powerful technique for laying bare the underlying physiological constraints on memories and processes.

5.9 CONCLUSION

In view of the enormous amount of research that has been done on human memory during the past twenty years, the prospect of attempting an overview of that field from an information-processing point of view was intimidating. I am not sure that the retrospect is any more comforting. My account is at best a very limited sample of all of the topics that deserve to be considered. It is very far from a random sample. By necessity it is limited to the research and theories with which I am familiar, and no one, I expect, can claim today to be familiar with the whole of the literature in this field.

In selecting topics for inclusion, I have been guided by several criteria, in addition to familiarity. I have tried to select topics that would illustrate the method of inferring memory processes and structures from observable phenomena; that would deal with the most solidly based, or at least widely accepted, conclusions about the organization of human memory; that would illustrate the nature of some of the questions that are open today; and that would show how our growing understanding of those information-processing systems called computers is helping us to understand the information-processing system called man.

In my introduction, I spoke of the division of labor between information-processing psychologists and physiological psychologists, and of the need for cooperation between them. My list of conclusions about human memory can also be interpreted as a list of queries directed to physiological psychology. I have tried to describe a number of properties of the engram, and of the storage system that holds it, as they are inferred from the phenomena they produce. I would hope that this characterization of the engram in information-processing terms may provide some clues to the physiologist in his continuing search for the biochemical basis on which it operates and the place or places where it resides in the human brain.

ENVOI

In his comments on my paper (see Chapter 6), Professor Riley raises a number of questions about the crucial hypothesis that the human CNS contains clearly distinguishable short-term and long-term memories, in addition to memories specific to particular sensory modalities. While the multiple-memory hypothesis should not be elevated to a dogma, it is widely accepted in cognitive psychology today, and the impression should not be left that it can be easily disposed of. I should like, therefore, to reply briefly to the specified objections Riley raises against the hypothesis.

Riley questions first the "total-time hypothesis." Of course my brief account did not describe all of the detailed qualifications attached to the hypothesis by the processing models that incorporate it, but attention to those qualifications would dispose of most, if not all, of the counterexamples. The fixation time in question is the time available for attending to the learning task. Hence requiring simultaneous performance of other tasks increases the total time to fixation. As already mentioned, the role of subject strategies in altering what is learned is also well documented. Hence I cannot agree that the experiments cited by Riley are "in clear opposition" to the hypothesis, or that they raise serious problems for dual-store theories.

In Riley's second argument, he acknowledges that short-term and long-term memory appear to fit different mathematical functions, but then paradoxically concludes that this difference does not support a multiple-store hypothesis. If he had said "does not prove" rather than "does not support," we would not disagree.

The third argument, on the modality of encoding in STM, attacks an assumption I did not make. It is true that stimuli in the form of words or letters are commonly held in memory in acoustically encoded form. This does not imply that there is anything intrinsically acoustic about the structure of that memory. Indeed, a much more plausible hypothesis is that the chunks of STM are simply "pointers" to information (however encoded) stored in the part of LTM that I called "recognition memory." Hence Riley's third argument is irrelevant to the multiple-store hypothesis.

The fourth argument, like the second, rests on a misconception of what it means for two memories to be different. In a matter of a fraction of a second of stimulus exposure, sufficiently "strong traces" are created to allow four words to be stored in STM. Five to ten seconds of processing must be done for the storage in memory of each additional word beyond four. It is precisely this discontinuity in the acquisition function that, like the corresponding discontinuity in the forgetting function, argues for two distinguishable forms of memory.

Finally, Professor Riley and I attach rather different meanings to the phrase "explanatory power." To me, a concept such as proactive interference lacks explanatory power if it does not postulate a mechanism—which it does not.

These disagreements should not obscure the basic consensus between Professor Riley and me with regard to the vital importance of parametric studies of both man and other organisms—a point he illustrates cogently with the examples cited in the second half of his comments.

ACKNOWLEDGMENT

This research has been supported in part by Research Grant MH-07722 from the National Institute of Mental Health, and in part by the Advanced Research Projects Agency of the Secretary of Defense (F44620-70-C-0107), a contract monitored by the Air Force Office of Scientific Research. I am grateful to my colleague Chris Frederickson for helpful comments on a first draft of this paper.

REFERENCES

ANDERSON, J. R., and BOWER, G. H. 1973. *Human Associative Memory*. Washington D.C.: V. H. Winston & Sons.

BAYLOR, G. W. 1971. A treatise on the mind's eye: An empirical investigation of visual mental imagery. Unpublished Ph.D. dissertation, Carnegie-Mellon University.

BOWER, G. H. 1972. Mental imagery and associative learning. In L. W. GREGG, ed., *Cognition in Learning and Memory*. New York: John Wiley & Sons.

BRANSFORD, J. D., and FRANKS, J. J. 1971. The abstraction of linguistic ideas. *Cognitive Psychology* 2: 331–350.

BROOKS, L. R. 1968. Spatial and verbal components of the art of recall. *Canadian Journal of Psychology* 22: 349–368.

CHARNESS, N. 1974. Memory for chess positions: The effects of interference and input modality. Unpublished Ph.D. dissertation, Carnegie-Mellon University.

CHASE, W. G., and CLARK, H. H. 1972. Mental operations in the comparison of sentences and pictures. In L. W. Gregg, ed., *Cognition in Learning and Memory*. New York: John Wiley & Sons.

CONRAD, R. 1959. Errors of immediate memory. *British Journal of Psychology* 50: 349–359.

COOPER, L. A., and SHEPARD, R. N. 1973. Chronometric studies of the rotation of mental images. In W. G. Chase, ed., *Visual Information Processing*. New York: Academic Press.

DANSEREAU, D. 1969. An information processing model of mental multiplication. Unpublished Ph.D. dissertation, Carnegie-Mellon University.

FEIGENBAUM, E. A. 1961. The simulation of verbal learning behavior. In *Proceedings of the 1961 Western Joint Computer Conference*, pp. 121–132.

GREGG, L. W., and SIMON, H. A. 1967. An information-processing explanation of one-trial and incremental learning. *Journal of Verbal Learning and Verbal Behavior* 6: 780–787.

HINTZMAN, D. L. 1968. Explorations with a discrimination net model for paired-associate learning. *Journal of Mathematical Psychology* 5: 123–162.

HUNT, E. 1971. What kind of computer is man? *Cognitive Psychology* 2: 57–98.

HUNT, E. 1973. The memory we must have. In R. C. Schank and K. M. Colby, eds., *Computer Models of Thought and Language*. San Francisco: W. H. Freeman.

KINCAID, J. P., and WICKENS, D. D. 1970. Temporal gradient of release from proactive inhibition. *Journal of Experimental Psychology* 86: 313–316.

KINTSCH, W. 1970. *Learning, Memory, and Conceptual Processes*. New York: John Wiley & Sons.

LINDSAY, R. K. 1963. Inferential memory as the basis of machines which understand natural language. In E. A. Feigenbaum and J. Feldman, eds., *Computers and Thought*. New York: McGraw-Hill.

McLEAN, R. S., and GREGG, L. W. 1967. Effects of induced chunking on temporal aspects of serial recitation. *Journal of Experimental Psychology* 74: 455–459.

MILLER, G. A. 1956. The magical number seven, plus or minus two. *Psychological Review* 63: 81–97.

NEWELL, A. 1972. A theoretical explanation of mechanisms for coding the stimulus. In A. W. Melton and E. Martin, eds., *Coding Processes in Human Memory*. New York: John Wiley & Sons.

NEWELL, A. 1973. Production systems: Models of control structures. In W. G. Chase, ed., *Visual Information Processing*. New York: Academic Press.

NEWELL, A., and SIMON, H. A. 1972. *Human Problem Solving*. Englewood Cliffs, N.J.: Prentice-Hall.

NORMAN, D. A. 1969. *Memory and Attention*. New York: John Wiley & Sons.

PAIVIO, A. 1971. *Imagery and Verbal Processes*. New York: Holt, Rinehart and Winston.

PETERSON, L. R., and PETERSON, M. J. 1959. Short-term retention of individual items. *Journal of Experimental Psychology* 58: 193–198.

QUILLIAN, M. R. 1968. Semantic memory. In M. Minsky, ed., *Semantic Information Processing*. Cambridge, Mass.: MIT Press.

REITMAN, W., GROVE, R. B., and SHOUP, R. G. 1964. Argus: An information processing model of thinking. *Behavioral Science* 9: 270–281.

ROSENBERG, S. 1973. A theory of semantic memory. Unpublished Ph.D. dissertation, Carnegie-Mellon University.

ROSENBERG, S., and PARKMAN, J. 1972. Semantic memory: Aspects of storage and retrieval. C.I.P. Working Paper, no. 170, Carnegie-Mellon University.

RUMELHART, D. E., LINDSAY, P. H. and NORMAN, D. A. 1972. A process model for long-term memory. In E. Tulving and W. Donaldson, eds., *Organization and Memory*. New York: Academic Press.

SCHANK, R. C. 1972. Conceptual dependency: A theory of natural-language understanding. *Cognitive Psychology* 3: 552–631.

SHEPARD, R. N., and CHIPMAN, S. 1970. Second-order isomorphism of internal representations: Shapes of states. *Cognitive Psychology* 1: 1–17.

SIMON, H. A. 1972. What is visual imagery? In L. W. Gregg, ed., *Cognition in Learning and Memory*. New York: John Wiley & Sons.

SIMON, H. A. 1974. How big is a chunk? *Science* 183: 482–488.

SIMON, H. A., and FEIGENBAUM, E. A. 1964. An information processing theory of some effects of similarity, familiarity, and meaningfulness in verbal learning. *Journal of Verbal Learning and Verbal Behavior* 3: 385–396.

SIMON, H. A., and GILMARTIN, K. 1973. A simulation of memory for chess positions. *Cognitive Psychology* 5: 29–46.

SPERLING, G. A. 1960. The information available in brief visual presentations. *Psychological Monographs* 74 (11, whole no. 498).

UNDERWOOD, B. J. 1969. Attributes of memory. *Psychological Review* 76: 559–573.

WICKENS, D. D. 1970. Encoding categories of words: An empirical approach to meaning. *Psychological Review* 77: 1–15.

WINOGRAD, T. 1972. *Understanding Natural Language*. New York: Academic Press.

6

Comments on Simon's Paper, and Some Observations on Information Processing in Animals

DONALD A. RILEY

ABSTRACT These comments concern information-processing approaches to the storage of memory in humans and in animals. The first part of the paper restricts itself to one problem taken up in Professor Simon's paper: Are long-term memory and short-term memory in humans different? In the recent past, a number of different lines of evidence have been advanced in support of the proposition that short- and long-term memory do indeed obey different laws. Five different lines of evidence are here examined with recent data that cast doubt on each. These lines deal with (1) the role of exposure time or rehearsal frequency, (2) forgetting rates, (3) encoding differences, (4) memory-store size, and (5) determiners of memory loss. In each case, the evidence seems to be either ambiguous or against the two-store hypothesis. In view of these considerations, the two-store hypothesis seems unwarranted at the present time.

The second section of the paper deals with information-processing approaches to the study of information storage and short-term memory in animals. Such approaches and experimental preparations are of interest not only to individuals who analyze information storage in selective-attention and cognitive processes in animals but also to individuals whose concerns are with the fine-grain analysis of information storage even on a moment-to-moment basis. Three recently developed experimental preparations are briefly considered: (1) the maintained-discrimination task, in which the discriminative capacities of animals may be repeatedly examined under varying instructions and sets; (2) a matching-to-sample task that permits precise estimates of how long the organism must examine a stimulus in order to use it at later time; and (3) high-speed memory-scan tasks in monkeys. Each of these tasks examines performance in a steady state free of the contaminating effects of habit acquisition. They permit a detailed analysis of the animal's memory for specific events, a prospect that may interest those concerned with neural mechanisms of learning and memory.

I assume that when individuals such as myself, whose work is outside the general area of neural mechanisms in learning and memory, are invited to a conference such as this, it is in the hope that they will discuss developments from their own respective fields of research that may be of value to scholars working at some other level. The work that I have been engaged in recently has been concerned with a fine-grain analysis of selective attention in animals under steady-state conditions. My work, and the work of

DONALD A. RILEY, Department of Psychology, University of California, Berkeley

others following this general line, is quite analogous to human information-processing work that investigates selective perception and short-term memory in a steady state. This work differs from most work on animal selective attention in that it is concerned not with acquisition of attention or habit formation, but rather with discrimination of stimuli under various instructional conditions and with memory for the events of single trials. Because this work seems to provide a bridge between human memory research and research on the physiological bases of memory, a discussion of some recent methodological advances in this area may be both informative and valuable. Consequently, my remarks are in two parts. First, I shall make some comments supplementary to Herbert Simon's essay dealing with conceptual issues in human memory (see Chapter 5). Then I shall discuss some current advances in animal information processing.

At the outset, I would like to express my own appreciation for Simon's thoughtful comments concerning different levels of explanation. It's nice to have someone with sufficient background to understand in detail the problems in another discipline show that a direct parallel exists between problems in his own field and those in ours. I find his comments concerning "bridge" theories especially instructive—perhaps because I resonate to the conclusion that even when we have a bridge theory that provides an explanation of cognition in physiological terms, researchers will still go on using information-processing concepts in their analyses of more complex phenomena. Perhaps explanatory concepts several steps removed from the events to be explained do not have the intuitive utility of those that are closer. Ultimately, however, bridges do get made. When they do, the success of these bridges undoubtedly depends in part on advances that occur in the more molecular disciplines. However, success also depends in part on the sorts of conceptual structures that are suggested by findings in the less molecular disciplines. It is because of this reciprocity that I feel it important to comment briefly on some recent developments concerning evidence for multiple-memory theory.

6.1 EVIDENCE WHICH QUESTIONS THE MULTIPLE-MEMORY HYPOTHESIS

Simon has summarized a view of the memory system that assumes several different kinds of memories or stores. He points out in his opening comments that this conception of human memory is the way it looks to a growing number of psychologists who approach memory from the information-processing point of view. I agree; but it is also true that there has been resistance to this conception, and recent developments suggest that some supporters of this general model are beginning to have doubts. Of course, we all know that most data can be interpreted in more than one way. I do not find it unlikely that some version of a multiple-store theory will be required to account for the data and that facts which now seem to cause difficulties will be accommodated. Nevertheless, facts that do not fit well into the model have been emerging. I shall now mention some of these facts and the difficulties they raise.

In the remarks that follow, I shall draw freely upon two recent excellent reviews, one by Craik and Lockhart (1972), the other by Wickelgren (1973), which examine the multiple-store arguments. The first of these reviews is a thoughtful analysis of the evidence for and against multiprocess systems. The authors conclude that much of the evidence breaks down, and that a more fruitful way to think of the memory system might in fact be paraphrased by the old expression, "It ain't what you do, it's the way that you do it." They argue that the duration of a memory depends less on what assumed storage system it is in than on how it has been processed by the subject or, in their terms, on the level of processing. We shall return to some of their observations in a moment.

Both of these papers, and others sharing this view, are concerned with two quite distinct issues. One is the evaluation of the evidence that has been advanced in the past to support the assumption that there are two or three separate store systems with different laws. The other issue concerns the search for an alternative theoretical structure. While Craik, Lockhart, and Wickelgren seem to agree that most of the phenomena generally advanced in support of the short-term store/long-term store distinction either no longer support or are irrelevant to that distinction, their final solutions are different. Wickelgren concludes that there are three kinds of evidence that can still be advanced to support the distinction. Craik and Lockhart argue that all of the data are consistent with a position which assumes that the strength of a memory depends upon the processing operations that the subject performs. To discuss some of these issues briefly but concretely, let me now turn to some of the important distinctions described by Simon and briefly recount some

TABLE 6.1
Characteristics held to distinguish two postulated memory stores

Short-term memory	Long-term memory
Rapid acquisition	Slow acquisition (total-time hypothesis)
Rapid loss	Slow loss
Phonemic	Semantic
Limited store	Unlimited store
Loss unrelated to interference	Loss a function of interference

of the recent data that seem to raise difficulties for the discrete-store hypothesis.

Simon has presented the argument that the evidence suggests three discrete memory stores: a sensory, very brief, primarily visual memory; a short-term, limited-capacity memory, largely phonemic in character; and a long-term memory of large capacity, with the amount stored depending on total exposure time. A number of distinctions are either directly indicated or implied by those descriptions. I shall not attempt to deal with all of them. Also, in the interests of brevity, I shall restrict my remarks to alleged differences between the long-term memory (LTM) and the short-term memory (STM), more or less ignoring the sensory memory. Table 6.1 indicates some of the differences found in experiments to measure memory as a function of time that have suggested to various theorists the need for more than one kind of memory store.

First, let us consider the possibility that the strength of storage in LTM is a function of the total time per item rather than any arbitrary division of this time into exposures or trials. As Simon indicates, there is a substantial body of literature on this topic. Recently, however, this general proposition has come under assault. As long ago as 1965, Glucksberg and Laughery showed one sort of violation of the total-time hypothesis in a task requiring that subjects keep a running count of the number of times four different consonants appeared. This was continued sufficiently long to be a clear LTM task. Retention was much better under a condition in which stimuli appeared for 0.1 sec followed by 1.9 sec off than under one in which stimuli appeared for 1.9 sec followed by 0.1 sec off. Since total time was the same, some other factor must have produced the effect. More recently, Stoff and Eagle (1971) have shown that differences in the reported strategies used by subjects in free-recall learning affect their ability to recall. This effect appeared at only one of two tested trial durations. Clearly, then, such an interaction casts doubt on the total-time hypothesis.

Yet another assault on the total-time hypothesis comes from evidence concerning rehearsal in STM. Craik and Watkins (1973) have shown that neither the amount of time a subject is required to think about an item in an STM task nor the number of rehearsals in the STM task is predictive of subsequent efficiency of recall over longer periods of time. Such findings are in clear opposition to the total-time hypothesis and also raise problems for dual-store theories such as the Atkinson-Shiffrin (1968) model, which assumes that the function of rehearsal is to maintain an item to STM store so as to increase the probability of its transfer into the LTM store. Craik and Watkins present further evidence suggesting that effective long-term retention depends not on rehearsal, but rather on the nature of rehearsal: if the subject engages in "elaborative" activities that associate the item with other items, long-term memory will be facilitated. It is in this sense that they argue that processing can occur at different levels and that the memory-store assumption seems inadequate.

What of the fact that forgetting is rapid at first and slower later on? This argument in and of itself cannot, of course, be advanced as a reason for assuming more than one kind of memory store. Rather, the argument must be of the nature that certain operations are necessary if transfer from one store to another is to take place, and that if these operations do not occur, the item will disappear. We have seen the difficulties in the assumption that either time or rehearsal, as such, transfers items from a short-term to a long-term store. Wickelgren has argued that, given a number of assumptions, it may be possible to demonstrate that the mathematical formula describing the forgetting function over long periods of time differs from that over short periods of time. Basically, Wickelgren argues that studies of retention over very brief intervals (10–20 sec) can describe retention loss by a simple decay function, whereas studies involving long-term retention require the assumption of a continuously weakening trace that is increasingly resistant to further decay. Only time and persistence will allow the evaluation of this latter notion. I only wish to make the point that Wickelgren's analysis is different from one that assumes that changes in rate of forgetting, as such, support a multiple-store hypothesis.

One sort of argument for a multiple-store hypothesis that has received wide attention is that the form in which material is maintained in the different memories changes. When an individual reads a word, the initial sensory memory is visual, but the information is then changed to a short-term store which is primarily acoustic in character. Subsequently, the memory is stored in long-term semantic memory. Simon has alluded to the evidence supporting these distinctions, but they too have come under some attack. A number of writers have recently argued that the acoustic character of memories in STM tasks is not due to a transfer from a visual store to an acoustic store in some information-processing chain. Rather, they argue, acoustic representations are directly related to the subject's tendency to articulate what he sees. The point is that the acoustic encoding is not necessarily the property of a short-term memory. Instead, it is a reflection of the way in which the subject is likely to encode verbal stimuli if given only a very short time in which to encode. Various techniques have been used to demonstrate these effects. For example, Peterson and Johnson (1971) required subjects to count backward during the visual presentation of letter strings; Tell (1972) in a similar situation required subjects to say the words "three consonants" while a letter string of three consonants was presented; Estes (1973) had subjects either classify letters (first or second half of alphabet) or pronounce letters. All procedures preventing voicing of the letters reduced immediate retention, although Estes's data show the acoustically encoded and the nonacoustically encoded retention curves drawing together after about 30 sec. This study also demonstrated the acoustic-confusion effect (for letters that sound the same) only when the letters were pronounced. Finally, in Estes's work, the letters of the letter string were presented in rapid succession, with each one in the same visual location. Such a procedure might be expected to "wipe out" iconic representations of letters, but Estes's letter strings clearly persisted for a second or so. This observation suggests a continuity between the memories stored in immediate-memory experiments and those in STM experiments.

Using similar techniques, Kroll, Parks, Parkinson, Bieber, and Johnson (1970) have demonstrated the presence of a visual short-term memory that is both persistent over at least 25 sec (i.e., noniconic) and nonphonemic. They showed this effect by forcing subjects to shadow acoustically presented letters at a high rate and then to recall either a visually presented letter or an acoustically presented and shadowed letter. The latter was spoken in a different voice from the distractor message. Over the time span of the experiment, the visually presented letter was retained better than the acoustically presented letter, and only the latter showed any acoustic-confusion errors. Again, then, this experiment questions the argument that coding differences imply different memory stores. Schulman (1972) has demonstrated semantic confusions in STM experiments by requiring semantic encoding of words. So, in the same way, coding differences as a way of distinguishing short-term and long-term memory come under question.

My intent in this recitation of evidence is to show that the contents of the store do not necessarily reflect anything about the temporal order of events or the amount of time that a memory has existed. Rather, such effects appear to reflect the way in which subjects have treated the material. There is little doubt that subjects under different circumstances code material in different ways. Nor does it seem unlikely that different kinds of coding may affect the efficiency of storage, the persistence of a memory, and the likelihood of recovery of the memory at a later time. However, none of these considerations can any longer be taken as evidence for the existence of different kinds of stores.

One of the facts that has been most influential in fostering the idea of different memories is that of limited capacity. We know that subjects cannot take in more than a few chunks of information at a time. The meaning of this important fact has, however, remained elusive. Is it evidence for a short-term store? If it is, the nature of this store must be different than previously imagined. If, however, as Craik and Lockhart argue, traces are traces and their strength varies according to the elaborateness of the processing that has been done on them, then the capacity limitation merely reflects the fact that nonprocessed material is not retained. If the same material is processed by simple rehearsal, it will be retained for a brief period of time, and if it is processed in more elaborate ways, it will be retained for longer periods.

It would be wrong to conclude this cursory examination of some of the evidence relating to multiple memory without explicit recognition of one aspect of Wickelgren's position. Wickelgren has argued that most of the published evidence that has been marshaled in favor of the dual-store hypothesis is irrelevant to the argument, but there are three kinds of evidence that he does consider relevant. One I have already mentioned: differences in the shape of the LTM function as opposed to the STM function. Another line of evidence comes from patients (mainly with hippocampal damage) who exhibit normal verbal short-term memory coupled with an almost complete inability to remember the same material over longer periods of time. The reality of these effects cannot be denied. What can be questioned, however, is whether they do in fact provide overwhelming support for a multiple-store hypothesis. While some interpretations have assumed that these facts are powerful evidence for two stores, Warrington and Weiskrantz (1970, 1971) have shown that cues that restrict alternatives can facilitate long-term recall for such individuals and that at least some of the memory deficit is attributable to the interfering effect of prior learned material.

The third kind of evidence with which Wickelgren deals concerns the effects of interfering material. Wickelgren has focused on the role of similarity in retroactive interference. Numerous investigators have shown that retroactive inhibition in long-term memory is affected by the similarity between original and interpolated learning. Wickelgren finds no evidence for such interference in short-term memory. He suggests that this difference

may provide grounds for distinction between two different stores, but he also indicates that without further evidence conclusions of this sort would be premature.

It is of considerable interest that Melton (1970) has also regarded the role of interference in LTM and STM tasks as critical to the issue of two memory mechanisms versus one. Indeed, Melton argues that the principal reason why proponents of a single-mechanism hypothesis resist the notion of two separate stores is that the effect of the degree of similarity between the interfering and the to-be-remembered material appears to operate the same way in both LTM and STM tasks. Interestingly enough, however, the evidence that he cites is concerned with proactive rather than retroactive inhibition. Keppel and Underwood (1962) were the first to show that retention loss in short-term memory is a function of the number of prior learned lists. Subsequent investigators (e.g., Wickens, 1970) have shown that this proactive effect depends upon category similarity, and Noyd (cited in Melton, 1970) has shown that the forgetting is greatest when the interfering and to-be-remembered units have the same length. Noyd has further shown that the intrusion errors are also maximal in frequency when the preceding unit and the to-be-remembered unit are of the same length. Facts of this general sort were what originally established the phenomenon of proactive inhibition in long-term memory. The demonstration of similar sorts of lawful relationships in short-term memory would further call into question the advisability of positing separate stores with different laws governing their operation.

To conclude this part of my comments, I should emphasize again that I do not wish to assert that there are not multiple memory stores, only that much of the frequently recited evidence does not appear today to be as unambiguous in its support of a multiple-store hypothesis as it did a short time ago. There is much to be said for the multiple-store hypothesis as a heuristic device, and much has indeed been said and written about it. It should not, however, be rested on too heavily as a strong theoretical position.

6.2 INFORMATION-PROCESSING APPROACHES TO MEMORY STORAGE IN ANIMALS

I shall now turn to some comments on recent approaches in the animal memory literature. This work has been aimed at examining factors affecting the way animals store and remember individual stimulus events, and it is remarkably similar to some recent work on information processing in humans involving selective attention and the effects of information load and precuing on the one hand, and high-speed memory searches on the other. I mention this work not only because I have been interested in it myself, but because I believe that people working from an information-processing approach are more likely to make contact with physiological psychologists and physiologists the closer their paradigms come together, with the consequent increase in likelihood that each will see a way of applying the techniques of the other. My comments, then, are largely methodologically oriented rather than theoretically oriented, although I shall comment directly on matters of substance and theory.

As I have suggested, the work to be described has been inspired in one way or another by work on human information processing and perception. Rather than viewing research on the rat as a means of approaching problems of human learning, as was the custom thirty years ago, a number of psychologists are now reversing the trend, using tools and analytic procedures developed in research on humans as a source of fruitful insights for understanding how to go about doing research in animals.

I wish to describe three different paradigms, all of which study attention or memory in steady states in animals. The first sort of experimental design was developed by Donald S. Blough and is called a "maintained-discrimination task." He has used it in the study of selective attention in pigeons. It is well known to students of animal learning, but is, I suspect, less well known outside of that field. The second is a matching-to-sample task devised by students of mine and me at Berkeley. This task, in effect, asks how much time an animal needs to see a sample in order to identify it later, and what happens if the animal is given less time. We have called these experiments "looking-time" experiments. The third kind of experiment is an adaptation of the memory-scan reaction-time experiment developed by Sternberg (1966), here applied to animals. This research was done by Douglas Eddy (1973), then of Carnegie-Mellon University. The first two paradigms are basically psychophysical in nature; the third involves a reaction-time methodology. All are potentially of considerable value in studying the reception, encoding, storage, and retrieval of simple information in animals.

Blough's (1969, 1972) maintained-discrimination task in pigeons involves reinforcing pecks to a key only in the presence of a positive stimulus compound, defined by the positive values on two separate dimensions, but never in the presence of any of a number of negative compounds. The design and results can be made clear by examination of Figure 6.1, where we see that the positive compound was defined as a hue wavelength value of 582 nm and a tone of 3990 Hz. Other wavelength values varied in 1-nm steps down to 576 nm and in 100-Hz steps down

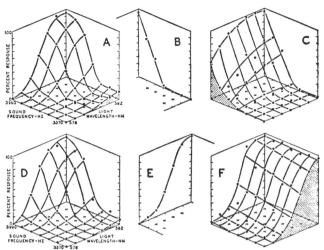

FIGURE 6.1 Discrimination data from a single bird. A: mean of the last two sessions on the baseline two-dimensional discrimination. B: last two sessions on auditory discrimination with the visual stimulus constant at its reinforced value (582 nm). C: first session on the baseline procedure after training with the visual stimulus constant. D: last two sessions on the second baseline series. E: last two sessions on visual discrimination with the auditory stimulus constant at its reinforced value (3990 Hz). F: first session on the baseline procedure after training with the auditory stimulus constant. From Blough (1969). Reproduced with permission from *Science* 166: 125–126. Copyright 1969 by the American Association for the Advancement of Science.

to 3370 Hz. The symmetrical nature of this display shows that Blough carefully chose the stimulus differences on the two dimensions to be equivalent. After the establishment of this discrimination, the variations along one dimension were removed from the design, and each value on the remaining dimension was paired only with the positive value on the removed dimension. The effect of further training in such a circumstance is shown in the second panel, where it is clear that discrimination improved markedly on the remaining dimension. On return to the full two-dimensional set, the improvement on the used dimension remained, but discrimination on the neglected dimension had deteriorated markedly. It should be emphasized that this is not a conventional retroactive-inhibition design. The animal has not learned competing responses in the presence of the same stimuli; rather, those stimulus variations on which the animal did so poorly in the last stage have been omitted from the design.

Blough's interpretation is that the animal selectively attends to and selectively processes information on one dimension only after prolonged single-dimension training. Support for this position comes from the fact that with further training on the full two-dimensional set, the discrimination on the neglected dimension returns but, as it does so, discrimination on the dimension that has been under training all along declines. These facts are consistent with the assumption that discrimination of small differences on the two dimensions at the same time exceeds the animal's capacity. Elimination of differences on one dimension allows the animal to restrict his attention to the other and thereby to improve that discrimination. Reintroduction of the full display again strains the animal's capacity, producing a deterioration in performance on one dimension as performance on the other improves.

As is usually the case with a first experiment using a novel procedure, alternative interpretations of Blough's data are possible. For example, all aspects of the reinforcement schedule are not constant from one condition to another. Perhaps more important, however, is that a response-competition or habit-interference interpretation may be made of the data. When the animal encounters stimuli varying on both dimensions from trial to trial, it is frequently confronted with a positive or near-positive cue on one dimension and a more clearly negative cue on the other dimension. Given such conflicting instructions, it may not be surprising that the animal makes mistakes which can be eliminated by training on one dimension alone.

Be that as it may, this general procedure appears to be an interesting and powerful way of studying multidimensional psychophysics in animals. It has the advantage over conventional learning experiments of being able to ask the animal the same question repeatedly while the animal is more or less in the same state. It has the additional advantage of being able to ask questions about how the animal perceives stimulus compounds. Can it neglect one element and process only another? If it processes both, does it treat the compound as some sort of a unified stimulus or does it evaluate each dimension separately? Blough (1972) attempted to ask about this second question by examining whether the changes in response probabilities imply a Euclidean metric (perceptually fused stimuli) or a city-block metric (discretely treated stimuli). I do not believe this second attempt has been very successful, but, to my knowledge, it is the first time that analytic techniques of this power have been applied to such perceptual problems with animals.

A directly complementary technique (also with pigeons) has been used in our laboratory to examine similar questions. Like some of the perceptual work in human information processing, we have asked whether a pigeon needs more time to examine two aspects of a compound stimulus than it takes to examine either aspect alone. The stimuli are vertical or horizontal white lines on a pecking key, or fully illuminated keys (either red or blue), or both the line and color at the same time. If either element is presented alone, it is followed by a test

of the two values on the relevant dimension. If the compound is presented (i.e., both line and color), then the animal is tested with either one dimension or the other. In the latter case, there is no prior information as to which dimension will be tested, and the animal must consequently process both to optimize performance. Maki, Leith, and Leuin have examined this question using both time and accuracy as the dependent variables (Maki and Leith 1973; Maki and Leuin, 1972). When time is used, a computerized version of the staircase psychophysical method is employed. When accuracy is used, various sample times are given either on the same day or on different days.

Results from these different procedures are substantially the same. It takes about twice as much time to store for later use values on two dimensions as it does a value on one dimension alone. (This is true when an intermediate criterion of performance—about 80 percent accuracy—is set.) Such results suggest serial processing of information. They are also quite consistent with the data from human research described by Lindsay (1970). Data from Maki and Leith's (1973) study are displayed in Figure 6.2, which shows percent correct responses for various sample times when the subjects are required to process one dimension (the open circles) and when they are required to process two dimensions (the closed circles). The assertion that it takes about twice as long to

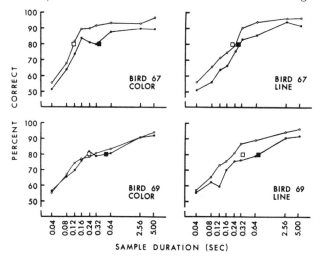

FIGURE 6.2 Matching to sample as a function of sample duration and number of features in the sample. For each bird the open circles show performance with one element only on the sample. The closed circles are for two elements (both line and color). The opened and closed squares are for element and compound samples, respectively, in an experiment by Maki and Leuin (1972) in which sample duration with a fixed criterion of 80%, rather than percent correct, was the dependent variable. From Maki and Leith (1973). Reproduced with permission from *Journal of the Experimental Analysis of Behavior* 19: 347. Copyright 1973 by the Society for the Experimental Analysis of Behavior, Inc.

process two dimensions as one comes from a comparison of the amounts of time needed to respond correctly on 80 percent of the trials when two dimensions are presented on the sample and when one dimension is presented on the sample. With shorter times or longer times, this relationship does not hold.

Two characteristics of these curves merit some comment. First, matching to elements is superior to matching to compounds, even at very short and very long sample times. Second, more looking time allows better matching, even with prolonged sample times. Why is the first observation of interest? In part because it says that even with only 40 msec of time, animals can extract some information from both dimensions—but not as much as from one. How do they do this? We do not know, but perhaps part of the answer may be that they can examine persisting sensory processes. Next, how at these very brief times do they extract information from both samples? Clearly they are not processing partial information in parallel, for two-dimension performance is not twice as good as one. Nor does it seem likely that they are pure serial processors, unless one is willing to entertain dimension-switching speeds so rapid that some testing on each dimension and switching can all occur in 40 msec. An examination of sensory aftereffects may perhaps also prove relevant to such speculations. One bit of evidence that it may comes from some exploratory work we have done to solve another problem. D'Amato and Worsham (1972) have reported that monkeys can perform almost perfectly on delayed matching-to-sample problems with a 40-msec sample. Perhaps, we thought (because our birds performed so poorly), our apparatus is different from D'Amato and Worsham's. To get a quick check on this problem, Lee Greene ran two graduate students as subjects in our apparatus. They performed almost perfectly with a 20-msec sample and a 1-sec delay. If, however, a white mask immediately followed the sample, performance dropped to slightly above chance. If humans and perhaps monkeys can use the aftereffects of stimulation so well, why not pigeons? We don't know, but we think it an interesting question.

Why does increasing time improve performance? Apparently, even looking times of as long as 5 sec are better than looking times of 2 sec or 1 sec. One possible answer comes from research of Farthing and Opuda (1973), who showed in a very similar task that if a pigeon is allowed to peck a sample key ten times, as opposed to once, his performance improves markedly. Now, our procedure does not require the bird to peck the sample key, but I can assure you that the bird does peck. Consequently, we have no way as yet of distinguishing looking times from the number of times the bird pecks the key. Whether Farthing and Opuda, by varying the number of pecks, were varying looking time, and looking time is the critical variable, or whether our paradigm which varies looking time is merely allowing more pecks, cannot be determined from the data that exist at the moment.

In evaluating Blough's paradigm I suggested that it does not readily distinguish response-competition effects from attentional effects. Our paradigm seems superior in this respect, for it does not present the animal with conflicting instructions in the test. Like Blough, we can give extensive testing with one dimension only to see if we get comparable selective attention effects—free, presumably, of possible response-competition interpretations. An experiment by Leith and Maki has done just this and has found, with extensive testing of just one of the two dimensions, that for the training dimension, performance improves both on element and on compound performance but the difference between them decreases (that is, the animal seems to be showing an attentional effect). On return to the standard condition in which both dimensions may be tested following a compound sample, the neglected dimension deteriorates to about the same extent that the attended dimension improves. Curiously enough, all of the improvement occurs at the longer sample times. It seems that animals always check both dimensions to some extent, perhaps merely because values on both vary from trial to trial, but it is only with an opportunity for relatively complete processing that selective-attention effects come into play.

Like Blough's experiment, this general approach appears to have considerable promise for studying simple cognitive functioning and information processing in animals. This procedure may be superior to Blough's in that it eliminates the response-competition factor to which I have previously alluded. On the other hand, Blough's task, formidable as it seems, may be simpler for animals such as pigeons to master than the matching-to-sample task. Lest anyone suffer from any illusions, however, I should hasten to say that both of these procedures are enormously expensive in terms of experimenter time. If they have a serious disadvantage, that is it.

In the matching-to-sample task, reduction in sample time correspondingly reduced successful performance. Possibly the lower performance with briefer samples reflects incomplete processing (that is, on some trials the processes involved in registration, encoding, and storage for subsequent use may not be completed because of the too brief sample time). Consequently, performance for any given sample time will represent different mixtures of completed and noncompleted tasks. Inferences about the locus of a selective-attention effect or other cognitive factors in such a situation may turn out to be exceedingly complex. It is for this reason that I was particularly interested to learn recently of the adaptation of Sternberg's (1966) high-speed memory-scan task, for in this task analysis is restricted to trials on which these processes *are* complete.

In its simplest form, Sternberg's general paradigm is as follows: The subject is required to memorize a small set of the possible digits from zero to nine; then on different trials he is presented with a digit which is either a member of the set or not a member of the set. Payoffs are weighted to emphasize high accuracy (i.e., completed processes), and errors are held to one to two percent. Major experimental variables include the number of items in the memorized set; whether the test item is a member of the set or not; whether the test stimulus is presented in intact form or degraded form; possible mental operations that a subject may be required to perform (such as adding one to each test item before searching the memory set); and of course the other variables that an experimenter might employ to influence the memory search (such as instructions to attend selectively to some items at the expense of others or to look for certain sorts of items in memory search).

The logic of Sternberg's experiment demands, at the minimum, a 2 × 2 factorial design. If two factors are shown to be additive, then they are held to affect different processes; if they are interactive, the inference is made that they affect the same stage. A typical result is that the average increase in reaction time for each additional item in the memory subset is constant. That is, if one item takes 300 msec and two items take 340 msec, then three items will take 380 msec and four items will take 420 msec. The assumed meaning of this simple additive result is that the test stimulus is compared sequentially with each of the items in the memory set. Typically, if the subject is presented with a test item not in the memory set, reaction time is slightly slower. But the effects are again linear. The fact that the negative set function parallels the positive set function permits the inference that only after search is completed does the subject make a decision as to whether the test item was or was not in the memory set. A negative decision for whatever reason takes slightly longer than a positive decision. Because these linear functions parallel each other, we can make the additional inference that the process is exhaustive rather than self-terminating; that is, the subject searches through the entire set before making a decision. Were this not the case, the function for positive test items would be flatter than for negative test items.

Suppose one finds an interaction between two factors, as, for example, between the number of possible alternative stimuli that are known by the subject to be in the total set and whether the stimulus is degraded or intact. (Such an interaction does indeed exist.) Sternberg would interpret this to mean that the effects of the number of alternatives and of stimulus degradation work on the same part or stage of the process. The logic of this argument should be clear. If degradation and the number of alternatives affect different processing stages, then the degradation of the stimulus should add to the effects of a small number of stimulus-response alternatives in the same way that it adds to a large number. The fact that it does not indicates that the degrading effects become more and more manifest as the uncertainty of the stimulus increases. Apparently both operations influence encoding.

This rather lengthy introduction may have been unnecessary for most readers, but it is essential if one is to appreciate the importance of Eddy's (1973) contribution, for he has adapted the Sternberg paradigm to monkeys and has obtained reaction-time data from stumptail macaques which show memory-search effects analogous to those reported by Sternberg. Eddy's monkeys were tested in a delayed matching-to-sample test. The memory set consisted of one, two, or three of four possible colors. The monkey could examine each item in a memory set in succession, determining the appearance of the next one by pressing a center panel. After the last item in the set appeared, there was a 500-msec interval, followed by two test items on lower side panels. If the animal pressed the panel associated with the correct item, he received a food reward.

Figure 6.3 shows results for two of his animals, with

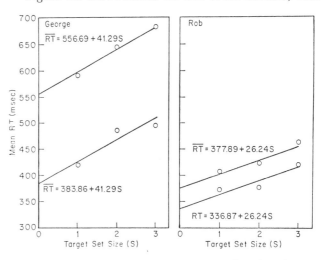

FIGURE 6.3 Mean correct reaction time as a function of target size and response window for two stumptail macaques. In each case the lower line represents the reaction times to the preferred windows; the upper lines are reaction times to the nonpreferred windows. Best-fitting, simultaneous lines having two intercepts and one slope are shown for each subject. From Eddy (1973). Reproduced with permission.

reaction time increasing linearly as a function of memory-set size. The data presented here are special in one sense: these two animals had position preferences. After finishing pressing the memory-set panel, they would wait in front of one of the two test panels until the test item appeared. If the item was correct, the animal pressed that panel. If not, the animal would press the other side. Because these two animals had strong position preferences, the press on the other side may be interpreted to mean that they had reached the decision that the item was not on their preferred side (that is, they had examined that test stimulus, searched their memory set, and arrived at a negative conclusion). The difference between the lower and upper curve for each animal, then, may be taken to represent the difference between a positive and a negative decision plus the time that the animal needs to get from one key to the other. The data, however, clearly support the hypothesis of an exhaustive search of memory for each sample. There are, of course, other possible interpretations, but the data are remarkably regular and this seems a reasonable interpretation. These are exciting data. They suggest the possibility of making detailed analyses of information processing in animals using much the same method now widely employed in human studies. They offer an opportunity for precisely pinpointing the stage in the information process at which the selective-attention effect in our paradigm occurs.

I am not quite sure what people interested in the neural basis of learning should do with the facts I have described. However, approaches such as those I have outlined hold the promise of a comparative psychology of information processing that will be able to discuss, not how much one species can learn relative to another, but how animals take in and use information and whether the processes have the same stages and the same interrelationships in different species.

ACKNOWLEDGMENT

Research for this paper was supported by NIMH research grant MH22153. I would also like to acknowledge with thanks conversations with Leo Postman and Saul Sternberg which have clarified my thinking on various issues discussed in this paper.

REFERENCES

ATKINSON, R. C., and SHIFFRIN, R. M. 1968. Human memory. A proposed system and its control processes. In K. W. Spence and J. T. Spence, eds., *The Psychology of Learning and Motivation*, Vol. 2. New York: Academic Press, pp. 89–195.

BLOUGH, D. S. 1969. Attention shifts in a maintained discrimination. *Science* 166: 125–126.

BLOUGH, D. S. 1972. Recognition by the pigeon of stimuli varying in two dimensions. *Journal of the Experimental Analysis of Behavior* 18: 345–367.

CRAIK, F. I. M., and LOCKHART, R. S. 1972. Levels of processing: A framework for memory research. *Journal of Verbal Learning and Verbal Behavior* 11: 671–684.

CRAIK, F. I. M., and WATKINS, M. J. 1973. The role of rehearsal in short-term memory. *Journal of Verbal Learning and Verbal Behavior* 12: 599–607.

D'AMATO, M. R., and WORSHAM, R. W. 1972. Delayed matching in the capuchin monkey with brief sample durations. *Learning and Motivation* 3: 304–312.

EDDY, D. R. 1973. Memory processes in *Macaca speciosa*: Mental processes revealed by reaction-time experiments. Unpublished Ph.D. dissertation, Carnegie-Mellon University.

ESTES, W. K. 1973. Phonemic coding and rehearsal in short-term memory for letter strings. *Journal of Verbal Learning and Verbal Behavior* 12: 360–372.

FARTHING, G. W., and OPUDA, M. J. 1973. Selective attention in matching-to-sample in pigeons. Paper presented at the Eastern Psychological Association meetings, Washington, D. C., May 1973.

GLUCKSBERG, S., and LAUGHERY, K. R. 1965. Sequential memory as a function of total time of information exposure and availability of information processing strategies. In *Proceedings of the 73rd annual convention of the American Psychological Association*, pp. 79–80.

KEPPEL, G., and UNDERWOOD, B. J. 1962. Proactive inhibition in short-term retention of single items. *Journal of Verbal Learning and Verbal Behavior* 1: 153–161.

KROLL, N. E. A., PARKS, T., PARKINSON, S. R., BIEBER, S. L., and JOHNSON, A. L. 1970. Short term memory while shadowing. Recall of visually and orally presented letters. *Journal of Experimental Psychology* 85: 220–224.

LINDSAY, P. H. 1970. Multichannel processing in perception. In D. I. Mostovsky, ed., *Attention: Contemporary Theory and Analysis*. New York: Appleton-Century-Crofts, pp. 149–171.

MAKI, Jr., W. S., and LEITH, C. R. 1973. Shared attention in pigeons. *Journal of the Experimental Analysis of Behavior* 19: 345–349.

MAKI, Jr., W. S., and LEUIN, T. C. 1972. Information processing by pigeons. *Science* 176: 535–536.

MELTON, A. W. 1970. Short- and long-term postperceptual memory: Dichotomy or continuum? In K. Pribram and D. E. Broadbent, eds., *Biology of Memory*. New York: Academic Press, pp. 3–5.

PETERSON, L. R., and JOHNSON, S. T. 1971. Some effects of minimizing articulation in short-term retention. *Journal of Verbal Learning and Verbal Behavior* 10: 346–354.

SCHULMAN, H. G. 1972. Semantic confusion errors in short-term memory. *Journal of Verbal Learning and Verbal Behavior* 11: 221–227.

STERNBERG, S. 1966. High speed scanning in human memory. *Science* 153: 652–654.

STOFF, M., and EAGLE, M. N. 1971. The relationship among reported strategies, presentation rate, and verbal ability and their effects on free recall learning. *Journal of Experimental Psychology* 87: 423–428.

TELL, P. M. 1972. The role of certain acoustic and semantic factors at short and long retention intervals. *Journal of Verbal Learning and Verbal Behavior* 11: 455–464.

WARRINGTON, E. K., and WEISKRANTZ, L. 1970. Amnesic syndrome: Consolidation or retrieval? *Nature* 228: 628–630.

WARRINGTON, E. K., and WEISKRANTZ, L. 1971. Organizational aspects of memory in amnesic patients. *Neuropsychologia* 9: 67–73.

WICKELGREN, W. A. 1973. The long and short of memory. *Psychological Bulletin* 6: 425–439.

WICKENS, D. D. 1970. Encoding categories of words: An empirical approach to meaning. *Psychological Review* 77: 1–15.

Neural Modeling
and Memory

7

Neural Models and Memory

MICHAEL A. ARBIB, WILLIAM L. KILMER, AND D. NICO SPINELLI

ABSTRACT This paper tries to provide an overall framework for thinking about the problem of memory. It thus starts with a review of the notion of an "internal model of the world" as providing the necessary memory structure for an adaptive system which must interact with a complex world. Then, within this general framework, it analyzes a number of models of the ways in which a neuron will change its behavior (as well as its connections) over time on the basis of its input-output history and assesses how, given the adaptive nature of its neurons, a network must be structured if the cooperative effect of change in the individual neurons is to yield improvement, in some sense, of the function of the overall network.

Two basic schemes for neural learning that are reviewed are the perceptron scheme, in which the behavior of neurons changes as a result of reinforcement, and the Hebb scheme, which is a scheme of "learning without a teacher." We show how the Hebb scheme can be adapted to explain some of the effects of early visual experience upon the connections in cat visual cortex. The companion paper by Cowan shows how the Hebb model may be used to explain some adaptation phenomena.

Since one of the most fascinating aspects of animal memory is the widely different types of learning of which different animals are capable, we provide a study of "Why Rats Can't Learn Birdsong"—both by assessing ethological elements that delineate the reasons for some of the species-specific learning capacities, and by looking at a theory of computation in neural networks which shows how the structure of a network may limit the tasks that it is capable of performing, no matter what plastic changes in the individual neurons may occur. Finally, we look at some of the beautiful neuroanatomy of the hippocampus, which has long been known to play a pivotal role in the process of relating sensory and motor events, and has been implicated by many workers in memory processes. Unfortunately, in a system as far from the periphery as the hippocampus, the significance of the input and output firing patterns is virtually unknown, and its anatomy has proved something of a Rorschach test for neural modelers. Nonetheless, we review a number of models which are consistent with the known anatomy, and which provide important concepts for those who would try to design experiments and to explore change within this fascinating neural system.

Our basic aim here is to analyze models that bridge the gap between studies of changes in the behavior or overall function of an organism (the psychology of learning) and the study of changes in properties of neurons (as afforded by the neuroanatomy of synaptic change and single-cell neurophysiology). We seek to understand how the brain enables an organism to interact with its world in an adaptive way.

In trying to provide a perspective on neural models and memory, we might have adopted any one of the following strategies:

i. To provide an exhaustive review of models of neural nets;

ii. To review models of different parts of the brain, and suggest ways in which they might be refined by incorporating memory mechanisms; or

iii. To provide a "top-down" approach, in which a major effort is placed on what memory models *should* do, rather than review what current models can do.

Our strategy is a compromise between (i) and (iii): Sections 7.1 and 7.3 provide a perspective of kind (iii), while the other sections provide a fragment of the exhaustive review called for under (i). Special attention is given to neural modification in visual cortex, to ethological evidence for learning predispositions, and to models of hippocampal adaptation.

7.1 A PERSPECTIVE

If a neural network is to change its overall behavior, individual neurons of the network must change, at least in their connections. Thus the problem of training a network can be broken, somewhat crudely, into two parts:

1. What formulas describe the way in which a neuron will change its behavior (including its connections) over time on the basis of its input-output history? (I.e., how may we represent a neuron as an adaptive system?)

2. Given the adaptive nature of its neurons, how must a network be structured if the cooperative effect of change in the individual neurons is to yield improvement, in some sense, of the function of the overall network?

Of course, these questions reflect but two levels in a hierarchy. The neurochemist will ask what changes in membrane/transmitter/DNA/RNA characteristics cooperate to yield the neuronal changes of (1); and the neuropsychologist must seek to characterize what constitutes adaptive change in one brain region when it only affects the organism's overt behavior in concert with

MICHAEL A. ARBIB, WILLIAM L. KILMER, and D. NICO SPINELLI, Computer and Information Science, and Center for Systems Neuroscience, University of Massachusetts, Amherst, MA

many other brain regions (as will be suggested by our brief mention of Luria below). We focus on (1) in Section 7.2 and (2) in Section 7.3. Then in Section 7.4 we commingle the two questions as we examine learning schemes posited for hippocampus. (For a more general perspective on neural modeling, less focused on memory problems, see Arbib, 1975).

It is inadequate to view an organism as simply responding to a succession of stimuli; rather, the internal state of the organism will determine, in great part, to what it will attend (its input) and how it will act upon its environment (its output). An organism, then, must also *model* the salient features of its environment and place its activity in the context of dynamic interaction. Below, we shall develop the "slide-box" metaphor for internal models, which—with its picture of many slides continually interacting and being updated, with no single locus of exclusive serial processing—will serve to emphasize our need to understand how computations can take place in a highly parallel network of dynamically interacting subsystems. Such an understanding may also help us probe the effect of brain damage upon behavior.

In 1929 Karl Lashley published *Brain Mechanisms and Intelligence*, in which he reported that the impairment in maze-running behavior caused by removing portions of a rat's cortex did not seem to depend on what part of the cortex was removed. He thus formulated two "laws": *the "law" of mass action* (that damage depends on the amount of brain removed), and *the "law" of equipotentiality* (that every part of the brain can make the same contribution to problem solving). Such data have seemed to many irreconcilable with any view of the brain as a precise computing network, but we may effect a reconciliation if we stress (with Luria; see below) the notion of a computation involving the cooperation of many subroutines that work simultaneously and in parallel. Often, a computation can be effected by a subset of the routines. In general, removing subroutines will lower efficiency, though for some tasks the missing subroutines may be irrelevant, so that their removal saves the system from wasting time on them when other tasks are to be done.

Thus equipotentiality is really only valid if we use rather gross measurements of changes in behavior; the underlying reality would seem to be that the removal of various subsystems can make quite different contributions to the level of performance on a given task. The brain theorist may thus find intriguing the notion of *neuroheuristic programming*, i.e., structuring a heuristic program in terms of concurrently active subsystems, with anatomical correlates. In this context it is worth recalling Luria's (1973) statement that the concept of localization of function has come to refer to a network of complex dynamic structures or combination centers, consisting of mosaics of distant points of the nervous system, united in a common task. Function is understood to be a complex and plastic system performing a particular adaptive task and composed of a highly differentiated group of interchangeable elements. The fact that the elements are interchangeable would allow transfer of function to occur. He goes on to state that the smooth execution of each act or function requires a series of both simultaneously and successively excited connections.

One of Luria's case studies was of a woman who had lesions, probably bilateral, involving predominantly the parieto-occipital region. She could neither copy letters of the alphabet nor write them from dictation, but she was able to write letters if they were included in whole, well-assimilated words. She could also write the alphabet correctly. In our computer jargon, we might say that the patient could no longer go from the name of a subroutine to its entry point, but could still use the subroutine in those programs that already included the entry point, rather than requiring explicit generation of the entry point each time the routine was required. The vividness of this metaphor encourages our interest in developing models of distributed computation appropriate to brain function.

Within this general context, we may now consider the memory structures required by any system that is to be capable of perception. For example, a human knows that if he presses his hands in a downward direction at a fairly high velocity toward a rectangular surface (a table top) that he has sensed only visually, his hands will not go through the surface, and a noise will ensue. But it is no trivial task to program a computer to take such little visual information and make predictions not only about the trajectory (which it could do with its effectors), but also about the resultant feedback, constraints, and sound. Such predictions are the essence of perception: extrapolating from partial sensory information to information about modalities other than those sensed that will be relevant to action.

Here, then, is the by now well-known idea of a long-term model of the world (see, e.g., Craik, 1943; Gregory, 1969), something which tells us that when we see surfaces of a certain kind, they are associated with certain textures, feelings, constraints on action, etc. We further posit a short-term memory containing information representing our model of the *current* state of the environment. Thus, instead of every millisecond having to recognize the scene anew, we notice only discrepancies, and use this greatly reduced information flow to update the short-term model that guides our activities. It is the long-term model, in turn, which allows us to build up these short-term models, using partial information to gain access to far more information relevant to action. (This is an *analysis-by-synthesis* view of perception.)

Our crucial thesis is that perception is inseparable from memory, which in turn is meaningless without reference to the action of the organism—or, more properly, the interaction of the organism with its environment. Perception can be seen as the construction of a partially predictive internal (short-term) model, using long-term memory to incorporate information about action possibilities and about sensory information from modalities besides those cuing. Perception is *dynamic*, both in that current information tends to be treated in the context of an existent short-term model, and also in that the extant model "unfolds" with time.

Clearly, then, information—save at such high levels as are involved in human linguistic activity—must be continually referred to what we shall call the *action frame*, namely, the frame of reference induced by the postural and effector mechanisms of the organism, the former serving to stabilize the frame offered by the latter. The repertoire of possible actions of an organism, and of possible questions it may ask, helps to determine the most appropriate neural representation of information. In particular, the organism may encode stimuli in different ways on different occasions depending on the questions prevailing at the time.

Perhaps some more insight into our notions of models of the world may be gained by a metaphor drawn from the making of movie cartoons (Arbib, 1972). Drawing each frame individually is too inefficient, and so instead, use is made of the layering technique. For example, a whole minute of the cartoon might go by without the background changing, so one could draw it just once. Or, in the middle ground, there might be a tree about which nothing particularly changes during a certain period of time except its position relative to the background. It could thus be drawn on a separate layer, which could then be displaced for succeeding frames. Finally, in the foreground, one might well be able to draw most portions of the actors for repeated use, and then position the arms, facial expressions, etc., individually for each frame. The layers can then be photographed appropriately by positioning them in a slide box for each frame, with only a few parameter changes and minimal redrawing required between frames.

A similar strategy for obtaining a very economical description of what happens over a long period of time might be used in the brain, with a long-term memory (LTM) corresponding to the slide file and short-term memory (STM) corresponding to the slide box. The act of perception might then be compared to using sensory information to retrieve appropriate slides from the file to replace or augment those already in the slide box, experimenting to decide whether a newly retrieved slide fits sensory input "better" than one currently in the slide box. Also, part of the action of the organism in changing its relationship with the environment might be viewed as designed to obtain input that will help update the STM, by deciding between "competing" slides, as well as helping update the LTM, by "redrawing" and "editing" the slides.

The theory and modeling that will occupy us in the rest of the paper focuses on neural adaptation in circumscribed regions of the brain. The fact that we shall close with little feeling for how to "wire up" a neural "slide-box system" is a measure of how much further we have to go if we are to understand the neural mechanisms of memory (but see note added in proof, p. 132). Time and again we shall be struck by the question of how changes which should be effected at the level of organismic behavior can in fact be yielded by appropriate changes at the neural level. To put it in crude terms, we should continually ask ourselves, *"What is in it for the neuron?"* Unfortunately, we shall be able to do little more than suggest how synaptic changes might be able to yield adaptive changes in the behavior of a single neural network—the other levels of discussion must be left to other papers in this volume. However, before we turn to the organizational principles that give meaning to the overall behavior within which the activity of such neural networks must be imbedded, it is perhaps worth noting that vertebrate strategies of learning by the *organism* may be *essentially* different from those of invertebrates. Thus studies of learning in such invertebrate preparations as *Aplysia* may only contribute to mammalian studies at the level of determining the mechanisms of neural modification, rather than at the level of seeing how such modifications may contribute to change in network behavior. Even at the level of component mechanisms, we may run into some trouble since one may caricature the difference between invertebrates and mammals by stressing the uniqueness of cells in *Aplysia* and the essentially layered structure of cell *tissues* in mammals. However, it may be that the visual systems of fly and octopus provide an appropriate bridge between the two.

One final comment needs to be made about the problem of *level*, as we try to relate the overall function of an organism to changes in the individual neurons: there is quite obviously a gross difference in time scale, in that a human may learn complex intellectual structures on a scale from seconds to years, whereas the individual actions of neurons are on a millisecond scale. We shall get *some* feel for this when we look at the convergence schemes for perceptrons in the next section, but it must be stressed that a full understanding of human learning cannot proceed without ideas whose faint glimmerings are seen in the data structures being evolved by workers in artificial intelligence (e.g., Schank and Colby, 1973).

7.2 TWO BASIC SCHEMES FOR NEURAL LEARNING

In this section we shall study two mathematical models of neural change. To focus the discussion we consider the system shown in Figure 7.1. The *preprocessor* is a mechanism that extracts from the environmental input a set of d real numbers. The set will be called a pattern, and the numbers will be called components of the pattern. The *pattern recognizer* then takes the pattern and produces a response which may have any of N distinct values, where there are N categories into which the patterns must be sorted.

The two classic learning schemes for McCulloch-Pitts-type formal neurons are the Hebb (1949) scheme (strengthen an active synapse if the efferent neuron fires) and the perceptron scheme of Rosenblatt (1961) (strengthen an active synapse if the efferent neuron fails when it should have fired; weaken an active synapse if the efferent neuron fires when it should not have fired).

The Hebb scheme has been elaborated by Brindley (1969), whose ideas have been developed by Marr (1969, 1970, 1971) in models of cerebellum, hippocampus (see Section 7.4), and neocortex. Marr's models provide ingenious mechanisms of codon selection, adjustment for level of background activity, etc. While these constitute an important contribution to our growing array of tools for the *synthesis* of neural networks with specified properties, we remain skeptical of their value as an *analysis* of the given regions of brain. Grossberg has made many studies of learning networks, with components ranging from the neural to the psychological, which make rich contact with studies of conditioning and of motivation (e.g., Grossberg, 1972). Kilmer and Olinski's 1974 study of learning in hippocampus (Section 7.4) is especially interesting for its use of developmental stages in tuning up the system.

The Hebb model has also been used by von der Malsburg (1973; see also Perez, Glass, and Schlear, 1975) in his model of the development of line detectors

in cat visual cortex. He uses a normalization rule and lateral inhibition to stop the first "experience" from "taking over" all "learning circuits"; these were used earlier by Spinelli (1970) in his OCCAM model of spinal-cord-like circuitry for an associative memory. In fact, Hirsch and Spinelli (1970) have shown that cat visual cortex is not restricted to line detectors, but can take the imprint of a specific visual experience, at least if the kitten sees only one or two things. We shall consider the work of Spinelli and von der Malsburg in Section 7.2.1.

The perceptron model was put on a firm mathematical footing by Block (1962) and has been embedded in a good textbook treatment of *Learning Machines* by Nilsson (1965). We shall study the perceptron convergence theorem in Section 7.2.2. Minsky and Papert (1969) have shifted attention from convergence questions to "What can a given network learn?," a question that has an interesting relationship to the network-complexity studies of Winograd (1965) and Spira (1969). We shall place their work in the context of network predisposition in Section 7.3.2.

The hologram as a mechanism for associative memory, and the whole range of Fourier optics, has provided much stimulus for neural modelers, although we shall not develop it in detail here (see, for example, Gabor, Kock, and Stroke, 1971; Willshaw, Buneman, and Longuet-Higgins, 1969; Kohonen, 1971; and Westlake, 1970). However, we think that those who, like Pribram (1974) or Pollen and Taylor (1974), expect the whole gamut of mathematical techniques to carry over from optics to neural nets—"the visual system makes a Fourier transform"—are mistaken. Such a view seems ill suited to handle our ability to perceive the world as made up of independently moving objects. Again, the reconstructibility of the hologram differs from our act of perception as a preparation to act, as distinct from a means of storing a veridical image. Blakemore, Campbell, and others have stressed the role of spatial frequency in the visual system (e.g., Blakemore, Nachmias, and Sutton, 1970; Campbell and Robson, 1968); but it seems to us that while frequency can provide cues (e.g., for texture) that augment cues such as contour, a total frequency transform is not made prior to "pattern recognition." However, we shall not develop the holography theme further in this article.

7.2.1 Learning without a teacher

In this section we consider Hebb-type schemes in which synaptic weights are adjusted without explicit reinforcement.

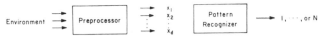

FIGURE 7.1 Environmental energies are transduced by the preprocessor into a pattern $(x_1, x_2, \ldots, x_d)$, which provides the input to the pattern recognizer, which in turn classifies the pattern into one of N classes.

EXPERIMENTS ON VISUAL MEMORY. It has been recently discovered that by limiting the visual experience of kittens to one or two simple visual patterns, it is possible to "fill up" their visual cortex with receptive fields whose shapes resemble the patterns in one or more details; some receptive fields are even recognizable, though blurred, representations of the image seen by the cat (see Chapter 18, this volume). Atrophy from disuse or misuse of visual mechanisms is well known in the clinic. Moreover, the experiments of Hubel and Wiesel (1962, 1970) have shown that monocular suturing of the eyelids or squint causes loss of binocularity of cells in the visual cortex of cats, whereas binocular suturing does not. These findings combine to suggest that by having kittens view a pattern of (three, say) vertical lines through one eye and a pattern of horizontal lines through the other during the critical period of development, one might be able to cause loss of binocularity for cells with vertically and horizontally oriented receptive fields as they are fed discordant information. To rephrase: the vertically exposed eye is expected to have a "hole" in the distribution of orientations for verticals. Appropriate "holes" in the behavioral repertoire, testing one eye at a time, should betray the function of the missing units.

The effects that this simple procedure has on the functional properties of visual-cortex cells are of astonishing magnitude (Hirsch and Spinelli, 1970, 1971). There are, in fact, only two types of units in the visual cortex of a kitten so deprived:

1. *Units uncommitted to specific visual features.* These units do not have a receptive field mappable by Spinelli's automated method and do not show any selectivity to lines and edges under manual control.

2. *Units with elongated receptive fields.* There are only two orientations. Units with vertical orientation can be mapped and respond to vertical lines only through the eye that has seen the three vertical bars; units with horizontal orientation can be mapped and respond to horizontal lines only through the eye that has seen the three horizontal bars.

Even more astounding are a few units with receptive fields that look like a carbon copy of the stimuli viewed during development! This almost photographic reproduction of images seen by the kittens weeks before suggested to Hirsch and Spinelli that they might be dealing with memory traces. Three possibilities had then to be examined:

1. The various classes of receptive fields one finds in the adult are genetically preprogrammed. Presence at birth, maturation after birth, or the necessity of environmental stimulation for the genome to express itself, are all subsumed in this hypothesis and can in various de-grees appear either in the same species for various classes of units or in different species. The hypothesis can then be made that the unstimulated units atrophy, fail to mature, or are not expressed. This hypothesis demands clear and predictable behavioral deficits from the kittens described above. It also predicts that once the damage is done, it should be permanent, i.e., letting the kittens have further, normal experiences after the critical period should not change the physiological picture. Furthermore, the set of available classes can be reduced but not *changed*.

2. Cells are genetically preprogrammed as in (1); however, during the critical period partial or total re-programming under environmental control can take place if needed. This would insure that the animal has feature detectors optimal for the environment in which it finds itself, and that it at least has the set of detectors that has proved most helpful to its species through natural selection. The transience of the critical period would be an advantage since it would be impossible for the rest of the brain to interpret information from de-tectors whose coding properties change over time (cf. Kilmer's core vs. noncore scheme for training hippo-campal circuitry, in Section 7.4). This hypothesis has essentially the same predictions as the one above, i.e., clear behavioral deficits for tasks that demand nonex-isting detectors and permanence of the physiological effects; however, it differs in that, even though there are limits, it allows for the property of generating receptive fields totally different from the ones originally prepro-grammed.

3. This might be called a memory hypothesis, i.e., that there are no genetically programmed detectors: what is programmed is an adaptive network capable of storing, in a very direct fashion, elementary visual experiences. The receptive-field shapes one maps in an adult cat would thus be bits and pieces of what the animal has seen in its past. This hypothesis predicts changes in the physiological picture, if new experiences are allowed, and also predicts no behavioral deficits, or perhaps only slight ones, since learning capacity does decrease with age.

In real life, of course, these three possibilities would be present in various ratios, depending on the animal.

Shortly after the Spinelli-Hirsch experiment appeared in the literature, Blakemore and Cooper (1970) pub-lished a similar experiment, though with notable dif-ferences. They raised two kittens in the dark except for a few hours every day when one kitten was put in a cylinder painted with vertical stripes and the other in one with horizontal stripes. Recording from the visual cortex after development showed that cells responded best to vertical lines, or lines close to vertical, in the vertically exposed kitten and to horizontal lines, or close to it, in the horizontally exposed kitten. Units were binocularly activated.

It is Spinelli's working hypothesis at this time that the experience-shaped receptive-field map represents nothing less than the engram for which Lashley searched in vain so long ago: to prove or disprove this hypothesis vis-à-vis other possible interpretations, and to understand the adaptive structure that brings it about, is the goal of his ongoing experiments. We now turn to models related to this phenomenon.

MODELS OF VISUAL MEMORY. Spinelli's (1970) OCCAM (a computer model for an Omnium-gatherum Core Content-Addressable Memory in the central nervous system) suggests a scheme for how memories might be multiply stored in discrete neural networks. The basic neural circuit is reminiscent of spinal mechanisms: there a specific, prewired input pattern (e.g., an itch) elicits a specific, prewired behavior (e.g., a scratch reflex). In OCCAM things are similarly organized except that both the input and the output pattern are arbitrary and determined by experience. Furthermore, the model specifies how inputs "find their way" to the appropriate memory trace; i.e., the OCCAM networks are *content-addressable*. Very little, if any, preprocessing of sensory activity is assumed. The model posits that the simplest and safest thing for an organism to do is to "store" information as it arrives, with the "selection" of "meaningful" stimuli accomplished by biasing memory at the time of action. Anything can thus become important and facilitate its own subset of memories.

Consider, then, the memory networks of Figure 7.2, addressed in parallel by stimuli entering the CNS. We shall see how they may form a content-addressable memory, wherein providing the system with part of a chunk of information will enable the system to play back the whole chunk.

The different columns are connected by collaterals from receiving cells and match cells which carry lateral inhibition to other input cells in nearby networks. It is assumed that only one interneuron per column is active at any time, and that different temporal segments of a pattern will be switched in a regular fashion through different interneurons. (In motor nerves, where individual fibers fire at about 10 per second, smooth contractions are obtained by regular phasing in and out of motor units.) A crucial assumption is that the synaptic conductivity tends in the limit to be directly proportional to the activity going through the synaptic junction itself, so that if a given quantity of activity is presented to the same synapse over and over again, an asymptote will be reached such that the conductivity will represent faithfully the amount of activity that produced it.

We then assume that whenever a synaptic connection is activated, the amount of excitatory potential generated is proportional to the synaptic conductivity (not to the activity that has generated it). If a temporal pattern is presented to a network repeatedly, it will be stored in the synaptic conductivity of the interneurons, which will thus cause the output cell to play out a better simulacrum of the input pattern.

The match-cell output provides a measure of correlation in the activity of the input cell and the output cell from which it receives collaterals. The pattern is presented to all networks in parallel. But eventually one cell will have a somewhat better adjustment than its neighbors, the activity in its match cell will rise and (thanks to the lateral-inhibition mechanism) turn down the input to nearby networks—i.e., the network that gets ahead, by chance, draws the pattern to itself and prevents the other networks from learning it. The number of networks that learn the same pattern is thus determined by the extent of the lateral inhibition. To ensure that the lateral inhibition "gets there in time," it is assumed that each time a cell is activated, an afterdischarge occurs—and that the longer the afterdischarge, the more the synaptic conductivity will be changed. Thus the longer the afterdischarge, the faster the learning—and this afterdischarge will be cut off by lateral inhibition if another "column" has already learned the pattern.

When one or more patterns have been stored, it is desirable that if new patterns are to be stored, this be done by networks that have not been previously used. To do this a given match cell becomes harder to activate if its network has been used often before. Then a pattern would have above-chance effect on a network in which it is already stored, reasonable effect upon an "uncommitted" network, and little effect on a network containing a well-learned pattern.

Since a portion of a pattern correlates well with the

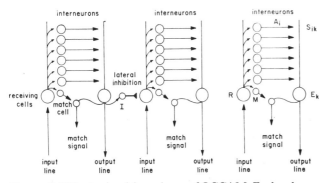

FIGURE 7.2 The basic wiring scheme of OCCAM. Each column learns a temporal sequence, with lateral inhibition blocking learning of a given sequence by too many columns.

whole output pattern, the match cell can signal which output cell is playing back the pattern of which the input is a fragment. A stimulus might then lead to the playing back of a sequence that includes both receiving the stimulus and making the adequate response. It should be pointed out that memory will also contain sequences in which the organism performed a response that led to undesirable consequences, and this is where the power of content-addressable memories comes in: a bias for the desired event will facilitate sequences that contain it. An acceptable match indicates what portion of the input pattern must match the output pattern for the correlation to be significant.

Pribram, Spinelli, and Kamback (1967) have suggested that presentation of a stimulus will generate a playback of the whole sequence: recognition of the stimulus; the appropriate behavior that goes with the stimulus; and finally expectation of the consequences of that behavior. The less stimulus presented, the more information there is in the playback, and the more risk there is in using it. (Of course, an animal might generate certain actions as an experiment to see if the present situation accords with the recalled details of the stimulus before reacting to the stimulus per se.) Ideally, then, the acceptable-match parameter should be set for the minimum value that allows unequivocal recognition of the stimulus, and thus the playback of the rest of that memory package containing information about what to do or not to do with it and what to expect.

The model assumes that while visual memory contains primarily visual information, it also contains enough nonvisual information to allow the readdressing of the system by the visually triggered memories so that auditory, somatic, gustatory, etc., strings are subsequently called into play. The internal addressing of the memory by internal states that would be part of the string—for example, hunger and the disappearance of hunger—would activate or facilitate all those memory strings containing such information, and therefore produce a partial level of match. This would then make available to the rest of the brain strings containing pertinent information about feeding behavior.

The following is the *key* to how such a memory structure can serve the adaptive behavior of the organism: If other parts of some strings are available in the environment, a higher level of match will be achieved for certain strings, and the connected behavior can then be played back if the acceptable level of match is reached or exceeded. Memory is thus continuously addressed by three agencies: internal states, external stimuli, and recently activated memories. It is the interplay of these three factors that gives behavior its continuity, variety, and purposefulness.

How would OCCAM differentiate patterns that are very similar but have different meanings? "Key" endings to the two patterns would of course make them different. Perhaps this is the way in which reinforcers act—behaviorally and neurally two patterns which may look identical are really different because their consequences, which are part of the same memory package, are different.

Reinforcers could also act to decrease lateral inhibition and increase learning speed, so that an organism would learn faster and more redundantly those strings whose information has survival value. Such reinforcers as pain and food might be permanently wired in, while others act on memory only through the software, as parts of existing programs or plans (see Pribram, 1969).

Whereas the OCCAM model of 1970 had a temporal-spatial converter to enable it to record temporal patterns, the von der Malsburg model (1973) is closer to the spirit of the results on visual-pattern memory mentioned earlier in this section. It was formulated to determine whether a simple circuit, possessing only a few characteristics of the cat's visual system, would organize itself into the "simple-cell" receptive-field patterns found by Hubel and Wiesel in area 17 of cat visual cortex, each cell having one preferred orientation to which it responds maximally. Von der Malsburg thought that genetically specified patterns of lateral excitatory and inhibitory influences in the geniculostriatal system might highly predispose this system toward its columnar organization. He also thought that a loose genetic specification of the details of the retinogeniculostriatal projection could be coupled with plastic synaptic mechanisms in the projection so as to enhance the columnar organizational tendencies of the striatal system.

His model to test these ideas consisted of a retina of 19 binary elements, a geniculostriatal manifold of 169 excitatory cells (E cells) and 169 inhibitory cells (I cells), interconnected according to a simple geometric specification. (The inhibitory interconnections serve much the same role as the lateral inhibition in OCCAM, with the E cells being both the "match cells" and the "output cells" since "recognition" rather than "temporal playback" is the task here.) The connection from each retinal cell A_i to each E cell E_k is through a Hebb synapse of strength S_{ik} which is modified by $\Delta S_{ik} > 0$ for each "modification time step" if A_i is active *and* if E_k fires. In this case the magnitude of ΔS_{ik} is proportional to the firing rate of E_k.

Given a suitable choice of units, the firing rate of any E or I cell is equal to the amount by which the excitation state H_k of the cell exceeds its threshold θ_k. Defining H_k^* as H_k if $(H_k - \theta_k) > 0$ and as 0 otherwise, the equation for H_k is

$$\frac{d}{dt} H_k(t) = -\alpha_k H_k(t) + \sum_{i=1}^{338} W_{ik} H_k^*(t) + \sum_{i=1}^{19} S_{ik} X_i(t),$$

where

α_k = decay constant of H_k,

W_{ik} = synaptic strength from E or I cell i to cell k,

$X_i(t)$ = 1 if A_i is active and 0 otherwise.

Since all ΔS_{ik} are positive, von der Malsburg had to renormalize his circuit to return $\sum_{i,k} S_{ik}$ to C (a constant) after each "modification time step" in order to keep his H_k bounded. He presented each retinal input with his model in a relaxed initial state, and then waited until all states H_k reached equilibrium (which always happened within about twenty steps) before he designated the next time step as a "modification time step."

He used nine different retinal inputs, each corresponding to a "line" of different orientation. He presented them in an appropriately mixed order, and after 100 modification times froze the ΔS_{ik} and checked the retinal input orientations that elicited maximal responses in each E cell. Figure 7.3 shows the result. The clustering of units responding to a given orientation is strikingly reminiscent of Hubel and Wiesel's columnar mapping results. Von der Malsburg's model actually did organize itself, with the help of a very restricted set of retinal inputs, because intially the preferred orientation map was chaotic and not at all like Figure 7.3. Though von der Malsburg got clusters of high E-cell activity from his intrinsic geniculostriatal dynamics before any S_{ik} adjustments were made, his high orientation specificity was accomplished by S_{ik} learning.

Von der Malsburg's model has rather severe limitations that are understood at this stage only qualitatively. His scheme is based on a highly restricted set of retinal inputs. His E-to-I and I-to-E influences are additive, nonplastic, and spatially arranged according to simple geometric rules. In reality, the brain's ubiquitous lateral connections must often convey signals that exert subtle logical effects (for example, in the frontal granular cortex of primates, where signals from all over the rest of the brain are brought together). Also von der Mals-

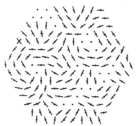

FIGURE 7.3 Each bar of this view onto the cortex indicates the optimal orientation of the E cell. Dots without a bar are cells that have never reacted to the standard set of stimuli. From von der Malsburg (1973).

burg does not use any evaluative criteria for changing his synaptic strengths, other than Hebb's rule which tends only to further entrench learning that has already occurred. His model could never, for example, reverse an already well learned response pattern.

Both the OCCAM and von der Malsburg schemes provide local, but multiply represented, storage. Both will store *whatever* comes in, not just the lines that von der Malsburg used in his test.

Lateral inhibition, which was not mentioned in the basic experiments of Hubel and Wiesel, plays a crucial role in the models, so that different "experiences" are stored in different units. In such systems feature detectors arise only to the extent that they respond to commonly occurring aspects of the animal's experience.

As new experimental findings accumulate, they will tell us how to merge the various models into one that will account for what is known. In the meantime models are a continuing source of inspiration for new experiments, and experiments are a continuing source of inspiration on how to improve models. This process of successive approximations is bringing us closer and closer to understanding how real brains work. Sharp theories and good experiments, combined with simulation to provide testability now that we can trace the effects of experience, will certainly unravel these adaptive neural networks that evolution took so long to develop.

7.2.2 The perceptron

In the terms of Figure 7.1, a pattern recognizer is a function $f: \mathbf{R}^d \to \{1, \ldots \mathcal{N}\}$. The points in $\mathbf{R}^d$ are thus grouped into at least $\mathcal{N}$ point sets, which we shall assume can be separated from each other by surfaces called *decision surfaces*. We shall assume for almost all points in $\mathbf{R}^d$ that a slight motion of the point does not change the category of the point. This is a valid assumption for most physical problems. The additional problem still exists of the category that is represented in more than one region of $\mathbf{R}^d$. For example, a, A, *a*, *A*, are all members of the category of the first letter of the English alphabet, but they would probably be found in different regions of a pattern space. In such cases it may prove to be necessary to establish a hierarchical system involving a computer apparatus that recognizes the subsets, and a separate system that recognizes that the subsets all belong to the same set. At any rate, let us avoid this problem by assuming that the decision space is divided into exactly $\mathcal{N}$ regions, eliminating split categories.

We call a function $g: \mathbf{R}^d \to \mathbf{R}$ a *discriminant function* if the equation $g(x) = 0$ gives the *decision surface* separating two regions of a pattern space. A basic problem of pattern recognition is the specification of such functions. Unfortunately it is virtually impossible for a human to "read out" the function he uses (not to mention *how* he uses it) to classify patterns. What, for example, is your intuitive idea of the appropriate surface to discriminate A's from B's? Thus a common strategy in pattern recognition is to provide a classification machine with an adjustable function and to "train" it with a set of patterns of known classification that are typical of those that the machine must ultimately classify. The function may be linear, quadratic, or polynomial depending on the complexity and shape of the pattern space and the necessary discriminations. Actually the experimenter is choosing a class of functions with adjustable parameters, which he hopes with proper adjustment will yield a function that will successfully classify any given pattern. For example, the experimenter may decide to use a linear function of the form

$$g(x) = w_1x_1 + w_2x_2 + w_3x_3 + \ldots + w_dx_d + w_{d+1}$$

in a two-category pattern classifier. The equation $g(x) = 0$ gives the decision surface, and thus training involves adjusting the coefficients $(w_1, w_2, \ldots, w_d, w_{d+1})$ so that the decision surface produces an acceptable separation of the two classes. We say that two categories are *linearly separable* if in fact an acceptable setting of such linear weights exists.

The reader may regard adaptive training as a case of the identification problem—it is as if we were trying to find a model of a black box that classifies the patterns on the basis of some samples of its input-output behavior.

Consider the case of a twofold classification effected by using a threshold logic unit (= McCulloch-Pitts neuron) to process the output of a set of binary feature detectors (Figure 7.4). We then have a set R of input lines (to be thought of as arranged in a rectangular "retina" onto which patterns may be projected) for a network which

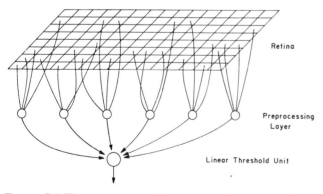

FIGURE 7.4 The perceptron wiring scheme. Connections from the retina to the preprocessing layer are fixed, but connections from the preprocessing layer to the linear threshold unit are variable via the adjustment scheme specified in the text.

consists of a single layer of neurons whose outputs feed into a threshold logic unit with adjustable weights. We want to analyze what classifications of input patterns can be realized by the firing or nonfiring of the output of such an array given different weight settings. Such a net is an example of what Rosenblatt (1961) calls a perceptron, a mechanism used to classify patterns on the retina into those which yield an output 1 and those which yield an output 0. The question asked by Rosenblatt and answered by many others since (an excellent review is in Nils Nilsson's monograph on *Learning Machines*) is: "Given a network, can we 'train' it to recognize a given set of patterns by using feedback on whether or not the network classifies a pattern correctly to adjust the 'weights' on various interconnections?"

The answers have mostly been of the following type: "If a setting exists which will give you your desired classification, I guarantee that my scheme will eventually yield a satisfactory setting of the weights."

We now give one of the perceptron convergence schemes. First some notation: With each predicate ψ we shall associate the binary function

$$\ulcorner\psi(x)\urcorner = \begin{cases} 1 & \text{if } \psi(x) \text{ is true,} \\ 0 & \text{if } \psi(x) \text{ is false.} \end{cases}$$

We recall, too, that for two vectors $\mathbf{x} = (x_1, \ldots, x_n)$ and $\mathbf{w} = (w_1, \ldots, w_n)$, we use $\mathbf{x} \cdot \mathbf{w}$ to represent the scalar product $(x_1w_1 + \ldots + x_nw_n)$.

Suppose, then, that there are d feature detectors in the preprocessing layer, so that the input to the linear threshold unit is a vector $\mathbf{x} = (x_1, \ldots, x_d)$. Let us augment $\mathbf{x}$ by adding a $(d+1)^{st}$ component set to 1 to obtain $\mathbf{y} = (x_1, \ldots, x_d, 1)$. Then if we let $\mathbf{w} = (w_1, \ldots, w_d, -\theta)$, which is the weight vector augmented by minus the threshold, we see that our equation for the response r of the unit can be abbreviated from

$$r = 1 \quad \text{iff} \quad \sum_{i=1}^{d} w_ix_i \geq \theta \quad \text{iff} \quad \sum_{i=1}^{d} w_ix_i - 1 \cdot \theta \geq 0$$

to the simple form

$$r = \ulcorner\mathbf{w} \cdot \mathbf{y} \geq 0\urcorner .$$

Consider a finite set y_1 of augmented vectors corresponding to category 1, and a finite set y_2 of augmented vectors corresponding to category 2. In assuming that the two categories are linearly separable, we guarantee that there exists at least one $(d+1)$ weight vector $\hat{\mathbf{w}}$ such that

$$\hat{\mathbf{w}} \cdot \mathbf{y} \geq 0 \quad \text{if} \quad \mathbf{y} \in y_1,$$
$$\hat{\mathbf{w}} \cdot \mathbf{y} < 0 \quad \text{if} \quad \mathbf{y} \in y_2.$$

We start with an arbitrary weight vector $\mathbf{w}$, which presumably misclassifies many patterns, and try to adjust it by repeated application of some error-correction training procedure. The procedure we shall study works repeatedly through the patterns in y_1 and y_2, testing each to see if the latest $\mathbf{w}$ classifies it correctly. If $\mathbf{w}$ classifies the current $\mathbf{y}$ correctly, we leave $\mathbf{w}$ unchanged and move on to the next $\mathbf{y}$. If the classification is incorrect, however, we change $\mathbf{w}$ to $\mathbf{w}'$, where

$$\mathbf{w}' = \begin{cases} \mathbf{w} + \mathbf{y} & \text{if } \mathbf{y} \text{ belonged to category 1,} \\ \mathbf{w} - \mathbf{y} & \text{if } \mathbf{y} \text{ belonged to category 2.} \end{cases}$$

The idea is as follows: If $\mathbf{y}$ is in category 1 but $\mathbf{w}$ misclassified it, then we had $\mathbf{w} \cdot \mathbf{y} < 0$ where we should have had $\mathbf{w} \cdot \mathbf{y} \geq 0$. Since $\mathbf{y} \cdot \mathbf{y} > 0$ for any nonzero vector, we have that

$$(\mathbf{w} + \mathbf{y}) \cdot \mathbf{y} = \mathbf{w} \cdot \mathbf{y} + \mathbf{y} \cdot \mathbf{y} > \mathbf{w} \cdot \mathbf{y}$$

and so—even if we do not have $\mathbf{w}' \cdot \mathbf{y} \geq 0$—we at least have that $\mathbf{w}'$ classifies $\mathbf{y}$ "more nearly correctly" than $\mathbf{w}$ does. Similarly for the category-2 correction.

Unfortunately, in classifying $\mathbf{y}$ "more correctly" we run the risk of classifying another pattern "less correctly." However, it can be proved (see, e.g., Nilsson, 1965) that our procedure does *not* yield an endless seesaw, but will eventually converge to a correct set of weights *if one exists*.

We close this section by noting that Minsky and Papert (1969) have revivified the study of perceptrons by responding to such convergence schemes with the basic question: "Your scheme works when a weighting scheme exists, but when does there exist such a setting of the weights?" In other words, they ask, "Given a pattern-recognition problem, how much of the retina must each associator unit 'see' if the network is to do its job?" They analyze this question both for "order-limited perceptrons," in which the "how much" is the "number of input lines per component," and "diameter-limited perceptrons," in which the "how much" is the diameter of the input array from which each component receives its inputs. We shall say more about this in Section 7.3.2.

7.3 WHY RATS CAN'T LEARN BIRDSONG

In Section 7.3.1, a consideration of ethology shows how the neural networks of different animals are predisposed to handle different ranges of problems (rats can't learn birdsong), and to be differentially "tunable." Then in Section 7.3.2 we look at the pretheory of network predispositions, complexity, and tunability. A crucial area for neural modeling must be the study of *complexity of computation*—for instance, how long a network of given components must take to compute a certain function, or what the range of functions is that can be computed by

networks of a given structure. The mathematical theory cannot at present be "plugged in" to solve biological problems, but it may help us refine the questions we ask of the experimenter and suggest important new ways of interpreting his results.

7.3.1 Ethology of network predisposition

The relative role of genetic, predispositional, and learning factors in animal behavior is perhaps most clearly suggested by reviewing some results on the ontogeny of birdsong (Ploog, 1971; Tinbergen, 1972; Marler, 1973; Manning, this volume).

1. Some birds (e.g., domestic fowl) will produce the species-specific call even if deafened at birth prior to exposure to the call. This implies a prewired, genetically determined motor model for call production. There is no process of matching to an auditory input.

2. Some birds (e.g., song sparrows) can develop the normal song even though raised in isolation from it, but if deafened at birth, they fail to develop the normal song. This suggests that auditory feedback from their own song production is necessary, presumably for matching with a template.

3. In the third type of ontogeny, not only is auditory feedback necessary, but an external "model" of the correct song must also be presented to the developing bird. For example, chaffinches raised in isolation have abnormal songs which lack much of the structure that forms when they are exposed to the species-specific song during development.

4. Some birds are more open to environmental and sociological influences. An example is the young male bullfinch, which if raised in proximity to its father acquires its species-specific song, but if raised experimentally by a foster species will instead develop the foster species' song. Such mimetic learning is seen in many parasitic birds, which acquire the song of the host early in life, but there are some parasitic species, such as the European cuckoo, which remain "resistant" as fledglings and retain their own species song. Thus, in some species a complex interaction can occur between an innate susceptibility (which provides the basis for the elaboration of a song template and which in turn facilitates the development of a species-typical song pattern) and environmental influences in the form of exposure, learning, feedback stimulation (reafferentation) while singing, and acculturation or acquisition of a "local dialect." Other avian species show a lesser dependence upon such interacting ontogenetic influences.

We see from this that some animals are genetically predisposed to learn certain things at certain times during their lives. Spinelli's work—reviewed in Section 7.2.1—also shows that early learning may occur in nerve cells without any obvious reinforcement. The ethology of imprinting shows that some kinds of probably permanent learning occur within narrow time limits during the lives of individuals. This is often illustrated by noting that a young animal must establish a strong bond to its mother and be willing to put forth enormous efforts to follow her if it is to continue to receive the food, protection, and shelter she can provide.

We shall next give examples in support of the idea that each animal is genetically prepared to learn some things easily and other things, of about equal complexity by our standards, not at all.

Garcia and Koelling confronted rats with a sweet-tasting liquid and a light-sound stimulus, both paired with radiation sickness—a malaise characterized by stomach upset (Garcia, 1971). Only the taste, not the bright light or loud sound, became unpleasant to the rats. In the complementary experiment, they paired the sweet taste and the light-sound stimuli with electric shock. This time the rats associated the light-sound combination, not the taste, with the shock.

Rat pups behave similarly: they avoid nursing from a foster mother if made sick from an injection shortly afterwards, whereas if not made sick they will nurse freely and repetitively from their foster mother.

The above adult-rat experiment illustrates both ends of the learning-predisposition spectrum. The rats were genetically predisposed to associate taste with illness, and this association occurred in spite of the hourlong delay between the taste and the illness. But the rats were not predisposed—were perhaps negatively predisposed—to associate taste with electric shock and to link external events (light and noise) with nausea. The evolutionary advantage is obvious: animals that are poisoned by a distinctively flavored food and survive, do well not to eat that food again.

Garcia (1971) cites many other instances indicating learning predispositions (see also Garcia and Levine, this volume):

1. Thiamine-deficient rats will, if given the choice, concentrate upon eating thiamine-rich foods.

2. When feral rats are trained by associations of flavors and illness to become bait-shy of a particular food, and are then allowed to raise a litter, the offspring will also be bait-shy of that food (cultural transmission!).

3. The ability of animals to associate consumption of a meal with its later effects, even after all traces have vanished from the gastrointestinal system, and then to reject only *novel* items that have appeared in their diet, is a notable exception to the principle of immediate reinforcement.

The foregoing effects presumably have their anatomical basis in the nucleus of the fasciculus solitarius of the brainstem, where gustatory and visceral afferent fibers both terminate.

Rats are not the only animals that show genetically predisposed learning. Wilcoxon has reported that "the bobwhite quail, which uses visual cues to identify food and to guide its pecking, is able to relate visual cues to an illness delayed for 30 minutes" (Garcia, 1971). Also, Grzimek of Germany has

investigated the memory horses have for certain processes —in particular for the disappearance of food—by pouring oats into one of four covered boxes in front of a horse's eyes. The horse was then allowed to walk from its stand to the boxes and to eat the oats from the bok which had just been filled. Even to an experienced horseman it will be incomprehensible that a horse cannot immediately grasp what seems an obvious connection. My horses went as often to the other boxes as to the one into which the food had just been put. It took very lengthy and tedious training to induce the animals to open first the box which had just been filled in front of their eyes. When that lesson had sunk in, the horses were no longer allowed to approach and feed immediately from the boxes which had just been filled, but had to wait for varying periods of time. One horse could keep the newly filled box in mind for only six seconds; the second horse could remember it for sixty. After a longer interval, it would again try all the other boxes.

By contrast, experiments with dogs and ravens have shown that they remember for hours food which has been buried in their sight, and my wolves retained such a memory for days. It should not be concluded from such experiments that a horse has a much poorer memory in general; *only that it has a very short memory for these particular processes.* The hiding of food plays no part in the life of grazing animals, while prey often hides from the wolf, which is a hunter. It is probable that in respect of territorial recognition and dominance fighting, for example, the memory of grazers is incomparably better. (Grzimek, 1968)

In a different vein, noting how hard it is for rats to learn to press bars to avoid shock, and for pigeons to peck keys to avoid shock (but not to get grain), we conclude that to train an animal to avoid a painful stimulus, we must choose from among its species-specific repertoire of *defensive* actions, not from its appetitive repertoire. The extensions of this principle to other realms is apparent.

Humans are not exempt from the foregoing sorts of effects. As evidence, we quote from an article by Seligman and Hager (1972):

Some years ago, one of us (Seligman) went out to dinner. He had an excellent *filet mignon* with *sauce Béarnaise,* his favorite, and then he went off with his wife Kerry to see the opera *Tristan und Isolde.* Some hours later he became violently ill with stomach flu and spent most of the night in utter misery. Later, when he attempted to eat *sauce Béarnaise* again, he couldn't bear the taste of it. Just thinking about it nauseated him.

At first glance, his reaction seemed to be a simple case

of Pavlovian conditioning: a conditioned stimulus (the sauce) had been paired with an unconditioned stimulus (the illness), which elicited an unconditioned response (throwing up). So future encounters with the sauce caused a conditioned response (nausea). At second glance, however, he realized that the *sauce-Béarnaise* phenomenon had violated all sorts of well-established laws:

1. The interval between tasting the sauce and throwing up was about six hours. The longest interval between two events that produce learning in the laboratory is about 30 seconds.

2. It took only one such experience for him to associate the sauce with sickness; learning rarely occurs in only one trial in the laboratory [one-shot learning].

3. Neither the *filet mignon* nor the white plate on which it was served, nor his wife, became distasteful to him; he associated none of them with the illness, only the *sauce Béarnaise*. But, according to laws of Pavlovian conditioning, all events or objects that occurred along with the illness (the unconditioned stimulus) should have become unpleasant [specificity].

4. His reaction had no cognitive or "expectational" components, unlike most conditioning phenomena. When he found out that another close colleague got sick the same night, *he knew* that the sauce hadn't caused the malaise at all—stomach flu had caused it. But knowing that the sauce was not the culprit did not inhibit his aversion to it one bit.

5. Finally, his loathing of *sauce Béarnaise* stayed with him about five years, whereas associations formed by Pavlovian conditioning generally die out in about a dozen trials.

From the same article:

Phobias too are selective: we have phobias about heights, the dark, crowds, animals, and insects, but we do not have phobias about pajamas, electric outlets, or trees, even though the latter may accompany trauma as often as the former. Isaacs Marks of London's Maudsley Hospital related a typical case. A seven-year-old girl, playing one day in the park, saw a snake, but she was not particularly alarmed. Several hours later she accidentally smashed her hand in a car door, and soon thereafter developed a fear of snakes that lasted into adulthood. Notice that she did *not* develop a car-door phobia, which would have been more logical. Moreover, considerable time elapsed between her seeing the snake and having the accident.*

Turning now to mice for some other results on the nature of learning, we read in an article by Quadagno and Banks (1973) that

the procedure of cross-fostering [different species (wild and inbred) of mice pups to their respective mothers] at birth [does] not affect the ability of the cross-fostered male and female *Mus* to mate with a conspecific. [But

---

*Reprinted from *Psychology Today* Magazine, August 1972. Copyright 1972 by Ziff-Davis Publishing Company. All rights reserved.

such] cross-fostering [does affect] many other social behaviours such as allogrooming, aggressive behaviour and approach-avoidance behaviour [in the species in question]. This implies that, in [some] mice, sexual behaviour may be firmly fixed by the genotype and that it is released by the presence of a conspecific. Other social behaviours are more labile and easily changed by manipulating the early experience of these rodents.

Another early developmental result reported in the same book is that

chicks of either sex reared in partial isolation (non-contactual) establish a dominance order in a matter of hours when assembled at the age at which group-reared controls form a peck-order. These results suggest that the age at which peck-rights form is determined essentially by processes of maturation rather than of learning only.

Another study (Hongan, 1971) has shown that pecking in newly hatched chicks begins as a simple response to a stimulus. Within a few weeks, though, pecking is differentiated into pecking for food and simple pecking (ground scratching) in response to nonfood stimuli. Presumably, later on the state of the gizzard and other internal conditions would also influence the responses.

On naturally predisposed habituation, Fox (1973) reports that among

certain birds, habituation seems to be involved in the differentiation of predators from friendly birds. Laboratory investigations indicate that ducklings give a crouching response to any object overhead. After a period of time, the response to objects seen frequently, e.g., leaves or friendly birds, habituates. On the other hand, hawks are seen infrequently and the response never habituates. Thus, as the result of selective experience, the crouching response occurs in the presence of hawks but not in response to familiar, friendly birds.

... Habituation could prove nonadaptive if it occurred readily to all stimuli, including stimuli that occasionally signalled danger. In at least some cases, animals exhibit a resistance to habituation to such stimuli. For example, sparrows fail to habituate to an owl or a model of an owl; this failure occurs even in hand-reared varieties in which other experiential variables have apparently been controlled.

For another perspective, we turn next to wolves, a particularly well studied type of social carnivore whose behavior enables us to see with special clarity the extent to which complex learning often involves comparatively simple elaborations of essentially "innate" response patterns. In the following discussion we should note from ethology that every phenotypic feature is influenced by instructions contained in the genes, and that a behavior is "genetically determined" if it differs among individuals of different genotypes but of the same experiences (assuming the latter to be possible). A "learned" behavior is one which differs among individuals of the same geno-type who have had the same experience except as regards the learned behavior. The modern ethological conception is that some behaviors are more environment-resistant (that is, less susceptible to environmental influence) than others. The less environment-resistant behaviors are the more "learnable" ones.

Fox (1972) cites many examples of highly predisposed learning in wolves. Wolves are weaned at ten to twelve weeks, and between six and twelve weeks each learns on its own to catch, kill, carry, defend, and eat small prey such as mice. Species-typical motor patterns such as leaping, forepaw stabbing, digging, overturning feces for bugs, and shaking prey held in the mouth, are built in and only await the appropriate stimuli for their release. What are learned are various sophistications and elabo-rations of these patterns. By three to six months a wolf cub has also learned to respond properly to its parents' moods, has learned which animals are familiar and which should be shied from as strangers, has "imprinted" the features and terrain of its home range, and has begun to socialize properly in accordance with the dominance relations of its pack. Between one and two years cubs learn the techniques of cooperative hunting during group play (e.g., cutting off, ambushing, prey testing, group stalking, herding, cornering, harassing, fatiguing, mass attacking, and decoying). This learning never occurs in individuals raised in isolation, only in groups of three or more free to play with each other and free to trail along on adult hunts. By three years wolves are fully integrated into their complex pack structures, having successfully reckoned with alpha males and females, siblings, parents, seasons, new births and deaths, and complicated individ-ual relations.

All this reminds one of the stages of human childhood, the proverbial seven ages of man, "teen-age gangs" of wild horse colts, and many other developmental parallels in the mammalian kingdom. One wonders, for example, how closely Piaget's "sets-of-sets" thinking (Piaget, 1967), which emerges at the age of about twelve in humans, is linked to the socialization stage of adolescence in all social mammals. At this stage sets of social relations must be recognized and observed. Are there regular sequences of types of learning that are always followed in mammalian brains?

At least among humans, there is evidence that this is so in natural language learning, since children seem to learn language the same way the world over. So far, among eighteen languages studied (Slobin, 1972), children progress through the same two-, three-, many-word grammatical stages, talking about the same sub-jects and rectifying the same category confusions at each

stage until mature adulthood. Recent studies also suggest that chimps undergo a similar series of cognitive develop-ments, but they have so far been taught little of man's language capability (Slobin, 1972).

Note, too, the close parallel between man and chim-panzees in spatial thinking and memory ability. Cogni-tive psychologists have noted that a human can more easily memorize a long sequence of items by imagining himself walking around a familiar building, and creating in the successive places that he passes visual images of the things he wants to remember. This is based on the fact that human beings seem to possess specialized and power-ful mechanisms for reasoning about spatial relationships, which form the basis of visual perception. Helmholtz referred to them as processes of "unconscious inference." These ideas relate to an experiment of Menzel (1973), who reports that

juvenile chimpanzees, carried around an outdoor field and shown up to 18 randomly placed hidden foods, remembered most of the hiding places and the type of food that was in each. Their [food-collection paths, taken after they were released (to retrieve the food)], approx-imated optimum [routes] and they rarely rechecked a place they had already emptied of food.

Obviously their spatial memory was excellent.

To add another perspective, we note that selective breeding and training in domesticated canids (espe-cially dogs) brings out (or, by affecting thresholds, makes more accessible) certain behavioral traits which can be modified, shaped, or redirected through training. Guarding (with or without barking), herding, leading or guiding, and retrieving are examples of traits that have been bred to very low response thresholds in certain breeds. Animal trainers, of course, must exploit these predispositions.

For yet another perspective, Schneider has found that in newborn hamsters subcortical pathways between the tectum and the thalamus are implicated in pattern dis-crimination (Anon., 1974). But in adult hamsters, pattern discrimination seems to take place in the cortex. This suggests many possible migrations of functions dur-ing ontogeny in mammalian brains. On a similar tack, Section 7.4 notes McLardy's position that mammalian hippocampus may be more important for survival during the formative period of behavior.

Still further afield, child-beating mothers are remark-ably likely to have been beaten by their own mothers as children (Stoll, 1970). Here a model of behavior is "learned" in early life but is not expressed until adult-hood. This reminds us of the chaffinches who were kept in auditory isolation after being caught their first sum-mer, and who then sang the song of their species for the first time the following spring (Nottebohm, 1972). This returns us full circle to the opening topic of this subsection, and with this we turn to the beginnings of a mathematical theory of network complexity and predisposition.

7.3.2 A pretheory of network predisposition

In Section 7.2.2, in our study of training a perceptron to make binary classification, we noted that if a linear separation exists, the training algorithm will reach it. We now turn to Minsky and Papert's (1969) study of when it is possible to combine the information in a given preprocessing layer to perform a given pattern-recognition task. We suggest that their work be considered as one phase of a pretheory for the questions of "predisposition" of neural networks raised in the ethological sampler of our previous subsection.

We are going to be interested in pattern predicates ψ such that $\psi(X)$ is true for some patterns X and false for others (e.g., X is connected, or X is of odd parity), and we shall ask such questions as, "How many inputs are required for the preprocessing modules of a one-layer perceptron?" Of course, we can always get away with using a single element, computing an arbitrary Boolean function, and connecting it to all the squares. So the question that really interests us is, "Can we get away with a small number of squares connected to each of the input neurons?"

Minsky and Papert show that if a predicate is unchanged by various permutations, then we may use this fact to simplify its coefficients with respect to the set of masks—and that this simplified form will often enable us to place a lower bound on the order of the predicate. Rather than giving the theory, we shall try to clarify the approach by a simple example.

Consider the simple Boolean operation of addition modulo 2 (Figure 7.5). If we imagine the square with vertices $(0, 0)$, $(0, 1)$, $(1, 1)$, and $(1, 0)$ in the Cartesian plane, with (x_1, x_2) being labeled by $x_1 \oplus x_2$, we have 0s at one diagonally opposite pair of vertices and 1s at the other diagonally opposite pair of vertices. It is clear that there is no way of interposing a straight line such that the 1s lie on one side and the 0s lie on the other side. In other words, it is clear in this case—from visual inspection— that no threshold element exists which can do the job of addition modulo 2. However, we shall prove it mathematically in order to gain insight into a general technique that Minsky and Papert use over and over again.

Consider the claim that we wish to prove wrong—that there actually exists a threshold element θ with weights α and β such that $x_1 \oplus x_2 = 1$ if and only if $\alpha x_1 + \beta x_2$ exceeds θ. The crucial point is to notice that the function of addition modulo 2 is symmetric, so that we must also

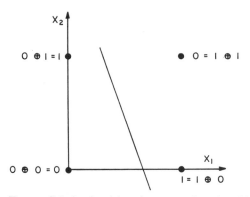

FIGURE 7.5 An intuitive demonstration that binary addition cannot be realized by a threshold element—no single line can separate the 0s from the 1s.

have $x_1 \oplus x_2 = 1$ if and only if $\beta x_1 + \alpha x_2$ exceeds θ, and so, adding together the two terms, we have $x_1 \oplus x_2 = 1$ if and only if

$$\frac{\alpha + \beta}{2} x_1 + \frac{\alpha + \beta}{2} x_2 > \theta.$$

Writing $(\alpha + \beta)/2$ as γ we see that, by using the symmetries of addition modulo 2, we have reduced three putative parameters α, β, and θ to a pair of parameters γ and θ such that $x_1 \oplus x_2 = 1$ if and only if $\gamma(x_1 + x_2)$ exceeds θ. We now set $t = x_1 + x_2$ and look at the polynomial $\gamma t - \theta$. It is a degree-1 polynomial, but note: at $t = 0$, $\gamma t - \theta$ must be less than zero; at $t = 1$, it is greater than zero; and at $t = 2$, it is again less than zero. This is a contradiction. A polynomial of degree 1 cannot change sign from positive to negative more than once. We thus conclude that, in fact, there is no such polynomial, and thus we must conclude that there is no threshold element which will add modulo 2.

We now understand a general method used again and again by Minsky and Papert: Start with a pattern-classification problem. Observe that certain symmetries leave it invariant. (For instance, for the parity problem or the simple case of addition modulo 2, any permutation of the points of the retina would leave the classification unchanged.) Use this to cut down the number of parameters describing the circuit. Then lump items together to get a polynomial and examine actual patterns to put a lower bound on the degree of the polynomial, fixing things so that this degree bounds the number of inputs to the one-layer perceptron. For a proof of this *group-invariance theorem* the reader may refer to Minsky and Papert's book.

One application of the group-invariance theorem shows that to tell whether or not the pattern of activated squares is connected requires a number that increases at least as fast as the square root of the number of cells in the retina. These results are most interesting, and point the way toward further insight into the functioning of the nervous system, but they are restricted to highly mathematical functions instead of the complex perceptual problems involved in the everyday life of an organism. We might note, too, that any full model of perception must not have the purely passive character of the perceptron model, but must involve an active component in which hypothesis formation is shaped by the inner activity of the organism and related to past and present behavior (see the discussion of internal models in Section 7.1).

We have already stressed the interest, in the study of complexity of computation, in trade-offs between time and space. Minsky and Papert asked, "If we fix the number of layers in the network, how complicated must the elements become in order to get a successful computation?" We close this section by noting that Winograd and Spira have tackled the complementary problem of how, if we bound the number of inputs per component, we can proceed to discover how many layers of components we require. More specifically, they studied algebraic functions (e.g., group multiplication) instead of looking to the problem of classifying patterns. Winograd (1967), and later Spira and Arbib (1967) and Spira (1969), studied networks whose components were limited in that there was a fixed bound on the number of input lines to any component. In what follows, each module is limited to have at most r input lines. We are once again assuming a unit delay in the operation of all our modules.

The Winograd-Spira theory is based on the simple observation exemplified by Figure 7.6. Here we see that if there are two inputs per module and if an output line of a circuit depends on 2^3 input lines, then it takes at least three time units for an input configuration to yield its corresponding output.

This apparently trivial observation has surprisingly powerful consequences: Winograd and Spira proved for certain mathematical functions that no possible scheme

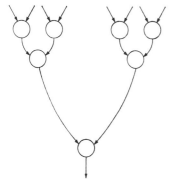

FIGURE 7.6 The quickest possible path from 2^3 inputs to an output in a configuration where each module receives two inputs.

of wiring neurons can compute the function in less than a certain time delay, intimately related to the structure of the function. In particular, they showed how to go from the structure of a finite group to a minimal time for a network computing the group multiplication. Furthermore, Spira (1969) was able to provide for any group a network that is essentially time-optimal, in that it produces its output within one time unit of the time specified by the theorem.

We thus have an extremely important result for any theory of neural networks: for a certain type of restricted component we can show how to build a network that is optimal with respect to the time required for computing. However, to appreciate the full complexity that lies ahead of the automata theorist who would contribute to the study of information processing in the nervous system, we must make several observations. First, to achieve time optimality in his network, Spira had to use an extremely redundant encoding for the input and output to ensure that "the right information would be in the right place at the right time." The flavor of this can be given by the observation that we can multiply numbers far more quickly if they are given in prime decomposition, for example,

$$(2^2 \cdot 3^4 \cdot 5^2 \cdot 7^1) \times (2^1 \cdot 3^0 \cdot 5^1 \cdot 7^2) = (2^3 \cdot 3^4 \cdot 5^3 \cdot 7^3),$$

than if they are given in decimal form, for in the former case we need only add exponents ($2 + 1 = 3, 4 + 0 = 4, 2 + 1 = 3, 1 + 2 = 3$) instead of going through the lengthy computation of decimal multiplication.

This observation reminds us of the organization of the cat visual system, where a million optical fibers feed 540 million cells in the visual cortex. Thus, as we move up into the visual cortex, what we reduce is not the number of channels, but rather the activity of the channels, as each will respond only to more and more specific stimuli. The result is a network with many, many neurons in parallel, even through the network is rather shallow in terms of computation time. It might well be that we could save many neurons, at the price of increased computation time, both by narrowing the net while increasing its depth and by using feedback to allow recirculation of information for a long time before the correct result emerges. We see here the need for a critical investigation of the interplay between space and time in the design of networks.

The ganglion cells in the retina of a frog seem fairly well suited to a life spent living in ponds and feeding on flies, since the brain of the animal receives specific information about the presence of food and enemies within the visual field (Lettvin et al., 1959). But the price the animal pays is that it is limited in its flexibility of response because its information is so directly coded.

A cat (Hubel and Wiesel, 1962), on the other hand, has to process a greater amount of information if it is to find its prey—but it can eat mice instead of flies. A cat cannot compute its appropriate action as quickly, perhaps, as the frog can, but it makes up for that by having extra computational machinery enabling it to predict and make use of previous experience in developing a strategy for governing its action.

We see that to model the behavior of the animal completely, we must make an adequate model of its environment and take into account structural features of the animal. It is not enough to work out an optimum network whereby a frog can locate a fly; we must also compute whether it is optimal to couple that network to the frog's tongue, or to have the frog bat the fly out of the air with its forelimb, or to have the frog jump up to catch the fly in its mouth. Clearly the evolution of receptors, effectors, and central computing machinery was completely interwoven, and it is only for simplicity of analysis that we concentrate here on the computational aspects, holding many of the environmental and effector parameters fixed. Again, we shall ignore the interesting pattern-recognition problem of determining the most effective features to be used in characterizing a certain object in a given environment. For instance, to characterize a mouse one could go into many details including the placement of hairs upon its back, but for the cat it is perhaps enough to recognize a grey or brown mobile object with a tail and within a certain size range. It should be clear that the choice of features must depend upon the environment: if there exists a creature that meets the above prescription for a mouse but happens to be poisonous, then it will clearly be necessary for a successful species of cat to have a perceptual system that can detect features differentiating the poisonous creatures from the edible mice.

We should further note that Winograd and Spira's best results were for groups, where we can make use of the mathematical theory elaborated over the past hundred years. It will be much harder to prove equally valuable theorems about functions that are not related to classical mathematical structures. If we were to replace the very simple limitation on number of inputs by an assumption limiting the actual types of functions that the neurons can compute, we would have to expect a great increase in the complexity of the theory. Some would conclude from this analysis that automata theory is irrelevant to the study of the nervous system, but we would argue that it shows how determined our study of automata theory must be before we can hope to understand fully the function of the nervous system.

Another kind of learning limitation that can be best treated in the terminology of Section 7.1 on interacting sets of active subsystems has been discussed by Geschwind, Luria, and others with respect to language functions in the brain. We quote a case description by Geschwind (1970) given in support of his disconnection-syndrome hypothesis:

This syndrome was described in 1892 by Dejerine. His patient suddenly developed a right visual field defect and lost the ability to read. He could, however, copy the words that he could not understand. He was able, moreover, to write spontaneously, although he could not read later the sentences he had written. All other aspects of his use and comprehension of language were normal. At postmortem Dejerine found that the left visual cortex had been destroyed. In addition, the posterior portion of the corpus callosum was destroyed, the part of this structure which connects the visual regions of the two hemispheres. Dejerine advanced a simple explanation. Because of the destruction of the left visual cortex, written language could reach only the right hemisphere. In order to be dealt with as language it had to be transmitted to the speech regions in the left hemisphere, but the portion of the corpus callosum necessary for this was destroyed. Thus, written language, although seen clearly, was without meaning.

Apparently, if interacting subsystems of the brain are not richly enough connected, information bottlenecks arise that are sufficient to make some affective knowledge ineffable and some visual sensations useless, as well as to preclude the learning of varying associations (as we documented in Section 7.3.1).

7.4 A CASE STUDY: THE HIPPOCAMPUS

In Section 7.2 we examined studies of adaptation schemes for individual neurons; and in Section 7.3 we saw that different networks can learn different things, both because of the basic pattern of their internal connectivity and because of their place in the overall flux of information.

In this section we shall review a few attempts to model some memory mechanisms in the mammalian hippocampal formation. One reason for choosing hippocampus is that more neurophysiological research on memory has been associated with it than with any other mammalian structure. Other reasons are that its circuitry is clearly organized and comparatively simple; that rats and cats, our most studied mammals, have large and easily accessible hippocampi; that hippocampal responses appear to correlate about as well with motor as with sensory events (O'Keefe and Dostrovsky, 1971; Ranck, 1973; Segal and Olds, 1973; and Vinogradova, 1970), suggesting that the hippocampus pays a pivotal role in the vitally important sensorimotor relationship process; and, finally, that the hippocampus seems closely related to several common human diseases (McLardy, 1973a, b, c, d).

Our task in the remainder of the section will be to find memory models consistent with the neural connectivity of the hippocampus. However, we shall see that in a system as far from the periphery as the hippocampus, the significance of its input and output firing patterns is virtually unknown, which makes it hard to specify which changes in neural connectivity are "desirable"! As a result, the anatomy has proved something of a Rorschach test for neural modelers.

For example, Stanley and Kilmer (1975) took as the point of departure for their model of dentate gyrus the general observation that successful animal behavior must involve decisions and actions integrated in time. In order to help model such decisionary activity they considered a memory network that was designed to learn sequences of inputs separated by various time intervals and to repeat these sequences when cued by their initial fragments, the structure of the model being based on the anatomy of the dentate gyrus. Like the hippocampus, the model comprised a number of arrays of cells, called lamellae. Each array consisted of four lines of *neuromimes* (i.e., model neurons, or "neuron mimics") coupled in a regular fashion to neighbors within the array and with some randomness to neuromimes in other lamellae. The neuromimes were described by first-order differential equations. Two of the neuromime lines in each lamella were so coupled that sufficient excitation by a system input generated a wave of activity that moved slowly along the lines away from the point of excitation. Such waves effected dynamic storage of the representation via connections between lamellae. When an input was again presented to the memory, waves were excited, and these moved through the system as before to generate the next input's representation after the proper time interval. The system thus implemented a process of associative chaining. Stanley and Kilmer plan to develop the memory circuit to allow an existing decisionary circuit to process sequences rather than single inputs, and to learn to ignore repeated nonsignificant inputs (i.e., to habituate).

Olds (1969) compared the crisscross TA-to-GD, GD-to-CA3, and CA3-to-CA1 connections to the connection grid of a random-access magnetic-core computer memory. While he exploited his analogy between hippocampal circuitry and core memory arrays very well, perhaps the greatest weakness of his model was its representation of neurons by simple magnetic switches.

In Sections 7.4.1 and 7.4.2, we shall develop two other models due to Marr and Kilmer, respectively. It seems to us valuable to add all these schemes to the neural modeler's armamentarium, as a challenge to theorist and experimentalist alike to design experiments that are more relevant to understanding the nature and mechanism of hippocampal action.

7.4.1 The Marr model

David Marr (1971) proposed an elegant model for the GD-CA3 subsystem of hippocampus (see Figure 7.7) based on the following fundamental premise: Assume that the model receives every input event E_k of a set of such events at least once, in some arbitrary order with respect to the other input events. Every E_k is presented as a binary n-tuple of 1s and 0s containing exactly M 1s. A randomly specified subset of L of these n-tuple lines feeds each codon c_i of a set of codons $c_1,...,c_l$. The codons represent GD granule cells. Connections between input lines and codons are made through Brindley synapses, each of which contains an unmodifiable excitatory component and an excitatory component that is strengthened by each simultaneous pre- and post-synaptic activation (1 = activation, 0 = quiescence). A codon emits a 1 if the sum of its input excitations exceeds its threshold, otherwise it emits a 0. Thus an often-presented E_k will be able to excite some codons to such a degree that even a "fragment of E_k," having 0s in place of some of E_k's 1s, will fire many of them. Marr regulates his codons with supplementary inhibitory G and S cells that cause about the same number of codons to fire in response to any input, no matter what fragment of an E_k it is. The codon rank, therefore, tends to respond to a fragment of any E_k just as it first did to the most presented E_k that is sufficiently similar to it. In this sense the codon rank possesses a simple memory of all the E_k.

Randomly chosen subsets of c_i connect through Brindley synapses to each PQ_j, where PQ_j represents a CA3 pyramidal cell. Let E_k' be any fragment of E_k. Then the function of PQ_j is to compute approximately the

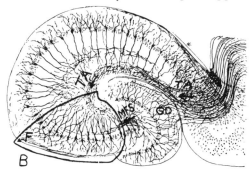

FIGURE 7.7 A cross section of the hippocampus. Region B is that modeled by Kilmer and Olinski. TA = temporoammonic pathway. GD = gyrus dentatus. MFS = mossy fiber system. F = output to fornix. From Krieg (1966).

conditional probability $P(\Omega_j \mid E'_k)$ that the consequences of E'_k, as fed into $P\Omega_j$, imply that the "completion" of the input event to E_k lies in class Ω_j. This partition is mechanized by the modifiable Brindley synapses connecting the c_i to the $P\Omega_j$. The idea is that a codon-rank output that fires $P\Omega_j$ hard will strengthen synapses in such a way that similar codon-rank outputs will also fire $P\Omega_j$, thereby adumbrating Ω_j. (Marr's [1970] neocortical model uses a simple reinforcement signal R telling when $P\Omega_j$ is to fire to define the Ω_j classes in an arbitrary way. This requires a different type of synapse between the c_i and $P\Omega_j$.)

$P\Omega_j$ approximately computes $P(\Omega_j \mid E'_k)$, which is given by a term of the type $A[\sum_i P_i - B]/n_k$, where A and B are constants, n_k is the number of codons firing in response to E'_k, and P_i is the probability that the completion of E'_k to E_k belongs to Ω_j given that the output of c_i is 1. Marr inputs to $P\Omega_j$ an approximation to n_k by adding divisively inhibitory D cells, which he argues convincingly should be interpreted as basket cells. As in the codon rank, Marr also adds S and G cells to provide subtractive inhibition to regulate the level of principal output, now coming from the $P\Omega_j$. This inhibition inputs to $P\Omega_j$ an approximation to B in the $P(\Omega_j \mid E'_k)$ formula. The P_i of that formula are approximated by Brindley synaptic strengths, and A is a scale factor.

Marr's full GD-CA-3 model, if augmented with D cells in his GD portion, would contain representatives of every major cell type in GD-CA3, with nothing extra included. Note that he essentially *derives* the need for all but the c_i and $P\Omega_j$. His model proves that an abundance of simple, randomly connected components with plastic synapses could be put to powerful use in brains as simple classifiers of past experience.

It is a shame to have to omit Marr's detailed mathematics in this review, because the exact power of his results is contained in his theorems. Nevertheless, one can bypass the mathematics and still study by computer simulation all but Marr's optimality theorems and his limiting cases containing indefinitely large numbers of elements.

James Stanley did some computer simulation of Marr's model at the University of Massachusetts, and he found that extremely large numbers of components would probably be needed to make the model perform at all well. While in principle this is no drawback for a brain model, in practice it makes the model difficult to refine. Some refinement seems desirable because neurons are far from codons or $P\Omega_j$ computers, and nervous connectivity is far from random.

Marr's model has enough in common with the percep-

tron and von der Malsburg models of Section 7.2 to invite comparison to each of them. Marr's codon rank corresponds to the perceptron's feature-detection layer and to von der Malsburg's E-cell layer. Note, though, that the perceptron's feature detectors do not have any inhibitory feedback for tonic regulation, but Marr's codons and von der Malsburg's E cells do. Von der Malsburg's cortical cells each can be thought of as corresponding to the perceptron's output unit, and each of Marr's $P\Omega_j$ units could be converted into a perceptron-like output unit by adding a threshold and then quantizing each output signal as either 1 or 0 depending on whether or not $P\Omega_j$'s output exceeded this threshold. Marr's inhibition of $P\Omega_j$ cells, which is needed to compensate for his use of Brindley synapses and large number of $P\Omega_j$ units, would still remain as an important difference; Marr's formation of Ω_j classes without the aid of external reinforcement is akin to von der Malsburg's approach, and distinct from the perceptron.

7.4.2 The Kilmer model of CA3

Kilmer and Olinski (1974) caricatured the known anatomy, physiology, and functional organization of CA3 hippocampus, and augmented the result with some plausible memory mechanisms. Their first goal was to obtain a circuit model of CA3 that would enable them to study by computer simulation some possible CA3 memory processes involving interneurons (neurons whose axons do not leave the hippocampus proper). Because so little is known about CA3 intracellular physiology, only those processes associated with probable intercellular connection plasticities were considered.

Figure 7.8 outlines the connection scheme of the mod-

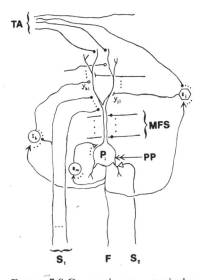

FIGURE 7.8 Connections to a typical pyramid of Kilmer-Olinski simulation. See text for further details.

el, which represents only one transverse section. Extrinsic inputs to the model are interpreted as representing temporoammonic (TA), mossy-fiber-system (MFS), septohippocampal-reinforcement (S_2), and septohippocampal-data (S_1) inputs. The extrinsic model inputs are binary and feed pyramidal neuromimes, P_i, each of which represents a pool of perhaps a hundred pyramidal neurons of CA3. Each P_i computes, with unit latency, an output pulse-repetition rate x_i given by

$$x_i = P_i(\mu) + P_i(E) + P_i(I) + P_i(PP) + P_i(q) + P_i(B),$$

where

$P_i(\mu)$ is a trainable nonlinear function of five non-S_2 extrinsic inputs to P_i;

$P_i(E)$ is a sum of excitations produced by the set of excitatory interneuromimes E_j feeding P_i;

$P_i(I)$ is a sum of inhibitions produced by the set of interneuromimes I_k feeding P_i;

$P_i(PP)$ is a nonlinear function of P_i-to-P_i inputs arising from functionally similar P_i units;

$P_i(q)$ is a trainable Markovian predictive function which is positive if the probability q (that x_i should be large based on the model's response to its previous input) is high, and is negative if q is low; and

$P_i(B)$ is a divisively inhibitory basket-cell interneuronal input to P_i.

The $P_i(\mu)$ functions are fully defined in Kilmer and Olinski (1974). The x_i function is only meant to approximate the effects of the various kinds of influences acting on each pyramidal-cell pool. The $P_i(\mu) + P_i(B)$ part of the equation is intended to correspond closely in effect to the $P\Omega_j$ output equation of Marr. The other terms have no counterpart in Marr's equation.

Each I_k (or E_j) in the full model (Figure 7.9) represents a pool of perhaps ten inhibitory (or excitatory) interneurons, whereas B_m represents a basket-cell inhibitory influence on P_i which regulates by negative feedback P_i's baseline firing rate. I_k computes at each time step a nonlinear function of the inputs feeding it to produce an output burst or not, and inhibits the many P_i into which it bursts in proportion to the magnitude of the connecting synaptic strength y_{ki}. The same holds for each E_j except that it excites the P_i into which it bursts. The y_{ji} associated with each P_i are adjusted by successive incre-

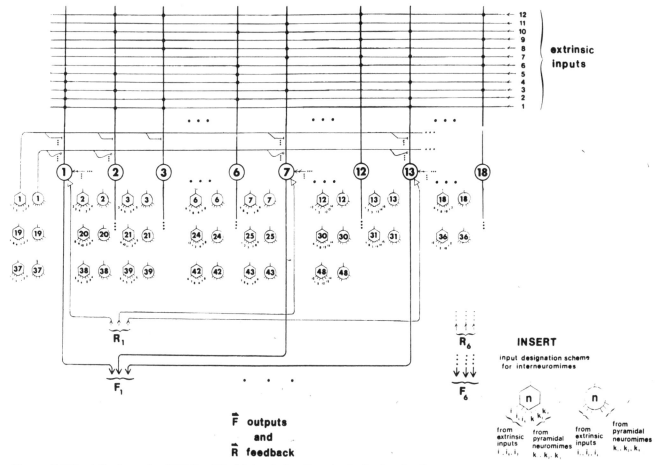

FIGURE 7.9 Overall schematic of Kilmer-Olinski simulation. See text for further details.

ments, on the basis of criteria signaled over S_2, in order to enable the model's output to improve with experience. The PP input to P_i represents direct pyramidal-to-pyramidal effects in CA3. F represents the fimbria-fornix output pathway of CA3. No commissural representation has been included.

All connections in Figure 7.8 have been biologically confirmed or corroborated at least in kind, but distressingly little experimental evidence is available for magnitudes and interpretations. Single neuromimes in the model represent pools of CA3 neurons in order to accommodate better the electrophysiological data of Ranck (1973) and others. Extrinsic inputs are binary, and simply provide information on which the neuromimes of the model compute. The complete computer-simulated model contains 18 P_i neuromimes; 96 each of the I_k and E_j interneuromimes; a total of 12 extrinsic input lines of the MFS, S_1, and TA types; and one S_2 line per P_i. With noted exceptions, these numbers are not intended to reflect closely corresponding proportions in the hippocampus. The resulting distortions, which are hopefully innocuous, arise from our desire to keep the model as small as possible (e.g., by letting pyramidal cells "pool" their interneurons).

A fundamental idea in constructing the model was that, because interneuronal axons do not leave the hippocampus, the only direct way that interneurons can improve the quality of hippocampal output (transmitted over pyramidal axons, corresponding to F in Figure 7.9) is to raise or lower pyramidal firing rates.

From a successive-snapshot viewpoint of hippocampal operation, and holding all of the model's plastic mechanisms constant, the model of Figure 7.9 operates as follows: First, an overall extrinsic input consisting of twelve binary signals in parallel is presented and fixed. Second, each P_i computes a nonlinear $P_i(\mu)$ response to the five extrinsic inputs it receives, where the five in question are randomly selected during the model's specification. This response is then modified by the addition of $P_i(PP)$, $P_i(q)$, and $P_i(B)$ quantities. Each P_i output is limited to between 20 and 80 pulses per second. Third, each interneuromime computes from its extrinsic and P_i inputs a nonlinear decision to burst or not. As part of the model's specification, for each interneuron three extrinsic inputs were selected at random and three P_i inputs were counted off from a regular succession (see the insert on Figure 7.9). Fourth, the former output of each P_i is modified by the addition of $P_i(E)$, which is the sum of all the y_{ji} connected to E_j that are firing, and the addition of $P_i(I)$, which is minus the sum of all the y_{ki} connected to I_k that are firing. Finally, the interneuromimes recompute their outputs in response to their

new P_i inputs. This gives rise to a more or less different set of E_j and I_k firing into P_i. After several go-arounds in the P_i-to-interneuromime-to-P_i loop, an essentially stable P_i output pattern and a nearly constant interneuromime firing pattern is converged upon. These patterns are maintained until a new extrinsic input is presented to the model. A complete simulation sequences through 50 overall inputs to the model in the foregoing manner.

The goal of training the model is to ensure that for each overall extrinsic input the stable P_i output pattern is uniformly "desirable." Since input-output specifications of hippocampus have been little probed by experimentalists (Ranck's work provides an encouraging start in remedying this deficit), there is no biological evidence as to what is, indeed, "desirable," and so we simply specified ad hoc whether the "desired" P_i output for each overall input was either 20 or 80, before the model was simulated.

The full model contains two types of plasticity. The first type is associated with functions computed by the neuromimes, and the second type consists of modifiable y_{ji} excitatory and y_{ki} inhibitory synaptic strengths. We shall summarize our interpretation of these two types of plasticity in biological terms, noting that the validity of the model requires only that this interpretation be approximately correct.

Kilmer and McLardy (1971) have posited, mostly on the basis of circumstantial evidence, that pyramidal cells of mammalian hippocampus are diffusely innately programmed, and that after birth "hippocampal instincts" are quickly sharpened through experience, and then later sophisticated and elaborated in play and mimicry. The circuitry that is close to maturity at birth we have denoted "core circuitry." We envision a corresponding hippocampal process whereby at first a relatively small number of innately programmed pyramids in the core make contact with clusters of interneurons, probably under septohippocampal-reinforcement criteria. Then other pyramids are trained—i.e., become programmed through experience—and they in turn form cell clusters whose interneurons are partially coextensive with those in the core. Cluster after cluster is trained in this way, each to compute part-novel decisions on part-novel variations of previous hippocampal input patterns. This process diminishes in importance by postadolescence.

Now back to the model. We assumed a prespecified core of P_i-interneuromime circuitry which had no postdevelopmental plasticity. The core in Figure 7.9 consists of all the circuitry computing F_1, F_2, and F_3.

After the core of the model had been determined, we wanted to train the rest so as to correspond to the developmental and learning process described above, whereby cell clusters become functional one after another. We therefore grouped our 18 P_i into 6 subsets of 3 P_i each (see Figure 7.9) and required each kth subset to compute a go/no-go decision F_k as follows: if the average firing rate over the three P_i computing F_k exceeds 50, $F_k =$ "go"; otherwise, $F_k =$ "no-go." (We might interpret $(F_1 =$ go) as triggering a freeze, etc.) With this F_k scheme, of course, the a priori specifications of the P_i functions computing each F_k had to be identical.

We next supposed that our core circuitry computed F_1, F_2, and F_3, and that a neuromime cluster-by-cluster engagement process would train F_4, F_5, and F_6 one after another. A major advantage of our stage-by-stage training plan is that although each F_i is trainable using only positive and negative reinforcement, in the end the entire circuit is able to produce the desired six-dimensional output vectors $\mathbf{F} = (F_1, F_2,..., F_6)$.

Because animals can learn relatively arbitrary things within the predispositional constraints of Section 7.3, like turning left for food when a square appears and turning right when a triangle appears, criteria must be provided to any learning circuit that will allow it to select best responses from a large repertoire to each of many different input stimuli. That CA3 can do this seems likely from the experiments of Segal and Olds (1973), Hydén, Lange, and Seyfried (1973), and others. That the requisite CA3-reinforcement information arises largely in the septal and medial forebrain bundle regions also seems plausible (Stein and Wise, 1971; Antelman, Lippa, and Fisher 1972; Stevens, 1973; Akiskal and McKinney, 1973; Ito and Olds, 1971). We believe it likely that signals from the TA system selectively boost and depress subsets of pyramidal cells as a way of setting generalized aim, purpose, and attention information into CA3's operating program (recall that the TA system originates in entorhinal cortex [Hjorth-Simonsen, 1973], which is directly supplied by secondary association areas all over the rest of the brain [Van Hoesen, Pandya, and Butters, 1972]). Thus we interpret the $\mathbf{R}$ reinforcement information in Figure 7.9 as arriving mostly over septohippocampal fibers in the fimbria-fornix.

We have confirmed by simulation that each F_i stage can be well trained according to the above plan by simulating the following sequence of steps:

1. Train the P_i and interneuromime functions, then train the y's .To train the y's, let each P_i's neutral output be taken as 50 pulses per second, and each desired P_i output for each overall input to the model be set a priori to either 20 or 80 pulses per second. Then, to a first approximation, an I_k can, on the average, improve a

P_i's output by being connected to it if, over all those times that I_k fires, P_i's output exceeds 50 less often than not. In this case the strength of the y_{ki} synapse should vary monotonically with the number of helpful minus the number of harmful influences. Thus, if I_k fires into P_i 8 times over the entire sequence of 50 overall inputs, and if for 6 of these 8 times P_i's desired output is less than 50, y_{ki} might best be made $(6-2)/8 = 0.5$. We have adopted a generalized version of the y_{ki} formula that this example suggests. Our model's formula includes the constraint that no y_{ki} magnitude ever exceed 0.5. The main purpose of this constraint is to prevent an excessive influence in those few cases where it produces an effect in the wrong direction. Also, all y_{ki} that are minus according to a straight generalization of the formula in the example are set to 0. This is tantamount to requiring that I_k not be connected to P_i if, on the average, such a connection would be harmful. Every possible connection between an I_k and a P_i not prohibited by the (minus $y \rightarrow 0$) rule is realized with the appropriate positive y_{ki} value. Mutatis mutandis, the same conventions apply to the excitatory y_{ji} connections between the E_j and the P_i. In the above, assume that a negative reinforcement over $\mathbf{R}$ implies that the F_i being trained is in error, and that a positive reinforcement implies that this F_i is correct. This assumption is not always valid, but when it is not the effects of the error will always be corrected in step 3. In step 1, interpret the training of interneuromime functions as the neurological development of a statistically random set of cell functions whose only notable characteristic is that they don't fire very much.

2. To develop some terminology, suppose interneuromime I_k is firing and that it is connected to m P_i neuromimes for which n have a desired output exceeding 50 and $(m - n)$ have a desired output less than 50. We say then that I_k "helps" in $(m - n)$ places and "harms" in n places. Similarly, with appropriate changes, we have "helps" and "harms" for excitatory interneuromimes. In step 2, we modify interneuromime functions so that those firings in step 1 that were almost as harmful as helpful (i.e., $(m - n - 1) \le n$) are deleted, and also so that all kth interneuromime quiescences (nonfirings) in step 1 that can be transformed into firings that are helpful at every nonzero y_{ki} are so transformed. Helpful or harmful influences are recognizable at every such y_{ki} if it is always assumed that a negative reinforcement fed back over $\mathbf{R}$ to the currently operative part of the model (the core, plus those clusters either trained or now in training) is attributable to a mistake in the F_i currently being trained. Plausible neural mechanisms for representing the modifications in this step might easily be based on reinforcement effects at synapses.

3. Finally, retrain the y's to correspond to the modified interneuromime functions. If an incorrect assumption about F_i's correctness was made in step 1, causing F_i to be trained wrongly there, the same assumption in this step will cause F_i to be reversed and thereby corrected.

With our three go/no-go F_i bits engaged one after another, starting with F_4, we simulated the hippocampus using this model to determine what percent, over all 50 inputs to the model, of F_i outputs were correctly go or no-go as a function of the number of interneuromimes used. This was to answer the question how many interneuromimes are required in order almost always to ensure more helpful than harmful y_{ji} and y_{ki} influences at each P_i under the best possible conditions of P_i input to interneuromimes.

In repeated simulation with varying numbers of interneurons, we found that about 200 interneurons should be connected to each P_i unit in order to reduce the model's output errors to less than 1 percent after training. Random interneuron functions constrained only by the requirement that they not fire very often were found to yield excellent and perhaps even best possible results. About three passes around the P_i-interneuron-P_i loop were found necessary for each model input before the mode's output F_i bits stabilized.

The essential assumptions upon which our model is based are as follows.

1. CA3 hippocampus contains numerous excitatory and inhibitory interneurons. An appreciable fraction of the inhibitory interneuronal output is provided by basket cells, and this fraction is important mainly for tonic regulation of pyramids. The remaining interneurons receive both extrinsic and pyramidal inputs in significant proportions.

2. To a reasonable first approximation, nonbasket interneuronal inputs to each pyramidal pool sum nearly algebraically to influence the pool's output in direct proportion to this sum.

3. Nonbasket interneurons fire infrequently over a typical day in the life of an unrestrained animal, and the relative firing patterns of these interneurons are not well correlated, at least after theta-wave and other macrorhythmic effects have been eliminated. Such randomness may be attributable to the way in which CA3 organizes its own impulse codes, or to factors affecting interneuronal growth and development, or to some mixture of the two.

4. The efficacy of nonbasket interneuronal influences on pyramids is plastic, is equivalent to synaptic efficacy, and is established under control of an extrahippocampal positive/negative reinforcement effect.

5. Pyramids and interneurons are drawn cluster by cluster into CA3 operation under the control of diffuse positive/negative reinforcements.

Future work will attempt to match the foregoing model's P_i output patterns to Ranck's recordings from single units in freely moving animals (Ranck, 1973) when the model is fed inputs from a habituation version of Stanley's GD model, which in turn is fed inputs from entorhinallike units as described by Ranck. A major question will be the extent to which interneuronal feedback potentiates *sequences* of CA3 response instead of just momentary decisionary outputs.

ACKNOWLEDGMENT

Preparation of this paper was supported in part by Public Health Service grants 5ROI NS 09755–03 COM from NINDS and 7ROI MH 25329–01 from NIMH.

REFERENCES

AKISKAL, J. S., and McKINNEY, JR., W. T. 1973. Depressive disorders: Toward a unified hypothesis. *Science* 182: 20–29.

ANDERSEN, P., and LØMO, T. 1969. Organization and frequency dependence of hippocampal inhibition. In H. Jasper, A. Ward, and A. Pope, eds., *Basic Mechanisms of the Epilepsies*. Boston: Little, Brown.

ANDERSON, P., BLISS, P.T.V., and SKREDE, K. K. 1971. Lamellar organization of hippocampal excitatory pathways. *Experimental Brain Research* 13: 222–238.

ANON. 1974. If you must fall on your head, do it while you're young. *New Scientist* 54 (May 25): 422.

ANTELMAN, S. M., LIPPA, A. S., and FISHER, A. E. 1972. 6-hydroxydopamine, noradrenergic reward, and schizophrenia. *Science* 175: 919–923.

ARBIB, M. A. 1972. *The Metaphorical Brain*. New York: Wiley-Interscience.

ARBIB, M. A. 1975. From automata theory to brain theory. *International Journal of Man-Machine Studies* 7: 279–295.

BLAKEMORE, C., and COOPER, G. F. 1970. Development of the brain depends on the visual environment. *Nature* 228: 477–478.

BLAKEMORE, C., NACHMIAS, J., and SUTTON, P. 1970. The perceived spatial frequency shift: Evidence for frequency-selective neurons in the human brain. *Journal of Physiology* 210: 727–750.

BLOCK, H. D. 1962. The perceptron: A model for brain functioning. I. *Reviews of Modern Physics* 34: 123–135.

BRINDLEY, G. S. 1969. Nerve net models of plausible size that perform many simple learning tasks. *Proceedings of the Royal Society (London)* B 174: 173–191.

CAMPBELL, F. W., and ROBSON, J. G. 1968. Application of Fourier analysis to the visibility of gratings. *Journal of Physiology* 197: 551–566.

CRAIK, K. J. W. 1943. *The Nature of Explanation*. London: Cambridge University Press.

DIDDAY, R. L., and ARBIB, M. A. 1975. Eye movements and visual perception: A "two visual system" model. *International Journal of Man-Machine Studies* (in press).

FOX, M. W. 1972. *Behavior of Wolves, Dogs and Related Canids*. New York: Harper & Row.

FOX, M. W., ed. 1973. *Readings in Ethology and Comparative Psychology*. Monterey, Calif.: Brooks / Cole.

GABOR, D., KOCK, W. E., and STROKE, G. W. 1971. Holography. *Science* 173: 11–23.

GARCIA, J. 1971. The faddy rat and us. *New Scientist* 49 (Feb. 4): 254–256.

GESCHWIND, N. 1970. The organization of language and the brain. *Science* 170: 940–944.

GREGORY, R. L. 1969. On how so little information controls so much behavior. In C. H. Waddington, ed., *Towards a Theoretical Biology. 2. Sketches.* Edinburgh: Edinburgh University Press, pp. 236–247.

GROSSBERG, S. 1972. Neural expectation: Cerebellar and retinal analogs of cells fired by learnable or unlearned pattern classes. *Kybernetik* 10: 49–57.

GRZIMEK, B. 1968. On the psychology of the horse. In H. Fredrich, ed., *Man and Animal: Studies in Behavior.* New York: St. Martin's Press, pp. 37–45.

HEBB, D. O. 1949. *The Organization of Behavior.* New York: John Wiley & Sons.

HIRSCH, H. V. B., and SPINELLI, D. N. 1970. Visual experience modifies distribution of horizontally and vertically oriented receptive fields in cats. *Science* 168: 869–871.

HIRSCH, H. V. B., and SPINELLI, D. N. 1971. Modification of the distribution of receptive field orientation during development. *Experimental Brain Research* 13: 509–527.

HJORTH-SIMONSEN, A. 1973. Projection of the lateral part of the entorhinal area to the hippocampus and fascia dentata. *Journal of Comparative Neurology* 146: 219–232.

HONGAN, J. 1971. Development of hunger system in young chicks. *Behavior* 39: 127–201.

HUBEL, D. H., and WIESEL, T. N. 1962. Receptive fields, binocular interaction and functional architecture in the cat's visual cortex. *Journal of Physiology* 160: 106–154.

HUBEL, D. H., and WIESEL, T. N. 1970. The period of susceptibility to the physiological effects of unilateral eye closure in kittens. *Journal of Physiology* 206: 419–436.

HYDÉN, H., LANGE, P. W., and SEYFRIED, C. 1973. Biochemical brain protein changes produced by selective breeding for learning in rats. *Brain Research* 61: 446–451.

ITO, M., and OLDS, J. 1971. Unit activity during self-stimulation behavior. *Journal of Neurophysiology* 34: 264–273.

KILMER, W. L., and McLARDY, T. 1971. A diffusely preprogrammed but sharply trainable hippocampus model. *International Journal of Neuroscience* 2: 241–248.

KILMER, W. L., and OLINSKI, M. 1974. Model of a plausible learning scheme for CA3 hippocampus. *Kybernetik* 16: 133–144.

KOHONEN, T. 1971. A class of randomly organized associative memories. *Acta Polytechnica Scandinavica* E125: 1–19.

KRIEG, W. J. S. 1966. *Functional Neuroanatomy,* 3rd ed. Evanston, Ill.: Brain Books Inc.

LASHLEY, K. S. 1929. *Brain Mechanisms in Intelligence.* Chicago: University of Chicago Press.

LETTVIN, J. Y., MATURANA, H., McCULLOCH, W. S., and PITTS, W. 1959. What the frog's eye tells the frog's brain. *Proceedings of the IRE* 47: 1940–1951.

LURIA, A. R. 1973. *The Working Brain.* Translated by Basil Haigh. New York: Basic Books.

MARLER, P. 1973. Developments in the study of animal communication. In Fox (1973).

MARR, D. 1969. A theory of cerebellar cortex. *Journal of Physiology* 202: 437–470.

MARR, D. 1970. A theory for cerebral cortex. *Proceedings of the Royal Society (London)* B 176: 161–234.

MARR, D. 1971. Simple memory: A theory for archicortex. *Philosophical Transactions of the Royal Society (London)* 262: 23–81.

McLARDY, T. 1973a. Schizophrenia and temporal lobe epilepsy interrelations. *International Research Communications System* March (73-3) 16-14-2.

McLARDY, T. 1973b. Deficit and paucity of dentate granule-cells in some schizophrenic brains. *International Research Communications System* March (73-3) 16-1-1.

McLARDY, T. 1973c. Gyrus dentatus granule-cell pathology in chronic alcoholism. *International Research Communications System* March (73-9) 16-8-6.

McLARDY, T. 1973d. Dentate granule-cell sensitivity to proximity of blood vessels in chronic alcoholism. *International Research Communications System* September (73-9) 39-8-2.

MENZEL, E. W. 1973. Chimpanzee spatial memory organization. *Science* 182: 943–945.

MINSKY, M. L., and PAPERT, S. 1969. *Perceptrons: An Introduction to Computational Geometry.* Cambridge, Mass.: MIT Press.

NILSSON, N. J. 1965. *Learning Machines.* New York: McGraw-Hill.

NOTON, D., and STARK, L. 1971a. Scanpaths in eye movements during pattern perception. *Science* 171: 308–311.

NOTON, D., and STARK, L. 1971b. Eye movements and visual perception. *Scientific American* 224(2): 34–43.

NOTTEBOHM, F. 1972. The origins of vocal learning. *American Naturalist* 106: 116–135.

O'KEEFE, O., and DOSTROVSKY, J. 1971. Directed threat response. *Brain Research* 34: 171–175.

OLDS, J. 1969. The central nervous system and the reinforcement of behavior. *American Psychologist* 24: 114–132.

PEREZ, R., GLASS, L., and SCHLEAR, R. 1975. Development of specificity in the cat visual cortex. *Journal of Mathematical Biology* 1: 275–288.

PIAGET, J. 1967. *Six Psychological Studies.* New York: Random House.

PLOOG, D. 1971. The relevance of natural stimulus patterns for sensory information processes. *Brain Research* 31: 353–359.

POLLEN, D. A., and TAYLOR, J. H. 1974. The striate cortex and the spatial analysis of visual space. In F. O. Schmitt and F. G. Worden, eds., *The Neurosciences: Third Study Program.* Cambridge, Mass.: MIT Press, pp. 239–248.

PRIBRAM, K. H., SPINELLI, D. N., and KAMBACK, M. C. 1967. Electrocortical correlates of stimulus response and reinforcement. *Science* 157: 94–96.

PRIBRAM, K. H., 1969. Four Rs of remembering. In K. H. Pribram, ed., *On the Biology of Learning.* New York: Harcourt Brace Jovanovich, pp. 193–225.

PRIBRAM, K. H. 1974. How is it that sensing so much we can do so little? In F. O. Schmitt and F. G. Worden, eds., *The Neurosciences: Third Study Program.* Cambridge, Mass.: MIT Press, pp. 249–261.

QUADAGNO, M., and BANKS, E. M. 1973. The effect of reciprocal cross-fostering on the behaviour of two species of rodents, *Mus musculus* and *Baiomys taylori ater,* david. In Fox (1973).

RAMÓN Y CAJAL, S. 1911. *Histologie du Système Nerveux de l'Homme et des Vertébrés,* Vol. 2. Paris: Maloine.

RANCK, J. 1973. Studies on single neurons in dorsal hippocampal formation and septum in unrestrained rats. *Experimental Neurology* 41: 461–555.

ROSENBLATT, F. 1961. *Principles of Neurodynamics: Perceptrons and the Theory of Brain Mechanisms.* Washington, D.C.: Spartan Books.

SCHANK, R. C. and COLBY, K. M. 1973. *Computer Models of Thought and Language.* San Francisco: W. H. Freeman.

SEGAL, M., and OLDS, J. 1973. Behavior of units in hippocampal circuit of the rat during differential classical conditioning. *Journal of Comparative and Physiological Psychology* 82: 195–204.

SELIGMAN, M. E. P., and HAGER, J. L. 1972. The *sauce Béarnaise* syndrome. *Psychology Today* (August): 59–87.

SLOBIN, D. 1972. Children and language: They learn the same way all around the world. *Psychology Today* (May): 71–82.

SPINELLI, D. N. 1970. OCCAM: A computer model for a content addressable memory in the central nervous system. In K. H. Pribram and D. E. Broadbent, eds., *Biology of Memory*. New York: Academic Press, pp. 293–306.

SPINELLI, D. N., HIRSCH, H. V. B., PHELPS, R. W., and METZLER, J. 1972. Visual experience as a determinant of the response characteristics of cortical receptive fields in cats. *Experimental Brain Research* 15: 289–304.

SPIRA, P. M. 1969. The time required for group multiplication. *Journal of the Association for Computing Machinery* 16: 235–243.

SPIRA, P. M., and ARBIB, M. A. 1967. Computation times for finite groups, semigroups, and automata. In *Proceedings of IEEE 8th Annual Symposium on Switching and Automata Theory*, pp. 291–295.

STANLEY, J. M., and KILMER, W. L. 1975. A wave model of temporal learning and habituation in the dentate gyrus of the mammalian brain. *International Journal of Man-Machine Studies* 7: 395–412.

STEIN, L., and WISE, C. D. 1971. Possible etiology of schizophrenia: Progressive damage to the noradrenergic reward system by 6-hydroxydopamine. *Science* 171:1032–1036.

STEVENS, J. R. 1973. An anatomy of schizophrenia? *Archives of General Psychiatry* 29: 177–189.

STOLL, E. 1970. The abused child. *The Sciences* (New York Academy of Science) 10(May): 5–8; 29–32.

TINBERGEN, N. 1972. Functional ethology and the human sciences. *Proceedings of the Royal Society (London)* B 182: 385–410.

VAN HOESEN, G. W., PANDYA, D. N., and BUTTERS, N. 1972. Cortical afferents to the entorhinal cortex of the rhesus monkey. *Science* 175: 1471–1473.

VINOGRADOVA, O. S., 1970. Registration of information and the limbic system. In G. Horn and R. A. Hinde, eds., *Short-Term Changes in Neural Activity and Behaviour* London: Cambridge University Press, pp. 95–140.

VON DER MALSBURG, C. 1973. Self-organization of orientation sensitive cells in the striate cortex. *Kybernetik* 14: 85–100.

WESTLAKE, P. R. 1970. The possibilities of neural holographic processes within the brain. *Kybernetik* 7: 129–153.

WIESEL, T. N., and HUBEL, D. H. 1965. Comparison of the effects of unilateral and bilateral eye closure on cortical unit responses in kittens. *Journal of Neurophysiology* 28: 1029–1040.

WILLSHAW, D. J., BUNEMAN, O. P., and LONGUET-HIGGINS, H. C. 1969. Non-holographic associative memory. *Nature* 222: 960–962.

WINOGRAD, S. 1965. On the time required to perform addition. *Journal of the Association for Computing Machinery* 12: 277–285.

WINOGRAD, S. 1967. On the time required to perform multiplication. *Journal of the Association for Computing Machinery* 14: 793–802.

ZIMMER, J. 1971. Ipsilateral afferents to the commissural zone of the fascia dentata, demonstrated in decommissurated rats by silver impregnation. *Journal of Comparative Neurology* 142: 393–416.

Note added in proof: For a more formal treatment of the slide-box metaphor, see the theory of *schemas* in M. A. Arbib, "Segmentation, schemas, and cooperative phenomena," in S. Levin, ed., *Studies in Biomathematics* (Washington, D.C.: Mathematical Association of America, 1976).

8

Are There Modifiable Synapses in the Visual Cortex?

JACK D. COWAN

ABSTRACT This paper is concerned with the question of what types of synaptic modification can account for certain figural aftereffects, in particular for human habituation or adaptation to sinusoidally modulated visual contrast patterns—sine-wave gratings. It is shown that homosynaptic mechanisms such as cellular fatigue cannot account for these effects, nor can heterosynaptic mechanisms unless they are of a certain type, equivalent to a modified form of what is known as the Hebb synapse, i.e., a synapse that requires concurrent presynaptic and postsynaptic activity for facilitation to occur. Two contrasting theories of the functional organization of the visual cortex are discussed in relation to such synaptic models. It is also suggested that presumed changes in the visual cortex of young kittens exposed to special stimuli can be accounted for in terms of similar changes of Hebb-type synapses.

8.1 INTRODUCTION

Model neural nets comprising excitatory and inhibitory elements with simple threshold and refractory properties, connected together in a many-to-many fashion, have been shown (and reshown) by many theorists to be capable of detecting, storing, and retrieving simple patterns (see Arbib, Kilmer, and Spinelli, this volume), provided they contain modifiable synapses.

Brindley (1967, 1969) has provided a fairly comprehensive classification of the various possible ways in which synaptic changes could be used to store information. He lists ten possible synaptic mechanisms, of which six are variants of a basic four, proposed (respectively) by Hebb (1949), Shimbel (1950), Eccles (1953), and Burke (1966). The Hebb synapse is modified by concurrent presynaptic and postsynaptic activity, the Shimbel synapse by postsynaptic activity, and the Eccles synapse by presynaptic activity; the Burke synapse utilizes presynaptic facilitation of presynaptic activity.

As Brindley notes, all but the Hebb synapse are rather inefficient as information-storage mechanisms. On the one hand, if modification of a synapse depends only on postsynaptic activity that reaches all relevant postsynaptic elements, then the synapses to a given cell do not constitute independent stores of information. On the other hand, if modification depends only on presynaptic

activity that reaches all relevant presynaptic sites, then all synapses from a given cell are modified together, and also do not constitute independent stores of information. The Hebb synapse does not suffer from such limitations, however, since modification depends upon both presynaptic and postsynaptic activity, and individual Hebb synapses can therefore function as independent stores of activity. It follows that mechanisms such as posttetanic potentiation (Larrabee and Bronk, 1947), posttetanic depression (Evarts and Hughes, 1957), and low-frequency depression (Lloyd, 1949; Eccles, 1964; Kandel and Tauc, 1965a) do not provide efficient ways of storing information. Such mechanisms have been termed *homosynaptic* (Kandel et al., 1970) in that a single cell, which can be presynaptic or postsynaptic, determines modification. The Hebb synapse is an example of *heterosynaptic* facilitation of excitatory postsynaptic potentials (EPSPs) in that two cells, one presynaptic and one postsynaptic, are involved in a synaptic modification.

Strictly speaking there is no direct evidence to support the Hebb synapse. However, Kandel and Tauc (1965a) have described heterosynaptic facilitation in *Aplysia* neurons that is not inconsistent with such a synapse. Figure 8.1 shows some of the details. EPSPs produced by stimulation of genital nerve are facilitated by concurrent stimulation of another pathway to the neuron, from the siphon nerve. It will be observed that this modifying stimulation actually fires the neuron, and the synapse could thus be of Hebb type. Against this, a further analysis by Kandel and Tauc (1965b) showed that facilitation could be produced by modifying stimuli that did not fire the neuron, and suggested that presynaptic facilitation (or inhibition) was responsible, i.e., that the synapse was of Burke type. Nonetheless, postsynaptic activity as a causative agent is not ruled out, and in fact on any time scale for modification that is long compared to the duration of a single impulse (as is the case in vertebrates), there is no practical difference between subthreshold postsynaptic activity at the trigger-zone and the time-averaged rate of firing of cells, and either could function as a modifier.

Marr (1969, 1970, 1971) has employed various heterosynaptic modification mechanisms in a most penetrating

JACK D. COWAN, Department of Biophysics and Theoretical Biology, University of Chicago, Chicago, IL

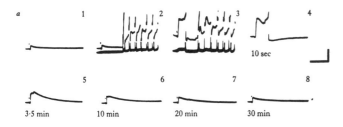

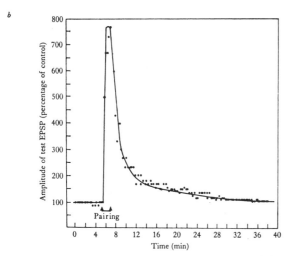

FIGURE 8.1 (a) Heterosynaptic facilitation in an *Aplysia* neuron: (1) Test EPSP produced by stimulation of genital nerve before pairing. (2) First of nine pairing trials of test EPSP and response to priming stimulus (6/sec train of 1-sec duration to the siphon nerve). (3) Seventh pairing trial. Note accompanying depolarization and increase in test PSP. (4–8) Test PSP 10 sec, 3.5, 10, 20, and 30 min after pairing. The lower traces in (2) and (3) are lower gain records. The voltage calibration is 10 mV for the upper and 100mV for the lower trace. The time calibration is 500 msec. (b) Time course of heterosynaptic facilitation. Same experiment as in (a) but a different run. The amplitude of the test EPSP is plotted as a function of time and of pairing; the period of pairing is indicated by arrows. From Kandel and Tauc (1965a). Reproduced with permission.

analysis of the neurotechnological requirements for the construction of nets capable of classifying, storing, and retrieving simple patterns, including both Hebb synapses and a synapse, similar to the *Aplysia* type, that requires presynaptic "climbing-fiber" activity to facilitate EPSPs and that will henceforth be referred to as a Marr synapse. Marr (1970) noted the utility of the Brindley synapse, a Hebb synapse with a constant unmodifiable component. The Brindley synapse can be thought of as a Marr synapse with a common origin for modifiable and modifying afferents.

8.2 MODIFIABILITY OF THE VISUAL PATHWAY

It will be seen that there are numerous ways in which

synapses can be modified and very little evidence, particularly in vertebrate pathways, to support any but the simpler homosynaptic possibilities (Eccles, 1961; Wickelgren, 1967; Bliss and Lømo, 1970; Lømo, 1970; Spencer and April, 1970; Wall, 1970). Pettigrew (see Chapter 18, this volume) has described numerous experimental observations of cells in the kitten visual cortex, the receptive fields of which appear to be modified by early exposure to patterned stimuli. Of particular interest are the observations of Spinelli and Hirsch (1971), who report the existence of "grating detectors"—cells whose receptive fields are trimodal—when kittens are exposed early to three-stripe gratings. Pettigrew's conclusion that such effects clearly imply a modification of the connections to individual cells, rather than some cellular attrition process, is consistent with synaptic modification.

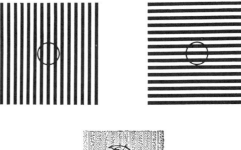

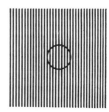

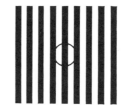

FIGURE 8.2 Subjective demonstration of spatial frequency-specific "channels," which may correspond to single-cell spatial selectivity in the cat. If the reader views this figure from a distance of about 3 m he or she will see, in the center, a person holding an umbrella. The superimposed lowcontrast vertical grating represents "rain." Now view, for about 60 sec, the high-contrast vertical grating of the same spatial frequency as the "rain," in the upper left, by letting the point of fixation wander around the circle. (This eye movement is required to prevent development of an afterimage of the grating.) After this adapting period, fixate the person's head and it will be noted that the "rain" has stopped, although it returns again after some seconds. Repeat the experiment, but this time fixate the horizontal grating in the upper right. A negative result is obtained. This is also the case if either of the lower gratings, of very different spatial frequency to that of the "rain," is viewed during the adapting period. From Blakemore and Campbell (1968). Reproduced with permission.

Unfortunately these experiments, unlike those in *Aplysia* and other invertebrates, do not allow the detailed analysis of synaptic transmission that would permit the elimination of possible mechanisms.

There is, however, another set of experimental observations, psychophysical in nature, that may help to narrow down possibilities. Ever since Gibson (1933) first described certain figural aftereffects—e.g., the straightened appearance of curved lines viewed continuously for a minute or so—there have been many experiments along similar lines, each utilizing one or more of the stimulus parameters now known to be detected by single cells in the visual cortex (see Chapter 18, this volume). A particularly pertinent set of experiments are those of Blakemore and Campbell (1968) on adaptation to spatial gratings. Figure 8.2 shows a dramatic example of such an adaptation experiment in which the reader can test his or her own adaptability. As is now well known to students of vision, the human visual system has been shown to be differentially sensitive to different spatial frequencies (measured in cycles per degree of visual angle) (Campbell, 1965). Thus, if one views a sinusoidally modulated grating, rather than the square-wave-modulated ones shown in Figure 8.2 (see Cornsweet, 1970, for details), through a fixed aperture, and if this grating is of constant luminance but varying spatial frequency, the modulation or contrast threshold at which one can just perceive the pattern is lowest around 4 to 6 c/deg and rises on either side of this frequency. The reciprocal function of such thresholds is termed the *modulation transfer function* (MTF).

A typical MTF obtained under such conditions is shown in Figure 8.3. It was shown by Campbell and Green (1965) that the high-frequency falloff (increase of threshold) is not caused by optical aberrations of the lens system, but is neural. The low-frequency falloff has been presumed to be caused by lateral inhibition, as in *Limulus* (Ratliff, 1965). If it is assumed that near threshold the visual system operates in a linear fashion, Fourier analysis can be utilized to compute the system response to various patterns. It follows that the Fourier transform of the MTF generates the so-called *line-spread function* (Cornsweet, 1970), i.e., the response of the system to a single line, from which the responses to most other patterns can be computed. Figure 8.4 shows such a function, obtained by Fourier-transforming the MTF shown in Figure 8.3. It will be seen that this function resembles the activity profile or *receptive field* of individual neurons of the visual pathway (see Bishop, Coombs, and Henry, 1971), but, of course, on a different spatial scale. Jung (1972) distinguishes between the two, calling the human line-spread function a *perceptive field* to distinguish it from the receptive fields of single cells.

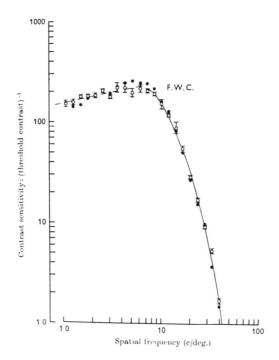

FIGURE 8.3 The contrast-sensitivity function for one human subject (F.W.C.). Contrast sensitivity is plotted on an arbitrary logarithmic scale against spatial frequency. The open circles and vertical bars show initial threshold estimates with 1 S.E. ($n = 6$). The filled circles are repeat determinations at the end of the series of adaptation experiments. The continuous curve is the function e^{-f}, and the interrupted portion was fitted by eye to the low-frequency data points. During threshold determinations the pattern was turned on and off twice per second, without changing mean luminance. From Blakemore and Campbell (1969). Reproduced with permission.

Blakemore and Campbell (1969) carried out a series of adaptation experiments similar to that depicted in Figure 8.2, with sinusoidally modulated gratings. Figure 8.5 shows the results of adaptation to a 7.1-c/deg grating. There is a contrast-threshold elevation over a rather narrow range of frequencies, centered on the adapting-stimulus frequency. If the *relative threshold elevation* (RTE) is plotted separately, as shown in Figure 8.5, it can be fitted with a curve that is strikingly similar to the MTF of a single cell of cat visual cortex of the

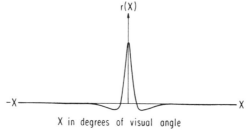

FIGURE 8.4 Fourier transform of the modulation transfer function shown in Figure 8.3, generating the human "perceptive field."

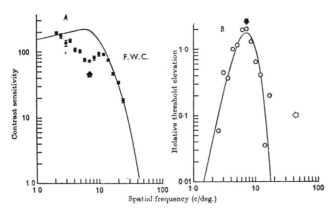

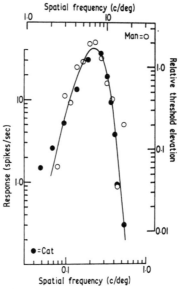

FIGURE 8.5 The effect of adapting at 7.1 c/deg. (A) The continuous curve from Figure 8.3 is reproduced. The filled circles and vertical bars are the means and S.E. ($n = 6$) for redetermination of contrast sensitivity at a number of spatial frequencies while F.W.C. was continuously adapting to a grating of 7.1 c/deg, 1.5 log units above threshold. The exact procedure is described in the text. (B) The depression in sensitivity due to adaptation at 7.1 c/deg is plotted, with open circles, as relative threshold elevation against spatial frequency. The vertical difference between each point and the smooth curve in Figure 8.5 A is the ratio of sensitivity before to that after adaptation. The relative threshold elevation is the antilogarithm of this difference minus one, so that no change in threshold would give a value of zero on the ordinate. The continuous curve is the function $[e^{-f^2} - e^{-(2f)^2}]^2$, fitted by eye to the data points. The filled arrows show the adapting frequency of 7.1 c/deg. The open arrow marks the value on the ordinate for a threshold elevation equivalent to $2\sqrt{2}$ times an average S.E. for determining contrast sensitivity. From Blakemore and Campbell (1969). Reproduced with permission.

FIGURE 8.6 Response of a "simple" field cortical neuron to a spatially modulated sinusoidal grating, compared with visual-threshold elevation in man produced by a similar stimulus. The closed circles are the responses (spikes/sec) of an orientation-specific cortical neuron from a cat. The sinusoidal-grating stimulus had a contrast of 0.5 and was drifting in the preferred direction, so that one bar of the grating passed over the receptive field each second. The open circles are the relative threshold elevations in man produced by adapting to a sinusoidal grating of contrast 0.7 and spatial frequency 7 c/deg. From Blakemore and Campbell (1969). Reproduced with permission.

"simple" type (Hubel and Wiesel, 1959, 1962). Figure 8.6 shows this in striking fashion.

Blakemore and Campbell (1969) suggest that this concurrence is not adventitious, and that the adaptation to sinusoidally modulated gratings is produced by the fatiguing of a set of simple cortical cells specifically tuned to a narrow band centered on the adapting frequency. Taken together with adaptation experiments such as those of Sullivan, Georgeson, and Oatley (1972), in which adaptation to a narrow bar is shown to produce a more or less uniform threshold elevation, somewhat similar to the frequency spectrum of the bar stimulus, and with quite different experiments related to the visibility of square-wave gratings (Campbell and Robson, 1968), the results have led to the suggestion that the visual cortex functions as a spatial Fourier analyzer (see Pollen and Taylor, 1974).

Such a suggestion has far-reaching implications. Area 17 (and perhaps area 19) of the visual cortex, instead of consisting of cells set up to detect local features such as edges, bars, slits, and corners, would have to be thought of as comprising sets of cells set up to detect the spatial

frequencies of stimulus patterns, a much more "global" operation, distributed rather than local in character, and implying much longer ranged connections in a secondary visual cortical area (e.g., inferotemporal cortex) to detect and combine the responses to individual frequencies. In view of all the experimental results obtained since Hubel and Wiesel (1955, 1962) first described oriented receptive fields in the cat cortex (see Bishop and Henry, 1971), such a view seems implausible. In the rest of this paper I shall outline an alternative interpretation of the adaptation experiments, based on the idea that there is a reorganization of cortical connectivity during adaptation (similar to that proposed by Pettigrew to account for the supposed development of receptive fields during a sensitive postnatal epoch) and that this reorganization of connectivity is produced by Brindley synapses.

8.3 A MODEL FOR VISUAL ADAPTATION

The idea that synaptic modification, not fatigue, is responsible for grating adaptation was originally proposed by my colleague H. R. Wilson (1975). In what follows I shall briefly describe Wilson's original model, together with recent extensions and generalizations (Cowan and Wilson, in preparation) that seem likely to provide an even better fit to the observations.

The starting point is to consider the way in which perceptive fields can be constructed from simpler elements. The simplest way follows Rodieck's (1965) construction of a retinal-ganglion receptive field as the difference of two line-spread functions, $k_e(x - x')$ and $k_i(x - x')$, as shown in Figure 8.7. Here k_e represents the spread of "excitation" in response to a line stimulus, and k_i the associated spread of "inhibition." Thus the response $r(x)$ at a point x in the visual system to a line $l(x')$ at a point x' in the visual field (the line-spread function shown in figure 8.4) is

$$r(x) = k_e(x - x') - k_i(x - x'), \tag{1}$$

and the response to an arbitrary stimulus $s(x')$, present over the whole visual field, can be written as the integral equation

$$r(x) = k_e(x) \otimes s(x) - k_i(x) \otimes s(x), \tag{2}$$

where

$$k(x) \otimes s(x) \equiv \int k(x - x') s(x') dx'. \tag{3}$$

Equation (2) can be Fourier-transformed into the algebraic equation

$$R(k) = K_e(k) S(k) - K_i(k) S(k), \tag{4}$$

where k is spatial frequency in cycles per degree of visual angle. It follows that if $s(x')$ is a sine wave, then

$$R(k) = \pi \alpha [K_e(k) - K_i(k)], \tag{5}$$

where α is the contrast or modulation depth of the sine wave. $R(k)$ in effect is the MTF as plotted in figure 8.3. Figure 8.8 shows a schematic representation of the resulting model of the visual system, in which the excitation and inhibition summate spatially to produce a response

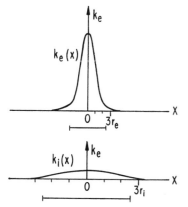

FIGURE 8.7 Excitatory and inhibitory line-spread functions, the difference of which provides a model for the human perceptive field shown in Figure 8.4.

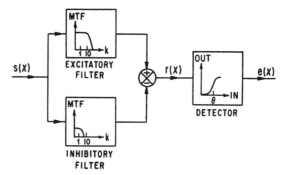

FIGURE 8.8 Schematic diagram showing the structure of the "single-channel" feedforward model for human contrast detection.

whose amplitude can trigger a "peak detector" to signal the presence of a suprathreshold stimulus. Such a model is said to be a "single-channel" model (Graham and Nachmias, 1971).

To account for the adaptation it is assumed that there is a strengthening of the inhibition (see Wickelgren, 1967; Wall, 1970), i.e., that

$$k_i(x - x') \rightarrow k_i(x - x')[1 + \lambda w(x,x')], \tag{6}$$

where λ is a constant and $w(x,x')$ is given by the time integral

$$\int_0^t r(x,t') s^*(x',t') e^{-\alpha(t-t')} dt',$$

s^* being the complex conjugate of s. (Thus, functionally, k_i increments as a leaky Brindley synapse.) Now, in obtaining the adaptation effect it is necessary to maintain a constant mean luminance, in order to eliminate afterimages, which would produce spurious results. This is usually obtained by phase modulation of the stimulus (Blakemore and Campbell, 1969; Klein and Stromeyer, 1974). Under such conditions it can be shown that $w(x, x')$ reduces to the convolution $r(x - x') \otimes s^*(x - x')$ (Cowan and Wilson, in preparation), and so the adapted line-spread function is given by the equation

$$r_a(x) = k_e(x - x') - k_i(x - x') \\ - \lambda k_i(x - x')[r_a(x - x') \otimes s_a^*(x - x')] \tag{7}$$

and the adapted MTF by the equation

$$R_a(k) = \pi \alpha [K_e(k) - K_i(k)] - \lambda' K_i(k) \otimes [R_a(k) S_a^*(k)]. \tag{8}$$

If $s_a(x)$, the adapting stimulus, is a sinusoid, as in the Blakemore-Campbell experiments, or a line, as (approximately) in the Sullivan-Georgeson-Oatley experiments, Equations (7) and (8) can be solved in closed form. The results are shown in Figure 8.9, in which RTE curves are shown for a number of adapting-stimulus frequencies. The theoretical curves provide a good fit to the experimental results on the high-frequency side, but do not do so well on the low-frequency side. Similar results obtain

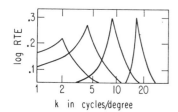

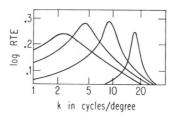

FIGURE 8.9 Relative-threshold-elevation curves, recomputed from Wilson (1975), obtained from a single-channel feedforward model, following adaptation to sinusoidally modulated gratings.

FIGURE 8.11 Relative-threshold-elevation curves obtained from a single-channel feedback model, following adaptation to sinusoidally modulated gratings.

$$R_a(k) = \pi\alpha K_e(k) - K_i(k)R_a(k)$$
$$- \lambda'K_i(k) \otimes [R_a(k)R_a{}^*(k)]R_a(k). \quad (12)$$

for adaptation to narrow bars or lines, in that there is a uniform threshold elevation at high frequencies, consistent with the observations of Sullivan, Georgeson, and Oatley (1972). However, the low-frequency side does not fit the observations too well.

There are, in fact, numerous reasons to suppose that the simple feedforward model outlined above is not as good a fit to the MTF as a feedback model would be. For example, at low luminance levels there is little low-frequency falloff in the MTF (van Meeteren and Vos, 1972). Moreover, the MTF can be fitted with a curve derived from a feedback model (Kelly, 1975; Wilson and Hines, in preparation). It follows that the simple feedback model depicted in Figure 8.10 ought to provide a better fit to both the unadapted and the adapted MTFs, given a suitable choice of the spread functions k_e and k_i. Equations (2) and (4) now become, respectively,

$$r(x) = k_e(x) \otimes s(x) - k_i(x) \otimes r(x) \quad (9)$$

and

$$R(k) = K_e(k)S(k) - K_i(k)R(k), \quad (10)$$

and if $s(x')$ is a sine wave, the MTF is now given by the expression

$$R(k) = \frac{\pi\alpha K_e(k)}{1 + K_i(k)} \quad (11)$$

and the adapted MTF by the equation

Once again, if $s_a(x)$ is a sinusoid, this equation can be solved for $R_a(k)$. The results are shown in Figure 8.11. Note that the fit to the experimental observations compares well with the feedforward case, so far as the shapes of the curves are concerned. Similar results obtain for adaptation to a single line.

Thus the modifications in perceptive fields produced by adaptation to simple one-dimensional visual stimuli can be accounted for in part by postulating Brindley synapses facilitating inhibition in either a feedforward or feedback model of the visual system.

8.4 PERCEPTIVE AND RECEPTIVE FIELDS

There remains the problem of accounting for the genesis and modification of perceptive fields in terms of the receptive fields of neurons in the visual pathway. As I have noted, Blakemore and Campbell (1969) remarked on the similarity between RTE curves and the MTFs of single cells in the cat cortex. Figure 8.12 shows the Fourier transform of the function used by Blakemore and Campbell to fit the threshold observations. It will be seen that the transform does indeed look like a receptive-field profile, although on an extended spatial scale. Thus the idea that a population of cells with such a receptive-field characteristic is fatigued during adaptation is quite plausible, and it is consistent with the theory proposed by Campbell and Robson (1968), on the basis of observa-

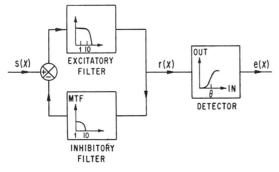

FIGURE 8.10 Schematic diagram showing the structure of the "single-channel" feedback model for human contrast detection.

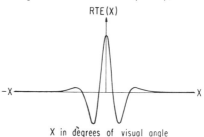

FIGURE 8.12 Fourier transform of the function $[e^{-k^2} - e^{(2k)^2}]^2$, used by Blakemore and Campbell (1969) to fit threshold-elevation data (see Figure 8.5).

tions on square-wave-modulated gratings, that the visual system consists not of a single channel, but of multiple, more or less independent channels, each tuned to a different pass-band of spatial frequencies and having a separate contrast threshold (see Figure 8.13). The overall MTF can then be thought of as the envelope of such a set of band-pass spatial filters, and the perceptive field as a summation over many cells with receptive fields of different sizes and sensitivities, each homogeneously distributed over large regions of the visual field (see Wiesel, 1960). Recent observations by Campbell and Maffei (1970) of human evoked potentials generated by the viewing of gratings seem to support such a theory, as do numerous more complex psychophysical experiments. In such a setting the fatiguing of a tuned population of cells seems quite plausible. However, there are a number of other observations which suggest that the theory as outlined above is not quite correct.

Measurements of human visual acuity—for example, the ability to resolve two points in the visual field (Mandelbaum and Sloan, 1947; Weymouth, 1958; Westheimer, 1972)—show that the minimum angle of resolution increases monotonically with visual eccentricity measured from the center of the fovea. If visual acuity at a given eccentricity is related to the spatial-frequency filtering characteristics of cells localized at corresponding points in the visual pathway, as seems to be the case, then the "channels" of the Campbell-Robson theory cannot be homogeneously distributed over the visual field, but must be somewhat localized, with channels tuned to higher spatial frequencies more centrally represented and low-frequency channels more peripherally represented. There is, in fact, evidence that the receptive fields of cat and monkey retinal ganglion cells, and subsequent cells, increase in size with retinal eccentricity (Fischer, 1973). This suggests that maximum sensitivity to spatial frequencies may be encoded in terms

of position in the visual field, mainly by virtue of a systematic variation in receptive-field sizes of retinal ganglion cells, a suggestion originally made by van Doorn, Koenderink, and Bouman (1972). Thus the channels may be spatially organized. Are they independent? Observations by Tolhurst (1972) on adaptation to square-wave gratings indicate that there is mutual inhibition between channels, as do similar observations by Stecher, Sigel, and Lange (1973).

Such details suggest that the visual system is organized in a fashion that parallels the auditory system, in which there is an early encoding of temporal frequencies into neural position coordinates at the basilar membrane (the "place" theory of sound encoding), with inhibition operating at higher levels of the system (see Whitfield, 1967). A quantitative theory of the visual system, similar to the above, is under development (Cowan and Wilson, in preparation). However, it should be recognized that a "spatial-frequency-into-place" encoding system is not a Fourier analyzer, but is, rather, merely the by-product of a system set up to detect edges and bars, with, perhaps, similar sensitivities in different parts of the visual field.

In such a locally addressed system, cellular fatigue as an adapting mechanism is not nearly so plausible a possibility as it is in the more globally addressed system contemplated by Campbell and Robson. It is difficult, for example, to see how more or less uniform RTE curves following adaptation to narrow bars (Sullivan, Georgeson, and Oatley, 1972) could be obtained in a locally addressed system by means of any fatigue mechanism, although the Brindley synapse works fairly well. In any case there are a number of observations and inferences which suggest that the fatigue theory is not viable. Wilson (1975), for example, notes first that the relaxation times for figural aftereffects following prolonged exposure are much longer than any simple fatigue model would warrant. Second, RTE curves become narrower at higher adapting spatial frequencies. According to the Campbell-Robson theory this implies that the visual system should be more sharply tuned to higher spatial frequencies, a conclusion at variance with experimental studies (Campbell, Nachmias, and Jukes, 1970). Third, Maffei, Fiorentini, and Bisti (1973), neurophysiologically, and Sharpe (1974), psychophysically, have shown that it is possible to adapt units that have not been directly stimulated. In addition, there is also the theoretical inference that any linear theory that uses homosynaptic modification mechanisms, either presynaptic or postsynaptic (e.g., fatigue), can be ruled out. It is easy to show that any kind of phase modulation of $s(x)$ or $r(x)$ alone will remove all spatial frequencies except zero. But on any linear theory, if the adapting stimulus $s(x')$ is a sinusoidally modulated grating then $r(x)$ will also be

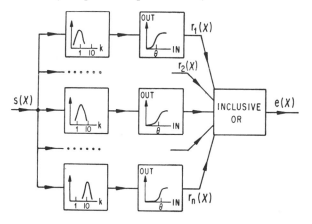

FIGURE 8.13 Schematic diagram showing the structure of a "multiple-channel" model for human contrast detection.

sinusoidally modulated, and so its phase average will simply reflect the background luminance. Any changes in the MTF produced by such an average cannot reflect the adapting frequency. In some ways this parallels Brindley's conclusion that homosynaptic modifications are not very efficient information stores. The Brindley synapse, as an example of the class of Hebb-type synapses, is able to store frequency information by virtue of its correlation structure.

It follows that, on such a place theory, there is still a simple and direct relationship between perceptive fields and receptive fields, as in the Campbell-Robson theory, except that the relationship is local, different locations having different sets of receptive fields. However, there is no simple and direct relationship between such location-dependent perceptive fields and the MTF, since Fourier methods cannot be used in the analysis of spatially inhomogeneous systems, at least not in any direct fashion. A full discussion of the ramifications of this problem as it applies to RTE curves is beyond the scope of this paper, and in what follows I shall simply assume that the visual system is locally isoplanatic (i.e., spatially homogeneous), so that the single-channel synaptic adaptation model holds, while recognizing that it will have to be modified somewhat to take account of spatial inhomogeneity. (In fact, such modifications are required to produce a good fit of both the relative amplitudes and shapes of RTE curves in the synaptic adaptation model.)

8.5 NEURAL REALIZATIONS OF THE MODEL

The model can now be made neurologically more specific. Since Maffei, Fiorentini, and Bisti (1973) have shown that grating adaptation occurs no more peripherally in the visual pathways than at the simple-cell cortical level, it will be assumed that interneurons in the visual cortex are the primary sites of modification. In this respect it is of interest to consider recent models of the cortical structures responsible for the generation of simple receptive fields. For example, Figure 8.14 shows a model for simple-cell receptive-field organization, due to Bishop, Coombs, and Henry (1971), in which there are numerous interneurons, both excitatory and inhibitory, acting as target sites for specific visual afferents. It was originally suggested that the deep pyramids of layer V are Hubel and Wiesel's "simple" cells (Hubel and Wiesel, 1962). However, recent studies of cortical neurons identified with intracellular stains have shown that simple cells are mostly stellate cells of layer IV (van Essen and Kelly, 1973). Brooks and Jung (1972) comment that some layer-V pyramids may still be simple cells, functioning as "target neurons" (Eccles, 1971) for the integration of stellate activity and for contrast enhancement. Whatever

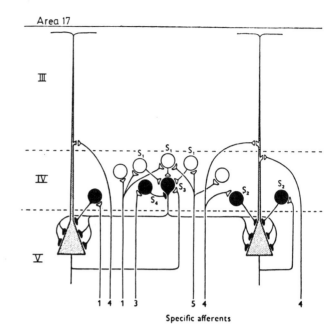

FIGURE 8.14 Possible neuronal circuits in a hypothetical model for simple-cell receptive-field organization in area 17. Stippled cells are pyramidal cells and the remainder are various kinds of stellate cells, with specific afferents numbered corresponding to the b matrix. S_1, S_2, and S_4 are Golgi type-II cells, and S_3 is a basket cell. Open boutons and cell bodies: excitatory synapses and neurons. Filled cell bodies and boutons: inhibitory neurons and synapses. From Bishop, Coombs, and Henry (1971). Reproduced with permission.

the facts turn out to be, there is ample evidence to support the idea that layer-IV (and perhaps layer-V) interactions are basic elements in the generation and modification of simple-cell responses. (See Marr, 1970, and Szentágothai, 1972.)

This being the case, there are essentially four possible models that, at the present stage of sophistication in experimental techniques, seem capable of fitting the data reasonably well. Figure 8.15 shows the four models, two of which are feedforward, and two feedback, systems. Models 1 and 3 employ Brindley synapses that facilitate IPSPs; models 2 and 4 employ Brindley synapses that facilitate EPSPs. It is not possible as yet to distinguish between the models on any experimental basis, although models 2 and 4 seem more natural.

8.6 DISCUSSION

The main point of this paper has been to try to make the case, not only for the *sufficiency* of the Hebb or Brindley synapse in the construction of modifiable nets, but also for its *necessity*. To do so I have had to sketch theories concerning the overall functional organization of that part of the visual system concerned with the simplest

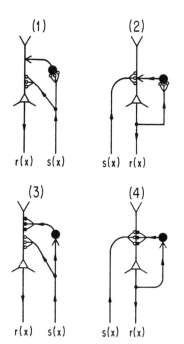

FIGURE 8.15 Possible cortical circuits mediating habituation or adaptation to maintained spatial patterns. Open circles: excitatory unmodifiable synapses. Arrow heads: modifiable Brindley synapses.

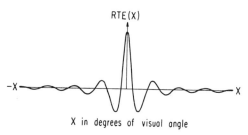

FIGURE 8.16 Fourier transform of the relative-threshold-elevation curve for adaptation to eight cycles per degree, as shown in Figure 8.9.

metric properties of stimuli, in order to provide a context within which questions of mechanism could be discussed. Psychophysical theories can help to provide this necessary context within which neurophysiology can operate.

It is of considerable interest that the Hebb and Brindley synapse has recently been used by many theorists as a way to encode orientation selectivity into initially nonoriented receptive fields (Cooper, 1974; von der Malsburg, 1973; Perez, Glass, and Schlear, 1975; see Arbib, Kilmer, and Spinelli, this volume, for details). It should be evident that the two-dimensional extension of the theory outlined in this paper, perhaps with facilitation of excitatory as well as inhibitory Brindley synapses, can serve as a useful model for the development of such fields and for many other psychophysical and neurophysiological phenomena. Preliminary calculations on the orientational selectivity of RTE curves in a two-dimensional generalization of the simple feedforward model support this idea (Wilson, 1975).

In this respect it is of interest to compare the Fourier transform of the RTE curves fitted by Blakemore and Campbell with that obtained from the synaptic model. Figure 8.12 and 8.16 show the two transforms. As expected, the first transform looks like the activity profile of a simple-cell receptive field, whereas the second one reflects the structure of the adapting stimulus, an infinite cosine wave. Thus, on the synaptic-modification hypothesis, adaptation to a periodic stimulus will result in a

change in neural connectivity directly related to the stimulus itself. The grating detectors observed by Spinelli and Hirsch (1971) could be generated, with suitable modification, by the same mechanism, i.e., by facilitating according to a rule similar to that given in Equations (6) and (7) or (12), EPSPs arising in simple cells or in their associated circuitry. On such a postulate, random eye movements would be required to produce that phase modulation which is necessary to store spatial organization in Brindley synapses, as shown in Section 8.2. A secondary consequence is that large numbers of cells must be involved in such a process, since phase modulation in effect creates an ensemble. One wonders whether the current paradigm that single cells are the functional units of behavior (see Chapter 18, this volume) is really apposite for anything other than the behavior of single cells.

ACKNOWLEDGMENTS

I should like to thank my colleague H. R. Wilson for helpful comments on the manuscript, S. Muka for computational services, and Ms. A. Pasley for secretarial services in the production of this manuscript. I should also like to thank Drs. P. O. Bishop, C. Blakemore, F. W. Campbell, E. R. Kandel, the Physiological Society (London), and the Syndics of the Cambridge University Press for permission to reproduce a number of figures in the text of this paper. Finally, I should like to acknowledge partial support from the Alfred P. Sloan Foundation and the National Institutes of Health for the work reported in this paper, and the hospitality of the Aspen Center for Physics, where parts of this work were completed.

REFERENCES

BISHOP, P. O., COOMBS, J. S., and HENRY, G. H. 1971. Interaction effects of visual contours on the discharge frequency of simple striate neurones. *Journal of Physiology* 219: 659–687.

BISHOP, P. O., and HENRY, G. H. 1971. Spatial vision. *Annual Reviews of Psychology* 22: 119–160.

BLAKEMORE, C., and CAMPBELL, F. W. 1968. Adaptation to spatial stimuli. *Journal of Physiology* 200: 11P–13P.

BLAKEMORE, C., and CAMPBELL, F. W. 1969. On the existence of neurones in the human visual system selectively sensitive to the orientation and size of retinal images. *Journal of Physiology* 203: 237–260.

BLISS, T. V. P., and LØMO, T. 1970. Plasticity in a monosynaptic cortical pathway. *Journal of Physiology* 207: 61P.

BRINDLEY, G. S. 1967. The classification of modifiable synapses and their use in models for conditioning. *Proceedings of the Royal Society (London)* B 168: 361–376.

BRINDLEY, G. S. 1969. Nerve net models of plausible size that perform many simple learning tasks. *Proceedings of the Royal Society (London)* B 174: 173–191.

BROOKS, B., and JUNG, R. 1972. Neuronal physiology of the visual cortex. In R. Jung, ed., *Handbook of Sensory Physiology*, VII/3B. Berlin: Springer-Verlag, pp. 325–440.

BURKE, W. 1966. Neuronal models for conditioned reflexes. *Nature* 210: 269.

CAMPBELL, F. W. 1965. Visual acuity via linear analysis. In *Proceedings of the Symposium on Information Processing in Sight Sensory Systems*. Pasadena, Calif.: California Institute of Technology, p. 177.

CAMPBELL, F. W. 1974. The transmission of spatial information through the visual system. In F. O. Schmitt and F. G. Worden, eds., *The Neurosciences: Third Study Program*. Cambridge, Mass.: MIT Press, pp. 95–103.

CAMPBELL, F. W., and GREEN, D. C. 1965. Optical and retinal factors affecting visual resolution. *Journal of Physiology* 181: 576–593.

CAMPBELL, F. W., and MAFFEI, L. 1970. Electrophysiological evidence for the existence of orientation and size detectors in the human visual system. *Journal of Physiology* 207: 635–652.

CAMPBELL, F. W., NACHMIAS, J., and JUKES, J. 1970. Spatial frequency discrimination in human vision. *Journal of the Optical Society of America* 60: 555–559.

CAMPBELL, F. W., and ROBSON, J. E. 1968. Application of Fourier analysis to the visibility of gratings. *Journal of Physiology* 197: 551–566.

COOPER, L. N. 1974. A possible organization of animal memory and learning. In *Proceedings of the Nobel Symposium on Collective Properties of Systems*. Aspenasgarden, Sweden.

CORNSWEET, J. 1970. *Visual Perception*. New York: Academic Press.

ECCLES, J. C. 1953. *The Neurophysiological Basis of Mind*. Oxford: Oxford University Press.

ECCLES, J. C. 1961. The effects of use and disuse on synaptic function. In J. F. Delafresnaye et al., eds., *Brain Mechanisms and Learning*. Oxford: Blackwell Scientific Publications.

ECCLES, J. C. 1964. *The Physiology of Nerve Cells*. Berlin: Springer-Verlag.

ECCLES, J. C. 1971. Functional significance of the arrangement of neurones in cell assemblies. *Archives für Psychiatrie Nervenkrankheiten* 215: 92–106.

EVARTS, E. V., and HUGHES, J. R. 1957. Relation of post-tetanic potentiation to subnormality of lateral geniculate potentials. *American Journal of Physiology* 188: 238–244.

FISCHER, B. 1973. Overlap of receptive field centers and representation of the visual field in the cat's optic tract. *Vision Research* 13: 2113–2120.

GIBSON, J. J. 1933. Adaptation, after-effect and contrast in the perception of curved lines. *Journal of Experimental Psychology* 16: 1–31.

GRAHAM, N., and NACHMIAS, J. 1971. Detection of grating patterns containing two spatial frequencies: A comparison of single-channel and multiple-channel models. *Vision Research* 11: 251–259.

HEBB, D. O. 1949. *The Organization of Behavior*. New York: John Wiley & Sons.

HUBEL, D., and WIESEL, T. N. 1959. Receptive fields of single neurones in the cat's striate cortex. *Journal of Physiology* 148: 574–591.

HUBEL, D., and WIESEL, T. N. 1962. Receptive fields, binocular interaction and functional architecture in the cat's visual cortex. *Journal of Physiology* 160: 106–154.

JUNG, R. 1972. Visual perception and neurophysiology. In R. Jung, ed., *Handbook of Sensory Physiology*, VII/3A. Berlin: Springer-Verlag, pp. 1–100.

KANDEL, E. R., CASTELLUCCI, V., PINSKER, H., and KUPFERMANN, I. 1970. The role of synaptic plasticity in the short-term modification of behavior. In G. Horn and R. A. Hinde, eds., *Short-Term Changes in Neuronal Activity and Behaviour*. London: Cambridge University Press.

KANDEL, E. R., and TAUC, L. 1965a. Heterosynaptic facilitation of neurones of the abdominal ganglion of *Aplysia depilans*. *Journal of Physiology* 181: 1–27.

KANDEL, E. R., and TAUC, L. 1965b. Mechanism of heterosynaptic facilitation in the giant cell of the abdominal ganglion of *Aplysia depilans*. *Journal of Physiology* 181: 28–47.

KELLY, D. H. 1975. Spatial frequency selectivity in the retina. *Vision Research* 15: 665–672.

KLEIN, S., and STROMEYER, C. F. 1974. Adaptation to complex gratings: On inhibition between spatial frequency channels. *Vision Research* (in press).

LARRABEE, M. G., and BRONK, D. W. 1947. Prolonged facilitation of synaptic excitation in sympathetic ganglia. *Journal of Neurophysiology* 10: 139–154.

LLOYD, D. P. C. 1949. Post-tetanic potentiation of response in monosynaptic reflex pathways of spinal cord. *Journal of General Physiology* 33: 147–170.

LØMO, T. 1970. Some properties of a cortical excitation synapse. In P. Anderson and J. Jansen, Jr., eds., *Excitatory Synaptic Mechanisms*. Oslo: Oslo University Press.

MAFFEI, L., FIORENTINI, A., and BISTI, S. 1973. Neural correlate of perceptual adaptation to gratings. *Science* 182: 1036–1038.

MANDELBAUM, J., and SLOAN, L. L. 1947. Peripheral vision acuity, with special reference to scotopic illumination. *American Journal of Ophthalmology* 30: 581–588.

MARR, D. C. 1969. A theory of cerebellar cortex. *Journal of Physiology* 202: 437–470.

MARR, D. C. 1970. A theory for cerebral neocortex. *Proceedings of the Royal Society (London)* B, 176: 161–234.

MARR, D. C. 1971. Simple memory: A theory for archicortex. *Philosophical Transactions of the Royal Society (London)* B 262: 23–81.

PEREZ, R., GLASS, L., and SCHLEAR, R. 1975. Development of specificity in the cat visual cortex. *Journal of Mathematical Biology* 1: 275–288.

POLLEN, D. A., and TAYLOR, J. H. 1974. The striate cortex and the spatial analysis of visual space. In F. O. Schmitt and F. G. Worden, eds., *The Neurosciences: Third Study Program*. Cambridge, Mass.: MIT Press.

RATLIFF, F. 1965. *Mach Bands: Quantitative Studies on Neural Networks in the Retina*. San Francisco: Holden-Day.

RODIECK, R. W. 1965. Quantitative analysis of cat retinal

ganglion cell response to visual stimuli. *Vision Research* 5: 583–601.

SHARPE, C. R. 1974. The colour specificity of spatial adaptation: Red-blue interactions. *Vision Research* 14: 41–51.

SHIMBEL, A. 1950. Contributions to the mathematical biophysics of the central nervous system with special reference to learning. *Bulletin of Mathematical Biophysics* 12: 241.

SPENCER, W. A., and APRIL, R. S. 1970. Plastic properties of monosynaptic pathways in mammals. In G. Horn and R. A. Hinde, eds., *Short-Term Changes in Neuronal Activity and Behaviour*. London: Cambridge University Press.

SPINELLI, D. N., and HIRSCH, H. V. B. 1971. Genesis of receptive field shapes in single units of cat's visual cortex. *Federation Proceedings* 30: 615.

STECHER, S., SIGEL, C., and LANGE, R. V. 1973. Spatial frequency channels in human vision and the threshold for adaptation. *Vision Research* 13: 1691–1700.

SULLIVAN, G. D., GEORGESON, M. A., and OATLEY, K. 1972. Channels for spatial frequency selection and the detection of single bars by the human visual system. *Vision Research* 12: 383–394.

SZENTÁGOTHAI, J. 1972. Synaptology of the visual cortex. In R. Jung, ed., *Handbook of Sensory Physiology*, VII/3B. Berlin: Springer-Verlag, pp. 269–324.

TOLHURST, D. J. 1972. Adaptation to square-wave gratings: Inhibition between spatial frequency channels and human visual systems. *Journal of Physiology* 226: 231–248.

VAN DOORN, A. J., KOENDERINK, J. J., and BOUMAN, M. A. 1972. The influence of the retinal inhomogeneity on the perception of spatial patterns. *Kybernetik* 10: 223–230.

VAN ESSEN, D., and KELLY, J. 1973. Correlation of cell shape and function in the visual cortex of the cat. *Nature* 241: 403–405.

VAN MEETEREN, A., and VOS, J. J. 1972. Resolution and contrast sensitivity at low luminances. *Vision Research* 12: 825–833.

VON DER MALSBURG, C. 1973. Self-organization of orientation sensitive cells in the striate cortex. *Kybernetik* 14: 85–100.

WALL, P. D. 1970. Habituation and post-tetanic potentiation in the spinal cord. In G. Horn and R. A. Hinde, eds., *Short-Term Changes in Neural Activity and Behaviour*. London: Cambridge University Press.

WESTHEIMER, G. 1972. Visual acuity and spatial modulation thresholds. In D. Jameson and L. M. Hurvich, eds., *Handbook of Sensory Physiology*, VII/4. Berlin: Springer-Verlag, pp. 170–187.

WEYMOUTH, F. M. 1958. Visual sensory units and the minimal angle of resolution. *American Journal of Ophthalmology* 46: 102–113.

WHITFIELD, I. C. 1967. *The Auditory Pathway*. Baltimore: Williams & Wilkins.

WICKELGREN, B. G. 1967. Habituation of spinal motoneurons. *Journal of Neurophysiology* 30: 1404–1423.

WIESEL, T. N. 1960. Receptive fields of ganglion cells in the cat's retina. *Journal of Physiology* 153: 583–594.

WILSON, H. R. 1975. A synaptic model for spatial frequency adaptation. *Journal of Theoretical Biology* 50: 327–352.

Varieties of Animal Learning
and Adaptation:
Ethological and
Experimental Approaches

9

Animal Learning: Ethological Approaches

AUBREY MANNING

ABSTRACT This paper reviews the ethological approach to
learning, which has been to regard it as one type of behavioral
response to the environment. Ethologists have always been
impressed by the variety of adaptive mechanisms exhibited by
animals. They are thus well prepared to accept the breakup of
traditional learning theories which aimed at the construction
of behavioral laws with wide generality.

Diverse forms of learning and their possible course of evolution are briefly discussed. Any rigid categorization into types is
rejected. A review of constraints on learning imposed by an
animal's structure and mode of life is organized under three
headings: (1) Sensory and motor bias, (2) prepared and contraprepared responses, and (3) the inherited predisposition to
learn. This latter category includes a number of beautiful
examples showing the subtle interplay between genetic predisposition and the environment during development.

The conclusion—simple enough—is that while a biological
approach to learning as a mode of adaptation can, as yet, tell us
little about neural mechanisms, it is an important prerequisite
for their study. We must know the range of the phenomenon we
are trying to explain, and the ethological approach is increasingly contributing to the study of learning in its own right.

9.1 INTRODUCTION

Learning has not traditionally been regarded as a major
interest of ethologists. This view is, however, only partly
justified, since a number of the classic ethological studies
—for example, Tinbergen's work in the 1930s on the
orientation of the wasp *Philanthus* to its nest (see Tinbergen, 1972)—are almost exclusively concerned with
this topic. Nevertheless, it is true that few ethologists
deliberately set out to investigate learning for its own
sake, and for this reason much of their work has an at-
titude which strongly contrasts with that of experimental
and comparative psychologists.

I certainly do not wish to reconstruct barriers between
the two schools of animal behavior which have recently
been demolished. The final echoes of the battle triggered
by Lehrman's (1953) critique can still be heard; however, for most purposes one cannot now simply identify
people as ethologists and then expect to know the approach they will take on behavioral issues and the techniques they will use. For example, we now have workers

AUBREY MANNING, Department of Zoology, University of
Edinburgh, Edinburgh, Scotland

with impeccable ethological pedigrees using operant-
conditioning techniques to investigate the motivation of
sticklebacks during their courtship displays (Sevenster,
1973)!

If I had to choose one feature that characterizes the
ethological *approach* (which is now shared by many psychologists), it would be the conviction that we cannot
fully understand behavior until we know its function in
the animal's environment and are thus able to suggest
how it came to evolve. For this reason much that is
highly relevant to the topic of this conference emerges
from ethological studies. While there is no highly consistent body of information on learning, per se, through
the animal kingdom, there is much information about
the means animals use to cope with the problem of survival—learning being one varied aspect of their diverse
solutions.

Lorenz's original view on the interaction between
instinct and learning—which he discusses in his 1966
essay on the evolution and modification of behavior—
was one of "intercalation" (*Instinkt-Dressur-Verschränk-
ung*): there are inherited fixed action patterns of motor
coordination and an inherited responsiveness to particular stimulus patterns or releasers; learning operates so
as to modify the times and contexts at which these inherited elements come into play and increases or decreases the range of stimuli that are effective. Lorenz's
emphasis has been on analyzing the adaptiveness of
animal behavior. As a result, he and some other ethologists still tend to stress the distinction between the inherited and learned elements of behavior. Recognizing the
role of the environment in the expression of genes during
development, they nevertheless feel that any further
analysis of behavior requires one to know whence came
the information mediating the adaptiveness of the patterns we observe. Did it come from the genome in the
usual course of development or from the individual's
own experience (learning or some other interaction with
its environment)?

I accept that formally it may be possible to answer this
question, but I cannot see that it is always a useful exercise, particularly if one is interested in learning as it is
conventionally defined. The elemental structure of

behavior which we derive from such an approach might bear little relationship to the actualities of development or of evolution. Thus inquiries into the source of information for the elements of the songs of chaffinches (*Fringilla coelebs*) or white-crowned sparrows (*Zonotrichia leucophrys*) would yield mixed answers since genes and environment interact so subtly at almost every stage. Further, this type of development has itself evolved to suit the particular modes of life of these two species—in other species song develops in different fashions.

However, even if I reject some aspects of Lorenz's argument, there can be no doubt that his view that learning only operates within constraints imposed by the inherent structure of an animal's behavior has been abundantly justified by recent research.

In a recent survey of constraints on learning, Hinde (1973) refers to that period of "heroic optimism" during the 1930s and 1940s when psychologists sought to construct a comprehensive theory of behavior. Included within this theory were certain laws of learning such as the universal capacity to associate any conditioned stimulus with any unconditioned response and the universal capacity for any reinforcer to increase or decrease the rate of any emitted response. There is no call for an ethologist to batter away at the crumbling structures of the great learning theories. This is going on rigorously from within psychology itself (see especially Seligman, 1970; Garcia, Clarke, and Hankins, 1973; and the collections of papers edited by Seligman and Hager, 1972, and Hinde and Stevenson-Hinde, 1973). It is impossible not to shed a few tears at the passing of these theories. Ill-founded generality is no use in the end, I recognize, but there are now so few major generalities of any kind to be made in animal behavior that one feels conceptually naked at times. It seems that the one secure concept to which we *can* hold is that of evolution by natural selection. Ethologists have always studied a wide range of highly diverse animals and have always regarded learning as one means of securing adaptiveness. Few of them felt that the rules governing key-pecking in pigeons were of any relevance in the field situation even if they were studying how birds acquire new responses in feeding. Hence they come "prepared"—in Seligman's sense—to welcome the new recognition of the diversity of learning specializations and restraints.

How is one to approach the study of animal learning? One way is to build up a phylogenetic scale of learning ability and look for the evolution of intelligence. In their different ways this has been followed by Bitterman (1965 a, b) and by Harlow (1958). There are considerable drawbacks to this approach that are well discussed by Hodos and Campbell (1969) and Anderson (1972).

First, there is the insuperable problem of constructing phylogenies from living representatives of the different phyla. We have no sound reason for regarding a modern teleost fish as representing the fish stage through which the higher vertebrates once evolved, and so on. More seriously, we have no grounds for assuming that learning ability has any common axis along which we can measure evolutionary progress toward the apes and man. To take such a view is, once again, to impose a generality which ignores the diversity of animal forms and adaptations. As the paleontologist A.S. Romer was wont to remind us, an animal cannot spend its time being a generalized ancestor; it must constantly adapt to its own environment and the problems posed by that environment. This statement is as true for behavior as for morphology, and any ethological approach to learning must look for the specializations that have evolved to cope with a particular mode of life. The astonishing development of associative-learning capacity in the Hymenoptera (of which more later) is a good example.

Within the vertebrates we do have more justification for our evolutionary constructs. At least we are dealing with a single phylum. Harlow's and Bitterman's use of learning-set formation to measure different levels of learning ability has a certain force here. This is especially true within the mammals themselves since their great period of adaptive radiation was, in geological terms, very recent. It is certainly possible to produce a scale of learning ability (speed of set formation, number of ambiguity stages which can be dealt with, and so on) which discriminates between the mammalian orders and puts the primates at the top, (e.g., Warren, 1965). Eventually we may be able to correlate this scale of abilities with brain structure and cautiously (remembering that the carnivores are *not* on the insectivore-primate line, for example) study the evolution of brain function. This hope must have spurred on the founders of the journal *Brain, Behavior and Evolution*.

9.2 TYPES OF LEARNING

Insofar as ethologists have studied learning capacities, I think many of them have been influenced by the classification of learning types used by Thorpe (1963) in his book—one of few recent works which have tried to review the literature on learning throughout the animal kingdom. Thorpe used six categories of learning: (1) habituation, (2) conditioned reflex type 1 (Pavlovian or classical conditioning), (3) conditioned reflex type 2 (equivalent to trial-and-error), (4) latent learning, (5) insight learning, and (6) imprinting. Of course any such classification is open to a host of criticisms, but it can be undeniably useful for descriptive purposes. However, twelve years on, Thorpe's six categories no longer look quite the same, and I need to discuss the present situation briefly.

Imprinting, it is now generally recognized, is characterized by its context rather than its content. During their early life many young animals rapidly come to form attachments, often without conventional reinforcement, whose results are very persistent and sometimes permanent. However, we can now see that the features which once seemed so unique are to be found elsewhere: speed, lack of apparent reward, and resistance to extinction are all familiar in other contexts. Imprinting clearly involves associative conditioning, but it also involves inherited predispositions to respond to potential "mother figures," sensitization, arousal, maturation of the central nervous system, and a variety of other features which show that it is not *just* a category of learning. Nor perhaps are any of the other apparently logical operations we classify as learning.

Habituation remains as a broad phenomenon which can be observed from the level of the synapse right through to the whole animal. Thorpe's definition, "the relatively persistent waning of a response as the result of repeated stimulation which is not followed by any kind of reinforcement," lacks rigor, but is probably the best we can do. There is no realistic boundary between what is commonly regarded as sensory adaptation and habituation, but one retains a time-scale criterion in the definition of the latter in order to draw attention to some of its features which may relate to central nervous phenomona.

Ethologists have been universally aware of the role of habituation in the natural habitat. Small animals that are commonly preyed upon show considerable habituation to frightening stimuli. Nereid worms cease to respond to a repeated shadow stimulus (Clark, 1960) since it probably "means" waving seaweed and not a predator. Small birds are not impressed by scarecrows for long. In such cases the fleeing response returns after an hour or so, or if the stimulus changes. However, there are some puzzling examples of the very persistent waning of a response, and the relationship of these phenomena to more typical habituation is obscure.

Thus Hinde (1954a, b) found that a single 30-minute exposure to an owl caused a drastic and permanent waning of alarm calling and other types of mobbing response by caged chaffinches. The response recovered rapidly to about 50 percent, but it then remained unchanged for months; nor did this time course change if a chaffinch was "hurt" by the owl (held right against the owl and some feathers pulled out!). It might be expected that the responses of prey animals to predators would always recover rapidly, for predators can never be safely ignored. Perhaps it was the length of presentation of the owl which caused the permanent depression. Predators in the wild are usually perceived briefly and infrequently, and the prey animal's habituation processes are adapted to this kind of contingency. Certainly abnormal constancy in a stimulus greatly reduces responsiveness. Researchers have found that they cannot use model fish as stimuli for quantitative tests of aggression or courtship in sticklebacks. The famous sign-stimuli described by Tinbergen (1951) work at first, but the response wanes rapidly unless a live fish is used. Perhaps the same phenomenon accounts for the ultimate ineffectiveness of playing the species' alarm calls to scare birds from buildings or airfields.

Habituation can, in principle, be related to neural events without much trouble. No such secure relationship is yet possible for associative learning, for all the plethora of models we have. Looking over the wide range of nervous systems from annelids, arthropods, molluscs, and vertebrates that can mediate unequivocal associative learning, perhaps it is profitable to think in terms of logical operations rather than neural events. There is a very real sense in which the classical conditioning of a honeybee to the smell of peppermint and that of a dog to the sound of a metronome are "the same."

I leave it to others better qualified than I to tell us whether the distinction between classical and operant conditioning must now disappear. Certainly the recent upsurge of interest in autoshaping (see particularly Moore, 1973) has vindicated an old ethological rule applied to the Skinner box. Pigeons will come to peck a lighted key that is contiguous with the presence of food, even if they are not rewarded for doing so. This fact would have emerged on the charts of the automatic recorder (once someone was unconventional enough to think of trying it), but it was, in fact, only by *watching* the animal in the experimental situation that it became evident. The pigeon "eats" the key, using motor patterns identical with those employed when it pecks at grain. If water is the reward being used, the bird "drinks" the key, keeping its bill closed and making typical water-swallowing movements.

At the very least, such observations show us that the pigeon brings its own natural repertoire of feeding or drinking responses into the Skinner box. Sevenster's work with operant conditioning in sticklebacks, discussed below, also shows a conditioned-stimulus object coming to be treated as part of the unconditioned situation. In general, autoshaping appears to be less readily elicited from mammals, although Moore (1973) records examples of rats chewing the bars that deliver food. The Brelands (1961) also describe various mammals performing unrewarded elements of their natural repertoire (rooting by pigs, food-washing by raccoons, etc.) in operant situations.

While habituation is a property of all nervous systems, associative conditioning is probably not achieved until the annelid level of central nervous development. In logical terms it marks a huge leap forward, but we can only speculate about its evolution. Wells's (1974) argument that associative learning developed from the phenomenon of sensitization is an attractive one. Sensitization involves a period of enhanced responsiveness to many types of stimulation following reward or punishment. It can give rise to an appearance of conditioning: for example, pairing light and food leads to the emergence of tube-living worms in response to light alone, but worms just fed also show enhanced responsiveness to subsequent light flashes. Wells discusses the balance that must be struck between habituation and sensitization in different types of invertebrates. The balance will be very different in a herbivorous snail, which must browse more or less continuously on encrusting algae, from that in an active carnivore. Among the invertebrates, it is almost always the carnivores which show the best development of associative learning. In evolution, associative learning emerged when animals began to discriminate between stimuli that occurred contiguously with reinforcement and those that did not. Sensitization may have provided the basis for this discrimination.

Thorpe's remaining two categories—latent learning and insight learning—have never been as satisfactory as the others. They have evaded suitable definition and can never be observed in isolation from other forms of learning. Thus all the famous experiments by Köhler and Maier on insight and reasoning depend on animals having considerable familiarity with, and associatively conditioned responses to, a situation before they are given their novel task. This extensive literature is well reviewed by Munn (1950) and by Thorpe (1963).

The latent-learning situation was rather important in that it forced psychologists to make a reassessment of conventional reinforcement and drive reduction and their role in learning. The Hullian supposition was that a rat, satiated with food and water, which explores a new maze attached to the side of his cage, will learn nothing about it. No drive is there to be reduced, so no learning can occur. Needless to say rats do not conform to this hypothesis, nor would any field naturalist expect them to do so. Knowledge of the home environment is a matter of life and death to predator and prey alike.

The young tawny owls (Strix aluco) studied by Southern (1954) systematically explored the area around the nest where they were reared. Each night they expanded their area of familiarity, but if driven to its edge they invariably turned back to keep within familiar ground. Exploration is not an easy drive to bring within a framework of learning theory, but we must accept that it is a vital factor in the survival of wild animals and a key means of early learning.

In general I feel that, with the possible exceptions of habituation and associative conditioning, attempts to classify learning are not very profitable. Animal learning studies must always bear in mind the way the animal lives in its natural environment. Only in this way shall we discover what kinds of problems are relevant to it and how its specializations of sensory and motor performance affect the way it learns.

9.3 ETHOLOGICAL CONSTRAINTS ON LEARNING: SOME EXAMPLES

I should now like to discuss some examples of these ethological constraints on learning under three headings, which cannot be rigidly exclusive: sensory and motor "bias"; prepared and contraprepared conditioned responses; and inherited predispositions to learn.

9.3.1 Sensory and motor bias

It is obvious enough that its sensory capacities will determine what an animal can learn. We should remember that classical conditioned-discrimination tests have been widely used to investigate just what those capacities are. Sensory bias may make such investigations more difficult because, even if we work within an animal's capacities, it may not respond maximally. Pigeons respond most readily to the hue of a visual stimulus, cats to its brightness. Honeybees have their own hierarchy of responsiveness, attempting to use first hue, then figural intensity (i.e., richness of contour), and finally shape, during a visual discrimination task. Along some of these dimensions they have a scale of preference which appears not to be affected by experience—thus they prefer high figural intensity to low—but all such preferences can be readily overcome by conditioning. However, a bee's ability to discriminate shape is very poor, and it will use this dimension only when no other visual cues are provided (Anderson, 1972).

Even where sensory capacities are generally assumed to be equivalent, animals may not approach objects in the same way. Devine (1970) tested rhesus and Cebus monkeys in the Wisconsin General Test Apparatus for the formation of visual learning sets. He observed that the rhesus tended to respond to the base of the objects presented, sliding across the floor to reach them. Cebus never did this; they stretched up on their legs and viewed the objects from above. Devine noted that they preferred objects which could be grasped by the apex. It is tempting to relate these behavioral differences to the normal ground-living habits of rhesus as contrasted with the much more arboreal *Cebus*. Certainly they mean that comparisons of the learning ability of New and Old World monkeys should be made with caution.

Motor bias is usually detected by what animals cannot learn rather than by what they can. Here we can see the force of Lorenz's assertions on the ineffectiveness of learning to overcome innate predispositions. Perhaps the most dramatic example of this was provided by Dilger (1962) when he hybridized two species of love bird (*Agapornis*). The hybrids inherited dispositions to perform two incompatible patterns of nest building. One parent species carried single pieces of nest material in the bill, the other tucked several pieces into the rump feathers. Hybrids tucked material but omitted to open their bill after tucking, so that they ended up with the piece of material still held in the bill. This they then dropped, to collect more and begin another abortive tucking sequence. Parrots are intelligent birds which learn rapidly in other situations, but Dilger found that it took many hundreds of trials extending over months for the hybrids to acquire a means of carrying nest material. Eventually the birds learned not to drop material and carried it up to the nest, but they never eliminated an abbreviated tucking procedure before carrying.

Such a situation reminds one of the Brelands' (1961) account of chickens which could not be prevented from scratching on the ground even though such actions delayed their getting a food reward. Similarly, Lorenz and others have pointed out the extreme conservatism which restricts all ground-nesting birds to retrieving eggs outside the nest cup in precisely the same way. The neck is extended and hooked over the egg which is then rolled back. This method is grotesquely inefficient for wading birds with slender bills, but they never use their feet, which would seem to be well adapted for the task. There is clearly a strong phylogenetic bias to retrieve with the bill, but presumably few birds are exposed to eggs outside the nest more than once or twice in a breeding season. There may be an inability to unlearn, but the natural situation will not normally provide much force for change.

9.3.2 Prepared and contraprepared conditioned responses

Seligman's (1970) terms "prepared" and "contraprepared" are most useful for drawing attention to the limitations of contiguity and reinforcement as sufficient factors for learning to take place. Some of the best examples of preparedness have come from laboratory and

field studies which Garcia and Levine (this volume) deal with in more detail. They emphasize two particular constraints: (1) stimuli and reinforcers are not associated at random, and (2) not all reinforcements are appropriate for any given response. The first constraint has been revealed and analyzed extensively though the work of Garcia and others on rats. Sickness as a reinforcer is most likely to be associated with taste stimuli occurring up to a couple of hours prior to its onset. There is increasing evidence of the persistence of such associations, even without any further reinforcement (see Garcia, McGowan, and Green, 1972).

These results coincide beautifully with our knowledge of the way in which predators learn to avoid distasteful prey. Many insects have evolved warning coloration associated with distastefulness. Often their color patterns show convergent evolution, so that different distasteful groups resemble one another—orange (or yellow) and black is a familiar combination—a phenomenon known as Müllerian mimicry. Brower and his associates have shown that toads and jays begin with no inborn response to warning coloration but acquire their aversion, often after a single trial. This aversion may develop following immediate reinforcement—a toad stung when capturing a bumblebee, for example—but it may also develop in a manner closely resembling Garcia's conditioning paradigm. Thus jays learn to avoid the monarch butterfly following an experience in which, some minutes after eating, they develop illness and vomiting lasting for about half an hour. The effect is so strong that jays have subsequently been seen to retch when simply shown a monarch (see Brower, 1971).

Clearly the whole evolution of warning coloration depends on the remarkable "preparedness" of predators to make this association of color with sickness. Garcia's rats specifically did not make visual associations—only taste was involved—but rats are not visual hunters. In birds, reptiles, and amphibia, visual cues are paramount in feeding, and the delayed associations of sickness and food intake can be based on visual cues alone (Brower, 1971; Wilcoxon, Dragoin, and Kral, 1971).

Field studies of bees have shown that their remarkable learning ability is very situation-dependent. Bees seem to learn when it is necessary to do so, but they will not form associations simply because stimulus and reward are presented together. In some of my early studies on the foraging behavior of bumblebees I worked with two contrasted flowering plants, *Cynoglossum officinale*, hound's-tongue, which has small inconspicuous flowers, and *Digitalis purpurea*, foxglove, whose flowers are very conspicuous. With both species, individual bees returned again and again to the same group of plants; they had clearly learned the general area where they were growing. However, the bees' foraging strategy within the groups was not the same. Bees visiting *Cynoglossum* learned the site of individual plants, especially when these were somewhat separate—more than 2 m—from the others. If such a plant was removed after a bee left, on its next visit the bee would fly to and briefly hover at the empty site before moving on. Bees visiting a group of *Digitalis* did not behave this way. They learned much less about the sites of individual plants and used vision to guide them. Removing the flowers from a *Digitalis* plant almost eliminated the visits it received, but a similar procedure had no effect—in the short term—with *Cynoglossum*. Not only did the bees learn the sites of individual plants, they also learned the general form of the plants and searched in the axils of the leaves where the flowers are borne.

Bees foraging on *Cynoglossum* often left a group of plants by making what I called a "searching flight." A bee would fly in broad sweeps about 0.5 m above the ground, frequently retracing its path. Such flights ended if it located a new *Cynoglossum* plant. It would then visit the flowers of the new plant and, as it left, make a brief circling orientation flight lasting perhaps 15 sec. This was enough to fix the site, for if the plant was removed, the same bee would hover there at its next visit. Searching flights were rarely observed with *Digitalis* bees: they found new plants readily enough and were guided to them visually from at least 4 m (Manning, 1956).

These observations show that bees do not necessarily associate the most conspicuous stimuli with reinforcement. They modify their learning according to the situation, "switching in" their learning system when it is required: one might also say that they learn no more than they have to.

The elegant work of Menzel (1968) provides another example of the extreme learning specializations of bees when visiting flowers. It had been known for some time (Opfinger, 1931) that honeybees learn color during the approach and alighting phase of flower visit; if the color is changed during feeding or as the bee leaves, this has no effect. Menzel showed that this learning process is both rapid and extremely restricted. He trained bees to visit a food source whose color could be varied second by second. Following a training visit the bees could be presented with two alternative sources on a subsequent test visit, and their choice would indicate which association they had made during training. Menzel found that a bee formed the color association during a 4-sec period which extended from 2 sec *before* to 2 sec *after* its tongue touched the sugar solution as it alighted. Color changes outside this period, even though they were equally "rewarded" (all bees were allowed to feed for 20 sec),

were not effective. However, reward and repetition were both important for retention. After one training visit with reward, bees retained the association for more than a day, but it disappeared beyond this time. Following three training visits the association was retained undiminished for at least fourteen days. Such learning characteristics are adaptive in that the bees will forget a casual visit to a food source which is not consistent, but will return repeatedly once a good flower crop has been located.

It seems probable that more detailed investigation of the learning capacities of any animal will reveal comparable specializations. These certainly have a genetic component and cannot reasonably be distinguished from other types of genetic predisposition to be discussed below.

The same is true of the incompatibilities between reinforcement and response which Garcia's type of work has revealed. Psychologists have probably met this phenomenon most often during avoidance-conditioning studies. Bolles (1970) has reviewed some of the problems encountered in shuttle boxes, where some types of rodents will freeze rather than run and thus appear to learn slowly. Even within a species, we meet the same differences: inbred mouse strains vary in shuttle-box performance as in so many other behavioral traits; C3H freeze and learn to avoid with difficulty, while C57 run much more readily (Duncan, Grossen, and Hunt, 1971). Bolles emphasizes how important it is to have sufficient knowledge of a species' typical defense and flight responses before approaching a study of avoidance learning.

Avoidance as a reinforcer seems particularly difficult for animals to associate with motor patterns from other functional parts of their behavioral repertoire. It is now well recognized how difficult it is to train pigeons to peck a key or cats to lick in order to avoid shock. As Shettleworth (1973) and others have pointed out, when one introduces an unusual reinforcement into a behavioral situation, one may gain some control over certain behavior patterns, but normal causal factors will still be present and are likely to affect the response. Reinforcers that are compatible with the response will obviously be most effective: Kruijt (1964) could not condition his jungle fowl to perform their courtship displays for food rewards, but they rapidly performed the required patterns when given access to a female as a reinforcement.

Such a result as Kruijt's has considerable importance for ethologists, because it could imply that the fowl has a good degree of "voluntary" control over the performance of individual courtship patterns. Since these patterns are believed to have evolved by the ritualization of conflict postures of various types, their voluntary performance might indicate that control of the display is now quite distinct from the conflicts that may have been its historical source—i.e., the displays are emancipated (Tinbergen, 1952). Before we can conclude this, however, we must know to what extent there was an element of classical conditioning in the jungle fowl's response. When the male performed the required courtship display in Kruijt's study, a basket covering the female was raised. Perhaps the basket came to elicit the display directly through conditioning; if so, we cannot necessarily conclude that a display can be performed in the absence of sexual stimuli.

Some recent work by Sevenster (1968, 1973) on instrumental conditioning of courtship and aggression in sticklebacks is of particular interest in this connection. It reveals a striking form of learning constraint and clearly shows that classical conditioning is occurring. Sticklebacks can be quite readily trained to swim through a ring suspended in their territory when given the opportunity to attack another male as reinforcement. (The rival is revealed behind a glass screen for 10 sec.) A 10-sec opportunity to court a female similarly presented is also an effective reinforcer. In both cases sticklebacks swim through the ring at regular and quite short intervals: 20 to 30 sec from the end of one reinforcement period to swimming through the ring again.

Sevenster also used a second type of operant response which required the stickleback to bite the green tip of a rod suspended in its territory just as the ring had been in the previous experiment. Now a significant difference appeared between the two reinforcement situations. That involving exposure to a rival male was unchanged: sticklebacks rapidly swam from displaying aggressively at the rival behind the glass to bite at the rod and then return to displaying. This was not the case when a female was the reward. The fish were more difficult to train in the first place and the intervals between responses became very long and more variable (3 to 75 minutes was an average interval). The behavior of males during these intervals was particularly interesting and provides one more reason to eschew automatic recording. Their behavior was intensely rod-orientated; to quote Sevenster, "The fish would approach the rod, and start circling around it with zigzag-like jumps and often with open mouth, sometimes making snapping movements at the tip or softly touching it." The zigzag dance is, of course, the stickleback's courtship display, and Sevenster used other tests also to show conclusively that the rod comes to act as a sexual stimulus which, particularly after a bout of courtship, inhibits biting. Only when his intense sexual arousal has had some time to decay can the male bring himself to bite the rod. Sevenster has been able to utilize this operant technique to investigate the time course of interactions between aggressive and sexual tendencies in a way that extends the usual range of ethological methods.

Investigation of the effects of different types of reinforcements on species-typical fixed action patterns has scarcely begun. It would seem to be a promising field for research for it may yield information both on the basis of learning constraints and on the accessibility and modifiability of fixed action patterns and their "normal" causal factors. Shettleworth (1972) and Stevenson-Hinde (1973) have reviewed what literature there is. Shettleworth (1973) herself provides one of the first systematic studies in which the effects of a standard reinforcer (food) on a whole range of a species' responses have been explored. She finds, for example, that food reinforcement will increase the frequency with which hungry hamsters perform rearing, digging, and scrabbling (scraping and exploring the surface of the substrate) but has little effect on face-washing. This latter pattern is the only one not associated with natural food gathering, and it is not surprising that it is less accessible to modification by food reward. Shettleworth describes a number of ways in which the exact form of digging, scrabbling, etc., is modified during the reinforcement period; in general hamsters are apt to perform very curtailed forms of so-called fixed action patterns. Ethologists have also observed curtailed patterns during conflict situations, when they may appear as "displacement activites"; we might look for possible common causal factors here.

9.3.3 Inherited predispositions to learn

All learning has an inherited basis, but under this heading I include evidence that some animals are "prepared" genetically for very specific learning tasks. It must be admitted from the outset that no real genetic evidence can be produced. We are dealing with specific types of learning that are shared by all members of a species. We might infer that because the environment does not seem capable of providing the specific information which such learning requires, then the genome must do so. Such an argument—it is that of Lorenz (1966), already discussed—is persuasive but not rigorous. Genetics depends upon there being differences, and genetic analysis cannot be applied when animals share the qualities under examination.

The strengths and weaknesses of the argument are exemplified by comparing the extent to which various sea birds learn the characteristics of their eggs and young. The eggshell pattern of gulls and terns varies greatly between individuals, and transfer experiments by Tinbergen (1953) and Cullen (1957) have shown that neither herring gulls (*Larus argentatus*) nor kittiwakes (*Rissa tridactyla*) are disturbed by exchanging their eggs for those of another pair. It is presumed that they do not recognize them: certainly they are far more attached to the nest site than to the pattern of the eggs. The obvious conclusion is that since eggs do not normally move, nest-site attachment is sufficient to ensure that birds incubate their own eggs and no egg learning is required. This conclusion is strengthened by the Buckleys' (1972) study on the royal tern (*Sterna maxima*). These terns nest in remarkably dense colonies; there are an average of 7.5 nests per square meter! Since the nest is no more than a scrape and on fairly featureless terrain, nest-site recognition is not easy. The Buckleys found that egg patterning is particularly variable in this species, in which a bird usually lays a single egg, and that when eggs are exchanged, the majority of terns will choose to incubate their own egg on the wrong site. They clearly learn to identify their individual egg and give it priority over the nest site, although they show some signs of disturbance on the wrong site. Tschanz (1959) has also found that the guillemot (*Uria aalge*) learns to recognize its own egg. Guillemots lay on flat ledges and build no nests. The eggs are closely packed together and can shift as birds leave or arrive, although their sharply conical shape minimizes the risk of their rolling off the ledge. They are strikingly variable both in ground color—pink, green, or white—and degree of black blotching.

Variations in what is learned cannot be ascribed to differences in the birds' abilities to discriminate patterns. The down markings of herring-gull chicks are comparable to those of the eggs. Chick transfers are not possible beyond the third day from hatching; by then parents have learned to identify their own young. The same is true of royal terns, although individual voice recognition is more involved here. Again this makes adaptive sense, in that chicks can wander out of the nest site and take shelter elsewhere. A final telling point is that kittiwake chicks, which cannot wander since they are hatched on isolated cliff nests, can be transferred between nests right up to the time of fledging—the parents do not discriminate against foreigners.

Through all these findings there is a strong suggestion, as we saw previously with foraging bees, that animals learn no more than makes adaptive sense. Since few of these sea birds will ever have had the chance to test out for themselves the wisdom of learning or not learning their eggs or chicks, and since all members of a species behave similarly, this does constitute strong circumstantial evidence for an inherited predisposition.

No genetic work is in prospect here unfortunately, but one example that *is* ripe for genetic analysis concerns differences in the learning of visual landmarks by two races of the honeybee, the Italian race *Apis mellifera ligustica* and the Canton (Austria) race, *A. m. carnica*, studied by Lauer and Lindauer (1971). The differences are more strikingly revealed when the bees are learning to feed at a food source on a table in the open air. The source is marked with a black star some 50 cm across, and around the table can be placed various large artificial landmarks (towers, etc.). Lauer and Lindauer performed a series of experiments comparing the rates of learning and what is learned in such a situation. They found that both races use three types of visual cue: (1) a sun-compass reaction which gives them the general bearing of the food source with respect to the hive, (2) landmarks (trees, the towers, etc.) close to the food source, and (3) details of the source itself (the black star contrasting with the surface of the table). The principal interracial differences relate to emphasis placed on category (2). *Carnica* bees learn much more about local landmarks than do *ligustica* and consequently are more disturbed by alterations to them. *Ligustica* rely more upon the sun compass to bring them within visual range of the food source, and they then respond directly to the source. If the local landmarks remain constant, *carnica* will at first ignore a move in the food source's position and respond to the site where it was last found; *ligustica* find the new site more quickly.

Lauer and Lindauer suggest that these differences are genetically determined, and certainly they are very constant within races and are unaffected even when mixed colonies consisting of worker bees of both races are tested. The differences make some adaptive sense: *ligustica* evolved in regions of high sunlight and forages only in sun, when the sun compass is always reliable; *carnica* is adapted to duller weather and will forage under cloudy skies, where concentration on visual landmarks will serve it well.

Koltermann (1973) has found other striking differences between the races of honeybee. He has studied the scent preferences of various Western races and compared them with those of the Eastern honeybee *Apis cerana*. All bees rapidly learn to associate scent with food, but the various races give preference to scents emanating from flowers native to their own habitats in India, the Middle East, or Europe. As with visual learning, Koltermann reports that there is very little variation between different colonies of the same race.

The evidence for genetic control of these differences is as yet incomplete because hybridization is an essential feature of genetic analysis. One awaits this development with interest. (It will not be too difficult to achieve since artificial insemination is now a familiar technique with honeybees.)

These examples, and those on bumblebees given earlier, have presented special aspects of learning in bees. Yet in the most general terms it would seem certain that the extraordinary development of associative learning in the Hymenoptera has itself been specially evolved. The ants, bees, and wasps (which make up the greater part of the order), whether they are solitary or colonial, all construct nests in which to lay eggs and raise their young. This involves their returning repeatedly to the same spot after excursions to collect nesting materials or food. Accurate orientation to environmental features is essential, and orientation flights during which there is very rapid learning of visual features are characteristic of bees and wasps. Tinbergen's original study with *Philanthus*, a solitary wasp, showed how changes to the visual environment around the nest were detected on an inward flight to the nest and led to a fresh orientation flight when the wasp left again.

The interdependence of the bees and the flowering plants has led to the concurrent evolution of flower structure, scent, color, pattern, and shape and the reactions of bees to all these attributes. Their responsiveness to color and scent is, in part, inborn, but their hour-to-hour responses are conditioned by their experience on the different flower crops. To this end their learning capabilities are highly specialized to match the physiology of the flowers on which they feed. Thus honeybees can learn to visit different flowers at different times of day according to the circadian rhythm of nectar secretion. Koltermann (1970) has shown experimentally that bees will readily learn to visit up to nine different dishes marked with scents at particular times of day. (Thus, for example, they will learn time-dependent cues such that geraniol is attractive between 0900 and 1000, orange-blossom scent between 1030 and 1130, and so on.) By contrast, Anderson (1972) was able to show that bees are not capable of making even a single dependent discrimination using color as a secondary cue—but then flowers do not change their color through the day.

When one has evidence of such striking specificity in learning, one can suggest an inherited basis with some confidence. Some examples from vertebrate learning are perhaps less securely based. A number of studies on the development of behavior in mammals by Eibl-Eibesfeldt (well reviewed in his 1970 book) show very rapid learning in certain situations. Polecats learn to direct killing bites to the nape of their prey, squirrels learn to gnaw at the thinnest part of nutshells, and so on. In such cases Eibl-Eibesfeldt argues that there is an inborn tendency to respond to the object in each case, but the response is, at first, ill-directed. A learning predisposition then ensures a rapid adjustment to the optimum response. Such evidence is suggestive, but we know too little of the

kinds of intermediate reinforcements that may occur during the modification of such responses to rule out more conventional learning.

We are on surer ground with some of the results from imprinting studies. Here work on visual imprinting to foster-parent species in ducks (Schuz, 1965) and Oestrildine finches (Immelmann, 1969a) have shown in both cases that while males will readily imprint sexually upon foreign females, they do so less rapidly than to the natural parent. The superiority of the natural female is revealed, for example, by a male requiring a shorter period of exposure to produce a stable response.

This suggests either that males have some inherited information on the form of their own females (as the females certainly have for their own males, at least in ducks) or that they have some kind of learning predisposition to respond to the natural mother. Perhaps this is no more than saying the same thing in two ways. Such a learning predisposition might take the form of an inherited "template" against which incoming visual stimuli from the mother can be matched. Gottlieb (1965) has demonstrated a similar preference by chick and mallard ducklings for their own species' calls, which are learned more readily than those of foreign species. He was unable to modify such preferences by exposing the young birds to other calls when they were still in the egg.

Finally, the development of bird song, to which I have already referred, provides some excellent examples of learning predisposition. The very diversity of developmental stories we know from the species already studied indicates how the pattern of development may itself be subject to natural selection. Marler and his group have been particularly active in this work (see, for example, Marler, 1970, which provides full references).

There is clear evidence that some birds (and here we are speaking particularly of white-crowned sparrows, *Zonotrichia leucophrys* and chaffinches, *Fringilla coelebs*) inherit a neural template against which songs they hear are compared. Without any auditory experience this template will enable only the crudest of songs to be produced, but if an isolated bird can hear itself, it can develop a simple version of the normal song. The template can therefore act to shape the sounds produced by the isolated bird toward the species norm. However, given normal exposure to singing adults, the template itself becomes modified. Now when the bird comes to sing for itself, it develops the full song, with any local dialect features that may have been present in the songs it has heard.

Learning predisposition is particularly revealed by the fact that only a certain range of songs will modify the template. Only the species' own song is effective, or with the chaffinch, the song of one foreign species, the tree pipit (*Anthus trivialis*); other songs are ignored, and in their presence the simple song of an isolated bird is produced. The fact that tree pipits are copied by chaffinches indicates that a particular tonal quality is required, because to the human ear also tree pipits do match the tone of chaffinches very exactly, although they have a different song pattern.

The selectivity here is directed at particular characteristics of the species' song, but not all bird species give this the same priority. Immelmann (1969b) has shown a male zebra finch (*Taeniopygia guttata*) will learn the song of his *father*, even if the latter is a foster father of another species and his own species can also be heard singing in the same room. Thus he will give the father's song priority over the songs of other males which may have a more correct tonal quality. Admittedly, Immelmann has cross-fostered his zebra finches only to species whose songs are not too far removed from their own; the birds presumably cannot sing outside a certain tonal range.

We do not fully understand the evolution of song learning and the significance of all the variations that are known. Why do chaffinches and white-crowned sparrows cease to modify their song beyond their first spring, while Oregon juncos (*Junco oreganus*) and indigo buntings (*Passerina cyanea*) still learn during their second year? One advantage of continued learning probably lies in the opportunity it gives for dialects to develop. These are transmitted from generation to generation, and playback experiments in the field have shown that both male and female white-crowned sparrows answer and move toward loudspeakers transmitting their own dialect rather than others (Milligan and Verner, unpublished results, quoted in Marler, 1970). Nottebohm (1969) has suggested that such effects will assist local populations with special adaptations to local conditions to keep together. This conservation of a gene pool would be advantageous provided it was not too rigid, and it is unlikely to become so on this basis alone.

9.4 CONCLUSIONS

From this brief and selective survey of ethological approaches to animal learning, we can certainly see an animal's learning capacities as a very special part of its adaptive behavior. We must expect to find that every species will have special features in its learning repertoire and we must accept that they may not fit too easily into any logical categories we set up. Nobody has put it better than the Brelands (1961) when they wrote, "After fourteen years of continuous conditioning and observation of thousands of animals, it is our reluctant conclu-

sion that the behavior of any species cannot be adequately understood, predicted, or controlled without knowledge of its instinctive patterns, evolutionary history and ecological niche."

This conclusion suggests caution and a good biological approach, but is it yet possible to say more? In particular is it possible, in the context of this conference, to deduce anything about learning mechanisms? Seligman and Hager (1972, p. 97) suggest that we should be looking for physiological and psychological differences between prepared and unprepared associative mechanisms. They quote various pieces of work which suggest that prepared associations may indeed have a more "robust" neural and physiological structure than ordinary learning.

I find it very difficult to make any generalizations after surveying the range of learning phenomena and the nervous systems that mediate them. Perhaps we ethologists can find some consolation in the recognition that the same micromechanisms (discussed by others in this volume) may underlie the different macromechanisms we observe in our animals. Again, perhaps there is little difference between the genetic determination of the predisposition to perform a particular fixed action pattern, and that to learn a particular thing. Much inherited learning disposition (e.g., song learning) depends on some kind of template of the required result, and this must be based on specific patterns of neural interconnectivity and functioning.

However little we know of the mechanisms, as an ethologist I derive much satisfaction from the fact that the study of instinct, in the old sense, and that of animal learning have never seemed closer together. They have now become complementary ways of studying adaptiveness together with its developmental and evolutionary basis. As a spur to our research endeavor, I still pin my hopes on a speculation by Galambos (1961) in a book on learning mechanisms:

It could be argued, in brief, that no important gap separates the explanations for how the nervous system comes to be organized during embryological development in the first place; for how it operates to produce the innate responses characteristic of each species in the second place; and for how it becomes reorganized, finally, as a result of experiences during life. If this idea should be correct, the solution of any one of these problems would mean that the answer for the others would drop like a ripe plum, so to speak, into our outstretched hands.

REFERENCES

ANDERSON, A. M. 1972. Some aspects of learning in insects. Unpublished Ph. D. dissertation, University of Edinburgh.
BITTERMAN, M. E. 1965a. The evolution of intelligence. *Scientific American* 212(1): 92–100.

BITTERMAN, M. E. 1965b. Phyletic differences in learning. *American Psychologist* 20: 396–410.

BOLLES, R. C. 1970. Species-specific defense reactions and avoidance learning. *Psychological Review* 77: 32–48.

BRELAND, K., and BRELAND, M. 1961. The misbehavior of organisms. *American Psychologist* 61: 681–684.

BROWER, L. P. 1971. Prey coloration and predator behavior. In *BIO Source Book*. Section 6: *Animal Behavior*. New York: Harper & Row, pp. 360–370.

BUCKLEY, P. A., and BUCKLEY, F. G. 1972. Individual egg and chick recognition by adult royal terns (*Sterna maxima maxima*). *Animal Behaviour* 20: 457–462.

CLARK, R. B. 1960. Habituation of the polychaete *Nereis* to sudden stimuli. 2. Biological significance of habituation. *Animal Behaviour* 8: 92–103.

CULLEN, E. 1957. Adaptations in the kittiwake to cliff-nesting. *Ibis* 99: 275–302.

DEVINE, J. V. 1970. Stimulus attributes and training procedures in learning-set formation of rhesus and cebus monkeys. *Journal of Comparative and Physiological Psychology* 73: 62–67.

DILGER, W. C. 1962. The behavior of lovebirds. *Scientific American* 206 (1): 88–98.

DUNCAN, N. C., GROSSEN, N. E., and HUNT, E. B. 1971. Apparent memory differences in inbred mice produced by differential reaction to stress. *Journal of Comparative and Physiological Psychology* 74: 383–389.

EIBL-EIBESFELDT, I. 1970. *Ethology. The Biology of Behavior.* New York: Holt, Rinehart and Winston.

GALAMBOS, R. 1961. Changing concepts of the learning mechanism. In J. F. Delafresnaye et al., eds., *Brain Mechanisms and Learning*. Oxford: Blackwell Scientific Publications, pp. 231–241.

GARCIA, J., CLARKE, J. C., and HANKINS, W. G. 1973. Natural responses to scheduled rewards. In P. P. G. Bateson and P. H. Klopfer, eds., *Perspectives in Ethology*. New York: Plenum Press, pp. 1–41.

GARCIA, J., McGOWAN, B. K., and GREEN, K. F. 1972. Biological constraints on conditioning. In A. H. Black and W. F. Prokasy, eds., *Classical Conditioning II: Current Research and Theory*. New York: Appleton-Century-Crofts.

GOTTLIEB, G. 1965. Imprinting in relation to parental and species identification by avian neonates. *Journal of Comparative and Physiological Psychology* 59: 345–356.

HARLOW, H. F. 1958. The evolution of learning. In A. Roe and G. G. Simpson, eds., *Behavior and Evolution*. New Haven: Yale University Press, pp. 269–290.

HINDE, R. A. 1954a. Factors governing the changes in strength of a partially inborn response, as shown by the mobbing behaviour of the chaffinch (*Fringilla coelebs*). I. The nature of the response and an examination of its course. *Proceedings of the Royal Society* (*London*) B 142: 306–331.

HINDE, R. A. 1954b. Factors governing the changes in strength of a partially inborn response, as shown by the mobbing behaviour of the chaffinch (*Fringilla coelebs*). II. The waning of the response. *Proceedings of the Royal Society* (*London*) B 142: 331–358.

HINDE, R. A. 1973. Constraints on learning—An introduction to the problems. In Hinde and Stevenson-Hinde (1973), pp. 1–19.

HINDE, R. A., and STEVENSON-HINDE, J., eds. 1973. *Constraints on Learning*. New York: Academic Press.

HODOS, W., and CAMPBELL, C. B. G. 1969. *Scala Naturae*: Why there is no theory in comparative psychology. *Psychological Reviews* 76: 337–350.

IMMELMANN, K. 1969a. Über den Einfluss frühkindlicher Erfahrungen auf die geschlectliche Objektfixierung bei Estrildiden. *Zeitschrift für Tierpsychologie* 26: 677–691.

IMMELMANN, K. 1969b. Song development in the zebra finch and other estrildid finches. In R. A. Hinde, ed., *Bird Vocalization*. London: Cambridge University Press. pp. 61–74.

KOLTERMANN, R. 1970. Zeitgekoppelte Lernprozessen bei der Honigbiene. *Zoologische Anzeiger* (Supplement) 33: 205.

KOLTERMANN, R. 1973. Rassen-bzw. artspezifische Duftbewertung bei der Honigbiene und ökologische Adaptation. *Journal of Comparative Physiology* 85: 327–360.

KRUIJT, J. P. 1964. Ontogeny of social behaviour in Burmese red jungle fowl (*Gallus gallus spadiceus*). Bonaterre. *Behaviour Supplement* 12: 1–201.

LAUER, J., and LINDAUER, M. 1971. Genetisch fixierte Lerndispositionen bei der Honigbiene. *Abhandlungen der Akademie der Wissenschaften und der Literatur* 1: 1–87.

LEHRMAN, D. S. 1953. A critique of Konrad Lorenz's theory of instinctive behavior. *Quarterly Review of Biology* 28: 337–363.

LORENZ, K. 1966. *Evolution and Modification of Behaviour*. London: Methuen.

MANNING, A. 1956. Some aspects of the foraging behaviour of bumble-bees. *Behaviour* 9: 164–201.

MARLER, P. 1970. A comparative approach to vocal learning: Song development in white-crowned sparrows. *Journal of Comparative and Physiological Psychology* 71: 1–25.

MENZEL, R. 1968. Das Gedachtnis der Honigbiene für Spektralfarben. I. Kurzzeitiges und langzeitiges Behalten. *Zeitschrift für vergleichende Physiologie* 60: 82–102.

MOORE, B. R. 1973. The role of directed Pavlovian reactions in simple instrumental learning in the pigeon. In Hinde and Stevenson-Hinde (1973), pp. 159–188.

MUNN, N. L. 1950. *Handbook of Psychological Research on the Rat*. Boston: Houghton Mifflin.

NOTTEBOHM, F. 1969. The song of the chingolo, *Zonotrichia capensis*, in Argentina. Description and evaluation of dialects. *Condor* 71: 299–315.

OPFINGER, E. 1931. Über die Orientierung der Biene an der Futterstelle. *Zeitschrift für vergleichende Physiologie* 15: 431–487.

SCHUZ, F. 1965. Sexuelle Pragung bei Anatiden. *Zeitschrift für Tierpsychologie* 22: 50–103.

SELIGMAN, M. E. P. 1970. On the generality of the laws of learning. *Psychological Review* 77: 406–418.

SELIGMAN, M. E. P., and HAGER, J. L. 1972. *Biological Boundaries of Learning*. New York: Appleton-Century-Crofts.

SEVENSTER, P. 1968. Motivation and learning in sticklebacks. In D. Ingle, ed., *The Central Nervous System and Fish Behavior*. Chicago: The University of Chicago Press, pp. 233–245.

SEVENSTER, P. 1973. Incompatibility of response and reward. In Hinde and Stevenson-Hinde (1973), pp. 265–283.

SHETTLEWORTH, S. J. 1972. Constraints on learning. *Advances in the Study of Behaviour* 4: 1–68.

SHETTLEWORTH, S. J. 1973. Food reinforcement and the organization of behaviour in golden hamsters. In Hinde and Stevenson-Hinde (1973), pp. 243–263.

SOUTHERN, H. N. 1954. Tawny owls and their prey. *Ibis* 101: 384–410.

STEVENSON-HINDE, J. 1973. Constraints on reinforcement. In Hinde and Stevenson-Hinde (1973), pp. 285–296.

THORPE, W. H. 1963. *Learning and Instinct in Animals*. 2nd ed. London: Methuen.

TINBERGEN, N. 1951. *The Study of Instinct*. Oxford: The Clarendon Press.

TINBERGEN, N. 1952. "Derived" activities: Their causation, biological significance, origin and emancipation during evolution. *Quarterly Review of Biology* 27: 1–32.

TINBERGEN, N. 1953. *The Herring Gull's World*. London: Collins.

TINBERGEN, N. 1972. On the orientation of the digger wasp *Philanthus triangulum*. In *The Animal in its World*. Vol. I: *Field Studies*. London: Allen & Unwin.

TSCHANZ, B. 1959. Zur Brutbiologie der Trottelume (*Uria aalge aalge* Pont.). *Behaviour* 14: 1–100.

WARREN, J. M. 1965. Primate learning in comparative perspective. In A. M. Schrier, H. F. Harlow, and F. Stollnitz, eds., *Behavior of Nonhuman Primates*, Vol. I. New York: Academic Press, pp. 249–281.

WELLS, M. J. 1975. Evolution and associative learning. In P. Usherwood, ed., *"Simple" Nervous Systems*. London: Edward Arnold, pp. 445–473.

WILCOXON, H. C., DRAGOIN, W. B., and KRAL, P. A. 1971. Illness-induced aversions in rat and quail: Relative salience of visual and gustatory cues. *Science* 171: 826–828.

10

Learning about Learning: Methodological Considerations and Some Suggested Experimental Approaches

E. M. EISENSTEIN

ABSTRACT The importance of methodological factors in influencing our behavioral results and, accordingly, the inferences we draw about what is going on in the central nervous system is discussed. An example is considered in which the same human galvanic-skin-response data could be used to support incremental or all-or-none learning, depending on whether the response is measured so as to preserve its incremental character or is scored as an all-or-none event.

Model systems and the assumptions underlying their use in studies of learning and memory are also considered. Model approaches are discussed in terms of their usefulness for answering fundamental questions about the learning process. Aneural systems, such as protozoa, are considered for their possible usefulness in assessing intracellular contributions, unconfounded by intercellular factors, to the learning and memory process.

10.1 INTRODUCTION

I think it is fair to say that broad generalizations about modifiable behavior are not likely to be very accurate if they do not take into account genetic constraints imposed on a given animal, with respect both to sensory capacities and to innately organized patterns of behavior as exemplified by instincts.

This statement epitomizes a perpetual problem that all biologists, regardless of their field of endeavor, must face: the trade-off between being a General Biologist and being a Comparative Biologist. In the former role, one deals with questions posed in terms of similarities in function among different organisms; in the latter, with questions posed in terms of differences in function among different organisms. Thus a General Biologist might ask about the similarities among organisms in how their nervous systems handle learned information, whereas the Comparative Biologist might be concerned with the differences in how two animals handle such information. Which of these two positions one adopts—whether to look for similarities or for differences among systems—will determine the approach one takes for an experimental or theoretical investigation of a given problem.

E. M. EISENSTEIN, Department of Biophysics, Michigan State University, East Lansing, MI

Accordingly, if one makes the assumptions implied in an ethological approach (that is, that the more "natural" the context in which a given behavior is observed, the more likely it is to reveal something about how the behavior is "normally" organized and controlled), then one will adopt a method of research that will be quite different from that of an experimental psychologist who assumes that the laws of behavior transcend any specific context, and so adopt a method consisting of abstract, simplified, and highly contrived laboratory situations and behavior that bears little or no relationship to the animals' "natural" environment.

I would like to discuss some thoughts on learning and memory in terms of (1) some methodological problems inherent in research in this area and (2) some approaches that may be useful in attacking some of the funndamental questions about the coding and storage of learned information.

10.2 METHODOLOGICAL CONSIDERATIONS IN INVESTIGATIONS OF LEARNING AND MEMORY

I would like to suggest that the methodology used in demonstrating the phenomenon of learning may contribute markedly to the behavioral results obtained and correspondingly to the inferences drawn about the CNS processes underlying these results. As an example I shall consider the important question of whether associative strength develops gradually with reinforcement or in an all-or-none fashion. It has generally been assumed that associations develop gradually with succeeding reinforcements, but evidence has been accumulating that associations may in fact occur in an all-or-none way (Estes, 1960). Estes reasoned that if learning were gradual, the effect of each succeeding reinforcement would be to increase the probability of a subject responding even though the subject had not yet made an appropriate response; if it were all-or-none, each reinforcement would only give the subject another opportunity to form the association in an all-or-none fashion irrespective of how many previous reinforcements he has had. Estes therefore predicted that the percentage of unconditioned subjects demonstrating a particular association for the first time should increase with successive reinforcements if learning is gradual (since the probability of responding would then presumably increase with each reinforcement) and should remain constant if learning is all-or-none (since the probability of responding would not change gradually with reinforcement, but would remain 0 until the trial when it becomes 1). His results for both verbal learning and eyeblink conditioning were uniform in support of the all-or-none hypothesis.

Support for either view may depend on many factors, among which are the animal selected and the response system studied. I would like to suggest that whether a response is measured in a way that preserves differences in magnitude or as an all-or-none event may also be an important factor in determining which view of learning is supported. Studies employing all-or-none response measures, such as probability of correct recall (Estes, 1960; Kintsch, 1963; Rock and Steinfeld, 1963; Eimas and Zeaman, 1963), often provide support for all-or-none learning; those employing measures that preserve differences in response magnitude, such as latency, support a notion of gradual learning (Eimas and Zeaman, 1963; Williams, 1962). Although this relationship is not perfect,[1] it appears sufficiently suggestive to warrant further consideration.

To test this hypothesis I took the galvanic-skin-response (GSR) data from a human conditioning experiment I had done, treated them in two ways—one taking into account differences in response magnitude and the other noting only whether a response was above or below some arbitrary magnitude—and compared the results. In this case the results did support the view that how a response is measured can influence which hypothesis of the learning process is supported (Eisenstein and Eisenstein, 1965).

Individual curves, plotted from data in which differences in response magnitude were preserved, were examined (Figure 10.1).[2] The transducer properties of

[1]Using both probability of recall and response latency, Williams (1962) found evidence supporting gradual learning. When two different criterion latencies were chosen, she found the probability of achieving them for the first time on each item also increased as a function of successive trials. Thus, with the same measure (latency), she found support for gradual learning regardless of whether the response was measured in a continuous or dichotomous fashion. At present our results remain partially at variance, since I found evidence for gradual learning when the response measure was continuous and support for the all-or-none position when the same response measure was dichotomous.

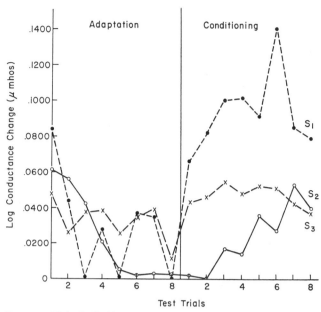

FIGURE 10.1 Individual curves for three subjects showing the gradual nature of GSR adaptation and conditioning (CS-UCS interval = 0.5 sec). Unpublished.

the apparatus clearly determine how the response is recorded. For these data the recorder followed faithfully the changes occurring in the response system studied. However, it is possible to treat these changes in an all-or-none fashion, considering only whether or not a response above a particular magnitude has occurred. The bar in a Skinner box is often set to work in this way.

[2]The galvanic skin response was recorded on male college students. The conditioned stimulus (CS) was a tone of 500 cps, 68 db, and 237.6 msec duration. The unconditioned stimulus (UCS) was an electric shock to the ankle of 244.0 msec duration. Response magnitudes were measured on eight interspersed CSs during adaptation and conditioning.

During adaptation all subjects (Ss) were treated identically. The UCS preceded the CS by 20 seconds, and the intertrial period varied between 60 and 90 seconds. For conditioning the Ss were divided into groups differing in the CS-UCS interval employed. The data from the experimental groups that showed conditioning (CS-UCS intervals of 0.25, 0.50, 0.75 and 1.0 sec) were pooled for the analyses in Table 10.1 A trace conditioning procedure was used.

Individual curves plotted from data in which differences in response magnitude were preserved were examined. In order to determine whether an individual curve showed evidence for gradual or one-trial learning, the number of increments between the response on the last adaptation trial and the maximum conditioned response was counted. In Figure 10.1, for example, S_1 shows five increments, while S_2 and S_3 show three each. Evidence for one-trial learning would be obtained if the subject showed one increment between response on the last adaptation trial and his maximum conditioned response. Of the 38 Ss, 1 showed no change from the last adaptation trial, 9 showed a one-step change, and 28 showed between 2 and 5 increments. The modal number of increments shown was 3.

TABLE 10.1

Percent of tested subjects whose first conditioned response occurred on one of the first four test trials

Test trial	Percent responding as a function of different cutoff points[1]		
	≥ 0.030[2]	≥ 0.035	≥ 0.038
1	39 (9/23)	26 (6/23)	26 (6/23)
2	14 (2/14)	18 (3/17)	12 (2/17)
3	14 (2/14)	6 (1/16)	12 (2/17)
4	17 (2/12)	27 (4/15)	27 (4/15)

1. Numbers in parentheses are the ratios of subjects responding for the first time on a given trial to those who have not responded before that trial. Occasionally data for a given trial is missing; thus $N = 23$ on trials 1 and 2, $N = 25$ on trial 3, and $N = 24$ on trial 4. Subjects whose data are missing on one trial may be available on the next trial, and the denominator reflects this fluctuation in N.
2. Log conductance change (in μmhos).

To produce such data, the individual data from all subjects showing evidence of gradual learning were dichotomized. Any response below an arbitrary level was given a value of 0, while any response equal to or above it was given a value of 1.

The dichotomized GSR data were then treated in the same way Estes had treated Gormezano's conditioned eyeblink data: (1) only Ss below the arbitrary cutoff point on the last adaptation trial, where the probability of responding is taken to be 0 before conditioning, were used; and (2) the percentage of unconditioned Ss responding for the first time on each of the first four test trials was noted.

The results for three different arbitrary cutoff points are shown in Table 10.1. They are all consistent in demonstrating no progressive increase in the percentage of first responses, which one would expect since the same data, in nondichotomized form, show evidence for gradual learning (Figure 10.1). Furthermore, with two of the cutoff points there is a marked similarity in the percentage of first responders shown on the first and fourth test trials.[3] While these results are more variable than those reported by Estes (probably due in part to the smaller N employed in this study), they are still more in line with an all-or-none than with a gradual interpretation of the individual learning process.

Thus the same body of data would appear to support either interpretation of the individual learning process, depending on whether the responses are recorded so as to preserve differences in magnitude or are scored as all-or-none events.

[3]On test trials the CS (tone) was given without the UCS (foot shock). In order to avoid having the subject know when the test trials would occur, they were not given at predictable times. Thus, for example, test trial 1 occurred after 1 CS-UCS pairing, while test trial 4 occurred after 7 CS-UCS pairings.

How is it possible for the same data to support either view of the learning process? Estes interpreted the fact that succeeding reinforcements yield a constant percentage of first responders as evidence supporting all-or-none learning. However, an alternative interpretation of this constancy based on an assumption of gradual learning is also conceivable. Figure 10.1 demonstrates that under the same conditions individuals vary in their rate of learning. The effect of succeeding reinforcements would be to bring those with progressively slower learning rates to the same level of responding. With a dichotomous (all-or-none) response measure, the impression could be gained that no learning had occurred until that trial when the response level rose above some arbitrary threshold. (Of the 25 subjects whose dichotomized data were considered in these analyses, for example, 9 failed to reach either the 0.035 or the 0.038 cutoff by the last conditioning trial; three other subjects who showed incremental changes did not show their first response within the first four test trials and were thus not included in the analysis.) Thus the percentage of first responders on succeeding trials might be constant even if individual learning is in fact gradual.

The present results suggest that, at least under certain conditions, the way a response is measured may influence conclusions drawn as to the nature of the learning process. It is important, then, that in work in this area, consideration be given to the extent to which support for the gradual or for the one-trial learning hypothesis reflects a property of the learning process per se, and the extent to which support of either view reflects a property of the way a response system is arbitrarily measured. Indeed, in view of the impact such methodological variables as procedure and apparatus can have on the results one obtains, it may be necessary to temper any conclusions drawn from a learning experiment with the caveat that the results may be due to many variables, only some of which are related to the CNS processes underlying learning.

10.3 MODEL SYSTEMS IN STUDIES OF LEARNING AND MEMORY

I would like to turn now from a consideration of methodological problems to one of experimental approaches. My own approach is that of the General Biologist. I am less concerned with those features of learning and memory that distinguish animals from one another than in those features that are common to all. Clearly there is a fundamental assumption here that there are in fact elements of learning and memory common to all animals. Being willing to make such an assumption makes it plausible to adopt a "model-system" approach to the problem.

The purpose of utilizing a biological model is to simplify the variables involved in the analysis. Fundamental to the use of a model system is the notion that the variables and their interaction in the model also apply to the intact and more complex biological system that is being modeled. One of the major reasons for going to phylogenetically simpler systems, which have been further simplified surgically, for investigations of, the macromolecular bases of learning and memory storage is a reduction in the complexity of interactions among the elements, particularly feedback loops.

The following hypothetical example may show how such a model-system approach can be useful in answering fundamental questions about the evolution of learning and memory networks. It would be desirable to know and to separate out, for example, the relative contributions that primary sensory input, motor output, efferent gating, and afferent feedback play in determining the final learning achieved.

Figure 10.2 attempts to schematize ways of experimentally separating out such contributions to learning and memory storage. If one were to record from the motor nerve directly and sever this distally from the effector (b), it should be possible to eliminate afferent feedback from the system. Correspondingly, if one stimulates primary sensory-nerve input directly, bypassing the primary receptor (c), it should be possible to separate

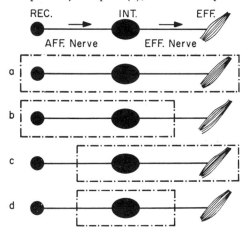

FIGURE 10.2 Conceptual preparations for studying learning phenomena. (a) The "usual" learning system of an intact organism, which may also serve as a model for part of an organism in which sensory and motor units are intact. (b) Bypassing of the effector and removal of afferent (proprioceptive) feedback from the system. (c) Bypassing of the receptor (and perhaps even the primary afferent neuron) and removal of efferent gating or control of primary input to the system. (d) Bypassing of both receptor and effector, thus eliminating from the system any efferent gating of sensory input or proprioceptive feedback from the effector response. REC.: receptor. INT.: integrator (ganglion or brain). AFF. Nerve: afferent nerve. EFF. Nerve: efferent nerve. EFF.: effector. From Eisenstein (1972).

out the effects of efferent gating on the system. By stimulating primary sensory input directly and recording the motor-nerve output (d), it should be possible to remove both sensory feedback and efferent gating. Thus such approaches as those shown in Figure 10.2 should make it possible to ascertain for a given system at any phylogenetic level what relative contributions these factors make to learning and memory storage. In principle, they allow us to ask as we ascend the phylogenetic scale whether or not and in what ways phenomena such as feedback and gating are involved in learning and memory storage. One might expect, for example, that at lower phylogenetic levels there is relatively little difference for a given system between stimulating the primary sensory nerve directly and recording from the motor nerve (d), and stimulating through its receptor and recording its effector output (a) (assuming that there is relatively little, if any, contribution from feedback and gating processes on learning in this system). However, as we ascend the phylogenetic scale, we may well expect to see marked differences in certain systems when we have eliminated their receptor and effector responses from consideration.

Another advantage of the approach shown in Figure 10.2 is that it allows us to do comparative studies of the relative integrative capacities with respect to learning and memory storage of different nervous systems at different phylogenetic levels. In addition, it becomes possible to do comparative studies of the relative integrative abilities of parts of the nervous system, one with respect to another, within the same animal.

One of the problems in comparative studies of learning and memory storage has been in assessing the effects of differences in the apparatus used and in the sensory and effector capabilities of different animals. Thus, for example, it has been difficult to compare meaningfully the learning of a maze by an octopus with bar-pressing learning in a rat, where both effector and sensory systems and the manipulations the animals perform are so different. How does one separate the specific contribution of the integrative capabilities of the nervous system per se from these other considerations?

Using such a schematic approach as I have described, one can monitor nervous output from a motor nerve and also put into the system direct electrical stimulation of sensory nerves and monitor what gets in. It now becomes possible to compare nervous systems directly. All inputs are measured in the same units, namely, some parameter of nerve discharges. It is thus possible to relate input and output directly. It also becomes possible to ask how the thoracic ganglia of a cockroach and of a crayfish compare in their ability to demonstrate Pavlovian or instrumental learning. One can use known sensory inputs, monitor motor outputs, and ask about rates of learning, retention, the discriminability of stimulus patterns (both spatial and temporal), as well as generalization—in fact, all the questions that are normally asked about learning, memory, and perception in any system—except that we now know exactly what is coming into and going out of the system and can talk about them in the same units. It then also becomes possible to correlate meaningfully the neuroantomy of these systems with their learning and memory capabilities.

With such simplified and carefully pruned systems it becomes possible to answer the question of how a biological system can encode in a three-dimensional structural way the various temporal sequences of events that form the basis of instrumental and Pavlovian learning procedures. Once such mechanisms in any simple system have been uncovered, we are then left with the empirical questions of what relationship, if any, the changes found in such a system have to normal learning in that system in the intact animal and what relationship, if any, such changes have to the bases of learning in other more complicated systems. If the bases of such temporal encoding can be established in any system, then we have a lever with which to look for specific changes in that same system in the intact animal and in other animals and to find, as we well may, that in some cases the results obtained from the pruned system fit what happens in the intact animal and in other cases they do not.

10.4 ANEURAL SYSTEMS IN STUDIES OF LEARNING AND MEMORY

One of the great simplifying aspects of aneural systems such as protozoans is that all events to be examined occur in one cell. Intercellular connectivities, which occur so profusely in neural systems and which are undoubtedly of great importance for their functions, are eliminated from consideration. Thus a great simplification can be achieved. However, as is apparent, this simplification is not without a price, since functions which in higher organisms occur in different cells, now all occur in one cell (Eisenstein, 1975). In more advanced systems, sensory transduction, integration, and initiation of behavior are relatively easy to separate since they occur in different parts of the animal. Such a separation is not so easy to observe in single-cell systems. One must be concerned with all three in any analysis of the mechanisms underlying behavior. One must not confuse miniaturization with simplification. While protozoa are miniaturized, they are not simplified to the same extent.

I believe that some of the most general and fundamental processes of living systems—transduction of an environmental event into a biological one, genetic control of behavior, coupling of stimulus input and behavioral output, as well as questions related to behavior modification—may be approachable for molecular studies at this phylogentic level in a way that they are not in more complex, neural systems. A major stumbling block in approaching these questions in neural systems—the role of any one cell in a complex matrix of cells—is bypassed.

The ciliates in particular would appear to be very promising for such studies. They show a variety of behaviors, and there is evidence in them for both habituation and sensitization. In addition, the ciliates respond to a large variety of stimuli, such as light, chemical changes (particularly pH changes in the medium), temperature, vibration, and electric shock. The larger ciliates such as *Spirostomum*, which may grow to 3mm, should be useful for single-cell studies of molecular changes underlying these behaviors.

This approach is based on the assumptions that mechanisms underlying learning can be separated into intra- and intercellular components and that nature has been parsimonious in solving the problem of information storage phylogenetically, so that intracellular findings at this level will apply at phylogenetically higher levels.

ACKNOWLEDGMENTS

Much of the research described in this paper was supported by NSF Grant GB 23371 to the author. I would also like to thank, belatedly, Professor M. A. Wenger, my major professor in psychology at UCLA, in whose laboratory I did work on Pavlovian conditioning in human subjects in 1959–1960 as part of my doctoral dissertation. At the time the work was supported by NIMH Grant MY-788 to Professor Wenger.

REFERENCES

Eimas, P. D., and Zeaman, D. 1963. Response speed changes in an Estes' paired-associative "miniature" experiment. *Journal of Verbal Learning and Verbal Behavior* 1: 384–388.

Eisenstein, E. M. 1962. Magnitude of conditioning as a function of CS-UCS interval: An attempt to condition several response systems concurrently. Unpublished Ph.D. dissertation, UCLA.

Eisenstein, E. M. 1972. Learning and memory in isolated insect ganglia. *Advances in Insect Physiology* 9: 111–181.

Eisenstein, E. M., ed. 1975. *Aneural Organisms in Neurobiology*. New York: Plenum Press.

Eisenstein, E. M., and Eisenstein, D. L. 1965. Some methodological considerations in the gradual vs. one-trial learning controversy. *American Zoologist* 5(no. 4) (abstract).

Estes, W. K. 1960. Learning theory and the new "mental chemistry." *Psychological Review* 67: 207–223.

Harris, J. T. 1971. Aspects of learning and memory in the cockroach. Unpublished Ph.D. dissertation, Tufts University.

HORRIDGE, G. A. 1962. Learning of leg position by the ventral nerve cord in headless insects. *Proceedings of the Royal Society* 157: 33–52.

KINTSCH, W. 1963. All-or-none learning and the role of repetition in paired-associate learning. *Science* 140: 310–312.

MILLER, P. L. 1970. Studies of learning in the insect central nervous system. In G. Horn and R. Hinde, eds., *Short-Term Changes in Neural Activity and Behaviour.* London: Cambridge University Press, pp. 475–498.

ROCK, I., and STEINFELD, G. 1963. Methodological questions in the study of one-trial learning. *Science* 140: 822–824.

WILLIAMS, J. P. 1962. A test of the all-or-none hypothesis for verbal learning. *Journal of Experimental Psychology* 64: 158–165.

11

Some Behavioral Approaches to the Study of Learning

ROBERT A. RESCORLA AND
PETER C. HOLLAND

ABSTRACT This paper attempts a characterization of situations commonly employed in the behavioral study of learning. The characterization is made in terms of differential experiences at one point in time resulting in differential behaviors at some later assessment time. Paradigms are segregated according to three different kinds of experiences: single stimulus presentation, exposure to relations among stimuli, and exposure to relations between responses and stimuli. Within each classification we identify various assessment techniques employed to indicate that the experience has modified the organism.

Although we point to a variety of behavioral changes attendant upon single stimulus presentation, our comments emphasize two: reduction in response evocation and decrement in trainability (ability to become a conditioned stimulus). In discussing exposure to relations among stimuli, we emphasize the advantages of a liberalized description of Pavlovian conditioning. We describe a particular theory that attempts to account for the sophisticated relations organisms learn. The role of intrinsic relations among stimuli is also discussed. Our comments are made in the context of two particular conditioning techniques, conditioned suppression and toxicosis, both of which emphasize the role of Pavlovian conditioning in emotional processes. Our discussion of the third paradigm, instrumental training, concerns only a few limited samples of modern concerns. We stress the complexity of instrumental training and suggest that it may be a poor paradigm for initial study of the biology of learning. We do suggest, however, that molar descriptions of behavior may prove as useful as molecular ones in studying the neural mechanisms of learning.

11.1 INTRODUCTION

The intention of this paper is to describe some currently studied issues and paradigms involved in the experimental investigation of animal learning. Since the elaboration of various biological and comparative aspects of learning is the domain of others here, we shall largely confine our discussion to behavioral studies with mammals. Furthermore, since the behavioral study of learning is a field which has occupied the energies of a large number of psychologists in this century, we shall by no means attempt an exhaustive review. Rather, we shall attempt to provide a sketchy overview of the field, emphasizing conceptual issues rather than data and dealing

ROBERT A. RESCORLA and PETER C. HOLLAND, Department of Psychology, Yale University, New Haven, CT

in depth with only a few selected issues of current interest.

Although it may appear to border on the sophistic, it is best to begin by attempting a characterization of those paradigms that the behavioral psychologist believes to involve learning. Such paradigms may be described in terms of the organism's experience and behavior at two different points in time. At t_1 the organism is exposed to some experience, normally produced by external stimulation, and then at t_2 the behavior of the organism is examined. The observation that the behavior at t_2 depends upon the experience at t_1 is the finding that is basic to the inference that learning has occurred.

Learning paradigms differ primarily in the kind of experience to which they expose the animal at t_1. Historically, three types of experience have predominated, and we shall organize the remainder of the paper around these treatments. The procedures may be casually described as exposing a subject to three different kinds of information about an external event: that it exists and has certain properties; that it bears certain relations to other events; and that it bears certain relations to the organism's behavior. These three options have been thought to describe the most elementary characteristics one can learn about an event.

Thus all three procedures involve the presentation of an external stimulus, S_1, to the organism; they differ in the circumstances of that presentation. The simplest is presentation of S_1 independently of the occurrence of other events. The issue is then whether simple exposure to a stimulus at t_1 produces differential behavior at t_2. It is in such paradigms that outcomes involving "habituation" have commonly been reported. For instance, presentation of a loud noise at t_1 reduces the likelihood that such a noise will evoke a startle response in a rat subject at t_2. A more complex procedure governing the presentation of the stimulus is described by the Pavlovian conditioning paradigm. In that paradigm the presentation of S_1 is dependent upon the occurrence of another event, S_2. In this context S_1 is labeled the unconditioned stimulus (US) and S_2 the conditioned stimulus (CS). Here the issue is whether the particular relation imposed upon two stimuli at t_1 produces differential behavior at

t_2. In the classical example, does the pairing of a tone with food at t_1 endow the tone with the ability to evoke salivation in a dog subject at t_2? The third procedure governing the occurrence of S_1 is that of instrumental training. In that paradigm the occurrence of S_1 is dependent upon the occurrence of some response by the organism. The issue then is whether the establishment of a relation between the occurrence of a response and that of a stimulus produces differential behavior at t_2. For instance, does the occurrence of a bar-press response followed by food at t_1 make it more likely that bar-pressing will occur at t_2?

Three comments should be made about this classification. First, the procedures as normally applied differ in ways other than those mentioned here. For instance, the kinds of stimuli employed as S_1 in the various paradigms can be quite different. Furthermore, the kinds of assessment procedures employed at t_2 will also differ. These issues will be dealt with in subsequent sections.

Second, the three procedures are not independent but tend, rather, to be embedded in each other. For instance, when a relation is arranged between S_1 and S_2, the organism must obviously receive simple exposure to those stimuli. Consequently, those processes responsible for change when the first paradigm is applied may also be operative in the second paradigm. Indeed, a major issue in the study of learning has been the development of techniques to unravel the relative contributions of the paradigms in any given experimental arrangement.

Third, it is important to note that this classification is made in terms of paradigms, not processes. In the discussion that follows we shall use this procedural commonality to organize a wide range of situations which differ substantially in both the stimuli employed and the organisms exposed to those stimuli. This does not involve a commitment to the idea that the same learning process is necessarily involved in all cases fitting a given paradigm. Grouping by paradigms, whatever the level of discourse, is a convenient starting place for analysis, but it is only that.

Of course, we all search for generality of process, whether our level of analysis is biological, chemical, or behavioral. Consequently, we shall often adopt a skeptical posture, biased in favor of demanding especially clear evidence when different processes are inferred from similar paradigms. Yet, from the outset, it seems unlikely that within a particular paradigm the entire range of results will be attributable to the same process. We may anticipate a range of outcomes from different applications of a paradigm. Eventually, we should see natural groupings of those outcomes such that some seem to require the inference of one process and others another process. Ultimately, we may hope for both a behavioral

theory and a biological mechanism that use both paradigms and outcome patterns to identify processes.

At the behavioral level this means that such terms as "association," "conditioning," etc., are theoretical entities and should not be identified in a one-to-one fashion with procedures; they are, rather, inferred from procedures and outcomes in the context of a theory. It is obviously one of the tasks of behavioral psychology to develop successful theories allowing the identification of such processes, but that task is far from complete, and the inference is correspondingly difficult.

It is the absence of well-formulated and accepted theoretical structures which has produced attempts to specify "learning" by definition. The primary function of such definitions (which are really based on inexplicitly stated theories) has apparently been to provide ground rules for certification of particular phenomena as "legitimate" examples of learning. Historically, such definitions have often taken the form of specification by exclusion, with the aim being to rule out such alternative "nonlearning" processes as fatigue, structural damage, etc. Although we feel that such arbitrary definitions are ultimately of little use, they have had an important impact upon what is studied in the learning laboratory. Examples of "associative" learning, such as those presumed to result from the second and third paradigms mentioned above, seem susceptible to relatively few alternative interpretations in terms of other known processes. By contrast, changes due to noncontingent stimulus presentation admit of interpretation in terms of a good many "nonlearning" processes. It is partly for this reason that "associative learning" has dominated American psychology while "habituation" and similar processes have received relatively less attention. It has even led to the anomaly that simple noncontingent stimulus presentation is frequently employed as a "nonlearning" control for associative learning.

Such definitions of learning have also favored the selection of some behavioral outcomes over others as indices of learning. For instance, increases in response from t_1 to t_2 seem less vulnerable to such nonlearning interpretations as fatigue, so they are usually preferred to response decrements. Similarly, behaviors at t_2 which are under the control of particular stimuli (such as the CS) are normally preferred to simple "state" changes. In the same spirit, it has been suggested that only if the change induced by experience is "relatively permanent," i.e., can be observed even if the interval between t_1 and t_2 is large, should learning be inferred from that change.

One important thing to remember about all such strictures is that they stem from inexplicitly stated primitive assumptions about learning. They serve in place of, and will eventually be replaced by, explicit theories of learning processes. Ultimately, whether a particular situation evidences learning is a decision to be made within a theory successfully describing the behavioral change in question. Until that time such commonly accepted guidelines may be useful but should hardly be treated as carrying the great moral weight that is sometimes attached to the word "learning."

11.2 NONCONTINGENT STIMULUS PRESENTATION

The most elementary experience to which an organism can be subjected at t_1 is the noncontingent presentation of a stimulus. In the extreme case we might be interested in the effects of a single event at that time; but more commonly the experience administered at t_1 consists of a set of presentations of the same event without regard to either the animal's behavior or the occurrence of other events.

Historically, psychologists have badly neglected the study of this sort of experience. Perhaps because of the long tradition of interest in associative learning in both philosophy and psychology, investigation of single event occurrence has been largely left to the biologist and physiologist. Many psychologists still have hesitations about including changes attributable to such exposure under the heading of "learning." Because experimental interest has so often focused on the associative changes, other changes have often been viewed with undeserved disdain. Whatever the historical reasons, the study of simple noncontingent event presentation has received considerably more attention in the last few years, and psychologists are beginning to attempt to catch up with their fellow scientists.

It is important to note one thing about our characterization of noncontingent-stimulus paradigms for the study of learning: the assessment as to the success of the t_1 experience in modifying the animal is made entirely in terms of the behavior at t_2. Historically, it has been more common to specify this paradigm in terms of the *change* in response of the animal between t_1 and t_2. For instance, it is common to infer habituation from a decrement in the response to S_1 between t_1 and t_2. We avoid this alternative specification for several reasons.

First, there are a great many influences upon the organism between t_1 and t_2, many of which are not under experimental control. These influences could work to produce either increments or decrements in behavior independently of the t_1 experience, thus masking or enhancing the effect attributable to stimulus presentation. Thus the critical observation is not a change in response, but differential behavior at t_2 depending upon differential experience at t_1. Furthermore, that dif-

ferential effect is equally identifiable whether it occurs against a generally rising or a generally falling baseline.

Second, specification of this paradigm in terms of a change between t_1 and t_2 artificially limits one to cases in which comparable observations can be made at the two times. It unduly restricts the t_1 experiences that we investigate to those contained in the t_2 assessment procedure.

Finally, the assessment at t_2 permits determination of the effects of various t_1 treatments under test conditions which are as similar as possible across different groups. As we shall see shortly, comparisons of the effects of various parameters upon noncontingent stimulus presentation have often inadvertently confounded the conditions of training with the conditions of testing. Making explicit the separation of training and test conditions emphasizes the need to arrange comparable test procedures for diverse treatments.

For these reasons, our discussion will be phrased in terms of procedures in which several organisms receive different experiences at t_1 and are then all subjected to a common assessment procedure at t_2. Typically, we shall be concerned with two groups of organisms, one of which undergoes simple stimulus presentation at t_1 while the other is subjected to a treatment that is similar but omits the stimulus presentation.

11.2.1 Assessment procedures and outcomes

Given the foregoing description of this paradigm, it becomes convenient to classify experiments according to the various assessment techniques employed at t_2 and the outcomes of those assessments. It turns out that quite different theoretical constructs have been inferred from those different outcomes despite considerable commonality of experience at t_1.

Probably the most common assessment technique involves the *elicitation power* of a stimulus. For instance, if S_1 initially evokes a response, then one may ask, what is the consequence of presentation of S_1 at t_1 for its ability to evoke a response at t_2? Not surprisingly, diverse outcomes have been reported, and contrary theoretical constructs have been formulated to account for those outcomes. The most usual finding is that such a procedure reduces the ability of S_1 to evoke a response at t_2, as compared to its evocative ability in a group that was not exposed at t_1. Typically, a theoretical construct of "habituation" is offered to account for this finding (see Groves and Thompson, 1970; Hinde, 1970; Thompson and Spencer, 1966, for recent reviews). It should be noted, however, that the term "habituation" is by no means employed uniformly by all investigators. Considerable confusion has resulted from the fact that some workers apply "habituation" to an outcome (response decrement), others apply it to a procedure (repeated stimulus presentation), while still others intend it to refer to a theoretical construct.

Despite the frequency with which response decrement results from repeated stimulus presentation, some investigators have also reported increases in the response to S_1. Such a finding, which is not uncommon in the early stages of repeated presentation (Groves and Thompson, 1970), is often used to justify the inference of a "sensitization" process. But there are also instances in which increase in response evocation is the major consequence of S_1 presentation. One particular case deserves mention because the response undergoes such a dramatic change and because it has generated a substantial literature of its own. This is the phenomenon of imprinting, in which, under appropriate circumstances, exposure to almost any S_1 will endow it with the ability to evoke a variety of responses at t_2. For instance, exposure of a newly hatched bird to a stimulus often gives that stimulus the power to modulate the emission of vocalizations, locomotor activity, and, later, sexual behavior.

In addition to changing response probability or amplitude, up or down, repeated stimulus presentation can also modify the topography of the response evoked by S_1. Of course, such a change can be represented as an increase in one set of responses concurrent with a decrease in others.

Presentation of S_1 may result in consequences not only for its own ability to elicit a response, but also for the ability of other stimuli to do so. In some cases this outcome encourages the inference of "stimulus generalization." This inference is most common when the response change is greatest for the presented S_1 and less for other, similar stimuli. For instance, in some response systems the greatest response decrement is produced to the stimulus that is most frequently presented, but some lesser decrement also accrues to related stimuli, presumably generalizing from the modification of S_1. On the other hand, there are instances in which S_1 presentation has greater consequences for the response provoked by some other stimulus than for its own ability to produce a response. This commonly occurs in the context of Pavlovian conditioning experiments, where the simple presentation of the US may dramatically change the response to the CS. In that context such an outcome results in the postulation of a "pseudoconditioning" or "sensitization" process. Unfortunately, because this sort of observation has been made in the context of investigation of the role of interevent relations, it has received little direct attention. But it is fully the equal of response decrement as an index of learning.

A more recently studied, but equally important, consequence of stimulus presentation is modification in the ability of the stimulus to function in subsequent learning paradigms. For instance, preexposed stimuli have recently been found to be less effective as signals in subsequent Pavlovian or instrumental-learning situations (see Lubow, 1973, for a review). This depression in effectiveness has been termed "latent inhibition," and various theoretical constructs have been suggested to deal with it. On the other hand, there are several literatures which suggest that preexposure may enhance the trainability of various stimuli. In some cases this enhancement has been viewed in terms of a general state change of the animal (e.g., Rosenzweig, Krech, and Bennett, 1960), while in others relatively specific "perceptual learning" has been inferred (e.g., Gibson and Walk, 1956).

Preexposure may modify not only the ability of a stimulus to be trained, but also its ability to train. Thus effective Pavlovian reinforcers may undergo either enhancement or depression of their reinforcing power as a result of prior exposure (e.g., Rescorla, 1973, 1974). Similarly, it has been argued that preexposure changes the novelty of stimuli and consequently modifies their instrumental reinforcing power (e.g., Butler, 1957; Glanzer, 1953). Finally, in the imprinting literature there is considerable evidence that exposure endows stimuli with positive instrumental reinforcing power (e.g., Hoffman et al., 1966).

This brief outline serves to emphasize an important point about the study of learning. If one wishes to conclude that an experience at t_1 has modified the animal, then *any* of these outcomes provides sufficient justification, as long as failure to administer the experience results in failure of the outcome. However, if one wants to go beyond that conclusion to describe the modification as "learning" and to detail the character of that learning, then one becomes involved in making an inference about theoretical processes. Furthermore, different kinds of assessment techniques will uncover different consequences of the same t_1 experience. Consequently, they will often lead to the inference of different underlying processes. That inference, however, is a fundamentally theoretical step; the terms postulated to account for these sorts of behavioral change are theoretical terms, and their use entails a more or less explicit commitment to a theory of learning.

11.2.2 Some sample data

Each of the above-mentioned outcomes of repeated stimulus presentation has generated a substantial literature of its own. Furthermore, in most cases those literatures have received thorough reviews over the last few years (Groves and Thompson, 1970; Hinde, 1970; Hoffman and Ratner, 1973; Lubow, 1973; Rosenzweig, Krech, and Bennett, 1960; Sluckin, 1964; Thompson and Spencer, 1966). Consequently, we shall not attempt to provide such a review here. Instead we shall mention some of the well-known effects of experimental variables upon two of the outcomes: decrement in elicitation power ("habituation") and depression in trainability ("latent inhibition"). We pick the former because of its prominence in the more biologically oriented literature and the latter because it is relatively unappreciated in that literature. We shall then make a few brief comments on some of the more behaviorally oriented attempts to theorize about these situations.

Consider the response-evoking power and the trainability of a given stimulus, S_1, at time t_2. One can ask, what are the conditions of the animal's experience at t_1 which differentially affect these measures at t_2? We mention six of the many variables.

Certainly the most widely studied variation in treatment at t_1 is the number of presentations of S_1. For both habituation and latent inhibition, it is clearly documented that the consequences for behavior at t_2 are an increasing function of the number of t_1 presentations. For instance, the magnitude of the startle reflex to a loud sound in rats at t_2 is a decreasing function of the number of prior presentations of that sound (e.g., Davis and Wagner, 1968). Similar observations have been made for a large number of other stimuli originally capable of evoking a response (see Spencer and Thompson, 1966; Hinde, 1970, for reviews). In parallel fashion, several investigators have found that interference with the trainability of a stimulus at t_2 is a function of the number of prior presentations (e.g., Domjan and Siegel, 1971; Lantz, 1973). Indeed, some authors have suggested that the occurrence of such effects be considered a prerequisite for an inference of the theoretical construct of "habituation."

A second variable of interest is the similarity of treatment at t_1 and t_2. For instance, the response to S_1 during the t_2 test will often be maximally affected by repeated presentations at t_1 of stimuli that are similar to S_1 (e.g., Coombs, 1938). Conversely, the trainability of S_1 is most disrupted by prior presentations of itself rather than other stimuli (Siegel, 1969). Again, this observation has often been taken as central to theoretical inferences. It indicates a kind of stimulus specificity which apparently rules out various state-change interpretations of the t_1 experience. It should be noted that the inference about stimulus specificity does not demand maximum effect when the t_1 and t_2 stimuli are identical; any function relating these two stimuli in a systematic way would be sufficient to rule out alternative "general" effects, although perhaps implying somewhat different theoretical conclusions.

An important exception to the above generalization

about stimulus similarity at t_1 and t_2 may appear when that similarity is manipulated by stimulus intensity, rather than by stimulus quality. Thus Davis and Wagner (1968, 1969) have reported two cases in which the attenuation of the response to S_1 at t_2 is maximal when stimuli other than S_1 have been presented at t_1. Using the startle response in the rat, they found that gradually increasing the intensity over trials toward the level of S_1 produced more habituation of the response to S_1 than did repeated presentation of S_1 itself. On the other hand, if a constant-intensity stimulus is to be repeatedly presented at t_1, then the response to S_1 at t_2 will be maximally disrupted by presentation of a stimulus more intense than S_1. There is a hint of a finding parallel to this latter outcome in a latent-inhibition experiment by Crowell and Anderson (1972). The technique suggested by Davis and Wagner for assessing the effects of different intensities of stimulation at t_1 upon a common test stimulus at t_2 is of immense general importance for the study of habituation. As they point out, a great many parametric studies of habituation confound the training experience with the testing procedure. They note in particular that studies of S_1 intensity have often drawn conclusions of questionable value by comparing the response reduction to two stimuli which differ in intensity at *both* the time of habituation treatment and the time of assessment.

Temporal aspects of t_1 presentation are also important in determining the consequences for behavior at t_2. A number of habituation studies indicate that maximum decrement in the reaction to S_1 at t_2 is produced by spaced, rather than massed, presentations of S_1 at t_1 (e.g., Davis, 1970). It is important to note that this occurs despite the observation that, during the t_1 exposure itself, the response to S_1 declines more rapidly for massed presentations. Apparently this latter result is partially attributable to a short-term performance decrement induced by proximity to the just-preceding S_1. So, as in the case of intensity, one may come to quite different conclusions about the effects of a parameter depending upon whether or not those effects are tested under comparable conditions. If tested by the response to S_1 at t_2, in which the interval between S_1 and the preceding S_1 presentation is similar in both groups, then spaced presentation produces more habituation; when tested in terms of the response to S_1 when the groups differ in the proximity to the just prior S_2, then massed presentation produces more (temporary) decrement. Similarly, Lantz (1973) has reported that spaced S_1 presentation at t_1 produces more latent inhibition at t_2 in a conditioned-suppression situation.

A historically important question has concerned the length of the interval between t_1 and t_2. Does the effect of an experience at t_1 diminish as that interval is lengthened? The available evidence suggests that although some diminution ("spontaneous recovery") may take place, there is often substantial retention of habituation over long intervals (e.g., Davis, 1972). In parallel fashion, latent inhibition is regularly assessed after 24 hours and has been reported to go undiminished for substantially longer periods (see Lubow, 1973). Again, some authors have suggested that the long-term retention of the t_1 experience should be a prerequisite for the identification of habituation or of latent inhibition.

Finally, it is worth mentioning that in some circumstances the presentation of a novel stimulus prior to the t_2 assessment will attenuate the effects of t_1 presentation. This effect, normally called dishabituation (after the parallel disinhibitory effect in Pavlovian conditioning), has been observed for both habituation and latent-inhibition assessment procedures (e.g., Groves and Thompson, 1970; Lantz, 1973). In some cases it has been described in terms of the novel stimulus introducing a dissimilarity between the presentations of S_1 at t_1 and t_2; in other cases it has been viewed as inducing an independent sensitization process which has little to do with the decrement induced by t_1 presentation.

One final point should be made for the case of the latent-inhibition assessment procedure. With this procedure the experimenter may elect to use any of a variety of training procedures to establish that S_1 is indeed less trainable. The most common are Pavlovian procedures, but instrumental techniques have also been employed. Apparently, S_1 presentation produces latent inhibition as measured by almost *any* subsequent learning experience the experimenter selects. This appears to apply to any relation to be learned between S_1 and a reinforcer, inhibitory as well as excitatory (see Reiss and Wagner, 1972; Rescorla, 1971).

Quite aside from the specific outcomes that such independent variables produce, two general comments are worth making. First, at several points we have noted that some authors suggest one outcome or another as being necessary for the inference of the occurrence of habituation or latent inhibition. Among those mentioned are permanence of the effect, stimulus specificity, and monotonicity of change with repeated presentation. Such restrictions are exactly the sort of definitional steps that we cautioned earlier can often retard, rather than advance, the building of a theory. They may eventually prove useful for ordering outcomes, but they ought not to become initial criteria which must be met before an outcome is studied.

Second, the availability of several assessment techniques for determining the consequences of t_1 events has a number of advantages. For instance, with some organisms or some stimuli, the demonstration and measure-

ment of a modification resulting from an exposure at t_1 may be better assessed by one technique than by another. Some authors have suggested that habituation is a primitive process which may occur in organisms not susceptible to modification by other learning procedures. Since the latent-inhibition phenomenon requires such susceptibility, changes in stimulus evocation would be a better technique in such cases. On the other hand, for stimuli that do not originally evoke an easily measured response, or on those occasions when it is advantageous to be able to select different responses as indices, reduction in trainability of the stimulus might be the method of choice.

Of course, these assessment techniques, while capable of demonstrating that the t_1 experience has generally modified the animal, may reflect different learning processes. Given that repeated stimulus presentation has, in different settings, been found to increase or decrease both the response-evocation power and trainability of stimuli, it would surely be rash to suggest that all such changes reflect the same process.

Even when behaviors fit a general pattern such as that described here for habituation or latent inhibition, the parametric details may vary greatly. Hinde (1970) has demonstrated the wide range of outcomes when such parameters are varied in habituation situations. As he notes, from a biological point of view it would be surprising if the range of changes resulting from repeated stimulus presentation in widely differing organisms all had the same neurological basis. But detailed identification of multiple processes awaits further analysis.

Thus the point of the above discussion is not so much to describe particular outcomes as to point to the kinds of observations that are typically employed. It is hoped that we can provide a common general framework in which diverse methodologies and techniques can be profitably discussed and compared.

11.2.3 Theories of latent inhibition and habituation

It is worth briefly mentioning some of the theoretical contexts in which results such as those of the preceding section have been placed. Actually, theory development has been much less vigorously pursued here than in the other learning paradigms we shall discuss; however, some efforts have been made. Without providing any detailed analysis, one can group these efforts into three categories. One group of theories attempts to understand the results of simple stimulus presentation in terms of the more elaborate Pavlovian or instrumental procedures. Various sources of associative learning are identified, and principles already available from associative experiments are employed. A second group of theories proposes new theoretical constructs, primarily concerned with perceptual processing of the stimuli presented. Finally, a third group of theories attempts to account for these changes in terms of biological levels of discourse.

Most of the attempts to account for habituation or latent inhibition in terms of associative processes have employed Pavlovian principles. For instance, Stein (1966) and Ratner (1970) have suggested similar theories. According to Stein, a stimulus onset initiates an excitatory process, whereas its termination initiates inhibitory rebound. When the stimulus is repeatedly presented, the rebound is regularly preceded by the stimulus initiation and so becomes conditioned to it. Consequently, after repeated presentation the stimulus evokes both excitation and competing inhibition and so generates a reduced response. Ratner's theory differs only in that the competing responses have their origin not in the inhibitory rebound, but in the responses evoked by situational stimuli immediately after the termination of S_1. Both of these theories were developed to account for habituation but could easily apply to latent inhibition as well.

A related approach to simple stimulus learning has been suggested for the case of imprinting by Hoffman and his collaborators (e.g., Hoffman and Ratner, 1973). They argue that certain aspects of stimuli, such as movement, have an innately positive value for newly hatched chicks. When an object is moved in front of the chick, Pavlovian conditioning results in the attachment of this positive value to other features of the object. As a consequence, these features have the ability to reward such index behaviors as following or pecking a pole (e.g., Hoffman et al., 1966); furthermore, the positive value may take the form of fear-reduction and thus enable these stimuli to inhibit distress calls (Hoffman et al., 1970; Hoffman, Eiserer, and Singer, 1972). Although theories of pseudoconditioning are rare, one suggested by Wickens and Wickens (1942) belongs to the present set. They argue that during simple US presentation, conditioning occurs between various aspects of the US, some of which are similar to the CS later tested. Finally, some authors have applied the notion of Pavlovian conditioned inhibition, especially to account for latent-inhibition phenomena. As we shall see in the next section, some stimulus relations yield inhibitions that share with latent inhibition reduced acquisition rates in subsequent excitatory conditioning.

All of these explanations have in common the feature that they describe what is apparently a single stimulus presentation as actually consisting of multiple stimuli bearing certain relations to each other. The automatic arrangement of the contiguity relation then provides the opportunity for the occurrence of interevent learning. When the power of data and theories of interevent learn-

ing are brought to bear upon such situations, a considerable portion of the data on habituation and latent inhibition seems to follow. For instance, the importance of stimulus similarity at t_1 and t_2, the role of the interval between S_1 presentations at t_1, and various other parametric features previously described may be deduced from known conditioning data.

An analogous case can be made for applying instrumental-learning principles to single-stimulus situations. For instance, in the case of habituation, the S_1 employed might have either positive or negative instrumental reinforcing power. Consequently, by engaging in activities which either accentuate or attenuate the reception of S_1, the subject would simultaneously modify the reinforcement power and the response magnitude evoked by S_1.

Detailed criticisms of such approaches in terms of differences in reactions to parameter values are not likely to prove very informative. It is simply very difficult to construct a Pavlovian or instrumental model of the habituation situation for which one can be sure of the appropriate values of such factors as US intensity, CS duration, CS-US interval, etc. Even such claims as the occurrence of habituation in organisms which otherwise do not show Pavlovian conditioning are vitiated by this inability to match parameters. The distressing feature of such theories, however, is that they attempt to account for what on the surface seems to be a simpler learning situation in terms of what is known about a more complex one. This is perhaps only natural since associative learning is better known and understood among psychologists. However, it seems likely that we shall ultimately have to develop theories about the learning of elements that can enter into associations. Perhaps the stimuli normally used in habituation experiments do not constitute such elements, but at some point we shall need a description of the constituents of an association and how the organism learns about them. Indeed, for many psychologists the interest in habituation stems from the hope that it might provide such a description.

The second set of suggested theories proposes a special process for the decrements of habituation and latent inhibition. For instance, a popular theory of the reduction in the orienting response has been put forth by Sokolov (1963). According to this theory each S_1 presentation results in a further buildup of an internal representation (neural model) of that event. Subsequent presentations of S_1 are then compared with the neural model, and the magnitude of the response depends upon the discrepancy between the two. As the model becomes more accurate, the discrepancy is reduced and hence the response magnitude decreases. A somewhat similar theory could be stated in terms of attention: repeated presentation might reduce the degree to which S_1 receives attention and so modify the response to it. This kind of approach has been especially common in accounting for the reduction in trainability observed in a latent-inhibition paradigm.

The third set of theories avoids the postulation of behavioral theoretical constructs and instead seeks an explanation at a more molecular level. For instance, Groves and Thompson (1970) have appealed to particular types of synapses which might be responsible for habituation. Similarly, Carlton (1963) has referred to biochemical changes. This form of theorizing, by direct reduction to neurological levels of discourse, is much more common for the present case than for associative learning. Perhaps this simply reflects the different backgrounds of those who have studied habituation and associative learning. In this approach to theory construction, one must be careful to avoid the impression that a phenomenon has been explained simply because the level of discourse has changed. For instance, the problems raised by trying to account for habituation in particular neurons are analogous to those of accounting for behavioral habituation. But, of course, there can also be considerable heuristic gain in shifting the problem to another theoretical and empirical domain.

In constructing and assessing theories such as these it may be useful to keep in mind a distinction that has proved fruitful in other learning contexts, namely, that between learning and performance. This distinction, although implicit in much of the foregoing discussion, is perhaps underappreciated in the present context. A complete theory would naturally specify both the product of learning and the means by which that product reveals itself in the organism's behavior. Unfortunately, theories that are adequate in characterizing the conditions for producing modification and in describing the product of those conditions are often inadequate in specifying how that learning is mapped into behavior. This distinction is especially applicable when organisms are exposed to a common experience at t_1 which is then assessed by different techniques at t_2. Instead of inferring different learning processes to account for the various results, we might consider in more detail the mapping of those processes onto different behaviors. Indeed, such widely disparate findings as response increase and response decrease may represent differences not in learning, but rather in how that learning generates behavior. This is obviously a matter for an adequate theory of noncontingent stimulus presentation to settle. But in trying to extend theories such as those described above to changes other than response decrement, we should

consider both learning and performance modifications. In any case, from the point of view of the behavioral psychologist the most severe shortcoming in the study of noncontingent stimulus presentation is its stunted theory development.

11.3 PAVLOVIAN CONDITIONING

Somewhat more complicated than the previous paradigm is the Pavlovian procedure. In this procedure some relation is arranged between S_1 and another stimulus S_2, at t_1, without regard to the organism's behavior. The consequences for that arrangement are then assessed at t_2. If arrangement of that relation between stimuli can be identified as responsible for differential t_2 behavior, one may say that Pavlovian conditioning has occurred. Historically, this procedure has been of considerable interest, partly because it can be viewed as a general model of associative learning. But until quite recently, American studies have slighted the Pavlovian paradigm in favor of the instrumental-learning procedure discussed in the next section. The reasons for this are multiple, but include such factors as the American concern for pragmatism and functionalism, with which instrumental behavior fits more neatly, and the ready availability of instrumental-learning techniques as compared to the technically complex procedures of Pavlov. Recently the development of convenient procedures for the study of Pavlovian conditioning, together with the realization that there is probably a Pavlovian component to the outcomes of instrumental-learning experiments, have served to reawaken interest in the Pavlovian paradigm.

Our characterization of Pavlovian conditioning as the learning of relations between events differs in many regards from traditional descriptions. It borrows more from the tradition of associationism in psychology than from that of reflexology in physiology. Thus we view conditioning more as the way in which the organism learns about the causal relations in his environment (what Tolman and Brunswik [1935] called the "causal texture") than as the transfer of control of a reflex from one stimulus to another. This emphasis has a number of important implications for the study of conditioning.

First, it suggests that a major focus of the study of conditioning is investigation of the range of relations to which the organism is sensitive. Traditional studies of Pavlovian conditioning have explored only an extremely narrow range of relations, but recent evidence suggests a much more sophisticated organism, sensitive to a wide variety of environmental relations. For this reason our discussion will concentrate upon several recent lines of evidence that explore this sensitivity. We shall omit discussion of many of the standard issues and experiments in Pavlovian conditioning in favor of indicating in depth the richness of the organism's ability to learn relations in the world.

Second, describing conditioning as the learning of environmental relations permits use of a broad range of assessment techniques at t_2 to determine whether the t_1 relation has indeed modified the organism. The most common technique examines the nature of the response evoked by a stimulus which has borne various relations to S_1 (the US) at t_1. That is, we typically ask whether the CS produces a conditioned response (CR). However, other, less commonly studied assessment techniques might also be useful. For instance, we could ask whether S_2 has acquired such other properties as the ability to serve as the reinforcer in either a Pavlovian or an instrumental paradigm as a result of its relation to S_1 at t_1. Such procedures are especially valuable in situations where it is difficult to measure the responses evoked by S_2 itself. Or we might ask about changes in the organism's t_2 behavior that are not occasioned by S_2 presentation. The simplest such case is that of "stimulus generalization," in which the response evoked by stimuli other than, but similar to, S_2 is investigated. But one may go further and ask whether the behavior of the organism is different at t_2 in the absence of any explicit stimulus presentation. If our interest is in identifying whether the organism has been modified by the event relations arranged at t_1, then *any* index behavior is acceptable.

Third, the study of relations among events need not be restricted to a particular subclass of events. Historically, it has been common to restrict Pavlovian conditioning studies to those S_1 events that evoke reflex responses and to those S_2 events that do not, prior to conditioning. As we shall note below, these restrictions seem to limit artificially the kinds of behavioral changes that we can hope to observe.

Thus, viewing Pavlovian conditioning in terms of learning about relations among events makes many of the familiar trappings of a conditioning experiment seem less important. Pavlovian conditioning is often described as selecting a stimulus that reliably evokes a response and pairing it with a neutral stimulus until that neutral stimulus also evokes the response. But few aspects of this description are critical to the present viewpoint. There is no reason to demand that S_1 reliably evoke a response or that S_2 fail to do so prior to conditioning. Nor should our index of conditioning necessarily be confined to response changes elicited by the CS, much less to responses that are similar to those evoked by the US. We shall even see that the specification of the rela-

tion normally employed in such descriptions—pairing—is misleading.

Of course, one may choose to restrict the word "conditioning" to some subset of the cases here discussed. We are free to place additional restrictions on the types of S_1 events and the types of behavioral changes that are acceptable instances of "conditioning." But then it will only be necessary to find another name for the many other instances of learning about relations that are currently being investigated. Moreover, in our view the placing of such supposedly pretheoretical restrictions can only serve to retard the development of an adequate theory of conditioning. Such restrictions may well grow out of a theory but surely should not precede it.

We should also mention an issue of continuing concern in studies of Pavlovian conditioning: what controls to run to ensure that we can identify the experience at t_1 as yielding "conditioning." It is important to realize that there are two quite different questions raised by this concern (see Seligman, 1969). The first is that of identifying a particular relation arranged between events as responsible for a particular change at t_2. Proposed relations can be evaluated in either of two ways: by comparison with other groups that omit the relation altogether or by examination of variations in behavior at t_2 when the relation is varied. The former procedure, which involves the identification of a "control" group, has been more popular, but probably falsely forces one to a commitment about a point of zero conditioning. Naturally, the particular control procedure that one adopts will depend upon the details of the relation that one wishes to assess. It is in this context that Rescorla (1967) has suggested the "truly random" control as useful for identifying the role of CS-US contingencies, as distinct from CS-US pairings. But this issue of the role of a particular relation in affecting behavior is an empirical one which may, at least in principle, be easily addressed.

The second issue, which it is important to keep separate, is the identification of a particular process as responsible for the behavior at t_2. Often one reads of attempts to identify the presence or absence of "associations" or "conditioning." The point to notice is that these are *theoretical* terms and that the identification of their occurrence can only be done within a particular theory. The very same operation may in some theories involve associations, while in others it may produce behavioral changes by quite different processes. The conclusion is that one can atheoretically provide controls for relations, but controls for learning processes involve theories. Of course, broad classes of theories often share assumptions in such a way that a common method can be used for similar inferences within those theories. Furthermore, as we shall see, there has recently been some progress toward adequate theories of conditioning. Nevertheless, it is important to keep separate those issues that are theoretical.

We turn now to a discussion of some of those relations that have proven successful in producing modifications. We first discuss two standard samples of Pavlovian relations—excitatory and inhibitory—and then turn to the role of intrinsic relations.

11.3.1 Excitatory relations: temporal

We consider first those relations that yield "excitatory" outcomes. Roughly speaking, excitatory relations are those in which two stimuli are learned as "going together" or "causally related." Two classes of excitatory relations have been extensively studied: those involving temporal variables and those involving "logical" or "informational" variables.

The most extensively studied temporal relation is that of the CS-US interval. One aspect of this relation is the sequence in which S_2 (the CS) and S_1 (the US) occur. Historically, conditioning has been thought to occur only with the particular sequential arrangement in which S_2 precedes S_1 (forward conditioning). Indeed, some authors have so incorporated this fact into the descriptions of conditioning that other orders are sometimes used as "control" procedures. More recent evidence suggests that this belief is not completely correct. Although they produce less conditioning than the forward arrangement, arrangements in which S_2 and S_1 are initiated together (simultaneous conditioning) or in which S_1 initiation precedes that of S_2 (backward conditioning) have been found to generate reliable learning in some preparations (e.g., Mowrer and Aiken, 1954; Heth and Rescorla, 1973). These demonstrations almost all share the feature that a relatively long US is employed, such that despite its initiation prior to the CS, the US completely overlaps the CS. Whether the use of that temporal relation will have similar results with all response systems remains unknown.

A second aspect of the study of the CS-US interval deals not with the sequencing of events per se but, rather, with the quantitative properties of the interval. Using the change in the response to S_2 at t_2 as the measure, a great deal of research demonstrates a gradient of conditioning as a function of the size of the CS-US interval at t_1. Virtually all conditioning preparations studied reveal some optimal CS-US interval at which the greatest response strength is observed, with shorter and longer intervals generating less responding. It was once widely believed that this optimal interval was the same (i.e., about 500 msec) for all conditioning situa-

tions, with a rapid loss as one departed from that value, but it is now evident that the function varies considerably from situation to situation. For example, while conditioning is observed only with very short intervals in eyelid (Gormezano, 1965), nictitating-membrane (Schneiderman and Gormezano, 1964), and leg-flexion (Wickens et al., 1969) preparations, jaw-movement conditioning seems to occur with somewhat longer intervals (Gormezano, 1972), and salivary and fear conditioning develop with intervals of several minutes (Kamin, 1965; Pavlov, 1927). Thus conditioning situations may share the form of the function relating the CS-US interval to the magnitude of conditioning, but they vary widely in the precise quantitative properties of that function.

A related situation is that of "temporal conditioning," in which S_1 is presented repeatedly with a constant interval between its occurrences. When using this arrangement, investigators typically treat the passage of time as being accompanied by a changing stimulus environment to which S_1 gradually produces conditioning. Temporal conditioning has received little investigation in its own right; it has been most often invoked as an explanation to account for such cyclic phenomena as the increase in activity in rats as the time of their daily feeding approaches (Bolles, 1967). In addition, some have wished to employ temporal conditioning as a model for explaining habituation within an associative framework.

11.3.2 Excitatory relations: logical

The discussion above indicates that the organism displays differential behavior at t_2 primarily when the S_1 and S_2 events have occurred in certain limited temporal relations at t_1. Recently, however, it has been suggested that the mere occurrence of these events in such temporal relations may not be sufficient to produce conditioning (e.g., Rescorla, 1967). Not only must a temporal relation be arranged between S_2 and S_1, but also a logical or informational relation must be obtained. To illustrate the sophistication of animals in learning such complex relations, we shall provide a detailed discussion below.

CORRELATION. One example of a logical relation is suggested by the notion of "contingency" or "correlation" between events. Note that the typical Pavlovian conditioning experiment arranges not only that the CS be followed by the US closely in time, but also that the US not occur frequently in the absence of the CS. Thus, not only are the events paired, they are also correlated in time in such a way that the CS provides information about the occurrence of the US.

Evidence that such logical relations play an important role in conditioning comes from conditioned-suppression experiments. In this situation subjects (typically rats) are first trained to perform some instrumental response, such as bar-pressing for food. They then receive Pavlovian conditioning relating certain signals to noxious USs, such as shock. The index of conditioning is the degree to which presentation of the signals modulates the performance of the instrumental response; excitatory, fear-eliciting CSs typically suppress the ongoing response. In one experiment using this situation, Rescorla (1968) presented rats with tones and shocks both randomly distributed in time, so that the probability of occurrence of the shock was equal in the presence or absence of the tone. (It is just this procedure, in which there is no CS-US correlation, that we have elsewhere argued provides an appropriate comparison for assessing the role of correlation as an operation producing behavioral change.) Subsequent testing with that tone showed that it produced little suppression of bar-pressing despite the previous exposure to a large number of close temporal pairings of tones with shock. However, when other groups received the same treatment but with the simple omission of those shocks programmed to occur in the absence of the CS, the tone developed substantial suppressive power. Notice that omitting those intertrial shocks introduces a logical-informational relation between the tone and shock while leaving the "pairings" the same.

There is now a large amount of subsequent research pointing to the importance of such correlations as determinants of conditioning (e.g., Benedict and Ayres, 1972; Dweck and Wagner, 1970; Rescorla, 1972). The greater the degree of the correlation, the more the conditioning. Note that this finding does not deny the importance of temporal relations; rather, it suggests an additional criterion which must be met for conditioning to occur. Loosely speaking, only those events occurring within a certain relatively narrow time band of the US which are also positively correlated with that event enter into the organism's determination of the "causal texture" of his environment. An animal is thus not easily misled by the occurrence of "accidental" contiguities that do not reflect true logical relations among environmental events.

RELATIONS INVOLVING MULTIPLE STIMULI. A great many other logical relations are introduced if we consider situations involving, not one, but multiple signals for S_1. A description of the effects of such relations can conveniently be presented within the framework of a recent theory of Pavlovian conditioning (Rescorla and Wagner, 1972) since that theory was explicitly formulated to deal with multiple-stimulus events. Although mathematical in form, we shall describe the theory only in casual terms here. The basic proposition is that the effectiveness of S_1

as a reinforcing event is not invariant, but depends upon the degree to which S_1 is "anticipated" or "signaled" by some other event. As in the theories of Hull (1943) or Bush and Mosteller (1955), a given US is viewed as being capable of establishing a maximum amount of "associative strength"; also as in those theories, the change in associative strength on a given trial depends upon the discrepancy between that maximum and the current strength of the stimuli being conditioned. However, the unique feature of the Rescorla-Wagner theory is that all stimuli present during a trial contribute to this discrepancy. That is, the amount of conditioning on a trial depends upon the discrepancy between the US's maximum and the accumulated current strength of *all* signals present on a trial. An anticipated US is modulated in effectiveness not only for the signal that provides the anticipation, but also for any other signal present; well-predicted USs are simply less effective reinforcers. This assumption enables the theory to describe the importance of various logical relations between CS and US.

One special feature of this theory is that it focuses on "associative strengths" rather than response probabilities. It makes explicit our earlier point that "conditioning" is a theoretical entity which has content only within the context of a theory.

The principal deduction from this model is that the amount of conditioning that occurs on a trial should depend upon the current strength of the stimuli present in the trial. The simplest application is to variations in the current strength of the target stimulus to which we measure the change in conditioning. It should be clear that, like the Bush-Mosteller model, this theory predicts a negatively accelerated acquisition curve for associative strength. Over trials as the CS becomes increasingly capable of predicting the US (i.e., as it gains associative strength), the US becomes increasingly less effective in augmenting the associative strength.

But the most interesting predictions are for cases in which the associative strength of one stimulus modulates the conditioning of other stimuli concurrently present. It is here that one sees the real power of the model to explicate the role of certain logical relations in conditioning. For instance, the model anticipates that if compound stimulus AX is being conditioned, the amount of conditioning to X should be affected by variations not only in the strength of X, but also in the associative strength of A. If A is especially strong at the time when AX receives reinforcement, then only a small discrepancy should result, and so X should gain little strength. That this occurs has been well documented in the "blocking" experiments of Kamin (1968, 1969). In the paradigmatic experiment, a group of rats was first given conditioned-suppression training in which A was followed by shock; subsequent addition of X

with continuation of the shock generated little conditioning to X. However, in groups without preconditioning to A, the AX-reinforced trials were quite adequate to establish conditioning to X. Despite the fact that X bore adequate temporal and correlational relations to the US in the experimental group, it was "blocked" from conditioning by the preconditioned A.

This kind of experiment illustrates the fact that conditioning depends not only upon the information that a signal provides about a US, but also upon the degree to which that information is new and not provided by other available stimuli. In other words, the organism may not attribute to the CS a causal relation with the US if he has already identified another causal agent. By describing the effective reinforcer as a discrepancy, the Rescorla-Wagner model points to a relatively simple mechanism for this sophisticated accomplishment.

Of course, alternative causal relations need not be established *prior* to the introduction of a signal in order to affect the amount of conditioning to that signal. Within the Rescorla-Wagner model, variations in the associative strength of A at the time of AX reinforcement may also be accomplished by some concurrent treatment of A. Two well-established conditioning results illustrate this point. The first is "overshadowing," in which comparison is made between the conditioning of one stimulus, X, when it is reinforced alone and when it is reinforced in conjunction with another neutral stimulus, A. The latter treatment generates less conditioning to X because A "overshadows" X. Speaking casually, A provides an alternative predictor for the US; more formally, within the Rescorla-Wagner model, over trials A too becomes conditioned and so contributes to the reduced discrepancy. A and X mutually block each other and so must share the associative strength.

A second example of the role of current information may be generated by a variation on the Kamin experiment. One may examine the effects of reinforcing AX when intermingled trials of A are treated in various ways. That is, instead of giving A associative strength by its prior history, we may give it value concurrently with the AX treatment. Two particular values are of interest. First, we may reinforce AX while not reinforcing A when it is presented alone. If we do that, X becomes well conditioned whereas A takes on little value; that is, we have eliminated A's overshadowing of X because X is now the only stimulus informative of shock. Second, we may reinforce both A and AX. This treatment makes X redundant and, as might intuitively be expected, eventually leads it to have little strength (Rescorla, 1972; Wagner, 1969b).

It is instructive to note that the Rescorla-Wagner model makes a somewhat intriguing prediction about such concurrent cases. Unlike the Kamin experiment, intermingling the A and AX trials means that the compound will sometimes be reinforced before A is fully conditioned; consequently, some conditioning of X should occur on early AX trials. However, as training proceeds, A will attain asymptotic strength due to the A-alone trials. An interesting thing then happens when an AX trial is presented: since A possesses the maximum strength the US will support and X also has strength, the total value of the compound is greater than this maximum. In the formal version of the model, such "overexpectations" generate negative discrepancies, and a loss of associative strength results. That this occurs has been documented by Rescorla (1970) and Wagner (1971). In the present context this means that X should lose strength. Eventually both A alone and the AX compound should approach the asymptote, forcing X to take on a zero value of associative strength. That is, the model correctly predicts that in this situation X should first gain strength and then lose it (Rescorla, 1972). Thus the model may not only make comprehensible the importance of logical relations, but may also provide an accurate trial-by-trial account of how they make contact with the organism.

This last account may be extended to include the CS-US correlational data previously reported. Although only one CS is explicitly presented, the situation contains background cues which can become conditioned. Rescorla and Wagner (1972) have illustrated how these background cues can convert such a situation into the kind of A/AX situation described above, and derive detailed parametric predictions which accord with the data. They also point out that the model then predicts some nonmonotonic acquisition functions, for which there is some evidence (Rescorla, 1972). Consequently, this model may also make understandable the importance of correlations without attributing to the organism the abilities of a statistician.[1]

Overall, these examples illustrate the sensitivity of the organism to a range of logical relations important in excitatory conditioning. It does seem to make sense to appeal to the intuition that an organism should be trying to decipher the causal relations among events in the world. The availability of a simple model that enables him to do this may make that intuition more palatable.

[1]This description also provides a good example of the distinction between the use of control groups to identify important relations and their use to identify theoretical terms such as association. The "truly random" control produces, according to the Rescorla-Wagner model, some initial conditioning followed by a return to zero associative strength. Consequently, within that theory it does not always provide an appropriate control for hypothetical processes of association. Yet it remains as a procedural control for identifying the role of CS-US correlations.

11.3.3 Inhibitory relations

All of the previously considered relations provide the animal with information that two stimuli "go together," i.e., are in some sense positively related in the environment. But it is reasonable to believe that the organism is also sensitive to relations in which stimuli do *not* go together, i.e., are negatively related. Just as Pavlovian conditioning might be the basis of the organism's discovery of causal relations in his environment, so it might provide information that certain events specifically preclude the occurrence of other events. This information is stored as various kinds of learned inhibition. Pavlov, of course, discussed such a conditioned-inhibition process at length, but it has only recently received extensive attention in America. We shall comment briefly on the definition and measurement of conditioned inhibition and then turn to the identification of those t_1 relations that produce it.

A conditioned inhibitor may be identified as a stimulus which through learning comes to control a tendency opposite to that of a conditioned excitor. Two aspects of this description should be emphasized. First, we are discussing learned inhibition, that is, inhibition dependent upon a particular set of t_1 experiences. Second, a conditioned inhibitor does not necessarily produce an overall decrement in behavior; rather, its consequence is to oppose the change otherwise observed in an excitor based upon the same US. For example, in the conditioned-suppression situation, conditioned excitation is reflected in a decrease in behavior; consequently, conditioned inhibition should oppose that and so produce an increase.

Unfortunately, the detection of this opposing tendency may be more difficult than the detection of excitation. For instance, in salivary conditioning, excitation is indexed by an increase in the probability of salivation following the CS. One would then expect the opposed inhibitory process to yield a decrease in that probability. However, the normal selection of signals that initially produce little salivation makes detection of any decrease impossible. It is therefore often difficult to differentiate between the absence of excitation and the presence of inhibition. Two assessment techniques have commonly been used to deal with this problem (Rescorla, 1969a). In the *summation test*, a suspected inhibitor is presented in conjunction with a known excitor. If the response to the compound is less than that which the excitor alone produces, then the stimulus is identified as an inhibitor. A *retardation test* involves using the suspected inhibitor as an S_2 in an operation known to produce excitatory conditioning. If acquisition of that S_2 is slowed relative to various control stimuli, it is identified as an inhibitor. Both to verify the presence of inhibition and to dis-

tinguish it from other processes, it may be necessary to employ several such assessment techniques for the same stimulus. However, it must be kept in mind that these techniques only assess the *presence* of inhibition and do not indicate whether that inhibition was acquired through a particular t_1 experience. That determination obviously involves other comparisons.

The question of most interest is what t_1 relations establish a stimulus as a conditioned inhibitor: What range of relations does the organism detect? The most obvious candidate, and the one advocated by Pavlov, is the pairing of a stimulus with nonreinforcement, that is, the simple occurrence of S_2 in the absence of S_1. However, the evidence indicates that simple presentation of a signal will not necessarily establish it as a conditioned inhibitor. We may consider two kinds of stimuli that can be subjected to such a treatment: neutral stimuli and previously trained stimuli. The repeated presentation of a novel stimulus constitutes the operation described in the previous section. We saw there that such a t_1 treatment does indeed make a stimulus more difficult to train in an excitatory t_2 test, thereby satisfying the retardation test. However, two additional results suggest that this "latent inhibition" is not the same as the conditioned inhibition described here. First, such a stimulus does not attenuate excitation in a summation test. Second, a repeatedly presented stimulus is retarded not only when subjected to excitatory conditioning, but also when subjected to treatments, described below, which are known to establish conditioned inhibition (Reiss and Wagner, 1972; Rescorla, 1971).

The second kind of stimulus for which repeated presentation has been described as establishing inhibition is a previously trained S_2. That is, extinction has been claimed to generate inhibition. There is no doubt that, after training, repeated nonreinforced presentation produces response decrement, but, even asymptotically, the procedure does not seem to yield a net conditioned inhibitor. Such an extinguished stimulus neither interferes with responding in a summation test nor is retarded in an acquisition test; indeed, reestablishment of excitation is often faster than initial training.

Relations that do generate inhibitors are suggested by the informational relations of the previous section. One suggestion is that a negative correlation between the CS and the US, in which the CS signals a time of reduced US likelihood, produces a conditioned inhibitor. A number of studies have indicated that this is so. For example, Rescorla (1969b) presented rats in a conditioned-suppression situation with tone CSs having different probabilities of shock in their absence; this generated different degrees of negative correlation between tone and shock. Subsequent summation and retardation tests of the tone stimuli found greater inhibition the more negative the correlation. Rescorla (1969a, b) has suggested that this negative correlation is a paradigmatic case for inhibition, from which many other cases may be generated.

Another set of informational relations producing inhibitors are specified by the Rescorla-Wagner model. In that model a conditioned inhibitor is described as a stimulus with negative associative strength to a US. The condition for the establishment of that negative strength is the occurrence of a negative discrepancy between the associative strength produced by a stimulus and that which the following US can maximally support. That is, associative strength of a stimulus is decremented whenever the presented US does not live up to what the stimulus led the organism to expect.

Several types of stimuli may be subjected to such negative discrepancies. The simplest example of a negative discrepancy occurs during extinction, when the signal produces considerable associative strength but is then followed by a US (nothing) which is capable of supporting a maximum of zero strength. Under these circumstances the associative strength of the signal will be decremented until it is in line with what the null event will support, i.e., until it is zero. But, in line with the available data, the model does not anticipate that the decremental process will proceed beyond zero, since at that point no discrepancy occurs.

More interesting cases of negative discrepancy occur with multiple stimuli. As in the case of reinforcement, the present model suggests that the concurrent presence of other stimuli will modulate the effects of nonreinforcement. For instance, if a previously trained stimulus, X, is nonreinforced in the presence of another stimulus, A, the associative strength of A will greatly affect the size of the decrements to X. If A is excitatory, then AX will generate a great negative discrepancy from the zero asymptote that the null event supports, and X should thus be especially decremented. Conversely, if A is inhibitory, then the AX compound will be less discrepant from zero, and little decrement should occur. Support for those predictions can be found in the experiments of Wagner (1969a) and Chorazyna (1962).

Likewise if the target stimulus, X, is a neutral stimulus, then its initially zero associative strength can be decremented in various amounts depending upon the current strength of any stimulus A in whose presence X is not reinforced. For instance, if AX is not reinforced while A alone is reinforced, the value of A will be high, thus resulting in substantial decrements to X on the nonreinforced trials. The initially neutral X will therefore develop a large negative associative strength. This paradigm will be recognized as the classical conditioned-inhibition procedure initially described by Pavlov. In it X, by countermanding the prediction of A, provides considerable information about the nonoccurrence of the US. Wagner and Rescorla (1972) indicate in detail how such other inhibitory paradigms as discrimination, inhibition of delay, and even the pairing of a signal with termination of the US, may be described within their model as special cases of this paradigm. Furthermore, by considering the presence of background cues to play the role of A, they argue that the negative-correlation paradigm can also be viewed as a special case.

Another feature of the Rescorla-Wagner model worth noting is that excitation and inhibition are not necessarily tied to reinforcement and nonreinforcement. Because it is the relationship between the US expected and that obtained that determines both the direction and magnitude of associative changes, one can arrange to separate inhibition from nonreinforcement. An example is given by Rescorla (1970) and Wagner (1971), who trained two stimuli, A and B, individually, to an asymptote with a given US. When these stimuli were presented together and followed by the same US, the consequences were decrements in the associative strengths of the elements and the compound. The two stimuli together led to "overexpectation" of the US, and reinforcement therefore yielded decrements.

These examples illustrate several important things about Pavlovian conditioning. First, the organism shows considerable subtlety in the kinds of relations about which he can learn. He learns not only when things go together but also when they are kept apart. Furthermore, he demands a high quality of evidence from the environment before he reaches these conclusions. Second, there does exist a model, which can be stated formally, that allows an integration of this learning. That model will undoubtedly prove inadequate eventually; but presently it provides a serviceable integration of the data. Furthermore, it suggests that a comparison process, evaluating US events in terms of current associative strengths, is central to the modification of Pavlovian behavior. Any search for the mechanism of Pavlovian reinforcement might well attend to this feature of the available behavioral data and seek neutral events that are not invariant but reflect such a comparison process.

11.3.4 The nature of S_1

Although all of the above relations may be arranged between a CS and almost any S_1, we should anticipate that the selection of S_1 is not irrelevant to the details of the behavioral change observed. At the most obvious level, selection of S_1 determines which response systems will normally be involved and guides the experimenter in his choice of responses to observe. At a more detailed level, variations in the parameter values of S_1 will produce variations in the level of conditioning observed. For instance, it is well documented that more intense, longer-lasting USs produce more substantial changes in the response to the CS (Gormezano, Moore, and Deaux, 1962; Sheafor and Gormezano, 1972). In the next section we shall discuss a broader claim that our choice of S_1 may not only affect the magnitude of conditioning, but actually encourage different learning processes.

One historically interesting question is whether an event must be "biologically significant"—i.e., identifiable as a "positive" or "negative" instrumental reinforcer (see below)—if it is to enter into learned relations as S_1. Or could S_1 be a neutral stimulus, by which is normally meant an event both without affective value and without ability to evoke a reflex?

The normal response-evocation measure of conditioning does not usually reveal evidence of a change in a response to S_2 when it is presented in a positive relation to a neutral S_1; however, psychologists have often attributed this failure to the assessment technique rather than to the learning. Consequently, the "sensory-preconditioning" paradigm (e.g., Brogden, 1939) has been developed to provide evidence for such learning. In this paradigm S_2 and S_1 are first presented in some relation. Then the neutral S_1 is modified, normally by pairing it with an effective Pavlovian US. Finally, S_2 is tested with the idea that any previously learned relation between S_2 and S_1 might now be revealed in differential S_2-evoked behavior. There is now a substantial literature on such paradigms, with a sufficient range of behaviors and control conditions to permit the conclusion that organisms do learn relations among "neutral" events. However, in line with the other data on S_1 potency, such effects are relatively small. Although some authors have attempted to characterize the results of such experiments as revealing a learning process which is qualitatively different from that of other Pavlovian preparations, the evidence for such a claim is sparse and remains unconvincing. In the absence of such evidence it seems prudent to continue viewing the learning about relations between neutral events as similar to the learning about relations between biologically significant ones.

A final issue raised by considerations of the S_1 event concerns which aspects of that event actually enter into the relations learned. Stimulus events are not unitary, but actually possess a variety of aspects or properties, any subset of which may enter into learned relations. Historically, psychologists working with conditioning have acknowledged only two major aspects of the S_1 event: stimulus and response aspects. The question of which aspects enter into learned relations has then taken the form of whether conditioning is S-S or S-R in nature. Although once the focus of lively controversy, the issue as stated in this form has been all but ignored recently.

However, a recent series of experiments in our laboratory seem to reopen that issue (Rescorla, 1973, 1974). In a conditioned-suppression situation we have attempted to modify the value of the US *after* conditioning is complete. Such postconditioning variation in the US value produces variation in the CR that the CS can subsequently evoke. This may be interpreted as indicating that some representation of the US is involved in the learned relation, and consequently as supporting an S-S view; however, parallel experiments within a Pavlovian second-order conditioning paradigm have suggested that response properties may also enter into relations (S-R learning). In this case postconditioning modification in the power of either the US or the first-order CS leaves second-order conditioning untouched (Rescorla, 1973). Thus some authors have suggested that the organism uses both stimulus and response properties of events in learning relations.

It may, however, be a historical anachronism to acknowledge only stimulus and response aspects of events. More generally, perhaps we should recognize that events have multiple properties about which organisms can learn. Presumably, much of that learning takes place simply as a result of presentation of these events, as suggested in an earlier section of this paper. But it may also be wise to consider the possibility that the organism makes use of a wide variety of these properties of events in learning about environmental relations.

11.3.5 Other relations among stimuli

We have characterized Pavlovian conditioning as the learning about relations among stimuli in the environment. In practice, however, the study of conditioning has explored only a highly restricted range of such relations. It seems likely that the organism is sensitive to many other so far uninvestigated relations; we mention here two that seem particularly good candidates.

SPATIAL RELATIONS The first is only a small step from those relations already mentioned: relations in space. Most of the previously discussed relations can be defined in terms of temporal features, but it seems equally plausible that the organism learns about relations among events in space. Certainly if we are to view Pavlovian conditioning as providing the animal with information about the causal texture of his environment, localization in space is an important aspect of that texture. Indeed, most discussions of the impression of causality involve reference to both space and time.

Perhaps it is the traditional choice of Pavlovian preparations and the stimuli employed in such preparations that has discouraged the investigation of learning about spatial relations. In many such preparations the stimuli are diffuse and without definite spatial localization; in others the decision to use reflex-eliciting events has constrained the choice of stimuli so as to make investigation of variation in spatial location difficult. Recent evidence that second-order conditioning is often a powerful phenomenon may remove such barriers, however. That procedure would permit the experimenter to select stimuli arbitrarily, with any spatial features he wishes, and to endow them with the power to serve as Pavlovian reinforcers.

There have been occasional suggestions that spatial features of stimuli interact with temporal Pavlovian relations (e.g., Köhler, 1947), but by and large the investigation of learning about space has been confined to instrumental preparations such as the maze. From the viewpoint of this paper, however, it seems reasonable to suggest that the learning about spatial relations among events in the environment be brought within the Pavlovian laboratory. Most of the questions that have historically been discussed in terms of temporal relations also apply to spatial relations. For instance, not only may we ask whether an organism can learn that two events occur in the same spatial locus, we can also study that learning as a function of physical proximity. We may also ask whether the organism can learn that two events always occur at separate points in the environment but never near each other. Such questions may be asked about events that are temporally uncorrelated (just as temporal questions have been asked largely without reference to spatial features of events), or they may be applied to events that have some fixed temporal relation. In the end it may turn out that spatial relations will be incorporated into a more global temporal framework by, for instance, demonstrating that contiguity in space works only because it is mediated by contiguity in time. Whether or not one thinks such a reduction is plausible, it is clear that we have badly neglected even the initial study of such relations.

INTRINSIC RELATIONS. A second kind of neglected relation requires more extensive comment. The relations among stimuli that we have so far discussed all share one feature: they can be arranged independently of the nature of the stimuli involved. For instance, one can abstractly describe the arrangement of temporal contiguity or contingency among stimuli without reference to the properties of those stimuli. This restriction to what might be called "extrinsic" relations agrees with the modern emphasis in the psychology of learning in which the actual stimuli fitting into a relation are viewed as arbitrary, to be selected for the convenience of the investigator.

But the characterization of Pavlovian conditioning given at the beginning of this section applies equally well to other relations whose arrangement *does* depend upon the nature of the items involved. These relations we shall term "intrinsic." Within the present framework, the exposure to *any* relation among items is of interest if it can be shown to be responsible for differential behavior at t_2. For instance, we can expose a subject at t_1 to two stimuli related by similarity; if we can then demonstrate that this exposure changes the behavior observed at t_2, as compared with that of a group not exposed to this relation, then we have produced the kind of change from which one might infer learning.

Traditionally, psychologists have taken extrinsic relations, such as contiguity, as primary and have attempted to investigate them independently of the properties of the individual events or the intrinsic relations among those events. However, one could just as readily ask whether exposure to intrinsic relations, such as similarity, produces a change independently of any particular extrinsic relation.

We have avoided the investigation of exposure to such intrinsic relations as similarity, membership in the same sensory system, or participation in the same organized response system, for several reasons. First, there is the suspicion that any changes observed might be attributable to presentation of the individual events, rather than to their relation. In that case the outcomes would be examples of the kinds of changes discussed earlier, and would not in any important way involve exposure to a relation. (Of course, experimental procedures could easily be devised to evaluate this possibility.) Second, intrinsic relations involve the structure of the organism; consequently, they take some power of experimental manipulation away from the investigator. The very nature of extrinsic relations is that the choice of events to be related is entirely at the disposal of the investigator. This has the value of permitting experimental arrangements which make implausible a variety of alternative accounts of the experimental outcomes in terms of innate features of the organism. With intrinsic relations, the properties of the events themselves constrain the relation, so that these alternatives may seem more viable and the assertion about learning less secure.

Perhaps for these reasons, there have been few recent experimental investigations with animals of the effects of exposure to intrinsic relations. Despite their inclusion in historical lists of conditions responsible for associations, such relations as similarity and resemblance have been largely neglected by modern investigators.

INTERACTION OF INTRINSIC WITH EXTRINSIC RELATIONS. There have appeared several lines of argument suggesting that intrinsic relations may *interact* with the standard extrinsic relations and thereby modulate their effectiveness. For instance, Razran (1957) argued that the relation between CS and US intensities modulates the results of arranging a CS-US contiguity; in addition to the separate effects of CS and US intensity, their ratio was argued to be important. Although Kamin (1965) found no evidence for this, his paper gave an early suggestion of such an interaction.

More recent and powerful evidence for interaction between intrinsic and extrinsic relations has come out of the "toxicosis" literature. In this procedure a Pavlovian paradigm is used in which the unconditioned stimulus, such as x radiation or poisoning, is capable of inducing illness. An early sample of such a procedure is the following experiment by Garcia (Garcia and Koelling, 1966), who has been largely responsible for popularizing the technique. Rats were first trained to lick at tubes for water, with each lick producing both a distinctive taste and the occurrence of an auditory-visual stimulus. After this exposure the rats were subjected to either x radiation or electric footshock. Subsequently they were permitted to drink under conditions such that each lick produced either the taste or the auditory-visual stimulus. The degree to which licking was suppressed was taken as an index of the conditioning to each stimulus. The finding of interest is that when shock was used, the most conditioning was shown by the auditory-visual stimulus, while when x-rays were used, the taste stimulus acquired more conditioning than did the auditory-visual stimulus.

This kind of result suggests that when an extrinsic relation (contiguity) is arranged between two stimuli, the behavioral change produced also depends upon the intrinsic relation between the stimuli. To predict the outcome it is insufficient to know the temporal contiguity or even separately what CS or what US was employed. Instead, the CS and US selections seem to interact so as to modulate the effects of their contiguity. One way to describe this is to note that the relative conditionability of a given CS depends upon the US employed. We are, of course, accustomed to the idea that different CSs have different saliences and different USs have different potencies. What is new here is that these apparently interact, so that relative CS saliences depend upon what US is employed. It is not just the properties of events but the relations of these properties that seem to be important.[2]

This result has led to a great deal of empirical work and theoretical controversy, most of which we shall not discuss. However, three issues should be mentioned in this context.

(1) First, a continuing concern has been whether the effects so observed are examples of "associative" learning or represent some "nonassociative" effects. Although this is ultimately a theoretical issue, attempts to answer it atheoretically employ a familiar experimental paradigm. Commonly, the extrinsic relation of pairing is selected, and one asks whether intrinsically related stimuli facilitate the behavior resulting from their pairing but fail to have a similar facilitative effect when no pairing relation is arranged. That is, does the intrinsic relation in fact interact with those extrinsic relations normally explored in conditioning? If so, it is deemed "associative"; if it has equivalent effects whether or not pairing is arranged, it is termed "nonassociative."

Two points should be made about this conclusion. First, it emphasizes the point that students of conditioning have made a major commitment to extrinsic relations. So committed are we to their primacy that we insist that only those intrinsic relations that interact with them are of interest. Our initial reaction to the revelation of any general effect of exposure to intrinsically related stimuli is to relegate the finding to "pseudo-conditioning." It is worth commenting that even if "association" were to be restricted to the learning of a small set of temporally defined relations, this would not preclude the possibility that exposure to other kinds of relations modifies the organism.

The second point is more technical: it turns out to require considerable experimental effort to demonstrate that intrinsic relations have effects that are confined to particular extrinsic-relation arrangements. Without detailing all of the logic, it is worth noting that many alternative interpretations can be avoided if the following two kinds of trials are both presented to the same organism: $A_1 B_1 \rightarrow US_1$ and $A_2 B_2 \rightarrow US_2$ (with appropriate counterbalancing in other groups). Here A_1 and A_2 share some intrinsic relation to US_1, whereas B_1 and B_2 share one with US_2. If, say, A_1 becomes more conditioned than B_1 whereas B_2 becomes more conditioned than A_2, then it seems reasonable to argue that the A dimension is especially associable with US_1 whereas B

—————————————

[2]This question is normally asked about positive correlations, but we could equally well ask whether it is especially easy to learn that two events are negatively correlated if they also bear some intrinsic relation such as similarity.

is especially associable with US_2. Because the same animal receives all six individual events, it is not easy to attribute such a pattern either to the exposure to the individual events or even to the simple exposure to any intrinsic relations per se. Thus interpretations in terms of "pseudoconditioning," or "sensitization," or differences in the potency of individual events, are made less plausible. But since A_1 becomes stronger than B_1 whereas the reverse is true of A_2 and B_2, the ordering of conditionability varies with the contiguous US, thus suggesting an interaction between intrinsic and extrinsic relations. Whether there is also a pure effect of the intrinsic relation cannot be answered from this design.

A number of experiments approximate this design, but none admit of unambiguous interpretation. For instance, Garcia and his colleagues (1968) used a discriminative conditioning paradigm consisting of two kinds of trials: $A_1B_1 \rightarrow US$ and $A_2B_2 \rightarrow 0$. For different groups the US was shock or x radiation. With one US, A_1 was more conditioned, while for the other B_1 showed more suppression. Although the response to A_2 and B_2 in this procedure provides evidence on the possibility of differential sensitization to the A and B dimensions, it leaves open other possibilities. For instance, the occurrence of a given US might affect which CS dimensions are particularly attended to on subsequent trials; e.g., animals who have been poisoned earlier may pay special attention to taste stimuli. Then any US presented on subsequent trials will give more conditioning to the taste stimuli. Although such an effect would be of interest, it would not represent the kind of special associability normally claimed for such preparations.

Related to the issue of whether such effects are "associative" is the possibility that they do not intimately involve learning at all. In these, as in most other learning experiments, it is common to employ only one assessment technique to measure the consequences of arranging the CS-US relation: the degree to which the CS evokes differential behavior. But any single assessment procedure may inadequately reflect the amount of learning because of the operation of a variety of other determinants of performance. Thus it is not impossible that CSs differ not in their associability with USs, but in their ability to evoke behavior based upon equal associations. If other assessment procedures were employed, perhaps considerable learning would be revealed to all CSs. For example, a CS declared nonconditioned by an evocation measure might reveal considerable learning if used to establish conditioning to another CS in a second-order conditioning paradigm. An outcome of just this sort has been observed in activity conditioning (Holland and Rescorla, 1975). Again, although interesting, such a

process has quite different implications for the interaction of intrinsic and extrinsic relations.

Thus a number of alternatives remain to be ruled out before we can conclude that intrinsic relations have their effects upon responding by interaction with extrinsic ones. It is to be hoped that future experiments will provide evidence on these alternative accounts since the question has been viewed as so important to theories of learning.

(2) A second, related issue is whether even such demonstrations of the effects of intrinsic relations might not eventually be reduced to the operation of known extrinsic parameters. The attempt to resolve this question has involved two experimental approaches. One approach seeks to uncover particular confounded extrinsic relations which might make appeal to intrinsic relations unnecessary. The other explores whether the operation of such extrinsic relations as contiguity are importantly modified by the presence of intrinsic relations. That is, are the laws of extrinsic relations the same when intrinsic relations are introduced and when they are absent; if not, then reduction of intrinsic to extrinsic relations would seem unlikely.

The first approach is well exemplified by a recent experiment of Krane and Wagner (1975). They noted that the USs most commonly employed in such studies, shock and stimulus-produced illness, may have quite different onset and duration patterns. The former is abrupt, usually brief, and typically administered immediately after the CS, whereas the latter is gradual in onset, of extended duration, and often delayed in its administration. Furthermore, the most investigated CSs in such experiments, taste and auditory-visual stimuli, may also have different durations and onset properties; the former may be functionally effective much longer than the latter. Thus, when a taste/external-stimulus compound is followed by shock or illness, the combinations of CSs and USs may differ in their effective temporal relations as well as in intrinsic relations. For instance, if the taste stimulus is effective for extended periods, then a brief shock administered early in that stimulus may leave most of the stimulus yet to occur (i.e., permit extinction) whereas an extended illness, whose onset is later, may have an effectively more favorable CS-US temporal relation. Krane and Wagner found evidence for this particular case by showing, with a taste CS, that delaying the onset of the shock actually increased the amount of conditioning that pairing produced. More generally, however, the point is that stimuli which have different intrinsic properties may also differ in traditionally studied parameters, the effects of which are well explored. Although such effects can often be subtle and difficult to detect, they may be responsible for much of the effect normally reported. If so, the need to appeal to intrinsic effects may not be so urgent on the basis of presently available evidence.

The second approach suggests that intrinsic relations should be viewed in the same framework as extrinsic ones. This approach attempts to demonstrate that effects known to occur in the absence of strong intrinsic relations also occur in their presence. Thus many of the variables we discussed earlier still have profound effects in those situations normally taken as subject to the operation of intrinsic relations. For instance, toxicosis conditioning has been found to display such phenomena as monotonic acquisition, extinction, blocking, overshadowing, latent inhibition, and conditioned inhibition (see Revusky, 1971). The one variable that has appeared to be outstanding is the temporal contiguity needed for conditioning. With toxicosis, delays between CS and US of many minutes, even hours, have proven to yield conditioning. Some authors have claimed that this is way outside the range to be anticipated on the basis of other forms of conditioning and thus should be taken as an indication of a fundamentally different learning process. Such authors overlook the variability in effective CS-US intervals within the traditionally studied conditioning paradigms. For instance, eyelid conditioning is difficult to obtain with intervals over a few seconds, but intervals of 5–10 minutes are easily successful with salivary or fear conditioning. Yet this difference in parameter values, which is fully as large as that between toxicosis and fear conditioning, has not been taken as an indication of fundamentally different learning processes. This is because there is a similarity in the *form* of the laws governing these types of conditioning. Even for the variable of CS-US interval, these situations all share a function in which conditioning first improves and then degenerates as the delay between CS onset and US onset increases. The available information on toxicosis is of the same type: conditioning is best with short delays between CS and US onsets but increasingly deteriorates as the time between onsets increases (e.g., Kalat and Rozin, 1971). Thus the present data do not support the conclusion that fundamentally different types of modification processes are at work.

(3) The third issue is that of the implications such findings on intrinsic relations might have for traditional theories of learning processes. Assuming that intrinsic relations could be shown to interact with traditional extrinsic relations, some authors have drawn Chicken Little-like conclusions, claiming severe limitations upon the generality of the phenomena of conditioning observed in other preparations. In light of the previous discussion, this may be a little overhasty. It seems unlikely that investigations of intrinsic relations will cause us to abandon the body of knowledge already built up using arbitrary stimulus events. It is, of course, entirely likely that future theories of conditioning will need to concede a role to such relations as they interact with traditionally studied variables; but such a concession may take the form of a simple addition to the list of variables known to affect conditioning.

On the other hand, the lasting impact of such studies may be more substantial and healthy. They may encourage us to realize that our study of conditioning has been restricted to a woefully small and inadequate range of relations among events. Certainly if we want to consider conditioning as a model situation in which we may explore how organisms learn interevent relations then we need to expand greatly the kinds of relations studied. Instead of insisting that intrinsic relations affect the operation of extrinsic ones in situations designed to study the latter, perhaps we should turn to the study of the alternative relations themselves.

11.3.6 Conditioning preparations

Some comments should be made about the preparations currently employed in the study of Pavlovian conditioning. Much of the previous discussion has used two relatively new techniques: conditioned suppression and toxicosis. In terms of sheer numbers these two techniques probably account for the bulk of current work with Pavlovian procedures. Indeed, their ease of use and ready accessibility to experimenters without special skills has been partly responsible for a resurgence of interest in the field of Pavlovian conditioning. By contrast, the traditional salivary preparation is slow in producing data and time-consuming to set up; consequently, this preparation accounts for only a small percentage of current experiments. However, it should be acknowledged that many other Pavlovian preparations are available, some of which are actively in use. The most obvious are like the suppression and toxicosis techniques in employing aversive USs: cardiac, eyeblink, and paw-flexion conditioning. Eyeblink conditioning in particular has produced a steady stream of data in American laboratories. More recently, two techniques that employ appetitive USs have been explored: jaw movement in the rabbit (e.g., Gormezano, 1972) and activity in the rat (e.g., Holland and Rescorla, 1975; Sheffield and Campbell, 1954). One final appetitive situation should also be mentioned, namely, "autoshaping." Recent evidence indicates that simply presenting in sequence a key light followed by access to grain leads pigeons to peck the key (Brown and Jenkins, 1968). This autoshaping procedure is of special interest because it demonstrates the control of one of the standard operant responses by a Pavlovian procedure.

Some of the techniques mentioned here, particularly the two we have emphasized, have met with resistance from some students of learning. It has been suggested on a number of grounds that they are not really examples of Pavlovian conditioning. This skepticism seems to stem from two sources. First, conditioned suppression and toxicosis do not comply with all of the ancillary requirements that some authors have introduced into the definition of conditioning. For instance, it may be difficult to identify the unconditioned response and even more difficult to argue that the conditioned response is similar to it. Our own position on this issue has already been stated: the meaningful imposition of such requirements depends upon commitment to a detailed theory, which unfortunately is not available.

Second, some authors feel that conditioned suppression and toxicosis are less direct than the indices of conditioning available in salivary or leg-flexion preparations. This feeling seems to have two sources: (1) both of these preparations involve the modulation of ongoing behavior, not the elicitation of a discrete response; (2) the behavior modulated is not reflex behavior, but instrumental behavior that has been explicitly trained by the experimenter. In our opinion these differences from other preparations are a matter of degree only; furthermore, the differences are not always to the disadvantage of the conditioned-suppression and toxicosis situations. In any experiment we must monitor behavioral change in an organism exhibiting ongoing behavior. No matter how artificially the investigator describes his data, concentrating on the trial periods and de-emphasizing the time between trials, the fact remains that the organism is continually behaving and the investigator is only modulating that behavior. Nor is it necessarily an advantage to select preparations in which the particular response being measured has an especially low probability in the absence of trial stimulation. Such situations may only result in low sensitivity in our ability to detect learning during its early stages. Indeed, a great deal may be happening prior to the first trial on which the experimenter is able to detect a change. Furthermore, response systems with zero base rates preclude a whole range of otherwise possible behavioral changes. The inability to measure initial decrements in behavior in such preparations makes especially difficult the study of inhibitory conditioning.

With regard to the claim that the modified behavior is actually instrumental in character, we feel even less defensive. Again, the expectation that one should measure reflex behavior is partly based upon pretheoretical conceptions. More importantly, as we shall argue in the next section, one of the important aspects of Pavlovian conditioning is precisely that it affects instrumental activity. From a psychological point of view, conditioning is important not only as a model of association, but also as a process that apparently has important motivational and emotional consequences for other behaviors. If conditioning were confined to what some have called "spit and twitches," it would lose much of its psychological interest. For this reason one may argue that it is precisely in the modulation of instrumental behavior that the most relevant studies of Pavlovian conditioning take place.

In the end, of course, the acceptance of particular techniques depends upon their usefulness for the study of particular problems. The track record of conditioned suppression and toxicosis for the study of sensitivity to relations among environmental events seems clearly to recommend their further use.

To summarize, then, in this section we have argued that Pavlovian conditioning should be viewed as the learning about relations among events. Furthermore, we have suggested that both temporal and informational relations are learned by our experimental organisms, which show surprising sophistication in their sensitivity to the detailed arrangement of events in the world. We have reviewed a theory of conditioning intended to explicate a way in which organisms can achieve such a level of sophistication. We have further argued that psychologists have restricted their study of the learning of relations to an artificially small set. The role of other, intrinsic relations among events forms an area that deserves extensive additional exploration. The sophistication of organisms in learning the relations already studied should encourage us in that exploration.

11.4 INSTRUMENTAL TRAINING

The final category of learning situations that have been studied by American psychologists is instrumental training or operant conditioning. We shall only provide a brief discussion of this set of procedures, for two reasons. First, this is historically the most studied of the learning procedures, and consequently the literature is vast, much too vast to permit even quick review here. Second, because of the complexity of the event relations with which an organism is presented in an instrumental-training procedure, they are probably the least useful for biological analysis. Although instrumental-learning procedures often provide fast and reliable behavior modifications, they contain within them both of the previously discussed procedures. Consequently, correlations with biological substrates necessitate constant dissection of the procedure to pinpoint the aspect responsible for a given biological change.

Instrumental-training procedures are all characterized by the arrangement of a relation between the organism's response and some event S_1. As in the case of Pavlovian conditioning, these situations may be separated along three dimensions: the nature of S_1, the relation between S_1 and the response, and the technique used to measure the resultant behavioral modification.

In this context, S_1 events are typically segregated into three classes: positive, negative, and neutral stimuli. This segregation is entirely circular since, typically, the impact of a stimulus upon preceding instrumental responses is what is used to make an assignment to one class or another. Most commonly, if S_1 increases the probability of a response that produces it, it is termed positive; if it decreases it, it is termed negative; if it leaves it unaffected, it is neutral. Historically, considerable experimental effort has been expended in an effort to find some property other than this response change that might characterize all positive reinforcers. Although this effort has largely been abandoned by psychologists, it has left a tradition in which learning theories designed to account for the effects of positive events are different from those intended to account for the effects of negative ones. Situations in which responses produce negative S_1s are often used in physiological studies of learning because of their rapid and powerful effects.

The second major dimension along which instrumental situations may be classified is the nature of the relation between the response and the reinforcement. Typically, two types of relations are employed: positive and negative correlations. With positive relations, the use of a positive S_1 results in response increases (reward) whereas the use of a negative S_1 results in decreases (punishment). Similarly, with negative response-S_1 relations, a positive S_1 results in response depressions (omission training) whereas a negative S_1 results in response increases (escape-avoidance). The theories for the learning of different kinds of relations have been no more uniform than have the theories for dealing with different kinds of S_1s.

Measures of the behavioral modification resulting from arranging the response-S_1 relations are more uniform in instrumental training than in the previous procedures. The almost universally measured behavioral change is variation in the occurrence of the response upon which S_1 is contingent. Various detailed measures, such as probability, latency, vigor, etc., are employed. Despite their logically equal status, learning is rarely assessed by measuring changes in nonreinforced responses. But if, when a relation has been arranged between R_1 and S_1, some feature of another response, R_2, changes, this is

evidence for the learning of the R_1-S_1 relation, even if there is no detectable change in R_1 itself. As in the case of Pavlovian conditioning, additional, possibly irrelevant, constraints have been placed on the measures used to assess the effectiveness of t_1 procedures. It may turn out to be informative to examine in detail responses other than the one being reinforced. For example, the failure of a response to change when a particular reinforcer is used may not indicate total insensitivity to the relation arranged if changes in other responses are observed.

Instead of pursuing in any detail specific examples of the kinds of learning produced by permuting these different dimensions, we shall make only a few general comments on three issues of current interest in instrumental training: the role of Pavlovian relations in instrumental learning; the issue of the optimum level of discourse for physiological comparison; and the consequences of intrinsic relations between responses and reinforcers.

11.4.1 The role of Pavlovian relations in instrumental learning

It is a common statement that any instrumental-learning situation has embedded within it the kinds of relations normally arranged in a Pavlovian experiment. Whenever we administer an S_1 contingent upon a prior response, we do so in the context of other external stimuli; this is especially obvious when we employ an external signal to indicate the appropriate time for the performance of the response. Furthermore, virtually all responses have either peripheral or central feedback to which the animal is sensitive. Either the external stimulus or the feedback stimulus can be thought of as a Pavlovian CS bearing a particular relation to the instrumental reinforcer S_1. Although the fact that the animal makes the response is partly responsible for the arrangement, nevertheless it remains true that there is arranged a Pavlovian relation between those stimuli and S_1.

This observation has resulted in two important issues for the analysis of instrumental behavior. One issue is experimental: How can one parcel out the contributions of the Pavlovian relation so as to expose the pure consequences of the relation arranged between response and stimulus? The other is more theoretical: What is the contribution of this normally embedded Pavlovian relation for the learning and performance of instrumental activities?

In principle the first question is easily answered. One would like to arrange an instrumental-learning situation in which, although the relation between response and S_1 is varied systematically, the features of the individual events, as well as the relations between S_1 and various stimuli, are kept constant. Any behavioral variation could then be identified as resulting from the response-S_1 relation. In practice this turns out to be a virtually impossible assignment.

The most sophisticated attempt has been the yoked-control procedure, which is clearly directed at separating out the Pavlovian relation. Consider a case in which we signal to the animal the availability of food upon bar-pressing and discover a rate increase during that regime. One might inquire whether the response-food relation is responsible for the increase or whether it is ascribable simply to the occurrence of food, or to that pairing of the signal with food which results from early "random" bar-presses. To assess this possibility one might run a yoked animal assigned to each instrumentally trained animal. The yoked animal would receive all of the same stimulus events: signal, food, etc., as the experimental animal, but his response would be irrelevant to the occurrence of food; rather, when the experimental animal made his response, both animals would receive food. Thus the two animals would be matched for the number of stimulus events, their distribution over time, and even their relationships; any resulting differences must be ascribed to the instrumental relation between response and reinforcer arranged for the experimental animal.

Although this is a serviceable procedure, it is not without its flaws. First, Church (1964) has provided an insightful discussion of ways in which the use of such a procedure could lead to logically wrong conclusions. In brief, he points out that the design confounds various sources of random error (including individual differences) with treatment effects, so that the results are necessarily ambiguous. For specific examples of difficulties that arise, we refer the reader to Church's article. Second, note that only some of the stimulus relations are actually matched in the two animals. There is no matching of the relation of the response-feedback stimuli to the reinforcer. Third, and most important, we must keep in mind that this is only a *procedural* control. While it might help us decide whether the instrumental response-reinforcer relation is critical for a certain kind of behavioral change, it does not necessarily single out the occurrence of "instrumental learning." As in Pavlovian conditioning, we need to distinguish between controls for procedures and controls for theoretical variables such as "instrumental learning."

The second consequence of acknowledging the embedding of Pavlovian procedures in instrumental-learning situations has proven to be more fruitful. Several authors have noted that this embedding produces Pavlovian conditioning of motivational and emotional tendencies (e.g., Rescorla and Solomon, 1967; Trapold and Overmier, 1972). Several important theoretical frameworks have emerged which acknowledge the role of underlying Pavlovian motivational conditioning in producing instrumental behavior.

This trend is particularly obvious in the case of avoidance learning. In a typical avoidance-learning situation a signal warns that a shock will occur if an instrumental response is not made. The regular sequence of that signal followed by shock on the early trials is argued to result in the conditioning of an emotional response, fear, to the signal. This fear is then described as having both response-activating properties when it increases and response-reinforcing properties when it decreases. This kind of two-process theory has been by far the most popular account of avoidance learning. It is capable of providing a detailed description not only of the acquisition of avoidance, but also of its special properties during extinction. There have been, however, a number of recent challenges to the adequacy of such a theory (Bolles, 1970; D'Amato, Fazzaro, and Etkin, 1970; Herrnstein, 1969; Seligman and Johnston, 1973). Without describing such challenges in detail, it is fair to make two comments about them. First, to a large extent they leave unchallenged the assertion that Pavlovian motivational conditioning occurs within the instrumental context; instead, they question the completeness of that process in accounting for the avoidance behavior. Second, in some cases the attacks upon the two-process account result from an insufficient appreciation of the complexity of Pavlovian conditioning. We described in Section 11.3 the sophisticated information an organism is capable of learning about Pavlovian relations; when that description replaces the rather dated account of Pavlovian conditioning with which many psychologists are familiar, considerable power is added to the two-process approach.

Of course, reward situations also arrange the conditions for Pavlovian motivational conditioning. Such "incentive" motivation has been incorporated into many recent accounts of appetitively maintained instrumental activity. Precursors to such an approach can be found in Tolman's notion of expectancy and in the Spence-Hull r_g-s_g mechanism. Much current theorizing reveals the elaborateness of the contribution of such theoretical Pavlovian mechanisms to instrumental behavior. Unfortunately, it remains true that modern information about the Pavlovian conditioning process is rarely fully incorporated into such theorizing.

Particularly in the case of appetitive reinforcers, it has been argued that the sole function of the relation arranged between response and reinforcer is to provide the occasion for a particular sort of Pavlovian conditioning. For instance, Sheffield (1966) argues that the instrumental situation is simply a case of Pavlovian conditioning of anticipatory consummatory activity to feedback from instrumental responses, due to the regular following of such feedback by the reward (food). That conditioning then allows response feedback to operate in a positive feedback manner to guide cybernetically the performance of instrumental activity. Similar notions have been suggested by Miller (1963) and by Mowrer (1960). These ideas have proven difficult to evaluate because of the close tie between responses and their feedback; however, a series of experiments by Taub and his associates (e.g., Knapp, Taub, and Berman, 1958) suggest that the feedback at issue cannot be peripheral in character.

In any case, it has become increasingly popular to acknowledge within theories of instrumental behavior the possible role of Pavlovian conditioning of motivational and emotional processes. One implication of this is that attempts to uncover the biological basis of learning might well avoid the instrumental situation. If one is seeking the neurological events related to learning, it would be best to employ a learning situation in which the fewest kinds of relations can be responsible for the behavioral change.

11.4.2 Level of behavioral discourse

A second issue raised by the instrumental-learning literature concerns the level of discourse appropriate for seeking correspondence with physiological data. This is a general issue which of course extends well beyond the case of instrumental training but it is particularly well illustrated in this context. It is commonly assumed that the more detailed the analysis behavioral psychologists can provide, the better will be the climate for investigation of the biological basis of learning. For instance, it would seem to favor biological attempts to understand the response-reinforcement relation if we could provide precise temporal data describing the individual events and their relations necessary to produce certain behavioral outcomes. Certainly the attempt to analyze behavior at an ever more molecular level seems an integral part of the entire enterprise of understanding how learning occurs and affects behavior. And, historically, this is an approach that has produced many positive accomplishments.

However, some authors have suggested that there are instances in which readily reproducible global descriptions of learned behavior have resisted such analysis. For instance, within the operant-conditioning tradition, investigations of choice behavior have generated the "matching law" (see, e.g., Herrnstein, 1970). Over a wide variety of conditions, if an organism is given a choice of two responses to make but is reinforced at different rates for his efforts, he will match his relative rate of responding to the relative rate of reinforcement. The

resulting mathematical function has been investigated over such a wide variety of conditions that it has come to be viewed as one of the fundamental facts of operant behavior; indeed, much of what is known in the instrumental literature could be redescribed in terms of that function. Furthermore, it permits precise quantitative description, the parameters of which suggest important roles for various psychological variables. Thus, when behavior is viewed in this molar fashion, summarizing over relatively large chunks of time, highly regular and reproducible laws result. Yet this situation has repeatedly resisted analysis in terms of the more molecular moment-to-moment events that produce the molar function. Attempts to uncover the individual temporal and sequential relations that generate this performance have proven uniformly unsuccessful. Herrnstein (1969) has argued that there is a similar problem in the analysis of avoidance learning. There, too, macroscopically regular behavior does not arise from any identified regularity of molecular events.

One may argue, of course, that the search has simply been insufficiently thorough. And, indeed, despite some claims to the contrary, most of us believe that more detailed descriptions will eventually prove possible. But that is not the issue. Rather, the point is that in seeking biological underpinnings for learning, it may prove fruitful in some cases to look for mechanisms corresponding to much more macroscopic laws. If there is regularity at the macroscopic level, it surely has a correspondence in the biology of the organism. In some cases it may prove valuable to look directly for that correspondence without expending too much effort on the intervening detailed behavioral analysis. Certainly this is a kind of argument that has proven successful in the investigation of the biological basis of visual processes. There too it has seemed useful to search for organizational principles in biology that correspond to organizational principles in psychology, despite the absence of a detailed understanding of how the latter results. It may be that the biology of learning can occasionally take a similar step.

11.4.3 Intrinsic response-reinforcer relations

A third issue of current interest concerns the nature of relations between responses and reinforcers. Like traditional studies of Pavlovian conditioning, investigations of instrumental training have emphasized extrinsic relations between responses and reinforcers—relations which may be described with little reference to the actual events playing the role of response and of reinforcer. That is to say, to a large extent psychologists have behaved as though there were an interchangeability among responses and among reinforcers such that the same laws will result from investigation of any arbitrarily selected pair. It is this assumption that has encouraged the extensive investigation of a few "representative" instrumental-learning situations.

Of course, it has from the outset been admitted that some responses are more trainable than others and that some reinforcers are more potent. And some historically important criticisms, such as those of Premack (1965, 1971), have even suggested that one cannot partition the world into events that are reinforcers and events that are responses. That is, events vary in strength to such an extent that what is a reinforcer for one response may be insufficiently strong to reinforce another; indeed, there may be an even stronger event that could serve to reinforce the reinforcer. However, the notion has survived that once responses have been ordered for their reinforceability by one reward, that ordering is not modified when another reinforcer is employed. It is just this assumption that has recently come under attack, primarily from investigators interested in the innate organization of the behaviors to be trained.

For instance, one of the most commonly trained instrumental responses with food reinforcement—barpressing—has proven to be very difficult to train with shock-avoidance. Bolles (1970) has investigated a variety of responses in a shock-avoidance situation and suggested that they vary widely in trainability. He argues that the differences reflect the involvement of these responses in the normal defense reactions of the organism. Similarly, Shettleworth (1973) has investigated the reinforceability by food of various behaviors in hamsters. It turns out that some responses, such as digging, are easily trained whereas others, such as face washing, are highly resistant to training. As a third example, Sevenster (1973) has found it differentially difficult to train fish to swim through a ring and to bite a bar as a function of whether the reinforcer is the presentation of a male or female of the same species. He argues that this outcome is related to the involvement of these responses in the aggressive and courting activities encouraged by the reinforcers. Finally, we should mention the first such example to gain the attention of experimental psychologists, that of Breland and Breland (1966). These investigators found, upon training arbitrary responses for various reinforcers, that the organism's normal activities in the presence of the reinforcers intruded. For instance, raccoons trained to put chips in a slot for food reward instead increasingly rubbed the chips together in the manner normally employed for washing food. Examples such as these have received considerable attention and have encouraged some authors to suggest that reinforcers are not interchangeable.

Of course, there are a large number of reasons why a given reinforcer may fail to increase the likelihood of a particular response. Not all of these reasons are of equal interest to those investigating learning processes. For instance, as noted earlier, the existence of differences in the trainability of responses and in the potency of reinforcers has been generally recognized. Indeed, one of the traditional justifications for distinguishing between Pavlovian conditioning and instrumental learning involves just such an admission of differential susceptibility to reinforcement. Some responses are claimed to be insensitive to instrumental reinforcers, while others are insensitive to Pavlovian USs. Consequently, failure to obtain a change in performance with a particular response-reinforcer pair must be accompanied by evidence both that the response in question is trainable and that the reinforcers can otherwise train. The simplest way to accomplish this is to introduce another response and another reinforcer in such a way as to show the original response to be modified by the same relation to the new reinforcer, and vice versa. In light of Premack's arguments about the importance of initial event probabilities, the new events should be matched for probability of occurrence with the original events.

Even if one is assured that he has both a potent reinforcer and a trainable response, failure of the pair to produce a behavioral change need not reflect a difficulty in learning their relation. For instance, either the motivational state necessary to make the reinforcer potent or the occurrence of the reinforcer itself may encourage the production of behaviors incompatible with the target response. The presence of a hunger state or the presentation of food to a hungry animal may greatly affect the probability of the response to be trained, perhaps by encouraging responses that are incompatible with it. This would not only prevent the investigator from viewing the response once learned, it might actually affect the organism's treatment. The occurrence of such incompatible responses may prevent adequate exposure to various aspects of the response-reinforcer contingency and so induce differences in the opportunity to learn.

A related, but somewhat more subtle, result can be produced by the Pavlovian conditioning inherent in any instrumental-training procedure. If the reinforcer is adequate to condition various motivational and emotional responses through Pavlovian processes, as well as to train instrumental behaviors, it becomes important to know the relations between these "anticipations" and the responses to be trained. For instance, in the case of shock-avoidance training in rats, it is common to argue that there is Pavlovian conditioning of an anticipatory fear reaction. That reaction may in turn produce freezing, which differentially competes with possible instrumental responses. Again, both performance of the activity and exposure to the reinforcement contingencies would be differentially affected for different instrumental activities, but this may not reflect inherent differences in ability to learn the relation between those responses and the reinforcer.

We have mentioned only some of the more obvious ways in which responses and reinforcers may not be entirely interchangeable (cf. Shettleworth, 1973). Although all of these are of interest in deciphering the behavior of the organism, they do not have equivalent implications for the study of learning. Furthermore, it has not proven easy to separate out these possibilities from the most interesting alternative, namely, that there is a differential ability to learn the relations of certain responses and reinforcers. But interest in this possibility is just emerging, and we can anticipate more and more adequate analytic experimentation along these lines. If we should convince ourselves that such intrinsic response-reinforcer relations affect trainability, then we face the task of characterizing those relations in such a way as to provide more than just a list of pairs that are especially related. A number of suggestions are available, but as yet these seem little more than circular descriptions.

We have to this point discussed only the possibility of intrinsic relations between responses and reinforcers. But the presence of a stimulus in most instrumental-learning situations also raises the possibility of intrinsic relations between that stimulus and both the response and the reinforcer. We should acknowledge that some authors have pointed to such possibilities. For instance, Konorski has argued that for certain stimulus dimensions it is especially easy to train certain instrumental responses, whereas for other dimensions other instrumental responses are favored (Dobrzecka, Szwejkowska, and Konorski, 1966; Konorski, 1967). Although the experiments to support this claim are flawed, the suggestion is an intriguing one. Similarly, some authors have pointed to a stimulus-reinforcer specificity in instrumental training similar to the one we have noted for Pavlovian conditioning. Perhaps the best experiment was done by Foree and LoLordo (1973), who trained pigeons to treadle in the presence of an auditory-visual signal either to avoid shock or to gain food. When shock was used, the auditory signal gained control over treadling; when food was used, the visual signal gained control. Such demonstrations, although still requiring analysis to rule out some of the analogous kinds of alternatives mentioned above, encourage the idea that there may be special relations among all three of the events normally entering into instrumental-learning situations.

The experimental analysis of these possibilities and their theoretical implications for the study of learning is one of the most exciting areas in the current study of learning. It is to be hoped that the experimentation carried out will soon catch up to the speculative theorizing that has so often predominated.

11.5 CONCLUSION

We have characterized learning situations as ones in which some experience at t_1 produces differential behavior at t_2. The experiences at t_1 have been separated into those involving noncontingent stimulus presentation, those involving relations among stimuli, and those involving relations between responses and stimuli. Within this framework we have identified a number of different assessment procedures that can be employed at t_2; indeed, we have urged the application of a variety of such procedures by a given investigator. Throughout we argued for the importance of being clear about which inferences from the data are fundamentally theoretical in character.

The discussion of noncontingent stimulus presentation centered around two different outcomes of such procedures: decrement in response evocation and decrement in trainability. We urged, however, the importance of developing general theories that will account for the diverse outcomes of such procedures when different assessment techniques are employed.

The discussion of Pavlovian conditioning centered around its description in terms of learning about relations among stimulus events. We argued that this description has an important liberalizing effect upon our thinking about conditioning. Using a specific theory of conditioning, we summarized some examples of the sophistication organisms reveal in deciphering causal relations. Finally, we noted that two specific conditioning paradigms, conditioned suppression and toxicosis, have dominated such studies of conditioning; we applauded that domination because of their role in both emotional and instrumental behavior.

Only three loosely related issues were described in our discussion of the instrumental-conditioning procedure: the involvement of Pavlovian conditioning in instrumental behavior; the suggestion that macroscopic laws of behavior might be a basis for comparison with biological data; and the role of intrinsic event relations in modulating instrumental learning. We argued that instrumental learning may be sufficiently complex as to discourage its initial use in the search for biological correlates of learning.

REFERENCES

BENEDICT, J. O., and AYRES, J. J. B. 1972. Factors affecting conditioning in the truly random control procedure in the rat. *Journal of Comparative and Physiological Psychology* 78: 323–330.

BOLLES, R. C. 1967. *Theory of Motivation*. New York: Harper & Row.

BOLLES, ·R. C. 1970. Species-specific defense reactions and avoidance learning. *Psychological Review* 77: 32–48.

BRELAND, K., and BRELAND, M. 1966. *Animal Behavior*. New York: Macmillan.

BROGDEN, W. J. 1939. Sensory pre-conditioning. *Journal of Experimental Psychology* 25: 323–332.

BROWN, P. L., and JENKINS, H. M. 1968. Autoshaping of the pigeon's keypeck. *Journal of the Experimental Analysis of Behavior* 11: 1–8.

BUSH, R. R., and MOSTELLER, R. 1955. *Stochastic Models for Learning*. New York: John Wiley & Sons.

BUTLER, R. A. 1957. The effect of deprivation of visual incentives on visual exploration motivation in monkeys. *Journal of Comparative and Physiological Psychology* 50: 177–179.

CARLTON, P. L. 1963. Cholinergic mechanisms in the control of behavior by the brain. *Psychological Review* 70: 19–39.

CHORAZYNA, H. 1962. Some properties of conditioned inhibition. *Acta Biologiae Experimentalis* 22: 5.

CHURCH, R. M. 1964. Systematic effect of random error in the yoked control design. *Psychological Bulletin* 62: 122–131.

COOMBS, C. H. 1938. Adaptation of the galvanic response to auditory stimuli. *Journal of Experimental Psychology* 22: 244–268.

CROWELL, C. R., and ANDERSON, D. C. 1972. Variations in intensity, interstimulus interval, and interval between preconditioning CS exposures and conditioning with rats. *Journal of Comparative and Physiological Psychology* 79: 291–298.

D'AMATO, M. R., FAZZARO, J., and ETKIN, M. 1968. Anticipatory responding and avoidance discrimination as factors in avoidance conditioning. *Journal of Experimental Psychology* 77: 41–47.

DAVIS, M. 1970. Effects of interstimulus interval length and variability on startle-response habituation in the rat. *Journal of Comparative and Physiological Psychology* 72: 177–192.

DAVIS, M. 1972. Differential retention of sensitization and habituation of the startle response in the rat. *Journal of Comparative and Physiological Psychology* 78: 260–267.

DAVIS, M., and WAGNER, A. R. 1968. Startle responsiveness after habituation to different intensities of tone. *Psychonomic Science* 12: 337–338.

DAVIS, M., and WAGNER, A. R. 1969. Habituation of the startle response under an incremental sequence of stimulus intensities. *Journal of Comparative and Physiological Psychology* 67: 486–492.

DOBRZECKA, C., SZWEJKOWSKA, G., and KONORSKI, J. 1966. Qualitative versus directional cues in two forms of differentiation. *Science* 153: 87–89.

DOMJAN, M., and SIEGEL, S. 1971. Conditioned suppression following CS preexposure. *Psychonomic Science* 25: 11–12.

DWECK, C. S., and WAGNER, A. R. 1970. Situational cues and correlation between CS and US as determinants of the conditioned emotional response. *Psychonomic Science* 18: 145–147.

FOREE, D. D., and LoLORDO, V. M. 1973. Attention in the pigeon: Differential effects of food-getting versus shock avoidance procedures. *Journal of Comparative and Physiological Psychology* 85: 551–558.

GARCIA, J., and KOELLING, R. A. 1966. Relation of cue to con-sequence in avoidance learning. *Psychonomic Science* 4: 123–124.

GARCIA, J., McGOWAN, B. K., ERVIN, F. R., and KOELLING, R. A. 1968. Cues: Their effectiveness as a function of the reinforcer. *Science* 160: 794–795.

GIBSON, E. J., and WALK, R. D. 1956. The effect of prolonged exposure to visually presented patterns on learning to discriminate them. *Journal of Comparative and Physiological Psychology* 49: 239–242.

GLANZER, M. 1953. The role of stimulus satiation in response alternation. *Journal of Experimental Psychology* 45: 387–393.

GORMEZANO, I. 1965. Yoked comparisons of classical and instrumental conditioning of the eyelid response; and an addendum on "voluntary responders." In W. F. Prokasy, ed., *Classical Conditioning: A Symposium*. New York: Appleton-Century-Crofts.

GORMEZANO, I. 1972. Investigations of defense and reward conditioning in the rabbit. In A. H. Black and W. F. Prokasy, eds., *Classical Conditioning II*. New York: Appleton-Century-Crofts.

GORMEZANO, I., MOORE, J. W., and DEAUX, T. 1962. Supplementary report: Yoked comparisons of classical and avoidance conditioning under three UCS intensities. *Journal of Experimental Psychology* 64: 551–552.

GROVES, P. M., and THOMPSON, R. F. 1970. Habituation: A dual process theory. *Psychological Review* 77: 419–450.

HERRNSTEIN, R. J. 1969. Method and theory in the study of avoidance. *Psychological Review* 76: 49–69.

HERRNSTEIN, R. J. 1970. On the law of effect. *Journal of the Experimental Analysis of Behavior* 13: 243–266.

HETH, C. D., and RESCORLA, R. A. 1973. Simultaneous and backward fear conditioning in the rat. *Journal of Comparative and Physiological Psychology* 82: 434–443.

HINDE, R. A. 1970. Behavioral habituation. In G. Horn and R. A. Hinde, eds., *Short-Term Changes in Neural Activity and Behaviour*. London: Cambridge University Press.

HOFFMAN, H. S., EISERER, L. A., and SINGER, D. 1972. Acquisition of behavioral control by a stationary imprinting stimulus. *Psychonomic Science* 26: 146–148.

HOFFMAN, H. S., STRATTON, J. W., NEWBY, V., and BARRET, J. E. 1970. Development of behavioral control by an imprinting stimulus. *Journal of Comparative and Physiological Psychology* 71: 229–236.

HOFFMAN, H. S., and RATNER, A. M. 1973. A reinforcement model of imprinting: Implications for socialization in monkeys and men. *Psychological Review* 80: 527–544.

HOFFMAN, H. S., SEARLE, J. L., TOFFEY, S., and KOZMA, Jr., F. 1966. Behavioral control by an imprinted stimulus. *Journal of the Experimental Analysis of Behavior* 9: 177–189.

HOLLAND, P. C., and RESCORLA, R. A. 1975. Second-order conditioning with food unconditioned stimulus. *Journal of Comparative and Physiological Psychology* 88: 459–467.

HULL, C. L. 1943. *Principles of Psychology*. New York: D. Appleton-Century.

KALAT, J. W., and ROZIN, P. 1971. Role of interference in taste-aversion learning. *Journal of Comparative and Physiological Psychology* 77: 53–58.

KAMIN, L. J. 1965. Temporal and intensity characteristics of the conditioned stimulus. In W. F. Prokasy, ed., *Classical Conditioning: A Symposium*. New York: Appleton-Century-Crofts.

KAMIN, L. J. 1968. Attention-like processes in classical conditioning. In M. R. Jones, ed., *Miami Symposium on the*

Prediction of Behavior: Aversive Stimulation. Miami: University of Miami Press.

KAMIN, L. J. 1969. Predictability, surprise, attention, and conditioning. In R. Church and B. Campbell, eds., *Punishment and Aversive Behavior.* New York: Appleton-Century Crofts.

KNAPP, H. D., TAUB, E., and BERMAN, A. J. 1958. Effect of deafferentation on a conditioned avoidance response. *Science* 128: 842–843.

KÖHLER, W. 1947. *Gestalt Psychology.* New York: Liveright.

KONORSKI, J. 1967. *Integrative Activity of the Brain.* Chicago: University of Chicago Press.

KRANE, R. V., and WAGNER, A. R. 1975. Taste aversion learning with a delayed shock US: Implications for the "generality of the laws of learning." *Journal of Comparative and Physiological Psychology* 88: 882–889.

LANTZ, A. 1973. Effect of number of trials, inter-stimulus interval, and dishabituation during CS habituation on subsequent conditioning in a CER paradigm. *Animal Learning and Behavior* 1: 273–277.

LUBOW, R. E. 1973. Latent inhibition. *Psychological Bulletin* 79: 398–407.

MILLER, N. E. 1963. Some reflections on the law of effect produce a new alternative to drive reduction. In M. R. Jones, ed., *Nebraska Symposium on Motivation: 1963.* Lincoln, Neb.: University of Nebraska Press.

MOWRER, O. H. 1960. *Learning Theory and Behavior.* New York: John Wiley & Sons.

MOWRER, O. H., and AIKEN, E. G. 1954. Contiguity vs. drive-reduction in conditioned fear: Temporal variations in conditioned and unconditioned stimulus. *American Journal of Psychology* 67: 26–38.

PAVLOV, I. P. 1927. *Conditioned Reflexes.* London: Oxford University Press.

PREMACK, D. 1965. Reinforcement theory. In D. Levine, ed., *Nebraska Symposium on Motivation: 1965.* Lincoln, Neb.: University of Nebraska Press.

PREMACK, D. 1971. Catching up with common sense, or two sides of a generalization: Reinforcement and punishment. In R. Glaser, ed., *The Nature of Reinforcement.* New York: Academic Press.

RATNER, S. C. 1970. Habituation: Research and theory, In J. H. Reynierse, ed., *Current Issues in Animal Learning.* Lincoln, Neb.: University of Nebraska Press.

RAZRAN, G. 1957. The dominance-contiguity theory of the acquisition of classical conditioning. *Psychological Bulletin* 54: 1–46.

REISS, S., and WAGNER, A. R. 1972. CS habituation produces a "latent inhibition effect" but no active "conditioned inhibition." *Learning and Motivation* 3: 237–245.

RESCORLA, R. A. 1967. Pavlovian conditioning and its proper control procedures. *Psychological Review* 74: 71–80.

RESCORLA, R. A. 1968. Probability of shock in the presence and absence of CS in fear conditioning. *Journal of Comparative and Physiological Psychology* 66: 1–5.

RESCORLA, R. A. 1969a. Pavlovian conditioned inhibition. *Psychological Bulletin* 72: 77–94.

RESCORLA, R. A. 1969b. Conditioned inhibition of fear resulting from negative CS-US contingencies. *Journal of Comparative and Physiological Psychology* 67: 504–509.

RESCORLA, R. A. 1970. Reduction in the effectiveness of reinforcement after prior excitatory conditioning. *Learning and Motivation* 1: 372–381.

RESCORLA, R. A. 1971. Summation and retardation tests of latent inhibition. *Journal of Comparative and Physiological Psychology* 75: 77–81.

RESCORLA, R. A. 1972. Informational variables in Pavlovian conditioning. In G. Bower, ed., *The Psychology of Learning and Motivation,* Vol. 6. New York: Academic Press.

RESCORLA, R. A. 1973. Effect of US habituation following conditioning. *Journal of Comparative and Physiological Psychology* 82: 137–143.

RESCORLA, R. A. 1974. Effect of inflation of the unconditioned stimulusvalue following conditioning. *Journal of Comparative Physiological Psychology* 86: 101–106.

RESCORLA, R. A., and SOLOMON, R. L. 1967. Two process learning theory: Relationships between Pavlovian conditioning and instrumental learning. *Psychological Review* 74: 151–182.

RESCORLA, R. A., and WAGNER, A. R. 1972. A theory of Pavlovian conditioning: Variations in the effectiveness of reinforcement and nonreinforcement. In A. H. Black and W. F. Prokasy, eds., *Classical Conditioning II.* New York: Appleton-Century-Crofts.

REVUSKY, S. 1971. The role of interference in association over a delay. In W. K. HONIG and P. H. R. JAMES, eds., *Animal Memory.* New York: Academic Press.

RIZLEY, R. C., and RESCORLA, R. A. 1972. Associations in second-order conditioning and sensory preconditioning. *Journal of Comparative and Physiological Psychology* 81: 1–11.

ROSENZWEIG, M. R., KRECH, D., and BENNETT, E. L. 1960. A search for relations between brain chemistry and behavior. *Psychological Bulletin* 57: 476–492.

SCHNEIDERMAN, N. and GORMEZANO, I. 1964. Conditioning of the nictitating membrane of the rabbit as a function of CS-US interval. *Journal of Comparative and Physiological Psychology* 57: 188–195.

SELIGMAN, M. E. P. 1969. Control group and conditioning: A comment on operationism. *Psychological Review* 76: 484–491.

SELIGMAN, M. E. P., and JOHNSTON, J. C. 1973. A cognitive theory of avoidance learning. In F. J. McGuigan and D. B. Lumsden, eds., *Contemporary Approaches to Conditioning and Learning.* New York: John Wiley & Sons.

SEVENSTER, P. 1973. Incompatibility of response and reward. In R. A. Hinde and J. Stevenson-Hinde, eds., *Constraints on Learning: Limitations and Predispositions.* New York: Academic Press.

SHEAFOR, P. J., and GORMEZANO, I. 1972. Conditioning the rabbit's (*Oryctolagus cuniculus*) jaw-movement response. *Journal of Comparative and Physiological Psychology* 81: 449–456.

SHEFFIELD, F. D. 1966. A drive-induction theory of reinforcement. In R. N. Haber, ed., *Current Research in Motivation.* New York: Holt, Rinehart and Winston.

SHEFFIELD, F. D., and CAMPBELL, B. A. 1954. The role of experience in the "spontaneous" activity of hungry rats. *Journal of Comparative and Physiological Psychology* 47: 97–100.

SHETTLEWORTH, S. J. 1973. Food reinforcement and the organization of behavior in golden hamsters. In R. A. Hinde and J. Stevenson-Hinde, eds., *Constraints on Learning: Limitations and Predispositions.* New York: Academic Press.

SIEGEL, S. 1969. Generalization of latent inhibition. *Journal of Comparative and Physiological Psychology* 69: 157–159.

SLUCKIN, W. 1964. *Imprinting and Early Learning.* London: Methuen.

SOKOLOV, Y. N. 1963. *Perception and the Conditioned Reflex.* Oxford: Pergamon Press.

STEIN, L. 1966. Habituation and stimulus novelty: A model

based on classical conditioning. *Psychological Review* 73: 352–356.

THOMPSON, R. F., and SPENCER, W. A. 1966. Habituation: A model phenomenon for the study of the neuronal substrates of behavior. *Psychological Review* 73: 16–43.

TOLMAN, E. C., and BRUNSWIK, E. 1935. The organism and the causal texture of the environment. *Psychological Review* 42: 43–77.

TRAPOLD, M. A., and OVERMIER, J. B. 1972. The second learning process in instrumental training. In A. H. Black and W. F. Prokasy, eds., *Classical Conditioning II*. New York: Appleton-Century-Crofts.

WAGNER, A. R. 1969a. Stimulus selection and a "modified continuity theory." In G. Bower and J. T. Spence, eds., *The Psychology of Learning and Motivation*, Vol. 3. New York: Academic Press.

WAGNER, A. R. 1969b. Stimulus validity and stimulus selection. In W. K. Honig and N. J. MacKintosh, eds., *Fundamental Issues in Associative Learning*. Halifax: Dalhousie University Press.

WAGNER, A. R. 1971. Elementary associations. In H. H. Kendler and J. T. Spence, eds., *Essays in Neobehaviorism: A Memorial Volume to Kenneth W. Spence*. New York: Appleton-Century-Crofts.

WAGNER, A. R., and RESCORLA R. A. 1972. Inhibition in Pavlovian conditioning: Application of a theory. In R. A. Boakes and S. Halliday, eds., *Inhibition and Learning*. New York: Academic Press.

WICKENS, D. D., NIELD, A. F., TUBER, D. S., and WICKENS, C. D. 1969. Strength, latency, and form of conditioned skeletal and autonomic responses as a function of CS-US intervals. *Journal of Experimental Psychology* 80: 165–170.

WICKENS, D. D., and WICKENS, C. D. 1942. Some factors related to pseudoconditioning. *Journal of Experimental Psychology* 31: 518–526.

12

Learning Paradigms and the Structure of the Organism

JOHN GARCIA AND MICHAEL S. LEVINE

ABSTRACT Rescorla and Holland's presentation of behavioral paradigms is critically evaluated for neurobehavioral science. The usefulness of any theory based primarily on the causal texture of the environment is questioned, for while successful organisms must conform to environmental pressure, molar description of their coping behavior gives little information concerning the central mechanisms by which the organism adapts. Environmental contingencies can force superficial behavioral conformity through different mechanisms, just as convergent evolution produces gross anatomical similarity in widely divergent species. In addition, it is pointed out that conditioning should not be considered merely in terms of the acquisition of information, since its most powerful effects are due to motivational changes. The neurobehaviorist must examine the causal structure of the behaving organism. The nature of stimuli depends upon the structure of afferent systems, the effectiveness of incentives for homeostatic mechanisms, and the topography of responses in motor systems. Finally, it is pointed out that a truly neurobehavioral theory is emerging from detailed observation of functional processes of neural structures in the behaving animal.

12.1 SOME LIMITATIONS OF BEHAVIORAL THEORY

Rescorla and Holland (this volume) have discussed the strategies of behavioral-training procedures in an orderly way, using these procedures to construct a theory of behavior in the traditional manner of learning theorists. They began with the simple situation in which a single stimulus is presented to a laboratory animal for the first time and the arousal and orienting responses that occur to the stimulation are observed. Next they discussed the complications of this simple procedure that are caused by habituation, which is a result of the repeated presentation of the same stimulus. Theoretical complexities became apparent when the effects of habituation upon subsequent training procedures were considered. For example, after habituation the power of the stimulus to evoke arousal and orientation gradually wanes. After habituation the stimulus also becomes an ineffective signal in new training procedures. Are these two separate functional processes? To those theorists who base

JOHN GARCIA, Department of Psychology, University of California, Los Angeles, and MICHAEL S. LEVINE, Department of Psychiatry, University of California, Los Angeles

their constructions upon training procedures, this question is apparently a meaningful one, but is it meaningful for those who seek to explain behavior in terms of neurological mechanisms?

Historically, the purpose of psychology has been to define the elements of behavior and the laws of their association. This search continues to this day. If the goal were feasible, then behavioral theory might indeed point the way to the neural mechanisms. Unfortunately, the "laws" of behavioral theory are overturned with disconcerting regularity by changes in training procedures. In this section we shall consider some of these basic concepts and their sensitivity to procedural changes.

12.1.1 Behavioral elements and their bonds

Rescorla and Holland went on to discuss more complex associative procedures, as when two events are paired in conditioning paradigms. The association of two events has often been considered the hallmark of true learning (see Rescorla, 1967). In classical (Pavlovian) conditioning, one event is a signal (CS) and the other is a stimulus (US) of consequence to the coping animal. In instrumental (Thorndikian or Skinnerian) conditioning, the coping animal's response is followed by the consequential stimulus. So strong has been this insistence upon an association that habituation is often considered a response change that is reinforced by the fact that nothing of consequence happens to the organism after the signal (MacKintosh, 1973).

The association bond between the two behavioral events has been of central concern to learning theorists during the last century, whether they considered these two events to be a stimulus and a response (S-R) or two stimuli (S-S). Conceptually, theorists have attempted to deal with the S-R bond in isolation, as dependent solely upon the intensity of the two events and the temporal proximity of their pairing. Even the apparently incremental growth in the strength of the conditioned response due to frequency—that is, to repeated S-R trials—has been considered a statistical artifact by diverse theorists (Estes, 1960; Krechevsky, 1938). These theorists have viewed the association as an "all-or-none" affair observable in the performance of an individual subject coping with a unitary element or "bit" of the problem. They therefore treated incremental learning curves as artifacts generated by averaging group performance on problems containing many bits. Ideally, a bit might be the occurrence of an isolated S-R bonding event, which is compatible with the axonal "all-or-none" law.

Unfortunately, the analysis of the behavioral situation into isolated bits has been proved impossible. For example, Rescorla (1967) logically extended the Pavlovian paradigm to include the notion of *correlation* between CS and US events and thus removed the limitations imposed by the traditional notion of *contingency* pairing of the CS and US. Essentially, he kept the number of CS-US pairings (tone-shock) constant for all groups of rats, but some groups received unpaired tones or unpaired shocks randomly distributed throughout training, and this was found to degrade the information value of the signaling tone. This procedure reduced the correlation between CS and US while maintaining the absolute number of contiguous CS-US pairings. Conditioning was found to be dependent upon correlation, i.e., the probabilistic relationship between many CS and many US events. Temporal pairing of individual CS and US events was not enough. To use Brunswik's (1955) terms, Rescorla "untied" correlational and contingency variables to extend the paradigm, and thus made the "all-or-none" behavioral law untenable.

Animals as "simple" as an ant are sensitive to the probabilistic nature of cues and signals (Fleer, 1972; Garcia, Clarke, and Hankins, 1973). Even the emission of a single response by the individual animal has to be viewed as the culmination of many factors, and this makes any match between behavioral bits and neurological bits extremely difficult, if not impossible. Here again, changes in training procedures have forced a complete change in basic theoretical notions concerning behavioral elements and their associations.

12.1.2 The demise of reinforcement

The bond between the two behavioral events in learning has usually been considered to be formed and strengthened through the action of a class of stimuli called reinforcers. This reinforcement process has been given a unique status in learning since Thorndike (1913) proclaimed the Law of Effect. The law explained how associations were "stamped in" by the action of the satisfiers (rewards) or annoyers (punishments) that motivated the animal's behavior in the laboratory apparatus.

Reinforcement maintained its unique position even after Premack (1965) convincingly demonstrated that responses and reinforcers are interchangeable. He showed that rats will run in order to drink under one set

of experimental conditions, but under another set of conditions, they will drink in order to run. Running and drinking are two behaviors; either one can be the instrumental coping activity or the consummatory goal activity. Either behavior can be the reinforcer, i.e., the second activity, of a contingent pair of behavioral events in a conditioning setup, which usually terminates the trial. Reinforcers are not a unique, finite class. Reinforcement is merely a procedural relationship set up between behavioral events. Once again, changes in training procedures have negated the notion of classes of elemental units in the associative process.

Reinforcement, particularly in operant formulations, has an almost mystical urgency. It has to be applied immediately after the response that it reinforces, for it can lose potency within a few seconds of that response. If a reinforcement effect is observed to occur over a longer time span, it is assumed that it has worked through a "chain" of adjacent behavioral elements to reach the more distal elements. An enormous amount of data collected in T mazes, discrimination tests, and Skinner boxes has shown that under the usual procedures, delay of reinforcement makes S-R association bonding unlikely. With immediate reinforcement, the bonded S-R elements can presumably be stored in memory and retrieved for use in the next trial. This process is not simply memory, since the animal can obviously remember an unreinforced signal for days, as habituation studies demonstrate. (Parenthetically, we note that conceptualizing habituation as a process reinforced by nothing of consequence happening to the animal makes an unreinforced signal impossible.) In any case the bonded S-R compound would seem to be the engram that has been the major objective of memory research.

Recently, however, Bow Tong Lett (1973) has demonstrated that the apparent necessity for immediate reinforcement is an artifact attributable to a confounding of temporal intervals and experimental situations in traditional experiments. Table 12.1 illustrates the issue. Normally, signals (S), responses (R), and reinforcers

TABLE 12.1

The position of the long interval in the temporal sequence of events in three learning paradigms

	Trial N (animal in test apparatus)	The long interval (animal in home cage)	Trial N + 1 (animal back in test apparatus)
Traditional	S-R-reinf.	———	S-R-reinf.
Lett (1973)	S-R	———	reinf.
Capaldi (1967) and Revusky (1974)	S	———	R-reinf.

(reinf.) occur with brief intervals on any given trial (N) in an apparatus such as the T maze. Then the animal spends a longer intertrial interval in the home cage. On the next trial (N+1), it is returned to the T maze for another S-R-reinf. sequence. Lett rearranged the sequence, placing the long interval in the cage between the S-R and the reinforcing events. She allowed her rat to assess the cues (S) and make its choice (R), and then immediately removed it from the T maze to a holding cage. After a waiting interval, she returned it to the stem of the T maze (blocking the choice point) and there provided it with contingent food reinforcement. The rat learned despite the fact that reinforcement was delayed for an hour after it had made its choice.

Table 12.1 compares Lett's procedures with traditional procedures and with another disrupted sequence similar to hers. Capaldi (1967) reinforced animals for running on alternate days and found that running speed depended upon whether the rat had been reinforced the day before. In this case the cue (S) to whether the end box contained food was an event twenty-four hours prior to the response (R). Revusky (1974) employed black and white runways, and the only cue (S) indicating contingent reinforcement for the rat was the color of the maze on the previous trial. Again, the rats learned even though the long interval was interposed between the cue and the reinforced response.

The problem confronting an animal in a Skinner box has also been critically discussed recently (Garcia, Hankins, and Rusiniak, 1974). An animal is usually continuously behaving—sniffing, walking, rearing, and manipulating features of the box. In operant conditioning one "bit" of this stream of behavior is arbitarily designated as correct and contingently reinforced. If the reinforcement is delayed, how can the animal decide which behavioral bit is correct? It may remember the bit well, but simply not be able to retrieve it in order to relate it to the reward. If reward follows immediately after a behavioral bit, however, that bit is *flagged* for future retrieval. Lett has shown that removing the animal from the context of the maze is another way to *flag* the response. When she returns the rat to the maze, it is able to relate the contingent reinforcement to the last behavioral bit it performed in the maze. All intervening behavior is flagged to another context, namely, the holding cage. These experiments indicate (1) that contextual cues are important for the retrieval of memories, and (2) that the psychological effect of time depends upon where and how the time is spent.

The demise of reinforcement deprives the neurophysiologist of an important marker event in his search for memory mechanisms. Heretofore he could assume that only his experimental group learned, for only that group received signals and made responses followed by contingent reinforcement. He could then look for synaptic changes, protein synthesis, or the neurophysiological memory process of his choice in the experimental group and make the appropriate comparison with the control group, which did not learn. Now the neurophysiologist must assume that control groups also learn, for all signals are processed and related to whatever follows, and behavioral events can be reinforced by long-delayed consequences. He is forced to search for a specific neurophysiological mediator of the specific bit of learning or memory in his experimental animals and to differentiate that mediator from other similar mediators associated with otherbits of learning or memory in his controls. Needless to say, this is a much more difficult task.

12.1.3 The causal texture of the environment

Rescorla and Holland have described conditioning as a process in which animals gather information concerning environmental contingencies, noting that the causal texture of the environment shapes behavior (cf. Tolman and Brunswik, 1935). However, there is a limit to what behavioral description of the "causal texture" of the environment can do for the researcher interested in neural mechanisms of learning. Animals can adopt similar behavioral strategies to cope with a variety of environmental pressures, but they may use entirely different neural mechanisms to achieve the same behavioral end. One of the more popular illustrations of this fact employed by zoologists is the gross similarity of form seen in the shark, the ichthyosaur, and the porpoise. The liquid environment of the sea has molded the general shape of these swift predatory organisms into similar streamlined forms, but their internal structures and their evolutionary histories are vastly different. Zoologists therefore reject the gross similarity as superficial and emphasize the differences in internal anatomical structure.

Behaviorists sometimes do just the opposite. Take Skinner's (1959) well-known example in which he points to the cumulative records of several organisms on the same fixed-interval reinforcement schedule. The Skinner box, which records only depressions of the lever and the periodic reinforcements, forces similar behavioral patterns in pigeon, rat, and monkey. All three organisms produce similar records because of the environmental pressure of the behavioral test. In contrast to the zoologist, however, Skinner rejects the obvious differences in anatomical structure and seeks his behavioral principles in the environmental pressures.

In a similar way, Fleer (1972) has demonstrated that ants placed in a series of reversal problems yield data that can be superimposed on data generated by rats in reversal problems. However, Fleer points out that the ants are achieving this adaptation with microscopic brains, called mushroom bodies, which are quite different from the mammalian brain of the rat. A neurobehavioral theory is required to explain behavioral similarities in the face of divergent anatomical structures as well as differential behaviors due to divergent structures of input-output systems.

12.1 BEYOND STIMULUS-RESPONSE-REINFORCEMENT

Paradigms set out in stimulus-response-reinforcement terms give us little information even about the functional properties of temporal intervals. For example, contextual variables can be "traded off" for time in the delayed-reaction paradigm. When this problem is set up in the traditional learning laboratory, an animal is presented with two choices directly in front of him. A light may signal the correct choice, but it goes out before he is allowed to make his response. Most animals, including monkeys, have a difficult time with this problem, particularly if their bodily orientation toward the locus of the now-absent cue is disrupted during a wait interval of a few seconds. However, if the same problem is carried out under "field conditions," animals have no such difficulties. One can throw a bone for a dog, spin him around and release him, and he heads in the appropriate direction. Show a dozen bits of banana hidden in a field to a chimp, and when he is returned to the field, he systematically finds them all with no wasted search motions (Menzel, 1973). In a richly variegated context, delaying the reaction for long time periods and disrupting the animal's orientation has little effect. No theorems or postulates from learning theory explain why the difficult delayed-reaction paradigm becomes simple when animals are taken out of the narrow confines of the laboratory problem box and tested in a broad field.

12.2.1 The causal structure of the organism
The specific nature of the signaling events and the reinforcing events are of extreme importance in determining whether an animal succeeds or fails in a given paradigm. For example, observe a cat learning a two-way avoidance in a shuttle box. He is given a visual signal, and if he does not move to the other compartment, a noxious stimulus is applied. He then moves to the safe compartment, and at a specified time he gets the signal again followed by punishment unless he returns to the original compartment. The procedure is repeated until the cat learns to shuttle back and forth on cue, avoiding the punishment with incessant movement. If the signal is an electric light and the punishment is electric shock,

many cats have a difficult time learning to shuttle. However, if the signal is water seeping into the back of the compartment and the punishment is cold, wet feet, most cats learn the shuttling response in a few trials. To say that water is a natural stimulus for cats and electricity is an artificial one is not much of an explanation. Perhaps in the course of evolutionary history natural selection has designed cats to perceive water and cold, wet feet as an entity to be avoided. Alternatively, it may be that kittens learn by experience that the clear liquid will chill their feet.

This is the classic and fruitless nature-nurture question, which impels students of human performance in their endless attempts to apportion individual differences to either heredity or environment through an analysis of variance. The question is fruitless because behavior can neither occur in an environmental vacuum nor be disembodied from inherited structure. Both Lorenz (1965) and Skinner (1966) agree that the causal textures of past environments have prepared organisms to cope with the causal texture of the present environment. For example, when the laboratory ferret encounters the laboratory rat in a confined space for the first time, the confrontation takes on an age-old pattern. The ferret attempts to separate the rat's head from its body by biting the back of the neck. This is the classic tactic of most butchers and executioners. The rat curls upright with its spine to the wall in a position to counterattack with teeth and claws. The ferret feints, darts, and nips to disrupt the defensive posture, but will only fasten its death grip on the back of the rat's neck where the rat cannot counterbite. Both animals appear to be making use of ancestral memory, but it is obvious from their youthful play activity that each individual animal of both species has an opportunity to discover the classic tactics empirically; indeed, the environment in which an individual behaves must be basically similar to the one in which the species evolved, for otherwise survival would be impossible. Whenever and wherever an individual behaves and learns, it can only develop some potential inherent in its behavioral machinery of bone, muscle, and nerve. Empirical environmental inputs alter the structural machinery of behavior as surely as do genetic mutations. The task of the neurobehaviorist is to describe the structure of the behavioral machinery, not to search for the ghost in the machine (Koestler, 1968).

A neurobehavioral theory should begin by taking into account the rudimentary facts concerning receptor systems in accordance with the Müller-Helmholtz doctrine of the specific energies of nerves. This doctrine proclaimed over one hundred years ago that the structure of the sensory system defines the nature of the stimulus, and that notion is still crucial for the understanding of conditioning today. For example, a signal or CS is not just any stimulus; one normally signals a laboratory animal through its head receptors. The eyes and the ears set in tandem pairs in the head perched on a swiveling neck are designed to pick up a signal in the distance and locate it in space via the "orienting reflex." These receptors are capable of operating over an enormous spectrum of energy and enchancing contrast phenomena and contours through lateral inhibition. The remarkable capacity of these special receptors to adapt without discomfort to ambient levels ranging from virtually zero energy to many orders of magnitude makes them ideal channels for the "neutral" signal or CS in conditioning experiments. The auditory system is the favored channel for defensive signals in avoidance paradigms because the signal is received no matter which way the head is turned. In effect, audition forms a defensive sphere completely surrounding the animal.

In contrast to the adaptive, wide-ranging, head receptor systems, which accept most types of CS stimulation, the US is presented via receptor systems that are not nearly so tolerant. The "comfort range" is much narrower in these receptors, and they do not adapt so readily to repeated stimulation; they can therefore be reliably used to goad the laboratory animal into action, trial after trial. Food or water contacting the mouth of a deprived animal is a good US or reinforcer, but electro-cutaneous shock is also popular because of the ease of control and instrumentation. Moreover, shock is extremely effective because it attacks an inner defense perimeter completely surrounding the animal. Electro-cutaneous shock can be conveniently described in physicalistic terms, but this may be deceptive when we consider questions related to the structure of the organism. Is the shock stimulating superficial "bright-pain" receptors calling for movement away from the contact area? Is the current shunting through tendon and muscle receptors, which call for immobility? Behavioral reactions to shock, not dial settings, are of primary importance in specifying intensity.

Although the vast majority of such studies employ the auditory stimulus as the CS and shock as the US, it is possible to reverse this, using a mild shock to signal a loud blast from a speaker. Such an experiment demonstrates that behavioral theories can be devised in terms of input-output relationships without regard to peripheral channels or central mechanisms. It is precisely for this reason that theoretical models based on behavior are relatively useless to guide neurophysiological research. A neurobehavioral theory must be sensitive to neurophysiological variables as well as behavioral variables.

In the past these sensory systems have been studied mostly by varying the classical physical parameters of the energy source. But most organisms in their natural situations are not subjected to intense, brief flashes of either light or pure tones. Natural visual and auditory signals consist of organized patterns of light and sound, facts which hint at the operating characteristics of the receptor systems. Progress has been made recently because pattern, position, movement, contrast, shape, and size have replaced amplitude and frequency as stimulus variables. Intensity, frequency, and recency of stimulation, the classical behavioral parameters, have proved to be inadequate in the study of central function.

Finally, it is becoming clear that needs, drives, and motivations are also empirical variables operating via the action of internal receptors. These internal need receptors have the narrowest comfort range. Small deviations from the optimal setting of an internal homeostatic receptor call for persistent reactions by changing the hedonic tone of external stimuli. For example, if the core temperature of the body is low, a heat source is pleasant and stimulates approach reactions. If the core temperature is higher by a few degrees, the same heat source is unpleasant and avoidance reactions are evoked. Similar mechanisms operate for calories, vitamins, water, and sex (Garcia, Hankins, and Rusiniak, 1974).

The abstract, disembodied notions of stimulus-response-reinforcement are inadequate even when our subject is the mythical generalized organism dealt with by most behavioral theories. This inadequacy becomes monumental when we consider genuine living animals. How can we generalize when the same organism changes its structure and its capacity to deal with environmental contingencies during development? How can we generalize from one species to another when each species is specialized to deal with the environmental contingencies in a particular niche? The answer is a direct one. We look for common structures and common mechanisms *within* animals with the traditional methods of comparative neurophysiology and biomedical research. This is the only way to generalize from one creature in one situation to another creature in another situation.

12.2.2 The modification of incentives
The unfortunate dichotomizing of behavior into nature *or* nurture has often obscured genuine breakthroughs in behavioral research. Take, for example, Breland and Breland's (1961) notion of *instinctual drift* (which may be an unfortunate choice of terminology). They found that the instrumental acts of animals commercially trained for amusement parks break down in a curious way after many months of working in the same exhibit.

For example, a pig might be required to put a token in a slot in order to obtain a food reinforcer. After many trials at asymptotic performance levels, the pig becomes reluctant to release the token into the slot. It begins to root the token around as if it were food. The raccoon's instrumental training also breaks down. It acts as if it is washing the token and cracking it open, as raccoons characteristically do to crayfish. The Brelands noted that these animals' instrumental behavior drifted toward instinctive species-specific behavior. But the more significant aspect of this phenomenon is that *the token has taken on the property of food*, i.e., the pig and the raccoon treat the token as food. This change resembles that described in the older social-psychology literature under the rubric *functional autonomy*, where "habits become drives" and "means become ends." After spending a great part of one's life working and saving money for necessities, the work and the money become valuable in themselves, despite the fact that all necessities are provided for. Neither the phenomenon nor its label is as important as the finding that conditioning procedures result in a modification of incentives.

Other investigators have demonstrated that a pigeon in a Skinner box does not merely peck at the key instrumentally to obtain grain; it acts as if it is eating the key, with precisely the same crisp pecks it uses to pick up grain. If the pigeon is reinforced by water, it acts as if it is drinking the key, with the same pumping action it uses to drink water (Jenkins and Sainsbury, 1969; Jenkins and Moore, 1973; Moore, 1973). In fact, the pigeon develops these responses toward the signaling key whenever it is associated with food, even if pecking the key *restricts* its access to the food (Brown and Jenkins, 1968). The significance of these findings is not that natural behavior is somehow more powerful than nurtured behavior, but rather that incentives have been modified, i.e., consummatory responses formerly directed to food objects are now redirected toward objects signaling food. This motivational shift is the essence of classical conditioning. Conditioning is not merely the acquisition of environmental contingencies as Rescorla and Holland imply.

The Brelands (1961) demonstrated that the incentive value of tokens changes after prolonged operant training. The flavor-toxicosis paradigm indicates that incentives can be modified in one or two trials if the appropriate reinforcer is applied. In this paradigm the animal is presented with a distinctive flavor; then, later, it is made ill by exposure to x rays or injection of a sublethal dose of toxin. (The dose can be so small that it is difficult to detect illness symptoms.)

This aversion procedure has been tried with a wide variety of laboratory animals and has yielded two remarkable conclusions. First, taste stimuli are the most effective CS with mammals, and the US must be an internal illness. Second, conditioning can occur in one trial even though the CS-US interval is an hour or more. The adaptive value of this mechanism for animals foraging for food is obvious and has been recently discussed in detail (Garcia, Hankins, and Rusiniak, 1974). The point we wish to stress here is that after conditioning, animals show disgust reactions to flavors they once enjoyed. Rats dig the flavored food out of their food cup just as they do when the food is adulterated with quinine. Sheep-killing coyotes, after one or two treatments with lamb meat followed by lithium illness, are still apt to charge a lamb, but they will retch and retreat from their prey rather than consume the now disgusting lamb (Gustavson et al., 1974).

Laboratory studies with rats indicate that conditioned aversions are curiously independent of instrumental responses. If a rat is first instrumentally trained to obtain saccharin water, and is then given aversion conditioning, his instrumental approach responses are not inhibited immediately. He is apt to work for the saccharin water and then refuse to drink it for many trials (Garcia, Kovner, and Green, 1970; Holman, 1974). Thus it is not descriptively accurate to say that an animal has acquired knowledge of environmental contingencies; rather, it acts as if the incentive for which it is working has been adulterated without its knowledge.

The behavioral-contrast paradigm is another example of how incentives can be changed by training procedures (Reynolds, 1961; Premack, 1969). For example, an animal can be trained on task A according to one reinforcement schedule and on alternate days on task B according to another reinforcement schedule. If the "payoff" in task A is then reduced, responding on task B is correspondingly increased even through the payoff in task B is kept constant. Degrading the reinforcement in one task seems to increase the relative incentive value of the reinforcement in the other task. The fact that parametric manipulations in one situation affect responding in another situation on the next day without obvious mediating chains or stimulus gradients should be disturbing to behavioral theoreticians. However, most of them accept the findings without abandoning the theoretical crutches of chains and gradients for learning within the conditioning sequence.

Another example of the changes in incentive values brought about by training procedures is the schedule-induced-polydipsia paradigm (Falk, 1969). A hungry rat satiated on water is placed on a fixed-interval schedule and soon learns that it must wait for the periodic delivery of food. If a water bottle is placed in the cage, the rat will drink copious amounts of water which it does not need. The rat needs food but must wait, and so it engages in "displaced drinking," apparently because the water is there and food is not. This form of displaced behavior has been observed in a number of species engaged in a variety of activities.

Consider the difficulty this produces for investigators observing the behavioral effects of brain stimulation from electrodes placed near the motivational areas of the hypothalamus (Valenstein, 1970). Even if the electrode placement is fixed to the site where a specific behavior is controlled, motivated, or elicited, that specific behavior may be blocked in the situation, and displaced behavior may be observed in response to "demand features" of the test situation. This may account for many of the different responses observed to the same electrode placement.

Dealing conceptually with incentive changes has often been difficult for behavioral theorists. Seligman and Hager (1972) have provided examples from Thorndike's early research on the instrumental conditioning of cats in the problem box. When a lever or string was attached to a door latch, hungry cats soon learned to escape from the box to obtain a food reinforcer. At the beginning of training, the successful response was repeated in a stereotypic way; but with repeated trial and error, the response topography became more efficient as unnecessary components dropped out according to the least-effort principle. Thorndike also tried to reinforce grooming and self-scratching responses by releasing the door and allowing the hungry cat to get the food. He found that it was more difficult to train these responses with food; and when he did succeed in reinforcing self-scratching responses with food, he found that the response topography quickly changed into a mere vestige of the natural self-scratching pattern. Thorndike wrote that he was at a loss to explain why this change in response topography took place. In retrospect, the explanation seems obvious. The original self-scratching response was intrinsically motivated and reinforced. The cat's chin was itching, and scratching the area provided relief, probably via some lateral-inhibition mechanism. The itch provided the incentive to scratch and shaped the response to that end. When access to food outside the box was made contingent upon scratching, this new incentive shaped the response topography to a new end. The cat oriented toward the food, and the scratching stopped when the door of the box opened and made the food available, again according to the least-effort principle.

Intrinsic motives and incentives (e.g., an itch) and intrinsic reinforcers (e.g., itch reduction) are troublesome to anyone interested in *control* of behavior because they are difficult to manipulate. For example, socially approved behavior can be shaped in disturbed patients, such as autistic children, by operant techniques employing external reinforcers, but these children are apt to revert to their original disturbed behavior patterns when the external contingencies are terminated. Patterns, such as repetitive rocking to and fro, seem to be intrinsically rewarding to the children, and these responses are therefore difficult to bring under operant control. A method of modifying these intrinsic rewards is needed (Lovaas, Litrownik, and Mann, 1971). Behavioral research has demonstrated that incentives can be modified many ways, and this approach may be the most powerful way to modify instrumental behavior.

12.3 THE EMERGENCE OF NEUROBEHAVIORAL THEORY

Neurobehavioral theory is emerging out of its Darwinian context on the basis of research combining neural structure with behavioral function. Historically, the most frequently used experimental technique to study the relationships between learning and brain function has been to remove portions of the brain and observe the consequent alterations in behavior. The use of this approach has recently been reviewed by Thomas, Hostetter, and Barker (1968), and it is elegantly discussed in historic perspective by Isaacson (this volume). We shall merely emphasize some general problems encountered when lesion effects are assessed behaviorally.

Lesion studies have in the past been used to determine reasonable functional categories as opposed to fanciful notions derived from human social behavior, as when Flourens refuted phrenology through his experimental lesion research. However, the method is limited. Whenever broad behavioral tasks are studied, the brain seems to function with *mass action* and *equipotentiality*, as Lashley (1950) described. For example, a rat uses a variety of sensory systems in an equipotential way to master a maze. If any given subset of cues is denied him, he will use whatever cues remain to solve the maze with reduced efficiency. If a single score is used to quantify the maze performance of animals denied different subsets of cues, then mass action and equipotentiality are *necessarily* observed in the "mental process" of maze performance. But these decremental effects which can be obtained by simply masking out the cues peripherally do not tell us much about brain action. As Isaacson points out, brain lesions can even improve performance in specific tasks. In our laboratory, septal lesions and hippocampal lesions disrupted buzzer-shock conditioning but enhanced flavor-illness conditioning (McGowan, Hankins, and Garcia, 1972). These results seem paradoxical only if we assume a general S-R reinforcement process subject to mass action. If we assume that the skull houses a variety of discrete (but interrelated) input-output systems, these results do not seem so strange; they merely reflect the oft-repeated axiom that lesions tell us very little about the functions of the destroyed area. Lesions tell us more about what the animal can do without the area destroyed than about how the lesioned area functioned.

It is tempting to view the brain as an aggregation of centers each controlling a given set of behavioral functions. However, the brain's intricate complexity makes proof of functional centers extremely difficult, if not impossible. If, on the one hand, deficits in the learning or retention of a specific behavioral task are observed after brain damage, it is not possible to conclude that the damaged neural areas participate in the analysis of information concerned with learning the specific task. The damaged areas may simply be transmitting information that is processed in other areas. If, on the other hand, deficits in learning and/or retention are not observed after the occurrence of brain damage, it is still not possible to conclude that the specific area damaged does not participate in processing information concerned with the behavioral task. Neural systems may contain redundant elements organized in a parallel fashion, so that damage to one part of the system leaves the behavioral functions essentially unaltered. Nevertheless, although lesion studies have not revealed details of information processing, they have provided us with a gross outline of the functional neural systems.

Another historical approach has been focused on information processing. These studies of the neural mechanisms of learning and memory have concentrated on disturbing memory processes by presenting a gross insult after the occurrence of the behavioral event. Such experiments have differentiated what has been called "short-term memory," which can retain information up to a few hours, from "long-term memory," which may last from days and months to years (McGaugh, 1966). Presumably, events in short-term memory are somehow transferred to long-term memory. The short-term memory may involve neuronal firing, while long-term memory involves some chemical or synaptic change.

This research hinges on the assumption that some change in neural activity (i.e., activity in reverberating circuits) outlasts the behavioral event. Presumably, treatments such as electroconvulsive shock or direct electrical stimulation of the brain through chronic indwelling electrodes disrupt the orderly changes in neural activity that occur during *memory consolidation*. To date, there have been no direct demonstrations that neural activity is altered in this hypothesized manner or even that discrete neural systems are involved in the laying down of memory traces. The theory of consolidation

dates back to Müller and Pilzecker (1900). However, recent studies have demonstrated that asphyxia, which produces isopotential electroencephalograms, does not interfere with short-term memory (Baldwin and Soltysik, 1966). While the direct electrophysiological activity of single neurons was not measured in these studies, they did provide evidence contrary to the hypothesis that "consolidation" depends upon ongoing electrical activity. Specification of the neural mechanisms of memory might be advanced if, in fact, it could be demonstrated that the activity of single neurons is altered during periods of consolidation.

12.3.1 Electrical correlates of behavioral functions

Classically, as we have just described, the study of neural mechanisms of learning and memory has been concerned with the ways in which learning and memory can be manipulated by interfering with the functioning of large areas of the brain. With the advent of effective technologies for recording the electrical activity of the brain, a different approach has become possible: a correlative approach designed to reveal the neural changes accompanying behavioral changes. In quest of the neural mechanisms supporting learning and memory, it is now possible to trace electrophysiologically the neural changes associated with behavioral changes. Early studies concentrated on recording electroencephalographic activity that occurred during learning (John and Killam, 1959; Adey, Dunlop, and Hendrik, 1960).

More recently, a great deal of effort has been spent determining how individual neurons respond during organized behavioral sequences. Examples of this approach can be found in recent studies by Woody (1974) and by Olds and co-workers (1972). Woody has mapped electrophysiologically the neural pathways involved in the acquisition of a conditional eyeblink response to an auditory stimulus. These studies have correlated changes in neural activity with behavioral changes that occur during conditioning. Some of the more recent experiments (Woody and Black-Cleworth, 1973) have provided evidence of specific changes in neurons in the motor cortex being correlated with acquisition of the conditional response. Olds and his associates have attempted to track the arrival of a stimulus through the brain by recording changes in the firing patterns of single neurons produced by the occurrence of the stimulus. By this method, it is possible to trace the course of the single stimulus through the brain in time and space and to determine if the patterns of neuronal firing are altered by making the stimulus more or less significant through a pairing with reinforcement. These systematic studies of changes in neurophysiological activity hold the most promise for elucidation of the brain mechanisms in learning and memory.

12.3.2 Neurobehavioral analysis of sensory inputs

Any neurobehavioral theory should begin by taking into account the analysis of input to the organism. After all, the first step in the learning process is the detection of relevant units of information by the organism. Lesions were the first tool used for analysis of the neural processing of sensory information. More recently, recordings of changes in the firing patterns of individual neurons have provided insight into how sensory systems are organized. The visual system is a prime example. Early studies of the responsiveness of single neurons in the visual system concentrated on the effects of varying the more obvious dimensions of the physical stimulus—intensity, frequency, and location. These variations appeared to affect the neuronal activity of a great many neurons in "lower" centers of the visual system (retina, lateral geniculate nucleus) without affecting the "higher" cortical areas. Since most organisms are not in their natural environments subjected to intense, brief, pure stimuli, it is not surprising that the major cortical elements of the sensory systems do not encode such information. Natural stimuli usually consist of moving organized patterns of contours of different intensities. Therefore, the use of such stimuli challenges the evolved capacity of the organism to detect and analyze information. With the studies of Hubel and Wiesel (1959, 1962, 1963, 1965), Lettvin and co-workers (1959), Wurtz (1969), Barlow (1953), and many others, a picture of the molecular functional organization of the visual system has developed. Two principles of organization of the visual system have emerged from these studies. First, in at least the cat and monkey, more complex coding of stimuli occurs at the higher cortical loci in the system; second, the responsiveness of the system is not fixed at birth, but can be altered by environmental processes.

In the lower visual centers, most neurons in the cat and monkey have receptive fields with antagonist centers and surrounds (Hubel and Wiesel, 1961; Kozak, Rodieck, and Bishop, 1965; Wiesel and Hubel, 1966). On the other hand, neurons in the visual cortex appear to be sensitive to stimulus orientation, movement, length, and width. The cortical neuronal network appears to be arranged in a columnar form. Within columns of cortical tissue, all cells are responsive to stimuli having the same orientation. Hubel and Wiesel (1959, 1963, 1965) have described three types of cortical cells with different complexities of visual fields: simple cells, complex cells, and hypercomplex cells. In the visual-association cortex located on the inferior convexity of the temporal lobe (inferotemporal cortex), some neurons respond to even more specific properties of the stimulus. One monkey cortical neuron responds to the silhouette of a monkey's hand (Gross, Bender, and Rocha-Miranda 1969).

In short, the nervous system appears to be more receptive to units of meaning than to the classical physical parameters of the stimulus. However, these sensory elements are by no means fixed at birth. Research concerned with the development of the specific receptive-field characteristics of many of these visual cortical neurons has been reviewed at this conference by Pettigrew (see Chapter 18, this volume). Briefly, the receptive-field characteristics of visual cortical neurons may be changed with experience (Hirsch and Spinelli, 1970; Wiesel and Hubel, 1965). This plasticity appears to have a critical period in development after which the system is set and no longer responds to such manipulations. The building blocks of the visual system, and probably other sensory systems, appear to be somewhat undifferentiated at birth and only later take on the characteristics of the adult. These diverse elements are put together during development.

12.3.3 Neurobehavioral analysis of motivation

Ablation and stimulation techniques have been applied to neural mechanisms controlling motivated behavior. Some progress has been made, but as in the case of the behavioral analysis of motivation, difficulties have arisen. In particular, research concerning motivational function of the lateral hypothalamus has led to conflicting interpretations. For quite some time it has been known that large lesions of the area known as the lateral hypothalamus, which includes the medial forebrain bundle and the many ascending and descending tracts coursing through it, produces a "motivationally inert" animal (Teitelbaum and Epstein, 1962). Such animals do not eat or drink, appear hypokinetic, and are generally unresponsive to their environment. While these animals generally recover when carefully nursed, they will usually die if left to their own resources.

A parallel set of findings indicate that electrical or chemical stimulation of the same region of the brain will produce an animal that engages in various organized behavioral sequences (Valenstein, Cox, and Kakolewski, 1969a). For example, electrical stimulation can produce eating, drinking, directed attack, object carrying, etc., in virtually all species of animal tested. Similarly, chemical stimulation with putative neurotransmitters can produce eating, drinking, directed attack, etc. The behaviors that are produced have been termed "stimulus-bound" because they can be turned on and off by the application of the eliciting stimulus. Many investigators have assumed that these behaviors result from the activation of associated "drive" states such as hunger, thirst, sexual arousal, etc., by the electrical or chemical stimulation. This notion was of considerable interest in view of the classical "drive-reduction" learning theories. Theoretically the stimulation produced a drive, which was reduced by the appropriate consummatory response. Thus many of the early research endeavors in this field were aimed at demonstrating that animals would work to receive the goal object when brain stimulation was applied.

However, the same hypothalamic electrode that produces stimulus-bound behavior can be used for self-stimulation in the now-classical method of Olds and Milner (1954). The animal operates the electronic switch to shock its own brain, as though the stimulation were pleasant. Since the same electrode placement in the same animal yields both reinforcing effects and drive effects, it is difficult in "drive-reduction" terms to understand why an animal would "self-stimulate" to make itself hungry. Glickman and Schiff (1967) have postulated that the elicitation of stimulus-bound behavior is itself rewarding. Perhaps different neurons at the same lateral hypothalamic site are concerned with different aspects of behavior. Some neurons play a role in the "appetitive" or searching phase of behavior and others in the "consummatory" phase of behavior. Some of these ideas have been confirmed in subsequent correlative studies (Hamburg, 1971; Linseman and Olds, 1973) in which changes in the firing patterns of neurons in the lateral hypothalamus were correlated with changes in behavior.

Hoebel (1969) has advanced another thesis on the basis of his research. A site that produces a stimulus-bound consummatory behavior, e.g., feeding, may be a rewarding site for self-stimulation before the animal engages in that consummatory act of feeding. After the consummatory act is completed, stimulation of that same area becomes aversive. This notion is attractive because of studies such as Cabanac's (1971), which demonstrated that glucose is pleasant to subjects whose blood sugar is low, and unpleasant to subjects whose blood sugar is high. The thesis that many internal (drive) receptors guide the coping behavior of animals by changing the hedonic quality of stimuli received by peripheral receptors has been recently reviewed (Garcia, Hankins, and Rusiniak, 1974).

It has been a popular assumption that motivational mechanisms are organized in the lateral hypothalamus and related areas in a system of relatively specific and differentiated neural circuits. Different systems of neurons are concerned with the control of the different types of behavior. For example, there is an eating system, a drinking system, a copulatory system, and so forth. These ideas of separate but overlapping systems have been somewhat paralleled by the data from studies of discrete lesions. Some lesions produce more severe adipsia, while others produce more severe aphagia; still others produce impairments in sexual behavior.

In sharp contrast to this fixed-neural-circuit hypothesis, Valenstein, Cox, and Kakolewski (1970) have interpreted their research to support the alternative hypothesis, namely, that motivational mechanisms operate through a single nonspecific plastic mechanism capable of producing different and normally independent responses through learning processes. Examination of the literature on stimulus-bound behavior certainly indicates that a considerable amount of overlap exists in the anatomical sites of the different stimulus-bound responses. More than one behavior can be elicited from the same stimulating electrode. Valenstein, Cox, and Kakolewski (1968) have demonstrated that the behavior elicited by hypothalamic stimulation can be changed without any modification of stimulus parameters. For example, if a rat initially eats in response to electrical stimulation of the lateral hypothalamus, removal of food is followed in time by emergence of a second behavior—generally, drinking or wood-gnawing. Subsequently, if the animal is tested with both stimuli present, both behaviors appear with approximately equal frequencies. These behavioral shifts are not restricted to oral behavior. Digging may be substituted for eating and drinking. Male sexual behavior and eating have been elicited from the same electrode (Caggiula, 1970). Similarly, von Holst and von St. Paul (1963) have demonstrated that in the domestic fowl several different responses may be produced by stimulation of the same electrode site at different times.

Wise (1968) has offered another explanation for these controversial findings; he suggests that the shifting "stimulus-bound" behavior may be due not to a plasticity of the neural circuitry, but to the stimulation of separate but overlapping systems having different thresholds of activation. The second behavior emerges because of a gradual decrease with time in the threshold to activation of the neural system responsible for it. Therefore, Valenstein's findings may still be viewed in terms of the existence of "fixed neural circuits." Valenstein, Cox, and Kakolewski (1966) answered Wise's objections by pointing out that high-intensity stimulation, which should activate several "circuits," does not produce the second behavior in the presence of the initially preferred goal object. Additionally, after the removal of the preferred goal object, the higher-intensity stimulation gradually acquires the ability to elicit the new behavior. Immediate elicitation would be expected if the new behavior were due simply to activation of a different neural substrate with a higher threshold.

We have already pointed out the relevance of Falk's

schedule-induced polydipsia for Valenstein's thesis. Hungry animals waiting for food on a fixed-interval schedule will drink if water spouts are presented. Falk (1969) has presented evidence against either a "dry-mouth" or "adventitious-reinforcement" explanation. He considers the increase in drinking as a form of "displacement" or "adjunctive" behavior. If water is not available, other behaviors occur. When an animal is prevented from reaching a goal object, several other behaviors may occur, depending upon the demand characteristics of the environment for the driven animal. This phenomenon appears to be a behavioral analogue to Valenstein's plasticity hypothesis, but it does not exclude the possibility that fixed neural circuits exist which are interconnected in such a way that the whole hierarchy of functional systems can be stimulated from one given anatomical site.

Determination of whether the neural mechanisms of motivation are fixed or plastic circuits awaits a new line of evidence. One possibility of resolution remains. By recording neural activity and correlating changes in such activity with changes in behavior, it should be possible to determine whether neurons reflect "fixed" or "plastic" circuitry. Through use of this approach it would be possible to begin to determine whether a single neural system exists that is responsive under many different behavioral conditions, or whether different types of motivated behavior are subsumed by different but overlapping neuroanatomical circuits. Such an experiment has to our knowledge not been attempted as yet, but there are reports in the literature of manipulations of the firing patterns of hypothalamic neurons during different motivational conditions. Neurons in the lateral hypothalamus appear to be "turned off" or inhibited during the occurrence of consummatory behaviors such as eating or drinking (Hamburg, 1971). However, the question of whether the same neuron is turned off by many different behaviors remains to be answered. These neurons appear to be "turned on" or excited when an animal is searching for a goal object or performing instrumental behaviors directed toward the goal object (Olds, 1973; Linseman and Olds, 1973). While more systematic studies are necessary to determine the precise properties of the stimulus or the response that are crucial for evoking changes in unit activity, these studies at least provide a background for answering the question of whether "fixed" or "plastic" neural circuits are concerned with motivation.

12.3.4 Neurobehavioral analysis of motor outputs
In addition to the characteristics of the input and motives, neurobehavioral theories should also be able to account for the output of the organism. Our view of behavior is that, like the molecular organization of sensory systems, motor responses can be reduced to their molecular components, and the neural substrates of these components can be studied in relation to learning. In essence, these studies have already begun with the work of both Woody (1974) and Olds and co-workers (1972).

Furthermore, the developmental plasticity of sensory systems (at least the visual system) suggests that environmental manipulations that reorganize these systems might be used in a similar manner to reorganize and manipulate response systems. For example, Held and Hein (1963) have shown that sensory restriction in neonatal kittens affects their motor responding late in development. Future work might advantageously seek to determine alterations in specific neural systems concerned with elicitation of the components of the responses. However, before such work can be done, the normal course of development of response components must be determined. We have begun to study the course of development of motor-response components in neonatal kittens by measuring their gross somatomotor activity and the component movements that are associated with it. Briefly, this work indicates that some components of motor activity in kittens develop gradually, while other components appear to increase markedly in frequency at specific developmental periods. This suggests possible differences in the maturation rates of neural systems concerned with different components, and provides a temporal basis for determining if environmental manipulations can alter the subsequent frequency of occurrence of the component responses.

In summary, it is obvious that a truly neurobehavioral theory is emerging from detailed observations of neural functions in the behaving animal. The nature of afferent inputs and appropriate units of stimulation are being specified in terms of their effectiveness in challenging central neural units. The nature and the dynamic interrelations of motivational systems are under scrutiny by direct interventions, which elicit and modify characteristic patterns of motivated behavior in a variety of species. The topography of responses and the appropriate units for analysis of behavior are also becoming apparent. Behavioral paradigms that give precise control over the animal under observation are of vital importance to neural scientists, but formal behavioral theories are not very useful. A broad Darwinian functionalism is guide enough. The details of a neurobehavioral theory will become clear as some study neural mechanisms with an eye on behavior and others attempt to explain behavioral phenomena in neurological terms.

REFERENCES

ADEY, W. R., DUNLOP, C. W., and HENDRIK, C. E. 1960. Hippocampal slow waves: Distribution and phase relationships in the course of approach learning. *Archives of Neurology* 3: 74–90.

BALDWIN, B. A., and SOLTYSIK, S. 1966. The effect of cerebral ischaemia resulting in loss of EEG on the acquisition of conditioned reflexes in goats. *Brain Research* 2: 71–84.

BARLOW, H. B. 1953. Summation and inhibition in the frog's retina. *Journal of Physiology* 119: 69–88.

BRELAND, K., and BRELAND, M. 1961. The misbehavior of organisms. *American Psychologist* 16: 681–684.

BROWN, P. L., and JENKINS, H. M. 1968. Auto-shaping of the pigeon's key peck. *Journal of the Experimental Analysis of Behavior* 11: 1–8.

BRUNSWIK, E. 1955. Representative design and probabilistic theory in functional psychology. *Psychological Review* 62: 193–217.

CABANAC, M. 1971. Physiological role of pleasure. *Science* 173: 1103–1107.

CAGGIULA, A. R. 1970. Analysis of the copulation-reward properties of posterior hypothalamic stimulation in rats. *Journal of Comparative and Physiological Psychology* 70: 399–412.

CAPALDI, E. 1967. A sequential hypothesis of instrumental learning. In K. Spence and J. Spence, eds., *The Psychology of Learning and Motivation: Advances in Research and Theory*. Vol. 1. New York: Academic Press, pp. 67–156.

ESTES, W., 1960. Learning theory and the new "mental chemistry." *Psychological Review* 67: 207–223.

FALK, J. L. 1969. Conditions producing psychogenic polydipsia in animals. *Annals of the New York Academy of Science* 157: 569–593.

FLEER, R. 1972. Some behavioral observations on the ant with special reference to habit reversal learning. Unpublished Ph.D. dissertation, State University of New York at Stony Brook.

GARCIA, J., CLARKE, J., and HANKINS, W. 1973. Natural responses to scheduled rewards. In P. Bateson and P. Klopfer, eds., *Perspectives in Ethology*. New York: Plenum Press.

GARCIA, J., HANKINS, W., and RUSINIAK, K. 1974. Behavioral regulation of the milieu interne in man and rat. *Science* 185: 824–831.

GARCIA, J., KOVNER, R., and GREEN, K. 1970. Cue properties vs. palatability of flavors in avoidance learning. *Psychonomic Science* 20: 313–314.

GLICKMAN, S. E., and SCHIFF, B. B. 1967. A biological theory of reinforcement. *Psychological Review* 74: 81–109.

GROSS, C. G., BENDER, D. B., and ROCHA-MIRANDA, C. E. 1969. Visual receptive fields of neurons in inferotemporal cortex of the monkey. *Science* 166: 1303–1306.

GUSTAVSON, C., GARCIA, J., HANKINS, W., and RUSINIAK, K. 1974. Coyote predation control by aversive conditioning. *Science* 184: 581–583.

HAMBURG, M. D. 1971. Hypothalamic unit activity and eating behavior. *American Journal of Physiology* 220: 980–985.

HELD, R., and HEIN, A. 1963. Movement produced stimulation in the development of visually guided behavior. *Journal of Comparative and Physiological Psychology* 56: 872–876.

HIRSCH, H. V. B., and SPINELLI, D. N. 1970. Visual experience modifies distribution of horizontally and vertically oriented receptive fields in cats. *Science* 168: 869–871.

HOEBEL, B. 1969. Feeding and self-stimulation. *Annals of the New York Academy of Science* 157: 758–777.

HOLMAN, E. 1974. The effects of need and appetite on consum-

matory and instrumental behavior in rats. *Learning and Motivation* (in press).

HUBEL, D. H., and WIESEL, T. N. 1959. Receptive fields of single neurons in the cat's striate cortex. *Journal of Physiology* 148: 574–591.

HUBEL, D. H., and WIESEL, T. N. 1961. Integrative action in the cat's geniculate body. *Journal of Physiology* 155: 385–398.

HUBEL, D. H., and WIESEL, T. N. 1962. Receptive fields, binocular interaction and functional architecture in the cat's visual center. *Journal of Physiology* 160: 106–154.

HUBEL, D. H., and WIESEL, T. N. 1963. Shape and arrangement of columns in cat's striate cortex. *Journal of Physiology* 165: 559–668.

HUBEL, D. H., and WIESEL, T. N. 1965. Receptive fields and functional architecture in two nonstriate visual areas (18 and 19) of the cat. *Journal of Neurophysiology* 28: 229–289.

JENKINS, H., and MOORE, B. 1973. The form of the auto-shaped response with food or water reinforcers. *Journal of the Experimental Analysis of Behavior* 20: 163–181.

JENKINS, H., and SAINSBURY, R. 1969. The development of stimulus control through differential reinforcement. In N. J. MacKintosh and W. K. Honig, eds., *Fundamental Issues in Associate Learning*. Halifax: Dalhousie University Press.

JOHN, E. R., and KILLAM, K. F. 1959. Electrophysiological correlates of avoidance conditioning in the cat. *Journal of Pharmacological and Experimental Therapeutics* 125: 252–274.

KOESTLER, A. 1968. *The Ghost in the Machine.* New York: Macmillan.

KOZAK, W., RODIECK, R. W., and BISHOP, P. O. 1965. Responses of single units in lateral geniculate nucleus of cat to moving visual patterns. *Journal of Neurophysiology* 28: 19–47.

KRECHEVSKY, I. 1938. A study of the continuity of the problem-solving process. *Psychological Review* 45: 107–133.

LASHLEY, K. S. 1950. In search of the engram. *Symposia of the Society for Experimental Biology* 4: 454–482.

LETT, B. T. 1973. Delayed reward learning: Disproof of the traditional theory. *Learning and Motivation* 4: 237–246.

LETTVIN, J. Y., MATURANA, H. R., McCULLOCH, W. S., and PITTS, W. H. 1959. What the frog's eye tells the frog's brain. *Proceedings of the Institute of Radio Engineers* 47: 1940–1951.

LINSEMAN, M. A., and OLDS, J. 1973. Activity changes in rat hypothalamus, preoptic area, and striatum associated with Pavlovian conditioning. *Journal of Neurophysiology* 36: 1038–1050.

LORENZ, K. 1965. *Evolution and Modification of Behavior.* Chicago: The University of Chicago Press.

LOVAAS, O., LITROWNIK, A., and MANN, R. 1971. Response latencies to auditory stimuli in autistic children engaged in self stimulatory behavior. *Behavior Research and Therapy* 9: 39–49.

MacKINTOSH, N. 1973. Stimulus selection: Learning to ignore stimuli that predict no change in reinforcement. In R. A. Hinde and J. S. Stevenson-Hinde, eds., *Constraints on Learning.* New York: Academic Press.

McGAUGH, J. L. 1966. Time-dependent processes in memory storage. *Science* 153: 1351–1358.

McGOWAN, B., HANKINS, W., and GARCIA, J. 1972. Limbic lesions and control of the internal and external environment. *Behavioral Biology* 7: 841–852.

MENZEL, E. W. 1973. Chimpanzee spatial memory organization. *Science* 182: 943–945.

MOORE, B. 1973. The role of directed Pavlovian reactions in simple instrumental learning in the pigeon. In R. A. Hinde and J. S. Stevenson-Hinde, eds., *Constraints on Learning*. New York: Academic Press.

MÜLLER, G. E., and PILZECKER, A. 1900. *Experimentelle Beiträge zur Lehre vom Gedächtniss*. Leipzig.

OLDS, J., DISTERHOFT, J. F., SEGAL, M., KORNBLITH, C. L., and HIRSH, R. 1972. Learning centers of rat brain mapped by measuring latencies of conditioned unit responses. *Journal of Neurophysiology* 35: 202–219.

OLDS, J., and MILNER, P. 1954. Positive reinforcement produced by electrical stimulation of septal area and other regions of rat brain. *Journal of Comparative and Physiological Psychology* 47: 419–427.

OLDS, M. E. 1973. Short-term changes in the firing pattern of hypothalamic neurons during Pavlovian conditioning. *Brain Research* 58: 95–116.

PREMACK, D. 1965. Reinforcement theory. In D. Levine, ed., *Nebraska Symposium on Motivation: 1965*. Lincoln, Neb.: University of Nebraska Press, pp. 123–180.

PREMACK, D. 1969. On some boundary conditions of contrast. In J. Tapp, ed., *Reinforcement and Behavior*. New York: Academic Press.

RESCORLA, R. 1967. Pavlovian conditioning and its proper control procedures. *Psychological Review* 74: 71–80.

REVUSKY, S. 1974. Long delay learning in rats: A black and white discrimination. *Bulletin of the Psychonomic Society* (in press).

REYNOLDS, G. S. 1961. Behavioral contrast. *Journal of the Experimental Analysis of Behavior* 4: 107–117.

SELIGMAN, M. E. P., and HAGER, J., eds. 1972. *Biological Boundaries of Learning*. New York: Appleton-Century-Crofts.

SKINNER, B. F. 1959. A case history in scientific method. In S. Koch, ed., *Psychology—A Study of a Science*. New York: McGraw-Hill.

SKINNER, B. F. 1966. The phylogeny and ontogeny of behavior. *Science* 153: 1205–1213.

TEITELBAUM, P., and ESPTEIN, A. N. 1962. The lateral hypothalamic syndrome. *Psychological Review* 69: 74–90.

THOMAS, G. J., HOSTETTER, G., and BARKER, D. J. 1968. Behavioral functions of the limbic system. In E. Stellar and J. M. Sprague, eds., *Progress in Physiological Psychology*, Vol. 2. New York: Academic Press, pp. 230–311.

THORNDIKE, E. 1913. *The Psychology of Learning* (Educational Psychology II). New York: Teachers College.

TOLMAN, E. C., and BRUNSWIK, E. 1935. The organism and the causal texture of the environment. *Psychological Review* 42: 43–77.

VALENSTEIN, E. S. 1970. Stability and plasticity of motivational systems. In F. O. Schmitt, ed., *The Neurosciences: Second Study Program*. New York: Rockefeller University Press, pp. 207–217.

VALENSTEIN, E. S., COX, V. C., and KAKOLEWSKI, J. W. 1968. Modification of motivated behavior elicited by electrical stimulation of the hypothalamus. *Science* 159: 1119–1121.

VALENSTEIN, E. S., COX, V. C., and KAKOLEWSKI, J. W. 1969a. The hypothalamus and motivated behavior. In J. Tapp, ed., *Reinforcement and Behavior*. New York: Academic Press, pp. 242–285.

VALENSTEIN, E. S., COX, V. C., and KAKOLEWSKI, J. W. 1969b. Hypothalamic motivational systems: Fixed or plastic neural circuits? *Science* 163: 1084.

VALENSTEIN, E. S., COX, V. C., and KAKOLEWSKI, J. W. 1970. Re-examination of the role of the hypothalamus in motivation. *Psychological Review* 77: 16–31.

VON HOLST, E., and VON SAINT PAUL, U. 1963. On the functional organization of drives. *Animal Behaviour* 11: 1–26.

WIESEL, T. N., and HUBEL, D. H. 1965. Extent of recovery from the effects of visual deprivation in kittens. *Journal of Neurophysiology* 28: 1060–1072.

WIESEL, T. N., and HUBEL, D. H. 1966. Spatial and chromatic interactions in the lateral geniculate body of rhesus monkey. *Journal of Neurophysiology* 29: 1115–1116.

WISE, R. A. 1968. Hypothalamic motivational systems: Fixed or plastic neural circuits? *Science* 162: 377–379.

WOODY, C. D. 1974. Aspects of the electrophysiology of cortical processes related to the development and performance of learned motor responses. *Physiologist* 17: 49–69.

WOODY, C. D., and BLACK-CLEWORTH, P. 1973. Differences in excitability of cortical neurons as a function of motor projection in conditioned cats. *Journal of Neurophysiology* 36: 1104–1116.

WURTZ, R. H. 1969. Visual receptive fields of striate cortex neurons in awake monkeys. *Journal of Neurophysiology* 32: 727–742.

Ontogeny of Learning
and Memory

13

The Ontogenesis of Learning and Memory

BYRON A. CAMPBELL AND XENIA COULTER

ABSTRACT The aim of this chapter is to review and analyze the ontogenesis of learning and memory in animals and man. First comes a discussion of the phenomenon of infantile amnesia—the total lack of recall, in humans, of the first few years of life—and a brief description of some of the empirical research that has been done on that phenomenon. Next is a detailed analysis of the ontogenesis of the learning process, with emphasis on infrahuman species. The major conclusion of this section is that very young organisms are capable of learning a wide variety of responses, provided the perceptual-motor requirements are appropriate to the age studied. This is followed by a review of research on the ontogenesis of long-term memory. Here the evidence indicates that memory in infrahuman mammals is much poorer in young animals than in adults, extending the concept of infantile amnesia to phylogenetically less developed species.

The next section reviews some of the possible causes of the poor memory of infancy. Two broad classes of variables are discussed, psychological and neural. Under the first category are considered the possible effects of retroactive and proactive experience, stimulus generalization, changes in information processing, and the emergence of species-specific behaviors. Under the second category are discussed the possible effects on long-term memory of continued neural growth, synaptogenesis, myelination, and other developmental changes in brain structure and function.

In the final section maturation of the central nervous system of rat and man are compared and related to the ontogenesis of long-term memory. By and large it is observed that the emergence of long-term memory parallels functional maturation of the central nervous system in both species.

The typical adult human has, at best, only a few fragmented memories of his first years of life. Even that master of recall, Sigmund Freud, was unable to discover, in himself or others, any remembrance of early childhood. For centuries this seemed to be an entirely normal situation, a natural corollary of the immaturity of the child's mind. But on closer examination of the developing child, many questions and paradoxes arise concerning the nature and course of this universal lack of recall, appropriately described by Freud as "infantile amnesia." It is clear from even the most casual observations that very young children are completely capable of registering and recalling memories, naming ob-

jects, and recognizing places and people seen sometimes only very briefly. The clarity of these memories has often been a subject of astonishment, probably because of the adult's near-total amnesia for that period of life. Darwin (1965), for example, cited the following instance:

I do not know whether it is worth mentioning, as showing something about the strength of memory in a young child, that this one when 3 years and 23 days old on being shown an engraving of his grandfather, whom he had not seen for exactly 6 months, instantly recognized him and mentioned a whole string of events which had occurred whilst visiting him, and which had never been mentioned in the interval. (p. 125)

Without doubt all parents have had similar experiences. Perhaps more astonishing, at least from a scientist's point of view, is that after several years it becomes apparent that the child, now growing up, has forgotten events and circumstances it was once perfectly capable of recalling.

Attempts to explain or even describe infantile amnesia have been sadly lacking in both scope and depth. Freud, of course, had the most colorful explanation. He believed that the primitive libidinal, selfish, and destructive impulses of infancy become so distressing to the developing child that they are repressed simultaneously with the resolution of the Oedipus complex. Little evidence has accumulated to support this view, and it now seems that other, more mundane phenomena are the basis of infantile amnesia.

The little research that has been done on infantile amnesia has focused on the ability of college students to recall their first few years of life. By and large the first event recalled in these studies occurred between the third and fourth year of life, although for some the earliest memory came from as late as age nine (Waldfogel, 1948). Of interest are the lack of a positive correlation between age of earliest memory and intelligence score, and the variety, in terms of emotional content, of first events recalled (Dudycha and Dudycha, 1941). For most young adults, memories of early childhood begin to achieve some clarity in kindergarten or first grade, with the sharpness of memory continuing to increase through the primary-school years.

BYRON A. CAMPBELL and XENIA COULTER, Department of Psychology, Princeton University, Princeton, NJ

During the thirties, when the concept of infantile amnesia was in vogue due to the omnipresence of Freud, a number of alternatives to Freud's "repression" theory were put forth. These have been summarized by Allport (1937) as follows:

1. Infant experiences are not verbalized and, therefore, cannot be held as concepts in consciousness.

2. The areas of the cortex involved in conscious memory are not myelinized and, therefore, are unable to hold "traces" of experience.

3. The apperceptive context of early life is so different from that of adulthood that events occurring in it cannot be recalled.

As is the case for much of our analysis of the memory process, little progress has been made in understanding the basis of infantile amnesia since these formulations were introduced. The most visible advance in recent years has been the proliferation of possible explanations of the poor memory of infancy (Campbell and Spear, 1972), a tradition we shall continue here. The major aim of the chapter will be to review and analyze the ontogenesis of learning and memory in animals and man and to discuss the neural and behavioral processes that might underlie the age-dependent differences in these phenomena.

13.1 THE ONTOGENESIS OF LEARNING

The first question that arises in regard to any type of amnesia is whether the inability to retain material can be attributed to some kind of deficit in the quality of the original learning. References to poor memories in children, such as those by Rousseau (1965), often assume the cause to arise from the initial learning process:

Although memory and reason are wholly different faculties, the one does not really develop apart from the other. Before the age of reason the child receives images, not ideas; and there is this difference between them: images are merely the pictures of external objects, while ideas are notions about those objects determined by their relations. . . .

I maintain, therefore, that. . .children. . .have no true memory. They retain sounds, form sensations, but rarely ideas, and still more rarely relations. . . .All their knowledge is on the sensation-level, nothing has penetrated to their understanding. Their memory is little better than their other powers, for they always have to learn over again when they are grown up what they learnt as children. (p. 83)

In the adult, there is certainly every indication that degree of original learning is an important determinant of memory. In fact, in one of the most recent theories of memory (Craik, 1973), an important learning variable,

depth of analysis, is made to play an almost exclusive role in determining subsequent retention. If young organisms truly are deficient in learning capacity, this alone might be sufficient to account for their subsequent inability to remember.

Unfortunately, learning capacity in immature organisms is extremely difficult to assess. This is so because it is adult performance that is used as a standard of comparison. As several writers have pointed out (Campbell, 1967; Zimmerman and Torrey, 1965), the need to equalize all conditions except age makes adult-young comparisons almost methodologically impossible. This is particularly true of motivation. Furthermore, the assessment problem is compounded by the very real question of whether such comparisons, even if possible, are appropriate. The use of adult behavior as a yardstick presupposes, as Kessen (1965) has expressed it, that the child is merely a reduced adult. Rather than asking whether learning capacity develops, the notion that the child is father to the man assumes that it does and ignores the possibility that learning by immature organisms may occur without any necessary relationship to adult learning. As a result, it is sometimes difficult to evaluate adequately much of the developmental-learning literature.

13.1.1 Learning capacity: Neonatal studies

One common approach to assessing infantile learning is to ask whether an immature organism can learn a given task at all. Questions of "capacity" (Zimmerman and Torrey, 1965) are particularly relevant in neonatal-learning research, that is, in studies where the chief behavioral characteristic of the ages studied is a severely limited sensory and response repertoire (relative to subsequent development). The absence at these ages of much of the behavior typically used to measure learning in adults has suggested to some writers not only that particular tasks cannot be learned, but that newborns may not be able to learn at all (Preyer, 1965; Spitz, 1959). Several reports of attempts to condition even such apparently simple responses as leg flexion in newborn dogs (Cornwall and Fuller, 1961; Fuller, Easler, and Banks, 1950; James and Cannon, 1952) have lent support to the idea that learning cannot take place until after a certain amount of postnatal neural maturation. Even habituation, considered by some to be a very simple form of learning, has been reported by several investigators to require some degree of postnatal development (Nikitiva and Novikova, cited by Lynn, 1966; Scott and Marston, 1950). Thus, in various descriptive or theoretical accounts of development, the first appearance of the ability to learn per se is frequently cited as an important signpost in the course of development (Bronson, 1965; Fox, 1965; Scott, 1968; Thompson, 1968).

In contrast to such views, there have been a growing number of reports, especially during the last ten years, suggesting that many forms of learning can be observed in animals at much younger ages than had previously been thought possible. Although Harlow (1959) and others (e.g., Mason and Harlow, 1958a) demonstrated quite early that responses by newborn monkeys could be classically conditioned, it is the more recent work by Lipsitt and Papousek with human infants that seems to have had the greatest impact in this area. In a series of studies, Lipsitt (1969) has provided dramatic evidence that newborn infants can be readily habituated to novel stimuli, and that they can also respond rapidly and efficiently to both Pavlovian and operant-conditioning contingencies. Concurrently, a number of investigators have reported similarly dramatic evidence for learning at very early ages in other altricial species.

In the albino rat, Caldwell and Werboff (1962) have shown that a vibrotactile CS can be aversively conditioned on the first day of life. More recently Thoman, Wetzel, and Levine (1968) have reported that tube-fed rat pups produce anticipatory conditioned responses by day three. Similarly, in puppies, Fox (1971) has reported that both habituation to odors and conditioning to odor cues can be established within five days of birth. Furthermore, Stanley et al. (1963) have demonstrated both appetitive and aversive Pavlovian conditioning to taste cues by day nine. Extending these early findings, Stanley and his collaborators have since shown that instrumental behavior can also be demonstrated in neonatal puppies. One- to seven-day-old beagles will learn to approach a cloth or wire stimulus for milk reinforcement (Stanley, Bacon, and Fehr, 1970); by day nine, puppies can learn to avoid a cloth-towel CS paired with a cold-air-blast UCS after five days of training (Bacon and Stanley, 1970a); and puppies less than two weeks of age not only will learn an appetitive discrimination reversal, but will also improve in reversal learning over a seven-day period (Bacon and Stanley, 1970b). Very recently Bacon (1973) has begun to test neonatal kittens in situations similar to those used with puppies, and he reports that instrumental avoidance learning can be seen in cats, as in dogs, by the third day of life.

A somewhat different approach to the same question is represented by the work of Rosenblatt and his colleagues with newborn kittens. Taking issue with those who argue that much of early behavior is innately organized (Kovach and Kling, 1967; Ewer, 1961), Rosenblatt (1971) has tried to show that newborns are not only capable of learning, but also exercise this capacity in the normal course of activity during the first few days, even hours, of life. In a series of studies, he has provided evidence that it is the learning of various olfactory, tactile, and thermal discriminations that accounts for the ability of newborn kittens to locate a pathway to the mother and to identify and grasp a particular nipple (Rosenblatt, 1972). Similar observations of neonatal learning have been presented for puppies by Fox (1971). Analogously, although relevant to a somewhat older age group, Galef and Clark (1971) have suggested that rat pups learn what foods they can safely eat from cues supplied by adults.

In sum, the latest evidence indicates that learning can and does take place in neurologically undeveloped organisms. Successes have been sufficient to suggest to Lipsitt (1971) that the capacity to learn may be at its peak at this point in development. Failures to obtain evidence of neonatal learning in earlier studies may be related to the fact that in those studies neonatal behavior was assessed in relation to adult behavior, a tactic which has been largely abandoned by later investigators. That is, failures occurred when responses to be conditioned were not yet in the animal's repertoire (see Rosenblatt, 1972), or when stimuli were employed that the animals could not yet perceive (see Cornwall and Fuller, 1961). Given that the task demands are appropriate to the neonatal state, learning apparently occurs without difficulty. The results of the more recent studies could possibly warrant the conclusion that learning "derives from a fundamental property of living matter and therefore does not necessarily require special complex neuronal circuits" (Hernández-Peón, 1966, p. 18). Whether or not one accepts this view of learning, it still seems unlikely that retention failures by young organisms can be attributed to some fundamental deficiency in their capacity to learn.

13.1.2 Learning rate: Juvenile studies of simple tasks

Even if young organisms are capable of learning, they may be unable to learn efficiently, that is, the strength of what they have learned may be insufficient to enable them to retain material for any length of time. Questions of learning strength are typically studied by comparing animals at different ages in the rate of acquisition of some particular task. If it takes young animals longer to learn than adults, it can be assumed that learning is in some way more difficult for the younger animal. Since the "rate" approach (Zimmerman and Torrey, 1965) requires that the animal be capable of performing the task, research in this area frequently involves juvenile organisms, which, while not yet physically or neurologically fully developed, are not observably limited in either sensory or response capability. The tasks used for these studies vary considerably in their complexity.

SIMPLE APPROACH AND ESCAPE. Conceptually, one of the simplest types of learning tasks has as its only requirement that the animal learn a particular response-reinforcement contingency. This might involve simple appetitive tasks such as running down an alley or pressing a manipulandum for food, or aversive tasks such as running or jumping to escape a noxious stimulus. There are surprisingly few age-related studies employing only such contingencies. Most simple approach or escape studies involving immature animals have been concerned with demonstrating that some learning does take place or with exploring the use of new types of reinforcements uniquely adapted to a very young organism (e.g., Stanley and Elliot, 1962; Bacon and Stanley, 1963; Stanley, Morris, and Trattner, 1965). One reason why there are so few studies with this simple paradigm may be that in these tasks learning is typically assessed in terms of response speed, a measure which could put the very young (or very old) organism at a disadvantage. This problem can be avoided if a trials-to-criterion measure is used, or if there are alternative goals such that learning can be measured in terms of the number of trials it takes the animal to choose consistently the correct goal.

Both such procedures were used by Stone (1929a, b) in one of the earliest adequately controlled studies of developmental learning. He trained rats ranging in age from 30 to 700 days to escape shock by jumping to a platform, or to one of three platforms, or to approach food in a maze. The overall results indicated that these tasks are learned at the same rate regardless of the age at which training takes place. In fact, older rats were, if anything, somewhat inferior.

Of the very few more recent studies using only approach tasks, nearly all have been concerned with the inferior performance of older rats, that is, with the effects of aging rather than development. Thus the youngest rats used in these studies have typically been no less than 60 to 90 days of age (Botwinick, Brinley, and Rabbin, 1962; Goodrick, 1968; Birren, 1962). One exception is a study by McGaugh and Cole (1965), who compared maze-bright and maze-dull rats at 150 days of age with those around 30 days of age. Using a Lashley III maze and two different intertrial intervals, they found that both young and old maze-bright rats learned at the same rate at either interval, but that young maze-dull rats learned more slowly than adults at the longer (30 min) interval.

It is surprising that young rats have been so seldom studied in such tasks, particularly since Kirkby (1967) has reported that they are less likely than adults to switch choices in a T maze after the first trial. Since a typical procedure in maze-training is to designate the alley opposite the first choice, arbitrarily, as the correct goal, one might expect young animals to do more poorly. With monkeys, in any event, this does not seem to be a problem. Mason and Harlow (1958b) found no differences between 15- and 45-day-olds in the speed with which they learned to approach the correct end of a Y maze. Both ages learned without difficulty in about six to nine trials.

There have been considerably more developmental rate studies using simple escape tasks. Crockett and Nobel (1963) found no difference between 21- and 90-day-old rats in the speed with which they learned to escape light. With mice of six different strains, Meier (1965) trained seven age groups ranging from 21 to 147 days of age to escape from a three-choice water maze. In nearly all strains on all measures, including reversal learning, the youngest mice learned at the fastest rate. Slower rates of learning always occurred in the older animals. Similar although less dramatic results have been reported by Smith (1968) with rats. Using shock as the noxious stimulus, he trained rats of 25, 100, and 175 days of age to escape by running to one of four possible goals. Again, only the oldest rats showed an impairment in learning rate. It is interesting that Birren (1962), studying rats in a water maze similar to Meier's, attributed the poorer performance of older rats to the fact that they may have greater dependence upon body-orientation cues than younger rats because they are less sensitive to other perceptual cues. By designing a task in which body orientation was the most salient cue, he was able to eliminate all age differences in learning the task.

Since rats older than 20 days are clearly able to learn simple aversive tasks at optimal rates, some investigators have begun to examine the abilities of somewhat younger animals. For example, Campbell et al. (1974) studied rats ranging from 15 to 35 days of age trained to escape shock in a single-choice T maze. They noted that the 15-day-old rats appeared to learn somewhat more slowly than the 17-, 20-, or 25-day-olds. This difference, however, was very small and resembled a similarly slow rate of learning by the 35-day-old group. According to Nagy and Murphy (1974), escape-learning deficits occur at ages much younger than those examined by Campbell's group. Testing mice pups of 5, 7, 9, and 11 days of age, Nagy and Murphy found that they could learn to escape when they were 9 days of age, but not earlier. However, these investigators defined escape learning as a reduction in turning in response to shock, and it is not clear that this type of response can be properly classified as escape. The behavioral change that normally defines escape learning is a reduction in response latency. It seems apparent that latency changes in a runway situation require a certain level of motor development since they cannot be observed in either rats (Misanin et al., 1971) or mice (Nagy and Misanin, 1973) until almost 15 days of age. Thus the deficit reported by Nagy and Murphy for younger animals may simply reflect an age-dependent change in reactivity to shock. Similarly, another report of early deficiencies in escape learning (James and Binks, 1963) can also be attributed to perceptual-motor deficits rather than to learning differences. In this study it was shown that chickens cannot learn to escape shock until the second day after hatching. However, Peters and Isaacson (1963) found that if cold water is used as the aversive stimulus, newborn chickens are as capable of learning to escape as 2-, 5-, 7-, or 10-day-olds. Thus the ability to acquire an escape contingency was apparently not deficient at any age, indicating that in James and Binks's study it was the ability to perceive or respond to a particular type of stimulus that changed with age.

In sum, the available evidence suggests that a certain level of maturity is not a necessary condition for animals to acquire the basic response-reinforcement contingencies that characterize simple approach or escape tasks. Where performance deficits have been found, they often seem to have been caused by age-related perceptual-motor deficiencies rather than by an inability to learn the required contingency. Nonetheless, the number of studies related to this issue have been remarkably few, and this conclusion must necessarily be somewhat tentative.

SPATIAL AVOIDANCE AND CER. Another conceptually simple task requires the animal to learn not that a response and a reinforcer are contiguous, but that a contingency exists between a stimulus (CS) and a reinforcer (UCS). Learning, or conditioning, is then assessed in terms of an altered level of responding to the CS. In some cases this change in responsiveness is represented by the development of highly specific anticipatory or preparatory behavior, such as a change in heart rate, salivation, leg flexion or eyeblink. Such responses have been used most often in studies assessing neonatal learning (e.g., Mason and Harlow, 1958a: Caldwell and Werboff, 1962). One briefly described study used this molecular type of response change for comparing rats 1, 3, 5, and 10 days of age (Gray and Yates, 1967), but with too few subjects to make any age-related conclusions possible. Much more frequently, different ages have been compared by means of a more general type of molar response

change, specifically the degree to which the presentation of a CS changes some already established ongoing behavior. A common example, particularly with rats, is the conditioned-emotional-response (CER) paradigm, in which, after being exposed to a certain number of stimulus-shock pairings, rats stop bar-pressing or drinking in response to the stimulus alone. Another common task used with rats is spatial avoidance, in which the animal suppresses its normal tendency to approach a particular location (usually a darkened compartment) that has previously been associated with noxious stimulation (usually shock).

Some accounts of the effects of age on the acquisition of stimulus contingencies suggest that younger rats may require more CS-UCS pairings than older rats to acquire stable conditioning. For example, Brunner, Roth, and Rossi (1970) reported that after one CS-UCS pairing, 50- and 120-day-old rats show significant amounts of lick-suppression, whereas 25-day-old pups do not. Similarly, Wilson and Riccio (1973) found that with three CS-US pairings, 23-day-old rats condition less well than 30- and 90-day-olds. In contrast, conditioning studies with many CS-US pairings have not shown any significant age differences. For example, Snedden, Spevack, and Thompson (1971) report that with thirty CS-US pairings, 26-day-old rats acquire lick-suppression as well as 37- and 72-day-olds. Also, Campbell and Campbell (1962), with fifteen CS-US pairings, and Coulter and Collier (unpublished data) with twelve, found no differences in suppression between young (23- to 25-day-old) pups and adults.

Investigators who have directly measured the number of pairings necessary for suppression to occur have not been able to find any age-related effects. Frieman et al. (1971) observed that, if anything, 18-day-old pups required fewer trials (7.7) than adults (8.8) to attain 90 percent suppression to three successive presentations of the CS. Similarly, Green (1962) found no differences in rate of acquisition among monkeys 1, 30, and 300 days of age; ongoing activity was equally suppressed in all three age groups after only a few CS-US presentations.

It is possible that the deficits observed by Brunner, Roth, and Rossi (1970) and Wilson and Riccio (1973) were due, not to the number of CS-US pairings, but rather to the use of brief intertrial intervals. Frieman, Warner, and Riccio (1970) exposed young and adult rats to what would seem to be an adequate number of trials (12 CS presentations and 15 presentations of the US). However, the one-second US (shock) was presented intermittently during the one-minute CS (tone) at a relatively rapid rate. Interestingly enough, the pups failed to acquire as much suppression as did the adults. It has occasionally been suggested that young rats may learn best with long intervals between trials, on the premise that immature organisms require more time for memory consolidation than adults (Thompson, 1957; Doty and Doty, 1964; Doty, 1966; Dye, 1969). Although the effect of varying the length of intertrial intervals with different age groups has never been tested with simple stimulus-contingent tasks, Caldwell and Werboff (1962) have reported on the effects of increasing the time between stimuli in such a task with newborn rats. They noted that pups appear to condition quite rapidly with longer interstimulus intervals than are optimal for adults, an effect that they also attributed to slow rates of memory consolidation in young animals. Some data from our laboratory may also bear upon this issue; we have found that three CS-US pairings, at 23, 30, and then 37 days of age, culminates in complete suppression of bar-pressing, whereas three CS-US pairings spaced minutes apart normally results in only slight suppression, even with adult rats (Coulter, 1974).

The results of spatial-avoidance studies do not provide much information regarding possible age differences in the acquisition of stimulus contingencies, since in none of these studies has the number of trials or the time between trials been systematically examined. In general, young animals have been shown to learn spatial avoidance as well as adults (Campbell and Campbell, 1962). Although Rohrbaugh and Riccio (1968) found that 18-day-olds avoided the compartment in which they had been shocked somewhat less than adults, this difference was very small; furthermore, the parameters in this study were almost identical to those of a subsequent study (Frieman, Rohrbaugh, and Riccio, 1969) in which no differences between pups and adults were observed.

In conclusion, the apparently simple question of whether young animals can learn stimulus contingencies at the same rate as adults requires a conditional answer. Under most circumstances young rats easily condition as well as adults. In those instances when they do not, it is not clear whether it is because young rats require more trials than adults or because they learn best with a particular set of temporal parameters. There is so little relevant data, however, that at this point it is difficult to assert that any real deficiency exists in younger animals, particularly since stimulus-contingent tasks have been used with such success for demonstrating efficient learning by neonatal animals.

ACTIVE AVOIDANCE. Unlike simple approach and escape tasks, or tests of spatial avoidance or CER, active avoidance is a task that is fairly difficult to characterize. It differs from escape learning in that some type of warning precedes the onset of the noxious stimulus, so that the animal can avoid the noxious consequences altogether.

In keeping with its procedural simplicity, at least one contemporary investigator conceptualizes the task in terms of simple response-reinforcement learning, in which, as in escape, the reinforcing consequence is a reduction in noxious stimulation (Herrnstein, 1969). In contrast, other investigators have treated this task as if it represented another example of stimulus-contingency learning (e.g., Hull, 1943). In this view avoidance, like suppression, is a molar change in behavior that results from the pairing of a warning signal (CS) with noxious stimulation (US). Most students of learning, however, consider active avoidance to be a task in which the animal is required to learn both types of contingency (see Kimble, 1961). In this view one might expect age-related differences, if they exist, to become accentuated by the increased requirements of the task.

Nonetheless, of the large number of studies using simple active avoidance as a means for studying developmental changes in learning, none has reported age effects any greater than those so far described. The history of these studies is, however, instructive. In six studies reported between 1958 and 1966, all but one (Kirby, 1963) showed that the youngest age group takes longer to learn avoidance than adults, and "young" in these studies referred to rats no less than 25, and in one case 50, days of age. (Denenberg and Kline, 1958; Denenberg and Smith, 1963; Doty and Doty, 1964; Thompson, Koenigsberg, and Tennison, 1965; Doty, 1966). Yet, in nine studies described in the literature since 1967, not one has replicated this deficit (Porter and Thompson, 1967; Goldman and Tobach, 1967; Riccio, Rohrbaugh, and Hodges, 1968; Fiegley and Spear, 1970; Klein and Spear, 1969; Riccio and Marrazo, 1972; Brennan and Riccio, 1972; Parsons and Spear, 1972). Animals over 20 days of age now learn to avoid just as rapidly as adults. On the other hand, of these recent studies, the three in which rats younger than 20 days were included all report deficits in the current youngest age group: at 19 days of age (Riccio, Rohrbaugh, and Hodges, 1968), 16 days (Klein and Spear, 1969), and even 10 days of age (Goldman and Tobach, 1967). Are young albino rats becoming more intelligent as time progresses, or is it possible that experimenters are becoming more proficient at arranging optimal conditions for learning at younger ages?

Learning to avoid by running, as is true of all these studies, demands a certain level of motor development, particularly since the response must be made within a very short period of time (typically, 5 seconds). Bolles (1970) has recently argued that the task is quickly learned by adult rats because experimenters have designed it so as to capitalize upon an innate response to aversive stimulation. If this type of response undergoes changes during development, it should not be surprising that younger rats appear to have difficulty in learning its requirements. Furthermore, the CS itself can be an inappropriate one for younger animals. Bacon (1973), for example, studying avoidance learning in neonatal kittens, found that when the CS was a cloth-lined compartment, 3- to 7-day-old kittens could not learn to avoid, whereas they could learn when the compartment was made of plastic mesh.

Thus it would seem that even when younger animals appear to learn avoidance more slowly than older animals, it is not necessarily because they are deficient in their ability to learn the required associations. Experimenters can eliminate these "learning deficiencies" merely by using stimuli or requiring responses more appropriate to the age studied. One must therefore conclude that even though such learning may involve both response and stimulus contingencies, young animals can learn active avoidance just as readily as they can learn simpler approach and escape tasks, spatial avoidance, and CER, and that under the proper conditions they can learn as rapidly as adults.

13.1.3 Learning rate: Juvenile studies of more complex situations

Thus far the evidence suggests that young organisms do not seem to be deficient in their ability to form associations between responses and reinforcements or between stimuli. When we turn to studies of developmental differences in rates of learning more complex tasks—that is, those involving either new kinds of contingencies or several contingencies at one time—the evidence is more difficult to assess. In particular, the effects of inappropriate perceptual-motor requirements become aggravated by complexity, and it becomes increasingly difficult to disentangle these effects from possible deficiencies in the ability of young animals to acquire the necessary contingencies.

DISCRIMINATIONS. One kind of added complexity is seen whenever discriminations are required. To learn a discrimination task the animal must first of all be capable of distinguishing between two stimuli. Several studies suggest that young animals require more experience with stimuli than do adults before they are able to distinguish between them. Certainly with monkeys, a species most often studied in this respect, visual discriminations are learned increasingly more rapidly during the first month of life (Zimmerman and Torrey, 1965). Furthermore, adult rates for learning different types of visual discriminations are achieved at different times throughout this period. Although Zimmerman (1961) and Harlow et al. (1960) present somewhat different age functions, both agree that adultlike rates of learning are first attained for simple spatial-discrimination tasks, followed by brightness discriminations, then simple-form, and finally complex-form discriminations.

No other species has been studied as systematically. Fox (1971) has described a study of black-white discrimination learning with puppies aged 5, 8, 12, and 16 weeks of age. He reports that older dogs tend to learn more rapidly than younger dogs, although not significantly more so. If puppies less than 5 weeks of age could have been tested, or if a more difficult discrimination had been required, the difference would probably have been significant. With rats, there are practically no studies of the development of discriminative abilities. Thompson (1957), although he presents no data, does mention that young rats are slower at acquiring pattern discriminations than adults, and Roberts (1966) has stated that visual discriminative capacities in rats improve up to about 40 days of age. Since rats are not highly dependent upon vision, it would be of interest to know whether there is a developmental sequence of discriminative ability, analogous to that observed in monkeys, within a sensory system of greater importance to the rat, such as olfaction. To date no such data are available.

When they are observed, age differences in the rates of learning various kinds of discriminations can be interpreted to indicate merely that perceptual abilities, like motor abilities, improve with age. The fact that a young rat makes a particular discrimination with difficulty may be no more relevant to how rapidly it can learn a particular contingency than the fact that a young rat locomotes with difficulty. However, discrimination deficiencies are important in that they may penalize a younger subject, so that the animal appears to be deficient in learning. Even if the perceptual requirements of the task seem to be simple, certain species, particularly subprimates, may be responding to cues unnoticed by the experimenter and there may be developmental differences in how well these uncontrolled aspects of the task are perceived.

One way to test for stimulus control is to use a generalization test (Terrace, 1966). The more the animal is under the control of the stimulus specified by the experimenter, the more its performance is disrupted as that cue is altered. Interestingly enough, in at least three studies that have compared young and adult animals in terms of stimulus generalization (Rohrbaugh and Riccio, 1968; Frieman, Rohrbaugh, and Riccio, 1969; Frieman, Warner, and Riccio, 1970), the older animals have consistently shown less stimulus control (i.e., greater generalization). The significance of these findings is not at all clear.

Given that an animal is able to discriminate between two stimuli, a discrimination task also requires the animal to learn a particular contingency that is relevant to one stimulus (S+ with response-reinforcement contingencies; CS+ with stimulus-contingent tasks) and not to another (S− or CS−). This requirement clearly makes the task more difficult regardless of age. Doty (1966), for example, compared simple avoidance to discriminated avoidance; in the latter task rats could avoid shock only if they ran to a lighted compartment rather than to an unlighted one. She found that introducing discrimination caused the performance level to drop by half in both adult and young rats. Although the younger rats learned both tasks more slowly than adults, the discrimination requirement did not enhance this deficiency. It is interesting that in a later study of discriminated avoidance, Doty (1968) found that if younger rats were handled for 20 days prior to training, they then learned the task faster than adults. A similar handling effect has been reported by Denenberg and Smith (1963), although with somewhat older animals. In general, however, most investigators have found that, regardless of difficulty, both young and adult rats acquire the discriminative contingency at the same rate, whether with discriminated avoidance tasks (Thompson, 1957; Dye, 1969) or with appetitive tasks such as running for water (D'Amato and Jagoda, 1960) or running, jumping or bar-pressing for food (Kay and Sime, 1962; Fields, 1953; Campbell, Jaynes, and Misanin, 1968).

Even if no differences in rate of learning are directly observed, there may be developmental differences in how a discrimination contingency is learned. As Jenkins (1965) has suggested, there are at least two strategies possible with a discrimination task: the animal may learn only to pay attention to the positive stimulus (following the rule, respond to S+, otherwise do nothing), or the animal may respond to S+ and also actively inhibit responding to S−. Just as with positive stimuli, negative-stimulus control can be assessed by means of a generalization test, but in this case performance should be disrupted in a direction opposite to that resulting from a test of S+. Bacon (1971), for example, trained two-week-old puppies to approach one set of tactile cues and not another, and then he exposed the animals to a variety of tactile cues. As the cues increasingly differed from S+, the young animals approached the goal more slowly; but as the cues increasingly differed from S−, the puppies did not tend to approach them more. Thus he found no evidence for negative-stimulus control in this task. Since no other ages were tested, it is impossible to know how this might compare with older animals in the same situation. Paré (1969) trained rats of four different ages in a discriminated CER situation

in which one tone was paired with shock (CS+) while another was explicitly not paired with shock (CS−). He observed that during acquisition older animals generalized more from CS+ to CS− than did younger animals, which could mean that they were attending more to the negative stimulus than were the younger animals. However, the strengths of the two stimuli were not explicitly tested. On the other hand, Brennan and Riccio (1972) examined the effects of Pavlovian discrimination training upon subsequent responding to altered values of a CS+ in an active-avoidance situation. Both 18-day-old pups and adults made increasingly fewer avoidance responses as the test values approached the CS−, in comparison to animals without CS− experience. Thus, in this instance, young animals appeared to learn as much about the negative stimulus as did adults.

In sum, it seems evident that while discriminative abilities, like motor abilities, develop with age, young animals do not appear to be particularly deficient in their ability to learn the discriminative contingencies required by a given task. However, the degree of this control may still differ at different ages. Even if they do, it is not clear whether such differences would arise from subtle discrimination deficiencies in the young animals or from a difference in learning strategy. Only more data will clarify these issues.

Passive avoidance and delayed responding. One skill which most investigators agree is difficult for young animals is the ability to inhibit previously established responses. We have reviewed the history of this idea elsewhere (Campbell, Riccio, and Rohrbaugh, 1971) and shall only remark again that the notion that inhibitory control develops slowly and only after excitatory control is established has been with us since the days of Hughlings Jackson. It is a particularly attractive hypothesis because it has physiological as well as behavioral implications. The behavioral evidence of inhibitory deficits early in development has arisen in part from studies of passive avoidance, a task in which animals must learn not to make a response (in particular, not to run from one compartment to another) in order to avoid noxious stimulation. In every study in which young rats have been compared to older rats on this task, whether the pups have been 10 (Riccio and Schulenberg, 1969), 15 (Riccio, Rohrbaugh, and Hodges, 1968; Schulenberg, Riccio, and Stikes, 1971), 20 (Brunner, 1969; Riccio and Marrazo, 1972), or 25 days of age (Fiegley and Spear, 1970), they have consistently learned with significantly greater difficulty than adults. Since pups at the same age do not have comparable difficulty learning active avoidance (that is, running from one compartment to another), investigators have attributed the difference to the fact that a response must be inhibited.

A similar interpretation has been applied to results arising from studies of the delayed-response task. In this task the animal is shown the location of a reinforcement, which is then covered from view for a given amount of time before the animal is permitted to obtain it. To perform this task successfully the animal may have to orient itself toward the goal during the delay, a requirement that young animals could have difficulty meeting. In fact, the length of time that they can withhold, or inhibit, their normal activity changes drastically as they grow older. Monkeys of less than 5 months of age perform very poorly with delays even as short as 5 seconds, and it is not until they are 8 or 9 months of age that they can respond well with delays up to 40 seconds (Harlow et al., 1960). Similar data have been reported by Fox (1971) for dogs, except that the deficit exists over a much shorter period of time. At 4 weeks the puppies can tolerate delays only up to about 3 seconds, but by 12 weeks they can perform as well as adults, with delays as long as 120 seconds. Surprisingly, no such deficit has yet been demonstrated in kittens (Wikmark, 1974); if it exists in cats, the inability to tolerate delays must occur well before weaning, much earlier than has been found in dogs.

If, indeed, young animals are deficient in their ability to inhibit responding, one could argue that this deficiency does not necessarily relate to the animal's ability to learn. As we have already suggested several times, age-dependent motor deficits should be considered separately from the assessment of an organism's ability to acquire contingencies. However, despite the attractiveness and simplicity of attributing response-inhibition deficits to young animals, this explanation may not be sufficient or even likely to account for the results of developmental studies of passive avoidance or delayed responding.

First of all, it is essentially not true that young animals always experience difficulty in response inhibition. Newborn babies will immediately inhibit sucking when confronted with a novel stimulus (Lipsitt, 1971). Habituation to that stimulus consists in overcoming what appears to be a very strong, natural tendency to withhold responding. Furthermore, as we have already mentioned, young animals do not have difficulty acquiring CER, a behavior that is assessed exclusively in terms of the animal's ability to inhibit ongoing responses. Even more to the point, passive-avoidance deficits by young animals are not seen at all times or in all species. For example, Grote and Brown (1971) have shown that rat pups are perfectly capable of learning passive avoidance in a single trial when licking is paired with poison.

With dogs, Fox (1971) trained 5-, 8-, and 12-week-old puppies to approach a human observer who then shocked the animals on the ear. In this instance the 5-week-old puppies rapidly learned to stop approaching the observer, whereas the oldest group could not learn to inhibit the approach response. Thus no inhibitory deficits were observed at an age at which they should have been most pronounced.

In addition to the fact that inhibitory deficits are not always seen in young animals, there is no real evidence to indicate that the difficulties experienced in learning passive avoidance are positively correlated with comparable difficulties in learning delayed-response tasks. In one of the few studies of delayed responding by rats (Doty, 1966), 20-, 150-, and 730-day-old rats were required to wait 5 seconds after the offset of the CS before running to a lighted compartment to avoid shock. Performance relative to simple active avoidance was very poor in all age groups, although the 150-day-old animals did avoid consistently more often than either the youngest or oldest animals. However, the difficulty experienced by the extreme age groups appeared to be unrelated to the delay per se because, in this study at least, both the 30- and 730-day-old rats were inferior to the 150-day-old animals on all tasks, and only one involved a delay. Thus no convincing data exist to suggest that rats show age-related deficits in delayed responding even though they have shown very marked age effects with passive avoidance. Even more striking, Fox's studies indicate that with puppies the ability to learn the two types of task is, if anything, inversely related.

An alternative explanation that has sometimes been applied to the results of passive-avoidance and delayed-response studies attributes difficulties in learning not to general deficits in a young animal's ability to inhibit responses, but to specific age-related differences in the strength of motivation underlying the response to be inhibited. For example, Fox (1971) argues that older dogs are unable to learn to inhibit an approach to humans because human goal objects are more reinforcing at that age than at younger ages; thus it is more difficult for older dogs to overcome a strong tendency to approach people. Analogous arguments can be applied to the results of passive-avoidance studies with rats (Campbell, Riccio, and Rohrbaugh, 1971), only in this case to account for poor performance by the youngest age groups. As has been shown by Moorcroft, Lytle, and Campbell (1971), young rats are dramatically more active than adults, particularly at the ages when they also show marked deficits in learning passive avoidance. Randall (1974) has shown that if young rats are tested in groups, activity level drops precipitously, suggesting that excessive activity by rat pups may reflect their response to isolation. Thus, in the typical passive-avoidance task, an isolated rat pup may be more motivated to run than a similarly isolated adult. However, several investigators (e.g., Riccio, Rohrbaugh, and Hodges, 1968) have pretested young and adult rats to determine the number of times they typically cross between the two compartments of the passive-avoidance apparatus, and they report that young animals do not cross over any more often than adults. In general, then, there is no independent evidence to suggest that differential response strengths account for passive-avoidance or delayed-response learning deficits. By and large, it is the deficit itself which is used to posit differences in underlying response tendencies.

There is yet another explanation that could account for passive-avoidance deficits. In passive avoidance animals are taught to inhibit a response by means of punishment, and it could be that they are truly deficient in their ability to learn the appropriate association between response and punishment. It is interesting that the behavioral results of spatial-avoidance and passive-avoidance procedures are the same (i.e., the avoidance of a particular compartment), yet young pups learn easily in one situation but not in the other. Spatial avoidance is a stimulus-contingent task in which the rat learns that a particular location is associated with a noxious event, whereas in passive avoidance the rat must learn that a particular response results in punishment. Thus the essential difference between the two procedures is not in the required response, but in the contingency that must be learned. Two studies have been mentioned in which young animals did not experience difficulty in learning passive avoidance (Grote and Brown, 1971; Fox, 1971), and it is noteworthy that in both cases the animals could have been learning stimulus contingencies. Although Grote and Brown (1971) considered their task as one in which licking was punished by poisoning, many investigators would consider it to have been a stimulus-contingent task in which animals learned to associate a particular taste with a noxious stimulus. Similarly, in Fox's study, it may well be that the dogs learned, not that an approach response was being punished, but that the human observer was associated with shock.

One relevant set of data has been reported recently by Riccio and Marrazo (1972), who compared 18- to 20-day-old pups and adult rats in their ability to learn a passive-avoidance task after first being trained in active avoidance in the same apparatus. As expected, they found that young animals learned to inhibit active-avoidance responses more slowly than adults. However, they also examined the effect of delaying the punishing consequences of running, which should have weakened the contingency between response and punishment. They found that as the delay between entering the unsafe compartment and shock increased, the performance of adults declined as expected (Kamin, 1959), but, surprisingly, the performance of the younger animals did not. In fact, there was some indication that the pups learned to avoid more rapidly as the delay increased, so that at the longest delay tested (10 seconds), pups learned to avoid as rapidly as the adults. If a procedure known to weaken a contingency has no effect upon the acquisition of that contingency, it is a reasonable possibility that the contingency is not being learned. It is interesting to note that as Riccio and Marrazo increased the time interval between running into the unsafe compartment and shock, they made the task more and more similar to that of spatial avoidance. That is, the delay enabled the animals to associate the compartment with shock, a stimulus-contingent task that we already know young animals are quite capable of learning.

If passive-avoidance deficits by young animals arise from an inability to associate punishment with their responses, then age-related deficits in delayed responding, in which no punishment is involved, must be accounted for independently. How to account for these deficits is still quite unclear. Besides requiring the animal to inhibit normal activity, delayed-response tasks also make demands upon short-term and long-term memories (Fox, 1971). If, however, the inability of young animals to tolerate delays reflects some kind of learning deficit, the nature of the associative failure is simply not understood.

We are left then with the real possibility that the ability to associate response and punishment, unlike other types of associative tasks, may require a certain level of development. The ability to learn delayed-response tasks also seems to require a certain maturity, but it is not clear why. It is also possible that both tasks are sometimes difficult for young animals because they both require responses to be inhibited. However, as we have pointed out, the evidence that links these two types of deficits to response inhibition is not particularly compelling.

To conclude this review of juvenile-learning studies, it is clear that as the learning requirements of any task become more complex, as discriminations, delays, and other features are added, young animals have been observed to learn with greater difficulty than adults. It should be noted, however, that increasing the complexity of a learning task also increases the perceptual-motor demands of the task and makes it more difficult to specify or control other task-related variables, such as motivation. Thus, even with consistent reports of "learning" deficits in complex tasks, it is not always possible to determine the true source of difficulty. It is also clear from this review that in those cases where the contingencies and task requirements are relatively easy to specify, young organisms seem to show no difficulty in learning, except possibly for contingencies involving punishment. Specifically, young organisms learn as rapidly as adults whenever the tasks involve contingencies between responses and reinforcement, or between stimuli, or a combination of both. When they have been observed to learn more slowly (or even more rapidly) than adults, simple changes in task parameters have been sufficient to eliminate those differences. In sum, as long as the perceptual-motor requirements are appropriate to the age studied, there seems to be no major underlying deficit in the ability of young organisms to learn simple but fundamental associative tasks. Implicit in this conclusion is the assumption that those aspects of the central nervous system necessary to mediate the relevant perceptual-motor processes are also functionally mature.

13.2 THE ONTOGENESIS OF MEMORY

From the preceding discussion it is evident that young mammals can and do learn a great many things with ease, limited of course by their sensory and motor capacities. The permanence of this early learning is another question. As noted in the introduction, a striking aspect of human development is the total lack of recall of one's early, formative years. While there is much to be said about the permanent and pervasive effects of early experience, our concern here is with the emergence of long-term memory per se.

Parenthetically, we see no logical inconsistency between the apparent poor memory of infancy and the permanent effects of the cumulative experiences of infancy. A child, for example, may develop normally under the care of one parent for the first few years of life, but have no specific recollection of that parent if separated from it and subsequently reared in another family setting. Yet the parental care given during those first few years is crucial for normal development. Most early-experience studies indicate that early caretaking alters the behavioral potential of the infant, an effect which clearly does not depend upon the child's ability to remember those experiences. As we have suggested elsewhere (Campbell and Spear, 1972), it is possible that the memory of actual events of infancy, when it is observed, occurs only for events repeatedly experienced throughout the developmental period.

13.2.1 Neonatal studies of memory
During the first half of this century there were numerous

ontogenetic studies of learning as part of an effort to understand and define intelligence, but little attention was focused on long-term retention despite the then-current interest in early-childhood memory. This is particularly true for the neonatal period both then and now. To our knowledge, there are only a few animal studies of long-term retention and none on human infants. While Lipsitt (1969), Papousek (1967), and many others have shown that the extent and quality of learning in the first few months of life is quite amazing, no effort has been made to see how these behaviors persist. As Lipsitt (1969, p. 28) has said, if "the newborn human creature is about as competent a learning organism as he can become," then some estimate of its ability to retain such learning is sadly overdue.

In one of the few retention studies in primate neonates, Mason and Harlow (1958a, b) conditioned monkeys by exposing them to tone-shock pairings in a stabilimeter cage for 30 days starting on the third day of life. Following this training, the monkeys were taught to approach food in a runway for 12 days, during the last 6 days of which the investigators presented the tone to determine if the CS altered the approach response; they found no effect. The following day the monkeys were tested for retention of the CS in the original training situation and showed no memory of conditioning. Because of the interpolated experience with tone alone, it is difficult to determine whether the monkeys' lack of response to the CS during the retention test was a true memory failure or the result of extinction. Green (1962), for example, found that although young monkeys acquire responses to the CS as well as older monkeys, they extinguish more rapidly. He, too, found poorer retention by the youngest age group, but again after much experience with the tone alone.

Rosenblatt (1971) described an intriguing study by Ivanitski with baby rabbits. With 5 days of conditioning, 1- to 5-day-old rabbit pups learned to lift their head in response to an odor associated with nursing. Then, after a 5-day period in which the odor was not presented, it was reintroduced. Interestingly enough, the rabbits no longer responded to the odor by lifting their heads; instead they ran toward the odor, a response quite appropriate to their level of development at that point. Although this study does not assess true long-term retention, it does suggest that infantile-memory failures, when they occur, cannot necessarily be attributed to changes in response patterns due to development. If memory of early learning exists, animals are apparently capable of responding to this memory even if they must do so in a more mature fashion.

13.2.2 Juvenile studies of memory
Despite the obvious importance of studying the retentive

capabilities of very young organisms, nearly all attempts to study and describe the phenomenon of infantile amnesia have concentrated upon juvenile animals, primarily rat pups. The need to study younger animals over a wider range of species is clearly urgent. Nonetheless, despite the limitations of the data that exist to date, it is striking how consistently investigators, at least in recent years, have demonstrated that young animals even with extensive behavioral repertoires remember less well than do adults.

ESCAPE AND APPROACH. Some years ago, however, it was believed that young animals had better memories than adults. Stone (1929a, b), one of the first to study the effect of age upon learning was also one of the first to put age-related retention expectations to empirical test. Unfortunately, his studies of the retention of simple approach and escape tasks were not well designed for examining memory per se. In particular, some of the necessary controls for the study of memory were overlooked. For example, no effort was made to equate the different age groups in terms of the strength of their initial learning; as a result, it is not surprising that he found young rats remembering more than adults, since he also reported that they learned more.

A more important problem, both in Stone's work and n several other age-related studies of the retention of simple approach and escape learning, is the age of the "young" animals at the start of the retention interval. Either the youngest rats have been no less than 60 to 90 days of age at the beginning of training (e.g., Goodrick, 1968) or, even if the animals were initially young, the training procedure lasted so long that the animals were adults by the time the retention interval began (e.g., Crockett and Nobel, 1963). It may be possible to determine something about a young animal's learning ability even if it matures during the course of acquisition; however, in an age-related study of retention, it is essential that the animal still be immature when the acquisition period ends.

This criterion can best be met if the task can be learned rapidly, as with escape training. Two such studies have been reported, and in both cases the results unequivocally demonstrated poor retention by the youngest animals tested. Smith (1968) trained rats of 25 and 100 days of age to escape shock in such a way that all animals attained criterion with 3 days of training. Even though both groups learned equally well, 75 days after the end of training rats that were 25 days of age when training began took significantly more trials to relearn the task than rats trained as adults. Extending this study to younger animals, Campbell et al. (1974) trained rat pups to escape shock at 15, 17, 20, 25, and 35 days of age.

Again, they found that after a 7- or 14-day delay the three youngest age groups remembered much less than the older animals. However, in contrast to Smith's study, the 25-day-olds remembered as well as the 35-day-olds (which presumably are like adults). It is possible that if retention had been tested after a substantially longer delay, the 25-day-old group in Campbell's study might also have shown a significant retention loss.

STIMULUS-CONTINGENT TASKS. Retention of spatial avoidance was first examined by Campbell and Campbell (1962) with rats ranging in age from 18 to 100 days. After conditioning five different age groups, they tested groups of animals either immediately after training or 7, 21, and 42 days later. Animals trained when over 30 days of age avoided the compartment in which they were shocked regardless of when tested, whereas animals trained at 18 or 23 days of age showed increasingly less avoidance the longer the time between training and testing. With the longest delay, neither of the two youngest showed any memory of original conditioning.

Using a CER procedure, Campbell and Campbell also found that rats trained at 25 days of age showed less lick-suppression after a 42-day delay than did rats trained as adults; however, the retention loss was considerably less than that observed with spatial avoidance. Following this up, Coulter, Collier, and Campbell have since found that if pups are given tone-shock pairings even as early as at 17–19 days of age, they in fact show no loss of suppression 42 days after conditioning (data in preparation). However, if they are conditioned at 14–16 days of age, rapid forgetting of CER does occur. Even with suppression at asymptote 5 days after these young pups are conditioned, 28 days after the last tone-shock pairing CER has been completely forgotten.

In a taste-aversion paradigm Alberts (1974) also found excellent retention after 28 and 56 days by rats that had been exposed to a particular taste paired with lithium chloride at 18 days of age. However, he found that extremely rapid forgetting of the aversion could be observed if original conditioning took place at 10 days of age. Somewhat less rapid forgetting was observed in a group conditioned at 12 days of age and, again, virtually no forgetting by those conditioned at 15 days of age.

Thus, with stimulus-contingent tasks, an interesting pattern of results can be seen. Young animals have been consistently shown to remember less well than older animals, but only when trained at much younger ages than that required to demonstrate retention losses of response-reinforcement contingencies. Furthermore, the nature of the stimulus-contingent task itself determines just how young the animals must be when conditioned if forgetting is to be subsequently seen. It would appear that as the task becomes easier to learn, susceptibility to forgetting can be observed only if animals are trained at increasingly younger ages. It would be of interest to determine whether response-reinforcement contingencies more easily acquired than those so far studied might also be susceptible to forgetting, only at much younger ages.

ACTIVE AVOIDANCE AND DISCRIMINATION. Kirby (1963) was the first to perform an ontogenetic study of the long-term retention of active avoidance. He trained rats to traverse a 30-inch runway at 25, 50, and 100 days of age and then tested them for retention 1, 25, or 50 days later. Just as with escape learning, the youngest age group again remembered least well 25 or 50 days after training. With the same age groups and retention intervals, Thompson et al. (1965) tried to compensate for changes in the perceived size of the environment brought about by growth by increasing the size of the apparatus for the two youngest age groups when testing them for retention. This procedure did eliminate all differences in retention among the different age groups. Unfortunately, the data also indicated that the task was forgotten by all age groups, so it is difficult to determine whether changing the apparatus was a help or a hindrance.

In actual fact, it is probably impossible to compensate for perceptual changes in developing animals, since there is no way to ascertain just what aspect of the changed situation may be important to a rat. Fiegley and Spear (1970), for example, also increased the size of their apparatus when testing the retention of rats trained 25 days earlier at 23 or 100 days of age. In this case the younger rats still forgot more than the adults. Oddly enough, with the same apparatus but without changing its size during the retention test, Parsons and Spear (1972) have failed to obtain significant differences in retention between the same two age groups. However, the young rats learned more quickly than the adults and then relearned somewhat more slowly, so that the direction of difference in the memory test was in the predicted direction.

In contrast to these studies, Doty (1968) found that with an avoidance task in which rats were required to learn a brightness discrimination, pups trained at 23 days of age showed better retention than adults when relearning the task 60 days later. However, this effect occurred only if the rats had been exposed to extensive handling prior to training. Without such handling, retention by the younger animals was significantly poorer than by adults. Since the retention test required substantial learning by all animals and early handling has been shown to enhance learning ability, the savings displayed by the handled subjects might be attributable

to a change in the learning skills of the younger animals rather than to a better memory. Somewhat different results were reported by Fox (1971), also with a brightness-discrimination task; he found that puppies ranging in age from 5 to 16 weeks when originally trained, all relearned the task at the same rate. Unfortunately, however, the puppies were explicitly extinguished during the retention interval, which could easily have eliminated any possible memory effects. When testing solely for the retention of a brightness-discrimination task, Campbell, Jaynes, and Misanin (1968) did observe marked forgetting by rats trained to a bar-pressing task at 23–26 days of age, whereas excellent retention was evident in rats trained as adults. Not only did the young rats show increasing forgetting of the discrimination with longer delay periods, but it also appeared that they were less able than adults to retain the bar-press response.

With active avoidance, then, greater retention losses have again been reported for animals trained when young than for those trained as adults; however, the results have not been as consistent as those reported for escape tasks, spatial avoidance, CER, and taste aversions. Nonetheless, in the active-avoidance studies described, the investigators have all examined the retention capabilities of rats trained at well over 20 days of age. Since active avoidance is learned as easily as stimulus-contingent or response-contingent tasks, one would expect to see consistent forgetting only in animals trained at younger ages than have so far been studied. Interestingly enough, with a discrimination task, which as indicated earlier is relatively difficult to learn, retention losses even by rats trained at 30 days of age were substantial relative to that seen in adults, especially over long retention intervals (e.g., 180 days).

PASSIVE AVOIDANCE. Remarkably consistent age-related retention differences have been reported for tasks in which responses are punished during training, even with a variety of procedural manipulations. In a simple version of passive avoidance, Campbell et al. (1974) punished 16-, 20-, 25-, and 100-day-old rats when they stepped into the dark compartment of a two-compartment apparatus. Retention, as measured by latency to enter the black compartment, was assessed either immediately after the animals attained a given criterion of learning or 1, 7, and 21 days later. Forgetting by the younger rats was consistently greater than by adults. After 21 days they showed virtually no memory at all of the original task, whereas adults showed virtually no forgetting. Fiegley and Spear (1970) used three different shock intensities for punishing separate groups of 25-day-old pups or adults in a similar step-through passive-avoidance task. Retention was improved in all groups by higher levels of punishment, yet the younger animals, regardless of shock intensity, always remembered less than adults 28 days after training. Similarly, Schulenburg, Riccio, and Stikes (1971) examined the retention of rats trained at 15, 21, and 100 days of age with the same task, only in this case they varied the duration of shock. As in Campbell's study, adults showed virtually no forgetting of the task 6, 12, or 24 days after training. However, the younger two age groups, even though they remembered more with the longest duration of shock, still showed significantly less retention than adults. With dogs, Fox (1971) examined the retention of another variant of passive avoidance, in which three groups of puppies ranging in age from 5 to 13 weeks were punished for approaching a passive human observer. After 7 or 14 days, the youngest group showed virtually no memory of the original task, whereas the older two groups maintained the same level of performance they had attained earlier.

Throughout this discussion we have tried to emphasize that infantile amnesia is probably not dependent upon deficiencies in learning. To make this point convincing it is important that age-related retention studies use tasks that are as easily learned by young animals as by adults. Since, as was discussed earlier, young animals, particularly rats, have greater difficulty learning passive-avoidance tasks than adults, passive-avoidance retention studies do not meet an important criterion for the study of infantile amnesia. However, it must be noted that young animals do eventually learn passive avoidance, and in the studies described they were always trained to the same criterion as adults. Since they take longer to learn, younger animals were exposed to more training than adults, and it can be argued that learning differences were in some sense turned to the younger animal's advantage. Furthermore, in at least one instance (Fox, 1971), the younger animals actually learned the task far more rapidly than the older animals; yet the same pattern of forgetting was observed. Finally, the size of the retention deficits that have been reported with passive avoidance is far out of proportion to the size of the original learning deficit.

To the extent that age-related retention deficits can be shown to be independent of speed of learning, relative rates of learning may ultimately be viewed as irrelevant to the phenomenon of infantile amnesia. Although we have been concerned here with the fact that a particular task is difficult for young animals to learn, it is important to note that retention deficits have been seen even when the task is considerably easier for younger animals than for adults. Training adult wolves to respond to humans without fear is extremely difficult, whereas socialization is easily achieved with immature wolves (Fox, 1971).

Nonetheless, once adult wolves are socialized, they remain so, even if they have no contact with humans for long periods of time. In marked contrast, young wolves rapidly regain their fearfulness unless they are repeatedly exposed to humans during the remainder of their development.

Thus passive-avoidance studies do not need to be excluded from consideration merely because of age-related differences in learning, interesting as they may be in their own right. Along with retention studies of other tasks, they produce the same pattern of results: no matter how well an immature animal can and does learn, long-term memory for the events of infancy is either poor or nonexistent.

13.3 DETERMINANTS OF INFANTILE AMNESIA

In the preceding sections we have shown that infantile amnesia is a demonstrable phenomenon in a number of species and that it seems to be independent of the ability of young animals to learn. Apart from its inherent interest as a phenomenon with which we are all familiar, infantile amnesia provides a scientific challenge which, in the course of its solution, may yield useful insights into the fundamental mechanisms of memory storage and retrieval.

Two types of processes, psychological and those arising from neurological maturation, are known to influence memory storage and retrieval, but at this stage of scientific evolution the relative contributions of these two kinds of processes to the poor memory of infancy are simply not understood. The following discussion describes what little is known about the determinants of infantile amnesia and speculates at length about the mechanisms that may possibly underlie that phenomenon.

13.3.1 Psychological processes
Psychological processes can be observed at any age but may be strengthened by the events that occur during development. By and large, these processes are dependent upon an organism's interaction with its external environment and can be viewed as resulting from "experience."

RETROACTIVE AND PROACTIVE INTERFERENCE. Responses that are acquired either before (proactive interference) or after (retroactive interference) the learning of a particular response are known to impair retention of that response. The extent of interference depends upon a vast array of conditions, ranging from the similarity of the items learned and the setting in which they were acquired to the frequency with which they were experienced.

In the context of developmental psychology, the following question remains to be answered: What are the relative contributions of retroactive and proactive interference to the basic phenomenon of poorer memory in infancy? According to the simplest model of proactive interference, older animals should forget more rapidly simply because they have lived longer and have thus acquired more learned habits that can interfere with the retention of more recently learned material. But as the data cited above indicate, this prediction is contrary to fact.

Retroactive interference remains a somewhat more viable candidate as a basis for the rapid forgetting of infancy. One could conceivably argue that the young of all species have to learn a great deal about the spatial-perceptual-social characteristics of the environment as they move about; the more they approach, interact with, and withdraw from stimuli in different ways and under varying conditions, the more they learn. In contrast, older individuals, inactive and maintained in a familiar environment, learn much less. Given this analysis, it follows that retroactive interference from learning occurring during the retention interval is likely to be higher in young than in adult animals.

On balance, however, it appears difficult to develop an interference model that can parsimoniously explain the differential rates of forgetting in infancy and adulthood. In the one experimental test of this hypothesis, Parsons and Spear (1972) found that housing infant and adult rats in enriched environments during a 60-day retention interval accelerated forgetting relative to animals housed in isolation, but that the younger rats were no more susceptible to retroactive interference than were the adults. At the human level it is equally difficult to understand how this simple model could predict, on either a quantitative or a qualitative basis, the poor memory of infancy. It appears to us that an enormous amount of learning occurs during all stages of development, from infancy through adolescence, and that memories for all of one's childhood should therefore be interfered with, not just those for the first few years of life. Further, one would predict that as life and adult development progressed, the continued learning would gradually erode all recollection of one's early life. To single out one stage in that complex developmental sequence as producing more retroactive inteference, on the basis of information currently available, is impossible.

Perhaps the most compelling evidence for the effects of retroactive interference as a general degrader of memory stems from the literature on amnesic patients suffering from consolidation deficits. In the classic case of H.M., it appears from the reports available to date that he has a clearer recollection of the events of 20 years ago than do most normal adults of his age and intellectual capacity. It seems reasonable to assume that the continued acquisition of new knowledge over a period of time would interfere with a normal person's memories of the past, but there is no apparent reason why this should impair memory for early childhood more than for any other period.

STIMULUS GENERALIZATION. By definition, stimulus events are never reproduced completely; consequently, performance on each successive trial in a learning task, regardless of intertrial interval, is determined by the perceived similarity of the ongoing trial to previous trials and by the strength of the acquired response. In well-trained adult animals little decrement of stimulus generalization occurs from trial to trial, even over long retention intervals, but in young animals the possibility exists that growth-induced changes in body and physiological makeup substantially alter the perception of the test environment, resulting in a performance decrement.

By far the most commonly considered source of age-induced decrement in stimulus generalization is the change in perceived size of the environment that is thought to occur as an animal matures. From this it follows that to a young rat, a maze may look like a great cavern from which escape requires a massive effort, but on retest after a retention interval, the same apparatus may appear much different because the visual angles from which the apparatus is viewed have changed or because the size of the apparatus, relative to the animal's body size, is now much smaller. Similarly, the child's viewpoint changes from one in which the world is populated by giants and distinguished by spots of gum underneath tabletops, to the adult view of the world as we know it. This hypothesis is so intuitively appealing that some psychologists have considered this the major mechanism underlying forgetting in infancy. Perkins (1965), for example, states in reference to Campbell and Campbell's (1962) report showing poorer retention of fear in infancy that "the stimulus situation to which fear was learned may be so altered by stimulus changes resulting from growth that there is nearly complete generalization decrement resulting from maturation-induced changes" (pp. 46–47).

Just as perceptual changes occur as a result of physical growth, response patterns can be similarly affected. If the original response required precise movements with respect to the environment, exact replication of these movements at a later time, when the child or animal is physically larger, would certainly be inappropriate, at least in the same environment. One can easily imagine that it might well be impossible to ride a tricycle at age 10 with the same response patterns necessary at age 3.

It is difficult to deny the importance of both stimulus generalization and response-change decrements in those situations where the original event has been defined in terms of environmental parameters such as size, location, or distance. In many animal studies these parameters are indeed important, both in the original task and in the retention test. However, forgetting has also been demonstrated for tasks that depend largely upon the memory of visual cues, such as brightness, or auditory or gustatory stimuli. It is difficult to see how these aspects of the environment can be affected by mere physical growth. We also have noted instances where memory of specific molecular responses has not been required, either in the original task or later. Avoidance, for example, can be executed in whatever manner is appropriate to the age; logically it should occur automatically if the animal remembers the significance of the stimulus. Certainly infantile amnesia is not a selective phenomenon, occurring only for spatial events; the kind of memory failure we are interested in seems to occur for all kinds of events.

In any case, if physical growth is a critical source of forgetting, one would expect to see forgetting throughout the developmental period. Children continue to grow beyond age 7; similarly, rats grow beyond 30 days of age. Once more, as in the case of retroactive interference, to the extent that infantile amnesia is confined to only one period of development, one can hardly account for it entirely by such general processes as stimulus generalization or response differentiation.

MATURATION OF SPECIES-SPECIFIC BEHAVIOR. During the normal course of development, many drastic changes take place in the animal's behavioral repertoire. Some are learned, some are contingent upon changes in physical capability, some are preprogrammed in unknown ways such that they emerge at a particular stage when the proper stimulus appears, and still others are hormonally dependent. Male preweanling rats respond to the dam by rooting and suckling; at sexual maturity the same rat responds to the same female by copulating. Similarly, pain produces withdrawal and flight in the young animal and attack in the adult (Hutchinson, Ulrich, and Arzin, 1965), and unfamiliar environments may elicit more fear in older animals (Candland and Campbell, 1962; Sluckin, 1965). These age-related modifications of behavior can act to interfere either permanently or temporarily with the performance of a previously learned response.

As a hypothetical example, we suspect it would be possible to train an immature female ring dove to peck at a ring dove egg in a nest for food reinforcement, and that the dove would show good retention of the response over long time periods. But if the bird is brought into broodiness by parturition or other means, it seems quite likely that it would now respond to the eggs by brooding rather than pecking, resulting in a measured loss in retention of the pecking response.

If this dominance of unlearned behavior over learned behavior did develop, it would then be of further interest to see if the learned behavior reappears when the hormonal or other conditions controlling the unlearned behavior are removed. In short, there must be many situations in which an emerging unlearned response takes precedence over a previously learned response to a given stimulus. The extent of this interference is undoubtedly proportional to the animal's repertoire of unlearned behaviors and is thus unlikely to be a major source of forgetting in man.

MATURATIONAL CHANGES IN INFORMATION-PROCESSING MECHANISMS. As a corollary to the above observation that emerging species-specific behaviors may interfere with previously learned responses, it seems reasonable to consider the possibility that changes in mode or style of information processing may also interfere with the retrieval of previously learned material. In higher mammals such as man, enormous changes take place in the way in which sensory information is encoded and responded to. The most obvious changes involve the use of language. To a preverbal child a book is simply another object in the environment; later the object is verbally labeled "book"; still later it is responded to by reading either overtly or covertly the title; and finally the title evokes a variety of emotional or evaluative responses ranging from interest to aversion.

Observations such as these again raise the question of the effect of such changes on memory. Is memory for a task learned at an early stage of development less accessible because stimulus information of that type is now processed in a different fashion? This is an intriguing possibility because the greatest changes in information processing appear to take place during the preschool and early school years, the transition period between complete amnesia for the events of early life and the beginnings of recall for childhood events. Language and the development of other cognitive skills may indeed play a role in what is remembered about one's childhood, but it is clear from the animal studies that infantile memory is also poor in animals that do not pass through such an obvious transition.

The juxtaposition of these two notions suggests a two-factor theory of foregetting during ontogenesis. Early in development, long-term memory may be poor due to the immaturity of the central nervous system; later in development, psychological transitions such as changes in the way in which information is processed may play a significant role, particularly in man and higher primates.

13.3.3 Neurological processes: General considerations

EMERGENCE OF LONG-TERM MEMORY IN RAT AND MAN. In the rat, emergence of long-term memory does not appear to be a unitary process. While we did not emphasize differences in the age at which long-term memory develops for various types of learned behavior in our review earlier in this chapter, significant and meaningful differences do appear to occur. On the basis of several experiments in our laboratory and others, it now seems that the emergence of long-term memory in the rat is complete at least as early as 15 days for learned aversions and as late as 30 to 40 days for passive avoidance. Development of long-term memory for other tasks appears to reach adult levels within these rather broad limits, and in no particular sequence.

The rates at which memory for learned aversions and passive-avoidance tasks develop are schematized in the left panel of Figure 13.1. The slopes of the curves and the points of origin and asymptote are derived from the studies described in Section 13.2. The functions are, of course, entirely hypothetical and inferential, but they do depict within reasonable limits the ages at which long-term memory for these two tasks becomes mature. Further research is necessary to elucidate the basis for these differences, and to determine if there are meaningful differences in the development of long-term memory for other classes of learned behavior.

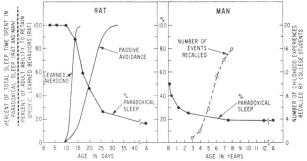

FIGURE 13.1 Comparison of the emergence of long-term memory in rat and man with one index of CNS maturity: percent of total sleep time spent in paradoxical sleep. The paradoxical-sleep data for rat are from Jouvet-Mounier, Astic, and Lacote (1970); those for man are adopted from Roffwarg, Muzio, and Dement (1966). The number of events recalled by college students of their early childhood is from Waldfogel (1948), and the theoretical functions describing development of memory in the rat are derived from research described in the text.

In man, the situation is even more uncertain. For reasons that are most puzzling, child-development psychologists have simply not studied memory over long time intervals. Although they have shown great interest in determining the age at which various tasks and responses can be acquired, they have displayed little or no concern with how long those things learned in infancy and early childhood are remembered. Because of the absence of experimental data on the emergence of long-term memory in the child, our best estimate stems from the retrospective studies of early-childhood memories described earlier in this chapter.

In the most quantitative of these studies, Waldfogel (1948) determined the number of events recalled from different childhood years by college students. These data are reproduced in the right panel of Figure 13.1. What is readily apparent from this study is that young, intelligent individuals are totally incapable of recalling anything of their infancy and early childhood. Even for age eight, the average number of events recalled is only sixteen, suggesting that for most people the clarity of recall continues to increase through the early school years. Evidence demonstrating that this increase is a true developmental phenomenon and not a function of decreasing retention interval can be found by asking any 50-year-old about his college days. Recall of those formative years is legendary, if somewhat exaggerated.

The differences between these indices of long-term memory in children and those used to study memory in the developing rat cannot be overemphasized. In the human studies man is being asked to recall the events of early childhood in the absence of any stimuli associated with that era, while the rat is returned to a highly distinctive setting and asked to reproduce a specific response acquired there early in development. If these same procedures were used with man, it seems quite likely that evidence for long-term memory would appear much earlier. What we are certain of, however, is that long-term memory in man increases enormously during the course of ontogenesis, and that one of the last and most complex phases of this developmental sequence is the disappearance of infantile amnesia.

We might also expect that long-term memory for different types of learning, as in the rat, would reach adult levels over a fairly long developmental span, but as of this time we have little notion of that time period, nor of the sequence in which adult memory capacities would appear.

CENTRAL-NERVOUS-SYSTEM DEVELOPMENT AND ITS RELATION TO LONG-TERM MEMORY. That some degree of central-nervous-system maturity is necessary for the complex processes of memory storage and retrieval is self-evident. The embryonic neural tube is simply not capable of "learning," at least in the way in which we characterize that process in the adult. The issue instead is to determine the extent to which the phenomenon of infantile amnesia is due to neural immaturity. As we have seen, most young mammals pass through a stage in which their ability to learn approximates that of the adult, yet their ability to remember is markedly inferior.

In the rat, the ontogenetic period associated with poor long-term memory parallels a period of rapid CNS development (Campbell and Spear, 1972). This close correlation does not necessarily imply a causal relationship, however, since the period is also marked by dramatic changes in the animals' behaviors, which could also impair retention through psychological processes such as those described in the preceding section.

The strongest experimental support for the importance of neural maturation as a critical substrate for the emergence of long-term memory stems from a recent study comparing the development of long-term memory in neonatal rats and guinea pigs (Campbell et al., 1974). The rat and guinea pig are both rodents, and they have similar histories of breeding for laboratory use. They differ, however, in one critical dimension: maturity of the central nervous system at parturition. The guinea pig, after a 65-day gestation period, is born with an almost fully developed central nervous system. Myelination is nearly complete, neural transmitters approximate adult levels, cellular differentiation is advanced, and cerebral electrical activity is similar to that of the adult, as are most other indices of brain function. In contrast, the rat is born after a 21-day gestation period and its brain is extremely underdeveloped in both structure and function. It is not until the rat is 20–30 days postpartum that its central nervous system approximates that of the newborn guinea pig.

Behaviorally, both animals are naive. Neither is familiar with its physical or social environment and both will learn a great deal about those conditions in the first few months of life, providing an opportunity for the variables described in the preceding section to impair memory more in infancy than in adulthood. Yet when memory for tasks learned equally easily by young and adults of both species is determined, only the young rat shows rapid forgetting. Thus the guinea pig's capacity for long-term memory appears to be fully developed at birth while the rat's is not. Because of the similarity in the experiences both will undergo during the course of development, it seems likely that the rapid forgetting shown by the neonatal rat is due primarily to immaturity of its central nervous system, rather than to extraexperimental learning that occurs during the course of development.

The ways in which neural maturation might impair

long-term memory and yet leave the ability to learn relatively unaffected are diverse. First, in the tradition of Hughlings Jackson (see Taylor, 1931, 1932), learning in the young animal could be mediated by earlier-maturing brain centers. Then, as development proceeded, later-maturing structures could assume dominance over the early-maturing regions and simultaneously prevent access to previously learned responses.

Inferential support for this hypothesis stems from the well-documented analysis of the disappearance of many reflexes during the normal course of ontogenesis and their reappearance following cortical injury or senile brain disease. The suckling and rooting reflexes of infancy, for example, are actively inhibited by the functional maturation of the cortex, and damage to that area results in their reappearance. It is not unreasonable to postulate a similar developmental pattern for the disappearance of memories acquired in infancy.

Unfortunately, the clinical literature on this question is incomplete and ambiguous. There are many descriptions of behavioral regression in senile brain disease, but there is no compelling evidence documenting the reappearance of forgotten childhood memories during senescence. In childhood, cerebral injury often induces regression to preverbal levels or to a lower level of functioning (i.e., from fifth grade to first grade), but again it is not apparent from the available reports that there is a corresponding reappearance of memories previously associated with that period of development (e.g., Blau, 1936).

In animals, a comparable state of affairs exists; there are simply no reports of the reappearance of behaviors acquired but subsequently forgotten early in development following cerebral insult. A study showing that a specific response, such as passive avoidance of a dark compartment acquired in infancy and forgotten during the normal course of development, could be reinstated by one or more types of CNS dysfunction would be a most informative and a useful tool for further research.

This line of reasoning is, of course, not limited to the sequential development of major cerebral structures; it can also be applied to intrastructural development. The neurons of the cerebral cortex, for example, start out as primitive, undifferentiated cells without synaptic junctions. As development proceeds, the dendritic and axonal structures become increasingly complex, and the number of synaptic junctions increases astronomically. As Marcus Jacobson (1970) puts it, "Why are the memories of infancy beyond recall? Are they obliterated by the growth of dendrites and development of synapses that occur in the cerebral cortex during the first years after birth?" (p. 344). Intuitively this is probably the most intriguing neural explanation of infantile amnesia, but unfortunately there is no supporting evidence whatsoever.

Cerebral development could also influence retrieval of childhood memories as a result of the striking change in the rate at which sensorimotor information is processed. Conduction velocity in the immature, unmyelinated axon is markedly slower than in the adult (Purpura et al., 1964). In addition, the refractory period of immature cells to repetitive stimulation is much longer (Scherrer, 1967). As a result, the amount of information the central nervous system of the young animal can process is much less than that of the adult.

If the central nervous system can process only limited amounts of information early in development, then the amount of information encoded in a stimulus sequence preceding the elicitation of a criterion response is necessarily less in infancy than in adulthood. Consequently, when an animal is tested for retention after a period during which neurological growth has occurred, the amount of information processed per unit time in the test environment should be greater than it was during the original learning. This change could conceivably result in a generalization decrement leading to poorer performance. Similarly, changes in speed of transmission per se could produce a generalization decrement. Proprioceptive feedback, for example, is more rapid in the adult than in the young rat.

Another way in which the immature central nervous system could differ from that of the adult lies in the memory-consolidation process. There is now considerable evidence available suggesting that some aspects of memory consolidation may span days or even years. In man, retrograde amnesia can extend backwards in time for months or even years following cerebral insult, suggesting that the consolidation of older memories has been continuous, with the result that they are more resistant to trauma than recent memories. Perhaps the immature organism is deficient in this ability.

Within the central nervous system, consolidation has been most often associated with the limbic system. In man, surgical resection of the hippocampus and alcohol-induced damage of the mammillary bodies (Korsakoff's syndrome) both produce severe anterograde amnesia (see Rozin, this volume, for a full discussion of these syndromes). Ontogenetically, these structures may mature relatively slowly (Altman, 1967), and this gives some support to the hypothesis that long-term consolidation is impaired in young mammals.

These are, of course, only some of the ways in which continued neural development could impair long-term memory. Our purpose in this brief discussion has been to focus attention on the possibility that continued neural growth may not only lead to development of the organism's full, adult intellectual capabilities, but in that process it may also obliterate or obscure many or most of the memories acquired during that period.

13.3.4 Neural processes: Relationship of CNS development in rat and man to the emergence of long-term memory

Both rat and man are born with immature central nervous systems, and both are deficient in long-term memory. Furthermore, psychological processes alone do not appear able to account for the phenomenon of infantile amnesia. In view of the strong possibility that the improvement of long-term memory that occurs during development in the two species is due at least in part to the maturation of the central nervous system, it is appropriate to compare the course of CNS development in rat and man to see if the emergence of long-term memory can be linked to either general or specific indices of CNS maturation.

An obvious hazard in this kind of analysis is the fact that little has been empirically established about the locus or necessary substrates of memory storage. Hence it is not yet possible to examine the development of specific brain regions or pathways in man or rat to see if growth of long-term memory parallels specific changes in brain structure or function. In the meantime all one can do is to compare the overall maturation of rat and human brain in order to see if the emergence of long-term memory coincides with cerebral development in the two species.

FORMATION OF SYNAPTIC JUNCTIONS. When the mechanisms of memory storage and retrieval are fully understood, the synapse is almost certain to be an essential component of that process. Therefore, the appearance and functional maturation of synaptic junctions is likely to be a useful index of the ability of any given region of the central nervous system to store and encode information.

Unfortunately, there are as yet few comparative studies of synaptic-junction formation using the recently developed electron microscopic techniques that allow visualization and counting of the number of junctions per unit volume of tissue (Bloom and Aghajanian, 1966). In an elegant and often cited study, Aghajanian and Bloom (1967) estimated the number of synaptic clefts in the molecular layer of the rat's parietal cortex at different ages from 10 days to adulthood. Their results are reproduced in the right panel of Figure 13.2. Beginning at 10 days of age, the number of visible junctions per cubic millimeter increases rapidly, reaching adult levels by about 30 days postnatally. It seems quite reasonable to assume that this same pattern of develop-

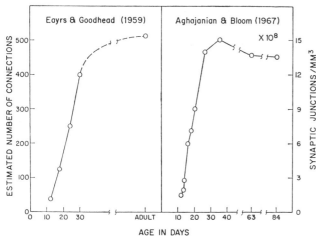

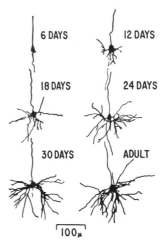

FIGURE 13.2 Estimated number of synaptic junctions per mm³ in rat cerebral cortex during postnatal maturation based on Golgi-Cox stains (from Eayrs and Goodhead, 1959) and electron microscopy (from Aghajanian and Bloom, 1967).

FIGURE 13.3 Changes with age in the appearance of pyramidal cells in the layer V of rat cerebral cortex. From Eayrs and Goodhead (1959).

ment occurs in other mammals and other brain regions, but at different rates postnatally. Spinal-cord and brainstem structures, for example, undoubtedly acquire their full complement of synaptic junctions long before the cortex is fully developed, even though direct data on this point is lacking.

As noted earlier, it is unfortunate that comparable studies on the formation of synaptic junctions are not yet available for the human cerebral cortex. Golgi stains of developing cortical cells are perhaps almost as useful, however, and there are numerous studies in both rat and man using this technique. For the rat, a study by Eayrs and Goodhead (1959) appears to be most valuable in the present context. They studied development of pyramidal cells in the ganglionic layer (layer V) of the rat cerebral cortex using a Golgi-Cox stain, and found that dendritic arborization proceeds rapidly between 10 and 30 days of age (see Figure 13.3). At birth, the pyramidal cells of the cortex are small and densely packed, the cortical layers are not yet differentiated, and there are few visible dendrites, either apical or basal. As development proceeds, dendritic arborization becomes increasingly complex until it approximates the adult structure by around 30 days of age. In a second phase of this study, Eayrs and Goodhead attempted to estimate the number of synaptic junctions present at different ages by counting the number of times dendrites of a given cell appeared to make axonal contact. The results obtained with this technique are reproduced in the left panel of Figure 13.2. Their findings are remarkably similar to those obtained by Aghajanian and Bloom in the molecular layer. Even though these two layers probably mature at different rates in the rat, as they do in man (Schadé and Van Groeningen, 1961), and the tissue samples were taken from somewhat different areas

within the parietal cortex, the overall correspondence between electron microscopic and Golgi-stain estimates of synaptogenesis suggests that dendritic arborization is a reasonable predictor of the number of synaptic junctions present at different developmental ages.

Numerous Golgi-Cox studies have been done on human brains at different levels of development and it has been found, not surprisingly, that the maturation of the human pyramidal cell proceeds in a similar fashion to that of the rat. At birth, pyramidal cells of the human brain are typically somewhat more developed, but subsequent dendritic growth proceeds in a comparable fashion. The time course, however, is much slower in man than in rat: the human pyramidal cell takes two to four years to approximate the complex arborization of the adult, as compared with 25–30 days in the rat (Schadé and Van Groeningen, 1961; Conel, 1939).

The sequence of pyramidal-cell development in two layers of the human cortex is depicted in Figures 13.4

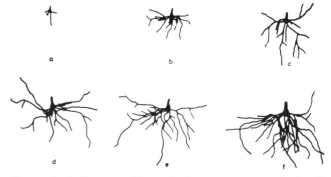

FIGURE 13.4 Changes with age in the appearance of the basal dendritic plexus of pyramidal cells in layer III of human cerebral cortex: (a) newborn; (b) 3 months; (c) 6 months; (d) 15 months; (e) 24 months; (f) adult. Camera lucida drawings from Schadé and Van Groeningen (1961). Reproduced with the permission of S. Karger AG, Basel.

and 13.5. Cells in layer III (Figure 13.4) are considerably less developed at birth than those in layer V (Figure 13.5), but by two years of age both approximate adult structure. However, it should be emphasized that Conel (1939) has reported dendritic growth as visualized by Golgi stains to continue slowly in most cortical regions for at least the next four or five years. This continuing growth is undoubtedly accompanied by synaptogenesis, but in the absence of electron microscopy the rate of synaptic formation is simply unknown.

The relationship of dendritic arborization to the emergence of long-term memory in rat and man is ambiguous. Casual examination of the Golgi-stained cortical pyramidal cells suggests that at 2 to 4 years of age the human brain is at approximately the same level of neural development as the 25- to 30-day-old rat. The same is not true for the emergence of long-term memory in the two species, at least when the available measures of memory are compared. As noted earlier, long-term memory appears to reach adult levels by 30 to 40 days of age for most laboratory tasks in the rat, while in man it continues to develop at least through the early school years. The possibility exists, however, that the slow and subtle changes in dendritic structure occurring after age 4 play a critical role in the complex forms of memory evidenced by man in the disappearance of infantile amnesia.

Myelination. Flechsig (1896) was the first to observe that myelin was either absent or grossly deficient in neonatal mammals, a finding which led him to postulate that myelination preceded function. In man, for example, he believed that the ability to form associations did not appear until two to three months postnatally, the time at which myelin is first observed in the cortical association areas. In mammals, myelination proceeds in a roughly caudocranial order. Myelin first appears in

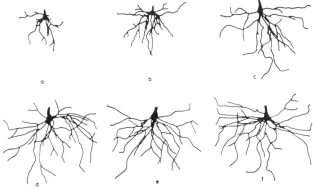

Figure 13.5 Changes with age in the appearance of the basal dendritic plexus of pyramidal cells in layer V of human cerebral cortex. Legend same as Figure 13.4. From Schadé and Van Groeningen (1961). Reproduced with the permission of S. Karger AG, Basel.

the spinal cord, then in the medulla, pons, and midbrain, and finally in the telencephalon. The cerebral cortex also myelinates sequentially starting at the projection centers and ending at the association centers (Jacobson, 1963).

In the rat, the first evidence of myelin appears in the ventral spinal roots at about 2 days postnatally, and it is not until the rat is about 10 days old that myelin begins to appear in the cerebrum. Within the telencephalon, thalamic fibers begin to myelinate between days 10 and 12 and are not fully myelinated until 40–50 days postnatally. In the cortex, myelination does not begin in many regions until 21 days and is not complete until the rat is approximately 60 days of age (Jacobson, 1963), with the period of most rapid deposition occurring between 30 and 40 days (Bass, Netsky, and Young, 1969).

In man, a similar sequence of myelinogenesis occurs, only at birth the human brain is considerably more mature than that of the rat. The ventral motor roots are fully myelinated, and there is visible evidence of myelin throughout the brainstem. Myelination proceeds rapidly, and by the end of the second year the infant brain is nearly completely myelinated except for the nonspecific thalamic radiations, cerebral commissures, and the cortex. Myelination in these regions continues slowly throughout the first decade and continues in the cortical association areas until the third or fourth decade of life (Yakovlev and Lecours, 1967).

There is little correlation between the development of memory and this index of CNS maturation in rat and man. Long-term memory in both species appears to be fully developed well before myelination is complete.

Inhibition of neonatal reflexive behaviors. As discussed earlier, learning in the neonate may be processed by phylogenetically primitive "lower" brain centers, which mature relatively early in the developmental sequence. Then, as maturation proceeds, later-developing structures could acquire "control" over those centers, and in that process access to information acquired earlier could be lost. This, of course, is Hughlings Jackson's view of CNS development. In the present context one might ask if the memories of infancy disappear simultaneously with the reflexes of infancy. In short, does functional maturation of the forebrain simultaneously inhibit reflexive behavior and the retrieval of information acquired prior to that time?

There is no simple answer to this question. The rooting and suckling reflexes, for example, disappear between the eighth and tenth month in man and between the fourteenth and sixteenth day in rat, considerably before long-term memory emerges in either species (Dekaban, 1970). There are, however, no studies involving long-term retention of conditioned suckling or conditioned inhibition of suckling extending through this transition period, leaving open the possibility that access to acquired information associated with these specific reflexive behaviors is blocked by maturation of the cortical regions inhibiting the reflexes.

The failure to find a correlation between one index of cerebral maturation, inhibition of reflexive behaviors, and the emergence of long-term memory does not rule out the Jacksonian possibility that continued cerebral growth inhibits access to previously learned material. Central-nervous-system growth continues long after the reflexes of infancy disappear, and this continued growth may inhibit access to earlier-acquired behaviors.

ONTOGENESIS OF CORTICAL ELECTRICAL ACTIVITY. Another functional measure of CNS development is the ontogenesis of spontaneous electrocortical activity. Since its discovery many years ago, changes in cortical electrical activity during development have been the subject of almost continual investigation. Such changes undoubtedly reflect maturation of neural structure and organization, and hence they are a useful and sensitive tool for studying the ontogenesis of cerebral function. As an index of general cerebral development, the electroencephalogram undoubtedly reflects subtle changes in functional neural development that may be difficult to detect with strictly morphological techniques.

In the rat, the cortex is electrically quiescent for the first 6–7 days postnatally, at which time weak signs of spontaneous electrical activity begin to appear. Developmental changes in both frequency and amplitude are slow from day 7 until approximately day 12, at which time rapid development begins and continues through days 20–25 (Deza and Eidelberg, 1967). By 30 days of age spectral analysis reveals no differences from the adult in terms of either frequency or amplitude.

In man, the course of development differs considerably. Human neonates show continuous spontaneous cortical electrical activity, with low-frequency components predominating, indicating considerably greater CNS maturity at parturition than found in the rat. As development proceeds, there is a shift to higher-frequency components. The biggest absolute changes occur during the first three years of life, but changes continue at a reduced rate until early adolescence. Eichorn (1970) has reviewed the results of several investigations of the frequency changes in alpha (waking) activity occurring during development. Her summary figure is reproduced as Figure 13.6.

Using this index of neural development, we find a closer parallel between the development of cerebral function and the emergence of long-term memory. In

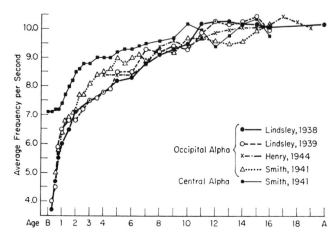

FIGURE 13.6 Development of the alpha rhythm in man. From Eichorn (1970).

the rat, memory reaches adult levels by 30–40 days of age, about the time that electrocortical activity assumes its adult characteristics. Similarly, in man, if we assume that the ability to recall past experiences continues to increase up to adolescence, there is also a close parallel between maturation of CNS function and the emergence of long-term memory.

ONTOGENESIS OF SLEEP. The final measure of CNS maturation to be discussed here is the development of normal sleep patterns. During the course of ontogenesis all nonprecocial mammals show a dramatic change in the relative amount of time spent in paradoxical sleep as opposed to slow-wave sleep. Not only do newborn mammals sleep more than adults, they also spend a greater percentage of time in paradoxical sleep than in slow-wave sleep. As development proceeds, paradoxical sleep decreases and slow-wave sleep increases, so that by adulthood a much higher percentage of time is spent in slow-wave sleep than in paradoxical sleep. This shift is generally interpreted as reflecting the caudal to rostral sequence of brain development, with the appearance and dominance of slow-wave sleep dependent upon functional maturation of the cerebral cortex (McGinty, 1971; Jouvet-Mounier, Astic, and Lacote, 1970).

Because of the ease and reliability with which the states of sleep can be measured, they are potentially a most useful index of CNS maturity. The simplest way to describe the ontogenesis of sleep is to plot the percentage of total sleep time spent in paradoxical sleep in rat and man from parturition to adulthood. Figure 13.1 shows this ontogenetic sequence and compares it to the development of long-term memory in the two species as described earlier.

What is immediately apparent from the figure is that the neonatal rat spends a much higher percentage of time in paradoxical sleep than does the human neonate, reflecting again man's higher level of maturity at birth. Paralleling the other measures of CNS maturation that we have described earlier, the rat shows a rapid change in CNS function between 10 and 25 days of age, with relatively little change thereafter (Jouvet-Mounier, Astic, and Lacote, 1970). In man, the most rapid development occurs during the first three years of life, followed by a slower rate of change for the next few years. Unfortunately, the data from which this figure was derived were based on children grouped together over fairly large age spans. The 7.5-year point, for example, included children from age 5 to age 9; thus any subtle changes in that period may have been obscured (Roffwarg, Muzio, and Dement, 1966).

When the development of paradoxical sleep is compared to the ontogenesis of long-term memory, it is apparent that in the rat long-term memory for all laboratory tasks investigated, ranging from learned aversions to passive avoidance, reaches maturity either before or at about the same time as the percentage of time spent in paradoxical sleep declines to its adult level. Similarly, in man, long-term memory, as measured by the ability to recall past events, increases rapidly as sleep patterns assume their adult characteristics.

CONCLUSIONS. This review of the developmental literature has failed to reveal the determinants of infantile amnesia. We are convinced, nonetheless, that neurological maturity, either because of the immature organism's inability to store or consolidate memories, or because of the subsequent neurological growth that occurs, is a major determinant of the poor memory of infancy.

The major support for this view stems from the close correlation between maturation of the central nervous system, particularly the cerebral cortex, and the development of long-term memory. This is true not only for rat and man, but for the guinea pig as well. The latter provides particularly compelling evidence since it is born with a nearly mature central nervous system and shows an adult capacity for long-term memory at birth. This finding suggests that experiential factors, at least in infraprimate mammals, play a minimal role in infantile amnesia. We must emphasize, however, that at this time there is no indication whatsoever as to which dimensions of neurological development are critical to the emergence of long-term memory in either rat, man, or guinea pig. More likely than not, it is an entire spectrum of interlocking neural processes that is responsible for adult levels of functioning, rather than the development of some critical component. This lack of a definitive answer to the causes of rapid forgetting in infancy is not unique, since there is currently little hard evidence available

concerning the locus and means of memory storage in the adult, a fact illustrated repeatedly elsewhere in this volume.

13.4 OVERVIEW

The purpose of this chapter has been twofold. In the first two sections we attempted to review in detail and with considerable care the empirical research concerned with the ontogenesis of learning and memory. We tried to show that the ability to acquire certain contingencies seems to be independent of age, and that the forgetting of early experiences is a demonstrable phenomenon which cannot be attributed to deficiencies in learning by young organisms. In the third section we attempted to describe critically and in depth some of the possible mechanisms by which one might account for infantile amnesia. We chose to consider these mechanisms under the somewhat arbitrary headings of "psychological" and "neurological" processes. These two categories are clearly not mutually exclusive since they undoubtedly underlie each other and interact in contributing to any behavioral phenomenon of interest. However, for those interested in determining the neural mechanisms of memory, the neurological accounts of infantile amnesia are of particular relevance. It is certainly possible that studies of development in immature organisms will provide investigators with a special tool for elucidating which neurological mechanisms determine memory in general and how they perform this function. If this is to happen, though, psychological processes that may contribute to the forgetting of early events must also be specified and controlled, a task that is particularly difficult in developmental research.

Hopefully we have made it clear just how far we are from understanding the neurological or psychological processes underlying the ontogenesis of long-term memory. It is, in fact, astonishing how few data exist, even at a simple descriptive level. We hope that our speculations regarding the possible determinants of infantile amnesia will suggest certain directions that research might take, and that this research will lead not just to greater insight into the nature of infantile amnesia but to a fuller understanding of memory processes at all ages.

REFERENCES

AGHAJANIAN, G. K., and BLOOM, F. E. 1967. The formation of synaptic junctions in developing rat brain: A quantitative electron microscopic study. *Brain Research* 6: 716–727.

ALBERTS, J. R. 1974. Ontogeny of learned aversions in the rat. Paper presented at the Eastern Psychological Association meetings, Philadelphia, April 1974.

ALLPORT, G. W. 1937. *Personality: A Psychological Interpretation.* New York: Henry Holt.

ALTMAN, J. 1967. Postnatal growth and differentiation of the mammalian brain, with implications for a morphological theory of memory. In G. C. Quarton, T. Melnechuk, and F. O. Schmitt, eds., *The Neurosciences: A Study Program*. New York: Rockefeller University Press, pp. 723–743.

BACON, W. E. 1971. Stimulus control of discriminated behavior in neonatal dogs. *Journal of Comparative and Physiological Psychology* 76: 424–433.

BACON, W. E. 1973. Aversive conditioning in neonatal kittens. *Journal of Comparative and Physiological Psychology* 83: 306–313.

BACON, W. E., and STANLEY, W. C. 1963. Effect of deprivation level in puppies on performance maintained by passive person reinforcer. *Journal of Comparative and Physiological Psychology* 56: 783–785.

BACON, W. E., and STANLEY, W. C. 1970a. Avoidance learning in neonatal dogs. *Journal of Comparative and Physiological Psychology* 70: 448–452.

BACON, W. E., and STANLEY, W. C. 1970b. Reversal learning in neonatal dogs. *Journal of Comparative and Physiological Psychology* 70: 344–350.

BASS, N. H., NETSKY, M. G., and YOUNG, E. 1969. Microchemical studies of postnatal development in rat cerebrum. I. Migration and differentiation of cells. *Neurology* 19: 258–268.

BIRREN, J. E. 1962. Age differences in learning a 2-choice water maze by rats. *Journal of Gerontology* 17: 207–213.

BLAU, A. 1936. Mental changes following head trauma in children. *Archives of Neurology and Psychiatry* 35: 723–769.

BLOOM, F. E., and AGHAJANIAN, G. K. 1966. Cytochemistry of synapses: A selective staining method for electron microscopy. *Science* 154: 1575–1577.

BOLLES, R. C. 1970. Species-specific defense reactions and avoidance learning. *Psychological Review* 77: 32–48.

BOTWINICK, J., BRINLEY, J. F., and RABBIN, J. S. 1962. Learning a position discrimination and position reversals by Sprague-Dawley rats of different ages. *Journal of Gerontology* 17: 315–319.

BRENNAN, J. F., and RICCIO, D. C. 1972. Stimulus control of shuttle avoidance in young and adult rats. *Canadian Journal of Psychology* 26: 361–373.

BRONSON, G. 1965. The hierarchical organization of the CNS: Implications for learning processes and critical periods in early development. *Behavioral Science* 10: 7–25.

BRUNNER, R. L. 1969. Age differences in one-trial passive avoidance learning. *Psychonomic Science* 14: 134.

BRUNNER, R. L., ROTH, T. G., and ROSSI, R. R. 1970. Age differences in the development of the conditioned emotional response. *Psychonomic Science* 21: 135–136.

CALDWELL, D. F., and WERBOFF, J. 1962. Classical conditioning in newborn rats. *Science* 136: 1118–1119.

CAMPBELL, B. A. 1967. Developmental studies of learning and motivation in infraprimate mammals. In H. W. Stevenson, E. H. Hess, and H. L. Rheingold, eds., *Early Behavior: Comparative and Developmental Approaches*. New York: John Wiley & Sons, pp. 43–71.

CAMPBELL, B. A., and CAMPBELL, E. H. 1962. Retention and extinction of learned fear in infant and adult rats. *Journal of Comparative and Physiological Psychology* 55: 1–8.

CAMPBELL, B. A., JAYNES, J., and MISANIN, J. R. 1968. Retention of a light-dark discrimination in rats of different ages. *Journal of Comparative and Physiological Psychology* 66: 467–472.

CAMPBELL, B. A., MISANIN, J. R., WHITE, B. C., and LYTLE, L. D. 1974. Species differences in ontogeny of memory: Support for neural maturation as a determinant of forgetting. *Journal of Comparative and Physiological Psychology* 87: 193–202.

CAMPBELL, B. A., RICCIO, D. C., and ROHRBAUGH, M. 1971. Ontogenesis of learning and memory: Research and theory. In M. E. Meyer, ed., *Second Western Symposium on Learning: Early Learning*. Bellingham, Wash.: Western Washington State College, pp. 76–109.

CAMPBELL, B. A., and SPEAR, N. E. 1972. Ontogeny of memory. *Psychological Review* 79: 215–236.

CANDLAND, D. K., and CAMPBELL, B. A. 1962. Development of fear as measured by behavior in the open field. *Journal of Comparative and Physiological Psychology* 5: 593–596.

CONEL, J. L. 1939–1959. *The Postnatal Development of the Human Cerebral Cortex*, 8 vols. Cambridge, Mass.: Harvard University Press.

CORNWALL, A. C., and FULLER, J. L. 1961. Conditioned responses in young puppies. *Journal of Comparative and Physiological Psychology* 54: 13–15.

COULTER, X. 1974. Long-term retention of CER: Effects of number of CS-US pairings. Unpublished Ph. D. dissertation, Princeton University.

CRAIK, F. I. M. 1973. A "levels of analysis" view of memory. In P. Pliner, L. Kramer, and T. M. Alloway, eds., *Communication and Affect: Language and Thought*. New York: Academic Press, pp. 45–63.

CROCKETT, W. H., and NOBEL, M. E. 1963. Age of learning, severity of negative reinforcement, and retention of learned responses. *Journal of Genetic Psychology* 103: 105–112.

D'AMATO, M. R., and JAGODA, H. 1960. Age, sex, and rearing conditions as variables in simple brightness discrimination. *Journal of Comparative and Physiological Psychology* 53: 261–263.

DARWIN, C. R. 1965. A biographical sketch of an infant. In W. Kessen, ed., *The Child*. New York: John Wiley & Sons, pp. 118-129.

DEKABAN, A. 1970. *Neurology of Early Childhood*. Baltimore: Williams & Wilkins.

DENENBERG, V. H., and KLINE, N. J. 1958. The relationship between age and avoidance learning in the hooded rat. *Journal of Comparative and Physiological Psychology* 51: 488–491.

DENENBERG, V. H., and SMITH, S. A. 1963. Effects of infantile stimulation and age upon behavior. *Journal of Comparative and Physiological Psychology* 56: 307–312.

DEZA, L., and EIDELBERG, E. 1967. Development of cortical electrical activity in the rat. *Experimental Neurology* 17: 425–438.

DOTY, B. A. 1966. Age differences in avoidance conditioning as a function of distribution of trials and task difficulty. *Journal of Genetic Psychology* 109: 249–254.

DOTY, B. A. 1968. Effects of handling on learning of rats. *Journal of Gerontology* 23: 142–144.

DOTY, B. A. and, DOTY, L. 1964. Effects of age and chlorpromazine on memory consolidation. *Journal of Comparative and Physiological Psychology* 57: 331–334.

DUDYCHA, G. J., and DUDYCHA, M. M. 1941. Childhood memories: A review of the literature. *Psychological Bulletin* 38: 668–682.

DYE, C. J. 1969. Effects of interruption of initial learning upon retention in young, mature, and old rats. *Journal of Gerontology* 24: 12–17.

EAYRS, J. T., and GOODHEAD, B. 1959. Postnatal development of the cerebral cortex in the rat. *Journal of Anatomy* 93: 385–401.

EICHORN, D. H. 1970. Physiological development. In P. H. Mussen, ed., *Carmichael's Manual of Child Psychology*, Vol. 1. New York: John Wiley & Sons, pp. 157–283.

EWER, R. F. 1961. Further observations on suckling behaviour in kittens together with some general considerations of the interrelations of innate and acquired responses. *Behaviour* 17: 247–260.

FIEGLEY, D. A., and SPEAR, N. E. 1970. Effect of age and punishment condition on long-term retention by the rat of active- and passive-avoidance learning. *Journal of Comparative and Physiological Psychology* 73: 515–526.

FIELDS, P. E. 1953. The age factor in multiple discrimination learning by white rats. *Journal of Comparative and Physiological Psychology* 46: 387–389.

FLECHSIG, P. 1896. *Gehirn und Seele*. Leipzig.

FOX, M. 1965. *Canine Behavior*. Springfield, Ill.: Charles C Thomas.

FOX, M. 1971. *Integrative Development of Brain and Behavior in the Dog*. Chicago: The University of Chicago Press.

FRIEMAN, J. P., FRIEMAN, J., WRIGHT, W., and HIGBERG, W. 1971. Developmental trends in the acquisition and extinction of conditioned suppression in rats. *Developmental Psychology* 4: 425–428.

FRIEMAN, J. P., ROHRBAUGH, M., and RICCIO, D. A. 1969. Age differences in the control of acquired fear by tone. *Canadian Journal of Psychology* 23: 237–244.

FRIEMAN, J. P., WARNER, L., and RICCIO, D. C. 1970. Age differences in conditioning and generalization of fear in young and adult rats. *Developmental Psychology* 3: 119–123.

FULLER, J. L., EASLER, C. A., and BANKS, E. M. 1950. Formation of conditioned avoidance responses in young puppies. *American Journal of Physiology* 160: 462–466.

GALEF, B. G., and CLARK, M. M. 1971. Poison avoidance in rat pups. *Journal of Comparative and Physiological Psychology* 75: 341–357.

GOLDMAN, P. S., and TOBACH, E. 1967. Behaviour modification in infant rats. *Animal Behaviour* 15: 559–562.

GOODRICK, C. L. 1968. Learning, retention, and extinction of a complex maze habit for mature, young and senescent Wistar albino rats. *Journal of Gerontology* 23: 298–304.

GRAY, P. H., and YATES, A. E. 1967. The ontogeny of classical conditioning in the neonate rat with varied CS-UCS intervals. *Psychonomic Science* 9: 587–588.

GREEN, P. C. 1962. Learning, extinction, and generalization of conditioned responses by young monkeys. *Psychological Reports* 10: 731–738.

GROTE, Jr., F. W. and BROWN, R. T. 1971. Rapid learning of passive avoidance by weanling rats: Conditioned taste aversion. *Psychonomic Science* 25: 163–164.

HARLOW, H. F. 1959. The development of learning in the rhesus monkey. *American Scientist* 47: 458–479.

HARLOW, H. F., HARLOW, M. K., RUEPING, R. R., and MASON, W. A. 1960. Performance of infant rhesus monkeys on discrimination learning, delayed response, and reversal learning. *Journal of Comparative and Physiological Psychology* 53: 113–121.

HERNÁNDEZ-PEÓN, R. 1966. Current concepts in the neurophysiology of learning. In *Deprivation in Psychological Development*. Washington, D.C.: Pan American Health Organization, publication no. 134, pp. 18–27.

HERRNSTEIN, R. J. 1969. Method and theory in the study of avoidance. *Psychological Review* 76: 49–69.

HULL, C. L. 1943. *Principles of Behavior*. New York: Appleton-Century-Crofts.

HUTCHINSON, R. R., ULRICH, R. E., and ARZIN, N. H. 1965. Effects of age and related factors on the pain-aggression reaction. *Journal of Comparative and Physiological Psychology* 59: 365–369.

JACOBSON, M. 1970. *Developmental Neurobiology*. New York: Holt, Rinehart and Winston.

JACOBSON, S. 1963. Sequence of myelinization in the brain of the albino rat. A. Cerebral cortex, thalamus and related structures. *Journal of Comparative Neurology* 121: 5–29.

JAMES, H. and BINKS, C. 1963. Escape and avoidance learning in newly hatched domestic chicks. *Science* 139: 1293–1294.

JAMES, W. T., and CANNON, D. J. 1952. Conditioned avoidance responses in puppies. *American Journal of Physiology* 168: 251–253.

JENKINS, H. M. 1965. Generalization gradients and the concept of inhibition. In D. I. Mostofsky, ed., *Stimulus Generalization*. Stanford, Calif.: Stanford University Press, pp. 55–61.

JOUVET-MOUNIER, D., ASTIC, L., and LACOTE, D. 1970. Ontogenesis of the states of sleep in rat, cat, and guinea pig during the first post-natal month. *Developmental Psychobiology* 2: 216–239.

KAMIN, L. J. 1959. The delay of punishment gradient. *Journal of Comparative and Physiological Psychology* 52: 434–437.

KAY, H., and SIME, M. E. 1962. Discrimination learning with old and young rats. *Journal of Gerontology* 17: 75–80.

KESSEN, W., ed. 1965. *The Child*. New York: John Wiley & Sons.

KIMBLE, G. A. 1961. *Hilgard and Marquis' Conditioning and Learning*. New York: Appleton-Century-Crofts.

KIRBY, R. H. 1963. Acquisition, extinction, and retention of an avoidance response as a function of age. *Journal of Comparative and Physiological Psychology* 56: 158–162.

KIRKBY, R. J. 1967. A maturation factor in spontaneous alternation. *Nature* 215: 784.

KLEIN, S. B., and SPEAR, N.E. 1969. Influence of age on short-term retention of active avoidance learning in rats. *Journal of Comparative and Physiological Psychology* 69: 583–589.

KOVACH, J. A., and KLING, A. 1967. Mechanisms of neonate sucking behavior in the kitten. *Animal Behaviour* 15: 91–101.

LIPSITT, L. P. 1969. Learning capacities of the human infant. In R. J. Robinson, ed., *Brain and Early Behaviour*. New York: Academic Press, pp. 227–245.

LIPSITT, L. P. 1971. Infant learning: The blooming, buzzing confusion revisited. In M. E. Meyer, ed., *Second Western Symposium on Learning: Early Learning*. Bellingham, Wash.: Western Washington State College, pp. 5–19.

LYNN, R. 1966. *Attention, Arousal, and the Orientation Reaction*. New York: Pergamon Press.

MASON, W. A., and HARLOW, H. F. 1958a. Formation of conditioned responses in infant monkeys. *Journals of Comparative and Physiological Psychology* 51: 68–70.

MASON, W. A., and HARLOW, H. F. 1958b. Performance of infant rhesus monkeys on a spatial discrimination problem. *Journal of Comparative and Physiological Psychology* 51: 71–74.

McGAUGH, J., and COLE, J. 1965. Age and strain differences in the effect of distribution of practice on maze learning. *Psychonomic Science* 2: 253–254.

McGINTY, D. J. 1971. Encephalization and the neural control of sleep. In M. B. Sterman, D. J. McGinty, and A. M. Adinolfi, eds., *Brain Development and Behavior*. New York: Academic Press, pp. 335–357.

MEIER, G. W. 1964. Differences in maze performance as a function of age and strain of house mice. *Journal of Comparative and Physiological Psychology* 58: 418–422.

MISANIN, J. R., NAGY, Z. M., KEISER, E. F., and BOWEN, W.

1971. Emergence of long-term memory in the neonatal rat. *Journal of Comparative and Physiological Psychology* 77: 188–199.

MOORCROFT, W. H., LYTLE, L. D., and CAMPBELL, B. A. 1971. Ontogeny of starvation-induced behavioral arousal in the rat. *Journal of Comparative and Physiological Psychology* 75: 59–67.

NAGY, Z. M., and MISANIN, J. R. 1973. Straight-alley escape behavior in infant mice: Effect of shock intensity. *Developmental Psychobiology* 6: 399–409.

NAGY, Z. M., and MURPHY, J. M. 1974. Learning and retention of a discriminated escape response in infant mice. *Developmental Psychobiology* 7: 185–192.

OLSEN, C. A., DELIUS, J. D., and HOCKEY, G. R. J. 1974. Brain temperature alterations and the retention of visual pattern discriminations in pigeons. *Physiology and Behavior* 257–260.

PAPOUSEK, H. 1967. Experimental studies of appetitional behavior in human newborns and infants. In H. W. Stevenson, E. H. Hess, and H. L. Rheingold, eds., *Early Behavior*. New York: John Wiley & Sons, pp. 249–277.

PAPOUSEK, H., and BERNSTEIN, P. 1969. The function of conditioning stimulation in human neonates and infants. In A. Ambrose, ed., *Stimulation in Early Infancy*. London: Academic Press, pp. 229–252.

PARÉ, W. P. 1969. Interaction of age and shock intensity on acquisition of a discriminated CER. *Journal of Comparative and Physiological Psychology* 68: 364–369.

PARSONS, P. J., and SPEAR, N. E. 1972. Long-term retention of avoidance learning by immature and adult rats as a function of environmental enrichment. *Journal of Comparative and Physiological Psychology* 80: 297–303.

PERKINS, JR., C. C. 1965. A conceptual scheme for studies of stimulus generalization. In D. I. Mostofsky, ed., *Stimulus Generalization*. Stanford, Calif.: Stanford University Press.

PETERS, J., and ISAACSON, R. 1963. Acquisition of active and passive responses in two breeds of chicken. *Journal of Comparative and Physiological Psychology* 56: 793–796.

PLOOG, D. W. 1966. Biological bases for instinct and behavior: Studies on the development of social behavior in squirrel monkeys. In J. Wortes, ed., *Recent Advances in Biological Psychiatry*. Society of Biological Psychiatry. Proceedings of the Annual Convention and Scientific Program, pp. 199–224.

PORTER, K. L., and THOMPSON, R. W. 1967. The effects of age and CS complexity on the acquisition of an avoidance response in rats. *Psychonomic Science* 9: 447–448.

PREYER, W. 1965. The mood of the child. In W. Kessen, ed., *The Child*. New York: John Wiley & Sons, pp. 134–151.

PURPURA, D. P., SHOFER, R. J., HOUSEPIAN, E. M., and NOBACK, C. R. 1964. Comparative ontogenesis of structure-formation relationships in cerebral and cerebellar cortex. In D. P. Purpura and J. P. Schadé, eds., *Progress in Brain Research*. Vol. 4: *Growth and Maturation of the Brain*. Amsterdam: Elsevier.

RANDALL, P. K. 1974. Ontogeny of amphetamine hyperactivity in the rat. Paper presented at the Eastern Psychological Association meetings, Philadelphia, April 1974.

RICCIO, D. C., and MARRAZO, M. J. 1972. Effects of punishing active avoidance in young and adult rats. *Journal of Comparative and Physiological Psychology* 79: 453–458.

RICCIO, D. C., ROHRBAUGH, M., and HODGES, L. A. 1968. Developmental aspects of passive and active avoidance in rats. *Developmental Psychobiology* 1: 108–111.

RICCIO, D. C., and SCHULENBERG, C. J. 1969. Age-related deficits in acquisition of a passive avoidance response. *Canadian Journal of Psychology* 23: 429–437.

ROBERTS, W. A. 1966. Learning and motivation in the immature rat. *American Journal of Psychology* 79: 3–23.

ROFFWARG, H. P., MUZIO, J. N., and DEMENT, W. C. 1966. Ontogenetic development of the human sleep cycle. *Science* 152: 604–619.

ROHRBAUGH, M., and RICCIO, D. C. 1968. Stimulus generalization of learned fear in infant and adult rats. *Journal of Comparative and Physiological Psychology* 66: 530–532.

ROSENBLATT, J. S. 1971. Suckling and home orientation in the kitten: A comparative developmental study. In E. Tobach, L. R. Aronson, and E. Shaw, eds., *The Biopsychology of Development*. New York: Academic Press, pp. 345–410.

ROSENBLATT, J. S. 1972. Learning in newborn kittens. *Scientific American* 227: 18–25.

ROUSSEAU, J. J. 1965. Emile, or on education. In W. Kessen, ed., *The Child*. New York: John Wiley & Sons, pp. 76–97.

SCHADÉ, J. P., and VAN GROENINGEN, W. B. 1961. Structural organization of the human cerebral cortex. I. Maturation of the middle frontal gyrus. *Acta Anatomica* 47: 74–111.

SCHERRER, J. 1967. Electrophysiological aspects of cortical development. In E. A. Asraytan, ed., *Progress in Brain Research*. Amsterdam: Elsevier, pp. 480–489.

SCHULENBERG, C. J., RICCIO, D. C., and STIKES, E. R. 1971. Acquisition and retention of a passive avoidance response as a function of age in rats. *Journal of Comparative and Physiological Psychology* 74: 75–83.

SCOTT, J. P. 1968. *Early Experience and the Organization of Behavior*. Monterey, Calif.: Brooks/Cole.

SCOTT, J. P., and MARSTON, M. V. 1950. Critical periods affecting the development of normal and maladjusted social behavior in puppies. *Journal of Genetic Psychology* 77: 25–60.

SEDLACEK, J., SVEHLOVA, M., Sedlackova, M., MARSALA, J., and KAPRAS, J. 1961. New results in the ontogenesis of reflex activity. In P. Sobotka, ed., *Functional and Metabolic development of the Central Nervous System* (Pilsen Symposium Suppl. 3). Prague: Charles University Press.

SLUCKIN, W. 1965. *Imprinting and Early Learning*. Chicago: Aldine.

SMITH, N. 1968. Effects of interpolated learning on retention of an escape response in rats as a function of age. *Journal of Comparative and Physiological Psychology* 65: 422–426.

SNEDDEN, D. S., SPEVACK, A. A., and THOMPSON, W. R. 1971. Conditioned and unconditioned suppression as a function of age in rats. *Canadian Journal of Psychology* 25: 313–322.

SPITZ, R. A. 1959. *A Genetic Field Theory of Ego Formation: Its Implications for Pathology*. New York: International University Press.

STANLEY, W. C., BACON, W. E., and FEHR, C. 1970. Discriminated instrumental learning in neonatal dogs. *Journal of Comparative and Physiological Psychology* 70: 335–343.

STANLEY, W. C., CORNWALL, A. C., PAGGIANI, C., and TRATTNER, A. 1963. Conditioning in the neonate puppy. *Journal of Comparative and Physiological Psychology* 56: 211–214.

STANLEY, W. C., and ELLIOT, O. 1962. Differential human handling as reinforcing events and as treatments influencing later source behavior in basenji puppies. *Psychological Reports* 10: 775–788.

STANLEY, W. C., MORRIS, D. D., and TRATTNER, A. 1965. Conditioning with a passive person reinforcer and extinction in Shetland sheepdog puppies. *Psychonomic Science* 2: 19–20.

STONE, C. P. 1929a. The age factor in animal learning. I. Rats in the problem box and the maze. *Genetic Psychology Monographs* 5: 1–130.

STONE, C. P. 1929b. The age factor in animal learning. II. Rats on a multiple light discrimination box and a different maze. *Genetic Psychology Monographs* 6: 125–202.

TAYLOR, J., ed. 1931. *Selected Writings of John Hughlings Jackson.* Vol. 1: *On Epilepsy and Epileptiform Convulsions.* London: Hodder and Stoughton.

TAYLOR, J., ed. 1932. *Selected Writings of John Hughlings Jackson.* Vol. 2: *Evolution and Dissolution of the Nervous System.* London: Hodder and Stoughton.

TERRACE, H. S. 1966. Stimulus control. In W. K. Honig, ed., *Operant Behavior: Areas of Research and Application.* New York: Appleton-Century-Crofts, pp. 271–344.

THOMAN, E. WETZEL, A., and LEVINE, S. 1968. Learning in the neonatal rat. *Animal Behaviour* 16: 54–57.

THOMPSON, R. W. 1957. The effect of ECS on retention in young and adult rats. *Journal of Comparative and Physiological Psychology* 50: 644–646.

THOMPSON, R. W. 1968. Development and the biophysical basis of personality. In E. F. Borgoth and W. W. Lambert, eds., *Handbook of Personality Theory and Research.* New York: Rand-McNally, pp. 149–214.

THOMPSON, R. W., KOENIGSBERG, L. A., and TENNISON, J. C. 1965. Effects of age on learning and retention of an avoidance response in rats. *Journal of Comparative and Physiological Psychology* 60: 457–459.

WALDFOGEL, S. 1948. The frequency and affective character of childhood memories. *Psychological Monographs* 62 (4, Whole No. 291).

WIKMARK, R. G. E. 1974. Maturation of spatial delayed response to auditory areas in kittens. *Journal of Comparative and Physiological Psychology* 86: 322–327.

WILSON, L. M., and RICCIO, D. C. 1973. CS familiarization and conditioned suppression in weanling and adult albino rats. *Bulletin of Psychonomic Science* 1: 184–186.

YAKOVLEV, P. I., and LECOURS, A. 1967. The myelogenetic cycles of regional maturation of the brain. In A. Minkowski, ed., *Regional Development of the Brain in Early Life.* Philadelphia: F. A. Davis, pp. 3–65.

ZIMMERMAN, R. R. 1961. Analysis of discrimination learning capacities in the infant rhesus monkey. *Journal of Comparative and Physiological Psychology* 54: 1–10.

ZIMMERMAN, R. R., and TORREY, C. C. 1965. Ontogeny of learning. In A. M. Schrier, H. F. Harlow, and F. Stollnitz, eds., *Behavior of Nonhuman Primates: Modern Research Trends,* Vol. 2. New York: Academic Press, pp. 405–447.

14

Organic Maturation and the Development of Learning Capacity

Joseph Altman and Fatma G. Bulut

ABSTRACT Infants differ from adults in their motivational status, peripheral sensorimotor development, and neural maturation. Therefore, when memory functions are studied in infant rats, it is necessary to select appropriate rewards or punishments, relevant signals or cues, and performance tasks that are part of the infant's motor repertoire and have a low threshold. It is only when these conditions are met that one can begin to study the maturation of the neural mechanisms underlying memory functions and their phenomenal characteristics in infants. In a pilot study, infant rats were rewarded by the opportunity to return to the home cage when mastering a simple two-choice discrimination with either position or a tactile stimulus used as the discrimination cue. The tasks were mastered gradually by pups started at 6 or 10 days of age, but 15-day-old rats showed an appreciable superiority over the younger animals. This superiority was eliminated by an x-irradiation treatment which selectively reduced the granule-cell population of either the cerebellar cortex or the hippocampal dentate gyrus in 15-day-old rats.

Intuitively, one might expect that the memory capacity of mammalian infants would match or surpass that of adults, not only because infants are embarking on a career of adapting themselves to the external world, which in mammals depends so much on the utilization of experience, but also because their "memory stores," if they exist at the outset, are less likely to be occupied than are those of adults. But, contrary to both this expectation and well-known psychoanalytic assumptions, available research (see Campbell, this volume) suggests that the mammalian neonate is unable to learn some problems and is handicapped not only in the time taken to acquire others, but also in the long-term retention of the problems mastered. To what extent are these learning handicaps due to such factors as the use of inappropriate incentives or the immaturity of sensory and motor systems, rather than to the underdevelopment of infantile memory mechanisms? Obviously we have to question on these grounds some of the available data regarding the apparent inadequacies of infant learning. The first question we should ask is this: Has the experimenter chosen an incentive that is appropriate to the infant at

JOSEPH ALTMAN and FATMA G. BULUT, Department of Biological Sciences, Purdue University, West Lafayette, IN

its particular stage of development? We do not have in mind such an obviously ill-chosen reward as offering solid food or water to a suckling neonate. But is, for instance, electric shock an appropriate form of punishment for an infant which is as yet unprepared for life in a hostile world but has to cope with life in the nest, where the major demands include competition for nursing sites and for the mother's attention in order to get cleaned, to be helped in micturition and defecation, and to be kept at the appropriate ambient temperature? The second question that we should ask is whether or not we have taken into consideration the infant's stage of sensory development when a conditioned stimulus or discrimination cue is presented. Again, we do not have in mind the obvious error of presenting a patterned visual stimulus to an infant whose eyes are not yet open; rather, we question the appropriateness of using an intense light flash, or an arbitrarily selected sound or smell, instead of the sounds, smells, and feels of the nest (of mother, siblings, nesting materials) where the life and training of the infant begins and continues for some time. In a similar vein we must consider the task set to the animal in terms of limitations of its motor capacities and the immaturity of its response repertoire.

14.1 MOTOR AND MOTIVATIONAL MATURATION

We tried to put some of these considerations into the design of a recently published set of experiments (Bulut and Altman, 1974). We wished to determine when young rats can begin to master a two-choice position and tactile discrimination in a modified Grice box. A previous study (Altman and Sudarshan, 1975) showed that rats aged 1–2 days tend to remain immobile in the open field, but from day 3 onward they spend an increasing amount of time in pivoting (Figure 14.1). This is a form of circular locomotion that results from movements of the forelimbs with the abdomen and hindlimbs acting as an anchor. Pivoting is maximal around days 6 and 7 and declines thereafter as the hindlimbs become involved and the animal begins to crawl (Figure 14.2).

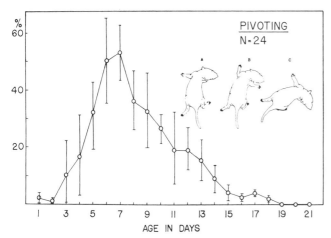

FIGURE 14.1 Mean percentage of time spent in pivoting in the open field. The decline in pivoting is associated with the emergence of coordinated quadruped progression with the entire trunk raised off the ground. Inset: tracings from motion picture of the three essential steps in "pivoting." A: The head is turned to the right. B: the right forelimb is pulled out from under the head and placed to the right. C: the shoulder region is pushed to the right by the left forelimb. Vertical lines represent 1 SD. From Altman and Sudarshan (1975).

If rats can pivot from day 3, it should be possible to determine whether or not they can locate and are drawn toward their home cage when removed from it. To test this the animals were placed in a circular wire enclosure; as indicated in Figure 14.3, they displayed from day 3 onward a significant tendency to orient their heads homeward. By day 8 all the animals were orienting themselves in that direction virtually all the time.

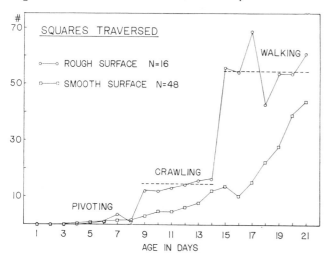

FIGURE 14.2 Mean number of squares (10 × 10 cm) traversed in a field (50 × 50 cm). On a rough (plywood) surface three activity levels are evident, associated with pivoting, crawling, and walking (or running) as successive stages in locomotor development. Exploratory activity is suppressed on a smooth (lucite) surface. Data were obtained by three observers and pooled. From Altman and Sudarshan (1975).

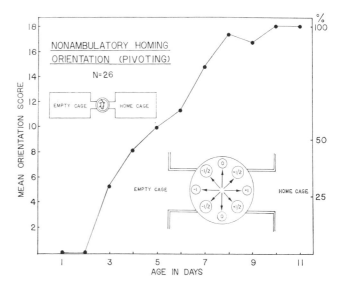

FIGURE 14.3 Orientation toward the home cage on a circular platform surrounded by a wire fence. Orientation of the animal was scored, as indicated in the inset, every 10 sec during a 180-sec daily observation period. From Altman and Sudarshan (1975).

However, few animals could reach home by day 8 in an apparatus where they had to traverse a 20-cm path over a 3-minute period (Figure 14.4). With increasing age, as they began to crawl, more and more animals were successful, and virtually all the animals homed successfully by day 14 or 15; this is the age when walking and running replace crawling (Figure 14.2).

The testing apparatus for learning is illustrated in Figure 14.5. The animals were 6, 10, or 15 days old at the beginning of the training procedure. One group of

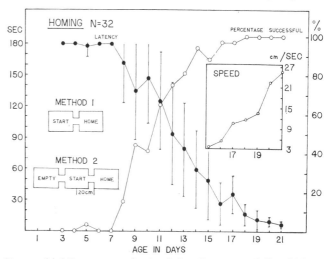

FIGURE 14.4 Percentage of animals homing successfully within 180 sec, and latency of responses. Data from the two methods shown are pooled. Speed of ambulation shown on insert is based on results from one group (method 1) during the period when all animals homed. Vertical lines represent 1 SD. From Altman and Sudarshan (1975).

ORGANIC MATURATION AND THE DEVELOPMENT OF LEARNING CAPACITY   237

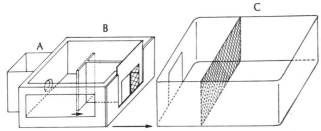

FIGURE 14.5 Apparatus (Grice box) used to study discrimination learning. A: start box. B: choice box. C: home cage. The two-alley choice box has two exits, one of which can be closed by means of a movable screen that does not interfere with penetration of odor from the home cage. The choice box is attached to the modified home cage (right) in which a wire screen prevents the mother from leaving the cage to retrieve the isolated pup. From Bulut and Altman (1974).

rats had to learn a position discrimination; half of these animals gained access to the home cage when they turned right, the other half when they turned left. Another group had to master a tactile discrimination; half of the animals had to traverse a rough-surfaced path, the other half a smooth-surfaced path. Errors were classified as those of omission (failing to move or get to the home cage) or commission (selecting the incorrect side). On the first two days of testing the 6-day-old animals failed to move much of the time. But if the missed choice opportunities are disregarded, they did not differ significantly, in terms of the actual number of errors committed before reaching a criterion level of learning, from the group whose training was started on day 10 (Figure 14.6). But the animals started on day 15 learned the position discrimination significantly faster than the younger groups. These results established that rats as young as 6 days, though handicapped as a result of loco-

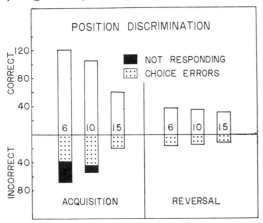

FIGURE 14.6 Position discrimination in three groups of animals aged 6, 10, and 15 days at the beginning of the experiment. The total number of trials to criterion was divided in each case into correct and incorrect responses; the latter were subdivided into errors of commission (choice errors) and omission (not responding). From Bulut and Altman (1974).

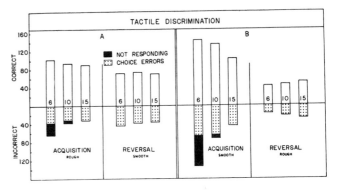

FIGURE 14.7 Mean percentage of trials to criterion (including failure to move) in a tactile discrimination task. A: rough surface correct in acquisition, smooth side on reversal. B: smooth surface correct in acquisition, rough surface on reversal. From Bulut and Altman (1974).

motor immaturity, can begin to learn a two-choice discrimination with position as a cue.

Somewhat more complicated results were obtained in the tactile discrimination task (Figure 14.7). Apparently, the younger the animal the greater the preference for a rough-surfaced floor, presumably because it provides better traction for crawling. This may explain why the 6-day-old subgroup that was trained to choose the rough floor (again disregarding the missed choice opportunities) was not inferior to the others in the number of actual trials to criterion. Learning to select the smooth-surfaced path was more prolonged for all groups, but the 15-day-old animals learned this task faster than the 6- and 10-day-old animals. Again this suggested that the two younger groups could learn the discrimination but that they were inferior to the animals whose training began on day 15.

14.2 NEURAL MATURATION

The lack of significant differences between the learning capacities of the 6- and 10-day-old rats, and the substantial improvement in the group started at the beginning of the third week, suggested the possibility that the maturation of some late-developing brain region might underlie the enhancement of learning capacity in the latter group. (As visual cues could not aid the animals in the discrimination, we disregarded the opening of the eyes as a possible factor). For some time we have been studying the postnatal development of the cerebellar cortex (reviewed in Altman, 1975) and hippocampus (reviewed in Altman and Bayer, 1975) in the rat. These are the two brain regions in which the granule cells, an important neuronal element, are predominantly or exclusively formed after birth. In conjunction with these normative ontogenetic studies, we have developed an

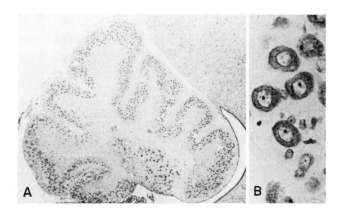

FIGURE 14.8 Photomicrograph of the cerebellar vermis of an adult rat that was irradiated several times after birth with 150–200r x rays. Note the predominance of Purkinje cells and the virtual absence of granule cells (A). Purkinje cells (shown enlarged in B) are not affected in terms of number or size of cell body. From Altman and Anderson (1972).

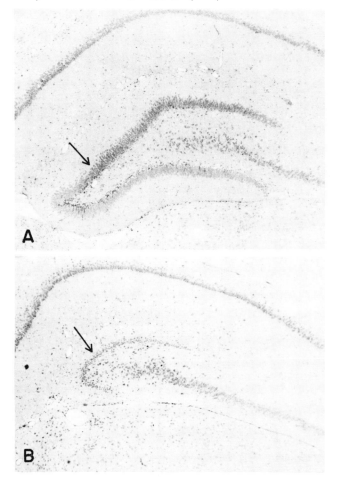

FIGURE 14.9 Photomicrographs of the dorsal hippocampus at 21 days in a normal rat (A) and a rat whose hippocampus was irradiated repeatedly during early infancy (B). Note reduction of dentate granular layer (arrows) in the irradiated animal. From Bayer et al. (1973).

experimental technique that allows us to prevent selectively the formation of these granule cells. This is accomplished by irradiating the region of the cerebellum (Figure 14.8) or of the hippocampus (Figure 14.9) after birth with low-level x-rays, which kill the multiplying cells that would subsequently differentiate as granule cells. Behavioral studies in adults indicate that experimental granule-cell agenesis in the cerebellar cortex (Brunner and Altman, 1973) or the hippocampal dentate gyrus (Bayer et al., 1973) results in syndromes comparable to those obtained with surgical removal of the cerebellum or hippocampus, respectively, implying an important functional role for these postnatally acquired elements.

Accordingly, we set out to examine in 15-day-old rats if irradiation of the cerebellum or the hippocampus interferes with the enhancement of learning capacity, with respect to the younger groups, that is seen in normal animals of this age. The results (Figure 14.10) indicate that irradiation of the hippocampus or the cerebellum with an x-ray schedule that prevents the formation of postnatally acquired granule cells significantly retards the acquisition and reversal of a position discrimination. In Figure 14.11 the results are summarized in terms of the number of daily sessions to criterion in the three normal age groups and the irradiated 15-day-old animals. The performance of the irradiated animals is somewhat superior in acquisition and inferior in reversal in comparison with that of the younger normal groups. (It should be noted that by the time the normal rats are reversed, they are all older than 15 days.)

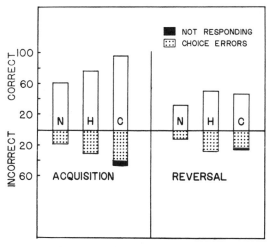

FIGURE 14.10 Position discrimination in three groups of animals (N = normal; H = hippocampus-irradiated: C = cerebellum-irradiated) that started training on day 15. The total number of trials were divided in each case into correct and incorrect responses; the latter were subdivided into errors of commission and omission (not responding). Revised from Altman et al. (1974).

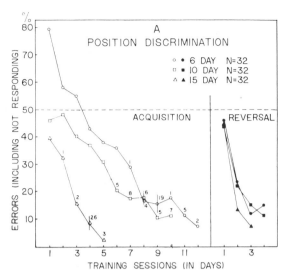

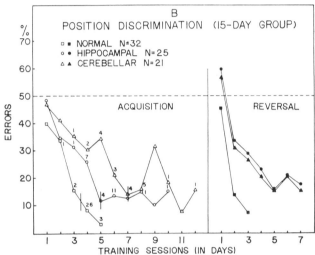

FIGURE 14.11 A: Mean percentage of errors (including failure to move and make a choice) on a position-discrimination task in animals that began training on days 6, 10, and 15. Numerals above scores indicate the number of animals that reached criterion on the day indicated; vertical bar is the mean for the group. B: Acquisition and reversal of the position habit in 15-day-old normal animals, and animals in which the development of the cerebellum or hippocampus was retarded with x-irradiation. From Altman et al. (1974).

These results indicate that interference with the development of either one of the selected late-developing brain regions, the cerebellum or the hippocampus, shifts the learning performance of older rats toward the level characteristic of younger animals. In retrospect, the results are somewhat surprising, since hippocampal damage in adults does not usually interfere with the acquisition of a simple two-choice discrimination (for a review, see Altman et al., 1973), and the old evidence (Lashley and Ball, 1929) suggests that the cerebellum is not involved in position discrimination. At the same time

the results are gratifying to us in that they lend some support to our speculation (Altman, 1967) that the postnatally acquired granule cells, which can be looked upon as "associative" neuronal elements, are somehow implicated in memory processes.

ACKNOWLEDGMENT

This research is supported by the National Institute of Mental Health, the National Institute of Child Health and Human Development, and the U.S. Atomic Energy Commission. We wish to thank Zeynep Kurgun-Chen and Kiran Sudarshan for their assistance.

REFERENCES

ALTMAN, J. 1967. Postnatal growth and differentiation of the mammalian brain, with implications for a morphological theory of memory. In G. C. Quarton, T. Melnechuk, and F. O. Schmitt, eds., *The Neurosciences: A Study Program.* New York: Rockefeller University Press, pp. 723–743.

ALTMAN, J. 1975. Effects of interference with cerebellar maturation on the development of locomotion. In N. A. Buchwald and M.A.B. Brazier, eds., *Brain Mechanisms in Mental Retardation.* New York: Academic Press, pp. 41–91.

ALTMAN, J., and ANDERSON, W. J. 1972. Experimental reorganization of the cerebellar cortex. I. Morphological effects of elimination of all microneurons with prolonged X-irradiation started at birth. *Journal of Comparative Neurology* 146: 355–406.

ALTMAN, J., and BAYER, S. A. 1975. Postnatal development of the hippocampal dentate gyrus under normal and experimental conditions. In R. L. Isaacson and K. H. Pribram, eds., *The Hippocampus: A Comprehensive Treatise.* New York: Plenum Press.

ALTMAN, J., BRUNNER, R. L., and BAYER, S. A. 1973. The hippocampus and behavioral maturation. *Behavioral Biology* 8: 557–596.

ALTMAN, J., BRUNNER, R. L., BULUT, F. G., and SUDARSHAN, K. 1974. The development of behavior in normal and brain-damaged infant rats, studied with homing (nest-seeking) as motivation. In A. Vernadakis and N. Weiner, eds., *Drugs and the Developing Brain.* New York: Plenum Press.

ALTMAN, J., and SUDARSHAN, K. 1975. Postnatal development in the laboratory rat. *Animal Behaviour* 23: 896–920.

BAYER, S. A., BRUNNER, R. L., HINE, R., and ALTMAN, J. 1973. Behavioural effects of interference with the postnatal acquisition of hippocampal granule cells. *Nature: New Biology* 242: 222–224.

BRUNNER, R. L., and ALTMAN, J. 1973. Locomotor deficits in adult rats with moderate to massive retardation of cerebellar development during infancy. *Behavioral Biology* 9: 169–188.

BULUT, F. G., and ALTMAN, J. 1974. Spatial and tactile discrimination learning in infant rats motivated by homing. *Developmental Psychobiology* 7: 465–473.

LASHLEY, K. S., and BALL, J. 1929. Spinal conduction and kinesthetic sensitivity in the maze habit. *Journal of Comparative Psychology* 9: 71–105.

15

Some Thoughts on the Ontogeny of Memory and Learning

MADGE E. SCHEIBEL AND
ARNOLD B. SCHEIBEL

ABSTRACT The purpose of this study is to document some of the structural changes that occur during the period of growth and development from birth to maturity. This is the period during which the organism learns most intensively about the world around him, and how to interact with that environment. It is also the time when the laying down of residues of these learning experiences and interactive techniques—called memory—is most active. While we do not understand the structural and functional mechanisms involved in the coding, storage, and retrieval of these traces, we feel intuitively that among the complex of developmental processes, some are undoubtedly involved in processes of learning and memory.

A broad range of developmental changes in structural organization has been identified, some of impressive dimensions. The dendrites (processes) of neurons in many parts of the nervous system regroup themselves into close aggregates or bundles. This change frequently occurs immediately preceding the appearance of a specific item or class of output phenomena from the area involved. It is suggested that the bundles may function as specialized zones where central programs for these outputs are coded.

Dramatic changes occur during the maturation of the cerebral cortex. One population of dendrite spines is lost, and another smaller species is substituted for them on the surface of most cortical pyramidal cells. While the vertically oriented dendrite branches of these pyramids are present at birth, the horizontal components do not appear till well into the postnatal period. As these develop, they form a dense horizontal plexus which becomes a candidate zone for a number of putative, horizontally organized coupling systems. This substrate may, in a sense, take the functional place of the thick, horizontal fiber layer just under the cortical surface which disappears at the same epoch.

Finally, the entire range of afferent fiber systems ascending to cortex from more caudal stations develop their final morphological patterns and establish definitive connections with nerve-cell systems as they mature. In other words, connections are progressively established or reworked as new cell systems come on line. The cerebral cortex can be taken as the ultimate model for the remainder of the central nervous system, developing, reshuffling connections, and remodeling structures as the repertoire of organismic responses becomes more complex and varied.

"It is not possible to demonstrate the isolated localization of a memory trace anywhere within the nervous system. Limited regions may be essential for learning or retention of a particular activity, but within such regions the parts are functionally equivalent. The engram is represented throughout the region."

K. S. Lashley (1950)

This introductory quotation from Lashley, summarizing 35 years of work and thought on the problems of memory and learning, seems an appropriate preface to the task at hand. For in serving as discussants to Byron Campbell's review (this volume), we are painfully aware that we must marshal data illuminating the ontogeny of processes which are still among the most mysterious of biological phenomena. But the pressing nature of the task, particularly for those of us who deal on a daily basis with the problems of psychiatric patients, emphasizes the need for attempts such as this, no matter how speculative—or ultimately wrong—our conclusions may be.

A bewildering variety of changes occur in developing brain tissue, and if in most forms the gross reproductive process among nerve cells is stilled at birth, the progression and increasing subtlety of maturative change certainly is not. Approximately ten years ago we had the opportunity to review some of the structural and functional changes that characterize postnatal development in the nervous system of mammalian vertebrates (Scheibel and Scheibel, 1964b). While the range of phenomena seems relatively limited by today's standards, it is interesting to note, retrospectively, how easily one can make a convincing case for each of these as being causally related to the ontogenesis of learning and/or memory.

Campbell has reconsidered several of these areas of change in the neural substrate, and the interested reader can easily acquaint himself with our previous article. In the meantime a burgeoning literature and a number of symposium volumes have appeared which consider in much greater detail recent work on neural ontogenesis. We shall therefore avoid the temptation to produce one more overview of an already well watched subject matter and shall concentrate instead on two maturative sequences. On intuitive grounds, each of these certainly falls within our purview, but to our minds at least there is more than that to recommend them, for they represent very different, perhaps antipodal, positions vis-à-vis the problems of storage and recall, and as such they may have paradigmatic value.

MADGE E. SCHEIBEL and ARNOLD B. SCHEIBEL, Departments of Anatomy and Psychiatry, University of California, Los Angeles

In the first section we shall trace the development of a specific structural complex, the dendrite bundle, which can be found in many portions of the central nervous system. Its appearance often seems time-locked to the initial development of a discrete item of output performance characteristic of the region in question. It is accordingly proposed as a putative program site coding certain types of repetitive or stereotyped output. Such a suggestion obviously recalls classic attempts to localize the engram anatomically. While similar in some respects to deterministic theories of memory, we feel there are positive points that commend such a notion to our attention.

In the second section we shall review certain aspects of the ontogenesis of the cortical ground substance, presented as the substrate vital to the higher-level processing and inscription of information (Bruner, Olver, and Greenfield, 1966). The multiple developmental phenomena that we propose to scan in a structure as cosmopolitan as the cerebral cortex will serve to epitomize a more modern position, i.e., that the acquisition and memorization "of a past experience is not represented deterministically by the activity of any single cell or group of cells in the population but is specified by the average activity of the population through time, reflecting alterations in the spatiotemporal pattern of discharge as a result of past experience" (John, 1967, p. 17).

15.1 DEVELOPMENT OF THE DENDRITE BUNDLE AS A STORAGE SITE FOR CENTRAL PROGRAMS

Over the past few years we have become interested in specialized configurations of dendrites which appear at rather specific epochs in ontogenesis at various sites along the neuraxis. The development of these bundles appears, in some cases, to be temporally correlated with the appearance of certain types of motor output of a stereotyped or repetitive nature, and a putative relationship has been suggested between the two. Because of the possibility that such bundle sites may represent storage loci for internal programs coding the specific item of output performance, a brief review of the sites as we know them seems indicated.

Studies by Romanes (1964) have shown that motoneurons in the ventral horn of the spinal cord are segregated into cell pools on the basis of the muscle innervated. However, study of sagittal and horizontal sections of Golgi-stained cord in young rodents, carnivores, and primates shows that the dendrites of these cells transcend cell-pool boundaries and mingle freely over much of their extent along the longitudinal axis of the cord (Scheibel and Scheibel, 1970a). In the newborn cat these

sagittally arranged dendrites show no particular morphological relationship to each other, but toward the end of the second week of postnatal life, many dendrite tips begin to cluster together to form short dendrite bundles. These complexes grow longer and more obvious with increasing dendrite length and are usually fully developed at the age of four to five months (Scheibel and Scheibel, 1970b; see Figure 15.1). Our attention has been particularly attracted to these structural complexes for two reasons. First, the dendrite shafts making up each bundle are derived from motoneuron pools innervating muscles of different, often antagonistic, function. Second, the bundle formations first begin to appear when the hind legs of the young kitten show initial evidence of weight-bearing, standing, and walking capabilities. By the fourth to fifth month of life, when the bundles appear to have achieved their ultimate growth, the young animal has gained its full repertoire of motor activities in the hind limbs, including the crouching, stalking behavior, and springing characteristic of mature feline activity. Electromyographic analysis of antagonist pairs in the hind limb, such as gastrocnemius and anterior tibial, strengthen the impression that reciprocal activity patterns, totally absent at birth, show traces of patterning at twelve to fourteen days and fully developed reciprocal sequencing at four months of age (Scheibel and Scheibel, 1970b).

The concept of central motor programs springs naturally from Graham Brown's observation that alternating sequences of flexor and extensor activity can be elicited following deafferentation (Brown, 1914). After reviewing this problem, Lundberg (1969) concluded that "the basic mechanism of the alternating activation of extensors and flexors in stepping is centrally programmed in the spinal cord and not provided exclusively by reflexes." His own conception of the substrate system, like that of Brown, favors paired half-centers made up of interneurons, one activating flexor and one extensor motoneuron, tied together by reciprocal lines of inhibition and modulated by supraspinal mechanisms (Jankowska et al., 1967). This is a classic circuit paradigm frequently invoked for output patterns that include alternating rhythms or sequences (e.g., respiration, etc.). It implies that central representation of an output that is repeated many times over may depend in part on impulse patterns circulating through well-defined and localizable circuits in the central nervous system. This idea has become less fashionable following the classic cortical-incision experiments of Lashley (1929, 1950).

The dendrite bundle appears to offer a relatively sheltered, and probably specialized, milieu where fragments or whole sequences of stereotyped or repetitive output programs may be coded along the facing mem-

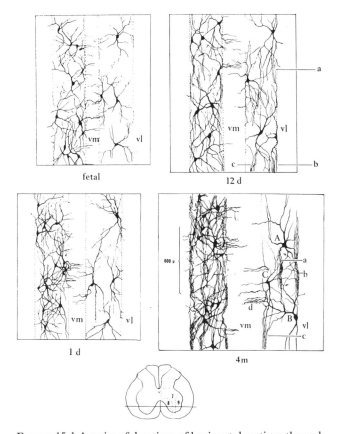

FIGURE 15.1 A series of drawings of horizontal sections through the ventral horn of the lumbosacral spinal cord to show development of motoneuron dendrites and dendrite bundles. In fetal cord, dendrites radiate without definite orientation. At 1 day of age the beginnings of sagittal orientation are already visible. At 12 days sagittal orientation is well advanced and the beginnings of bundle formation at a, b, and c are visible. At 4 months the motoneuron system is essentially mature, sagittal orientation of the dendrites predominates, and dendrite bundles at a, b, and c are well developed and project along the cord for relatively long distances. Neurons A, B, and C contribute dendrites to more than one bundle. Other abbreviations include vm, ventromedial white matter; vl, ventrolateral white matter; and d, small bundles of commissural dendrites which can be seen as early as the first postnatal day. Inset figure shows plane of section through cord. Drawn from sections of young cat spinal cord at various ages; stained by rapid Golgi variants. From Scheibel and Scheibel (1970b).

branes of dendrites sprung from the neurons supplying the muscle masses involved. Electron microscopic analysis of dendrite bundles in spinal ventral horn (Matthews, Willis, and Williams, 1971) and in cerebral cortex (Fleischauer, Petsche, and Wittkowski, 1972; Peters and Walsh, 1972) generally support the impression provided by Golgi impregnations.

While the relationship posited between dendrite bundles and motor output programs is entirely inferential, a possible test is provided by comparing the degree of structural maturation in lumbosacral and cervical cords. The newborn kitten has minimal control over its hind limbs except at the proximal (hip) joint. However, most full-term kittens are able to manipulate the maternal nipple zone during suckling with a characteristic, highly integrated treading motion of the forelimbs and feet almost immediately after birth. If our assumption linking dendrite-bundle development to items of stereotyped output involving flexor-extensor sequences is valid, evidence of dendrite bundles should be visible in cervical motoneuron pools at birth. Studies of such material show that sagittally organized motoneuron dendrites are at least 15 percent longer here than in the lumbosacral region and that dendrite bundles are already present. Such bundles are 50–100 μ long by the third to fourth postnatal day and up to 200 μ in length by the fourteenth day (Scheibel and Scheibel, 1971a), when bundles are first appearing in the lumbosacral ventral horn.

Recent Golgi studies have also indicated that dendrites crossing via the ventral commissure of Ramón y Cajal (1909–1911) from one anterior horn to the other are already organized into bundles at birth (Scheibel and Scheibel, 1973). These complexes include dendrites from motoneurons of many different cell pools on both sides as well as shafts from interneurons. We have tentatively identified these structures as possible program sites concerned with reflexive or stereotyped motor sequences involving the conjoint use of both extremities. Their precocious appearance may be related to the fact that the neonatal kitten is already capable of moving over a limited area, seeking the mother's flank, moving toward the nipple, etc. In this type of activity the hind limbs support no weight but are used, somewhat like the flippers of a sea mammal, to push the body forward. Such motion is undoubtedly of spinal origin, as can be shown briefly in exaggerated from in the acutely decapitated kitten (Scheibel and Scheibel, unpublished data).

Dendrite bundles have been found to develop at several places in the brainstem, notably in portions of the nonspecific (reticular) core, and they are presently under investigation in several cranial-nerve nuclei. Their development in the medullary and pontine reticular formation is of considerable interest insofar as it appears to be accompanied by at least partial loss of dendritic spines. The classic, sparsely branched, radiating pattern generated by dendrites of reticular neurons is well known from the studies of Ramón y Cajal (1909–1911) and from more recent work (e.g., Scheibel and Scheibel, 1958; Mannen, 1966; Ramón-Moliner and Nauta, 1966; Valverde, 1962). At birth the dendrite surfaces are covered by shaggy heteromorphic protospines, and there is a good deal of dendritic overlap. Successful Golgi impregnations of brainstem material from three- to four-month-old cats show two impressive changes: (1) the archaic spinal component has been almost entirely lost, leaving only small numbers of long spike-like structures; and (2) reticular-cell dendrites are now packed together in rather dense bundles for a large part of their trajectory (Scheibel, Davies, and Scheibel, 1973). As shown by Figure 15.2, the previous pattern of relatively straight single shafts is now at least partially replaced by bundles of dendrites curving around large fascicles of rostro-caudally running axons which make up a large portion of the reticular core. A number of dendrites from cells that are often quite distant from each other follow the same route for distances varying from fifty to several hundred microns. As with other bundle systems, dendrite shafts continue to join and leave the complex all along its course. As the direction of each bundle changes, its constituent elements also change, producing a coarse-woven, warp-and-woof appearance. As many as ten to fifteen shafts may be resolved in one bundle with the

light microscope, and the individual shafts may be so close that no space can be resolved between them, even with an oil-immersion objective.

The appearance and subsequent loss of protospines is an intriguing problem. In a recent communication (Scheibel, Davies, and Scheibel, 1973) we suggested that they might serve as postsynaptic targets for an archaic system of synaptic terminals that initially load the dendrite membrane with certain items of coded information in the late fetal and early postnatal period and are then resorbed. In a later section of this chapter we shall offer an alternative interpretation regarding the protospines of cerebral cortical pyramids. Both suggestions are, of course, highly speculative, and bear witness to the rudimentary state of the art.

The reshuffling of reticular dendrite systems constitutes a second challenging problem. It is conceivable that this change may be largely a consequence of compression caused by the growth of fiber masses traversing the reticular core. However, the resultant dendrite packing is still likely to be functionally significant. In line with our notions about dendrite bundles elsewhere, reticular dendrite bundles may also serve as sites for programs guiding rhythmic output sequences, such as respiratory rhythms or even the slower cadences of the rest-activity cycle. While such outputs are capable of autonomous activity, they are also responsive to override control by other systems that reflect moment-to-moment changes in the internal or external needs of the organism.

Golgi analysis had previously shown the nucleus reticularis thalami to form a grid or shell surrounding the anterior and lateral aspects of the thalamus, its dendritic systems arranged largely at right angles to the masses of thalamocortical axons, and its own axons recurrent upon the dorsal thalamus (Scheibel and Scheibel, 1966). In mature preparations we have recently found that dendrite systems in the ventrolateral portion of n. reticularis are compressed into bundle complexes similar in many respects to these structures elsewhere. Here, too, as in the reticular core farther downstream, the long and shaggy protospine system characteristic of the neonatal preparation is progressively lost as the dendrites rearrange themselves into bundles (Scheibel and Scheibel, 1972).

While the functional meaning of this structural figure is not clear, it is worth noting that its earliest appearance —between the eighth and twelfth days of life—coincides with the earliest appearance of thalamic spindles (T. L. Davies, R.D. Lindsay, M.E. Scheibel, and A.B. Scheibel, unpublished data). The characteristic discharge pattern of n. reticularis neurons consists of repetitive spike bursts (Negishi, Lu, and Verzeano, 1962), which appear temporally related to the development of thalamic spindles

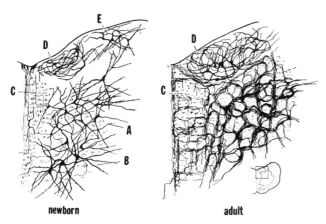

newborn   **adult**

FIGURE 15.2 A comparison of dendrite arrangements in the medullary reticular formation of the newborn and adult cat. In the neonate, neurons of the rostral part of nucleus reticularis parvocellularis (A) and of nucleus reticularis magnocellularis (B) are characterized by radiating dendrites bearing many spinelike excrescences. In the adult the dendrites appear to have been rearranged; they now are grouped in tightly packed bundles around the fascicles of myelinated axons running longitudinally through the reticular core. Surrounding structures include the medial longitudinal fasciculus (C), n. prepositus hypoglossi (D), and the medial vestibular nucleus (E). Rapid Golgi variant. From Scheibel and Scheibel (1973).

and may bear a causal relationship to them (Schlag and Waszak, 1970; Waszak, 1974). In line with our previous speculation on the role of dendrite bundles, it is possible that the repetitive-burst discharges of n. reticularis neurons are the major expression of the output programs coded in the bundle formations of this nucleus.

One other site of dendrite-bundle formation is worth noting. In neurally mature laboratory animals (rats and cats) and, on the basis of much less data, primates and man, the basilar dendrites of giant fifth-layer pyramids have long horizontal trajectories and are intermingled in bundle complexes (Figure 15.3). So far these basilar dendrite bundles appear limited to Betz cells in the primary motor area and to the giant cells of Meynert in primary visual cortex (Scheibel et al., 1974). There is virtually no intermingling with the basilar shafts of the surrounding medium or large-sized pyramids of layer 5. Using the Betz cells as a model, it is clear from studies of Golgi material in young and adult cats that basilar dendrite systems are still very short at birth (see Section 15.2), but between ten and fourteen days after birth these shafts begin to lengthen and appear to "seek each other out." In mature cats, individual shafts may extend for one millimeter or more and develop relationships with shafts from giant pyramids in surrounding cortical cell columns. In motor cortex Rosen and Asanuma (1972) have found that individual cell columns are similar to those described in sensory cortex (Powell and Mount-castle, 1959) and that each provides neural representation for a discrete element in the motor performance (Asanuma and Rosen, 1972).

The distribution of Betz cells is quite variable in the cat, where the average interval between such cells is $240 \pm 54 \ \mu$ (Scheibel et al., 1974), and even more so in man, where only 18 percent are found in visible cortex, with none at all in the lower half of area 4 (Lassek, 1954). In human cortex 75 percent of Betz cells are found in motor areas supplying the leg, with only 17.9 percent in the arm region and 6.6 percent in the head area (Lassek, 1954) despite the allocation of much larger cortical areas to head, arm, and hand than to leg. These differential counts suggest some sort of positive correlation with muscle mass, or antigravity status, or both.

The major antigravity activities of the biped are localized in the lower extremity and back. It may be that the typically phasic output of these large-axoned Betz cells (Evarts, 1967; Oshima, 1969: Takahashi, 1965) is selectively directed toward elicitation of flexor enhancement and extensor repression (Lundberg and Voorhoeve, 1962). Such a change in the status of the neuromuscular apparatus would seem intuitively necessary in order to allow superimposition of specific motor patterns on a background posture of supportive antigravity tonus.

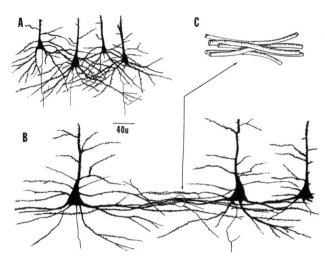

FIGURE 15.3 Details of dendritic organization in precruciate gyrus of adult cat showing disposition of basilar dendrites of third-layer pyramids (A) and fifth-layer pyramids (B). The latter are giant pyramidal cells of Betz which show the horizontal orientation, great length, and bundle formation characteristic of basilar shafts from these cells. C is an enlargement of the circled field in B, showing details of dendrite-bundle organization. A and B were drawn to the same scale. Golgi modifications. From Scheibel et al. (1974).

Actually, the demonstrably more rapid conduction of giant pyramidal cell axons (see, e.g., Evarts, 1967) can be conceived as initiating appropriate degrees of lysis in supportive activity across weight-bearing joints prior to onset of definitive motor patterns (Hore and Porter, 1972; Preston, Shende, and Uemura, 1967).

The basilar dendrite bundle systems that couple groups of adjacent Betz cells are conceived as repositories for central programs that sequence and modulate the phasic discharge patterns of Betz-cell groups. These are responsible, in turn, for initial patterns of downstream activity, setting the stage for the total motor act. Once again, as in previous examples cited, we conceive of this output program as essentially stereotyped and frequently repeated. While the range of output activities from motor cortex undoubtedly exceeds that inherent in a final common pathway system, we feel that the initial aspects of even the most complex and heterogeneous motor acts, those related to the initial regrouping of tension in anti-gravity-stressed muscles surrounding joints, are limited in number and may accordingly fall within the operational purview of a bundle complex.

We have obviously devoted considerable time to the development of this structural motif because of our conviction that the dendrite bundle may represent a significant site for the deposition and maintenance of certain types of memory. This group of examples does not exhaust the roster, and we are presently studying the structure in certain cranial-nerve motor nuclei and in parts of the basal ganglia. The code for each of these output programs is conceived to be inscribed along the glycoprotein shell (Pease, 1966), which extends appreciable distances out from each dendrite membrane (in the extended membrane concept of Lehninger, 1968) and may interact spatially with similar systems from adjacent dendrite shafts. In this manner the circumscribed extraneuronal space pool formed within each dendrite bundle may serve as a sheltered milieu harboring the output code specifying central programs peculiar to that neuronal constellation.

It seems likely that the type of memory with which we may be concerned here is of a special kind, perhaps best described as genetically programmed, instinctual, or endogenous. The output patterns are either delivered completely outside the realm of conscious participation (the programmed bursting of n. reticularis neurons, production of endogenous brainstem rhythms such as respiration, etc.) or else are continued in a more or less stereotyped fashion once they are triggered in the appropriate situation (standing, weight-bearing, walking, or running sequences, etc.). We might pose the additional question of whether certain activities that become virtually automatic through repetition (driving a car, the physical act of writing, some aspects of motor speech, etc.) also develop representation within such structural motifs. Our evidence is limited and is, so far, largely inferential. Note, however, that the type of function we have tentatively attributed to this structural paradigm is in some respects reminiscent of a category suggested by Bruner, Olver, and Greenfield (1966; see also Rozin, this volume), namely, the category of motor processing or encoding.

Before moving on, it is worth recalling that the concept of discrete loci for programming or program triggering is not without functional precedent. The command fiber of Wiersma (1952) and the command-interneuron concept developed by Wilson (1970) provide, in the invertebrate nervous system, a simple analogue of the dendrite system we have been considering. While the mechanisms involved in the initiation and performance of the stereotyped output are undoubtedly dissimilar, the command element provides a working model for a kind of localizable "motor memory" whose characteristics are subject to analysis.

15.2 SELECTED DEVELOPMENTAL PATTERNS IN THE CEREBRAL NEOCORTEX

The neocortex is, above all else, a multilaminate structure whose constituent elements show a high degree of constancy of arrangement. No matter what type of mammalian vertebrate we consider, the basic laminar arrangement is already obvious at birth, and with the exception of a few animal species (e.g., marsupials), all neurons—though not all neuroglia—have achieved their final division before birth. Within these constraints, however, the postnatal changes that occur are both numerous and profound. Not only are all neural elements significantly altered during postnatal maturation, the basic wiring diagram seems also to be changed between birth and maturity. Since it appears likely on an intuitive basis that many, if not all, of these changes have a bearing on the ontogeny of learning and memory processes, it would seem appropriate to review them. We shall concentrate on those visible with the light microscope and remind the reader that the changes which can be so defined may represent only the tip of the iceberg.

15.2.1 Postsynaptic elements

SPINES. Dramatic changes occur during the postnatal ontogenesis of cortical pyramids in all forms studied. We shall base our descriptions on kitten material, but the same comments will apply, with some allowance for temporal translation, to all mammalian vertebrates. In the newborn cat pyramidal-cell bodies are already arranged quite densely in laminae 2, 3, 5, and, to a lesser degree, 6. Apical shafts are present, and in most cases first-order bifurcations signaling the initial development of apical arches can be seen. The shafts tend to be nodulated and bear scattered groups of pleomorphic hairy structures from 3 to 10 μ in size. We have called them heteromorphic protospines on the basis of their appearance and precocious arrival (Scheibel and Scheibel, 1971b). These hairy structures are often quite densely clustered on the surface of the soma and on the proximal portion of the apical shaft, and to a lesser extent along the surfaces of the basilar dendrite anlage. Their role is not clear, but it is absolutely certain that they are lost during the process of maturation. Similar structures cover the Purkinje-cell body in the cerebellum at that period in ontogenesis when the climbing fiber makes initial contact with soma and the embryonic clump of Purkinje dendrites just beginning to sprout from the superficial surface of the cell. This early phase of climbing-fiber/Purkinje-cell development, called by Ramón y Cajal (1909–1911) the pericellular nest and capuchin stages, respectively, may provide some degree of clarification for our problem with the cerebral cortex.

The climbing-fiber/Purkinje-cell relationship is transient, soon to be followed by the development of synaptic interaction exclusively between climbing fiber and tertiary dendrites. Meanwhile the hairy silhouette of the

Purkinje soma is lost, and the mature synaptic relationship between basket-cell axons and Purkinje-cell bodies is established shortly thereafter. In a period of dynamic change in cerebellar cortex, with cell masses from Obersteiner's layer streaming downward into the subjacent granular layer (Obersteiner, 1883a, b; Ramón y Cajal, 1911), we suggest that the evanescent appearance of protospines on the surface of each Purkinje neuron may provide a better initial target for the growing climbing fiber. Whether this is strictly a physical process (i.e., providing a larger target), or is chemically mediated, or both, is obviously a question for tomorrow's neuroimmunology.

In returning to our consideration of protospines along the surface of pyramidal cells and the initial portion (100–250 μ) of the apical shaft, two facts are worth noting: (1) these are the only two parts of the pyramidal neuron that are routinely devoid of all spines in the neurally mature state; and (2) in the visual cortex of very young rabbits (Globus and Scheibel, 1967), and presumably in other mammals, the specific afferent (geniculostriate) radiation initially establishes synaptic contact with the central third of the apical shaft of the pyramid, just above this heavily protospined zone. We suggest that the protospine ensembles may aid in establishing an identifiable target for corticipetal afferent systems here, as they seem to do in cerebellum. Whether they serve this purpose primarily for the specific sensory afferent fibers that begin their terminal arborization just above this area, or whether they establish gradients for the ingrowing nonspecific afferents—whose growth is in some respects more like that of cerebellar climbing fibers —is not clear. In any case, these primitive systems are lost by the second postnatal week, and the typical densely packed, short, nodulated spines of mature cortex make their appearance. The new spine populations serve as specific postsynaptic coupling sites for the many synaptic terminals, from multiple sources, that converge upon each pyramid (Gray, 1959; Colonnier, 1964).

It remains to be determined whether a mature spine or spine cluster becomes a stable item of dendritic architecture, or whether it maintains capacity for plastic response. If disuse causes atrophy and loss (see, e.g., Globus and Scheibel, 1967; Valverde, 1967), does increased activity actually produce hypertrophy or branching, as suggested by Szentágothai (1971) and others, and if so, does this bear a significant relationship to learning and memory? Furthermore, does the normal wear and tear of synaptic usage produce spine turnover, with a resultant constant reshuffling of synaptic circuitry, or is there an element of hard wiring which increases with time, culminating only in the presumed neural deterioration that accompanies senility? These are clearly questions whose answers are already within reach.

DENDRITES. Even more impressive changes occur in the dendritic apparatus of pyramids in neonatal cats, the amount and tempo of change being determined in part by the cortical area. Using the visual area as an example, there are usually no well-developed basilar shafts at birth. Instead, a fringe of thick, whisplike protrusions extend from the sides and base of each pyramidal soma for distances of 10 to 50 μ. There may be as many as a dozen or more of these on each side, and a number may have blunt terminal enlargements reminiscent of axonal growth cones (Figure 15.4). During the first seven to ten days of postnatal life a few of these elements become progressively longer and develop side branches. The remainder disappear, probably through resorbtion. The entire basilar skirt achieves maturity by the third postnatal month. The total horizontal length of each branch may approach 200 to 300 μ, although in the case of giant pyramids of Meynert (and of Betz in the motor zone) the length may be three to four times as great. These are the elements that form dendrite bundles, as has been noted earlier.

The system of apical arches seldom shows extensive development until the second postnatal week, although most visual pyramids have already generated initial

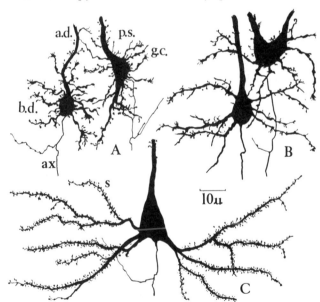

FIGURE 15.4 Cell bodies and basilar dendrites of pyramidal cells in the visual cortex of kittens at three postnatal epochs: A, 1 to 2 days; B, 7 to 10 days; C, approximately 90 days. Abbreviations: ax, axon; b.d., basilar dendrites; a.d., apical dendrites; p.s., pseudospines; s, mature spines; g.c., growth cones. Drawn from rapid Golgi material. From Scheibel and Scheibel (1971b).

bifurcation by the first or second day of life. As in the case of basilar shafts, the apical branches of visual pyramids are not fully developed until 60 to 90 days of age, with maturation coming latest in association areas. It is worth noting how progressive extension and branching of apical arches produces an extremely dense dendritic neuropil, perhaps the densest in the entire central nervous system (Scheibel and Scheibel, 1971b). Figure 15.5 illustrates in semidiagrammatic form how the three-dimensional domains produced by these terminal branches become progressively overlapped and interlocked. Because of the partial nature of Golgi impregnations, it is seldom possible to gain full appreciation of the density of this field, and of the resultant opportunities for interaction among the shafts crossing each other at various angles.

Some years ago Green and Petsche (1961) suggested that the densely packed hippocampal dendrites and the limited amount of intervening extraneuronal space might provide a satisfactory substrate for development of the hypersynchrony to which the hippocampus is prone. High concentrations of potassium temporarily trapped in these small "landlocked" interdendritic areas following initial hippocampal dendrite activity could encourage massive recurrent depolarization, leading to progressive extrasynaptic spread and further synchronization of hippocampal electrical activity.

The dense feltwork of apical arches characterizing the first layer of neocortex in the two- to three-month-old cat may provide a similar substrate, one that is essentially absent in newborn cortex. This may, in part, account for the well-known difficulty in detecting any form of cortical synchronous activity (spindles, alpha rhythm, recruit-

ment potentials, etc.) in newborn cortex (Scheibel and Scheibel, 1964a). Note also that several investigators (e.g., Spencer and Brookhart, 1961; Calvet, Calvet, and Scherrer, 1964) have drawn on cortical laminar analysis of synchronous waves to show that spindling and recruitment appear to be initiated in the distal portions of the apical shafts.

15.2.2 Presynaptic elements

Specific afferents such as the geniculocalcarine radiation have already moved into their final position at birth, although the axons are tenuous and the degree of terminal bifurcation is still restrained (Figure 15.6). While direct observation of Golgi impregnations obviously cannot furnish definitive data, studies using the electron microscope have been able to document the progressive development of axodendritic articulations during the first few weeks of life (Adinolfi, 1971), while interruption of the afferent system followed at suitable intervals by Golgi staining can locate the original position of such articulations along the middle third of the apical shafts of pyramids (see, e.g., Globus and Scheibel, 1967; Valverde, 1967). With the somewhat later maturation of fourth-layer stellate cells (see Altman and Bulut, this

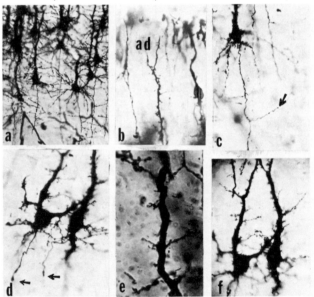

FIGURE 15.6 Details of developmental morphology from the visual cortex of a two-day-old kitten. (a) a general view of the layer of large pyramids in the fifth layer; (b) a simple terminal arch crowning an apical dendrite (ad) of a fifth-layer pyramid; (c) a developing recurrent collateral on the axon of a fifth-layer pyramid; (d) layer-3 pyramids showing the later development of the axons in these more superficial cells (arrows point to growth cones); (e) an apical shaft of a layer-5 pyramid showing protospines and developing oblique branches; (f) another view of the two pyramids in d shown at a different focus to reveal protospines on soma and larval dendrites on the first part of apical shafts. From Scheibel and Scheibel (1971b).

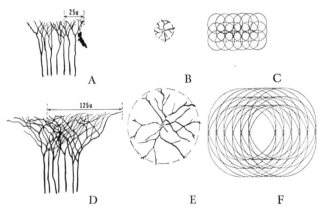

FIGURE 15.5 The growth of apical arches of pyramidal-cell dendrites in visual cortex of the young cat. A and D compare the spread of the apical-arch system at 2 and 90 days. B and E are drawn on the basis of tangential sections through the pial glial surface to show the approximate size of the two domains, while C and F show schematically how the domains interpenetrate each other at 2 and 90 days of age. Based on rapid Golgi material. From Scheibel and Scheibel (1971b).

volume), a second group of axodendritic connections is established between the specific visual afferents and these small neurons, without essential compromise of the earlier relationship. However, since most of the stellate-cell axons synapse, in turn, on adjacent pyramids, this later synaptological development, in effect, splices another neuron into the input-output circuit through cortex (Scheibel and Scheibel, 1964a, b). On intuitive as well as empirical grounds, this change in cortical circuitry can have profound implications for cortical function (Eccles, 1967).

Nonspecific afferents are also recognizable in many cortical areas at birth. The individual fiber is a long, relatively unramified branch ascending perpendicularly to the pial surface and often reaching the pial margin before turning or disappearing. Such a fiber actually makes up but one branch of the individual nonspecific fiber that breaks up in the subcortical white matter, producing a family of ascending branches. These generate a roughly cylindrical domain whose height is the total thickness of cortex and whose diameter is of the order of 1 mm. In the neurally mature cortex, each of the afferent fibers ascends along one apical shaft, or along an apical bundle. This prolonged axodendritic relation is reminiscent of the cerebellar climbing-fiber system, although the original fiber is not so frequently branched or reduplicated.

Over a considerable experience with several thousand Golgi-impregnated cortices, we have not been able to identify such physical relations between nonspecific afferent fibers and apical shafts, although each can be separately identified, until the tenth to fourteenth day of life (Scheibel and Scheibel, 1964a, b). Then, at the time when the mature spines begin to appear on the surface of the shafts, axodendritic contiguity can first be established. We have suggested the possibility of lateral migration of the nonspecific fibers, perhaps under some type of neurobiotactic force, to effect multiple synaptic contacts with the newly appearing spines. In view of what is now known about the impressive degree of plasticity in the neonatal nervous system (Caley, 1971), movement of this sort through the still considerable amounts of extracellular space does not seem unthinkable.

Aside from the putative role of nonspecific systems in tuning the membrane-sensitivity levels of cortical neurons, another function may be surmised for this fiber system. The columnar organization of cortical sensory and motor areas becomes physiologically demonstrable after these axodendritic articulations are established. Indeed, it may be more than coincidence that the average diameter of a cortical cell column (1 mm; see Powell and Mountcastle, 1959) is approximately the same as that of the terminal axonal domain generated by

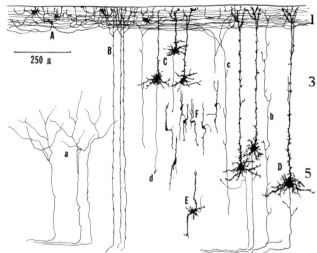

FIGURE 15.7 Representative elements in the visual cortex of perinatal kitten: (A) Cajal-Retzius cells and horizontal axons of first layer; (B) processes of ependymal glial cells reaching pial surface; (C) layer-3 pyramids; (D) layer-5 pyramids; (E) bipolar cells of layer 6; (F) very immature developing (bipolar) stellate elements (microneurons) of layer 4 (a, terminations of specific afferent fibers; b, a terminating nonspecific element; c, ascending fibers of uncertain origin which contribute to horizontal elements of first layer; d, developing axon and growth cone of a third-layer cell). Drawn from Golgi-stained material.

a single nonspecific fiber (Scheibel and Scheibel, 1958). The emergence of functionally discrete cortical cell columns, with all that this entails in terms of precise sensory mapping (Powell and Mountcastle, 1959) and molecular motor response (Asanuma and Rosen, 1972) may thus be directly related to the maturation of the nonspecific afferents.

15.2.3 Intrinsic elements

Among the many dramatic changes that take place in nonpyramidal cells within the cortex, we shall select two for consideration because of their possible pertinence to our area of interest. (These and other changes may be seen by comparing Figures 15.7 and 15.8 representing, respectively, the perinatal and mature visual cortex of the cat.)

1. Through the studies of Retzius (1893–1894) and Ramón y Cajal (1909–1911) it is fairly well known that the first layer in neocortex is characterized by a number of horizontal cells and large masses of fibers of various diameters running parallel to the pial surface. This axonal system disappears, pari passu, with the branching and spreading of the apical dendrite arches that eventually fill virtually the entire first layer.

2. Simultaneously with this change, another of even greater significance occurs deeper within the cortex. Maturation of stellate cells (short-axoned elements,

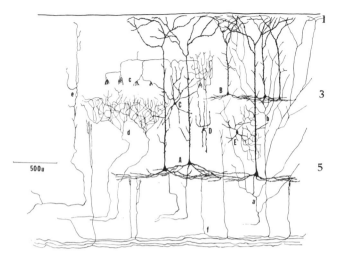

FIGURE 15.8 Representative elements in the mature visual cortex of the cat. This drawing does not reflect the very much larger proportion of stellate cells that are present in this type of sensory cortex. (A) Large fifth-layer pyramidal cells of Meynert showing the powerful horizontal groups of basilar dendrites that form bundles; (B), third-layer pyramids showing the shorter but still obvious horizontal masses of basilar dendrites; (C) an upper fourth-layer stellate cell whose axon terminates in a series of local perisomal basket formations; (D) a deeper fourth-layer stellate cell with ascending axon; (E) a deeper fourth-layer stellate cell with typical short-axon distribution (a, axon system and collaterals of large pyramid; b, axon system and collateral of third-layer pyramid; c, basket terminal system of a stellate cell; d, typical terminal arbors of a specific afferent projection; e, typical terminating element of a nonspecific projection; f, ascending terminals from corticocortical fibers running near the gray-white interface). Based on Golgi-stained preparations.

microneurons, etc.) is accompanied by elaboration of their local axonal systems. Most of these are of fairly limited extent, with the accent on vertical rather than horizontal dispersion. At the same time, the recurrent collateral systems of pyramidal cells also achieve their full expression. Here, too, much of the emphasis is placed on connectional patterns linking deeper with more superficial structures. The net result of all these axonal changes appears in a shift of dominant axon-mediated synaptic linkages from horizontal to vertical. (While axon-mediated horizontal linkages are being lost, basilar dendrite systems of pyramids in layers 2, 3, and 5 are setting up secondary horizontally coupled systems of their own.) Physiological studies support these structural observations. Purpura (1961) found that the superficial cortical response (SCR) can be evoked from relatively distant surface stations via slowly conducting but early-maturing paths. In the mature animal, where such distant responses are no longer easily obtained, careful laminar analysis using microstimulation and recording methods

(Asanuma and Rosen, 1973) shows that the flow of impulses is now predominantly vertical. Indeed, the characteristic developmental progression of the evoked cortical response, from long-latency surface negative to shorter-latency surface positive-negative (Ellingson and Wilcott, 1960), is almost certainly due to elaboration of pre- and postsynaptic neuropil, predominantly in the fourth layer.

15.3 A SUMMING UP

It is clearly premature to attempt interpretation of the significance of each of these sequences of ontogenetic change within the framework of development of learning and memory mechanisms. The following generalizations may be justified, however.

1. The postnatal maturative process is marked by an enormous increase in, and often a reshaping of, pre- and postsynaptic neuropil. Such changes are especially noticeable in the elaboration of basilar dendrites and apical arches of pyramids and in the development of recurrent collaterals of pyramidal-cell axons and the entire axonal system of stellate cells. The mustering or reshuffling of dendrites into bundles significantly exemplifies the amount of reshaping that is possible in neural tissue.

2. The surface morphology of pyramidal-cell dendrites shows significant change, with the development of mature spines in high density and their consistent articulation with very large numbers of presynaptic terminals from various sources. Sufficient data now exist to make it seem not improbable that spines remain plastically reactive through much of the life of the organism.

3. Cortical cell arrays are functionally organized in columns which are known to bear highly specified relations with peripheral sensory fields or motor elements.

4. The predominant direction of flow of axon systems shifts from essentially horizontal in the newborn to vertical in the mature cortex. The earlier type of organization, based largely on the massive axonal ensembles of the first cortical layer, is structurally reminiscent of the cerebellar parallel-fiber system. It is presumably organized to achieve maximal divergence of impulse patterns across ensembles of immature and still fairly densely packed neurons. The later-evolving pattern would appear to bring with it greater segregation of impulse sequences and their more intensive elaboration within territories of less densely packed neurons providing vastly enhanced synaptic surface.

On an intuitive basis, such an organizational model would seem well designed for iterative processing, elaboration, comparison, and extraction or isolation of the most general features of the information (the "universal"). Put another way, neonatal cortex recalls a random-access device. Mature neocortex might operate as a sorter of statistical invariances (Fair, 1963).

Evidence has already been presented here, and elsewhere in this volume, suggesting the relative ease with which visible substrate changes may be made to occur in a learning or "overload" situation. But the way becomes more difficult when we try to understand how such changes are generalized, coded, given introspective meaning, and organized for rapid retrieval. We have recounted the sequence of developmental changes that occur in neural tissue with the strong feeling that some, possibly all, are important for the problem we address. But we are still not ready to turn our back on some, point to others, and say "These are the ones!"

ACKNOWLEDGMENT

The personal studies on which this review has been based were supported by the following grants from the United States Public Health Service: NINDB 1056, NINDS 10567, and HD 00972.

REFERENCES

ADINOLFI, A.M. 1971. The postnatal development of synaptic contacts in the cerebral cortex. In M. B. Sterman, D. J. McGinty, and A. M. Adinolfi, eds., *Brain Development and Behavior*. New York: Academic Press, pp. 71–88.

ASANUMA, H., and ROSEN, I. 1972. Topographical organization of cortical efferent zones projecting to distal forelimb muscles in the monkey. *Experimental Brain Research* 14: 243–256.

ASANUMA, H., and ROSEN, I. 1973. Spread of mono- and polysynaptic connections within cat's motor cortex. *Experimental Brain Research* 16: 507–520.

BROWN, T. G. 1914. On the nature of the fundamental activity of the nervous centers together with an analysis of the conditioning of rhythmic activity in progression, and a theory of the evolution of function in the nervous system. *Journal of Physiology* 48: 18–46.

BRUNER, J. S., OLVER, R., and GREENFIELD, P. M. 1966. *Studies in Cognitive Growth*. New York: John Wiley & Sons.

CALEY, D. W. 1971. Differentiation of the neural elments of the central cortex in the rat. In D. C. Pease, ed., *Cellular Aspects of Neural Growth and Differentiation*. Berkeley: University of California Press, pp. 73–91.

CALVET, J., CALVET, M. C., and SCHERRER, J. 1964. Etude stratigraphique corticale de l'activité EEG spontanée. *Electroencephalography and Clinical Neurophysiology* 17: 109–125.

COLONNIER, M. C. 1964. The structural design of the neocortex. In J. C. Eccles, ed., *Brain and Conscious Experience*. New York: Springer-Verlag, pp. 1–23.

ECCLES, J. C. 1967. Postsynaptic inhibition in the central nervous system. In G. C. Quarton, T. Melnechuk, and F. O. Schmitt, eds., *The Neurosciences: A Study Program*. New York: Rockefeller University Press, pp. 408–427.

ELLINGSON, R. J., and WILCOTT, R. C. 1960. Development of evoked responses in visual and auditory cortices of kittens. *Journal of Neurophysiology* 23: 363–375.

EVARTS, E. V. 1967. Representation of movements and muscles by pyramidal tract neurons of the precentral motor cortex. In M. D. Yahr and D. P. Purpura, eds., *Neurophysiological Basis of Normal and Abnormal Motor Activities*. New York: Raven Press, pp. 215–253.

FAIR, C. M. 1963. *The Physical Foundations of the Psyche*. Middletown, Conn.: Wesleyan University Press.

FLEISCHAUER, K., PETSCHE, H., and WITTKOWSKI, W. 1972. Vertical bundles of dendrites in the neocortex. *Zeitschrift für Entwicklungs Geschichte* 136: 213–223.

GLOBUS, A., and SCHEIBEL, A. B. 1967. Synaptic loci on visual cortical neurons of the rabbit. The specific afferent radiation. *Experimental Neurology* 18: 116–131.

GRAY, E. G. 1959. Axo-somatic and axo-dendritic synapses of the cerebral cortex—an electron microscope study. *Journal of Anatomy* 93: 420–433.

GREEN, J. D., and PETSCHE, H. 1961. Hippocampal electrical activity. IV. Abnormal electrical activity. *Electroencephalography and Clinical Neurophysiology* 13: 868–879.

HORE, J., and PORTER, R. 1972. Pyramidal and extrapyramidal influences on some hindlimb motoneuron populations of the arboreal bush-tailed possum, *Trichosurus vulpecula*. *Journal of Neurophysiology* 35: 112–121.

JANKOWSKA, E., JUKES, M. G. M., LUND, S., and LUNDBERG, A. 1967. The effect of DOPA on the spinal cord. 6. Half-center organization of interneurons transmitting effects from reflex afferents. *Acta Physiologica Scandinavica* 70: 389–402.

JOHN, E. R. 1967. *Mechanisms of Memory*. New York: Academic Press, p. 17.

LASHLEY, K. S. 1929. *Brain Mechanisms and Intelligence: a Quantitative Study of Injuries to the Brain*. Chicago: University of Chicago Press.

LASHLEY, K. S. 1950. In search of the engram. *Symposia of the Society for Experimental Biology*. 4: 454–482.

LASSEK, A. M. 1954. *The Pyramidal Tract*. Springfield, Ill.: Charles C Thomas.

LEHNINGER, A. L. 1968. The neuronal membrane. *Proceedings of the National Academy of Science* 60: 1055–1101.

LUNDBERG, A. 1969. *Reflex Control of Stepping*. Oslo: Universitetsforlaget.

LUNDBERG, A., and VOORHOEVE, P. 1962. Effects from the pyramidal tract on spinal reflex arcs. *Acta Physiologica Scandinavica* 56: 201–219.

MANNEN, H. 1966. Contribution to the morphological study of dendritic arborization in the brain stem. In T. Tokizane and J. R. Schadé, eds., *Correlative Neurosciences*, vol. 1 (*Progress in Brain Research*, vol. 21). Amsterdam: Elsevier, pp. 131–162.

MATTHEWS, M. A., WILLIS, W. D., and WILLIAMS, V. 1971. Dendrite bundles in lamina IX of cat spinal cord. A possible source of electrical interaction between motoneurons. *Anatomical Record* 171: 313–328.

NEGISHI, K., LU, E. S., and VERZEANO, M. 1962. Neuronal activity in the lateral geniculate body in the nucleus reticularis of the thalamus. *Vision Research* 1: 343–353.

OBERSTEINER, K. 1883a. Beitrage zur Kenntniss von feinerem Bau der Kleinhirnrinde. *Sitzungsberichte der Kaiser Wilhelm Akademie das Wissenschaftlichkeit* 50.

OBERSTEINER, K. 1883b. Der feinere Bau der Kleinhirnrinde beim Menschen und Thieren. *Biologische Centralblatt* 3.

OSHIMA, T. 1969. Studies of pyramidal tract cells. In H. H.

Jasper et al., eds., *Basic Mechanisms of the Epilepsies*. Boston: Little, Brown, pp. 253–261.

PEASE, D. C. 1966. Polysaccharides associated with the exterior surface of epithelial cells: Kidney, intestine, and brain. *Journal of Ultrastructure Research* 15: 555–588.

PETERS, A., and WALSH, T. M. 1972. A study of the organization of apical dendrites in the somatic sensory cortex of the rat. *Journal of Comparative Neurology* 144: 253–268.

POWELL, T. P. S., and MOUNTCASTLE, V. B. 1959. Some aspects of the functional organization of the cortex of the postcentral gyrus of the monkey: A correlation of findings obtained in a single unit analysis with cytoarchitecture. *Bulletin of the Johns Hopkins Hospital* 105: 133–162.

PRESTON, J. B., SHENDE, M. C., and UEMURA, K. 1967. The motor cortex–pyramidal system: Patterns of facilitation and inhibition on motoneurons innervating limb musculature of cat and baboon and their possible adaptive significance. In M. D. Yahr and D. P. Purpura, eds., *Neurophysiological Basis for Normal and Abnormal Motor Activities*. New York: Raven Press, pp. 61–72.

PURPURA, D. P. 1961. Morphophysiological basis of elementary evoked response patterns in the neocortex of the newborn cat. *Annals of the New York Academy of Science* 92: 840–859.

RAMÓN Y CAJAL, S. 1909–1911. *Histologie du Système Nerveux de l'Homme et des Vertébrés*, 2 vols. Paris: Maloine.

RAMÓN-MOLINER, E., and NAUTA, W. J. H. 1966. The isodendritic core of the brain stem. *Journal of Comparative Neurology* 126: 311–335.

RETZIUS. 1893–1894. Die Cajal'schen Zellen der Grosshirnrinde beim Menchen und bei Säugethieren. *Biologische Untersuchungen* 5 and 6.

ROMANES, G. J. 1964. The motor pools of the spinal cord. In J. C. Eccles and J. P. Schadé, eds., *Organization of the Spinal Cord*. Amsterdam: Elsevier, pp. 93–119.

ROSEN, I., and ASANUMA, H. 1972. Peripheral afferent inputs to the forelimb area of the monkey motor cortex: Input-output relations. *Experimental Brain Research* 14: 257–273.

SCHEIBEL, M. E., DAVIES, T. L., LINDSAY, R. D., and SCHEIBEL, A. B. 1974. Basilar dendrite bundles of giant pyramidal cells. *Experimental Neurology* 42: 307–319.

SCHEIBEL, M. E., DAVIES, T. L., and SCHEIBEL, A. B. 1973. Maturation of reticular dendrites: Loss of spines and development of bundles. *Experimental Neurology* 38: 301–310.

SCHEIBEL, M. E., and SCHEIBEL, A. B. 1958. Structural substrates for integrative patterns in the brain stem reticular core. In H. H. Jasper et al., eds., *Reticular Formation of the Brain*. Boston: Little, Brown.

SCHEIBEL, M. E., and SCHEIBEL, A. B. 1964a. Some structural and functional substrates of development in young cats. In W. Himwich and H. Himwich, eds., *The Developing Brain* (*Progress in Brain Research*, Vol. 9). Amsterdam: Elsevier, pp. 6–25.

SCHEIBEL, M. E., and SCHEIBEL, A. B. 1964b. Some neural substrates of postnatal development. In *Review of Child Development Research*, Vol. 1. New York: Russell Sage Foundation, pp. 481–519.

SCHEIBEL, M. E., and SCHEIBEL, A. B. 1966. The organization of the nucleus reticularis thalami: A Golgi study. *Brain Research* 1: 43–62.

SCHEIBEL, M. E., and SCHEIBEL, A. B. 1970a. Organization of spinal motoneuron dendrites in bundles. *Experimental Neurology* 20: 106–112.

SCHEIBEL, M. E., and SCHEIBEL, A. B. 1970b. Developmental relationship between spinal motoneuron dendrite bundles and patterned activity in the hind limb of cats. *Experimental Neurology* 29: 328–335.

SCHEIBEL, M. E., and SCHEIBEL, A. B. 1971a. Developmental relationship between spinal motoneuron dendrite bundles and patterned activity in the forelimb of cats. *Experimental Neurology* 30: 367–373.

SCHEIBEL, M. E., and SCHEIBEL, A. B. 1971b. Selected structural-functional correlations in postnatal brain. In M. B. Sterman, D. J. McGinty, and A. M. Adinolfi, eds., *Brain Development and Behavior*. New York: Academic Press, pp. 1–22.

SCHEIBEL, M. E., and SCHEIBEL, A. B. 1972. Specialized organizational patterns within the nucleus reticularis thalami of the cat. *Experimental Neurology* 34: 316–322.

SCHEIBEL, M. E., and SCHEIBEL, A. B. 1973. Dendrite bundles in the ventral commissure of cat spinal cord. *Experimental Neurology* 39: 482–488.

SCHLAG, J., and WASZAK, M. 1970. Characteristics of unit responses in nucleus reticularis thalami. *Brain Research* 21: 286–288.

SPENCER W. A., and BROOKHART, J. M. 1961. A study of spontaneous spindle waves in sensorimotor cortex of cat. *Journal of Neurophysiology* 24: 50–65.

SZENTÁGOTHAI, J. 1971. Memory functions and the structural organization of the brain. *Symposia Biologica Hungarica* 10: 21–35.

TAKAHASHI, K. 1965. Slow and fast groups of pyramidal tract cells and their respective membrane properties. *Journal of Neurophysiology* 28: 808–824.

VALVERDE, F. 1962. Reticular formation of the albino rat's brain stem. Cytoarchitecture and corticofugal connections. *Journal of Comparative Neurology* 119: 25–54.

VALVERDE, F. 1967. Apical dendrite spines of the visual cortex and light deprivation in the mouse. *Experimental Brain Research* 3: 337–352.

WASZAK, M. 1974. Firing pattern of neurons in the rostral and ventral part of nucleus reticularis thalami during EEG spindles. *Experimental Neurology* 43: 38–59.

WIERSMA, C. A. G. 1952. Neurons of arthropods. *Cold Spring Harbor Symposium on Quantitative Biology* 17: 155–163.

WILSON, D. M. 1970. Neural operations in arthropod ganglia. In F. O. Schmitt, ed., *The Neurosciences: Second Study Program*. New York: Rockefeller University Press, pp. 397–409.

Effects of Differential
Experience on
Brain and Behavior

16

Enduring Brain Effects of Differential Experience and Training

WILLIAM T. GREENOUGH

ABSTRACT Since any learning event probably produces a number of transient physiological effects in addition to those involved in the storage of memory, it is suggested that a search for enduring consequences of information storage may be a fruitful experimental approach. Brain changes that regularly occur in situations in which lasting behavioral changes follow experience are the more likely "engram" candidates. Considerable data from studies of developing mammals suggest that relatively permanent brain effects may be produced by various aspects of the rearing environment. Alterations in behavior and brain physiology, chemistry, and anatomy have been reported following hormonal, social, sensory, and complexity manipulations. Of particular interest are alterations in the number and/or pattern of synaptic connections, which have been reported following all of these manipulations. The role of these changes remains to be determined.

Recent preliminary work has suggested that similar alterations may follow formal training in adulthood. An experiment is described in which mature rats exhibited slightly more neuronal dendritic branching in posterior dorsal cortex following extensive maze training than did handled controls. Continued examination of a range of developmental and adult paradigms may provide an excellent opportunity to establish relationships between brain changes and information storage in the nervous system.

In the most general sense, as investigators of memory, we are interested in relatively enduring processes that occur in conjunction with some environmental event and that mediate the effects of that event upon later behavior. However, for most of us, the use of the term "memory" implies a reasonably specific relationship between the earlier and later behavioral events. Thus we all readily accept that if an animal is given several rewarded trials in a T maze and then consistently chooses the rewarded alternative, it has formed a (short- or long-term) memory for the experience. Fewer of us might accept the development of visuomotor coordination with experience (as reported, e.g., by Held and Hein, 1963) as memory, probably because a specific relationship between earlier and later experiences is less clear (although it is becoming more so; see, e.g., Hein, Held, and Gower, 1970). Still fewer would accept the relationship between early

WILLIAM T. GREENOUGH, Department of Psychology, University of Illinois, Champaign, IL

visual experience and later visual ability as more than a parallel to memory processes as we view them in adults (see Chapter 18, this volume). And the relationship between early stressful events or endocrine activity and adult behavior is seen by most as a "developmental" rather than a "memorial" process.

An alternative is to view these examples in terms of a continuum of increasing specificity with regard to the relationship between experience and later behavior. As such, they may share some underlying mechanisms. To the extent that developmental information storage resembles the memory storage of adults, the more rapid changes in development may provide the researcher with a magnifying glass for the observation of their common substrates. The work described by Pettigrew, Spinelli, Rose, and others in this symposium and that discussed below indicates that experience during development may bring about rapid and profound alterations in the functioning of relatively well defined CNS subsystems. Such changes have been detected in behavioral, electrophysiological, biochemical, and anatomical measures. Furthermore, considerable evidence indicates that, once established, these environmental effects may be, like memory, relatively permanent. Whether developmental information storage shares with memory storage the susceptibilities and strengths described elsewhere in this symposium remains to be determined. One goal of this review is to examine several processes on a proposed development-learning continuum to determine the extent to which common biological correlates can be found.

At one level or another it appears that we have no choice but to look at the common aspects of processes that we believe involve the formation of memory. We cannot isolate a "pure" memory for study. Whenever memory of a conventionally—or unconventionally—accepted type is produced in an organism or in some isolated part of one, there are also produced a number of transient, and probably some enduring, changes which are not necessarily related to the storage of memory for the experience. Whole organisms experience stress, sensory stimulation, motor activity, etc., to at least some degree during any training experience. Parts of organisms must receive conceptually similar physiological or supraphysiological treatments if a change is to be established in the operating characteristics of the system under study. A "nonlearning" control cannot be given identical treatment or it, too, will learn. Moreover, to select as "controls" those subjects that did not learn a particular behavior in the same situation or number of trials (e.g., Shashoua, 1970) requires the unlikely assumption that these controls did not learn anything else —rather than that they may have learned behaviors other than those the experimenter has chosen to measure. And the use of controls for which the experimental contingencies are different from those for "properly trained" animals (e.g., yoked controls; see Machlus and Gaito, 1969) would also seem to assure that the controls learn something *different* from the latter group, and is also likely to subject the organisms to different degrees of stress (e.g., Weiss, 1968). Similar arguments can be applied to other control procedures which have been presented (Greenough and Maier, 1972), and it seems unlikely that a single experiment can be designed to isolate memorial and nonmemorial correlates of the learning or memory-formation process. Hence, whether we choose to examine memory from a developmental perspective or through the use of learning tasks, the approach would seem to require that we search for biological processes that occur across a broad range of behavioral situations. Moreover, we should be very careful in our decisions to rule out certain biological processes as potential memory substrates—decisions implicit in the choice of "controls." The use of a "resting," or home-cage, control makes it likely that a good deal of transient noise resulting from the training procedure will not be removed in the comparison. The use of inappropriate controls risks removal of the signal. Nevertheless, reference standards of some sort are necessary. The most reasonable solution seems to be to choose those groups that are maximally different in terms of memory, regardless of differences in "extraneous" aspects of the task, as our starting point.

If a sizeable proportion of the nonmemorial effects of training are in fact temporary, then examination of the enduring effects may hold more promise. The bulk of the work on CNS correlates of training has emphasized the immediate or short-term effects of the initial experience: macromolecular synthesis, short-term electrophysiological changes, etc. Relatively little effort has been directed at what one might term the "residue" of memory. Certainly we would agree that the ultimate engram must endure in one form or another for as long as the memory remains stable. The biochemical, electrophysiological, and anatomical work on longer-term consequences of

behavioral experience and training which is emphasized in this review seems a promising beginning in this direction.

16.1 A PRELIMINARY CAUTION: HORMONAL AND METABOLIC EFFECTS AS "DIFFERENTIAL EXPERIENCE" FOR THE NERVOUS SYSTEM

The fact that many of the differential-experience procedures to be discussed below may affect the levels of various hormones should not be overlooked. A large literature indicates that hormones have both transient and permanent effects upon behavior, brain chemistry, brain physiology, and brain anatomy. To a certain extent these hormonal effects provide us with models of the effects of extrinsic input upon the nervous system. However, there is no reason to believe that the brain stores information from hormonal inputs in anything like the same way that it stores information arriving through sensory channels. Thus the fact that hormones can affect a variety of brain measures, and the fact that behavioral stimulation can affect hormonal levels, should lead us to be cautious about the interpretation of neurological correlates of behavioral experiences. While an overwhelming number of transient effect of hormones on brain and behavior have been reported, this review will concern itself primarily with the enduring effects of these hormones on brain function. The bulk of the enduring effects have involved the administration or the withdrawal of hormones during development.

A number of studies have dealt with the effects of excessive or insufficient levels of hormones normally present in development. The absence of thyroxin, for example, results in a syndrome called "cretinism," which has been reported in animals (Davenport and Dorcey, 1972; Eayrs, 1961) and man (see, e.g., Turner and Bagnara, 1971; Wilkins, 1965). Both behavior and brain development are severely retarded in cretinism (Balázs et al., 1968; Eayrs, 1961, 1964a; Nicholson and Altman, 1972). Furthermore, overdoses of thyroid hormone during postnatal development may have equally devastating effects upon the brain (Nicholson and Altman, 1972; Pelton and Bass, 1973). The administration of small doses of thyroxin shortly after birth has been shown to enhance brain and behavioral development in rats, although the long-term consequence of this treatment seems to be the disruption of normal patterns of maturation (Eayrs, 1964b, c; Schapiro, 1968, 1971). The absence of growth hormone (GH) with hypophysectomy postnatally may reduce brain growth (Gregory and Diamond, 1968; Rosenzweig, Bennett, and Diamond, 1972c), while prenatal GH administration may enhance brain growth and behavioral ability (Block and Essman, 1965; Clendinnen and Eayrs, 1961; Zamenhof, Mosley, and Schuller, 1966). Perhaps because of the procedural approaches to date, the effects of these hormones appear to be relatively general, affecting regions of the brain in proportion to their current rates of development. There does not appear to be a great deal of information regarding the effects of these hormones on later stages of brain development.

In contrast, some recent data suggest that the effects of hormones upon postnatal brain development may occasionally be quite selective, and conceivably could provide us with models for the effects of extra-CNS influences upon the "wiring diagram" of the brain. Raisman and Field (1971, 1973) have examined the effects of testosterone upon regions of the basal forebrain associated (in lesion and implant studies) with sexual behavior. Previously it had been shown that the presence of testosterone during a short pre- or postnatal period determined much of the adult sexual behavior of a variety of mammalian species (Young, Goy, and Phoenix, 1964). Raisman and Field found that the dorsal preoptic area of female rats had more spine-type non-amygdaloid connections than did either males or testosterone-treated females. This suggests a relatively specific neuronal effect of testosterone which correlates temporally with its ability to alter behavior permanently. However, there is some reason to believe that testosterone may have comparatively widespread and enduring effects upon the nervous system. Pfaff (1966) has reported that females and neonatally castrated male rats have smaller neuronal nuclear and nucleolar cross-sectional areas in several subcortical areas than do normal male rats. Bubenik and Brown (1973) have reported similar size differences in the medial amygdaloid nucleus of monkeys. These effects may be more localized than those of thyroxin or growth hormone, however, since in both sex-hormone studies regions were found in which no size differences were apparent.

A third aspect of enduring hormonal effects upon the nervous system which is of importance both for the interpretation of behavioral results and as a potential memory model is the apparent involvement of hormones in mediation of the effects of early stressful stimulation upon the nervous system. It has been known for some time that a stressful event that occurs during roughly the first week of postnatal life of a rat can permanently alter its biological and behavioral responsiveness to stress (e.g., Denenberg, 1967; Levine and Mullins, 1966). Rats that have been stressed by handling, temperature extremes, electric shock, and other methods, show, as adults, enhanced active-avoidance learning, increased survival from severe physiological insults, reduced emotional behavior in novel environments, and more

finely graded hormonal responses to varying degrees of stress (Levine, 1956; Levine and Mullins, 1966, 1968; Weininger, 1953, 1956). The most commonly measured biological response to stress in such studies is the level of adrenal and circulating corticosteroid hormones. These hormones are regulated by blood levels of adrenocorticotrophic hormone (ACTH), which in turn is regulated by the neuronally controlled corticotropin releasing factor (CRF). More recent work indicates that GH levels can be increased by regular handling, at least in mature rats, while acute stress may reduce GH levels (e.g., Takahashi, Daughaday, and Kipnis, 1971). Hence both behavioral and biological components of the stress response seem to be under rather direct nervous-system control.

The modification of CNS control by an early experience may involve direct effects of the stressful stimulation upon the nervous system, indirect effects via changes in the levels of GH, CRF, ACTH, and possibly adrenocorticosteroids, or interactions among these processes. It seems clear that animals stressed during the first week of postnatal life are capable of an adrenocorticosteroid response (Haltmeyer et al., 1966; Levine and Mullins, 1968). Schapiro (1968) and his co-workers have examined some effects of administration of corticosteroid hormones during early postnatal life in the rat. Injection of 1 mg of cortisol acetate on postnatal day 1 (considerably greater than the amount that would be available naturally) had a clearly detrimental and generally retarding effect on biochemical, physiological, and behavioral measures of development. Cortisol-treated animals gained weight more slowly, their brain development was generally retarded in terms of both anatomical and electrophysiological measures, and their adult immunological response was depressed. In contrast, postnatally manipulated animals generally mature more rapidly than controls, in terms of both brain and behavioral development (Levine, 1962; Levine and Alpert, 1959; Levine and Mullins, 1968). Moreover, Schapiro and Vukovich (1970) found that early postnatal stressful stimulation (an overwhelming regimen, including electric shock, temperature extremes, handling, and other physical stresses) increased the number of synaptic spines on Golgi-stained neurons in the cerebral cortex, whereas the cortisol injections decreased spine density. Thyroxin administration during the same period accelerated spine formation (Schapiro, 1971). Schapiro (1971; see also Schapiro and Vukovich, 1970) suggests that hormonal changes do not directly mediate the effects of experience on the organization of the central nervous system but that, perhaps influenced by the environment, they may provide an optimal "biochemical climate" for the establishment of an appropriately connected nervous system. This view suggests that hormones, whether or not they have direct and selective effects on postnatal neural development, are modulated by experience and can modulate the effects of experience upon the developing nervous system. To the extent that these processes continue into later development in adult life, the role of hormones in bringing about changes following a training experience should not be discounted.

16.2 DIFFERENTIAL SENSORY EXPERIENCE

One aspect of the correspondence between behavioral indices of altered brain function and anatomical brain measures deserves a short elaboration (see also Chapter 18, this volume). Behavioral measures and electrophysiological measures indicate three "levels" of visual development. First, light deprivation during development has moderate to severe effects upon visual function in most mammalian species studied (e.g., Baxter, 1966; Gibson, 1969; Riesen, 1966; Tees, 1971; Walk and Walters, 1973). Second, adult or near-adult animals can show considerable recovery from the effects of binocular visual deprivation if they are exposed to normal light (Baxter, 1966; Riesen, 1966; Walk and Gibson, 1961; Walk and Walters, 1973). Third, sensitive measures have often shown that after deprivation, animals never reach the level of normal light-reared controls (Riesen, 1966).

One set of anatomical studies correlates well with this pattern of results. Valverde (1971; see also Valverde and Ruiz-Marcos, 1969) has described three classes of pyramidal-cell apical dendritic spine responses to visual experience in mouse visual cortex. The first type develops around the time of eye opening, about 12 to 15 days of age, and is seen whether or not visual experience is available. The second class of dendrites is vision-dependent, in the sense that spines appear whenever light is supplied, even if the time of eye opening is well past. This population correlates with recovery from visual deprivation. The third type develops normal spines if and only if visual experience is available at the normal time for eye opening; that is, it is both age- and experience-dependent. This "critical-period" class of spines correlates with the behavioral finding that the normally experienced animal may reach a level which the developmentally deprived animal cannot later achieve. From a memory-model standpoint, the second class of neurons is perhaps the most interesting, since it suggests the existence of a population of neurons that is "waiting," so to speak, to be modified (or made functional) by experience. Conceivably, similar neurons could lie waiting to encode experience in many regions of the brain.

16.3 DIFFERENTIAL SOCIAL EXPERIENCE

In one sense, the social situation in which an organism is reared (or living) represents just one aspect of its total environment and the stimulation that that environment provides. However, research has shown social stimulation to be a vital element in the emotional development of some social species, and in at least a few species the continuing presence of conspecifics in adulthood seems to be required for "normal" behavior. Since contact with other members of the species is often manipulated in studies of the effects of sensory and other environmental stimulation and training, a brief review of the effects of social conditions upon behavior and brain function is appropriate.

16.3.1 The "isolation syndrome"
Much behavioral work has centered upon the "isolation syndrome" in rodents, canines, and primates. Typically, animals kept in relatively small groups serve as controls. The measures that have been emphasized, and seemingly the syndromes themselves, differ quite markedly across species. For example, mice appear to be more susceptible to the effects of isolation in adulthood than do rats or, perhaps, most other species (Baer, 1971; Hatch et al., 1963; Sigg, Day, and Colombo, 1966; Wiberg, Airth, and Grice, 1966). It appears, however, that social isolation, during development or adulthood, can stress most higher mammalian species to at least some degree (Ader, 1965; Hatch et al., 1963; Meyer and Bowman, 1972; Sackler and Weltman, 1967). Fuller (1967) has suggested that isolated animals may be traumatized when subjected to environments containing higher levels or novel types of stimulation. The trauma may arise from at least two sources: (1) the organism becomes adapted to the comparatively low levels of sensory stimulation in the isolated environment (Melzack, 1959; Welch, 1967); and (2) the absence of peers, stressful to the organism, sensitizes it to further environmental stress (Moore, 1968; Plaut and Grota, 1971; Riege and Morimoto, 1970; Welch and Welch, 1968). In rodents, behavioral effects of isolation have been seen in appetitive and avoidance performance (e.g. Goeckner, Greenough, and Maier, 1974; Lovely, Pagano, and Paolino, 1972; Valzelli, 1973), exploratory activity (e.g., Ader and Friedman, 1964; Essman, 1966), sexual and aggressive activity (in mice: Charpentier, 1969; Lagerspetz, 1969; Scott and Fredericson, 1951; Valzelli, 1973), and various other measures of irritability and stress reactivity (e.g., Ader, 1965; Baer, 1971). In primates, similar effects have been reported in play, aggression, and sexual behavior (e.g., Harlow, 1962).

Many of the effects of isolation, particularly in adults,

appear to be transient, disappearing rapidly when grouped housing is restored (Bronson and Chapman, 1968; Conner and Gregor, 1973; Hatch et al., 1965; Plaut and Grota, 1971; Wood and Greenough, 1974). Other effects, particularly those associated with postnatal or postweaning isolation, may be quite difficult to reverse with later environment (e.g., Harlow, 1962; Mason, 1968; Prescott, 1971).

A variety of physiological and biochemical effects of social isolation have been reported. In the aggression literature, one pronounced effect is altered turnover of brain monoamines in both rats and mice (Valzelli, 1973; Valzelli and Garattini, 1968, 1972). Essman (1971a, 1972) has also reported decreased cortical cholinesterase and acetylcholinesterase activity after isolation in mice, as well as a differential effect of the cholinergic stimulant, nicotine, on avoidance learning in isolates. Valzelli (1973) has similarly reported enhanced avoidance performance in isolated mice following administration of the serotonin-synthesis inhibitor para-chlorophenylalanine. In general, these differences seem producible and reversible within a few weeks in mice of any age (Garattini, Giacalone, and Valzelli, 1969; Valzelli, 1973). Production and reversal of such effects may take somewhat longer in rats (Sigg, Day, and Colombo, 1966; Valzelli and Garattini, 1972). In contrast, some brain effects of isolation during development may be more permanent. Essman (1971b) has reported remarkably large reductions, in comparison with control groups, in the amount of DNA in the cerebellum, diencephalon, and cortex of mice isolated at various ages after weaning. This implies that many fewer neurons and glial cells are formed during this critical developmental period if animals are kept in isolation. Moreover, Essman (1971b, 1972) has reported that isolated mice have relatively higher glial RNA concentrations and relatively lower neuronal RNA concentrations than do grouped mice. The RNA differences are particularly large in synaptosomal fractions. Welch et al. (1974) have reported that, in rats, grouping for one year postweaning increased RNA concentration in brain, while DNA concentration appeared to vary with living space. Melzack and Burns (1965) have reported an electrophysiological hyperexcitability in dogs reared in isolation which may persist for some time after exposure to a testing situation. Essman (1971b) found that both natural and barbiturate-induced sleeping time was shorter in isolated than in grouped mice. Similarly, McGinty (1971) found that kittens reared in isolation slept less than their group-housed counterparts; when they were placed (at 23 weeks of age) in the group environment, their sleep increased beyond the level of group-reared cats. McGinty also reported that $4\frac{1}{2}$ hours' exposure to a novel stimulating environment increased isolated kittens' subsequent sleep time by 25 percent. (The review by Bloch, in this volume, hints at the value this increased sleep may have for the organism.)

Although these results do not all fit a clear pattern, Essman (1971b) and Prescott (1971) have suggested that much of the data is consistent with the hypothesis that social deprivation increases the excitability of the brain and of somatosensory regions in particular, since they have been deprived of normal environmental stimulation. The effects of the deprivation, if performed during development, appear not to be rapidly reversible by later environmental situations. Hence the "isolation syndrome" has aspects in common with sensory-deprivation syndromes and might be considered an independent component of the complex-environment paradigm described below.

16.3.2 Effects of overcrowding

A second aspect of social experience which needs to be mentioned if only briefly is the effect of high population density or group size on brain and behavior. The amount of work on this phenomenon is limited, compared to that on the effects of isolation. However, considerable evidence suggests that chronic overcrowding, especially during development, can act as a stressor in mammals. Animals kept in large groups have higher adrenal weight (e.g., Brain and Nowell, 1970; Christian, Lloyd, and Davis, 1965; Sassenrath, 1970), higher pituitary weight (Bell et al., 1971), altered activity patterns (Bell et al., 1971, Christian, 1955), reduced stamina (Anderson, Werboff, and Les, 1968), reduced reproductive potential (Christian and LeMunyan, 1958; Snyder, 1968), and behavioral changes including aggression and various bizarre patterns of social and reproductive behavior (Calhoun, 1962; Christian, Lloyd, and Davis, 1965; Sassenrath, 1970). In addition acquisition of complex appetitively and aversively motivated tasks is impaired, although no obvious deficits appear in simpler situations (Goeckner, Greenough, and Mead, 1973; Goeckner, Greenough, and Maier, 1974). Bell et al. (1971) assessed a variety of effects of group size and group density on mouse brain. They found that brain weight decreased with increasing group size in a fixed space (Goeckner, Greenough, and Mead, 1973, reported a tendency in this direction), but increased with group size at constant density. Whole-brain DNA and protein content (and concentration) decreased with increasing group size, regardless of density (in contrast to the results of Welch et al., 1974). RNA content decreased with density. No effects were seen on brain acetylcholinesterase or serotonin levels.

The research available, then, suggests that, just as

excessive visual stimulation may be damaging, at least in albino rats (e.g., Anderson and O'Steen, 1972; Noell and Albrecht, 1971), so, too, it may be possible to exceed the level of social stimulation that is required for the development and maintenance of social and other behavior. Taken together, the isolation and overcrowding studies suggest that normal brain and behavior development depends upon an optimal, rather than a maximal, level of environmental stimulation. The degree to which deviations from this optimum affect the organism, through stress and through diminished sensorimotor stimulation (and, indeed, the degree to which these are independent), has not been determined.

16.4 DIFFERENTIAL ENVIRONMENTAL COMPLEXITY

As any higher vertebrate matures, it acquires a great deal of both general and specific knowledge of its environment. While the degree to which a particular type of experience contributes may be debated, there is little doubt that interaction with the environment is required in the development of such capacities as visuomotor coordination (Hein, 1972; Held and Hein, 1963), perceptual constancies (e.g., Gibson, 1969), and fine motor skills (Adams, 1968). Later in development, the organism learns a variety of rules of its particular environment: locations of food and safety, sources of danger, social relationships and appropriate social behaviors, etc. Unlike the cases of early stress or visual development, many of these processes of information acquisition in later development do not seem to be tied to a critical period; thus they may represent a gradation between the utilization of ongoing neuronal growth during a critical period and the postdevelopmental memory of an adult, or they may include both types if they are basically different.

The development of some of these capacities may be studied in the environmental-complexity (EC) paradigm originated by Hebb (1947, 1949) and investigated extensively by Rosenzweig, Bennett, and Diamond (e.g., 1972a) and their collaborators. The bulk of this work has used rodents. Exactly what constitutes a complex environment differs widely across investigators. Hebb (1947) reared rats as pets in his home. Krech, Rosenzweig, and Bennett (1960) grouped rats with two of seven possible toys placed in their cage each day and began training them at about 60 days of age on maze and discrimination tasks. More recently, this group has examined a variety of complex rearing procedures. Our EC procedure (e.g., Volkmar and Greenough, 1972) exposes groups of animals to a daily selection from well over 100 different toys in their home cage and a free-

exploration box. With the possible exception of Hebb's (1947) conditions, the stimulation provided by such environments probably falls short of that available in the typical natural environment of a wild rat. However, they may provide significantly more stimulation than some other environments that are called complex or "enriched," in which groups of animals are housed undisturbed with the same small set of toys for several weeks (e.g., Henderson, 1970; McCall, Lester, and Dolan 1969). The choice of comparison groups has also varied across experimenters, the most common conditions being isolation and social housing in a laboratory cage (e.g., Rosenzweig, Bennett, and Diamond, 1972a; West and Greenough, 1972). Complexity and sociality necessarily covary in the experimental condition, and even the social controls in such experiments may be considered relatively restricted socially. Where conditions differ radically from those of Rosenzweig, Bennett, and Diamond, it will be noted in the following sections. Also, except as noted, the studies below involve animals exposed to environments at weaning or shortly thereafter.

16.4.1 Behavioral indications of altered brain function

A large number of investigations of the behavioral effects of complex environments have appeared since the original investigations of Hebb (1947, 1949). The evidence supports, in general, a conclusion that differential rearing yields behaviorally different animals, although the use of terms such as "intelligence" (Hebb, 1947) may be misleading. Differences on learning tasks may reflect emotional and motivational consequences of the environments as well as differences related to the processing and storage of environmental information. Some behavioral aspects of social isolation were described in the preceding section. Only a small amount of work has been directed toward the identification of particular behavioral capacities (e.g., attentional, memorial) that are affected by the differential environments. However, some cautious conclusions may be drawn from the more general tests of behavioral ability.

MAZE LEARNING. Perhaps the most consistent behavioral finding involves the superior performance of EC animals on complex mazes. Rodents reared in environments ranging widely in degree of complexity have outperformed rats raised in isolated (IC) or socially housed (SC) conditions (usually in terms of error scores) in a number of experiments (e.g., Bingham and Griffiths, 1952; Brown, 1968; Greenough et al., 1970; Hebb, 1947; Hymovitch, 1952; Rosenzweig, 1971). However, this finding has not been universal. LeBoeuf and Peeke (1969) and Peeke, LeBoeuf, and Herz (1971), for example, found no effect on Lashley III maze learning of a complex environment in which the same set of objects remained in a large group cage throughout the EC period (compared to isolated rats). The reasons(s) for the more general finding of enhanced maze performance is not clear. Maze tasks sample a variety of behavioral abilities. Fear or reactivity to the experimenter and test situation (McCall, Lester, and Dolan, 1969; Myers and Fox, 1963) in the isolated or socially housed animals could produce performance deficits, but although such differences may play a role, tests of this hypothesis have not been universally supportive (e.g., Greenough, Madden, and Fleischmann, 1972; Morgan, 1973; Rosenzweig, 1971). However, in light of the isolation effects reviewed above, this possibility must always be considered when isolated animals are included in the comparison. Similarly, the suggestion that differences in exploratory activity may yield maze differences (Zimbardo and Montgomery, 1957) has met with mixed experimental findings (Brown, 1968; Donovick, Burright, and Swidler, 1973; Forgays and Read, 1962; Forgus, 1954; Freeman and Ray, 1972; McCall, Lester, and Dolan, 1969). The suggestion that familiarity with environments similar to mazes may enhance performance in ECs (e.g., Bernstein, 1973; Forgus, 1954; Wilson, Warren, and Abbott, 1965) is probably correct, but not very useful for interpretation changes in behavioral capacity in ECs. Greenough, Wood, and Madden (1972) found that socially reared mice matched EC performance when Lashley III maze trials were spaced in time, but that the SCs fell to IC levels when trials were massed, suggesting a possible difference in information processing or storage capacity. Perhaps the most consistent finding is that EC animals may gain an advantage in maze learning through their tendency to use extramaze cues (Brown, 1968; Forgays and Forgays, 1952; Hymovitch, 1952). This suggests that the EC animals have learned that physically distant aspects of their environment can be important, which is generally not the case for animals reared in small cages. At the least, then, the maze-learning studies indicate that the differentially reared animals have learned different techniques for dealing with their environment.

OTHER APPETITIVELY MOTIVATED TASKS. Differences in performance on visual-discrimination tasks appear to be less consistent than on mazes. Bingham and Griffiths (1952), Krech, Rosenzweig, and Bennett (1962), and Nyman (1967) found no effects of complex environments in visual-discrimination learning. Krech, Rosenzweig, and Bennett did find differences in discrimination-reversal learning, and Morgan (1973) has reported that ICs were inferior in reversal learning in an object-manipulation task. Greenough, Yuwiler, and Dollinger (1973) have reported differences between EC and IC rats in an operant brightness discrimination. Donovick, Burright, and Swidler (1973) found no differences in alternation learning in a T maze with ECs that had been exposed to the same set of toys throughout rearing. However, John Ward and Tom Reh, in our laboratory, found significant differences between EC and IC rats in the rate of acquisition of an alternation pattern in a task in which the two choice alleys were adjacent. Nyman (1967) has also reported enhanced sequential-alternation performance after exposure to complex environments. Bernstein (1973) found both SC and EC rats superior to running-wheel isolates in T-maze learning. In contrast, Hymovitch (1952) found no differences on a ten-unit T maze among four groups reared in stovepipe cages, running wheels, group cages, or complex environments, although these animals had previously been trained (and showed environmentally induced differences) on a Hebb-Williams maze.

A very preliminary parallel might be drawn between the effects of restricted rearing and the effects of lesions of the hippocampus and other basal forebrain regions. Hippocampal damage has been found to retard performance on complex mazes, discrimination reversal, and alternation (e.g., Kimble, 1968; Isaacson and Kimble, 1972; Thomas, Hostetter, and Barker, 1968). While this correlation is based on limited data, further experiments along these lines would seem warranted (see Altman, Brunner, and Bayer, 1973). In this connection, Walsh et al. (1969) and Fleischmann (1972) have reported anatomical differences in the hippocampus between EC and IC rats.

AVERSIVELY MOTIVATED TASKS. A limited amount of work has examined effects of environmental complexity on avoidance learning. Edwards, Barry, and Wyspianski (1969) found ECs superior to isolates in a footshock-motivated brightness-discrimination task. Freeman and Ray (1972) reported an interaction between rat strain and rearing complexity on two-way shuttlebox performance and no difference on a light-dark Y maze discrimination. Freeman and Ray also found socially reared rats superior to ECs in passive-avoidance retention. Greenough et al. (1970), however, found EC mice superior to isolates in passive avoidance, and other work in our laboratory with rats has generally confirmed this, although we have not tested SCs on the tasks.

NOTES ON ENVIRONMENTAL VARIABLES AND SPECIES GENERALITY. A few studies have examined the effects of the degree of complexity of the environment upon behavioral performance. The problem of the sensitivity of the behavioral tests used in such studies is particularly evident here. For example, Bernstein (1973) found no effect of the addition of "toys" to a large-cage environment when animals were tested on a Lashley III maze and a T maze, while Forgays and Forgays (1952), using a Hebb-Williams maze, found a graded effect across seven levels of complexity. Again, the similarity between the environment and the test situation may play a role in such studies (Forgus, 1954). Studies of the generality of environmental-complexity effects on learning in nonhuman species other than rodents appear to have been limited to dogs, cats, and primates. A number of experimenters have found pet or socially reared dogs superior to restricted animals on visual- and spatial-discrimination tasks (Clarke et al., 1951; Fuller, 1966; Melzack, 1962; Thompson and Heron, 1954). The restricted groups in these experiments typically appear, from the descriptions, to have suffered from isolation stress. Initial work with monkeys failed to find effects of isolation rearing on discrimination tasks when relatively long pretraining periods were used (Griffin and Harlow, 1966). Recent work by Gluck, Harlow, and Schiltz (1973), however, indicates that effects of differential environmental complexity can be seen on complex oddity-discrimination tasks but not on simpler discriminations or delayed-response problems. Research using humans has been necessarily less precise. Nonetheless, experimental data have suggested that environmental stimulation has a major influence on the development of an array of behavioral skills (see, e.g., Gibson, 1969; Hunt, 1961; Paraskevopoulos and Hunt, 1971).

AGE DEPENDENCE AND PERMANENCE OF COMPLEX-ENVIRONMENT EFFECTS. A proportion of the behavioral effects of complex environments seem to be tied to relatively "critical" or "sensitive" periods in development. For example, the enhancement of maze learning was most pronounced in some early studies when the complexity experience occurred at or near the age of weaning in rats (Forgays and Read, 1962; Forgus, 1954; Hymovitch, 1952). In contrast, Nyman (1967) found the effects of complexity on sequential alternation to be maximal when a 10-day exposure began at 50 days of age. Rosenzweig (1971) has reported that EC rearing affects learning of visual-discrimination reversals only if the exposure period begins near weaning age, while maze performance is facilitated by exposure beginning at least as late as 60 days of age. He suggests that the reversal task is sensitive to early isolation, whereas maze performance may be facilitated by general exploratory experience, which can be gained at later ages. This two-component (age-dependent and age-independent) notion is appealing if one wishes to suggest exposure to

complex environments as a model for training. If we consider the potential limbic involvement suggested above, one can argue that the development of age-dependent limbic attention-inhibition systems (Isaacson and Kimble, 1972) may be more temporally sensitive to experience. A second component of the environmental-complexity effect may be similar to the learning of specific environmental events and contingencies, at least in the sense that it may occur at any age.

With regard to the enduring effects of EC on behavior, most investigators have found that the environmentally induced differences in appetitive-task performance persist as long as the animals remain in the differential environments (Forgays and Forgays, 1952; Forgus, 1954; Hymovitch, 1952; Rosenzweig, 1971). Forgays and Read (1962) reported that differences in Hebb-Williams maze performance induced by short post-weaning periods in complex environments endured to maturity when the rats spent the interval in small laboratory cages (whether the rats were grouped or isolated is not clear from their report), and similar findings occurred in other age-dependency studies described above. Rosenzweig (1971) found that differences on discrimination-reversal and maze learning tended to diminish during testing. On the other hand, at least three studies have reported differences on a second of two tasks following relatively extensive training on the first (Forgays and Forgays, 1952; Greenough et al., 1970; Greenough, Wood, and Madden, 1972), and unpublished data from our laboratory also support this finding. Hebb (1949) found that rats reared as pets improved more during testing than did those reared in laboratory cages. The extent to which the differences persist appears to depend upon the differences between the environments used, the similarity of the testing tasks, the age at which testing begins, and the degree to which the tasks are differentially sensitive to early exposure to complex environments.

16.4.2 Environmental-complexity effects upon brain physiology

Physiological assessment of differential brain function has been rare in environmental-complexity studies, in contrast to the extensive work on visual development (see Chapter 18, this volume). Edwards, Barry, and Wyspianski (1969) reported that the mean latency of three major component peaks in the cortical evoked potential to a light flash was shorter in ECs after four weeks of differential rearing. After eight weeks' rearing, significant effects were seen in only one component. Tagney (1973) reported that EC rats spent 56 percent of their time sleeping, compared to 46 percent for ICs, after about four weeks' differential rearing. The percentages of sleep time spent in REM sleep and slow-wave sleep did not differ. When IC rats were then transferred to the EC environment, their sleep increased toward the EC level. Most of the increase was in slow-wave sleep. Sleep patterns of EC rats transferred to isolation did not change. Tagney (1973) suggests extra sleep time may be necessary for macromolecular synthesis and restoration of brain function after higher levels of activity (see also Bloch, this volume). However, sleep time may be a function of social exposure, as noted by Essman (1971b; see also Section 16.3). Tagney's suggestion is compatible with McGinty's (1971) data, but the role of sleep vis-à-vis the environmental demand remains an open question. It is perhaps worth noting that "controls" in physiological studies of visual deprivation are typically cage-reared, often in isolation. To the extent that the above findings represent a closer approximation to "normal" development, the use of complex-environment controls in such studies of sensory-system development may be advisable.

16.4.3 Environmental-complexity effects upon brain chemistry

Biochemical work on differential environmental complexity can be loosely grouped in two classes: that which indicates differential levels of overall metabolic activity, and that which suggests selectively altered activity of a specific process that may affect behavior. Since weight in some brain regions differs between groups, chemical measurements relative to tissue weight (or to each other) may be a better index of changes in individual constituents independent of overall changes in brain.

GENERAL METABOLIC MEASURES. Perhaps the most striking effect of these differential rearing procedures on brain is the alteration produced in the weights of various brain regions. Since the original report of greater cortical weight in EC than in isolated rats (Rosenzweig et al., 1962), the phenomenon has been replicated in various ways by a number of other investigators (e.g., Altman et al., 1968; Geller, Yuwiler, and Zolman, 1965; Greenough, Yuwiler, and Dollinger, 1973; Henderson, 1970; LaTorre, 1968; Walsh et al., 1971), and extensively examined by Rosenzweig, Bennett, and Diamond (e.g., 1972a, b; Bennett et al., 1964; Rosenzweig, 1971). Dimensional differences, measured microscopically, are discussed below. The weight differences are greatest in occipital cortex in the rearing paradigm of Rosenzweig, Bennett, and Diamond (1972a), although significant effects are seen in somesthetic, remaining dorsal, and ventral cortex. Subcortical weight is slightly greater in IC rats. Socially reared rats tend to follow the IC weight pattern, except for subcortical weight, where they

follow the ECs (Rosenzweig, Bennett, and Diamond, 1972a), suggesting that isolation stress may be responsible for this subcortical effect. Rats exposed to the complex environment as young (105-day-old) or old (285-day-old) adults show similar cortical weight increases (Rosenzweig, Bennett, and Diamond, 1972a; Riege, 1971), although longer exposure periods are necessary to yield equivalent effects. Cortical-weight differences occur when rats are differentially reared in darkness or blinded, and the occipital region of the cortex continues to be the most affected (Rosenzweig et al., 1969). In experiments in which the rats are placed in the differential environments at weaning, the cortical-weight differences appear to reach maximal levels at 15 to 30 days of age and may then decline slightly to a persisting baseline difference (Bennett, Rosenzweig, and Diamond, 1970; Cummins et al., 1973; Rosenzweig, 1971; Walsh, Cummins, and Budtz-Olsen, 1974). The brain-weight differences are not a mere reflection of body-weight effects (although these may interact; see Rosenzweig, Bennett, and Diamond, 1972a). Typically, IC rats have heavier body weights than ECs (e.g., Greenough, Yuwiler, and Dollinger, 1973), as do SC rats in short-duration experiments from weaning (Rosenzweig, Bennett, and Diamond, 1972a). Tagney (1973) has reported that IC rats consume more food than ECs.

Measures of total protein, total RNA, dry weight of brain tissue, and the activity of hexokinase have suggested that the increase in cortical weight reflects real tissue growth, rather than increased fluid content or some similar nonanabolic swelling, process. All three measures closely followed measures of cortical weight (Rosenzweig, Bennett, and Diamond, 1972a, b). DNA per unit tissue weight was, however, lower in ECs, suggesting a relative increase in cellular size. An index of metabolic activation, the ratio of RNA to DNA, was significantly greater in EC than in IC rats (due primarily to an RNA increase in EC rats; see Bennett, this volume), and also greater in cyclic-light-reared than in dark-reared rats (Rosenzweig, Bennett, and Diamond, 1972a). Altman and Das (1964) reported increased synthesis of glial DNA in EC rats after 110 days of differential rearing.

Levitan, Mushynski, and Ramirez (1972) examined levels of metabolic activity in terms of the regional rates of incorporation of leucine into protein in various subcellular fractions in rats after sixteen postweaning days of EC or SC rearing. They reported a higher level of incorporation into or stabilization of nuclear proteins in EC subcortical brain regions (particularly hippocampus) and no differences in cortical or subcortical perikaryonal cytoplasmic fractions. In synaptosomal fractions, EC rats showed higher incorporation rates in subcortical regions, while SC rats (surprisingly, in terms of all other data in this section) showed higher rates of incorporation in cortical synaptosomal fractions. In a related examination of gene activation, Mushynski, Levitan, and Ramirez (1973) found no differences when competition-hybridization techniques were used to assess possible differences in the relative number of genes expressed in the RNA of EC and SC rats.

ENZYMATIC AND NEUROTRANSMITTER MEASURES. The bulk of enzymatic-activity measurement by Rosenzweig, Bennett, and Diamond (e.g., 1972a, b; Bennett et al., 1964; Rosenzweig, 1971) has involved acetylcholinesterase (AChE), cholinesterase (ChE), and choline acetyltransferase. In comparison with EC rats differentially housed for 80 days postweaning, the results for acetylcholinesterase have indicated an increase in activity in IC rats relative to tissue weight in the cortex and a slight decrease in the rest of the brain (cerebellum plus noncortical tissue through the medulla). Cholinesterase activity was relatively increased in the cortex and less so in the rest of the brain in the EC rats. The effects appear to result from isolation since, in general, socially housed rats follow the ECs on these measures. With shorter differential rearing, AChE reductions in EC rats were seen, but little change occurred in ChE. Both types of change could result from increases in amounts of glial tissue and perhaps from growth in noncholinergic neurons. Similar effects are seen when differential housing begins in early adulthood, except that SC values are more intermediate. In older rats, enzymatic measures appear to be less affected by differential housing. Choline acetyltransferase activity appeared to parallel AChE activity when it was measured, while acetylcholine measures revealed no differences.

Geller and Yuwiler (1968) reported directionally similar cortical AChE and ACh differences, as well as greater whole-brain absolute (not relative to weight) AChE activity in ECs. Cortical ChE activity, however, was slightly (not significantly) greater in IC rats. A mixed pattern of cholinergic enzyme and ChE changes was seen in various subcortical regions. Geller, Yuwiler, and Zolman (1965) reported no differences in whole-brain serotonin, dopamine, 5-HTP decarboxylase, or glutamic acid decarboxylase per unit protein. However, the IC rats showed a pattern of elevated whole-brain norepinephrine, increased liver transaminase activity, and increased adrenal weight, indicative of a possible reaction to isolation stress. Further work (Geller, 1971; Geller and Yuwiler, 1968) has indicated that the norepinephrine differences occur in their caudate-nucleus tissue sample, and that the relative increase in the IC occurs rapidly after the onset of differential housing. Riege and

Morimoto (1970) found a similar norepinephrine difference in a combined hypothalamus and caudate-nucleus sample, but norepinephrine levels in other brain regions were greater in ECs, so that the net difference, while favoring ICs, was not significant. Since tumbling stress increased EC norepinephrine values in combined caudate-nucleus and hypothalamus samples more than for ICs, one might conclude that the ICs were already suffering some isolation stress. However, adrenal weights were equivalent in nonstressed EC and IC rats in this experiment, although they increased more with stress in the ICs. Furthermore, differential stress did not appear to affect the AChE and ChE effects described above. It is not clear why the rats derived from the Tryon strains used in this and most other experiments by Rosenzweig, Bennett, Diamond, and their collaborators do not manifest the isolation syndrome detailed earlier.

16.4.4 Environmental effects on brain anatomy

GROSS DIMENSIONAL DIFFERENCES. Environmental-complexity-induced differences in the size or thickness of various brain regions have been reported by several investigators (e.g., Altman et al., 1968; Diamond et al., 1966; Walsh et al., 1969). Detailed studies by Diamond (1967; Diamond et al., 1972; Rosenzweig, Bennett, and Diamond, 1972a) have corroborated, with greater precision, the weight measures discussed above. As in the weight studies, the postweaning effects appeared greatest after about 30 days' differential housing and were maximal in occipital cortex (Diamond et al., 1972). Preweaning differential housing produced even greater effects (Malkasian and Diamond, 1971). In 30-day postweaning studies, Diamond et al. (1972) reported that EC rats' cortices were also thicker than those of IC rats in somesthetic, temporal, and frontomedial regions. Differences appeared to be slightly larger and more consistent throughout the cortex when differential housing began at 60 days of age rather than at weaning (with the rats housed socially up to this age). Similar differences were seen between EC and IC female rats, although these differences were slightly smaller than those found in males (Diamond, Johnson, and Ingham, 1971). After 80-day postweaning exposure periods, differences in cortex are apparently smaller than after 30-day periods and are restricted to frontal and occipital regions (Diamond, 1967; Walsh et al., 1972). Slightly smaller differences were seen in occipital cortex when 80 days' differential housing began at 105 days of age rather than at weaning (Diamond et al., 1972). Socially reared rats tend overall to be intermediate between ECs and ICs (Diamond et al., 1972), being close to ECs in temporal cortex and slightly more similar to ICs in medial occipital cortex. Altman et al. (1968) and Walsh et al. (1971) have reported greater overall cerebral length in adult animals exposed to environmental complexity. Walsh et al. (1969) also reported greater hippocampal thickness in EC than in IC rats; Rosenzweig (1971) indicated that similar differences in hippocampus have sometimes, but not consistently, appeared in his group's studies.

CELLULAR DIMENSIONS AND COMPOSITION. Diamond et al. (1966) reported that EC rats have a higher density of glial cells in occipital cortex than do ICs. Diamond (1967) also found greater perikaryonal and nuclear sizes in the occipital cortex of EC rats. The glial increase correlates with the Altman and Das (1964) report of an increase in DNA labeling in the glial cells of EC rats. Cellular dimensions were also increased in groups exposed to complex environments prior to weaning (Malkasian and Diamond, 1971).

DENDRITIC BRANCHING. Initially, Holloway (1966) reported that dendritic branching, in terms of dendritic intersections with multiple concentric circles at intervals around the cell body, appeared to be greater in layer-2 stellate neurons from EC-rat visual cortex than in those from ICs. Fred Volkmar and I followed this up with studies of four occipital-cortex cell types in EC, SC, and IC rats which were differentially reared for 30 days after weaning (Greenough and Volkmar, 1973; Volkmar and Greenough, 1972). The region we selected overlaps to a great extent with the one that has shown the greatest thickness differences in the studies of Diamond and her colleagues (e.g., Diamond et al., 1972). Camera lucida drawings of rapid-Golgi-stained neurons were analyzed (see Figure 16.1) in terms of the intersections between their dendrites and concentric rings (after Sholl, 1956) and in terms of the number and length of dendrites at each order away from the cell body or apical dendrite (after Coleman and Riesen, 1968). The results were remarkably consistent: in small, medium, and large pyramidal neurons and in stellate neurons, EC rats consistently had more higher-order dendritic branches than their IC littermates (24 of 24 cases in fifth-order branching). SC rats were intermediate, but tended to be closer to the ICs in higher-order branching (EC > SC in 19/24 cases; SC > IC in 17/24 cases). In pyramidal neurons, the bulk of branching differences occurred in basal dendrites, although sporadic differences occurred in some apical regions. Figure 16.2 shows typical results for layer-4

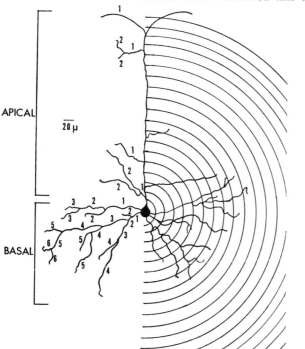

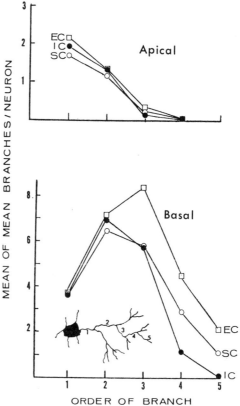

FIGURE 16.1 Analysis procedures for camera lucida drawings of Golgi-stained neurons. The right side of the neuron drawing illustrates the concentric-ring analysis, in which intersections between dendrites and rings are recorded. The left side shows branches numbered in terms of their order away from the cell body.

FIGURE 16.2 Mean number of branches at each order away from the cell body and apical dendrite in layer-4 pyramidal neurons from 6 triplet sets (N = 18) of rats reared for 30 days under complex (EC), social (SC), or isolated (IC) conditions.

pyramidal neurons. The lengths of branches at each order did not differ consistently across groups. The concentric-ring analysis confirmed the greater branching and indicated that the total volume occupied by neurons from the three groups did not differ to any great extent. It was estimated by omega-squared apportionment of the branching variance in the concentric-ring analysis that the environmental treatment accounted for 11 to 18 percent of the variance (depending upon the neuron population), while the litter from which the animals came and the interactions accounted for 7 to 24 percent. As much as half of the variance in some of the analyses was attributable to these two factors and their interaction.

We have also examined branching patterns in pyramidal cells of lateral frontal cortex and temporal cortex of rats reared in EC, IC, and SC for 30 postweaning days (Greenough, Volkmar, and Juraska, 1973). In the frontolateral area, which showed no thickness differences in the Diamond studies, we were not able to detect any differences resulting from differential rearing, although differences related to litter still appeared. In temporal cortex, smaller but reliable differences were seen in layer-4 pyramidal-cell basal dendritic branching. Again, differences among members of different litters were present.

The cortical regions in which we have to date found differences in dendritic branching correspond reasonably well to the pattern of weight and thickness differences described by Diamond et al. (1972). This suggests that differences in dendritic volume, along with differences in perikaryonal size and glial density, may account for much of the gross size difference.

The high amount of variance consistently associated with differences between the litters from which animals have come should not be attributed merely to genetic similarity among siblings. Rats are multiple ovulators, and it is highly unlikely that triplet members of a litter share the same genetic constitution, although they may be more similar than members of different litters (Ross, Ginsburg, and Denenberg, 1957). Moreover, littermates have shared the same environment from conception to weaning—an environment that includes nutritive differences among litters as well as differences in maternal and other environmental stimulation. The concordance between litters does suggest that, across environmental groups, equivalent sets of neurons are stained by the capricious Golgi staining technique.

Globus et al. (1973) have reported that EC rats have a higher frequency of synaptic spines on basal dendrites of occipital-cortex pyramidal neurons than do ICs. They have also reported, in agreement with our findings, minimal differences in the overall volumetric size of the dendritic tree. These findings, combined with ours indicating increased dendritic surface, suggest a considerably greater number of synapses per neuron in animals reared in complex environments. To attempt precise quantitative estimates of this difference would be premature, of course, but it is clear that the effects of postweaning environmental complexity at the neuronal level can be more than trivial.

MEASUREMENTS ON INDIVIDUAL SYNAPSES. Both Møllgaard et al. (1971) and West and Greenough (1972) have examined individual synapses in EC and IC rats with electron-microscopic techniques. Møllgaard et al. measured the length (two-dimensional estimate of area) of the postsynaptic opaque region in type-1 synapses from layer 3; the length averaged 52 percent greater in EC rats. (Bennett, this volume, describes more recent results.) West and Greenough measured postsynaptic thickening length, bouton diameter, and the length of the region of tight apposition of the pre- and postsynaptic processes in type-1 synapses in layers 1, 4, and 6 of occipital cortex. EC rats averaged about 14 percent longer in postsynaptic thickening length in layer 4. Other measures were not consistently statistically significant. Møllgaard et al. (1971) reported that the frequency of synapses in the tissue was one-third less in EC rats. We have observed much smaller frequency differences in the same direction (unpublished data), but we have tentatively attributed this to the fact that EC synapses in our study may have been larger on the average, so that the probability of appropriate orientation of the irregular surface of the synaptic cleft in a thin section would have been lower (synapses that could not be clearly measured were eliminated from our calculations).

These findings, as well as related work indicating increased synaptic size in some areas of the visual system with exposure to patterned light (Cragg, 1967; Fifková, 1970), appear to suggest that some synapses grow larger with environmental stimulation. However, the results should be interpreted with caution. The regions in which the larger synapses are seen are also regions in which new synapses form following the same treatments. It is quite possible that the new synapses are larger than those formed previously. For example, Larramendi (1969) and Rakic (1973) have described changes in cerebellar postsynaptic morphology after the contact has formed. If this is so, differences in average measures may merely reflect the new synaptic formation. Alternatively, newly formed synapses may be smaller than existing ones, in which case the averages would underestimate the degree to which existing synapses have grown larger. Finally, we really have little evidence to support the general assumption that synapses, once formed, remain connected indefinitely. We do know that when afferents are lost through damage, the vacated "sites" may be rapidly occupied by sprouts from other afferent populations (see, e.g., Raisman, 1969, and in this volume). It is not inconceivable that some synapses nondegeneratively regress and re-form, depending, perhaps, for their existence upon the occurrence of some preservative signal determined by the functional utility of the connection.

16.4.5 Permanence and age dependence of brain effects

Rosenzweig, Bennett, and Diamond (1972a; see also Bennett, this volume) reported that differences in cortical weight and thickness between EC and IC rats appeared to persist for as long as the animals were differentially housed. Cummins et al. (1973) reported that differential cortical dimensions were apparent after over 500 days of differential rearing, although Walsh et al. (1974) have reported a decrease in the size of the difference over time. Other work with longer periods of exposure (Geller, Yuwiler, and Zolman, 1965; Walsh et al., 1969) generally supports the conclusion that these cortical differences persist to some extent for as long as differential environments are maintained. Larger cortical-thickness differences at earlier periods may represent metabolic processes involved in the establishment of more enduring changes, such as increased dendritic length and synaptic spines. We have not yet completed studies on the permanence of the differences in dendritic branching. Differences in cholinesterase appear to follow a longer time course than do the weight effects (Rosenzweig, Bennett, and Diamond, 1972a). Krech, Rosenzweig, and Bennett (1962) reported that weight and chemical differences were attenuated by training experiences, possibly because the training provided both groups with stimulation to some extent equivalent to the complex environment.

The age of onset of differential housing may affect the magnitude of the cortical weight and thickness differences reported by Rosenzweig and co-workers, but such effects have been seen in older rats. Significant weight effects of differential rearing were found by Riege (1971) in rats housed at 285 days of age. Longer exposure periods appear to be necessary to produce maximal effects in older animals (Rosenzweig, Bennett, and Diamond, 1972a). In contrast to the behavioral findings, in which certain tasks may be affected only by differential rearing shortly after weaning, age-dependent qualitative differences in the brain have not been reported. The possible similarity between the behavioral effects of isolation rearing and those of limbic lesions suggests that effects of differential rearing in limbic

structures (Walsh et al., 1969; Fleischmann, 1972) may be age-dependent.

16.4.6 Differential rearing as a model for memory

Interpretations of the causes of the various brain effects include differential stress (e.g., Geller, Yuwiler, and Zolman, 1965; Hatch et al., 1963), hormonal or nutritive effects, differential sensory and motor stimulation, and differential rates of brain maturation to an asymptotic level or different levels. The possibility that hormonal or nutritive differences among the rearing groups bring about the brain or behavioral differences cannot be entirely discounted. Diamond, Johnson, and Ingham (1971) found that the thickness of female rat cortex was apparently increased during pregnancy, regardless of environment. The profound effects of hormones upon developing brain discussed earlier could conceivably underlie at least some of the environmental effects. On the other hand, Rosenzweig, Bennett, and Diamond (1972c) reported that hypophysectomized rats showed brain-weight effects after differential rearing, although the overall weight of both EC and IC brains was lower than in comparably treated intact rats. Moreover, the effects of the environment on brain anatomy occur only in certain regions (particularly in studies using older animals), whereas hormonal or nutritive effects might be expected to occur more generally throughout the cortex. With regard to stress and its associated hormonal consequences as a source of the anatomical effects, Riege and Morimoto (1970) reported that daily brief tumbling stress did not alter the EC-IC brain-weight pattern (although ChE increased in stressed ICs). With regard to both brain and behavioral effects, the "isolation syndrome" described above must almost certainly play some role, although it has been difficult for us to demonstrate it i nbehavior. Greenough, Madden, and Fleischmann (1972) compared the maze learning of EC rats with ICs that were either handled daily or left undisturbed except for minimal laboratory care. While some differences appeared in initial running of a straight alley (for water reward), there were no differences in maze errors between the two IC groups, while the EC group was superior to both. In unpublished work, Roger West, William E. Wood, and I have compared maze learning in EC and IC rats stimulated during the first or second postnatal week to that in an undisturbed control group. Across four replications we have seen no interaction between our version of Levine and Mullins's (1966) "emotional immunization" and the rearing environments. With regard to sensory stimulation, Rosenzweig et al. (1969) have reported that effects of differential rearing also occur in occipital cortex of blinded or dark-reared rats, although the effects are somewhat smaller.

(It is also interesting to note, in this regard, that the IC curve for layer-4 stellate-cell dendritic branching in rats from the 1972 Volkmar and Greenough study falls nearly on top of the corresponding 1968 Coleman and Riesen data for caged, light-reared cats, and curves for SC and EC rats fall above the IC curve.) Differential development may well account for some effects in young animals, but it cannot account for effects in adults. At this point, then, it seems reasonable to conclude that no unitary explanation of these sorts can account for the array of effects of differential rearing that have been reported.

If we assume that the effects of a complex environment on brain and behavior arise from more than one source, then we can consider some additional evidence for differential memory formation as one of the components. First, both behavioral and brain effects of environmental complexity appear to be potentiated by drugs that affect memory formation. Bennett, Rosenzweig, and Wu (1973) and Rosenzweig and Bennett (1972) have reported that daily administration of amphetamines and metrazol (but not strychnine) can potentiate the effects of environmental complexity upon their brain measures. LeBoeuf and Peeke (1969) and Peeke, LeBoeuf, and Herz (1971) have reported that the effects of a complex environment upon maze learning can be enhanced by daily strychnine administration. Whether these effects occur through facilitation of behavior in the free environment or through some more direct interaction with the environmental input upon the brain is not certain, but this is far from clear in experiments on drug-facilitated memory in general. Second, brain-weight effects of environmental complexity can occur after a very few days in the environment, on a time scale more compatible with that of learning and memory experiments (Bennett et al., 1974; Ferchmin, Eterović, and Caputto, 1970). Third, brain-weight differences occur even when exposure to environmental complexity is restricted to as little as two hours per day (for 30 days), a daily period somewhat more comparable to that of a learning experiment (Rosenzweig, Love, and Bennett, 1968). Fourth, behavioral effects seem to be greatest on tasks that are closer to the complex environment, especially mazes, although, as noted before, an age-dependent general process may be affected by early isolation. Similarly, considerable work has shown that experience with geometric forms can, under certain conditions, facilitate later form discrimination (see, e.g., Gibson, 1969), and the phenomenon of "latent learning" of various tasks seems reasonably well established (see, e.g., Mowrer, 1960, Chapter 2).

In a sense, it seems it would be much more difficult to argue that EC rats do *not* learn more than their IC and SC counterparts than it is to argue that they do. Perhaps

a more important problem is to determine which, if any, of the differences that have been measured in the brain are related to memory. The most reasonable approach, although not an exceptionally fruitful one to date, would seem to be to compare these environmental effects with those that occur in other environmental situations in which differential memory formation is arguably likely. The major advantage of the environmental-complexity paradigm as a starting point may be that its effects upon the brain are profound. Even if similar effects occur in other situations, they may be difficult to impossible to find. The two most promising approaches to this problem seem to be the use of model systems, in which the part of the nervous system undergoing training can be isolated for study, and whole-organism training situations, in which long-term training may result in enduring effects that are larger or more extensive than those of a relatively short behavioral experience.

16.5 ENDURING EFFECTS OF FORMAL TRAINING ON BRAIN MEASURES

In this section I wish to concern myself primarily with those brain effects of training procedures that are also seen in the EC-IC model and that appear to persist in time. Short-term biochemical and electrophysiological measures are discussed elsewhere in this symposium, and the results of model-systems studies have been recently reviewed elsewhere (e.g., Thompson, Patterson, and Teyler, 1972). This is not to suggest that the short-term biochemical effects described by Rose in this volume, as well as by other recent reviews (e.g., Booth, 1973; Glassman, 1969), do not persist, at least in part, or lead to persisting changes. However, the sorts of techniques used in these studies appear, due to the rapid metabolic turnover of the nervous system, to be limited in their application to relatively short training and measurement periods.

16.5.1 Enduring effects of training upon brain chemistry and physiology

The vast bulk of studies of the effects of training procedures on brain chemistry have assessed changes during and shortly after the training period (see, e.g., the reviews by Dunn and by Rose, this volume). Longer-term biochemical consequences of training have been reported in some studies. Among the earlier reports was a series of papers by Hydén and co-workers (e.g., Hydén and Egyházi, 1962, 1964) describing changes in the amounts, neuron-glial locations, and ratios of bases in rat brain RNA during and following motor learning tasks. The effects were quite large in regions presumably rather directly involved with afferent or efferent aspects of the training procedure. More recently, Hydén and Lange (1970a,b; 1972) reported short-term changes in regional amino acid incorporation and increases in hippocampal S-100 proteins following handedness-reversal training. Administration of antiserum to some of these brain-specific proteins interfered with handedness-reversal learning. Hydén and Lange (1972) also reported that leucine incorporation into brain protein was depressed during an extended handedness-training experience. Since S-100 proteins constitute a very small percentage of brain protein, the later results are not incompatible with the original findings.

A series of studies by Bogoch (e.g., 1968, 1973) has similarly focused upon changes in a select group of brain protein components. Bogoch has reported both short-term and enduring effects of training procedures upon glycoproteins in pigeon brain. Glycoproteins are associated with nerve membranes in the brain, and different groups have been associated with myelin, neuronal and glial cell bodies, and synaptosomes (Bogoch, 1968). There is evidence for systematic variation in the pattern of glycoprotein concentrations during development, and the gross disruption in glycoprotein chemistry in Tay-Sachs disease is associated with severe mental dysfunction (see Bogoch, 1968; White, Handler, and Smith, 1968). Bogoch (1968) reported short-term whole-brain increases in several glycoprotein groups following extended operant discrimination training in pigeons. Moreover, the glycoprotein fraction that has been associated with mitochondria and synaptosomes remained above untrained control levels for several months following training. The differences were remarkably large, as were differences in total brain protein content. Bogoch (1973) has further reported a positive relationship between the brain concentration of the synaptosome-associated glycoprotein group and correct performance on a difficult discrimination task; in short-term incorporation studies, the glycoproteins that had been increased during extended training (Bogoch, 1968) were more rapidly labeled in pigeons undergoing training than in resting controls. Bogoch (1968) suggested that the newly synthesized glycoproteins might selectively facilitate synaptic transmission. The association of certain glycoprotein groups with synaptic fractions, however, makes the data equally compatible, at this stage, with the notion that new synapses form during the training experience, or that some other anabolic change occurs with training. The findings of Bogoch and of Hydén's group, while preliminary, suggest that such measures might be usefully applied to environmental-complexity studies as well as to other species and training situations.

A few studies have investigated the effects of formal training procedures upon some of the enzymatic activi-

ties that have been altered following exposure to complex environments. Rosenzweig, Bennett, and Diamond (1972a) have indicated that their "total AChE" measure (weight × enzyme activity per unit weight) may be slightly affected by formal training while more profound changes, especially in weight, are brought about by deprivation and rehousing procedures prior to training. Brown (1971) has reported remarkably large (approximately 50 percent) differences in visual-cortex AChE and ChE activity between rats that were discrimination-trained or patterned-light-stimulated and yoked controls. The differences disappeared after three days of social housing. The data appear from the report to be highly variable across subjects, and the changes appear to occur in light-stimulated animals regardless of the training contingency. Izquierdo et al. (1973) reported that choline acetylase activity in dorsal hippocampus was reduced slightly during a pre-experimental food-deprivation period, but returned to pre-deprivation levels as the rats were straight-alley-trained. No changes were observed in AChE activity. In general, these studies have not shown a consistent pattern of cholinergic enzyme changes with training, although it appears that the cholinergic system may be affected by a variety of environmental conditions.

16.5.2 Enduring anatomical correlates of training

A limited number of studies have evaluated the effects of formal training on brain anatomy. Appetitive discrimination and maze training were originally included in the environmental-complexity treatment of Krech, Rosenzweig, and Bennett (e.g., 1960), but this addition "could be omitted without affecting the cerebral results" (Rosenzweig, Bennett, and Diamond, 1972a, p. 210). More recently, this group has begun to examine the effects of training alone on brain measures. Brief summaries of their results (Rosenzweig, Bennett, and Diamond, 1972a; Rosenzweig, 1971) report small but significant enzymatic differences (see above), but no effects upon the cortical-weight measures that are influenced by environmental complexity. Cummins et al. (1973) have reported that 500-day-old IC rats subjected to three weeks of daily Hebb-Williams maze training had significantly greater cortical length × width measures than did untrained ICs. Rosenzweig, Bennett, and Diamond (1972b), however, have reported that re-caging and water deprivation may bring about increases in weight measures, and these procedures were not carried out with controls in the Cummins et al. study.

Despite the long history of suggestions that memory may involve the formation of new synaptic connections, direct tests of the effects of formal training upon measures of connectivity have been rare. Smit, Uylings, and Veldmaat-Wansink (1971–1972) analyzed dendritic branching patterns in rabbit cortex and found that variation in higher-order dendrite segments occurred beyond the level predicted by models that did fit lower-order segments. They suggest that this variation may represent a substrate for plasticity in the adult brain. (It should be noted that, while Greenough and Volkmar, 1973, found no consistent differences between the lengths of higher-order branches in EC and IC rats, the number of complete branches in ICs was very small. Comparisons that included branches leaving the section showed no significant differences, but this measure would be quite biased against possibly longer higher-order dendrites in the more highly proliferated group.)

Rutledge (this volume) describes an experiment that appears to support this notion. Cats were trained to associate foreleg shock with an electrical-stimulation CS to the suprasylvian gyrus. Untrained cats received the electrical CS but no leg shock. The results of analysis of Golgi-stained tissue suggested two classes of "use" effects upon neuronal growth. First, apical regions of layer-2 and layer-3 pyramidal cells homotopically contralateral to the stimulated region (which received the callosal input) had significantly more dendritic branches, longer terminals, and more dendritic spines, regardless of UCS presentation. Second, greater numbers of vertical and oblique spines were seen in animals that had also received the UCS. The results depend upon comparisons between the stimulated and "receiving" hemispheres, and no unimplanted controls were run. However, Rutledge notes that the control (stimulated) side appeared comparable to normal material from their and other laboratories.

The Rutledge findings are of particular interest because of some recent findings from our laboratory involving the measurement of neuronal dendritic dimensions following training. We consider the results preliminary, but since a similar pattern has emerged in two entirely independent studies, we have reasonable confidence in them. In the study I shall describe in detail, Janice Juraska, Timothy DeVoogd, George Cybulski, Fred Volkmar, and I examined dendritic branching in male Sprague-Dawley albino rats which had been trained, beginning at 75 to 80 days of age, on a series of Hebb-Williams maze problems for water reward. Each rat learned a new problem (within a maximum of 24 trials) to perfection each day. On most days rats were also tested on previously learned problems. Since test performance was generally better than original acquisition, we assume that the rats remembered either specific problems or general properties of the maze over time. As a control group we used similarly water-deprived littermates that had been housed in the same cage with

their respective trained brothers until training was begun. During training all rats were housed individually in standard cages of sheet metal and wire mesh. Control littermates were removed from their cages, handled, and given a small amount of water, generally several times each day. At the end of the 26-day training period rapid-Golgi-stained sections were analyzed according to our usual procedures. Layer-4 (medium) and layer-5 (large) pyramidal and stellate neurons from posterior dorsal cortex (Krieg's areas 17 and 18) were examined. Except for stellates, 35 neurons of each type were drawn from each member of 7 pairs of rats. As in all of our anatomical studies, the animals were coded at the time of sacrifice so that the experimenters drawing and scoring neurons were unaware of treatments of individual animals.

Results of this study are shown in Table 16.1. The

TABLE 16.1

Mean numbers of pyramidal-neuron dendritic branches in maze-trained vs. control (handled) rats

	Layer 4			Layer 5		
	Trained	Handled	p	Trained	Handled	p
Apical branches						
Total dendrites	5.9	5.9	ns	6.7	7.4	ns
First- and second-order obliques	5.2	5.2	ns	5.9	6.5	0.05
Higher-order obliques	0.69	0.75	ns	0.9	0.9	ns
Concentric-ring intersections < 250 μ from the cell body	20.4	20.3	ns	20.7	21.0	0.01
Concentric-ring intersections > 250 μ from the cell body	3.9	2.7	0.001	10.1	8.8	0.005
Basilar branches						
Number of branches at each order from the cell body:						
1st	4.4	4.2	0.03	4.4	4.3	ns
2nd	8.2	7.7	0.01	8.1	8.0	ns
3rd	9.7	9.1	0.02	9.5	9.7	ns
4th	5.6	6.0	ns	5.6	6.0	ns
≥ 5th	1.7	2.0	ns	2.0	1.8	ns

p: statistical significance. ns: not significant.

concentric-ring analysis indicated small reliable effects in layer-4 and layer-5 pyramidal neurons. The effects were maximal some distance from the cell body. No consistent differences were detectable in basilar dendritic branching, or in the branching of stellate neurons. When the numbers of branches at each order from the apical dendrite and their lengths were analyzed, the differences in each measure for the most part fell short of significance (across the entire apical dendrite). However, a concentric-ring analysis of the apical dendrites only indicated that differences consistently occurred in the outer regions—beyond 200 microns from the cell body.

For these outer apical regions, the trained-handled difference was 46 percent for layer-4 pyramidal neurons (p < 0.001) and 15 percent for layer-5 pyramidal neurons (p < 0.005). A small, possibly "compensatory," 5 percent difference in the reverse direction appeared in the inner portion of layer-5 apicals (p < 0.01; we have not seen this effect in further work). The inner region of layer-4 apical dendrites, on the other hand, slightly favored the trained animals (3 percent; p < 0.10).

A problem with these data involves the way in which neurons are selected for drawing. Generally, we have attempted to pick out neurons with both apical and basal portions fairly well contained in the section. Hence some sacrifices must be made in both regions. Since the apical dendrite extends through a greater distance, the probability is greater that significant portions of its branches will travel off the section. If one uses oblique sectioning angles such that the entire apical dendrite runs off section, it can sometimes be drawn from an adjacent section. However, this is a laborious procedure, and we do not use it routinely. (There is still some loss of branches.)

An alternative is to select neurons on the basis of the completeness of the apical dendrite, regardless of losses in the basal area. In a replication on these same animals, we selected approximately 20 apical dendrites of layer-4 and layer-5 pyramidal neurons from each of the 14 animals in the study and analyzed them in the usual ways, except that the inner vs. outer cutoff point was 250 microns. (The second set of neurons was drawn and scored by experimenters who had not been involved with the initial sample. No attempt was made to exclude neurons from the first sample, except that the selection criteria probably reduced the overlap considerably.) The results for this sample, presented in Table 16.2, are even more clear-cut. Layer-5 pyramidal neurons, in the outer apical region, have more dendritic branching whether measured by the concentric-ring analysis or in terms of total dendritic length. The increase appears to occur at branch orders beyond the first branch from the apical shaft. In layer-4 pyramidal neurons the effects are somewhat less pronounced and seem to occur at less extreme

TABLE 16.2

Dendritic-branch measures in a replication study of pyramidal neurons in trained vs. handled rats

	Layer 4			Layer 5		
	Trained	Handled	p	Trained	Handled	p
Apical branches						
Total dendritic length	574.6	515.4	0.03	627.6	608.8	ns
First- and second-order obliques near the cell body	357.6	323.2	ns	430.6	433.4	ns
First- and second-order obliques distant from the cell body	176.6	162.4	ns	188.2	163.0	0.05
Higher-order obliques near the cell body	32.4	27.8	ns	8.0	6.8	ns
Higher-order obliques distant from the cell body	8.0	2.0	0.03	0.56	5.8	0.04
Concentric-ring analysis						
Intersections < 250 μ from the cell body	28.2	26.5	0.05	27.5	27.4	ns
Intersections > 250 μ from the cell body	15.0	13.7	ns	16.1	12.5	0.0001

distances from the cell body. Figure 16.3 shows the ring-by-ring analysis of apical dendrites in the two cell populations. The curves are arranged in terms of the relative average depth of their cell bodies in the cortex, measured from the pial surface. The points at which the curves for the trained and handled animals diverge are roughly comparable for the two populations in terms of cortical depth, suggesting that the training-correlated changes tend to occur in the same cortical layer or layers. Rough calculations (exact determination of layer boundaries is not possible in rapid-Golgi-stained material) suggest that the effects occur in layers 3 and 4.

These data have been corroborated in part by a study in which Timothy DeVoogd, Dorothy Flood, Fred Volkmar, Judy O'Brien, and I examined layer-4 and layer-5 pyramidal neurons of 40-day-old hooded rats trained on a series of visual-discrimination tasks. Again, water reward was used, and deprived handled littermates served as controls. In this experiment, however, the trained and control animals lived in a larger sawdust-floored cage with a third animal. Training consisted of 20 daily trials on a series of paired visual cues in an apparatus similar to that described by Grice (1948). Rats solved from 8 to 11 consecutive problems such as black vs. white, horizontal vs. vertical stripes, triangle vs. circle, etc., to a criterion of 18 out of 20 correct daily choices over a 35-day training period.

In this experiment, in which whole neurons were drawn, a 15 percent trained-untrained difference (p < 0.01) occurred in the outer half of the concentric-ring analysis of layer-5 pyramidal neurons. There were no consistent effects in basilar dendritic branching in layer-4 or layer-5 pyramidal neurons, and only sporadic significant effects appeared in layer-4 apical dendrites. We are currently investigating apical dendrites independently.

While these effects seem comparatively large in the context of the outer region of the apical dendrite, they are quite small when compared with the dendritic mass of the entire neuron, representing 1 or 2 percent of total dendritic length at best. Moreover, the findings are preliminary, and the reliability must be assessed through replication, which we are beginning. The results tentatively suggest that new synaptic connections may form during long-term training experiences. The effects were very much smaller than those observed after similar periods of postweaning environmental complexity, and they were not apparent in the basal dendritic region, which seemed to be most affected in the complexity studies. It could be argued that effects of this magnitude would be less easily detected in the more complex and extensive basilar portion of the pyramidal-cell dendritic tree. However, an alternative possibility is suggested by the occasional small differences seen in less carefully an-

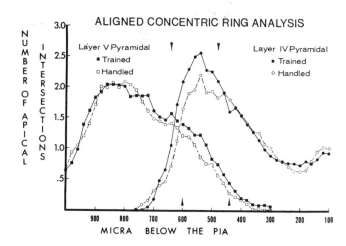

FIGURE 16.3 Ring intersections with apical dendrites of layer-4 and layer-5 pyramidal neurons in 7 littermate pairs of maze-trained and handled rats. Significant differences between groups tend to occur at about the same depth in the cortex in both types of neurons. Arrows indicate the range in which significant differences occurred between the groups.

alyzed apical dendrites in the complexity study (Greenough and Volkmar, 1973). It is possible that growth in the apical region corresponds to a component of the complex environmental experience that is similar to the training experience, while changes in basal dendrites correspond to other effects of environmental complexity on brain development. We are currently evaluating the apical dendritic effects of rearing complexity with more precision than in our earlier studies.

Of course, as noted above, any change in the brain that occurs after a training procedure need not be (and, judging from collective experience in this area, probably is not) related to the memory for the training. Miminal steps were taken to equate nonmemorial aspects of the experience for the groups compared. Thus, while we may be able to add long-term formal training to the growing list of experiences that can affect brain anatomy, we remain uncertain as to the functional role of these anatomical effects. It is hard to imagine that such alterations play no role in the functioning of the brain. Assessment of the role(s) will almost certainly require a more detailed knowledge of the circumstances under which such effects do and do not occur.

16.6 SUMMARY AND CONCLUSIONS

Several types of enduring biological correlates of differential and training experiences have been reported over the past decade and a half. A number of these correlates support—or are compatible with—the notion that such experiences produce changes in the number of synaptic connections in various brain regions. Anatomical data indicating new synaptic formation have been reported following stimulation in infancy, exposure of the visual system to environmental light, exposure to complex environments, "model" training procedures, and formal training. The consistency of this finding across several types of experience suggests that the formation of new synapses may indeed be involved in the mediation of the effects of behavioral experience upon later behavior in development and adulthood.

The bulk of other enduring changes that have been reported are consonant with the formation of new synapses. RNA and protein increases, as well as the increased numbers of glial cells, might provide metabolic support for the increased amount of neuropil. Enzymatic changes related to synaptic transmission might be expected with increased synaptic formation. Changes in various specific protein groups could play metabolic or structural roles. Short-term changes could reflect the metabolic aspects of the establishment of new connectivity which are not required in its maintenance.

On the other hand, we should keep in mind that memory for a single event, even in adults of a species, need not be a unitary process. Different cells could conceivably use different mechanisms to carry out their various roles in the formation of a memory. Certainly, if altered connectivity were a part of a cell's role in a memory process, a sequence of changes leading to the ultimate growth would be expected.

A question of some interest is whether environmentally stimulated alterations in connectivity occur on a time scale comparable to that indicated in studies of the consolidation of long-term memory. While estimates of memory formation time have varied with the technique used to examine it (see McGaugh and Gold, Flood and Jarvik, and Chorover, this volume), at least some synaptic alterations have been reported to occur within the longer temporal estimates. Valverde (1971) and Cragg (1967) have reported alterations in synapses within two days after initial exposure to light in rodents.

If we accept that the study of enduring changes—and particularly changes in synaptic connectivity—are memory-substrate candidates worthy of further pursuit, then I would suggest that the pursuit involve as wide a range of experimental paradigms as possible. Much of the research reviewed in this and other papers in this volume involves a single behavioral paradigm in which memory differences may or may not be a major component. The alternative course, to search for processes common to a variety of forms of differential experience, ranging from the earliest of hormonal and sensory experiences to the widest reasonable variety of formal training tasks, will certainly require more effort. But a search for the common consequences of experience seems a potentially fruitful approach to the understanding of its storage in the nervous system.

ACKNOWLEDGMENTS

Preparation of this chapter and the research contained in it that has not previously been reported has been supported by Grant HD 06862 from the National Institute of Child Health and Human Development. The assistance of John Conlee, James Crandall, and Terry Linden, in addition to those mentioned in the text, is gratefully acknowledged.

REFERENCES

ADAMS, J. A. 1968. Response feedback and learning. *Psychological Bulletin* 70: 486–504.

ADER, R. 1965. Effects of early experience and differential housing on behavior and susceptibility to gastric erosions in the rat. *Journal of Comparative and Physiological Psychology* 60: 233–238.

ADER, R., and FRIEDMAN, S. B. 1964. Social factors affecting emotionality and resistance to disease in animals. IV. Differential housing, emotionality, and Walker 256 carcinosarcoma in the rat. *Psychological Reports* 15: 535–541.

ALTMAN, J., BRUNNER, R. L., and BAYER, S. A. 1973. The hippocampus and behavioral maturation. *Behavioral Biology* 8: 557–596.

ALTMAN, J., and DAS, G. D. 1964. Audioradiographic examination of the effects of enriched environment on the rate of glial multiplication in the adult brain. *Nature* 204: 1161–1163.

ALTMAN, J., WALLACE, R. B., ANDERSON, W. J., and DAS, G. D. 1968. Behaviorally induced changes in length of cerebrum in rats. *Developmental Psychobiology* 1: 112–117.

ANDERSON, A., WERBOFF, J., and LES, E. P. 1968. Effects of environmental temperature, humidity, and cage density on body weight and behavior in mice. *Experientia* 24: 1022–1023.

ANDERSON, K. V., and O'STEEN, W. K. 1972. Black-white and pattern discrimination in rats without photoreceptors. *Experimental Neurology* 34: 446–454.

BAER, H. 1971. Long-term isolation stress and its effects on drug response in rodents. *Laboratory Animal Science* 21: 341–349.

BALÁZS, R., KOVÁCS, S., TEICHGRÄBER, P., COCKS, W. A., and EAYRS, J. T. 1968. Biochemical effects of thyroid deficiency on the developing brain. *Journal of Neurochemistry* 15: 1335–1349.

BAXTER, B. L. 1966. Effects of visual deprivation during postnatal maturation on the electroencephalogram of the cat. *Experimental Neurology* 14: 224–237.

BELL, R. W., MILLER, C. E., ORDY, J. M., and ROLSTEN, C. 1971. Effects of population density and living space upon neuroanatomy, neurochemistry, and behavior in the C57B1/10 mouse. *Journal of Comparative and Physiological Psychology* 75: 258–263.

BENNETT, E. L., DIAMOND, M. C., KRECH, D., and ROSENZWEIG, M. R. 1964. Chemical and anatomical plasticity of brain. *Science* 146: 610–619.

BENNETT, E. L., ROSENZWEIG, M. R., and DIAMOND, M. C. 1970. Time courses of effects of differential experience on brain measures and behavior of rats. In W. L. Byrne, ed., *Molecular Approaches to Learning and Memory.* New York: Academic Press, pp. 58–89.

BENNETT, E. L., ROSENZWEIG, M. R., DIAMOND, M. C., MORIMOTO, H., and HEBERT, M. 1974. Effects of successive environments on brain measures. *Physiology and Behavior* 12: 621–631.

BENNETT, E. L., ROSENZWEIG, M. R., and WU, S.-Y. C. 1973. Excitant and depressant drugs modulate effects of environment on brain weight and cholinesterases. *Psychopharmacologia (Berlin)* 33: 309–328.

BERNSTEIN, L. 1973. A study of some enriching variables in a free-environment for rats. *Journal of Psychosomatic Research* 17: 85–88.

BINGHAM, W. E., and GRIFFITHS, JR., W. J. 1952. The effect of different environments during infancy on adult behavior in the rat. *Journal of Comparative and Physiological Psychology* 45: 307–312.

BLOCK, J. B., and ESSMAN, W. B. 1965. Growth hormone administration during pregnancy: A behavioral difference in offspring rats. *Nature* 205: 1136–1137.

BOGOCH, S. 1968. *The Biochemistry of Memory.* London: Oxford University Press.

BOGOCH, S. 1973. Brain glycoproteins and learning. New studies supporting the "sign-post" theory. In W. B. Essman and S. Nakajima, eds., *Current Biochemical Approaches to Learning and Memory.* Flushing, N. Y.: Spectrum-Halstead, pp. 147–159.

BOOTH, D. A. 1973. Protein synthesis and memory. In J. A. Deutsch, ed., *The Physiological Basis of Memory.* New York: Academic Press, pp. 27–58.

BRAIN, P. F. and NOWELL, N. W. 1970. The effects of differential grouping on endocrine function of mature male albino mice. *Physiology and Behavior* 5: 907–910.

BRONSON, F. H., and CHAPMAN, V. M. 1968. Adrenal-oestrous relationships in grouped or isolated female mice. *Nature* 218: 483–484.

BROWN, C. P. 1971. Cholinergic activity in rats following enriched stimulation and training. Direction and duration of effects. *Journal of Comparative and Physiological Psychology* 75: 408–416.

BROWN, R. T. 1968. Early experience and problem-solving ability. *Journal of Comparative and Physiological Psychology* 65: 433–440.

BUBENIK, G. A., and BROWN, G. M. 1973. Morphologic sex differences in primate brain areas involved in regulation of reproductive activity. *Experientia* 29: 619–621.

CALHOUN, J. B. 1962. Population density and social pathology. *Scientific American* 206 (2): 139–148.

CHARPENTIER, J. 1969. Analysis and measurement of aggressive behaviour in mice. In S. Garattini and E. B. Sigg, eds., *Aggressive Behaviour.* Amsterdam: Excerpta Medica, pp. 86–100.

CHRISTIAN, J. J. 1955. Effects of population size on the adrenal glands and reproductive organs of male mice in populations of fixed size. *American Journal of Physiology* 182: 292–300.

CHRISTIAN, J. J. and LeMUNYAN, C. D. 1958. Adverse effects of crowding on lactation and reproduction of mice and two generations of their progeny. *Endocrinology* 63: 517–529.

CHRISTIAN, J. J. LLOYD, J. A., and DAVIS, D. E. 1965. The role of endocrines in the self-regulation of mammalian populations. *Recent Progress in Hormone Research* 21: 501–578.

CLARKE, R. S., HERON, W., FETHERSTONHAUGH, M. L., FOR

GAYS, D. G., and HEBB, D. O. 1951. Individual differences in dogs: Preliminary report on the effects of early experience. *Canadian Journal of Psychology* 5: 150–156.

CLENDINNEN, B. G., and EAYRS, J. T. 1961. The anatomical and physiological effects of prenatally administered somatotrophin on cerebral development in rats. *Journal of Endocrinology* 22: 183–193.

COLEMAN, P. D., and RIESEN, A. H. 1968. Environmental effects on cortical dendritic fields. I. Rearing in the dark. *Journal of Anatomy* 102: 363–374.

CONNOR, H. S., and GREGOR, G. L. 1973. Crowding and isolation: Determinants of agonistic and food seeking behavior in Norway rats. *Journal of Comparative and Physiological Psychology* 84: 593–597.

CRAGG, B. G. 1967. Changes in visual cortex on first exposure of rats to light. *Nature* 215: 251–253.

CUMMINS, R. A., WALSH, R. N., BUDTZ-OLSEN, O. E., KONSTANTINOS, T., and HORSFALL, C. R. 1973. Environmentally-induced changes in the brains of elderly rats. *Nature* 243: 516–518.

DAVENPORT, J. W., and DORCEY, T. P. 1972. Hypothyroidism: Learning deficit induced in rats by early exposure to thiouracil. *Hormones and Behavior* 3: 97–112.

DENENBERG, V. H. 1967. Stimulation in infancy, emotional reactivity, and exploratory behavior. In D. C. Glass, ed., *Neurophysiology and Emotion.* New York: Rockefeller University Press, pp. 161–190.

DIAMOND, M. C. 1967. Extensive cortical depth measurements and neuron size increases in the cortex of environmentally enriched rats. *Journal of Comparative Neurology* 131: 357–364.

DIAMOND, M. C., JOHNSON, R. E., and INGHAM, C. 1971. Brain plasticity induced by environment and pregnancy. *International Journal of Neuroscience* 2: 171–178.

DIAMOND, M. C., LAW, F., RHODES, H., LINDNER, B., ROSENZWEIG, M. R., KRECH, D., and BENNETT, E. L. 1966. Increases in cortical depth and glia numbers in rats subjected to enriched environment. *Journal of Comparative Neurology* 128: 117–125.

DIAMOND, M. C., ROSENZWEIG, M. R., BENNETT, E. L., LINDNER, B., and LYON, L. 1972. Effects of environmental enrichment and impoverishment on rat cerebral cortex. *Journal of Neurobiology* 3: 47–64.

DONOVICK, P. J., BURRIGHT, R. G., and SWIDLER, M. A. 1973. Presurgical rearing environment alters exploration, fluid consumption, and learning of septal lesioned and control rats. *Physiology and Behavior* 11: 543–553.

EAYRS, J. T. 1961. Age as a factor in determining the severity and reversibility of the effects of thyroid deficiency in the rat. *Journal of Endocrinology* 22: 409–419.

EAYRS, J. T. 1964a. Endocrine influence on cerebral development. *Archives of Biology* 75: 529–565.

EAYRS, J. T. 1964b. Effect of neonatal hyperthyroidism on maturation and learning in the rat. *Animal Behaviour* 12: 195–199.

EDWARDS, H. P., BARRY, W. F., and WYSPIANSKI, J. O. 1969. Effect of differential rearing on photic evoked potentials and brightness discrimination in the albino rat. *Developmental Psychobiology* 2: 133–138.

ESSMAN, W. B. 1966. The development of activity differences in isolated and aggregated mice. *Animal Behaviour* 14: 406–409.

ESSMAN, W. B. 1971a. Changes in cholinergic activity and avoidance behavior by nicotine in differentially housed mice. *International Journal of Neuroscience* 2: 199–206.

ESSMAN, W. B. 1971b. Isolation-induced behavioral modification: Some neurochemical correlates. In M. B. Sterman, D. J. McGinty, and A. M. Adinolfi, eds., *Brain Development Behavior*. New York: Academic Press, pp. 203–227.

ESSMAN, W. B. 1972. Contributions of differential housing to brain development: Some implications for sleep behavior. In C. D. Clemente, D. P. Purpura, and F. E. Mayer, eds., *Sleep and the Maturing Nervous System*. New York: Academic Press, pp. 99–107.

FERCHMIN, P. A., ETEROVIĆ, V. A., and CAPUTTO, R. 1970. Studies of brain weight and RNA content after short periods of exposure to environmental complexity. *Brain Research* 20: 49–57.

FIFKOVÁ, E. 1970. Changes of axosomatic synapses in the visual cortex of monocularly deprived rats. *Journal of Neurobiology* 2: 61–71.

FLEISCHMANN, T. B. 1972. Effects of differential rearing complexity on synapses of the rat hippocampus (Regio superior—CA-1). Unpublished M. A. thesis, University of Illinois, Champaign.

FORGAYS, D. G., and FORGAYS, J. W. 1952. The nature of the effect of free-environmental experience in the rat. *Journal of Comparative and Physiological Psychology* 45: 322–328.

FORGAYS, D. G., and READ, J. M. 1962. Crucial periods for free-environmental experience in the rat. *Journal of Comparative and Physiological Psychology* 55: 816–818.

FORGUS, R. H. 1954. The effect of early perceptual learning on the behavioral organization of adult rats. *Journal of Comparative and Physiological Psychology* 47: 331–336.

FREEMAN, B. J., and RAY, O. S. 1972. Strain, sex, and environment effects on appetitively and aversively motivated learning tasks. *Developmental Psychobiology* 5: 101–109.

FULLER, J. L. 1966. Transitory effects of experiential deprivation upon reversal learning in dogs. *Psychonomic Science* 4: 273–274.

FULLER, J. L. 1967. Experiential deprivation and later behavior. *Science* 158: 1645–1652.

GARATTINI, S., Giacalone, F., and VALZELLI, L. 1969. Biochemical changes during isolation-induced aggressiveness in mice. In S. Garattini and E. B. Sigg, eds., *Aggressive Behaviour*. Amsterdam: Excerpta Medica, pp. 179–187.

GELLER, E. 1971. Some observations on the effects of environmental complexity and isolation on biochemical ontogeny. In M. B. Sterman, D. J. McGinty, and A. M. Adinolfi, eds., *Brain Development and Behavior*. New York: Academic Press, pp. 277–296.

GELLER, E., and YUWILER, A. 1968. Environmental effects on the biochemistry of developing rat brain. In L. Jílek and S. Trojan, eds., *Ontogenesis of the Brain*. Prague: Charles University Press, pp. 277–284.

GELLER, E., YUWILER, A., and ZOLMAN, J. F. 1965. Effects of environmental complexity on constituents of brain and liver. *Journal of Neurochemistry* 12: 949–955.

GIBSON, E. J. 1969. *Principles of Perceptual Learning and Development*. New York: Appleton-Century-Crofts.

GLASSMAN, E. 1969. The biochemistry of learning: An evaluation of the role of RNA and protein. *Annual Review of Biochemistry* 38: 605–646.

GLOBUS, A., ROSENZWEIG, M. R., BENNETT, E. L., and DIAMOND, M. C. 1973. Effects of differential experience on dendritic spine counts in rat cerebral cortex. *Journal of Comparative and Physiological Psychology* 82: 175–181.

GLUCK, J. P., HARLOW, H. F., and SCHILTZ, K. A. 1973. Differential effect of early enrichment and deprivation on learning in the rhesus monkey (*Macaca mulatta*). *Journal of Comparative and Physiological Psychology* 84: 598–604.

GOECKNER, D. J., GREENOUGH, W. T., and MAIER, S. F. 1974. Escape learning deficit after overcrowded rearing in rats: Test of a helplessness hypothesis. *Bulletin of the Psychonomic Society* 3: 54–56.

GOECKNER, D. J., GREENOUGH, W. T., and MEAD, W. R. 1973. Deficits in learning tasks following chronic overcrowding in rats. *Journal of Personality and Social Psychology* 28: 256–261.

GREENOUGH, W. T., FULCHER, J. K., YUWILER, A., and GELLER, E. 1970. Enriched rearing and chronic electroshock: Effects on brain and behavior in mice. *Physiology and Behavior* 5: 371–373.

GREENOUGH, W. T., MADDEN, T. C., and FLEISCHMANN, T. B. 1972. Effects of isolation, daily handling, and enriched rearing on maze learning. *Psychonomic Science* 27: 279–280.

GREENOUGH, W. T., and MAIER, S. F. 1972. Molecular changes during learning: Behavioral strategy—a comment on Gaito and Bonnet. *Psychological Bulletin* 78: 480–482.

GREENOUGH, W. T., and VOLKMAR, F. R. 1973. Pattern of dendritic branching in occipital cortex of rats reared in complex environments. *Experimental Neurology* 40: 491–504.

GREENOUGH, W. T., VOLKMAR, F. R., and JURASKA, J. M. 1973. Effects of rearing complexity on dendritic branching in frontolateral and temporal cortex of the rat. *Experimental Neurology* 41: 371–378.

GREENOUGH, W. T., WOOD, W. E., and MADDEN, T. C. 1972. Possible memory storage differences among mice reared in environments varying in complexity. *Behavioral Biology* 7: 717–722.

GREENOUGH, W. T., YUWILER, A., and DOLLINGER, M. 1973. Effects of posttrial eserine administration on learning in "enriched"- and "impoverished"-reared rats. *Behavioral Biology* 8: 261–272.

GREGORY, K. M., and DIAMOND, M. C. 1968. The effects of early hypophysectomy on brain morphogenesis in the rat. *Experimental Neurology* 20: 394–414.

GRICE, G. R. 1948. The relation of secondary reinforcement to delayed reward in visual discrimination learning. *Journal of Experimental Psychology* 38: 1–16.

GRIFFIN, G. A., and HARLOW, H. F. 1966. Effects of three months of total social deprivation on social adjustment and learning in the Rhesus monkey. *Child Development* 37: 533–548.

HALTMEYER, G. C., DENENBERG, V., THATCHER, J., and ZARROW, M. X. 1966. Response of the adrenal cortex of the neonatal rat after subjection to stress. *Nature* 212: 1371–1373.

HARLOW, H. F. 1962. The heterosexual affectional system in monkeys. *American Psychologist* 17: 1–9.

HATCH, A. M., BALÁZS, T., WIBERG, T. S., and GRICE, H. C. 1963. Long-term isolation stress in rats. *Science* 142: 507.

HATCH, A. M., WIBERG, G. S., ZAWDIZKA, Z., CANN, M., AIRTH, J. M., and GRICE, H. C. 1965. Isolation syndrome in the rat. *Toxicology and Applied Pharmacology* 7: 737–745.

HEBB, D. O. 1947. The effects of early experience on problem-solving at maturity. *American Psychologist* 2: 306–307.

HEBB, D. O. 1949. *The Organization of Behavior*. New York: John Wiley & Sons.

HEIN, A. 1972. Acquiring components of visually guided behavior. In A. D. Pick, ed., *Minnesota Symposia on Child Psychology*, Vol. 6. Minneapolis: University of Minnesota Press, pp. 53–68.

HEIN, A., HELD, R., and GOWER, E. C. 1970. Development and segmentation of visually controlled movement by selective exposure during rearing. *Journal of Comparative and Physiological Psychology* 73: 181–187.

HELD, R. and HEIN, A. 1963. Movement-produced stimulation in the development of visually-guided behavior. *Journal of Comparative and Physiological Psychology* 56: 872–876.

HENDERSON, N. D. 1970. Brain weight increases resulting from environmental enrichment: A directional dominance in mice. *Science* 169: 776–778.

HOLLOWAY, R. L. 1966. Dendritic branching: Some preliminary results of training and complexity in rat visual cortex. *Brain Research* 2: 393–396.

HUNT, J. M. 1961. *Intelligence and Experience.* New York: Ronald Press.

HYDÉN, H., and EGYHÁZI, E. 1962. Nuclear RNA changes of nerve cells during a learning experiment with rats. *Proceedings of the National Academy of Sciences (USA)* 48: 1366–1373.

HYDÉN, H., and EGYHÁZI. E. 1964. Changes in RNA and base composition in cortical neurons of rats in a learning experiment involving transfer of handedness. *Proceedings of the National Academy of Sciences (USA)* 52: 1030–1035.

HYDÉN, H., and LANGE, P. W. 1970a. Correlation of the S100 brain protein with behavior. In R. E. Bowman and S. P. Datta, eds., *Biochemistry of Brain and Behavior.* New York: Plenum, pp. 327–345.

HYDÉN, H., and LANGE, P. W. 1970b. S100 brain protein. Correlation with behavior. *Proceedings of the National Academy of Sciences (USA)* 67: 1959–1966.

HYDÉN, H., and LANGE, P. W. 1972. Protein changes in different brain areas as a function of intermittent training. *Proceedings of the National Academy of Sciences (USA)* 69: 1980–1984.

HYMOVITCH, B. 1952. The effects of experimental variations on problem solving in the rat. *Journal of Comparative and Physiological Psychology* 45: 313–321.

ISAACSON, R. L., and KIMBLE, D. P. 1972. Lesions of the limbic system: Their effects upon hypotheses and frustration. *Behavioral Biology* 7: 767–793.

IZQUIERDO, J. A., BARATTI, C. M., TORRELIO, M., ARÉVALO, L., and McGAUGH, J. L. 1973. Effects of food deprivation, discrimination experience, and physostigmine on choline acetylase and acetylcholinesterase in the dorsal hippocampus and frontal cortex of rats. *Psychopharmacologia (Berlin)* 33: 103–110.

KIMBLE, D. P. 1968. Hippocampus and internal inhibition. *Psychological Bulletin* 70: 285–295.

KRECH, D., ROSENZWEIG, M., and BENNETT, E. L. 1960. Effects of environmental complexity and training on brain chemistry. *Journal of Comparative and Physiological Psychology* 53:509–519.

KRECH, D., ROSENZWEIG, M. R., and BENNETT, E. L. 1962. Relations between brain chemistry and problem-solving among rats raised in enriched and impoverished environments. *Journal of Comparative and Physiological Psychology* 55: 801–807.

LAGERSPETZ, K. M. J. 1969. Aggression and aggressiveness in laboratory mice. In S. Garattini and E. B. Sigg, eds., *Aggressive Behaviour.* Amsterdam: Excerpta Medica, pp. 77–85.

LARRAMENDI, L. M. H. 1969. Analysis of synaptogenesis in the cerebellum of the mouse. In R. Llinas, ed., *Neurobiology of Cerebellar Evolution and Development.* Chicago: American Medical Association Education and Research Foundation, pp. 803–843.

LATORRE, J. C. 1968. Effect of differential environmental enrichment on brain weight and on acetylcholinesterase and cholinesterase activities in mice. *Experimental Neurology* 22: 493–503.

LEBOEUF, B. J., and PEEKE, H. V. S. 1969. The effect of strychnine administration during development on adult maze learning in the rat. *Psychopharmacologia (Berlin)* 16: 49–53.

LEVINE, S, 1956. A further study of infantile handling and adult avoidance conditioning. *Journal of Personality* 25: 70–80.

LEVINE, S. 1962. The psychophysiological effects of infantile stimulation. In E. Bliss, ed., *Roots of Behavior.* New York: Harper & Row, pp. 246–253.

LEVINE, S., and ALPERT, M. 1959. Differential maturation of the central nervous system as a function of early experience. *Archives of General Psychiatry* 1: 403–405.

LEVINE, S., and MULLINS, JR., R. F. 1966. Hormonal influences on brain organization in infant rats. *Science* 152: 1585–1592.

LEVINE, S., and MULLINS, JR., R. F. 1968. Hormones in infancy. In G. Newton and S. Levine, eds., *Early Experience and Behavior.* Springfield, Ill.: Charles C Thomas, pp. 168–197.

LEVITAN, I. B., MUSHYNSKI, W. E., and RAMIREZ, G. 1972. Effects of an enriched environment on amino acid incorporation into rat brain subcellular fractions *in vivo. Brain Research* 41: 498–502.

LOVELY, R. H., PAGANO, R. R., and PAOLINO, R. M. 1972. Shuttle-box avoidance performance and basal corticosterone levels as a function of duration of individual housing in rats. *Journal of Comparative and Physiological Psychology* 81: 331–335.

MACHLUS, B., and GAITO, J. 1969. Successive competition hybridization to detect RNA species in a shock avoidance task. *Nature* 222: 573–574.

MALKASIAN, D. R., and DIAMOND, M. C. 1971. The effects of environmental manipulation on the morphology of the neonate rat brain. *International Journal of Neuroscience* 2: 161–170.

MASON, W. A. 1968. Early social deprivation in the nonhuman primates: Implications for human behavior. In D. C. Glass, ed., *Environmental Influences.* New York: Rockefeller University Press, pp. 70–101.

McCALL, R. B., LESTER, M. L., and DOLAN, C. G. 1969. Differential rearing and the exploration of stimuli in the open field. *Developmental Psychology* 1: 750–762.

McGINTY, D. J. 1971. Encephalization and the neural control of sleep. In M. B. Sterman, D. J. McGinty, and A. M. Adinolfi, eds., *Brain Development and Behavior.* New York: Academic Press, pp. 335–357.

MELZACK, R. 1959. The role of early experience in emotional arousal. *Annals of the New York Academy of Sciences* 159: 721–730.

MELZACK, R. 1962. Effects of early perceptual restriction on simple visual discrimination. *Science* 137: 978–979.

MELZACK, R., and BURNS, S. K. 1965. Neurophysiological effects of early sensory restriction. *Experimental Neurology* 13: 163–175.

MEYER, J. S., and BOWMAN, R. E. 1972. Rearing experience, stress, and adrenocorticosteroids in the rhesus monkey. *Physiology and Behavior* 8: 339–343.

MØLLGAARD, K., DIAMOND, M. C., BENNETT, E. L., ROSENZWEIG, M. R., and LINDNER, B. 1971. Qualitative synaptic changes with differential experience in rat brain. *International Journal of Neuroscience* 2:113–128.

MOORE, K. E. 1968. Studies with chronically isolated rats: Tissue levels and urinary excretion of catecholamines and plasma levels of corticosterone. *Canadian Journal of Physiology and Pharmacology* 46: 553–558.

MORGAN, M. J. 1973. Effects of post-weaning environment on learning in the rat. *Animal Behaviour* 21: 429–442.

MOWRER, O. H. 1960. *Learning Theory and the Symbolic Processes.* New York: John Wiley & Sons.

MUSHYNSKI, W. E., LEVITAN, I. B., and RAMIREZ, G. 1973. Competition hybridization studies on brain ribonucleic acid from rats reared in enriched and deprived environments. *Journal of Neurochemistry* 20: 309–317.

MYERS, R. D., and FOX, J. 1963. Differences in maze performance of group vs. isolation reared rats. *Psychological Reports* 12: 199–202.

NICHOLSON, J. L., and ALTMAN, J. 1972. Synaptogenesis in the rat cerebellum: Effects of early hypo- and hyperthyroidism. *Science* 176: 530–532.

NOELL, W. K., and ALBRECHT, R. 1971. Irreversible effects of visible light on the retina: Role of vitamin A. *Science* 172: 76–79.

NYMAN, A. J. 1967. Problem solving in rats as a function of experience at different ages. *Journal of Genetic Psychology* 110: 31–39.

PARASKEVOPOULOS, J., and HUNT, J. McV. 1971. Object construction and imitation under different conditions of rearing. *Journal of Genetic Psychology* 119: 301–321.

PEEKE, H. V. S., LeBOEUF, B. J., and HERZ, M. J. 1971. The effect of strychnine administration during development on adult maze learning in the rat. II. Drug administration from day 51 to 70. *Psychopharmacologia (Berlin)* 19: 262–265.

PELTON, E. W., and BASS, N. H. 1973. Adverse effects of excess thyroid hormone on the maturation of rat cerebrum. *Archives of Neurology* 29: 145–150.

PFAFF, D. W. 1966. Morphological changes in the brains of adult male rats after neonatal castration. *Journal of Endocrinology* 36: 415–416.

PLAUT, S. M., and GROTA, L. J. 1971. Effects of differential housing on adrenocortical reactivity. *Neuroendocrinology* 7: 348–360.

PRESCOTT, J. W. 1971. Early somatosensory deprivation as an ontogenetic process in the abnormal development of the brain and behavior. In E. Goldsmith and J. Morr-Jankowski, eds., *Medical Primatology, 1970.* Basel: S. Karger AG, pp. 356–375.

RAISMAN, G. 1969. Neuronal plasticity in the septal nuclei of the adult rat. *Brain Research* 14: 25–48.

RAISMAN, G. W., and FIELD, P. M. 1971. Sexual dimorphism in the preoptic area of the rat. *Science* 173: 731–733.

RAISMAN, G., and FIELD, P. M. 1973. Sexual dimorphism in the neuropil of the preoptic area of the rat and its dependence on neonatal androgen. *Brain Research* 54: 1–29.

RAKIC, P. 1973. Kinetics of proliferation and latency between final cell division and onset of differentiation of cerebellar stellate and basket neurons. *Journal of Comparative Neurology* 147: 523–546.

RIEGE, W. H. 1971. Environmental influences on brain and behavior of year-old rats. *Developmental Psychobiology* 4: 151–167.

RIEGE, W. H., and MORIMOTO, H. 1970. Effects of chronic stress and differential environments upon brain weights and biogenic amine levels in rats. *Journal of Comparative and Physiological Psychology* 71: 396–404.

RIESEN, A. H. 1966. Sensory deprivation. In E. Stellar and J. M. Sprague, eds., *Progress in Physiological Psychology*, Vol. 1. New York: Academic Press, pp. 117–147.

ROSENZWEIG, M. R. 1971. Effects of environment on development of brain and of behavior. In E. Tobach, L. R. Aronson, and E. Shaw, eds., *The Biopsychology of Development.* New York: Academic Press, pp. 303–342.

ROSENZWEIG, M. R., and BENNETT, E. L. 1972. Cerebral changes in rats exposed individually to an enriched environment. *Journal of Comparative and Physiological Psychology* 80: 304–313.

ROSENZWEIG, M. R., BENNETT, E. L., and DIAMOND, M. C. 1972a. Chemical and anatomical plasticity of brain: Replications and extensions. In J. Gaito, ed., *Macromolecules and Behavior*, 2nd ed. New York: Appleton-Century-Crofts, pp. 205–277.

ROSENZWEIG, M. R., BENNETT, E. L., and DIAMOND, M. C. 1972b. Brain changes in response to experience. *Scientific American* 226(2): 22–29.

ROSENZWEIG, M. R., BENNETT, E. L., and DIAMOND, M. C. 1972c. Cerebral effects of differential experience in hypophysectomized rats. *Journal of Comparative and Physiological Psychology* 79: 56–66.

ROSENZWEIG, M. R., BENNETT, E. L. DIAMOND, M. C., WU, S.-Y., SLAGLE, R. W., and SAFFRAN, E. 1969. Influences of environmental complexity and visual stimulation on development of occipital cortex in rat. *Brain Research* 14: 427–445.

ROSENZWEIG, M., KRECH, D., BENNETT, E. L., and DIAMOND, M. 1962. Effects of environmental complexity and training on brain chemistry and anatomy: A replication and extension. *Journal of Comparative and Physiological Psychology* 55: 429–437.

ROSENZWEIG, M. R., LOVE, W., and BENNETT, E. L. 1968. Effects of a few hours a day of enriched experience on brain chemistry and brain weights. *Physiology and Behavior* 3: 819–825.

ROSS, S., GINSBURG, B. E., and DENENBERG, V. H. 1957. The use of the split-litter technique in psychological research. *Psychological Bulletin* 54: 145–151.

SACKLER, A. M., and WELTMAN, A. S. 1967. Effects of isolation stress on peripheral leukocytes of female albino mice. *Nature* 214: 1142–1143.

SASSENRATH, E. N. 1970. Increased adrenal responsiveness related to social stress in rhesus monkeys. *Hormones and Behavior* 1: 283–298.

SCHAPIRO, S. 1968. Some physiological, biochemical, and behavioral consequences of neonatal hormone administration: Cortisol and thyroxine. *General and Comparative Endocrinology* 10: 214–228.

SCHAPIRO, S. 1971. Hormonal and environmental influences on rat brain development and behavior. In M. B. Sterman, D. J. McGinty, and A. M. Adinolfi, eds., *Brain Development and Behavior.* New York: Academic Press, pp. 307–334.

SCHAPIRO, S., and VUKOVICH, K. R. 1970. Early experience effects upon cortical dendrites: A proposed model for development. *Science* 167: 292–294.

SCOTT, J. P., and FREDERICSON, E. 1951. The causes of fighting behavior in mice and rats. *Physiological Zoology* 24: 273–309.

SHASHOUA, V. E. 1970. RNA metabolism during acquisition of new behavioral patterns. *Proceedings of the National Academy of Sciences (USA)* 65: 160–167.

SHOLL, D. A. 1956. *The Organization of the Cerebral Cortex*. London: Methuen.

SIGG, E. B., DAY, C., and COLOMBO, C. 1966. Endocrine factors in isolation-induced aggressiveness in rodents. *Endocrinology* 78: 679–684.

SMIT, G. J., UYLINGS, H. B. M., and VELDMAAT-WANSINK, L. 1971–1972. The branching pattern in dendrites of cortical neurons. *Acta Morphologica Neerla-Scandinavica* 9: 253–274.

SNYDER, R. L. 1968. Reproduction and population pressures. In E. Stellar and J. M. Sprague, eds., *Progress in Physiological Psychology*, Vol. 2. New York: Academic Press, pp. 119–160.

TAGNEY, J. 1973. Sleep patterns related to rearing rats in enriched and impoverished environments. *Brain Research* 53: 353–361.

TAKAHASHI, K., DAUGHADAY, W. H., and KIPNIS, D. M. 1971. Regulation of immunoreactive growth hormone secretion in male rats. *Endocrinology* 88: 909–917.

TEES, R. C. 1971. Luminance and luminous flux discrimination in rats after early visual deprivation. *Journal of Comparative and Phsyiological Psychology* 74: 292–297.

THOMAS, G. J., HOSTETTER, G., and BARKER, D. J. 1968. Behavioral functions of the limbic system. In E. Stellar and J. M. Sprague, eds., *Progress in Physiological Psychology*, Vol. 2. New York: Academic Press, pp. 229–311.

THOMPSON, R. F., PATTERSON, M. M., and TEYLER, T. J. 1972. The neurophysiology of learning. *Annual Review of Psychology* 23: 73–104.

THOMPSON, W. R., and HERON, W. 1954. The effects of restricting early experience upon the problem-solving capacity of dogs. *Canadian Journal of Psychology* 8: 17–31.

TURNER, C. D., and BAGNARA, J. T. 1971. *General Endocrinology*. Philadelphia: W. B. Saunders.

VALVERDE, F. 1971. Rate and extent of recovery from dark rearing in the visual cortex of the mouse. *Brain Research* 33: 1–11.

VALVERDE, F., and RUIZ-MARCOS, A. 1969. Dendritic spines in the visual cortex of the mouse. Introduction to a mathematical model. *Experimental Brain Research* 8: 269–283.

VALZELLI, L. 1973. The "isolation syndrome" in mice. *Psychopharmacologia (Berlin)* 31: 305–320.

VALZELLI, L., and GARATTINI, S. 1968. Behavioral changes and 5-hydroxytryptamine turnover in animals. In S. Garattini and P. A. Shore, eds., *Advances in Pharmacology*, Vol. 68. New York: Academic Press, pp. 249–260.

VALZELLI, L., and GARATTINI, S. 1972. Biochemical and behavioral changes induced by isolation in rats. *Neuropharmacology* 11: 17–22.

VOLKMAR, F. R., and GREENOUGH, W. T. 1972. Rearing complexity affects branching of dendrites in the visual cortex of the rat. *Science* 176: 1445–1447.

WALK, R. D., and GIBSON, E. J. 1961. A comparative and analytical study of visual depth perception. *Psychological Monographs* 75 (Whole No. 15).

WALK, R. D., and WALTERS, C. P. 1973. Effect of visual deprivation on depth discrimination of hooded rats. *Journal of Comparative and Physiological Psychology* 85: 559–563.

WALSH, R. N., BUDTZ-OLSEN, O. E., PENNY, J. E., and CUMMINS, R. A. 1969. The effects of environmental complexity on the histology of the rat hippocampus. *Journal of Comparative Neurology* 137: 361–366.

WALSH, R. N., BUDTZ-OLSEN, O. E., TOROK, A., and CUMMINS, R. A. 1971. Environmentally induced changes in the dimensions of the rat cerebrum. *Developmental Psychobiology* 4: 115–122.

WALSH, R. N., CUMMINS, R. A., and BUDTZ-OLSEN, O. 1974. Time course of environmentally induced changes in brain and body weights. Paper presented at 82nd Annual Convention of the American Psychological Association, New Orleans, La., September 1974.

WALSH, R. N., CUMMINS, R. A., BUDTZ-OLSEN, O. E., and TOROK, A. 1972. Effects of environmental enrichment and deprivation on rat frontal cortex. *International Journal of Neuroscience* 4: 239–242.

WEININGER, O. 1953. Mortality of albino rats under stress as a function of early handling. *Canadian Journal of Psychology* 7: 111–114.

WEININGER, O. 1956. The effects of early experience on behavior and growth characteristics. *Journal of Comparative and Physiological Psychology* 49: 1–9.

WEISS, J. M. 1968. Effects of coping responses on stress. *Journal of Comparative and Physiological Psychology* 65: 251–260.

WELCH, B. L. 1967. Invited discussion of aggression, defense, and neurohumors. In C. D. Clemente and D. B. Lindsley, eds., *Aggression and Defense*. Berkeley: University of California Press, pp. 150–164.

WELCH, B. L., BROWN, D. G., WELCH, A. S., and LIN, D. C. 1974. Isolation, restrictive confinement or crowding of rats for one year. 1. Weight, nucleic acids and protein of brain regions. *Brain Research* 75: 71–84.

WELCH, B. L., and WELCH, A. S. 1968. Differential activation by restraint stress of a mechanism to conserve brain catecholamines and serotonin in mice differing in excitability. *Nature* 218: 575–577.

WEST, R. W., and GREENOUGH, W. T. 1972. Effect of environmental complexity on cortical synapses of rats: Preliminary results. *Behavioral Biology* 7: 279–284.

WHITE, A., HANDLER, P., and SMITH, E. L. 1968. *Principles of Biochemistry*. New York: McGraw-Hill.

WIBERG, G. S., AIRTH, J. M., and GRICE, H. C. 1966. Methodology in long term toxicity tests. *Food and Cosmetic Toxicology* 4: 47–55.

WILKINS, L. 1965. *The Diagnosis and Treatment of Endocrine Disorders in Childhood and Adolescence*, 3rd ed. Springfield, Ill.: Charles C Thomas.

WILSON, M., WARREN, J. M., and ABBOTT, L. 1965. Infantile stimulation, activity, and learning by cats. *Child Development* 36: 843–853.

WOOD, W. E., and GREENOUGH, W. T. 1974. Effects of grouping and crowding on learning in isolation-reared adult rats. *Bulletin of the Psychonomic Society* 3: 65–67.

YOUNG, W. C., GOY, R. W., and PHOENIX, C. H. 1964. Hormones and sexual behavior. *Science* 143: 212–218.

ZAMENHOF, S., MOSLEY, J., and SCHULLER, E. 1966. Stimulation of the proliferation of cortical neurons by prenatal treatment with growth hormone. *Science* 152: 1396–1397.

ZIMBARDO, P. G., and MONTGOMERY, K. D. 1957. Effects of "free environment" rearing upon exploratory behavior. *Psychological Reports* 3: 589–594.

17

Cerebral Effects of Differential Experience and Training

EDWARD L. BENNETT

ABSTRACT Enduring brain differences can be found between animals kept in enriched (EC) or impoverished (IC) environments (differential environments). These include differences in cortical weight, cortical depth, size and number of asymmetric synapses, ratio of RNA to DNA, and certain enzymatic measures. Several of these measures of cerebral differences decrease in magnitude when rats are removed from EC and placed in IC. This convergence of EC toward IC values is slow, and differences have been found to persist for at least 50 days. The rate of convergence differs among cerebral measures; for example, the ratio of RNA to DNA converges more rapidly than does the ratio of cortical to subcortical weight.

Differential environments have been found to produce measurable cerebral differences within four days. Housing rats out of doors in a seminatural environment leads to enhanced cerebral differences. Alternative explanations of the EC-IC effects (e.g., attributing them to differential handling or stress) have been considered and rejected.

The goal of several investigators is to determine if any of these cerebral differences are closely associated with learning and memory mechanisms. We believe that differential environments are a useful tool for studying memory mechanisms. Many of the changes found undoubtedly represent the integrated or cumulative effects of a number of individual memorial processes. We believe that the explanation of long-term memory will ultimately be cast in terms of anatomical changes. We predict that further studies will demonstrate that brain changes resulting from differential experience are implicated as concomitants of memory mechanisms.

The excellent review of Dr. Greenough (this volume) on the enduring brain effects of differential experience has made my job as a discussant both easy and difficult at the same time: easy in that there is not an additional large number of significant papers in this area of research which must be summarized and referenced; difficult in that it will be hard to add many significant new ideas to those already discussed. As noted by Dr. Greenough, many behavioral, physiological, and biochemical differences have been found between animals raised in isolated or impoverished conditions (IC), standard colony conditions (SC), and enriched conditions (EC). Numerous investigators in this country and abroad have begun to study the effects of such differential environments.

EDWARD L. BENNETT, Laboratory of Chemical Biodynamics, Lawrence Berkeley Laboratory, University of California, Berkeley

The goal of many workers in this area is to determine if any of these differences are in fact closely associated with learning and memory mechanisms. We believe some brain changes may be quite closely related. It is our strong conviction that explanations of long-term memory will ultimately be cast in terms of anatomical changes. At the gross level, these are reflected in changes in measures of cortical weight and thickness and cell size. However, these relatively gross changes may reflect, in part, higher metabolic activity necessary for sustaining higher levels of cerebral (neuronal) activity and, in part, higher levels of biosynthetic activity required for making more subtle anatomical changes.

I would like to comment here on several of the areas that Greenough has reviewed, in the process adding new data, in some cases preliminary, from experiments in our laboratory. These comments will include updated results on synaptic differences produced by environmental complexity as studied by electron micrography, some additional observations on the permanence and persistence of EC effects, some observations on age dependence, and some recent work in our laboratory and in Switzerland on enhancement of EC effects. Then I would like to discuss some experiments in progress that attempt to relate EC-IC effects to neural processes concerned with memory. Along the way I would like to suggest several potential areas of future research using differential environments.

17.1 ANATOMICAL DIFFERENCES PRODUCED BY DIFFERENTIAL ENVIRONMENTS

We started looking for fine structural changes about a decade ago. Holloway (1966) first reported differences in dendritic branching on tissue prepared in our laboratories. We recently reported the higher frequency of dendritic spines on basal dendrites of occipital-cortex pyramidal neurons in rats raised in enriched environments when compared to littermates raised in impoverished conditions (Globus et al., 1973). Greenough has summarized some of his elegant studies on dendritic branching as well.

With respect to measurements on individual synapses

Table 17.1

EC-IC percentage differences in brain weights and body weights in experiments with different starting ages and with durations of 30 days or more (1960–1974)†

	Duration (days)							
	30	37	45	60	80	100	130	160
25 days of age at start								
N (pairs)	267	24	23		206	46	58	22
Occipital cortex	9.6***	6.1***	8.0***		7.3***	9.8***	8.5***	11.4***
Total cortex	5.2***	4.6***	6.4***		4.2***	6.6***	6.8***	2.5**
Rest of brain	0.1	0.9	2.6**		−0.8*	0.7	1.6*	−3.3**
Total brain	2.3***	2.4*	4.2***		1.2***	3.2***	3.7***	−0.9
Cortex/rest of brain	5.0***	3.6***	3.6***		5.1***	5.8***	5.2***	6.1***
Body weight	−8.9***	−4.7*	1.1		−7.7***	−4.8**	−7.5***	−6.8*
60 days of age at start								
N (pairs)	133							
Occipital cortex	7.2***							
Total cortex	5.5***							
Rest of brain	1.9***							
Total brain	3.4***							
Cortex/rest of brain	3.6***							
Body weight	−0.8							
105 days of age at start								
N (pairs)					45			
Occipital cortex					10.9***			
Total cortex					5.4***			
Rest of brain					1.7*			
Total brain					3.2***			
Cortex/rest of brain					3.7***			
Body weight					−0.1			
185 days of age at start								
N (pairs)	21			21				
Occipital cortex	6.0**			3.6*				
Total cortex	3.2**			4.7***				
Rest of brain	1.1			2.9***				
Total brain	2.0			3.6***				
Cortex/rest of brain	2.1**			1.7*				
Body weight	0.6			0.7				
290 days of age at start								
N (pairs)	21			23				
Occipital cortex	4.8***			9.6***				
Total cortex	2.7**			5.8***				
Rest of brain	0.2			2.1*				
Total brain	1.2			3.6**				
Cortex/rest of brain	2.5**			3.6**				
Body weight	−4.3			4.0				

†Percentages are 100 (EC − IC)/IC.
*p < 0.05. **p < 0.01. ***p < 0.001.

of occipital cortex, an updating of our results brings them more in line with Greenough's. While we originally reported a 52 percent increase in the length of the post-synaptic opaque region in type-1 synapses or asymmetrical axodendritic junctions from layer 3, and a frequency decrease of one-third (Møllgaard et al., 1971), we have not been able to replicate these findings. Our best present estimates based on thirteen complete sets of triplets are much more in agreement with those of Greenough: about a 5 percent EC-IC difference in length (p < 0.05) and an 8 percent decrease in frequency (ns) in layer 4 (Diamond et al., 1975). While it would have been nice to have been able to replicate the much larger differences, I feel that the important observation is that differential environments produce synaptic changes that can be detected by current anatomical methods. These are the types of changes that we feel are most likely to be closely associated with memory processes. Certainly this is an area of research that deserves much more intensive investigation. However, such investigations are restricted now by the laborious nature of the research—it requires a great deal of skill, patience, and many months of dedicated work to carry out refined quantitative work at the anatomical level. Ultimately, sufficient resources must be made available so that much of the quantitation can be automated and computerized. Marian Diamond, in collaboration with Leroy Kerth of the Lawrence Berkeley Laboratory, is now undertaking some feasibility studies of more automated quantitation using scanning equipment originally developed for research in high-energy physics.

17.2 THE PERMANENCE AND PERSISTENCE OF BRAIN EFFECTS

Greenough has raised the questions of the permanence and age dependence of brain effects of differential environments, and we have new data that bear on these questions.

While certain effects of complex experience may be transient or change in magnitude with time, I believe the conclusion is valid that differences in several cerebral measures are permanent: weight (Table 17.1) and thickness of cortex; ratio of cortical to subcortical weight, acetylcholinesterase activity and cholinesterase activity; and RNA/DNA ratio (Table 17.2; I shall discuss this measure in more detail shortly). By "permanent," I mean that these differences are maintained for as long as the animals are differentially housed.

A question related to permanence is that of the persistence of effects of differential housing when animals are removed from enriched conditions and placed in impoverished conditions. If some of the effects of dif-

Table 17.2

Permanence of EC-IC percentage differences of RNA/DNA ratio in the occipital cortex in experiments of different durations†

	Duration (days)					
	4	8	12 to 15	30	80	125
% difference	8.5***	6.0***	11.2***	11.2***	11.0***	4.9**
No. of pairs with EC > IC	41/44	26/30	43/44	34/35	18/20	33/41

†Experiments were begun at 25 days of age. Percentages are 100(EC − IC)/IC.
**p < 0.01. ***p < 0.001.

ferential environments are related to memory storage, we would expect that some cerebral differences would persist for a long time when animals are rehoused, while others, related to early steps in storage, would cease to differ relatively quickly.

Brown (1971) reported surprisingly large (and variable) differences in AChE and ChE activities produced by her version of an enriched environment. She claimed that these effects vanished within a few days after animals were placed into isolation. Under our conditions of EC, we have not found this to be the case—differences in cortical brain-weight measures and AChE activity fall but are measurable for at least seven weeks when our EC rats are placed into IC, and the fall is slower after 80 days of EC than after 30 days of EC (Bennett et al., 1974). The persistence of brain-weight measures is shown in Figure 17.1.

17.3 AGE DEPENDENCE OF THE CEREBRAL EFFECTS OF DIFFERENTIAL EXPERIENCE

Greenough has already noted that the postweaning age at which animals are housed in differential environments does not appear to be critical for producing differences

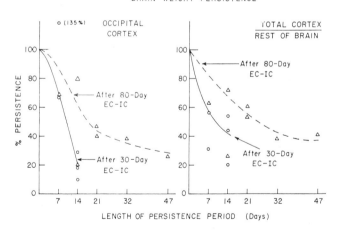

FIGURE 17.1 The persistence of cortical brain weight in rats transferred from an enriched to an impoverished environment after 30 or 80 days in EC. From Bennett et al. (1974). Reproduced with permission of *Physiology and Behavior.*

in certain cerebral measures, including cortical weight and depth. In fact, the differences in brain weights are remarkably similar in magnitude whatever the starting age of the rats, at least to one year of age (Table 17.1).

Only one study of which I am aware has investigated the cerebral effects of differential environments in pre-weaning rats. This is the study of Malkasian and Diamond (1971), who reported that young rat pups living in a multifamily enriched environment had significantly greater cortical depths and larger neuronal nuclear areas, in both the somatosensory and occipital areas of the cortex, than pups from rats raised under standard colony conditions. These authors concluded that these cortical differences demonstrated more plasticity in the neonate than in the young adult rat brain. To date, I know of no experiment in which the differential environments have been initiated at preweaning ages and then carried through for 30 days or more into post-weaning, and the resulting cerebral effects investigated. This may be a fruitful area for further research.

17.4 ENHANCED EC EFFECTS

When it is realized that an enriched environment can increase brain measures, it is only natural to ask if EC effects can be even further increased; that is, can a "super" EC condition be devised? We have recently shown that certain stimulant drugs can interact with the enriched conditions to produce enhanced cerebral effects (Bennett, Rosenzweig, and Wu, 1973; Rosenzweig and Bennett, 1972), but perhaps some purely environmental methods can be found.

It would appear from his description of procedures that Greenough uses a somewhat larger complement of toys than we do. Several years ago we became aware of a study by Ferchmin, Eterović, and Caputto (1970), who reported small but significant increases in cerebrum weight (total brain excluding cerebellum, medulla, and pons) after as few as four days of EC. They also reported an initial increase in total brain RNA and RNA/mg after four days of EC. However, after eight days of EC, RNA/mg differed only slightly between groups. We were fortunate enough to have Drs. Ferchmin and Eterović in our laboratory for two years, and in discussion it became quite apparent that their EC conditions were considerably more complex than ours. They rotate animals twice a day among four cages, some of which are considerably larger than ours and offer more opportunity for climbing. We have run a number of experiments comparing the effects of what we shall refer to as FEC (Ferchmin EC) to our regular EC and IC conditions.

I shall discuss the weight results first and come back to results concerning nucleic acids later. The most striking observation to be made is that significant weight effects can be found in occipital cortex and total cortex when four days of differential environments are begun at weaning (Table 17.3). Thus certain cerebral effects are shown with much shorter durations of differential environments than we had previously realized. The differences obtained by the Ferchmin EC are very similar to those obtained with the usual EC. A possible advantage of FEC over regular EC is seen only in the weight ratio of cortex to the rest of the brain at four and eight days (1.7 vs. 0.2 percent, and 2.6 vs. 1.7 percent).

Two Swiss investigators, Kuenzle and Knüsel (1974), have also attempted to enhance EC conditions in order to get increased cerebral differences. They housed a group of 70 rats in two large cages provided with varied stimulus objects and connected by tunnels. Each day for 29 days food was placed in one of the cages and water in the other, so that the rats had to shuttle back and forth between the two cages. Gradually the rats were made to solve problems and to climb ropes or jump from one platform to another in order to traverse the tunnels. Brain values of rats from this "superenriched environment" (SE) were compared with those of rats of the same strain kept for 29 days in a copy of our typical EC conditions. In three successive experiments SE rats were found to be significantly greater than ECs in cerebral length, weight of occipital cortex, and ChE/AChE ratio in occipital cortex; small but nonsignificant differences in the same direction were found in the RNA/DNA ratio in occipital cortex.

Another, quite different method by which we have tried to enhance the effects of differential environments is through the use of a "seminatural" environment.

TABLE 17.3
Comparison of EC-IC brain-weight differences obtained by Ferchmin EC and regular EC†

	Con- dition	Duration (days)			
		4	8	12	15
N (pairs)	FEC	72	24	12	
	EC	48	24	12	22
% difference from IC					
Occipital cortex	FEC	5.2***	5.4***	8.3***	
	EC	6.6***	7.1***	7.3**	10.4***
Total cortex	FEC	2.6***	2.0*	2.7**	
	EC	2.2***	2.8**	3.8***	6.4***
Total brain	FEC	1.7***	0.6	1.3	
	EC	2.0***	1.8*	2.4**	5.3***
Cortex/rest of brain	FEC	1.7***	2.6***	2.6**	
	EC	0.2	1.7*	2.3**	2.0**

†Experiments begun at 25 days of age.
*$p < 0.05$.   **$p < 0.01$.   ***$p < 0.001$.

Our seminatural-environment rats (SNE) live out of doors in 9-m² enclosures with a dirt floor 60 cm or so in depth. These animals are exposed to the rigors of Berkeley weather. Rats put into the seminatural environment at about 40 days of age have adapted well, and virtually all have survived. We now have nine experiments in which we can compare rats raised in a seminatural environment for 30 days to rats raised in regular EC conditions at the Field Station in the Berkeley hills. The seminatural environment does bring about moderate but significant increases in cerebral weight measures over the Field Station EC animals, which in turn are significantly different from IC littermates (Table 17.4). A limited number of additional control experiments indicate that Field Station EC animals are not significantly different from EC rats maintained in Tolman Hall. (All comparisons are against the appropriate littermate group run in the same experiment. However, different combinations of groups were run in different experiments; thus the overall difference from seminatural environment to Tolman IC cannot be obtained by adding differences of intermediate groups.) Thus, to date, raising rats in a seminatural environment appears to be a simple and effective way to obtain significantly larger EC effects than we have typically obtained. These results suggest that laboratory EC conditions are good but not optimal.

17.5 FACTORS PRODUCING CEREBRAL EFFECTS

In order to evaluate whether the effects of differential environments can be related to learning and memory mechanisms, we must have a more complete understanding of the factors that produce cerebral differences.

In a number of studies we have attempted to specify some of the factors in the EC condition that produce differences in cerebral measures. Several years ago we discussed possible alternative explanations of cerebral effects of differential experience (Rosenzweig, Bennett, and Diamond, 1972), and we have recently prepared a more thorough and up-to-date review of this question (Rosenzweig and Bennett, 1976). We have shown that neither the greater handling nor motor activity in EC seems to be crucial. EC-IC effects can be found in animals blinded or raised in the dark, although visual deprivation does produce its own effects; and studies by Riege and Morimoto (1970) have shown that stress is not a component of the EC effect. From results of numerous experiments we have also concluded that it is not essential to maintain the IC rats in a room separate from the EC rats: the ongoing laboratory activities associated with maintaining a large number of EC rats do not modify the cerebral measures of the EC rats. However, both social stimulation and stimulation from inanimate objects do contribute to the EC-IC differences.

Recently, while visiting our lab, Pedro Ferchmin performed an experiment for a quite different purpose which also very clearly ruled out many factors as possible contributors to EC effects. Ferchmin wished to test whether any EC effects would be induced by observation learning; that is, would effects be found in rats that were individually housed in small cages within the EC cage? These animals had the opportunity to observe the EC animals, were exposed to the smells and noises of the EC animals, and even had a limited amount of social contact. After 30 days the observer group showed no significant cerebral differences from the IC group but differed significantly from the EC littermates whose cages they shared in a limited way (Table 17.5). On measures of exploratory behavior taken during the last two days of the experiment, IC rats fell significantly below EC, and the observer rats were somewhat below IC. We conclude that actual contact with an enriched environment is necessary for the development of EC effects (Ferchmin, Bennett, and Rosenzweig, 1975).

17.6 ENRICHED ENVIRONMENTS AS A TOOL TO STUDY NEURAL MECHANISMS OF MEMORY

If we wish to relate some of the EC effects to memory mechanisms, it is highly desirable, if not essential, to produce at least some of the EC effects by what I shall term "formal training." In this connection, Greenough has reviewed some of his experiments in which tantalizing, and perhaps even significant, differences have been found in certain dendritic measures.

Over the past several years we also have been attempting to produce cerebral differences by formal

TABLE 17.4

Comparison of brain-weight differences produced by a seminatural environment (SNE), Field Station EC, and Tolman EC (% weight differences)†

	SNE vs. FS-EC	SNE vs. IC	T-EC vs. IC	FS-EC vs. T-EC
N (pairs)	105	59	33	23
Occipital cortex	5.4***	11.2***	9.4***	−1.4
Total cortex	3.8***	7.0***	4.1***	−1.2
Rest of brain	1.3**	0.9	−1.5	−0.4
Total brain	2.3***	3.5***	0.9	−0.8
Total cortex/subcortex	2.4**	6.1***	5.6***	−0.8
Body weight	−0.1	−7.7***	−7.7**	−1.6

†Comparisons made only between littermate groups.
**p < 0.01.   ***p < 0.001.

Table 17.5

Comparisons of brain weights and body weights among rats in three environmental conditions

	IC Means†	% Differences OC vs. IC	EC vs. IC	EC vs. OC
Experiment 1				
(N = 10 per group)				
Cortex				
Occipital	66.8	3.3	7.0*	3.6
Total	666.6	1.3	5.2***	3.9**
Rest of brain	885.2	0.2	1.2	1.0
Cortex/rest	0.753	1.1	4.0**	2.9*
Body weight	214.2	−1.4	−7.1	−5.7
Experiment 2				
(N = 12 per group)				
Cortex				
Occipital	71.4	0.2	4.7*	4.5*
Total	689.4	−0.1	3.4**	3.5**
Rest of brain	962.0	−0.3	0.3	0.6
Cortex/rest	0.717	0.2	3.1**	2.9**
Body weight	318.0	−5.2	−1.7	3.7
Experiments 1 and 2				
(N = 22 per group)				
Cortex				
Occipital	69.3	1.5	5.7**	4.1*
Somesthetic	57.3	−2.6	2.4	5.2**
Rem. dorsal	298.3	0.0	5.3***	5.3***
Ventral	254.0	1.5	2.9	1.4
Total	679.0	0.5	4.2***	3.7***
Rest of brain	927.1	−0.1	0.7	0.8
Total brain	1606.1	0.2	2.2**	2.0**
Cortex/rest	0.733	0.6	3.5***	2.9***
Body weight	270.8	−3.9	−3.7	0.2

†Units are mg for brain weights and gm for body weights.
*p < 0.05. **p < 0.01. ***0 < 0.001.

training, though our measures have been somewhat less refined than those used by Greenough. In our first experiments we trained rats on a series of bar-pressing tasks over a number of days with food reward. Small and marginally significant chemical differences were obtained in cortical samples.

We are now attempting two somewhat different training procedures in hopes of finding clearer effects. In one, the trained rats run for food reward on self-paced trials in an automatic Hebb-Williams-type maze. These rats can be compared to control rats that are equated for motor activity but only run a straight-alley runway for their food. In the first several experiments small differences in cortical weights were found in the expected direction. However, more recent experiments, conducted under what were intended to be more favorable conditions, have not yielded weight effects.

Our second training procedure we call the "group maze." In this procedure a plastic maze is inserted as a second floor inside the EC cage, and animals must go up and down to get food and water. The intervening partitions can be changed, and maze patterns of increasing complexity can be constructed. This is the complex maze (CM). Another group maze is similar except that a simple route leads through the maze from food to water, and this route is never changed; this is the simple maze (SM). Rats in these two conditions can be compared to rats in the regular EC condition, to rats housed twelve to a large empty cage (group condition—GC), as well as to the IC rats. To date we have completed six experiments with three to five conditions in each experiment. Since all experiments did not have all groups, the presentation of results is complicated, but a few general conclusions can be made (Table 17.6). It is clear that the rats raised in regular EC, CM, or SM had very similar cerebral measures, and all differed significantly from ICs. Naturally, we were disappointed that the animals in the complex group maze did not differ from those raised in the simple group maze. We next asked to what extent these differences could be due to the social effects of twelve rats living in a large empty cage, since we already knew that the rats we call "social controls," which live three to a relatively small laboratory cage, typically fall between EC and IC rats. Not unexpectedly, twelve rats living in a large empty cage fall about halfway between IC rats and EC rats, so social stimulation does play an important role but does not produce the whole effect.

17.7 BIOCHEMICAL EFFECTS OF DIFFERENTIAL ENVIRONMENTS

For a number of years we concentrated on measurements

TABLE 17.6

Percentage differences in brain-weight values between littermates in five conditions: enriched condition (EC), complex maze (CM), simple maze (SM), group condition (GC), and impoverished condition (IC)

	A. Occipital cortex				B. Total cortex				C. Total brain				D. Cortex/rest of brain			
	CM	SM	GC	IC	CM	SM	GC	IC	CM	SM	GC	IC	CM	SM	GC	IC
EC	-0.9	0.1	2.6*	6.7***	-0.2	1.1	2.7***	5.5***	0.1	0.7	1.8**	3.3***	-0.4	0.6	1.5**	3.9***
N (pairs)	47	59	47	47	47	59	47	47	47	59	47	47	47	59	47	47
CM		-0.1	3.8***	8.2***		0.5	2.8**	5.2***		0.1	2.1**	2.7***		0.7	1.1	4.3***
N (pairs)		68	44	68		68	44	68		68	44	68		68	44	68
SM			2.2**	8.2***			1.4*	4.6***			1.2	2.6***			0.5	3.6***
N (pairs)			56	68			56	68			56	68			56	68
GC				3.7**				2.4**				0.5				3.2***
N (pairs)				44				44				44				44

*p < 0.05. ** p < 0.01. *** p < 0.001.

of acetylcholinesterase and cholinesterase as indicators of biochemical (and anatomical) effects of differential environments. I shall not review the voluminous data that we have obtained in this area except to say that we have generally found an increase in total AChE activity in the cortex and an even larger increase in ChE activity (Rosenzweig, Bennett, and Diamond, 1972). This is particularly true after 80 days' exposure to the enriched environment. We have interpreted these results as indicating that an increase in glial function of the rat cortex resulted from the enriched environments (as compared to the impoverished controls). We then turned to an investigation of RNA and DNA content of the rat cortex in the usual EC-IC paradigm and also in animals raised in the light and in the dark. In both cases we found an increase in the RNA/DNA ratio of the more stimulated rat of the comparison pair (EC or light-raised) (Rosenzweig, Bennett, and Diamond, 1972). Our enthusiasm for pursuing such research was dampened at the time by the fact that the methods available for the analysis of brain nucleic acids in the midsixties were either inaccurate or laborious (or both).

Recently we have developed a new and more reliable method for determining nucleic acid content in brain tissue (Morimoto, Ferchmin, and Bennett, 1974). This method uses cetyl trimethylammonium bromide (CTAB) as the specific precipitant for nucleic acids. In a large number of experiments we have found a highly reproducible and significant increase in the RNA/DNA ratio of the cortex when animals are maintained in EC conditions and compared to their IC littermates. This is particularly true for the occipital and total-cortex measures (see Table 17.2, occipital cortex). Little or no change is found in the subcortex. Most of the increase in ratio is due to a decrease of DNA/mg, and this in turn is related to the increase in cortical weight in EC. With experiments of varied durations there first appears to be a small, transient, but significant, increase in RNA/mg

in favor of the EC groups, after which the RNA difference again approaches zero. With a short (4-day) exposure to EC an increase in total brain RNA has been found both by Ferchmin, Eterović, and Caputto (1970) and by ourselves. The increase in total RNA and in RNA/DNA in EC is found for experiments of all durations, from 4 days to 165 days.

17.8 THE SIGNIFICANCE OF ENVIRONMENTAL COMPLEXITY FOR STUDYING NEURONAL AND BIOCHEMICAL COMPONENTS OF MEMORY

As discussed by Rose, Hambley, and Haywood, and by Dunn (this volume), the results of numerous studies have suggested that an increased incorporation of precursors of RNA and protein into brain may be associated with training. Typically, the effects can only be monitored by highly sensitive radioactive-tracer experiments and represent only a transient and quite small increase in the total macromolecular synthesis. Our recent results have shown that the RNA/DNA ratio in the cortex of a rat maintained in EC is significantly and reproducibly larger than that of its IC littermate. The effect can be found within four days after exposure to EC, as shown by both the experiments of Ferchmin's group and our own experiments. Does this increase represent the integrated effect of many individual learning-memory events, which others have shown to cause an increased incorporation of RNA precursors? We would like to believe that this is the case. If so, we would predict several results: (1) RNA will respond more rapidly to altered experience than other brain measures; (2) the increase in RNA/DNA ratio will not persist for as long as the weight effects when EC rats are removed to an IC environment; and (3) eventually an appropriate paradigm clearly involving only training will increase the RNA/DNA ratio of selected brain areas, and this increase will

TABLE 17.7
Effects of successive environments on RNA and DNA measures (% differences)†

	Duration (days)		Occipital cortex			Dorsal (including somethetic) cortex		
	EC	IC	RNA/mg	DNA/mg	RNA/DNA	RNA/mg	DNA/mg	RNA/DNA
EC	45	0	−2.8*	−8.9***	6.7***	−1.4	−4.8**	3.6*
EC·IC	30	15	−4.5**	0.8	−5.3**	−2.8*	0.3	−3.1
EC	58	0	−2.2*	−7.5***	5.8***	−0.4	−5.0***	4.9**
EC·IC	30	28	−3.3**	−1.8	−1.6	−2.2**	−2.5	0.3
EC	109	0	−0.2	−6.2***	6.3***	0.2	−4.4**	5.1**
EC·IC	95	14	−3.1*	−2.2	−0.9	−1.9	−1.2	−0.8
EC	119	0	0.9	−4.7**	5.8***	0.8	−2.1*	2.9***
EC·IC	91	28	−3.8**	−0.5	−3.2*	−1.4*	2.0	−3.3**

†All experiments begun at weaning (25–28 days of age). Percentages are (EC − IC)/IC or (EC·IC − IC)/IC. Each value represents the average of 12 littermate comparisons.
*p < 0.05. ** p < 0.01. *** p < 0.001.

be detectable by nontracer methods. Data that we have just obtained show that, as predicted, RNA does respond sensitively to experience, and the persistence of RNA/DNA effects is much less than the persistence of weight effects (Table 17.7). As discussed above, we are still attempting to devise a series of formal training experiments that will reliably produce many of the cerebral differences Greenough and I have discussed. Ultimately, I believe we shall be successful in finding such differences, some of which will be important in elucidating memory mechanisms.

17.9 SUMMARY

Differential environments are thought to be a useful paradigm for the study of memory mechanisms. Some of the cerebral differences, such as cortical weight and the ratio of RNA to DNA, have temporal properties consistent with their involvement in memory storage. For example, cerebral differences can be found within four days, differences can be produced over a variety of starting ages and durations of differential environments, and differences persist for months when animals are removed from EC and placed into IC. Active participation in the EC environment is required, and larger differences can be produced when groups of animals are placed in a seminatural environment. Maze experience has produced cerebral differences in excess of those produced by a group of animals in a large empty cage. As Dr. Greenough has stated, "it would be much more difficult to argue that EC rats do *not* learn more than their IC and SC counterparts than it is to argue that they do." We therefore believe that ultimately a number of biochemical and anatomical changes will be found to result from differential environments. Many of these changes, we suggest, will represent the cumulative

effect of a number of memorial events taking place in EC conditions.

ACKNOWLEDGMENTS

The research summarized in this chapter has extended over a number of years, and contributions have been made by a number of individuals. These include Pedro Ferchmin, Marie Hebert, Hiromi Morimoto, Donald Dryden, Arun Prakash, and Jessie Langford. Essential support for our research has been most recently provided by NSF Grant GB-30368, and the U.S. Atomic Energy Commission through the Lawrence Berkeley Laboratory.

REFERENCES

BENNETT, E. L., ROSENZWEIG, M. R., DIAMOND, M. C., MORI-MOTO, H., and HEBERT, M. 1974. Effects of successive environments on brain measures. *Physiology and Behavior* 12: 621–631.

BENNETT, E. L., ROSENZWEIG, M. R., and WU, S.-Y. C. 1973. Excitant and depressant drugs modulate effects of environment on brain weight and cholinesterases. *Psychopharmacologia (Berlin)* 33: 309–328.

BROWN, C. P. 1971. Cholinergic activity in rats following enriched stimulation and training: Direction and duration of effects. *Journal of Comparative and Physiological Psychology* 75: 408–416.

DIAMOND, M., C., LINDNER, B., JOHNSON, R., BENNETT, E. L., and ROSENZWEIG, M. R. 1975. Differences in occipital cortical synapses from environmentally enriched, impoverished, and standard colony rats. *Journal of Neuroscience Research* (in press).

FERCHMIN, P. A., BENNETT, E. L., and ROSENZWEIG, M. R. 1975. Direct contact with enriched environments is required to alter cerebral weights in rats. *Journal of Comparative and Physiological Psychology* 88: 360–367.

FERCHMIN, P. A., ETEROVIĆ, V. A., and CAPUTTO, R. 1970. Studies of brain weights and RNA content after short periods of exposure to environmental complexity. *Brain Research* 20: 49–57.

GLOBUS, A., ROSENZWEIG, M. R., BENNETT, E. L., and DIA-
MOND, M. C. 1973. Effects of differential experience on dendritic spine counts in rat cerebral cortex. *Journal of Comparative
and Physiological Psychology* 82: 175–181.

HOLLOWAY, R. L. 1966. Dendritic branching: Some preliminary results of training and complexity in rat visual
cortex. *Brain Research* 2: 393–396.

KUENZLE, C. C., and KNÜSEL, A. 1974. Mass training of rats in a
superenriched environment. *Physiology and Behavior.*

MALKASIAN, D. R., and DIAMOND, M. C. 1971. The effects of
enrivonmental manipulation on the morphology of the neonate rat brain. *International Journal of Neuroscience* 2: 161–170.

MØLLGAARD, K., DIAMOND, M. C., BENNETT, E. L., ROSEN-
ZWEIG, M. R., and LINDNER, B. 1971. Qualitative synaptic
changes with differential experience in rat brain. *International
Journal of Neuroscience* 2: 113–128.

MORIMOTO, H., FERCHMIN, P. A., and BENNETT, E. L. 1974.
Spectrophotometric analysis of RNA and DNA using cetyl-
trimethylammonium bromide. *Analytical Biochemistry* 62:
436–448.

RIEGE, W. H., and MORIMOTO, H. 1970. Effects of chronic stress
and differential environments upon brain weights and biogenic amine levels in rats. *Journal of Comparative and Physiological Psychology* 71: 396–404.

ROSENZWEIG, M. R., and BENNETT, E. L. 1972. Cerebral changes
in rats exposed individually to an enriched environment.
Journal of Comparative and Physiological Psychology 80: 304–
313.

ROSENZWEIG, M. R., and BENNETT, E. L. 1976. Enriched environments: Facts, factors, and fantasies. In J. L. McGaugh
and L. Petrinovich, eds., *Knowing, Thinking, and Believing.*
New York: Plenum Press (in press).

ROSENZWEIG, M. R., BENNETT, E. L., and DIAMOND, M. C.
1972. Chemical and anatomical plasticity of brain: Replications and extensions. In J. Gaito, ed., *Macromolecules and
Behavior*, 2nd ed. New York: Appleton-Century-Crofts.

18

Effects of Early Sensory Experience on Brain and Behavior: A Summary of Presentations by J. D. Pettigrew and D. N. Spinelli

(The conference included a paper by J. D. Pettigrew, "The Single-Neuron Approach to Memory in the Developing Nervous System," and a discussion of this subject by D. N. Spinelli. In lieu of final drafts of their papers, and since a number of other participants refer to this interesting material in their chapters, the editors have prepared the following brief statement and list of references that will guide the reader into this topic.)

Differences in early visual environment can cause striking changes in the properties of receptive fields of single cortical neurons. Investigating these effects required first a careful mapping of the receptive fields. This was done by Hubel and Wiesel (1959, 1962) and others. Most cells in visual regions of the cortex show specificity for one or more of the following aspects of the stimulus: (1) position in the visual field; (2) orientation; (3) binocularity (ocular dominance and ocular disparity); (4) movement (direction and velocity); (5) size; and (6) color. Effects of early experience were first observed by Hubel and Wiesel (1963) when they sutured one eyelid in a group of kittens; they later found that most cortical cells responded preferentially, or only, to the eye that had been used. They eventually showed that there is a sensitive period for this effect in kittens, lasting from about the third week to the third month after birth (Hubel and Wiesel, 1970).

More specific effects were found when kittens were allowed only restricted visual experience. For example, kittens were fitted with goggles that allowed them to see only three vertical lines with one eye and three horizontal lines with the other. Later recording disclosed only vertical receptive fields in the eye exposed to vertical lines and only horizontal receptive fields in the eye exposed to horizontal lines (Hirsch and Spinelli, 1970; Spinelli et al., 1972). A few units had receptive fields consisting of three lines, which looked almost like a carbon copy of the original stimuli. Blakemore and Cooper (1970) reported similar results with kittens kept in the dark except for a daily period in a cylinder painted with either vertical or horizontal stripes. Exposing kittens to only small dots of light produced cells that responded

preferentially to small moving targets (Pettigrew and Freeman, 1973). Changes in the preferred stimulus of a cell have been produced during the course of recording by an acute conditioning procedure (Pettigrew and Garey, 1974).

These animal experiments have helped us to understand human defects arising from divergent gaze (amblyopia ex anopsia) or astigmatism. Recent research has shown that astigmatic adults have reduced acuity in the meridian of their impairment even when their refractive errors have been completely corrected with lenses (Freeman and Thibos, 1973; Pettigrew and Freeman, 1973). An astigmatic person is usually astigmatic from infancy, but it is a rare child in whom astigmatism is corrected during the first years of life. As a consequence, input is blurred in a particular orientation, and the development of the visual system suffers from a relative lack of stimulus input in that orientation. "Evidently, a complex nervous system does not develop to functional perfection solely through genetic control. There must be a period of plasticity during which [an individual's] experience helps to determine the connections of [his] neural network" (Freeman and Thibos, 1973, p. 878). Uncorrected astigmatism during childhood appears to result in neural defects which cannot be overcome by years of corrected vision during adolescence and adulthood. It is not known how early in life a child's vision must be corrected in order to prevent or repair the neurological defect, but Freeman and Thibos report, "Two subjects we have examined so far, who were corrected at 2 and 3 years of age, respectively, showed no orientation effects in spite of considerable astigmatism" (p. 878). In this case it appears that early detection and correction of an optical defect may prevent the development of a permanent neural defect.

What is the mechanism of the cortical modification? The restricted experience might be thought to allow the attrition of cells that do not receive stimulation, or it might be interpreted as arising through a modification of receptive fields. Evidence against the attrition hypothesis was provided by the failure to observe gaps or nonfunctional cells even in kittens with highly restricted inputs. On the other hand, the existence of cells with novel field properties indicates the possibility of a modification of fields. Further evidence for modification was found in the "recapture" experiments of Blakemore and Van Sluyters (1974)—whichever eye had been open for the three days preceding recording commanded the most cortical units. But the plasticity is not unlimited, and innate biases are found.

It has been suggested that the receptive fields of cells of the visual cortex represent engrams of what an animal has seen. Other investigators, without going this far, maintain that the techniques of these experiments will allow us to study how visual memories are stored.

REFERENCES

BLAKEMORE, C., and COOPER, G. F. 1970. Development of the brain depends on the visual environment. *Nature* 228: 477–478.

BLAKEMORE, C., and VAN SLUYTERS, R. C. 1974. Reversal of the physiological effects of monocular deprivation in kittens: Further evidence for a sensitive period. *Journal of Physiology* 237: 195–216.

FREEMAN, R. D., and THIBOS, L. N. 1973. Electrophysioiogical evidence that abnormal early visual experience can modify the human brain. *Science* 180: 876–878.

HIRSCH, H. V. B., and SPINELLI, D. N. 1970. Visual experience modifies distribution of horizontally and vertically oriented receptive fields in cats. *Science* 168: 869–871.

HIRSCH, H. V. B., and SPINELLI, D. N. 1971. Modification of the distribution of receptive field orientation in cats by selective visual exposure during development. *Experimental Brain Research* 13: 509–527.

HUBEL, D. H., and WIESEL, T. N. 1959. Receptive fields of single neurones in the cat's striate cortex. *Journal of Physiology* 148: 574–591.

HUBEL, D. H., and WIESEL, T. N. 1962. Receptive fields, binocular interaction, and functional architecture in the cat's visual cortex. *Journal of Physiology* 160: 106–154.

HUBEL, D. H., and WIESEL, T. N. 1965. Binocular interaction in striate cortex of kittens reared with artificial squint. *Journal of Neurophysiology* 28: 1041–1059.

HUBEL, D. H., and WIESEL, T. N. 1970. The period of susceptibility to the physiological effects of unilateral eye closure in kittens. *Journal of Physiology* 906: 419–436.

PETTIGREW, J. D., 1972. The importance of early visual experience for neurons of the developing geniculo-striate system. *Investigations of Ophthalmology* 11: 386–394.

PETTIGREW, J. D., 1974. The effect of selective visual experience on stimulus trigger features of kitten cortical neurons. *Annals of the New York Academy of Sciences* 228: 393–405.

PETTIGREW, J. D., and FREEMAN, R. D. 1973. Visual experience without lines: Effect on developing cortical neurons. *Science* 182: 599–601.

PETTIGREW, J. D., and GAREY, L. J. 1974. Selective modification of single neuron properties in the visual cortex of kittens. *Brain Research* 66: 160–164.

SPINELLI, D. N., HIRSCH, H. V. B., PHELPS, R. W., and

METZLER, J. 1972. Visual experience as a determinant of the response characteristics of cortical receptive fields in cats. *Experimental Brain Research* 15: 289–304.

WIESEL, T. N., and HUBEL, D. H. 1963. Single cell responses in striate cortex of kittens deprived of vision in one eye. *Journal of Neurophysiology* 26: 1004–1017.

WIESEL, T. N., and HUBEL, D. H. 1965. Comparison of the effects of unilateral and bilateral eye closure on cortical unit responses in kittens. *Journal of Neurophysiology* 28: 1029–1040.

Biochemical Approaches to
the Study of Memory

19

Neurochemical Approaches to Developmental Plasticity and Learning

STEVEN P. R. ROSE, JOHN HAMBLEY, AND
JEFF HAYWOOD

ABSTRACT Experience creates long-term changes in the functioning of the nervous system, and these changes must have cellular correlates. These changes are associated variously with ontogenetic specificity, developmental plasticity, and learning in the narrow sense. In addition, there are shorter-term, transient responses to environmental change. Devising experiments that separate out cellular events exclusive to, and necessary and sufficient for, learning, is not easy; there are both behavioral and biochemical "side effects" that present grave problems of control. Against this background, we review biochemical work from three laboratories: Glassman's group at Chapel Hill, Hydén's at Göteborg, and our own. We discuss evidence from our own work relating protein synthesis in rat visual-cortex neurons to the onset of visual stimulation, and experiments with the chick imprinting system which seem to show that increased incorporation of precursors into protein and RNA in the anterior forebrain roof is associated with the storage of new information per se, rather than with other consequences of exposure to a stimulus situation. In broad terms, we propose that changes in brain biochemistry in response to both specific learning situations and more general environmental events are associated with specific alterations in cellular structure that affect cell connectivity. We suggest that the mechanisms involved at the biochemical level are likely to be similar to those that occur during less specific developmental plastic responses but confined to a more delimited cellular set. We emphasize both the epistemological and experimental difficulties involved in testing such a model.

19.1 INTRODUCTION: THE THEORETICAL FRAMEWORK

The contributions in this volume share a common premise that changes in an organism's behavior associated with learning are accompanied by measurable changes in the brain at the anatomical, biochemical, and physiological levels. Moreover, most models of such changes assume that their major site is synaptic, that is, that in some way experiential events modulate synaptic connectivity, through the formation of new synapses or the activation or inhibition of old ones. There is nothing very new here, and we are not the only contributors to point out that such models have been around since before the

STEVEN P. R. ROSE, JOHN HAMBLEY, and JEFF HAYWOOD, Department of Biology, The Open University, Milton Keynes, United Kingdom

beginning of this century. However, the number of possible permutations of mechanisms for modulating synaptic connectivity is so large, and the techniques for distinguishing between them experimentally so primitive, that to pile on further speculation at this point would be not merely premature, but would actually retard the field. What is at issue is not the conceptual framework, nor indeed an experimental literature in which a variety of changes in brain biology have been revealed in association with a range of behavioral and environmental manipulations, but rigorous ways of interpreting the significance of such changes in terms of relatively specific processes at either the behavioral or the cellular level. Both the organism's responses to environmental or behavioral manipulation and the cellular events associated with these responses are so multifaceted that experimental designs and interpretations which attempt to explore causally linear, or one-for-one, correlations between the levels are almost certain to end in confusion.

The purpose of this paper is to discuss attempts that have been made to associate biochemical changes with relatively specific changes in the organism's behavior from which learning can be inferred. However, we shall argue, partly on theoretical grounds and partly by reviewing the experimental approaches to the question, first, that such simple associations are hard, if not impossible, to make, and second, that this is a ground for optimism rather than despair, for those changes and relationships which one can detect are much richer and more interesting than narrow reductionism presupposes. We must, therefore, begin by phrasing our question more generally: To what extent is the nervous system plastic and modifiable by experience?

Clearly a portion of the connections in the vertebrate nervous system, particularly those directly related to coding for sensorimotor information, may be genetically programmed; connections are made which are apparently specific (at least on the macroscale at which experimental observation has been possible) and independent of experience, and they do not appear to have a capacity for functional adaption (e.g., Sperry, 1944). A simple example of a consequence of such specificity is provided by the observation that rats reared for long periods in total darkness show startle responses and depth discrimination immediately upon exposure to light.

On the other hand, there are a large number of ways in which experience, especially during development, can result in long-term consequences at the behavioral, brain-structural, and neurophysiological levels—some of which are covered by others in this volume. The most extreme changes may be produced by undernutrition or hormonal imbalance, which perhaps scarcely count as "experience" in the sense we are discussing here, but which, if inflicted on laboratory animals or humans, especially during certain key periods of brain development, result in apparently irreversible deficits in cell number and brain weight (e.g., Dobbing and Smart, 1974). Functional deprivation (e.g., rearing animals in darkness) produces changes which are more germane here; when rats or mice are so reared, the neurons of the outer layer of the visual cortex are more closely packed, and there is a reduction in spines on the apical dendrites of visual-cortex pyramidal cells (Valverde, 1967, 1971) and in the number and density of synapses (Cragg, 1970). Lack or restriction of visual input also results in an alteration of the neurophysiological recognition properties of visual-cortex cells (see Chapter 18, this volume). Some of these changes may be reversed or reduced by subsequent exposure to "normal" light conditions (Valverde, 1971). At an even less extreme level comes the environmental manipulation of "enriched" versus "impoverished" environments and its consequences in terms of changes in cortical weight and enzyme levels (Greenough, this volume; Bennett, this volume). In such situations a variety of effects are occurring, and some of these will presumably represent learning as far as the animal is concerned, even though as investigators we have no ways of quantifying or manipulating this learning. But other effects are more properly regarded as examples of general developmental plasticity, that is, changes in the overall potentiality and responsiveness of the nervous system. These can be distinguished from learning in the narrow sense, by which we refer to the processes involved in acquisition and storage when a particular experience exerts a specific and relatively long-lasting effect on behavior. Is learning, then, merely a more specific and delimited form of developmental plasticity? It will be one argument of this paper that, at least at the level of the cellular correlates of learning, they are closely related.

However, learning is only one aspect of an animal's behavioral response to a new and particular situation; others, which may be involved to a greater or lesser extent, include sensory stimulation, locomotor activity, arousal, attention, and stress. These too may be expected (indeed, are known) to have cellular correlates—and not merely in the brain, but at the whole-body level—in terms of changes in blood-flow and hormonal levels and all their metabolic consequences. Can these be distinguished from the events particularly associated with learning? It would be reasonable to assume that such responses are, on the one hand, more general and less specific to the detailed characteristics of the stimulus concerned than are those of learning per se, and on the other that they are less long-lasting. By definition, long-term memory requires long-term changes in cell properties. However, one or all of these more general responses of the organism may be an inevitable—almost indissociable—correlate of learning, thereby confounding attempts to discriminate between mechanisms at the cellular level.

19.1.1 Cellular correlates of experience

We must, then, in studying the cellular correlates of experience and plasticity, expect to find four analytically, but not necessarily experimentally, distinguishable categories of events: (1) those associated with and determining the ontogenetic specificity of the nervous system; (2) those associated with, in broad terms, developmental plasticity; (3) those associated with the acquisition and storage of specific information, that is, learning; and (4) those associated with more general short-term responses of brain to environment, that is, transient changes of the type we have elsewhere described as "state-dependent" effects (Rose, 1974). In what follows we shall disregard category 1, and having made this one reference to ontogenetic specificity, we shall also ignore the question of how far the system is itself, of necessity, ontogenetically specified to be plastic. We shall consider some of the biochemical aspects of the remaining three categories, returning to the theoretical implications of these distinctions in the final section.

Having emphasized above the difficulty of establishing a specific effect at the behavioral level, we must point to the equivalent difficulty at the biochemical level. It is not merely that each of the four categories of events may mobilize a different type of biochemical response (in fact, we would argue that this is unlikely to be a problem, that there may well be a biochemical continuity among mechanisms which differ primarily in cell address and specificity rather than at the molecular level). Beyond this, the response itself may include a complex of changes, some of which are on the "direct line" of coding the change and others of which are secondary consequences. Thus, if a "direct-line" change involved enhanced lipid synthesis, this would in turn require more ATP, and hence more glucose metabolism, oxygen consumption, and blood flow. Enhanced blood flow could result in an increased flux of amino acids across the blood-brain barrier, and if labeled amino acid were injected as a protein precursor, this could further result in an increase in intracellular-pool specific radioactivity and hence an apparent enhancement of protein incorporation as well. But other factors could equally well lead to enhanced uptake of labeled amino acids. These factors include a change in the rate of protein synthesis, changed turnover, changed ion flux across the cell membrane, and conformational changes resulting in different parameters for active transport of the amino acid, to name but a few directly associated with the cell itself. In addition, events remote from the cell may result in secondary effects—such as changed hormonal levels or fluctuating tissue needs elsewhere in the system which deprive the cell of essential metabolites, In all probability several of these mechanisms are in operation, both in the cell itself and in its relations with other cells, and looking for *the* unitary biochemical response is thus likely to be as fruitless as looking for *the* unitary behavioral response.

Can one identify one or a number of biochemical changes that are both necessary for and exclusive to learning? As is well known, there are three broad classes of experimental approach: (1) to look for changes at the metabolic/biochemical level accompanying learning or environmental change; (2) to examine the effects of inhibitors of particular biochemical processes on learning or retention; and (3) to identify unique biochemicals which may "encode" memories. Only the third purports to describe an exclusive biochemical response that is both necessary *and* sufficient. As has been argued before (e.g., Rose, 1970), the attention to this type of process derives from the obsession of some molecular biologists, in the late 1950s and 1960s, with the biological significance of the punning relationship between brain memory and genetic and immunological "memories"; the approach falls outside the paradigms of this paper—and, we suspect, this meeting—and will not be discussed further.

The use of specific inhibitors of biochemical processes looks at first sight promising; it ought to be able to reveal necessary if not exclusive processes underlying learning. However, things are not so simple. Even assuming a single site of action for the inhibitor, and hence no side effects (as are known to occur, for instance, with puromycin), it does not follow that if blocking protein synthesis blocks retention, then protein synthesis is *the* biochemical correlate of learning. Instead, protein synthesis may support other biochemical processes which are themselves such correlates, or it may be a correlate of other aspects of the behavioral mix of which learning is a part. And above all, the blanket inhibition of protein or RNA synthesis—so fundamental an aspect of cell metabolism—cannot be used to tell us much, except at the most general level,

about the biochemistry of the changes we are interested in. The function of any of the proteins whose synthesis may be affected, their cellular localization, etc., are not determinable in this way. What the inhibitor experiments have done is to suggest something about the temporal relationships of acquisition, storage, retention, and recall; for this purpose, they have been a useful new tool.

We are left, therefore, with the task of cataloging the biochemical correlates of learning and environmental changes, in the hope that these can be assembled into some sort of a meaningful pattern and that to some extent it will be possible to disentangle the behavioral variables. This type of approach has been adopted by a number of groups over the past years, and although the animals studied, tasks given, and biochemical techniques used have differed, they do demonstrate certain common features. We shall talk, inevitably, most extensively about our own work, but in doing so it will be appropriate also to refer to other groups, notably those of Glassman at Chapel Hill, North Carolina, and of Hydén at Göteborg, Sweden. We review the work from the standpoint of its approach to two methodological problems: at the behavioral level, the problem of distinguishing learning from developmental and state-dependent changes, and at the biochemical level, that of interpreting the temporal sequence and metabolic mechanisms underlying complex observed differences.

19.2 VISUAL STIMULATION AND BIOCHEMICAL CHANGE

In order to review the biochemical problem critically, we begin by considering the data obtained in our laboratory with respect to the first exposure of dark-reared rats to the light. In these experiments we have been content to provide the animal with a strong functional stimulus, which is certainly going to affect its behavior (and learning) in a variety of ways, but without our being able to control or specify more precisely just which ways are involved. The consequences of such sensory deprivation followed by exposure to light in a somewhat novel environment are likely to include, at the behavioral level, the switching on of a whole series of adaptations and responses to objects the animal sees, whereas hitherto it has only smelled or felt their equivalents in its home cage. In addition, the activation of hitherto unused integrative systems probably occurs. At the cellular level this may mean both the switching on of a developmentally plastic sequence of neuronal differentiation and, in a synaptic model of learning, the creation of specific new pathways. Biochemically these processes may be identical (see the argument in Sections 19.1 and 19.5). And of course, in its new environment the animal is bound to be in a different state of stress and arousal than its littermate back in the dark again after the isotope injection. In passing, one may note the perhaps questionable nature of an experimental strategy that uses albino rats to study the effects of visual deprivation and stimulation, rather than, say, olfactory stimuli; the utility of the visual modality for these experiments lies in the great ease with which it can be controlled.

In any event, the simplicity and massive nature of the stimulus may be anticipated to evoke a comparably large response involving many brain regions. This allows us to concentrate on analyzing the biochemical responses with some chance of success. In our early experiments (Rose, 1967; Richardson and Rose, 1972) we were able to show that in rats reared for 50 days in the dark and then exposed to the light, there was a transient elevation of incorporation of [³H]lysine into protein in the visual cortex, lateral geniculate, and retina, as compared to dark controls. This increase, of up to 20–30 percent, occurred within 1–3 hrs of first exposure of the animals. It did not occur in the frontal ("motor") cortex or in liver.

19.2.1 Pools and the specificity of biochemical effect

An increase in incorporation does not necessarily mean increased net synthesis—or even increased turnover— a point that all precursor studies must take into account. It may be a secondary response reflecting an increased flux of radioactive amino acid across the cell membrane which raises the specific radioactivity of the pool, as hypothesized above; and this flux may itself result from a changed blood flow or changed uptake mechanisms. In addition, other factors such as a change in alternative paths of metabolism of the precursor, or an absolute change in the size of a precursor pool that is rate-limiting for synthesis, may occur. Indeed, several of these phenomena are known to take place. As far as blood flow is concerned, Bondy, Lehman, and Purdy (1974) have shown in a number of experiments with the avian visual system that deafferentation, or even just visual attention, can affect blood flow. There are several cases in which amino acid pools are known to be rate-limiting—plasma tryptophan uptake for brain serotonin synthesis is but one (Fernstrom and Wurtman, 1972). In sensory deprivation there are changes in brain free amino acid levels (Davis, Himwich, and Agrawal, 1969), and in our experimental situation an elevation of free pool amino acids in the visual cortex of dark-reared rats could be shown, which fell to the "normal" values on exposure to light (Rose, 1972). Finally, although our choice of lysine as precursor was motivated by the fact of its relatively exclusive metab-

olism to protein, it is now known that a rapid exchange of [³H] from amino acids to H_2O occurs prior to the entry of the amino acid into the cell. Therefore, water metabolism might in principle confound the results (e.g., Schotman, Gipon, and Gispen, 1974); in practice, it appears not to, as similar results may be obtained with [¹⁴C]precursors.

Of course, if one merely wishes to show a biochemical correlate of stimulation, these questions do not matter. There is no intrinsic reason why pool changes, for instance, should be less interesting than changes in macromolecular synthesis, except that the latter are more likely to be a mechanism for encoding the permanent responses of the cell. But the biochemical mechanisms are important—especially if they can be related to function. We must extend our biochemical models to take into account, rather than merely gloss over, such changes in pool size.

Classical precursor-product kinetics of the Zilversmit type would suggest that we need to relate protein specific radioactivity (or rather protein-lysine specific radioactivity) to precursor specific radioactivity. But what is the precursor? Most directly, it is aminoacyl tRNA, which is almost impossible to measure; more remotely, it is intracellular free amino acids, which are hard to measure, though free radioactivity is easy. Hence arises the practice of expressing results as relative radioactivities (bound/free radioactivity). We did this in our early experiments, as has Hydén and also the Chapel Hill group (see below).

We must distinguish between *size* and *specific radioactivity* of a precursor pool. Even if no changes occur in the rate of synthesis and degradation (i.e., turnover) of a macromolecule, if the specific radioactivity of a precursor increases, for whatever reason, there will be a higher amount of radioactivity incorporated into the macromolecule, and hence an apparent increase in synthesis. This does not automatically follow for an increase in the pool size in which the specific radioactivity of the precursor stays constant. Only if the pool is rate-limiting will increased synthesis occur. This is qualitatively different from the case above, however, because it is a real physiological response of the system.

Empirically the problem is to correct for possible artifacts due to changes in pool specific radioactivity while taking account of physiologically significant alterations in total pool size which are integral parts of the biochemical response. But even if the total as well as radioactive precursor is measured, and any changes in specific radioactivity are compensated for, the measure is still limited in the sense that while the incorporation of radioactivity into product is a cumulative measure (as little turnover is likely to occur if a brief period of labeling is used), the precursor specific radioactivity is an instantaneous "snapshot" at the end of the labeling period. Quite dramatic changes may occur early on but be disguised by later events (see, e.g., Oja, 1973; Marchisio and Bondy, 1974). Only if the specific radioactivity of the actual precursor in the compartment in which synthesis is occurring is known throughout the incorporation period will it be possible to distinguish strictly between the two hypotheses—changes in pool specific radioactivity or enhanced synthesis—on the basis of these data alone. Quite clearly this is an enormous constraint; indeed, we have evidence both in the rat and in the chick imprinting situation (see Section 19.4) that there are changes both in pool size and synthetic activity in different brain regions.

More fruitful ways of circumventing this problem in relation to the protein-synthesis question exist. In the first place, we can seek collateral evidence that processes supportive of protein synthesis are enhanced at times compatible with the presumed elevation in protein synthesis. For instance, enhanced protein synthesis may require enhanced RNA synthesis, and these changes —the incorporation of labeled RNA precursors—can be measured. Of course, such measures would also be affected by changes in blood flow, but the intracellular metabolism and compartmentation of RNA precursors such as orotic acid, uridine, or uracil are quite different from that of lysine. Changes in RNA incorporation over a prior or similar time course to changes in protein would support the synthesis interpretation. In the situation in which dark-reared rats are exposed to visual stimulation, such changes have indeed been obtained, in experiments analogous to ours, by Dewar and co-workers (Dewar and Reading, 1973; Dewar, Reading, and Winterburn, 1973).

Changes might also be presumed to occur in the enzyme RNA polymerase, and the assay of this enzyme in vitro cannot be directly dependent upon precursor-pool effects. But the problem with in vitro enzyme assays is the interpretation of the in vivo significance of an elevation in activity assayed under artificial and optimally activated conditions. Again, however, such changes are useful supporting evidence for the proposition that enhanced protein synthesis occurs—especially if the changes are organized in a temporal sequence such that they occur after the onset of the stimulus but before the elevation in incorporation of amino acid into protein. In the rat, Dewar and Reading (1973) have reported higher visual-cortex RNA polymerase activity in a sighted strain as compared to a strain with retinal degeneration, a situation possibly analogous but not

directly comparable to ours. We have studied RNA polymerase in our chick imprinting situation, and an analogous logic, presumably, lies behind the Chapel Hill group's study of nuclear phosphorylation.

There is, however, another approach to the question of the biochemical specificity of the protein changes found. If only certain proteins change in incorporation rate under the experimental condition, then it is difficult (though, granted the cellular heterogeneity of the brain, not impossible) to account for such changes in terms of generalized precursor effects. This argument prompted our attempt to fractionate retinal and visual-cortex proteins following labeling during first exposure to light (Richardson and Rose, 1973a,b). The experiments were done double-labeled, with [^{3}H] and [^{14}C] precursors in control and experimental animals, or vice versa, and the tissues worked up together to reduce error variability. Fractionation was done first in terms of soluble or particulate proteins, and then both protein fractions were run on polyacrylamide gels. Protein bands were cut out and counted and an average [^{14}C] / [^{3}H] ratio for all bands on the gel calculated; then each band was compared individually with the average. Those that differed significantly from the average (high differential-activity bands) were regarded as representing protein fractions whose labeling was disproportionately affected by the visual stimulation. In the visual cortex 2 out of 21 soluble protein bands and 7 out of 20 particulate ones showed such high differential activity. Elevations of the order of 50 percent in the two soluble protein bands occurred; in the particulate fraction the elevations were less, and one band showed a 40 percent depression. In the retinal proteins significant effects occurred in rather more fractions, both soluble and particulate, suggesting a more general and more complex response to light in this tissue.

This restricted effect seems to rule out the possibility that the protein-incorporation changes are artifacts related to the pool effects; they are responses to the environmental change in their own right. However, a problem with gel techniques of this sort is that while they are useful for indicative analytical purposes, they are not readily adapted to preparative work, subpurification routines, or assisting in ascribing functional roles to proteins. For these purposes, other means must be adopted.

19.2.2 Cellular and subcellular localization
In our first-exposure situation, we have therefore gone back to the whole visual cortex and attempted alternative fractionations. Subcellular fractionation reveals that most of the elevation in incorporation occurs in ribosom-

al and nuclear subfractions (Jones-Lecointe, Rose, and Sinha, 1974), and further subfractionation of these, using double-labeling techniques, is now under way.

Another possible fractionation technique is to separate the visual cortex into its cellular components, neuronal and neuropil (glial-enriched) fractions. This technique has enabled us to show that all of the elevation in incorporation that occurs during first exposure takes place in the neuronal proteins and none in the glial (Rose, Sinha, and Broomhead, 1973). Further subfractionation has shown that the neuronal proteins whose synthesis is enhanced on first exposure are water-insoluble. What is more, an interesting set of observations has enabled us to say something about the labeling kinetics of these proteins. In turns out that in all regions of the normal rat cortex (at least in the 50-day-old animals) incorporation into neuronal protein at short labeling times exceeds that into glial protein by a factor of about 1.6. As the labeling time is extended, neuronal-protein specific radioactivity falls and that of glial protein rises, so that the neuronal/glial incorporation ratio drops from 1.6 to about 0.5–0.6 at 4 hours and thereafter stays constant. We have interpreted this as indicating the presence of a rapidly labelled neuronal-protein fraction which migrates from the perikaryon over a period of hours (Rose and Sinha, 1974a). In the dark-reared animal's motor cortex, the kinetics of this process are as in the normal animal. However, in the visual cortex, even at short times after injection of precursor, the neuronal/glial incorporation ratio does not rise above about 0.7, although it increases toward the normal level if the animal is exposed to light. If the labeling of all protein fractions were generally suppressed in the dark-reared animal, one might assume that prolonging the labeling period to 4 hours should lower the neuronal/glial incorporation ratio still further—to around 0.2. However, this does not occur; at all labeling periods investigated, in the visual cortex of dark-reared animals the ratio remains more or less constant at around 0.7. This, we argue, is compatible with the hypothesis that in dark rearing the synthesis of rapidly labeled, rapidly transported particulate neuronal proteins is suppressed in the visual cortex, and that light exposure switches on their synthesis and export (Rose and Sinha, 1974b). Work is under way to fractionate these proteins further.

It is worth emphasizing that when the analysis has reached this stage, it is subject to severe methodological constraints. The visual-cortex area, from both hemispheres combined, may be equivalent to some 20 mg of protein. Subcellular fractionation yields some 0.5 percent of this in a ribosomal fraction. Cell fractionation yields about 5 percent in the neuronal fraction, some half of which is particulate. Unless one pools animals—a

dangerous procedure in behavioral experiments—one is committed to running protein fractionations with only a few hundred micrograms of protein as starting material, an amount which is far below what conventional methods can satisfactorily handle. The problem is particularly acute when what one is fractionating is not an enzyme activity or the equivalent, where cycling and other techniques can magnify effects, but a difference between two incorporation rates. Double labeling can only partially compensate at this point, where both expense and sensitivity of assay combine as obstacles to progress.

19.3 MORE DEFINED SPECIFIC-LEARNING SITUATIONS

19.3.1. The Hydén experiments

The discussion of the first-exposure experiments has concentrated on the biochemistry of a rather general environmental stimulus. It is now appropriate, against the background of the complexities thus introduced, to look at the attempts that have been made to refine the stimulus situation. Even here, however, it will not be possible to ignore the biochemical issues that arise. The work of Hydén and his collaborators at Göteborg has been a long search for ways of overcoming the scale problem referred to in the previous paragraph. To do this they have used microdissection techniques for individual cells and subsequent ultramicroanalytical techniques for determination of RNA and its base ratios and of precursor incorporation into specific protein fractions.

The research directions and techniques used by Hydén have evolved with the years, and it is often difficult to trace the thread of continuity that links the earlier and the later published results and the hypotheses that have been developed to embrace them. Our account will certainly not be able to do justice to all the models and sometimes surprising experiments which have emerged.

The Göteborg group was initially concerned with changes (both qualitative and quantitative) in RNA during and after the learning of a test which involved prolonged balancing to reach food. As compared to controls, which were caged animals with free access to food, or animals whose vestibular functions were stimulated by mechanically altering their orientation, the "learning" group showed qualitative changes, as determined by base ratios, in the neuronal RNA of Deiters's nucleus. This was superimposed upon a quantitative increase in RNA content of the nerve cells in both the learning group and the functional control group. The qualitative changes in neuronal RNA were found in the cell nucleus and not in the cytoplasm. In the same experimental situation the glial cells of Deiters's nucleus showed an even greater base-ratio change than did the neurons (Hydén and Egyházi, 1962).

In an attempt to control the learning task more closely, attention was then turned to a motor task, which has the advantage of requiring a discrimination. The task chosen involves a transfer of handedness; that is, the animal is trained to use its nonpreferred paw to reach food. Once an animal learns, that is, reverses its preference, this behavior remains stable for very long periods. Moreover, the left side of the brain can serve as a control for the right in this learning experiment. Before commenting on the biochemistry, we should note that these experiments, while concerned with the acquisition of a new skill, may not necessarily be exclusively measuring a correlate of learning. Might not any changes found reflect responses to situations that require, say, the animal's focused attention, but do not involve learning? For example, would a rat that is forced by suitable penalties or rewards to wait for a particular signal before responding —and is, hence, forced to maintain a high level of vigilance—show high rates of synthesis during performance as well as during acquisition? Nothing that has been done so far provides a clear answer on this point (Horn, Rose, and Bateson, 1973a). In addition, the choice of brain region for sampling biochemical changes may be less than obvious (Bateson, 1970). Whatever the behavioral response involved, however, the fact is that in these experiments not only was there an increase in overall RNA content in an area of sensorimotor cortex anterior to the bregma, base-ratio analysis revealed that there was also a striking change toward the production of RNA rich in adenine and uracil. The production of this so-called "DNA-like" RNA has been put forth as evidence for the production of a putative mRNA (Hydén, 1973b). One problem with this interpretation is that transcription of any *small* region of the genome may produce a specific mRNA with a base ratio quite unlike the average complementary DNA base ratio.

The small neurons that manifest the change in nuclear RNA in this cortical region have a scanty cytoplasm; thus the predominantly nuclear RNA response here is said to accord to some extent with cytological evidence. This cortical response, and a similar one in hippocampus, is contrasted with more general changes in the production of cytoplasmic ribosomal RNA, with its characteristic high guanine and cytosine content. Such general responses in RNA synthesis are shown, for example, by spinal motor neurons and other large neurons following intense motor activity. But it should be noted that while the small cortical neurons show an elevation of only 10 pg RNA/cell with training, this is a 40–50 percent increase in total RNA. This is, in fact, a greater response than most of the cytoplasmic RNA changes seen in

response to gross sensory stimulation, hormones such as ACTH, or general stress. This goes unmentioned in Hydén's discussions and perhaps undercuts his clear distinction between a small specific mRNA response in learning and a gross production of ribosomal RNA in response to general ("nonlearning") physiological stimulation. Nevertheless, the results do stand as testimony to the fact that a variety of training procedures can result in increased synthesis of some species of RNA, in both neurons and glia.

The conventional molecular biological wisdom suggests that RNA exists in order to promote the production of proteins. Hydén and his collaborators have been successful in exploring the biochemical consequences of their training procedure here too. Using the transfer-of-handedness paradigm, they measured the incorporation of [3H]leucine into protein in various small brain regions at different times during acquisition and also after the learning curve had flattened out (Hydén, 1973a). In these experiments "corrected specific radioactivities" were used as a measure of protein synthesis following one hour of labeling with intraperitoneally injected [3H]-leucine. A puzzling outcome was that trained animals had a lower incorporation relative to controls in all brain regions. What was done with the data was to compare, in each brain region, the ratios of the corrected specific radioactivities of trained animals to those of controls after different periods of training. The ratios in the cortex were initially of the order of 30 percent, but they increased to approximately 50 percent in animals still on the ascending portion of the learning curve, and fell back to the control values with overtraining. But in the limbic system, particularly the hippocampus, the ratios fell progressively from near 100 percent to about 25 percent with increasing training. A qualitative picture thus emerges which suggests that during acquisition there is a shift of leucine incorporation from predominantly limbic to cortical structures. With overtraining, all brain regions, except one thalamic nucleus, showed similar or lowered ratios compared to those found during the initial training.

The trouble with these experiments from a biochemical point of view is that we really cannot discount so easily the fact that in all brain regions trained animals showed perhaps only 30–40 percent of the incorporation of the control animals. This could not have been a performance effect because animals were matched by this criterion. Such a gross discrepancy once again highlights the problems of controls. Nevertheless, the kind of internal comparison that has been made in this experiment, especially in showing the decline in involvement of the hippocampus with increasing time of training, is perhaps a strategy that could be used more often as a tool in itself. Such regional shifts in metabolism and the influences that mediate them are very interesting aspects of the dynamics of the adaptation occurring during training, and they may yield useful information on the interaction of neural systems during learning not yet detected by other procedures. In this regard a task with a fairly long acquisition time, on the order of days, is perhaps to be desired.

In both the transfer-of-handedness and the balancing tasks, Hydén's results are clearest with respect to neural sites involved in, or promoting, acquisition rather than storage. In the further elaboration of the transfer-of-handedness paradigm, Hydén has emphasized the role of the limbic system, and especially of the hippocampus, its main integrating center. The biochemistry has centered around the brain proteins S-100 and 14-3-2. Previously S-100 was considered predominantly glial, but it has been found to be localized in neuronal nuclei in the hippocampus, and it is now thought to be an important component of the filamentous web below the nerve-cell membrane (Hydén, 1973c). The protein 14-3-2 is considered to be a soluble neuronal protein.

Using very elegant microtechniques, Hydén and his collaborators have been able to show that in the CA3 region of the hippocampus, there is an increase in the amount of both S-100 protein and Ca^{2+}. A new band appears on polyacrylamide gels in the S-100 region, and this has been interpreted in terms of an interaction between S-100 and Ca^{2+} which produces a conformational change in the protein (Hydén and Lange, 1968, 1970; Hydén, 1973a). The elevated Ca^{2+} levels are thought not to be due to tissue swelling since neither Na^+ nor K^+ show the effect, but where the extra Ca^{2+} comes from is not explained. While such sequestering actions, particularly of membrane proteins, would be expected to influence neuronal connectivity, there is no reason why this need be specifically related to long-term storage. In fact, it provides an ideal heuristic model for short-term memory! Nor, for that matter, do the investigators make clear the relationship between these results with Ca^{2+} and the demonstrated higher specific activity, and implied de novo synthesis, of S-100 in CA3 hippocampal neurons with training.

There is intriguing immunological evidence of the relationship of S-100 to learning. During acquisition, the antibody to S-100, applied intraventricularly, is claimed to reach the pyramidal cells of the hippocampus and thereby prevent further improvement in performance. This is not the case for S-100 antibody absorbed with its antigen, or for antibodies to conspecific γ-globulins (Hydén, 1973a). But such disruption of acquisition could be a function of processes other than the hypothesized impairment of connectivity. Nor is the exclusiveness of

these immunological responses to the hippocampus fully established. In fact, as far as we are aware, the enhanced synthesis and involvement of proteins other than S-100 and 14-3-2 have not been thoroughly investigated, and certainly not ruled out.

19.3.2 The Glassman experiments

In a long series of experiments, Glassman and his colleagues at Chapel Hill have examined the effects of avoidance training on several biochemical parameters in rat and mouse brain. Animals were trained to escape electric shock to the feet by jumping from the cage floor to a safe ledge when warned of the impending shock by a light and buzzer. This task is usually mastered within about ten trials, and because the training period was usually fifteen minutes, the animals were overtrained. Two types of control animals were used: one, a quiet control, was left in its cage throughout the experiment; the other was yoked to the trained animal. The yoked animal received the same stimulation from handling, shocks, lights, and buzzers as the trained, but had no safe ledge to which it could escape. The yoked control was included to provide a measure of the effects of stress in the absence of learning. However, as both Church (1964) and Bateson (1970) have pointed out, there are ambiguities in the use of the yoked control which can lead to positive behavioral differences between the trained and control animals in all cases. Moreover, the yoked control probably cannot compensate adequately for such phenomena as arousal and stress, since these may depend upon the attendant circumstances, which differ between the training and control situations.

RNA metabolism was investigated by measuring the incorporation of radioactively labeled uridine injected intracranially 30 minutes before a 15-minute training period. If the animals were killed immediately after training, there was a 28 percent increase in incorporation into nuclear RNA and a 40 percent increase into polysomes in the brains of trained versus yoked mice (Zemp et al., 1966; Adair et al., 1968). This increased incorporation was localized in the diencephalon (Zemp, Wilson, and Glassman, 1967), predominantly in the neurons (Kahan et al., 1970). The effect seemed to be associated primarily with the acquisition of new behavior; indeed, prior-trained animals injected before retest did not show any enhanced incorporation relative to yoked animals. However, those that had been yoked and were then trained, and also those that had been trained and then had the behavior extinguished, did show the increased incorporation of uridine into polysomes (Adair, Wilson, and Glassman, 1968; Coleman, Wilson, and Glassman, 1971). The absence of many of the hormones that have been shown to affect cerebral nucleic acid synthesis, e.g., ACTH (Jakoubek et al., 1972), did not alter these results (Adair, Wilson, and Glassman, 1968; Coleman et al., 1971). Using a similar training situation, Uphouse, MacInnes, and Schlesinger (1972) have also found increased precursor incorporation into polysomes in trained versus yoked animals, while the ratio of polysomes to monosomes also increased.

Glassman's group has regularly calculated incorporation data as the ratio of the incorporated radioactivity in a sample to that in uridine monophosphate (UMP) in an attempt to correct for pool size. This procedure has two drawbacks, the first being that the immediate precursor of RNA is UTP, not UMP, and the specific radioactivity of the two may differ appreciably, and the second being that their method of calculating the UMP specific radioactivity has resulted in their seriously miscalculating the size of the effects found. Entingh et al. (1974) and Dunn (this volume) have redetermined the specific radioactivity of the UMP in the brains of trained and yoked mice and found the UMP radioactivity of the trained animals to be 20 percent less than that of the yoked mice. This accounts for the whole of the increased labeling of nuclear RNA and a substantial proportion of that in polysomes. Such a reinterpretation serves to underline the absolute necessity for determining the true specific radioactivity of the precursor before any corrections are made, and in the absence of such a determination, it may well be better not to correct at all. However, in the Entingh study the injection route was also changed from intracranial to subcutaneous, perhaps because the former route is much more likely to be misplaced, can create local concentrations and abnormal precursor distributions, and has questionable effects in behavioral experiments, where the anesthesia and changed volumes of cerebrospinal fluid or extracellular fluid must create local traumas. (Its main advantage is, of course, the higher proportion of injected isotope incorporated in the brain and hence the lowered expense of experiments.) But it should be noted that there are differences in uptake rate and metabolism when intracranial and systemic injection routes are compared (Marchisio and Bondy, 1974; Schotman, Gipon, and Gispen, 1974).

In later experiments the Chapel Hill group has looked at the effects of training on protein and phosphoprotein metabolism (Machlus, Wilson, and Glassman, 1971a, b). With radioactive pyrophosphate as the labeled precursor, the degree of phosphorylation of nonhistone acid-extractable nuclear protein was found to be higher in the basal forebrain of trained animals than in that of either yoked or quiet animals; moreover, the absolute molar ratio of phosphoserine to serine was higher. Because no precursors were used in this latter measurement, it helps substantiate the incorporation data. However, it was not only training that produced the increased phosphorylation; merely placing a pretrained, but not yoked, animal in the training situation (i.e., "reminding" it of its previous trials) produced the same effect. Thus the increased phosphorylation that occurred after reminding would seem to be related not simply to stress, but also to the prior experiences of the animal.

Using [³H]lysine as the precursor for protein, Rees et al. (1974) have extensively examined the effects of training for 15 minutes and of each of the separate parameters of the training situation, such as buzzers or shocks, on lysine incorporation. Whereas the effects of training on uridine incorporation in the brain decreased with time, those on lysine incorporation did not; indeed, they increased slightly. This fits in well with the known metabolic sequence of protein synthesis, and it is similar to that found in our experiments (see Bateson, Horn, and Rose, 1972). Three measures were made: precursor acid-insoluble (i.e., incorporated) and acid-soluble (i.e., free pool lysine) radioactivities, and also relative radioactivity, which is the ratio of these two. Approximately equal increases in relative radioactivity (RR) in comparison with quiet controls were produced by training, 30 handlings, and 30 buzzers, while 20 shocks produced a slightly lower increase. However, such measures as RR mask the real complexity of the situation. For example, while handling did not affect the pool radioactivity but increased the incorporated radioactivity by 26 percent, buzzers increased both pool and incorporated radioactivity, but the resultant RRs were the same in both handled and buzzer groups. In the liver all treatments produced massively increased RRs without any increase in pool radioactivity. Thus the use of relative radioactivity as a measure can obliterate sharp differences in biochemical responses in different behavioral situations, and these may be crucial to an understanding of overall processes.

19.4 THE CHICK IMPRINTING SYSTEM

A few preliminary comments about the avian brain will be necessary before we start discussing our chick imprinting experiments ("our," in this context, refers to the collaborative work, begun in 1968, between the Open University group and Drs. Pat Bateson and Gabriel Horn in Cambridge). At first it might seem that the chicken brain is a poor system to investigate because it lacks the neocortex that appears in the pallial mantle and is characteristic of mammalian brain organization. But the striatal complex of the avian brain is comparable to the neocortex of mammals in that it is the major recipient of specific visual and auditory projections from the thalamus. In fact, on the basis of very careful comparative studies, Nauta and Karten (1970) suggest that it is not so much the striatal complex and the neocortex but the neurons within them that are homologous. It is the evolution of different morphogenetic forces in vertebrates that results in the same neurons taking on either a striatal or cortical arrangement in the higher integrating centers. Thus at the cellular level we may expect that the specification properties and potential plasticity of the striatal neurons of the avian forebrain would be the same in principle as those of mammalian cortical neurons.

The anatomy of the avian visual system, with its complete decussation of the optic tracts and a well-defined retinothalamohyperstriatal pathway (Meier, Mihailovic, and Cuenod, 1974), known from both behavioral and physiological work to be closely involved in visual-discrimination learning, is favorable to the further study of learning in the neonatal chick. Additional advantages are that posthatch cerebral growth represents cell enlargement rather than an increase in cell number (Zamenhof, Van Marthens, and Bursztyn, 1971), while at the practical level the blood-brain barrier is not yet formed in chicks at the age at which we use them, which greatly facilitates in vivo metabolic work with labeled precursors.

Young chicks learn rapidly, and simple sensory manipulations result in pronounced and long-term behavioral discriminations. While it has been argued that the imprinting process is unique and is not analogous to other forms of learning, especially in older animals, more recent opinion among ethologists and experimental psychologists has tended to reject this argument and to regard imprinting as merely a special case of more general learning phenomena (Bateson, 1971). The exposure to the imprinting stimulus (in our experiments, a flashing light) is the first significant visual experience of the birds, which are maintained in darkness until 18–24 hours after hatching. The period is also one in which a considerable amount of brain development is occurring. Therefore, the cellular effects of imprinting are likely to be intertwined with those of ontogenesis. Nevertheless, we feel that the young chick represents an animal model which gives a reasonable chance of success in mapping some of the cellular correlates of memory storage.

We shall not review our early experiments in detail here (they may be found in Bateson, Horn, and Rose, 1972; and Horn, Rose, and Bateson, 1973a, b). In these, we compared the incorporation of intracardiac-injected labeled precursors into protein and RNA in several brain regions: the midbrain, containing the optic tectum and most of the thalamic nuclei; the base of the forebrain, containing predominantly neo-, ecto-, and paleostriatum; and the forebrain roof, containing most of the hyperstriatum, part of which comprises the Wulst, and

the hippocampus. Thus the midbrain region contains cell systems dealing with primary visual input and the initial stages of information processing, while the forebrain roof is concerned with higher-order processing. In later experiments we have divided the roof into anterior and posterior regions—though it must be remembered that the dissections are somewhat arbitrary and far from anatomically precise.

In the early experiments we found that there was increased incorporation of [³H]uracil into RNA and [³H]lysine into protein in the forebrain roof of chicks that had been exposed to the imprinting stimulus for 78 and 105 minutes, respectively, but not in birds either exposed to a diffuse overhead light or kept in darkness. These changes were preceded by increased activity of RNA polymerase in the same region of the imprinted birds (Haywood, Rose, and Bateson, 1970). The results fitted into an anticipated temporal sequence of biochemical changes in which new protein synthesis followed the mobilization of new RNA synthesis on a DNA template.

These results raised three questions: First, were the changes directly related to the acquisition of the imprinted behavior? Second, were there measurable biochemical events which preceded the increased activity of RNA polymerase? And third, what were the end products of the biochemical sequence? To answer these questions we have used two different experimental approaches: one gives maximal behavioral information but restricts the biochemical techniques that can be used; the other allows more sophisticated biochemical manipulations to be performed while keeping the task as simple as possible, thus giving less behavioral data. In the former the birds are exposed to the stimulus in free-running wheels, from which information about their activity during exposure can be continuously monitored, and they are given a choice test at the end of this period between the imprinted and a novel stimulus. Using this method, we have tried to determine the relation of biochemical changes to behavior.

The problem of controls for "nonspecific effects" such as stress and motor activity constantly besets investigations of this kind. One way of minimizing the consequences of such effects is to use the animal as its own control. By surgically dividing the cerebral hemispheres, we prevented information obtained by one eye, and hence the contralateral hemisphere, from being transferred to the ipsilateral hemisphere. Increased incorporation of uracil into RNA was found in the contralateral (trained) as compared to the ipsilateral (control) hemisphere (Horn, Rose, and Bateson, 1973b). To a certain extent such a procedure minimizes general effects—for example, hormonal levels and precursor supply—but only insofar as they are independent of blood flow, which could differ between the two hemispheres during the exposure (e.g., Bondy, Lehman, and Purdy, 1974). There was no control for sensory stimulation. To approach the problem the effects of the duration of learning prior to the precursor incorporation were examined (Bateson, Rose, and Horn, 1973).

Birds were exposed to the stimulus for 20, 60, 120, or 240 minutes on the first day after hatching in the absence of precursor. On the second day they were injected with [³H]uracil and all exposed to the stimulus for 60 minutes. None of the groups differed from the others in stimulus preference when tested at the end of the second 60-minute exposure, but the incorporation into the anterior part of the forebrain roof was negatively correlated with the duration of exposure on day 1. That is, those birds with the least exposure on day 1—and therefore, we reason, the most to learn on day 2—showed the highest incorporation in the anterior forebrain roof. This was not due to a "carry-over" effect from the first day's treatment because the incorporation of precursor into birds kept in the dark on day 2 was identical irrespective of their treatment on day 1. This experiment would tend to rule out sensory stimulation per se as a trigger for the biochemical effects. However, it might be argued that the onset of visual stimulation on day 1 had initiated a process of neuronal differentiation which in the case of short-exposure birds was not complete by day 2, and that this process was not necessarily related to memory or learning; this possibility is not ruled out by the experiment.

The latest of this series of experiments used only trained birds. There is great variability between birds from the same hatch in their behavior toward the imprinting stimulus. Some respond very early in the exposure period and others much later; some develop a weak and others a strong preference for the familiar stimulus. Several measures of the birds' behavior, during both exposure and testing, were recorded, and we examined their correlation with the extent of incorporation in four brain regions (Bateson, Horn, and Rose, 1975). There were precursor-incorporation effects (depressions) in the whole brain which correlated with the latency of response to the stimulus, and there was a just-significant correlation between specific radioactivity in the anterior forebrain roof and a preference for the familiar, the measure of learning used in these experiments. When the depressions were accounted for by relating the incorporation in the two portions of the forebrain roof to that in the forebrain base and midbrain, there remained only one significant correlation, namely, between the incorporation in the anterior forebrain roof and the birds' preference for the familiar as opposed to a novel stimulus. To put it simply, the more the birds had

learned, the more they had incorporated in the anterior forebrain roof. No other behavioral measure of the battery we made could be related to an elevation in incorporation.

These three experiments very strongly suggest that the biochemical measures are directly related to the acquisition of the new behavior pattern. However, the biochemical mechanism of this is still unclear. In particular, the significance of depressions in incorporation is uncertain. Some later experiments suggest that such depression may be related to decreased precursor availability due to intense motor activity in birds exposed to the stimulus in free-running wheels. Motor activity is also known from other experiments to affect brain protein metabolism (Tiplady, 1972), and care is needed in controlling for this aspect of behavior.

Analysis of the data from this series of experiments suggested that, at the biochemical level, there were two distinct types of effect occurring, one in the precursor-pool radioactivity and one in the incorporation into protein, and that these two effects were only partially correlated. A further experimental series, in which the substantial effects of motor activity were limited by putting the birds in pens facing the flashing light rather than in free-running wheels during exposure, cast some light on this. In these, we looked again at the incorporation of [¹⁴C]lysine into protein, this time with a shorter labeling period (20 min). We looked for changes which might occur *subsequent* to exposure to the imprinting stimulus. While one hour of exposure to the imprinting stimulus is adequate to produce striking behavioral changes, we know that it is a cumulative rather than an instantaneous process; central brain changes presumably continue, as do measurable behavioral changes, beyond the actual time of exposure to the imprinting stimulus. Measuring incorporation over this later period has the advantage that direct responses to changing sensory stimulation, etc., are not occurring then. Both experimental and control birds are in identical conditions while incorporation is taking place, the only variable being prior experience. These experiments showed that when precursor was injected into birds returned to the dark after 60 minutes of exposure, there was an increased incorporation of lysine into cytoplasmic protein in one region—the anterior forebrain roof—in comparison with birds which had not been exposed. However, there were no differences if the period of exposure was reduced to 30 minutes or extended to 120 minutes.

When changes in precursor-pool radioactivity were examined in these experiments, it appeared that following one hour of imprinting stimulation of the exposed birds, free-pool radioactivity tended to increase in all brain regions, but total free lysine also increased in parallel. Thus the specific radioactivity of the pool lysine did not differ between experimental and control birds. Tissue swelling did not occur, and so cannot account for this increase, which may be an analogous phenomenon to the change in free-pool amino acids found in dark-reared rats (see Section 19.2.1). In any event, the change in lysine pool was *not* reflected in a changed incorporation rate into protein in every brain region, suggesting that the lysine concentration is not rate-limiting under these conditions, though there is a likelihood of this happening at times of increased synthetic demand—such as when intense motor activity depletes the precursor pool. As a check that the change in pool radioactivity is not in some way dependent upon intracellular metabolism of lysine, we have repeated the experiment using 2-aminoisobutyrate, which is not incorporated. It, too, showed enhanced uptake into all brain regions in animals that had been exposed to the imprinting stimulus for an hour and then placed back into the dark. Thus the question of changes in blood flow as an important factor in controlling regional shifts in neurochemical adaptation to specific sensory inputs by modulating precursor availability is very much open.

In experiments such as these we have been able to dissociate changes in the incorporation of precursor into RNA or protein in particular brain regions, apparently correlated with particular aspects of behavior that imply learning, from the rather more general biochemical consequences of other aspects of behavior, such as stress and arousal, which may affect metabolite supply. But these latter effects may be necessary for, even if not exclusive to, learning.

Other biochemical parameters that we have measured following exposure to the imprinting stimulus have not been associated with radioactive-substrate uptake and changes in pool size or specific radioactivities, but represent an alternative approach to the question of the biochemical precursors and consequences of enhanced protein synthesis. The increased activity of RNA polymerase in the forebrain roof of trained birds proved to be transient: after 15 minutes exposure it was lower than in birds exposed to diffuse light; it was higher than both dark-maintained and diffuse-light-exposed birds after 30 minutes and was back to control levels by 45 minutes (Haywood, Rose, and Bateson, 1975).

We reasoned that if, as the literature seemed to suggest, cyclic AMP was a possible link between electrical activity and metabolic adaptation, we might see an elevation of cyclic AMP preceding the major effect on RNA polymerase (Hambley, Rose, and Bateson, 1972). But at 15 minutes and other times of exposure, cyclic AMP levels were *lower* in the forebrain roof of birds exposed to the imprinting stimulus, whereas there were elevations in midbrain in birds exposed to either flashing or diffuse light relative to dark-exposed control birds. The major measurable effect of imprinting stimulation on cyclic AMP levels occured after one hour of exposure, when there was an elevation in the forebrain roof relative to dark- or diffuse-light-exposed birds. At the same time in this region there was an elevation in total adenyl cyclase activity. Given that such a change may reasonably represent an effect at the level of the postsynaptic membrane, and that the elevation in cyclic AMP occurs with longer rather than shorter periods of stimulation, it would seem less probable that the effect is an aspect of of the "switching on" of the RNA polymerase. Moreover, it does seem possible, on the basis of in vitro experiments, that cyclic AMP may affect protein synthesis by promoting amino acid uptake into the cells, and thus may be concerned with a translational rather than a transcriptional modulation of protein synthesis in response to polysynaptic visual input in the forebrain roof (Hambley, unpublished results).

Such results as we have obtained using uracil and lysine as precursors for RNA and protein, respectively, are difficult to interpret in terms of known cellular functions. Measuring the activity of RNA polymerase and adenyl cyclase gives us some information about specific biochemical processes, but these are still only inferentially associated with processes directly affecting connectivity. As an approach to this question, we have looked at the activities of two enzymes involved in acetylcholine metabolism. Chicks were exposed for one hour to the imprinting stimulus or kept in the dark (Haywood, Hambley, and Rose, 1973). They were then put back in separate pens in a dark incubator, and the activities of acetylcholinesterase (AChE) and choline acetyltransferase (ChAc) were measured in three brain regions at various times later. There was a transient increase in the activity of ChAc in midbrain of the exposed birds immediately after the end of exposure. The activity of AChE did not change until one hour later, at which time there was an increase in its activity in the forebrain roof of exposed birds. Six hours later there was a general brain increase in the activity of this enzyme in these birds. By twelve hours there was a depression in the midbrain of these same birds, and by twenty-four hours all differences between experimentals and controls had disappeared. The relationship between these transmitter changes and those of protein metabolism are unknown, as are the reasons for the apparent oscillations in activity levels. However, if the altered transmitter-enzyme activities were in fact due to their increased synthesis, then the delay in the appearance of their increased activity could have been simply a reflection of the time necessary for sufficient synthesis to permit detection to have occurred, and for transport to their site of action.

19.5 CONCLUSIONS

We shall now return to the questions which must preoccupy us at this conference:

1. To what extent do the experiments discussed in this review identify biochemical correlates of learning and developmental plasticity, as opposed to other, more general, responses of the organism to its environment?

2. What sort(s) of biochemical mechanism(s) can be proposed to interrelate the variety of diverse effects which have been reported?

These questions must be set in a framework that makes clear the limits of the biochemist's contribution. We would not argue (as do some advocates of simple systems) that to "solve" the problem of memory we need (merely) define the wiring diagram or the firing properties of all the cells used in learning a task. Such specification would be a mammoth biochemical task and a rather boring one. Rather, we are trying to identify general processes at the biochemical level in order to understand how a population of cells alters its *pattern of activity*.

In any event, in response to the first question, it is quite clear that no one of the experiments that have been so far described—ours or anyone else's—is completely capable of singling out *learning* as opposed to something more general; indeed, it must be asked whether it is even possible to design a single experiment in which the *only thing* that happens to the experimental, as compared to the control, animal is that it learns. We think probably not—but the question may in fact not be a meaningful one. Learning must involve a set of complex brain events, and to attempt, even at the behavioral level, to reduce it to a linear set of processes in which one, and only one, change occurs (storage) is surely to mislead. Perception, attention, and arousal are likely to be inevitable correlates of learning; perhaps muscular activity is too, for the types of animal learning usually studied. There are also bound to be complex brain and whole-body correlates, in terms of, for example, hormonal and blood-flow changes, which cannot be discounted. We must learn not to regard these as trivial or as "side effects." Indeed, the concept of a "side effect" (except insofar as it relates to an experimental artifact) is itself one we must struggle against. The point is that certain processes related to learning and memory may be theoretically distinct but not empirically separable in any one experiment. The very difficult task that lies in front of us is to devise a battery of sophisticated behavioral experiments with which to tease apart processes that are both necessary for and exclusive to learning from processes that represent only necessary conditions. In principle, this should be our goal—but the distinction having been made, it should be remembered that any adequate cellular theory must encompass the relationships between all the necessary events.

In terms of the categories described in Section 19.1.1, there is unlikely to be any learning without, at the cellular level, changes of the category-4 type—state-dependent transients—as well as changes in category 3—long-term modifications. In addition (at least in our experiments, though not, perhaps, in those of Hydén and Glassman), we must always expect that category-3 changes—those of learning per se—are going to be superimposed upon those of category 2—developmental plasticity of a more general kind. We shall argue below that while category-4 changes are likely to be different at the biochemical level, we must expect a degree of biochemical similarity in the mechanisms of events of types 2 and 3.

But can any of the changes we have discussed be reasonably securely marked as learning correlates? In all of the experiments, ambiguities in controls exist and alternative explanations of just which behavioral correlate is being examined may be advanced. Nevertheless, at a certain point, criticism of individual experiments becomes more pernickety than productive. Alternative explanations each time become distinct special pleading, and parsimony may reasonably be argued as a reason for rejecting such special explanations in favor of the more unifying one. When the evidence from the inhibitor experiments is combined with that from correlation experiments, it would seem unreasonable to deny that protein synthesis has been shown to be one necessary correlate of learning, and it looks very much as if there is a degree of selectivity in this process such that some proteins in particular brain cells are produced in increased quantities as learning takes place. Taken together, experiments that individually provide weak evidence of specificity may add up to something rather stronger.

When we turn to the question of the details of the biochemical processes, further uncertainty arises. Because the biochemical correlation studies are measures of events occurring during or shortly after learning, we cannot distinguish between category-3 and category-4 (long-term or transient) effects, except by "balance-of-probability" arguments. There is also the special case of category-2 responses being elicited or promoted by the characteristics of the training situation.

It may be that the precise biochemical events associated with storage may not be distinguishable in greater detail until more is known of the mechanisms of the recall process, which may provide further clues to the types of changes that storage involves. Yet we must be wary of assuming that biochemistry has anything to contribute to the study of recall, which is likely to be a problem of scale, address, and connectivity not itself involving the triggering of distinctive biochemical processes, and hence may be more readily approachable at the neurophysiological level.

Long-term memory storage probably requires a maintained alteration in brain cell structure, which suggests that changes in the synthesis of macromolecules are more likely to be involved than are changes in pool sizes or oscillatory shifts in enzyme activities. These latter effects can be interpreted in three ways:

1. as essential aspects (or consequences) of the metabolic mobilization associated with new protein synthesis;

2. as consequences of other aspects of the organism's response to the learning situation; and

3. as correlates of short-term as opposed to long-term memory storage.

The transient changes which have been found in RNA polymerase, cyclic AMP, amino acid pool size, and AChE could be fitted with varying degrees of certainty into one or several of these categories. For example, it would not be unreasonable to link RNA polymerase activity to the metabolic mobilization associated with protein synthesis; but while the changes in pool size and cyclic AMP levels may represent consequences of other aspects of the organism's response to the learning situation, they may nevertheless also be necessary for the storage process. That is, the above categories may not be mutually exclusive. It would be wrong to minimize, at a theoretical level, the interest or significance of such changes. As we argued in a different context above, they should not be dismissed as merely confounding factors in the analysis of effects of macromolecular synthesis.

In addition, we should consider the implication of the fact that in quite a number of studies there are data suggesting that depressions of precursor incorporation occur. This is true at certain stages following the first exposure of rats to the light (Rose, 1967; Richardson and Rose, 1972), following forced exercise (Tiplady, 1972), and in some of the chick imprinting experiments. Protein fractionation suggests that depressions may occur in incorporation into some proteins even when there is an overall elevation of incorporation (Richardson and Rose, 1973a, b). The causes and significance of such depressions may vary with specific aspects of the different training situations, such as intense motor activity. As Booth and Pilcher (1973) suggest, it would be wrong to dismiss the effects as trivial; however, it is clearly incorrect to argue, as they do, that because memory formation may involve the switching off of synapses (Mark, 1970; Rosenzweig et al., 1972), a depression of protein synthesis is a necessary correlate of such a "switching-off" mechanism. The switching off of a cell property such as a synaptic contact may well depend on the active synthesis of some agent which exerts its effect at either a pre- or a postsynaptic site.

In any event, to have shown that the enhanced synthesis of certain proteins is a *necessary* and perhaps exclusive correlate of learning does not prove that it is *sufficient* in the absence of information about other long-term metabolic changes, for instance in glycoprotein or lipid synthesis (Bogoch, 1968). The more positive approach would be to say something about the cellular localization and function of the new proteins that are produced. We are at the beginning of this road. It ought to be possible, once the specific proteins have been more firmly characterized, to ascribe to them both a localization and a function. (Are they axonally transported? synaptic membrane proteins? postsynaptic receptors? transsynaptic molecules? enzymes of transmitter metabolism?). The "signposting" theory of Bogoch (1973), in which the addition of sugar molecules to the surface membrane influences connectivity, is one of several models that can embrace all of these possibilities. But whether the biochemical machinery needed to perform such posttranslational control is present at the presynaptic membrane is open to question (Reith et al., 1972).

The methods by which such processes can be identified exist, and though their application will be laborious, we should not be pessimistic. In our view, moving in this direction is more likely to yield fruitful results than concentrating on the early stages of the modulation of protein synthesis. We may take it for granted that some type of intracellular second-messenger system will be involved, and that this system must be part of a general cellular mechanism routinely employed during ontogenesis for the orderly synthesis of specific proteins and the suppression of the synthesis of others. The question of the details of this mechanism is, we suggest, much better approached as an aspect of the general issue of control of transcription and translation during development of the brain than as a major issue in the biochemistry of learning.

The approach of studying the structural consequences of these metabolic changes makes acute the question of distinguishing between our category-2 and category-3 effects. Are there unique biochemical processes associated with learning which distinguish it from developmental plasticity? This is relatively unknown territory from the experimental point of view. But it seems to us that there is a plausible theoretical framework within which the question can be approached, and which argues from two general biological principles that seem to be of universal significance:

1. the evolution of specific systems from general ones; and

2. parsimony of biochemical mechanisms.

We propose that there is a continuity between developmental plasticity and learning in the nervous system and those mechanisms of plasticity and environmental response that, in evolutionary terms, emerged prior to nervous systems, such as hormonal signaling mechanisms (Horridge, 1968). Among all of these we would expect to find a basic similarity of process, becoming increasingly specific in its cell localization and range of effect. Thus the biochemical changes categorized as "developmental plasticity" are, we suggest, similar to those involved in learning, with the difference being primarily in scale (how many cells are involved), address (where in the nervous system the cells concerned lie), and connectivity.

As has been argued elsewhere (Horn, Rose, and Bateson, 1973a), changes occur in the morphological and functional properties of neurons during ontogeny. The direction of these changes is such that neurons progressively lose their plasticity. The factors responsible for the termination of plasticity may be local, remote but internal (as with changes in hormone levels), or external (as in visual experience).

A given neuron may be functionally connected to many others, but the number of connections may become restricted as a consequence of synaptic activity initiated by experience. The combinations of synaptic inputs necessary to terminate connectional plasticity may be expected to have varying grades of complexity. This view is based on studies in the mammalian visual and auditory systems, in which the features of external stimuli necessary to fire a cell are more complex as recordings are made successively from first-order to fifth-order sensory neurons. Some neurons involved with storage would have the necessary combinations of synaptic inputs provided by relatively simple external stimuli, so these neurons would cease to be plastic quite early in life. For other modifiable neurons, the necessary combinations of inputs may have such a low likelihood of occurrence that the connections remain plastic for a large part of the animal's life.

If experience modifies the connectivity of neurons in those parts of the CNS that are necessary for the detection of common features of the environment, such as lines and angles, the sensory capacities of the animal must be restricted. This occurs, for example, in cats reared in a limited environment (see Chapter 18, this volume). However, in other parts of the CNS perceptual or integrative changes may occur without any apparent restriction of sensory capabilities. This is the case with imprinting, where the characteristics of the stimulus are learned simply as a result of exposure at a particular stage of development. Thus we have at our disposal a model wherein early environmental events influence brain development in such a way as to promote learning.

The crucial question before us, of course, is how this influence is transmitted. We feel that the view we have presented here, of a continuum between developmental influences and learning and the implied analogy with cellular response provides a convenient conceptual paradigm (and, with imprinting, an experimental one) within which to work. (Greenough, this volume, also stresses similarities between developmental processes and learning.) The alteration of the properties of the classifying cells of the mammalian cortex by restriction of functional connections suggests things about neural mechanisms of memory which are not new. Thus the view of cellular changes in learning as the *selection* of particular patterns of synaptic connectivity has been promulgated by Young (1964) and refined by Mark (1970, 1974) to include synaptic repression specifically as a principle. If there is some degree of isomorphism between the dendritic fields of the classifying cells of, for example, the mammalian striatal cortex and the features of the environment they respond to, does environmental modification result in altered dendritic-tree geometry? Is this a morphological correlate of the functional elimination of synapses or another aspect of the process? Certainly dendritic morphology is altered by function (see Greenough, this volume). How then are dendrites organized in development? These are questions about which we know nothing, yet for the biochemist they represent urgent areas of investigation which, it is our contention, are of great relevance to the problem of memory.

If such mechanisms are common to both development and learning, we should not expect to find that unique biochemical changes are associated with learning, but rather that these changes are special cases—more limited in scale—of general responses. Coding for memory, then, would reside in the specificity of synaptic address rather than in a unique biochemistry. The coding potential of the nervous system (and its 10^{14} synapses in the human cerebral cortex) may allow for all the flexibility of development and learning on the basis of a small number of relatively simple and universal biochemical mechanisms.

ACKNOWLEDGMENTS

The ideas developed in this paper, and many of the experiments within it, are the result of ongoing work and discussion in the Brain Research Group at the Open

University, and particularly with Altheia Jones-Lecointe, Ken Richardson, and Arun Sinha; and with Dr. Pat Bateson (Sub-Department of Animal Behaviour, Madingley, Cambridge) and Dr. Gabriel Horn (Department of Anatomy, University of Cambridge). Research support from the Open University and the Medical and Scientific Research Councils is gratefully acknowledged. Comments by Dr. Bateson on the first draft of this paper are particularly appreciated.

REFERENCES

ADAIR, L. B., WILSON, J. E., and GLASSMAN, E. 1968. Brain function and macromolecules: IV. Uridine incorporation into polysomes of mouse brain during different behavioral experiences. *Proceedings of the National Academy of Sciences (USA)* 61: 917–922.

ADAIR, L. B., WILSON, J. E., ZEMP, J. W., and GLASSMAN, E. 1968. Brain function and macromolecules: III. Uridine incorporation into polysomes of mouse brain during short-term avoidance conditioning. *Proceedings of the National Academy of Sciences (USA)* 61: 606–613.

BATESON, P. P. G. 1970. Are they really the products of learning? In G. Horn and R. A. Hinde, eds., *Short-Term Changes in Neural Activity and Behaviour*. Cambridge: Cambridge University Press, pp. 553–564.

BATESON, P. P. G. 1971. Imprinting. In H. Moltz, ed., *The Ontogeny of Vertebrate Behaviour*. New York: Academic Press, pp. 369–387.

BATESON, P. P. G., HORN, G., and ROSE, S. P. R. 1972. Effects of early experience on regional incorporation of precursors into RNA and protein in the chick brain. *Brain Research* 39: 449–465.

BATESON, P. P. G., ROSE, S. P. R. and HORN, G. 1973. Imprinting: Lasting effects on uracil incorporation into chick brain. *Science* 181: 256–258.

BATESON, P. P. G., HORN, G., and ROSE, S. P. R. 1975. Imprinting: Correlations between behaviour and incorporation of ^{14}C-uracil into chick brain. *Brain Research* 84: 207–220.

BOGOCH, S. 1968. *The Biochemistry of Memory*. New York: Oxford University Press.

BOGOCH, S. 1973. Brain glycoproteins and learning: New studies supporting the "signpost" theory. In W. B. Essman and S. Nakajima, eds., *Current Biochemical Approaches to Learning and Memory*. New York: Spectrum-Halstead, pp. 147–157.

BONDY, S. C., LEHMAN, R. A., and PURDY, J. L. 1974. Visual attention affects brain blood flow. *Nature* 248: 440–441.

BOOTH, D. A., and PILCHER, C. W. T. 1973. Behavioural effects of protein synthesis inhibitors: Consolidation blockage or negative reinforcement? In G. B. Ansell and P. B. Bradley, eds., *Macromolecules and Behaviour*. London: Macmillan, pp. 103–112.

CHURCH, R. M. 1964. Systematic effect of random error in the yoked control design. *Psychological Bulletin* 62: 122–131.

COLEMAN, M. S., PFINGST, B., WILSON, J. E., and GLASSMAN, E. 1971. Brain function and macromolecules: VIII. Uridine incorporation into brain polysomes of hypophysectomized rats and ovariectomized mice during avoidance conditioning. *Brain Research* 26: 349–360.

COLEMAN, M. S., WILSON, J. E., and GLASSMAN, E. 1971. Brain function and macromolecules: VII. Uridine incorporation into mouse brain during extinction. *Nature* 299: 54–55.

CRAGG, B. G. 1970. Synapses and membranous bodies in experimental hypothyroidism. *Brain Research* 18: 297–307.

DAVIS, J. M., HIMWICH, W. A., and AGRAWAL, H. C. 1969. Some amino acids in the developing visual system. *Developmental Psychobiology* 2: 34–39.

DEWAR, A. J., and READING, H. W. 1973. A comparison of RNA metabolism in the visual cortex of sighted rats and rats with retinal degeneration. *Experimental Neurology* 40: 216–231.

DEWAR, A. J., READING, H. W., and WINTERBURN, A. K. 1973. RNA metabolism in subcellular fractions from rat cerebral cortex and from the visual cortex of rats with retinal degeneration. *Experimental Neurology* 41: 133–149.

DOBBING, J., and SMART, J. L. 1974. Vulnerability of developing brain and behaviour. *British Medical Bulletin* 30: 164–168.

ENTINGH, D., DAMSTRA-ENTINGH, T., DUNN, A., WILSON, J. E., and GLASSMAN, E. 1974. Brain uridine monophosphate: Reduced incorporation of uridine during avoidance learning. *Brain Research* 70: 131–138.

FERNSTROM, J. D., and WURTMAN, R. J. 1972. Brain serotonin content: Physiological regulation by plasma neutral amino acids. *Science* 178: 414–416.

HAMBLEY, J. W., ROSE, S. P. R., and BATESON, P. P. G. 1972. Effects of early visual experiences on the metabolism of cyclic AMP in chick brain. *Biochemical Journal* 127: 90 p.

HAMBLEY, J. W., and ROSE, S. P. R. 1973. Effects of early visual experience on adenyl cyclase in avian brain. In *Proceedings of the 4th Meeting of the International Society for Neurochemistry*, Tokyo, 1973 (Abstract).

HAYWOOD, J., HAMBLEY, J., and ROSE, S. P. R. 1973. Changes in acetylcholinesterase activity in chick brain following exposure to an imprinting stimulus. In *Proceedings of the 4th Meeting of the International Society for Neurochemistry*, Tokyo 1973 (Abstract).

HAYWOOD, J., HAMBLEY, J., ROSE, S. P. R., and BATESON, P. P. G. 1974. Effects of early visual experience on ^{14}C-lysine incorporation into the chick brain. *Transactions of the Biochemical Society* 2: 241–243.

HAYWOOD, J., ROSE, S. P. R., and BATESON, P. P. G. 1970. Effects of an imprinting procedure on RNA polymerase activity in the chick brain. *Nature* 288: 373–374.

HAYWOOD, J., ROSE, S. P. R., and BATESON, P. P. G. 1975. Changes in chick brain RNA polymerase associated with an imprinting procedure. *Brain Research* 92: 227–235.

HORN, G., ROSE, S. P. R., and BATESON, P. P. G. 1973a. Experience and plasticity in the central nervous system. *Science* 181: 506–514.

HORN, G., ROSE, S. P. R., and BATESON, P. P. G. 1973b. Monocular imprinting and regional incorporation of tritiated uracil into the brains of intact and "split-brain" chicks. *Brain Research* 56: 227–237.

HORRIDGE, G. A. 1968. *Interneurons*. San Francisco: W. H. Freeman.

HYDÉN, H. 1973a. Changes in brain protein during learning. In G. B. Ansell and P. B. Bradley, eds., *Macromolecules and Behaviour*. London: Macmillan, pp. 3–26.

HYDÉN, H. 1973b. RNA changes in brain cells during changes in behaviour and function. In G. B. Ansell and P. B. Bradley, eds., *Macromolecules and Behaviour*. London: Macmillan, pp. 51–75.

HYDÉN, H. 1973c. Organized complexities and protein response of brain cells. In *Proceedings of the 4th Meeting of the International Society for Neurochemistry*, Tokyo 1973 (Abstract).

HYDÉN, H., and EGYHÁZI, E. 1962. Nuclear RNA changes during a learning experiment in rats. *Proceedings of the National Academy of Sciences (USA)* 48: 1366–1373.

HYDÉN, H., and LANGE, P. 1968. Protein synthesis in the hippocampal pyramidal cells in rats during a behavioral test. *Science* 159: 1370–1373.

HYDÉN, H., and LANGE, P. 1970. S100 protein: Correlations with behavior. *Proceedings of the National Academy of Sciences (USA)* 67: 1959–1966.

JAKOUBEK, B., BURESOVA, M., HAKEJ, I., ETRYCHOVA, A., PAVLIK, A., and DEDICOVA, A. 1972. Effect of ACTH on the synthesis of rapidly-labelled RNA in the nervous system of mice. *Brain Research* 43: 417–428.

JONES-LECOINTE, A., ROSE, S. P. R., and SINHA, A. K. 1974. Subcellular localization of proteins labelled in visual cortex on first exposure of dark-reared rats to light. *Transactions of the Biochemical Society* 2: 238–239.

KAHAN, B., KRIGMAN, M. R., WILSON, J. E., and GLASSMAN, E. 1970. Brain function and macromolecules: VI. Autoradiographic analysis of the effects of a brief training experience on the incorporation of uridine into mouse brain. *Proceedings of the National Academy of Sciences (USA)* 65: 300–303.

MACHLUS, B. J., WILSON, J. E., and GLASSMAN, E. 1971a. Effects of brief experiences on the phosphorylation of acid-extractable proteins in brain nuclei. In *Proceedings of the 3rd Meeting of the International Society for Neurochemistry*, Budapest (Abstract).

MACHLUS, B. J., WILSON, J. E., and GLASSMAN, E. 1971b. Phosphorylation of nuclear proteins during avoidance behaviour of rats. In *Proceedings of the 1st Annual Meeting of the Society for Neuroscience*, Washington, D. C.

MARCHISIO, P. C., and BONDY, S. C. 1974. The kinetics of cerebral RNA synthesis in relation to the route of injection. *Experientia* 30: 335–336.

MARK, R. F. 1970. Chemospecific synaptic repression as a possible memory store. *Nature* 225: 178–179.

MARK, R. F. 1974. *Memory and Nerve Cell Connections*. Oxford: Clarendon Press.

MEIER, R. E., MIHAILOVIC, J., and CUENOD, M., 1974. Thalamic organization of the retino-thalamo-hyperstriatal pathway in the pigeon. *Experimental Brain Research* 19: 351–364.

NAUTA, W. J. H., and KARTEN, W. J. 1970. A general profile of the vertebrate brain with sidelights on the ancestry of the cerebral cortex. In F. O. Schmitt, ed., *The Neurosciences: Second Study Program*. New York: Rockefeller University Press, pp. 7–26.

OJA, S. S. 1973. Comments on the measurement of protein synthesis in the brain. *International Journal of Neuroscience* 5: 31–33.

REES, H. D., BROGAN, L. L., ENTINGH, D. J., DUNN, A. J., SHINKMAN, P. G., DAMSTRA-ENTINGH, T., WILSON, J. E., and GLASSMAN, E. 1974. Effect of sensory stimulation on the uptake and incorporation of radioactive lysine into protein of mouse brain and liver. *Brain Research* 58: 143–156.

REITH, M., MORGAN, I. G., GOMBOS, G., BRECKENRIDGE, W. C., VINCENDON, G. 1972. Synthesis of synaptic glycoproteins I. *Neurobiology* 2: 169–175.

RICHARDSON, K., and ROSE, S. P. R. 1972. Changes in ³H-lysine incorporation following first exposure to light. *Brain Research* 44: 299–303.

RICHARDSON, K., and ROSE, S. P. R. 1973a. Differential incor-

poration of lysine into retinal protein fractions following first exposure to light. *Journal of Neurochemistry* 21: 521–530.

RICHARDSON, K., and ROSE, S. P. R. 1973b. Differential incorporation of ³H-lysine into visual cortex protein fractions during first exposure to light. *Journal of Neurochemistry* 21: 531–537.

ROSE, S. P. R. 1967. Changes in visual cortex on first exposure of rats to light. *Nature* 215: 253–255.

ROSE, S. P. R. 1970. Neurochemical correlates of learning and environmental change. In G. Horn and R. A. Hinde, eds., *Short-Term Changes in Neural Activity and Behaviour*. London: Cambridge University Press, pp. 517–551.

ROSE, S. P. R. 1972. Changes in amino acid pools in the rat brain following first exposure to light. *Brain Research* 38: 171–178.

ROSE, S. P. R. 1974. Neuronal protein synthesis and environmental stimulation: State-dependent and longer term effects. *Transactions of the Biochemical Society* 2: 196–199.

ROSE, S. P. R., and SINHA, A. K. 1974a. Incorporation of amino acids into proteins in neuronal and neuropil fractions of rat cerebral cortex: presence of a rapidly-labelling neuronal fraction. *Journal of Neurochemistry* 23: 1065–1076.

ROSE, S. P. R., and SINHA, A. K. 1974b. Incorporation into a rapidly-labelling neuronal protein fraction in visual cortex is suppressed in dark-reared rats. *Life Sciences* 15: 223–230.

ROSE, S. P. R., SINHA, A. K., and BROOMHEAD, S. 1973. Precursor incorporation into cortical protein during first exposure of rats to light: Cellular localization of effects. *Journal of Neurochemistry* 21: 539–546.

ROSENZWEIG, M. R., MØLLGAARD, K., DIAMOND, M. C., and BENNETT., E. L. 1972. Negative as well as positive synaptic changes may store memory. *Psychological Review* 79: 93–96.

SCHOTMAN, P., GIPON, L., and GISPEN, W. H. 1974. Conversion of (4,5)-³H-leucine into ³H₂O and tritiated metabolites in rat brain tissue. Comparison of a peripheral and intracranial route of administration. *Brain Research* 70: 377–380.

SPERRY, R. W. 1944. Optic nerve regeneration with return of vision in anurans. *Journal of Neurophysiology* 7: 57–69.

TIPLADY, B. 1972. Brain protein metabolism and environmental stimulation: Effects of forced exercise. *Brain Research* 43: 215–225.

UPHOUSE, L., MacINNES, J. W., and SCHLESINGER, K. 1972. Effects of conditioned avoidance training on polyribosomes of mouse brain. *Physiology and Behavior* 8: 1013–1018.

VALVERDE, F. 1967. Apical dendrite spines of the visual cortex and light deprivation in the mouse. *Experimental Brain Research* 3: 337–352.

VALVERDE, F. 1971. Rate and extent of recovery from dark rearing in the visual cortex of the mouse brain. *Brain Research* 3: 1–11.

YOUNG, J. Z. 1964. *A Model of the Brain*. Oxford: Clarendon Press.

ZAMENHOF, S., VAN MARTHENS, E., BURSZTYN, W. 1971. Effects of hormones on DNA synthesis and cell number in the developing chick and rat brain. In M. Hamburgh and E. J. W. Barrington, eds., *Hormones in Development*. New York: Appleton-Century-Crofts, pp. 101–119.

ZEMP, J. W., WILSON, J. E., and GLASSMAN, E. 1967. Brain function and macromolecules. II. Site of increased labelling of RNA in brains of mice during a short-term learning experience. *Proceedings of the National Academy of Sciences (USA)* 58: 1120–1125.

ZEMP, J. W., WILSON, J. E., SCHLESINGER, K., BOGGAN, W. O.,

and GLASSMAN, E. 1966. Brain function and macromolecules. I. Incorporation of uridine into RNA of mouse brain during short-term training experience. *Proceedings of the National Academy of Sciences (USA)* 55: 1423–1431.

Note added in proof: The new addresses of Drs. Hambley and Haywood are as follows: John Hambley, Department of Behavioural Biology, Research School of Biological Sciences, Australian National University, Canberra, Australia; Jeff Haywood, Department of Biochemistry, University of Leeds, Leeds, United Kingdom.

20

Biochemical Correlates of Training Experiences: A Discussion of the Evidence

ADRIAN J. DUNN

ABSTRACT 1. The specificity of biochemical correlates of training is defined in terms of its chemical, anatomical, temporal, and behavioral aspects. The existing data are briefly assessed with regard to these different types of specificity.

2. An analysis of the kinetics of precursor uptake into brain RNA leads to the conclusion that it is difficult if not impossible to relate changes in the labeling of RNA with radioactive precursors to changes in RNA synthesis. There are thus at present no data indicating unequivocally that changes in RNA synthesis are correlated with training or learning.

3. The neurochemical responses that have been observed during training involve large areas of the brain, not the small number of discrete cells that might be predicted from current hypotheses of learning mechanisms. These responses involve, in particular, an increase in the incorporation of amino acids into brain protein that appears to be associated with stress and is possibly mediated by ACTH. It is suggested that the stress of a novel experience may increase certain anabolic functions in the brain, thereby enabling plastic changes to occur. In this model the specific location of the changes would be determined by anatomical-electrophysiological factors. The advantage of this model is that the anatomical-electrophysiological specificity does not need to be duplicated by chemical specificity or complex feedback circuitry. Evidence consistent with the model is discussed.

20.1 TYPES OF SPECIFICITY IN LEARNING

There is now a considerable body of evidence for changes in brain biochemical metabolism resulting from training procedures in rodents and chicks (Glassman, 1969; Horn, Rose, and Bateson, 1973; Dunn et al., 1974; Uphouse, MacInnes, and Schlesinger, 1974; Rose, Hambley, and Haywood, this volume). The major problem is that of specificity. It is ironic that specificity in this sense has been so often poorly defined, and I shall attempt to rectify this.

In training experiments there are four distinct types of specificity. These are chemical, anatomical, temporal, and behavioral, or in other words the answers to the questions:

WHICH chemicals are changed?

WHERE in the brain do the changes occur?

ADRIAN J. DUNN, Department of Neuroscience, University of Florida, College of Medicine, Gainesville, FL

WHEN during learning do the changes occur?

WHAT aspects of the experience are critical for the observed chemical changes?

Criteria for the analysis of these specificities have been defined elsewhere (Entingh et al., 1975). I shall summarize here the answers we now have to these questions.

20.1.1 Which chemicals are changed?

A list of the major groups of biochemicals in which changes correlated with training have been observed is given in Table 20.1. Clearly a number of different chemicals have been implicated in learning processes. This list is so long that one might ask whether all the changes may not be merely the result of a general disturbance of metabolism. This is especially plausible since many of the changes were detected by observing the incorporation of radioactively labeled precursors into the brain biochemicals. While this technique is very sensitive, it is unfortunately very susceptible to changes in blood flow or permeability. In fact, its limitations are such that the only conclusive deduction that can be made from an

TABLE 20.1
Brain biochemicals in which changes have been observed during training

Chemical	Experimenters
RNA	Hydén (1967)
	Glassman and Wilson (1970)
	Bateson, Horn, and Rose (1972)
	Matthies (1973)
	Izquierdo (1972)
Proteins	Beach et al. (1969)
	Hydén and Lange (1970a)
	Bateson, Horn, and Rose (1972)
	Rees et al. (1974)
Glycoproteins	Bogoch (1973)
	Damstra-Entingh et al. (1974)
Nuclear phosphoproteins	Machlus et al. (1974)
Synaptic phosphoproteins	Perumal et al. (1975)
Nucleotides	Entingh et al. (1974)
Gangliosides	Dunn et al. (1974)
Acetylcholine	Deutsch (1973)
Catecholamines	Seiden, Brown, and Lewy (1973)

observed change is that the metabolism of the precursor has been altered, which may or may not have been due to a changed synthesis of the product molecule. (See Rose, Hambley, and Haywood, this volume, for a discussion of this "pool" problem.) However, some of the changes have been detected without the use of isotopes, notably in the studies of Hydén and Izquierdo on RNA, of Machlus on nuclear phosphoproteins, and of Bogoch on glycoproteins.

To test for the presence of a general metabolic disturbance, an experiment was performed using [¹⁴C]-glucose as a precursor. Male C57B1/6J mice were injected with [U-¹⁴C]glucose and trained in the jump-up conditioned-avoidance task described by Zemp et al. (1966). The brains were analyzed for radioactivity in soluble, free amino acid, glycoprotein, and protein fractions. The results (Table 20.2) show no large effects. In particular, there was no effect on the uptake of ¹⁴C by the brain. The only significant change was an increase of approximately 10 percent in trained as compared to quiet or yoked animals in the incorporation into the trichloroacetic-acid-precipitated fraction. However, when this fraction was chemically fractionated by acid hydrolysis, no significant change was found in either hydrolysate or residue, or in the ratio of the two.

Better evidence that the changes in the different biochemicals are not a consequence of a gross metabolic disturbance arises from the differences in the behavioral characteristics of the various biochemical responses (see Section 20.1.4).

20.1.2 Where in the brain do the biochemical changes occur?

From our understanding of the way in which the brain functions electrically, it has always been assumed that memory is the result of changes in a few highly specific pathways. This would imply that the chemical changes associated with memory involve a small number of cells, probably distributed throughout the brain. However, the changes that have in fact been observed are rather gross and normally involve whole regions of brain tissue if not the whole brain (Entingh et al., 1975). Even in those cases where changes have been sought in single cells, the anatomical specificity has not been demonstrated. In Hydén's studies of Deiters's neurons (Hydén and Egyházi, 1964) and hippocampal CA3 pyramidal cells (Hydén, 1967; Hydén and Lange, 1970a), while he apparently observed changes between the neurons and the surrounding glia, he did not analyze other neurons in the same region and thus failed to show a specific localization. In fact, in a later study (Hydén and Lange, 1970b) changes were detected throughout the limbic system. An independent study performed in Hydén's laboratory also appeared to confirm gross changes throughout the hippocampus (Levitan, Ramirez, and Mushynski, 1972). Thus the results obtained in no way conform to the expectations, and if we believe that the gross changes are related to the specific changes we deem necessary for learning, the hypothesis must be radically altered if not discarded. I shall return to this point later.

20.1.3 When during learning do the biochemical changes occur?

This has been the least studied of the specificities. In general, changes have been observed during or shortly after training. It is pertinent that the changes in RNA/UMP labeling observed by Zemp et al. (1966) decreased

Table 20.2
Incorporation of [U-¹⁴C]glucose into fractions of mouse brain during conditioned-avoidance training

| Treatment | Radioactive Incorporation | | | | % of TCA-soluble in amino acids | % of TCA-ppt resistant to HCl |
	Blood (dpm/ml)	Whole brain (dpm)	TCA-ppt (dpm)	RR†		
Trained	1,050,000 ± 130,000	319,000 ± 26,000	18,300 ± 1,800	0.0605* ± 0.0016	68.6 ± 0.5	60.9 ± 0.5
Yoked	1,000,000 ± 90,000	305,000 ± 23,000	15,300 ± 700	0.0550 ± 0.0009	67.1 ± 1.3	60.0 ± 0.5
Quiet	967,000 ± 34,000	345,000 ± 34,000	17,600 ± 841	0.0540 ± 0.0024	69.2 ± 1.1	60.9 ± 0.5

†RR (relative radioactivity) = TCA-ppt/(whole brain − TCA-ppt).
*Significantly different from yoked (p < 0.02), and from quiet (p < 0.05) (two-tailed t-test).

Procedure: Three groups of four C57B1/6J mice (male, 6-week-old) were injected intraperitoneally with 10 μCi of [U-¹⁴C]glucose. Three minutes later one group was trained in the conditioned-avoidance task described by Zemp et al. (1966) (see also Glassman and Wilson, 1970) for 15 minutes; a second group was yoked to the trained animals, and the third group was left quiet. Two minutes later the mice were killed and their brains excised and fractionated. Trichloroacetic-acid-precipitated (TCA-ppt) counts were determined on paper discs as described by Mans and Novelli (1961). Amino acids were separated from the trichloroacetic acid supernatant on a Dowex 50 column (Dunn and Giuditta, 1971). The trichloroacetic acid precipitate was treated with 1M HCl for two hours at 80°C to hydrolyze the carbohydrate from glycoprotein and then filtered on glass-fiber filters.

very nearly true at this time after injection). The base composition of brain nuclear RNA is 21.5 percent uracil by weight (Balázs and Cocks, 1967); therefore, the uridine content of brain nuclear RNA is 321 nmoles per gram brain. Thus the relative specific radioactivity of the uridine in brain nuclear RNA at fifteen minutes is $0.32 \times 352 \div 321 = 0.35$. This would signify that 35 percent of the nuclear RNA is synthesized during the fifteen-minute pulse if we assume that the uridine nucleotides are of the same specific radioactivity throughout the pulse. In fact, of course, the initial specific radioactivity is zero, so we are grossly underestimating the proportion synthesized during the fifteen minutes; it is probably more like 70 or 80 percent. This result is not unique for uridine, and similar values may be obtained using the other nucleotides. This deduction assumes that the free nucleotide pools throughout the cells are homogeneous. If they are not, it would not substantially alter the result unless the pool of nuclear nucleotides is very much more radioactive than the mean. If the free nucleotide pool throughout the brain is not homogeneously labeled (which is probably the case), the result would not be affected, provided we assume that the rate of synthesis of nuclear RNA is similar for all the cells. Then "hot" areas would make "hot" RNA, but the averaging of both RNA and nucleotides throughout the brain would compensate for this. We are forced to conclude that at least a substantial part of brain nuclear RNA is being synthesized very rapidly; since it does not appear in any other fraction, it must also be rapidly degraded.

This conclusion of a rapid turnover of a part of nuclear RNA is not unique to the brain. Several years ago Harris (1963) came to the conclusion, on the basis of actinomycin D experiments and labeling studies, that nuclear RNA in liver cells turned over very rapidly indeed. In fact, he went so far as to suggest that hnRNA never enters the cytoplasm. While this extreme position is unlikely to be true, it is now generally accepted that hnRNA turns over very rapidly and that only a small fraction of it enters the cytoplasm, the rest being degraded in the nucleus (Soiero et al., 1968). Presumably some of it is a precursor to messenger RNA, but the function of the remainder is unknown. Thus, when brain RNA is examined following labeling with short pulses of radioactive precursors, one is studying a small class of poorly characterized RNA molecules of unknown function.

A further point is that with such a high turnover rate, the life expectancy of the RNA molecules is too short to be measured with pulses of radioactivity longer than a few minutes. Most probably, uptake of the precursors is so slow relative to the synthesis that the synthesis rate cannot be estimated even with very short pulses. Thus it is impossible to estimate the rate of synthesis of brain RNA accurately using these techniques; as a corollary, the rate of incorporation of tracer precursors into total brain RNA cannot be used as a meaningful index of the rate of RNA synthesis. It follows that changes in the labeling of RNA relative to that of precursors are more likely to be due to changes in precursor metabolism than to changes in RNA metabolism.

To illustrate this point let us reexamine the study of Zemp et al. (1966). In their experiments [³H]- or [¹⁴C]-uridine was injected intracranially. The RNA was then isolated from various subcellular fractions of the brain. To control for potential variability of the injection and the uptake of the uridine into the tissue, the radioactivity in uridine monophosphate (UMP) was also measured. (UMP rather than UTP was used since the biochemical techniques required to perform subcellular fractionation permitted the degradation of UTP, the direct RNA precursor, to UMP. Other uridine nucleotides such as UDP and the UDP sugars are probably also degraded to UMP.) The two-isotope design was used since neither the recovery of RNA nor that of UMP was quantitative. By homogenizing the two brains together, losses for each could be equalized, and the ratio of the RNA/UMP values for the pair took this into account. Unfortunately, inherent in this design is the impossibility of distinguishing whether an increase in the ratio is due to an increase in RNA radioactivity or a decrease in UMP radioactivity. The time parameters used in the experiments are important here. Both trained and yoked animals were treated similarly for the first 30 minutes of uridine incorporation and differently only for the subsequent 15 minutes. Thus a 25 percent increase in the RNA/UMP ratio in a trained animal would indicate a 75 percent increase in RNA labeling in the last 15 minutes, assuming the incorporation to be linear throughout the 45-minute pulse. In fact, the incorporation is not linear (Figure 20.2), so that the increase would be even greater. Since such a large change seems unreasonable, it is more likely that there was in fact a decrease in UMP labeling (possibly in addition to an increase in RNA labeling).

Dan Entingh and I set out to resolve these problems. I devised a quantitative method for determining the radioactivity of the RNA (Dunn, 1971). The recovery of UMP could be quantified by adding a standard amount of [¹⁴C]UMP to the homogenizing medium (see Entingh et al., 1974). Since we had also observed that intracranial injections and the ether anesthesia used for them impaired the behavior, and that the distribution of radioactivity following intracranial injections was poor and mostly periventricular (also reported by Kottler, Bowman, and Haasch, 1972, and Crockett and Quinton,

1973), we preferred to use peripheral injections. We determined that subcutaneous injections of [5-³H]-uridine gave higher incorporations of radioactivity into the brain with greater reproducibility than intraperitoneal injections, and that the results were consistent enough that we did not have to use a two-isotope procedure. Table 20.4 shows the results of such an experiment, typical of a number of experiments performed independently by Dan Entingh, Terri Damstra-Entingh, and myself (see also Entingh et al., 1974). There was no change in the labeling of RNA with subcutaneously injected [³H]uridine concomitant with training under the conditions used by Zemp. The Entinghs went on to show that there were, in fact, changes in the radioactivity of UMP in trained but not in yoked animals, and that these could account for the changes observed by Zemp (Entingh et al., 1974). However, this change in UMP labeling does not appear to account quantitatively for the changes observed by Adair, Wilson, and Glassman (1968) (or by Uphouse, MacInnes, and Schlesinger, 1972) in the labeling of polyribosomes (Entingh et al., 1974). It is also impossible to exclude the possibility that particular RNA species are undergoing changes in labeling, or that the changes in UMP might be a consequence of altered RNA metabolism.

In other instances there is evidence that alterations of precursor nucleotide metabolism could explain changes in the labeling of RNA in nervous tissue. Shashoua (1970) found changes in the ratio of the incorporation of [³H]-orotic acid into uridine and cytidine of goldfish brain RNA during acquisition of a swimming skill. However, changes in free pyrimidine nucleotides were also observed when the aquarium water was poorly aerated and were attributed to hypercapnia (Baskin, Masiarz, and Agranoff, 1972). Also, the increased incorporation of [³H]uridine into RNA observed following electrical stimulation of *Aplysia* R2 neurons has been shown to be dependent upon the uridine concentration in the incubation medium (Wilson and Berry, 1972). These precursor problems may also apply to other studies that have used radioactive precursors to estimate RNA synthesis.

TABLE 20.4
Incorporation of [5-³H]uridine into mouse brain during jumpbox training

Treatment	Total amount incorporated (dpm)	RNA (dpm)	RNA/soluble
Quiet	12,600 ± 890	2,170 ± 170	0.209 ± 0.005
Trained	12,700 ± 830	2,180 ± 120	0.203 ± 0.008

Procedure: Six C57Bl/6J mice (male, 8-week-old) were injected subcutaneously with 100 μCi [5-³H]uridine and trained in the jumpbox as in Zemp et al. (1966).

20.3 THE APPARENT STRESS-INDUCED INCREASE IN THE INCORPORATION OF AMINO ACIDS INTO BRAIN PROTEIN: IS IT UNRELATED TO LEARNING?

Rees et al. (1974) recently reported that after mice had been trained in the conditioned-avoidance task described by Zemp et al. (1966), there was an increase in the incorporation of [4,5-³H]lysine into brain and liver proteins. This response was observed when the amino acid was injected after training had been completed. A similar response was also observed with [4,5-³H]leucine and [1-¹⁴C]leucine as precursors (Brogan, unpublished observations). The response was not specific to training; it was also observed when the mice were subjected to a series of footshocks or loud buzzer soundings (Table 20.5). That the response may have been due to stress was indicated by an apparent habituation; that is, animals trained for several days sequentially showed diminished biochemical responses both in brain and in liver (Figure 20.3). These results resemble those of Altman and Das (1966) with exercise in rats.

Since such a response seemed very likely to have been due to corticosteroids secreted in response to stress, we repeated the experiments using adrenalectomized animals. The results shown in Table 20.6 indicate that the changes observed in both brain and liver also occurred in

TABLE 20.5
Incorporation of [4,5-³H]lysine into mouse brain and liver protein

Treatment	n	Brain RR (mean ± s.e.m.)	% increase over quiet	Liver RR (mean ± s.e.m.)	% increase over quiet
Quiet	48	0.127 ± 0.002	[0]	0.431 ± 0.013	[0]
Trained	14	0.149 ± 0.004	+17***	0.700 ± 0.032	+62***
Yoked	4	0.144 ± 0.008	+13*	0.607 ± 0.039	+41**
Buzzers	11	0.148 ± 0.005	+16***	0.639 ± 0.023	+48***
Shocks	11	0.143 ± 0.005	+12**	0.696 ± 0.046	+61***
Lights	6	0.132 ± 0.004	+4	0.570 ± 0.039	+32**

*p < 0.05. **p < 0.01. ***p < 0.001. (Two-tailed t-test.)
Procedure: C57Bl/6J mice (male, 6- to 8-week-old) were subjected to the behavioral treatment for 15 minutes. Twenty minutes later they were injected subcutaneously with 30 μCi of [4,5-³H]lysine. Ten minutes later they were killed and the radioactivity in brain and liver protein was determined. RR (relative radioactivity) = (radioactivity in protein)/(radioactivity in free lysine). For full details see Rees et al. (1974), from which these data are reproduced.

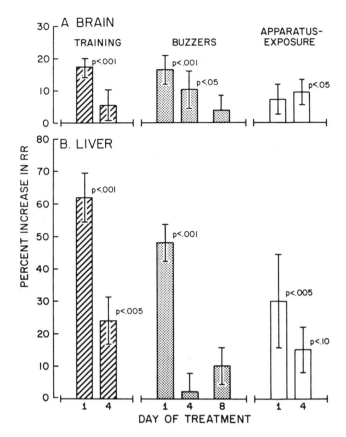

Effects of behavioral treatments on relative radioactivity of brain and liver protein in adrenalectomized mice

Group	n	Brain (mean ± s.e.m.)	% increase over quiet	Liver (mean ± s.e.m.)	% increase over quiet
Quiet	10	0.131 ± 0.006	[0]	0.552 ± 0.064	[0]
20 shocks	9	0.161 ± 0.005	+23**	1.025 ± 0.104	+86***
30 buzzers	9	0.154 ± 0.006	+18*	0.788 ± 0.058	+43*

*$p < 0.05$. **$p < 0.005$. ***$p < 0.001$. (Two-tailed t-test.) Adrenalectomized mice treated as described in Table 20.5 (data from Rees, 1972).

FIGURE 20.3 Habituation of the increased lysine incorporation into protein in response to repeated experiences. Mice were either trained or exposed to the apparatus, with or without random loud buzzer soundings, for 15 minutes each day. On days 1, 4, or 8 they were injected with [³H]lysine and treated as described in Table 20.2. From Rees et al. (1974). Reproduced with the permission of ASP Biological and Medical Press (Elsevier Division).

adrenalectomized animals, which were shown to have very low plasma corticosteroid levels. The results cannot, therefore, have been due to corticosteroids, but could have been due to adrenocorticotrophic hormone (ACTH). Preliminary data indicate that ACTH injected into intact animals does indeed produce a similar response (Table 20.7).

Other workers have shown that ACTH increases the incorporation of amino acids into brain protein. Semigonovsky and Jakoubek (1971) showed that high doses of ACTH increased the incorporation of [U-¹⁴C]leucine into protein of mouse brain. Rudman et al. (1974) showed a similar effect of ACTH and β-MSH (melanocyte-stimulating hormone) on the incorporation of L-[U-¹⁴C]valine, L-[U-¹⁴C]tyrosine, L-[U-¹⁴C]leucine, and L-[U-¹⁴C]lysine into mouse brain protein. Further, Reading (1972) showed that synthetic ACTH₄₋₁₀, a peptide fragment of ACTH that has very little adrenal activity, increased the incorporation of [¹⁴C]leucine

into rat brain protein. However, with the peptide synthesized with the phenylalanine residue at position 7 in the D (as opposed to the L) configuration, no such change was observed. Neither Reading nor Rudman et al. observed any changes in the liver.

Hypophysectomized rats display lower contents of RNA and ribosomes than normal rats (Gispen et al., 1970). Schotman et al. (1972) showed that chronic treatment of hypophysectomized rats with ACTH₄₋₁₀ stimulated the incorporation of [³H]leucine into brain protein. Moreover, treatment with ACTH₄₋₁₀(D-phenylalanine) decreased the incorporation. There is thus widespread support for the hypothesis that ACTH and similar peptides increase the incorporation of amino acids into protein without intermediate adrenocortical activity.

In a number of studies de Wied and his co-workers have shown that ACTH can restore to normal the impaired behavior of hypophysectomized rats (de Wied, 1974). These effects are observed in adrenalectomized animals and thus appear to be direct effects of ACTH, not mediated by adrenal steroids. Also, ACTH₄₋₁₀,

TABLE 20.7

Incorporation of [³H]lysine into mouse brain and liver protein

Injection	Brain (RR ± s.e.m.)	% increase over saline	Liver (RR ± s.e.m.)	% increase over saline
Saline	0.161 ± 0.010	[0]	0.576 ± 0.046	[0]
ACTH (0.1U)	0.216 ± 0.007	+24*	0.995 ± 0.209	73*
ACTH (1U)	0.223 ± 0.010	+29*	1.081 ± 0.154	88*

*$p < 0.05$. (Two-tailed t-test.)

Procedure: C57Bl/6J mice were injected with saline or ACTH. Fifteen minutes later they were injected with [4,5-³H]lysine for ten minutes as described in Table 20.5.

BIOCHEMICAL CORRELATES OF TRAINING EXPERIENCES   317

which has no adrenal activity, is fully active behaviorally. Notably, ACTH$_{4-10}$ retards the extinction of shuttle-box avoidance learning in normal rats, but ACTH$_{4-10}$ containing D-phenylalanine accelerates the extinction. ACTH$_{4-10}$ is also behaviorally active when implanted directly into the region of the parafascicular nucleus (van Wimersma Greidanus and de Wied, 1971). Gold has shown that ACTH also facilitates the acquisition of a passive-avoidance task in rats and in mice (McGaugh and Gold, this volume).

Other pituitary peptides may be behaviorally active. Lysine vasopressin has been reported to retard extinction of active and passive avoidance in rats (Bohus, Ader, and de Wied, 1972), and it is active when implanted directly into the brain in the same areas where ACTH$_{4-10}$ is active (van Wimersma Greidanus, Bohus, and de Wied, 1972). Lande, Flexner, and Flexner (1972) have reported that desglycinamide lysine vasopressin can reverse puromycin-induced amnesia in mice, and this probably accounts for the previously reported effect of corticotrophin gel in this respect (Flexner and Flexner, 1971). De Wied, Sarantakis, and Weinstein (1973) have speculated that these behavioral activities of peptides may explain the so-called transfer effects (Ungar, 1973).

There are other indications that ACTH may have direct effects on cells in the brain. Motta, Fraschini, and Martini (1969) have reviewed the evidence that elevated plasma ACTH stimulates electrical activity in areas of the septum, somatomotor cortex, thalamus, midbrain reticular formation, and amygdala, and inhibits activity in the median eminence, lateral hypothalamus, and hippocampus. These effects must not require adrenal activity since they appear in adrenalectomized animals, and corticosteroids often have opposite effects. Pfaff, Silva, and Weiss (1971) have also shown opposing effects of ACTH and corticosterone on the firing rate of dorsal hippocampal neurons.

20.4 HYPOTHESIS: HORMONAL INVOLVEMENT IN LEARNING

There is thus a body of evidence indicating that ACTH may have direct cerebral effects in both hypophysectomized and intact rats and mice, possibly including an increased rate of protein synthesis. I wish to suggest that these phenomena may play a role in learning, and that this could reconcile some of the existing data on biochemical correlates of learning with the expected small number of localized changes. Specifically, I propose that the novelty of a new experience is a stressor for the animal, and that the physiological reaction to this stress is the secretion of ACTH and possibly other pituitary

hormones (e.g., melanocyte-stimulating hormone, MSH). Besides acting on the adrenal cortex or other peripheral tissues, these hormones then directly alter cerebral metabolism, a process possibly manifested in an increased rate of protein synthesis. The biochemical responses might then facilitate the adaptation of the brain to the novel environment. This may take the form of an altered metabolic state that is conducive to the occurrence of plastic changes (e.g., connectivity changes). This effect would be anatomically widespread, as are the observed neurochemical changes. If we further postulate that plastic changes actually occur only at those precise locations where the electrophysiological state is favorable, we can explain how a general change in metabolic activity can result in a small number of specifically localized changes. Moreover, if the localization of the changes can be dictated by electrophysiological-anatomical factors, we no longer have to duplicate their specificity with a chemical-behavioral specificity.

The hypothesis is that hormones secreted in response to stress increase plasticity in order to facilitate adaptation to the response. This action of ACTH on the brain would then be consistent with its direct and indirect effects on other organs preparing the body to cope with stress. (For a similar hypothesis, but involving a number of neurotransmitters and hormones as well as ACTH, see Kety, this volume.)

Consistent with this hypothesis is the observation that acquisition is facilitated by prior footshock (Levine et al., 1973; Gold et al., 1973) and by ACTH. It also explains why hypophysectomized animals learn poorly and why this deficit can be restored by ACTH. Finally, it explains why, in training experiments, neurochemical responses are observed over such widespread regions of the brain. The fact that the increased incorporation of lysine into brain and liver protein habituates with repeated experience indicates that learning has occurred. Presumably the familiar experience is less stressful.

It is not suggested that ACTH is the only hormone that may have this action, nor that it is necessary for learning. It seems likely that lysine vasopressin and MSH act similarly. Other hormones may act on different regions, or subcellular locations, or with different metabolic responses. It is interesting in this regard that there appear to be differential responses of ACTH and MSH to different forms of stress (Sandman et al., 1973).

ACKNOWLEDGMENTS

Research reported here has been supported by grants from the National Institutes of Health (MH25486, NS07457, and MH18136), the National Science Foundation (GB 18551), and the Ciba-Geigy Corporation. I am grateful to Drs. Edward Glassman and John E. Wilson for the use of facilities and to Eleanor Brown, Mark Williams, and Byron Bergert for technical assistance. I am also indebted for many fruitful discussions to Dr. Dan Entingh, Dr. Terri Damstra-Entingh, Dr. John E. Wilson, and Dr. Edward Glassman, and especially to Dr. Howard D. Rees for kindly allowing me to reproduce some of his data and for reading this manuscript.

REFERENCES

ADAIR, L. B., WILSON, J. E., and GLASSMAN, E. 1968. Brain function and macromolecules. IV. Uridine incorporation during different behavioral experiences. *Proceedings of the National Academy of Sciences (USA)* 61: 917–922.

ADAMS, D. H. 1965. Some observations on the incorporation of precursors into ribonucleic acid of rat brain. *Journal of Neurochemistry* 12: 783–790.

ALTMAN, J., and DAS, G. D. 1966. Behavioral manipulations and protein metabolism of the brain: Effects of motor exercise on the utilization of leucine-H^3. *Physiology and Behavior* 1: 105–108.

BALÁZS, R., and COCKS, W. A. 1967. RNA metabolism in subcellular fractions of brain tissue. *Journal of Neurochemistry* 14: 1035–1055.

BASKIN, F., MASIARZ, F. R., and AGRANOFF, B. W. 1972. Effect of various stresses on the incorporation of [^{3}H]orotic acid into goldfish brain RNA. *Brain Research* 39: 151–162.

BATESON, P. P. G., HORN, G., and ROSE, S. P. R. 1972. Effects of early experience on regional incorporation of precursors into RNA and protein in the chick brain. *Brain Research* 39: 449–465.

BEACH, G., EMMENS, M., KIMBLE, D. P., and LICKEY, M. 1969. Autoradiographic demonstration of biochemical changes in the limbic system during avoidance training. *Proceedings of the National Academy of Sciences (USA)* 62: 692–696.

BOGOCH, S. 1973. Brain glycoproteins and learning: New studies supporting the "sign-post" theory. In W. B. Essman and S. Nakajima, eds., *Current Biochemical Approaches to Learning and Memory*. New York: Spectrum Publications, pp. 147–157.

BOHUS, B., ADER, R., and DE WIED, D. 1972. Effects of vasopressin on active and passive avoidance behavior. *Hormones and Behavior* 3: 191–197.

BONDY, S. C. 1966. The ribonucleic acid metabolism of brain. *Journal of Neurochemistry* 13: 955–959.

BOWMAN, R. E., and STROBEL, D. A. 1969. Brain RNA metabolism in the rat during learning. *Journal of Comparative and Physiological Psychology* 67: 448–456.

CROCKETT, R. S., and QUINTON, E. E. 1973. Distribution of 5-^{3}H-uridine incorporated into RNA of mouse brain as a function of injection route—Autoradiographic investigation. *Federation Proceedings* 32: 597.

DAMSTRA-ENTINGH, T., ENTINGH, D., WILSON, J. E., and GLASSMAN, E. 1974. Environmental stimulation and fucose incorporation into brain and liver glycoproteins. *Pharmacology, Biochemistry and Behavior* 2: 73–78.

DEUTSCH, J. A. 1973. The cholinergic synapse and the site of memory. In J. A. Deutsch, ed., *The Physiological Basis of Memory*. New York: Academic Press, pp. 59–76.

DE WIED, D. 1974. Pituitary-adrenal system hormones and behavior. In F. O. Schmitt and F. G. Worden, eds., *The Neurosciences: Third Study Program*. Cambridge, Mass.: MIT Press, pp. 653–666.

DE WIED, D., SARANTAKIS, D., and WEINSTEIN, B. 1973. Behavioral evaluation of peptides related to scotophobin. *Neuropharmacology* 12: 1109–1115.

DUNN, A. 1971. Use of cetyl trimethylammonium bromide for estimation of the *in vivo* incorporation of radioactive precursors into RNA. *Analytical Biochemistry* 41: 460–465.

DUNN, A. J., and GIUDITTA, A. 1971. A long-term effect of electroconvulsive shock on the metabolism of glucose in mouse brain. *Brain Research* 27: 418–421.

DUNN, A., ENTINGH, D., ENTINGH, T., GISPEN, W. H., MACHLUS, B., PERUMAL, R., REES, H. D., and BROGAN, L. 1974. Biochemical correlates of brief behavioral experiences. In F. O. Schmitt and F. G. Worden, eds., *The Neurosciences: Third Study Program*. Cambridge, Mass.: MIT Press, pp. 679–684.

ENTINGH, D., DAMSTRA-ENTINGH, T., DUNN, A., WILSON, J. E., and GLASSMAN, E. 1974. Brain uridine monophosphate: Reduced incorporation of uridine during avoidance learning. *Brain Research* 70: 131–138.

ENTINGH, D., DUNN, A., GLASSMAN, E., WILSON, J. E., HOGAN, E., and DAMSTRA, T. 1975. Biochemical approaches to the biological basis of memory. In M. S. Gazzaniga and C. B. Blakemore, eds., *Handbook of Psychobiology*. New York: Academic Press, pp. 201–238.

FLECK, A., and MUNRO, H. N. 1962. The precision of ultraviolet absorption measurements in the Schmidt-Thannhauser procedure, for nucleic acid estimation. *Biochemica et Biophysica Acta* 55: 571–583.

FLEXNER, J. B., and FLEXNER, L. B. 1971. Pituitary peptides and the suppression of memory by puromycin. *Proceedings of the National Academy of Sciences (USA)* 68: 2519–2521.

GISPEN, W. H., DE WIED, D., SCHOTMAN, P., and JANSZ, H. S. 1970. Effects of hyphophysectomy on RNA metabolism in rat brain stem. *Journal of Neurochemistry* 17: 751–761.

GLASSMAN, E. 1969. The biochemistry of learning: An evaluation of the role of RNA and protein. *Annual Review of Biochemistry* 38: 605–646.

GLASSMAN, E., and WILSON, J. E. 1970. The incorporation of uridine into brain RNA during short experiences. *Brain Research* 21: 157–168.

GOLD, P. E., HAYCOCK, J. W., MACRI, J., and MCGAUGH, J. L. 1973. Retrograde amnesia and the "reminder effect": An alternative interpretation. *Science* 180: 1199–1200.

HARRIS, H. 1963. Nuclear ribonucleic acid. *Progress in Nucleic Acid Research* 2: 20–59.

HORN, G., ROSE, S. P. R., and BATESON, P. P. G. 1973. Experience and plasticity in the central nervous system. Is the nervous system modified by experience? Are such modifications involved in learning? *Science* 181: 506–514.

HYDÉN, H. 1967. Biochemical changes accompanying learning. In G. C. Quarton, T. Melnechuk, and F. O. Schmitt, eds., *The Neurosciences: A Study Program*. New York: Rockefeller University Press, pp. 765–771.

HYDÉN, H., and EGYHÁZI, E. 1964. Changes in RNA content and base composition in cortical neurons of rats in a learning experiment involving transfer of handedness. *Proceedings of the National Academy of Sciences (USA)* 52: 1030–1035.

HYDÉN H., and LANGE, P. W. 1970. Protein changes in nerve cells related to learning and conditioning. In F. O. Schmitt, ed., *The Neurosciences: Second Study Program*. New York: Rockefeller University Press, pp. 278–289.

HYDÉN, H., and LANGE, P. W. 1970b. Protein synthesis in limbic structures during change in behavior. *Brain Research* 22: 423–425.

IZQUIERDO, I. 1972. Hippocampal physiology: Experiments on regulation of its electrical activity, on the mechanism of seizures, and on a hypothesis of learning. *Behavioral Biology* 7: 669–698.

KOTTLER, P. D., BOWMAN, R. E., and HAASCH, W. D. 1972. RNA metabolism in the rat brain during learning following intravenous and intraventricular injections of ³H-cytidine. *Physiology and Behavior* 8: 291–297.

LANDE, S., FLEXNER, J. B., and FLEXNER, L. B. 1972. Effect of corticotropin and desglycinamide⁹-lysine vasopressin on suppression of memory by puromycin. *Proceedings of the National Academy of Sciences (USA)* 69: 558–560.

LEVINE, S., MADDEY, J., CONNER, R. L., MUSKAL, J. R., and ANDERSON, D. C. 1973. Physiological and behavioral effects of prior aversive stimulation (preshock) in the rat. *Physiology and Behavior* 10: 467–471.

LEVITAN, I. B., RAMIREZ, G., and MUSHYNSKI, W. E. 1972. Amino acid incorporation in the brains of rats trained to use the non-preferred paw in retrieving food. *Brain Research* 47: 147–156.

MACHLUS, B., ENTINGH, D., WILSON, J. E., and GLASSMAN, E. 1974. Brain phosphoproteins: The effect of various behaviors and reminding experiences on the incorporation of radioactive phosphate into nuclear proteins. *Behavioral Biology* 10: 63–74.

MANDEL, P., and HARTH, S. 1961. Free nucleotides of the brain in various mammals. *Journal of Neurochemistry* 8: 116–125.

MANS, R. J., and NOVELLI, G. D. 1961. Measurement of the incorporation of radioactive amino acids into protein by a filter-paper disc method. *Archives of Biochemistry and Biophysics* 94: 48–53.

MATTHIES, H. 1973. Biochemical regulation of synaptic connectivity. In H. P. Zippel, ed., *Memory and Transfer of Information*. New York: Plenum Press, pp. 531–547.

McEWEN, B. S., and ZIGMOND, R. E. 1972. Isolation of brain cell nuclei. In. N. Marks and R. Rodnight, eds., *Research Methods in Neurochemistry*, Vol. 1. New York: Plenum Press, pp. 139–161.

MOTTA, M., FRASCHINI, F., and MARTINI, L. 1969. "Short" feedback mechanisms in the control of anterior pituitary function. In W. F. Ganong and L. Martini, eds., *Frontiers in Neuroendocrinology, 1969*. New York: Oxford University Press, pp. 211–253.

PERUMAL, R., GISPEN, W. H., WILSON, J. E., and GLASSMAN, E. 1975. Phosphorylation of proteins from the brains of mice subjected to short-term behavioral experiences. *Progress in Brain Research* 42: 201–207.

PFAFF, D. W., SILVA, M. T. A., and WEISS, J. M. 1971. Telemetered recording of hormone effects on hippocampal neurons. *Science* 172: 394–395.

READING, H. W. 1972. Effects of some adrenocorticotrophin analogues on protein synthesis in brain. *Biochemical Journal* 127: 7P.

REES, H. D. 1972. Brain protein metabolic correlates of sensory stimulation and behavior in mice. Unpublished Ph.D. dissertation, University of North Carolina, Chapel Hill.

REES, H. D., BROGAN, L. L., ENTINGH, D. J., DUNN, A., SHINK-

MAN, P. G., DAMSTRA-ENTINGH, T., WILSON, J. E., and GLASSMAN, E. 1974. Effect of sensory stimulation on the uptake and incorporation of radioactive lysine into protein of mouse brain and liver. *Brain Research* 68: 143–156.

RUDMAN, D., SCOTT, J. W., DEL RIO, A. E., HOUSER, D. H., and SHEEN, S. 1974. Effect of melanotrophic peptides on protein synthesis in mouse brain. *American Journal of Physiology* 226: 687–692.

SANDMAN, C. A., KASTIN, A. J., SCHALLY, A. V., KENDALL, J. W., and MILLER, L. H. 1973. Neuroendocrine responses to physical and psychological stress. *Journal of Comparative and Physiological Psychology* 84: 386–390.

SCHOTMAN, P., GISPEN, W. H., JANSZ, H. S., and DE WIED, D. 1972. Effects of ACTH analogues on macromolecule metabolism in the brain stem of hypophysectomized rats. *Brain Research* 46: 347–362.

SEIDEN, L. S., BROWN, R. M., and LEWY, A. J. 1973. Brain catecholamines and conditioned behavior: Mutual interactions. In H. C. Sabelli, ed., *Chemical Modulation of Brain Function*. New York: Raven Press, pp. 261–275.

SEMIGONOVSKY, B., and JAKOUBEK, B. 1971. Effects of ACTH on the incorporation of L-[U-¹⁴C]leucine into the brain and spinal cord in mice. *Brain Research* 35: 319–323.

SHASHOUA, V. E. 1970. RNA metabolism in goldfish brain during acquisition of new behavioral patterns. *Proceedings of the National Academy of Sciences (USA)* 65: 160–167.

SOIERO, R., VAUGHAN, M. H., WARNER, J. R., and DARNELL, J. E. 1968. The turnover of nuclear DNA-like RNA in HeLa cells. *Journal of Cell Biology* 39: 112–117.

UNGAR, G. 1973. Evidence for molecular coding of neural information. In H. P. Zippel, ed., *Memory and Transfer of Information*. New York: Plenum Press, pp. 317–341.

UPHOUSE, L. L., MacINNES, J. W., and SCHLESINGER, K. 1972. Effects of conditioned avoidance training on polyribosomes of mouse brain. *Physiology and Behavior* 8: 1013–1018.

UPHOUSE, L. L., MacINNES, J. W., and SCHLESINGER, K. 1974. Role of RNA and protein in memory storage: A review. *Behavior Genetics* 4: 29–81.

VAN WIMERSMA GREIDANUS, TJ. B., and DE WIED, D. 1971. Effects of systemic and intracerebral administration of two opposite acting ACTH-related peptides on extinction of conditioned avoidance behavior. *Neuroendocrinology* 7: 291–301.

VAN WIMERSMA GREIDANUS, TJ. B., BOHUS, B., and DE WIED, D. 1972. Effects of peptide hormones on behavior. In *Proceedings of the 4th International Congress on Endocrinology*, pp. 197–201.

VON HUNGEN, K., MAHLER, H. R., and MOORE, W. J. 1968. Turnover of protein and ribonucleic acid in synaptic subcellular fractions from rat brain. *Journal of Biological Chemistry* 243: 1415–1423.

WILSON, D. L., and BERRY, R. W. 1972. The effect of synaptic stimulation on RNA and protein metabolism in the R2 soma of *Aplysia*. *Journal of Neurobiology* 3: 369–379.

WILSON, J. E., and GLASSMAN, E. 1972. The effect of short-term training experiences on the incorporation of radioactive precursors into RNA and polysomes of brain. In R. Fried, ed., *Methods of Neurochemistry*, Vol. 2. New York: Marcel Dekker, pp. 53–72.

ZEMP, J. W., WILSON, J. E., SCHLESINGER, K., BOGGAN, W. O., and GLASSMAN, E. 1966. Incorporation of uridine into RNA of mouse brain during short-term training experience. *Proceedings of the National Academy of Sciences (USA)* 55: 1423–1431.

21

Biological Concomitants of Affective States and Their Possible Role in Memory Processes

SEYMOUR S. KETY

ABSTRACT The concept of a unitary nature of learning is challenged on the ground that so powerful an adaptation is not apt to depend upon a single modality. It is suggested that in any single species, especially one fairly well advanced in evolution, a variety of mechanisms are implicated. These may be very primitive at spinal synapses, while within the neocortex, the cerebellum, and the hippocampus the primitive processes are probably complemented by a consortium of neural and metabolic processes that accompany learning. A number of possible mechanisms are noted whereby an affective state that follows particular experiences and acts may operate to enhance the consolidation of the sensory and motor patterns preceding and accompanying the act, so that thereafter even a hint of the experience evokes the affective state and increases the probability of the response. A number of observations are examined that are compatible with the hypothesis that the norepinephrine and other biogenic amines, as well as the steroid and hypothalamic hormones, released in affective states may affect cortical synapses in the hemispheres, the cerebellum, and the hippocampus to enhance consolidation of the sensory, motor, or affective associations preceding the affective state. A number of behavioral, pharmacological, anatomical, and neurochemical findings bearing on affect and memory are accounted for by such hypotheses, although crucial evidence in their support is yet to be obtained.

There are few problems in psychobiology more challenging and at the same time more heuristic than that of memory, a remarkable process that underlies learning and has important and obvious implications for pedagogy. The unprecedented growth of knowledge in the neurobiological and psychological sciences which public support of fundamental research has made possible has elucidated many of the processes on which memory and learning appear to depend and has opened the way to an even fuller understanding. I should like to take this opportunity to reflect on some of the information that has been acquired and to speculate a bit on biological concomitants of learning which may be playing more than an incidental role in bringing it about.

21.1 IS LEARNING UNITARY?

There is a theme running through this conference and,

SEYMOUR S. KETY, Department of Psychiatry, Harvard Medical School and Massachusetts General Hospital, Boston, MA

in fact, through the whole field of memory which proclaims the unitary nature of learning. It is known to be a property of all animal species, and there is a belief that the same fundamental process is involved. It has even been suggested that this process is akin to the biological processes involved in the development of the nervous system. At one time, although apparently no longer, it was felt by many that the processes involved in memory were congruent with those involved in the storage of genetic information and represented in the coded sequences of macromolecules.

I should like to take issue with this notion. I have always been impressed with the prolific diversity of nature, and the unity of memory processes, like the unity of biochemistry, seems to be something of an oversimplification.

The ability to profit from experience, to alter subsequent behavior on the basis of previous challenges and their outcomes, is a remarkable and important adaptation for survival. It is certainly less wasteful and may be quite as important as natural selection. That process by which *the species* becomes better adapted or increases its probability of survival can operate only over very long time spans, resulting in adaptations to constant or slowly changing environmental vicissitudes. On the other hand, learning permits *the individual* to develop idiosyncratic adaptations to his own particular environment and to make rapid changes in his behavior. We come into the world with a genetic endowment based upon the experience of the species, and then by means of learning mechanisms we proceed to build upon it, developing highly specialized behavior patterns which are much more closely attuned to our individual experiences.

So profound and powerful an adaptation as learning or memory is not apt to rest upon a single modality. Rather, I suspect that advantage is taken of every opportunity provided by evolution. There were forms of memory before organisms developed nervous systems, and after that remarkable leap forward it is likely that every new pathway and neural complexity, every new neurotransmitter, hormone, or metabolic process that played upon the nervous system and subserved a learning process was preserved and incorporated.

Invertebrate learning has much to teach us, especially since it can be studied more rigorously than the processes occurring in the mammalian brain. We must be aware, however, that it gives us only one part of a remarkable concert of memory processes that are possible and that have come into play in nervous systems of greater complexity and with more varied behavioral options.

I would suggest that many different memory processes have adapted the large range of species for survival, and that in any single species, especially those that are later in evolution, a variety of mechanisms are employed. Primitive mechanisms may be employed at spinal synapses, whereas within the neocortex, the cerebellum, the hippocampus, and other functional systems the primitive processes are probably complemented by a consortium of neural and metabolic processes that accompany learning.

Most theories of memory and most of the models discussed at this conference have emphasized the requirement of repetitive activation of a pathway in the development of a persistent change in properties of component synapses. Chamberlain, Halick, and Gerard demonstrated in 1963 that a postural asymmetry produced by a unilateral cerebellar lesion and the resultant differential activation induced a persistent functional asymmetry at the level of the lower motor neuron in the spinal cord. Further experiments (Chamberlain, Rothschild, and Gerard, 1963) adduced evidence that stimulation or inhibition of RNA synthesis could facilitate or retard this process.

Rutledge, Greenough, and Davis (this volume) each cite evidence that repeated activation of a pathway produces functional and even morphological changes, providing specific and localized support for the earlier findings of Rosenzweig and Bennett (1969) on the effects of a generalized increase in sensory input on cortical weight and cholinergic enzyme activity, and of Globus and co-workers (1973) on the density of dendritic spines. Such processes, which appear to imply the establishment of new neuronal connections and circuits, require protein synthesis, as do more subtle types of long-lived synaptic facilitation, whether it be to form new synapses, to increase synaptic surface, to synthesize more receptors or more transimitter vesicles, or to augment the enzymatic machinery required for transmitter synthesis.

It is possible, however, that the adaptive efficacy of such mechanisms is remarkably enhanced in certain more complex types of neuronal interactions and in later evolutionary developments by the incorporation of special regulatory mechanisms that play upon this primordial process in a selective manner.

21.2 AFFECT AND LEARNING

It is common experience that memories associated with strong emotional states are more firmly established, as is the dependence of many types of learning on reward or punishment. There is, of course, obvious adaptive advantage in mechanisms that favor the consolidation of those experiences that are especially significant for survival. I should like to speculate about possible mechanisms by means of which an affective state that follows particular experiences and specific acts may so operate that even a hint of the experience will in the future evoke the affective state and increase the probability of the response. This could be done by enhancing the consolidation of the sensory and motor patterns preceding and accompanying the act.

Perhaps affect is not taken account of in most theories of learning because it does not enjoy a high degree of credibility among rigorous psychologists or neurobiologists. They think of it as a subjective state—what Skinner would call a "mentalism." But states of affect, such as anxiety, fear, anger, hunger, sexual arousal, satiety, or pleasure, are more than subjective experiences. They are also adaptive biological states associated with general and specific changes in autonomic, visceral, and endocrine function. There must also be appropriate changes in the central nervous system, and as a result of the rich developments in the neurobiological sciences over the past two decades, we are beginning to appreciate what some of these central changes may be. We have become aware of systems of neurons, employing special transmitters such as serotonin, dopamine, norepinephrine, or other substances that, like the peripheral autonomic system, have their origins in a relatively small number of neurons whose axons branch extravagantly to innervate most of the central nervous system. We have learned that many peripherally released hormones, notably the gonadal and adrenal steroids, readily enter the brain and may affect receptors within it. Recently, a series of polypeptides formed within the hypothalamus have been shown to act as modulators of the release of various pituitary hormones. They may have yet other functions, still undemonstrated, since some are found in the cerebral cortex and other areas quite remote from the hypothalamus or pituitary.

The peripheral biological components of these affective states play important roles in the survival of the individual or the species (e.g., the maintenance of blood flow to the brain, increased blood flow to the myocardium and skeletal muscle, or the mobilization of glucose), and it is highly likely that the central components will be found to play similarly crucial roles when we understand them.

There are types of learning, especially in man, that appear to involve more than a simple linkage between sensory perception and motor performance. An important affective component has been added which appears to serve a function in the acquisition of the learned behavior, to be associated in its retrieval, and to guide its performance. Campbell and Coulter (this volume) cite an interesting experiment by Ivanitskii, who conditioned rabbit pups for the first five days of life to lift their heads in response to an odor presented during suckling. Then, after five days without this olfactory stimulus, during which the pups acquired their normal patterns of locomotion, the odor was again presented. Now, instead of merely lifting their heads, they ran toward it in a behavioral response that had never been coupled with the odor before.

Obviously what had been learned was not a performance but an affective association (or, if you will, an appetitive drive). It would not be surprising if the odor could now be used as a positive reinforcement in an entirely new type of learning. Animals can be trained to work for tokens that can be exchanged for food. Some will hoard the tokens and display various forms of gratification in their simple acquisition. Such processes must occur very commonly in human learning, where affective states and their symbolic representations are piled one upon the other and the affective states become ends in themselves and reinforcements for further elaborations. Are there biological concomitants of these affective states which favor the persistence of the pathways that brought them about?

I have elsewhere suggested the possibility that in some kinds of learning, some of the biological concomitants of affective states may act to favor the persistence of the neural patterns preceding them (Kety, 1967) and, more specifically, that biogenic amines and hormones released in such states may modulate trophic processes occurring at recently activated synapses in order to promote selectively the persistence of those circuits that have led to reward or the relief of discomfort (Kety, 1970). The concept was derived from an ingenious learning machine developed by Widrow and Angell (1962), which is made up of conducting units called "memistors." Each memistor consists of a very thin strip of metal immersed in a solution of one of its salts. An independent input can bring about a change in the conductivity of the metal strip by changing the strength and polarity of a plating current applied to it, thereby increasing or decreasing the thickness of the conductive layer. If these units were wired together in a complex network, it is easy to see how the conductivity of a particular pathway could be permanently enhanced by the application of a plating current to its component units. Widrow and Angell's

model was actually more sophisticated, employing distributive properties of the array to achieve the memorization of a pattern. Its learning process had a number of interesting resemblances to learning by the central nervous system; acquisition and extinction occurred along a roughly exponential curve and were not dependent on particular components; and the engram could not be localized because it became the property of the array. However, how the memory trace is laid down geometrically is not as important as the resemblance of each unit to a synapse in which a long-lived change in conductivity may be imposed by an independent input.

It seems possible that the various cortical surfaces act like Widrow and Angell's arrays in a memorization process, that substances released and distributed over them in affective states may serve the function of the plating current to induce a long-lived change in the resistance of recently activated synapses, and that genetically endowed and experientially learned affective states take the place of the external decisions of the operator regarding when and how much plating current to apply.

One would expect that as a result of selective pressure, certain adaptive responses to commonly encountered stimuli from the environment could become genetically endowed; this would apply both to appetitive behavior to stimuli that in the history of the species have been associated with food, water, mating, safety, or relief of discomfort, and to aversive behavior to threatening or noxious stimuli. A species that did not possess such built-in responses would soon become extinct. The power of such processes would be greatly increased if, in addition to wiring in a particular aversive or appetitive response to each significant stimulus, capable of permitting survival before learning and development has occurred, there were also built in a central affective state capable of triggering a repertoire of aversive or appetitive reactions, the complexity of which depended on the state of development. If, in addition, these affective states were associated with the release of substances that might enhance the retention of the sensory and motor patterns immediately preceding or accompanying them, an additional survival advantage would result.

What one would look for would be mechanisms whereby affective states could affect synapses generally but with a greater effect on those recently activated and still displaying some reverberating or "hot-tube" quality. Under such circumstances, an affective state that regularly follows the activation of particular sensory and motor pathways might, with repetition, enhance those patterns in contrast to randomly activated patterns. This enhancement could occur by a process of algebraic summations similar to that which occurs in the computation of average transients.

21.3 RECENT RESEARCH SUPPORTING THE ROLE OF AFFECTIVE STATES IN LEARNING

Certain anatomical pathways and neurochemical processes have been suggested which may satisfy some of the requirements of such a model. In 1967 Scheibel and Scheibel described in some detail the disposition of the "unspecific afferents" in the cerebral cortex; they demonstrated that these long-climbing axons weave about the apical dendrites of pyramidal cells but have rather loose associations with the dendrites, in contrast to the large number of well-defined synapses established at the terminals of the "specific afferents." Shortly thereafter, Fuxe, Hamberger, and Hökfelt (1968) identified the terminations of norepinephrine-containing axons in the cortex, pointing out the similarities in their distribution to that of the unspecific afferents.

Such adrenergic or other amine-releasing terminals invading the millions of sensory-sensory and sensory-motor synapses of the cortex, may provide a remarkably effective mechanism whereby amines released in emotional states can affect a crucial population of synapses throughout the brain. The hippocampal and cerebellar cortex are also characterized by similar fibers, some of which contain norepinephrine. Reivich and Glowinski (1967) have demonstrated a concentration of ^{3}H-labeled norepinephrine about the apical dendrites of pyramidal cells in the hippocampal cortex. There is even rather compelling evidence that axons from the same adrenergic neurons in the brainstem may be distributed to cerebral, hippocampal, and cerebellar cortex as well as to hypothalamus and other areas (Andén, Fuxe, and Larsson, 1966.)

It is well known that affective states are associated in the periphery with both neurogenic and endocrine processes, and it is possible that their central components employ humoral as well as neurogenic modes. There may be an unappreciated but important adaptive function served by the tendency of apical dendrites and their synapses to lie close to the surface in a remarkably similar fashion in the cortices of the cerebrum, hippocampus, and cerebellum, and there may also be a reason why surface is so important in the evolution of the cortex that it is increased severalfold by the development of cortical convolutions. Although embryological and geometrical considerations have been invoked to explain this phenomenon, it is also possible that the position of these structures in close proximity to the cerebrospinal fluid permits substances carried in that medium to act on cortical synapses. Its constant flow from the ventricles over the whole cortical surface offers a means of superfusing the cortex with substances derived from the blood stream at the choroid plexus or released by various neuroendocrine terminals along its path. Diffusible substances injected into one ventricle or into the cisterna magna are thus rapidly distributed over the surface of the brain and penetrate its superficial layers.

The polypetide hormones of the hypothalamus, those from the pituitary, and the steroid hormones of the adrenal cortex, many of which are regularly secreted in states of arousal and stress, may thus have access to this rich population of synapses. Many of these substances have, in one system or another, displayed a capacity to affect the synthesis of RNA or of protein. Corticosterone has been found to restore tryptophan hydroxylase activity in the midbrain of adrenalectomized rats (Azmitia and McEwen, 1969). The steroid hormones and ACTH influence acquisition and extinction in reciprocal ways (de Wied, 1969; Levine and Brush, 1967). It is tempting to speculate upon the possibility that by the actions of adrenal steroids on cortical synapses, consolidation may be delayed during the anxiety of an unresolved situation and facilitated when a favorable outcome is achieved, so that the blood corticosteroid levels fall and ACTH secretion rises.

It is possible that processes of learning which are especially influenced by affective states occur in the various cortices, and that each cortex registers a particular kind of association. Thus sensory patterns and associations could be primarily consolidated in the neocortex, motor patterns in the cerebellar cortex, while in the hippocampus the association of these to the contigent affective states could be acquired.

One way to test the viability of a hypothesis is to examine its ability to predict or explain observations that did not contribute to its development. Several recent observations are compatible with this model, and sometimes it is useful in explaining apparent inconsistencies. Protein and RNA synthesis have both been found to be stimulated at sites of increased neuronal activity (Berry, 1969; Glassman, 1969), but not consistently, perhaps because a crucial affective state has not been contingent. That this is a possibility is suggested by the finding (Gardner et al., 1970) that an aversive stimulation is associated with increased incorporation of labeled uridine into rat brain RNA, but only when the element of novelty is present.

The possibility that some of the substances released in affective states and gaining access to cortical synapses may favor the consolidation of learning by stimulating protein synthesis, is compatible with recently acquired information on the actions of cyclic-3′5′-AMP in the brain. This substance is present in high concentration in the central nervous system, as is the enzyme responsible for its synthesis, adenylate cyclase. It is crucially involved in enzyme induction and protein synthesis in a wide variety of bacterial and mammalian cells and appears to increase the activity of a protein kinase in brain (Miyamoto, Kuo, and Greengard, 1969). There is good evidence that cyclic AMP may mediate the effects of norepinephrine on central neurons (Siggins, Hoffer, and Bloom, 1969), and it is not unlikely that it may intervene in the action of certain hormones in the brain, as it is known to do in peripheral tissues. It is interesting that the stimulation of protein kinase by cyclic AMP can be markedly potentiated by Mg^{++} or K^+ and inhibited by Ca^{++}, which suggests means whereby the effects of certain neurotransmitters or hormones could be differentially exerted on recently activated synapses.

There is evidence for the occurrence of protein synthesis at synapses and for its modulation by catecholamines and other substances. Droz and Barondes (1969) have demonstrated radioactive protein at nerve endings in the mouse cerebrum within fifteen minutes after the administration of labeled amino acids. Gilbert (1972) has adduced evidence for the synthesis of new protein by synaptosomal membrane fractions. There are some observations which are compatible with a stimulation of neuronal membrane synthesis by norepinephrine; at least that amine in relatively high concentrations stimulates the incorporation of labeled phosophorus into phospholipid in brain slices (Hokin, 1969) or in synaptosomal fractions (Sneddon and Keen, 1970).

If one or another substance presumably released in affective states serves to favor the consolidation of preceding experiences, then drugs or procedures that augment or diminish that release should have a corresponding effect on the consolidation of an antecedent training. Recent observations with a few such substances appear to be compatible with this prediction. Amphetamine is thought to increase the release and persistence of norepinephrine at central synapses, while caffeine may potentiate the postsynaptic activity of that amine by enhancing cyclic AMP concentration through its effect on its inactivating enzyme, phosphodiesterase. Both of these drugs, under some circumstances, appear capable of enhancing acquisition when administered immediately after training (Bignami et al., 1965; Oliverio, 1968). Recently, the ability of amphetamine or footshock to counteract the suppression of consolidation brought about by cyclohexamide has been reported (Barondes and Cohen, 1968). Amphetamine has also been found to accelerate markedly the consolidation of the postural asymmetry induced in the spinal cord by cerebellar lesions (Palmer, Davenport, and Ward, 1970). Dunn (this volume) has made observations compatible with the enhancement of consolidation by means of ACTH, while the effects on retention of that hormone as well as norepinephrine administered after training are alluded to by McGaugh and Gold (this volume).

Consolidation can be impaired by agents that deplete central synapses of certain amines. When reserpine, which causes a depletion of catecholamines and serotonin, is injected immediately after a training experience, it impairs retention (Dismukes and Rake, 1972). When the precursors of reserpine, dopa and 5-hydroxytryptophan—which would be expected to antagonize the depletion of catecholamines or serotonin by reserpine, respectively—are administered in conjunction with it, they appear to prevent the obliteration of active or passive avoidance, respectively (Allen, Allen, and Rake, 1974). Diethyldithiocarbamate, an inhibitor of dopamine-β-hydroxylase which is capable of depleting the brain of norepinephrine but not of serotonin or dopamine has been found to produce a significant amnesia when administered before or immediately after a training trial, but not when the administration is delayed for two hours (Randt et al., 1971). Quartermain (this volume) cites more recent observations by his group.

Lesions of the medial forebrain bundle, which would be expected to deplete the telencephalon of norepinephrine, serotonin, and dopamine, are reported to depress acquisition, among other effects (McNew and Thompson, 1966; Sheard, Appel, and Freedman, 1967), and lesions which are limited to the locus ceruleus bilaterally, which would deplete the neocortex of norepinephrine, have been reported to impair acquisition without disturbing other aspects of behavior (Anlezark, Crow, and Greenway, 1973).

Convincing evidence of a long-lived effect of one or another of these substances on transmission in central synapses has not been obtained. However, Libet and Tosaka (1970) have obtained such evidence in sympathetic ganglia, where brief exposure to dopamine produces facilitation of muscarinic depolarization persisting for two hours or more. They suggest "a long-lasting metabolic and/or structural change in the postsynaptic neuron induced by the initial action of the modulating transmitter, dopamine." Crow (1968) and I independently postulated a special role for the noradrenergic pathways of the brain in the facilitation of consolidation; I now believe it to be more reasonable that a number of the neurotransmitters and hormones that gain access to central synapses in affective states play similar roles. It is not difficult to suggest what these substances may be and how they may act, but more definitive information concerning their effects on memory consolidation and the specific neuronal processes by which these effects are brought about remains to be acquired.

ACKNOWLEDGMENT

Work on which this paper was based has been supported in part by research grant MH16674–06 from the National Institute of Mental Health.

REFERENCES

ALLEN, C., ALLEN, B. S., and RAKE, A. V. 1974. Pharmacological distinctions between "active" and "passive" avoidance memory formation as shown by manipulation of biogenic amine active compounds. *Psychopharmacologia (Berlin)* 34: 1–10.

ANDÉN, N. E., FUXE, K., and LARSSON, K. 1966. Effect of large mesencephalic-diencephalic lesions on the noradrenaline, dopamine and 5-hydroxytryptamine neurons of the central nervous system. *Experientia* 22:842–847.

ANLEZARK, G. M., CROW, T. J., and GREENWAY, A. P. 1973. Impaired learning and decreased cortical norepinephrine after bilateral locus ceruleus lesions. *Science* 181:682–684.

AZMITIA, JR., E. C., and MCEWEN, B. S. 1969. Corticosterone regulation of tryptophan hydroxylase in midbrain of the rat. *Science* 166:1274–1276.

BARONDES, S. H., and COHEN H. D. 1968. Arousal and the conversion of "short-term" to "long-term" memory. *Proceedings of the National Academy of Sciences (USA)* 61:923–929.

BERRY, R. W. 1969. Ribonucleic acid metabolism of a single neuron: Correlation with electrical activity. *Science* 166: 1021–1023.

BIGNAMI, G., ROBUSTELLI, F., JANKU, I., and BOVET, D. 1965. Psychopharmacologie. *Comptes Rendus de l'Academie des Sciences (Paris)* 260:4273–4278.

CHAMBERLAIN, T. J., HALICK, P., and GERARD, R. W. 1963. Fixation of experience in the rat spinal cord. *Journal of Neurophysiology* 26:662–673.

CHAMBERLAIN, T. J., ROTHSCHILD, G. H., and GERARD, R. W. 1963. Drugs affecting RNA and learning. *Proceedings of the National Academy of Sciences (USA)* 49:918–924.

CROW, T. J. 1968. Cortical synapses and reinforcement: A hypothesis. *Nature* 219:736–737.

DE WIED, D. 1969. Effects of peptide hormones on behavior. In W. R. Ganong and L. Martini, eds., *Frontiers in Neuroendocrinology*. New York: Oxford University Press.

DISMUKES, R. K., and RAKE, A. V. 1972. Involvement of biogenic amines in memory formation. *Psychopharmacologia (Berlin)* 23:17–25.

DROZ, B., and BARONDES, S. H. 1969. Nerve endings: Rapid appearance of labeled protein shown by electron microscope radiography. *Science* 165:1131–1133.

FUXE, K., HAMBERGER, B., and HÖKFELT, T. 1968. Distribution of noradrenaline nerve terminals in cortical areas of the rat. *Brain Research* 8:25–31.

GARDNER, F. J., DEBOLD, R. C., FIRSHEIN, W., and HEERMANS, JR., H. W. 1970. Increased incorporation of ¹⁴C-uridine into rat brain RNA as a result of novel electroshock. *Nature* 227:1242–1243.

GILBERT, J. M. 1972. Evidence for protein synthesis in synaptosomal membranes. *Journal of Biological Chemistry* 247:6541.

GLASSMAN, E. 1969. The biochemistry of learning: An evaluation of the rate of RNA and protein. *Annual Reviews of Biochemistry* 38:605–646.

GLOBUS, A., ROSENZWEIG, M. R., BENNETT, E. L., and DIAMOND. M. C. 1973. Effects of differential experience on dendritic spine counts in rat cerebral cortex. *Journal of Comparative and Physiological Psychology* 82:175–181.

HOKIN, M. R. 1969. Effect of norepinephrine on ³²P incorporation into individual phosphatides in slices from different areas of the guinea pig brain. *Journal of Neurochemistry* 16:127–134.

KETY, S. S. 1967. Intelligence, biology and social responsibility. In J. Zubin, ed., *Psychopathology of Mental Development*. New York: Grune & Stratton, pp. 193–201.

KETY, S. S. 1970. The biogenic amines in the central nervous system: Their possible roles in arousal, emotion and learning. In F. O. Schmitt, ed., *The Neurosciences: Second Study Program*. New York: Rockefeller University Press, pp. 324–336.

LEVINE, S., and BRUSH, F. R. 1967. Adrenocortical activity and avoidance learning as a function of time after avoidance training. *Physiology and Behavior* 2:385–388.

LIBET, B., and TOSAKA, T. 1970. Dopamine as a synaptic transmitter and modulator in sympathetic ganglia: A different mode of synaptic action. *Proceedings of the National Academy of Sciences (USA)* 67:667–673.

MCNEW, J. J., and THOMPSON, R. 1966. Role of the limbic system in active and passive avoidance conditioning in the rat. *Journal of Comparative and Physiological Psychology* 61:173–180.

MIYAMOTO, E., KUO, J. F., and GREENGARD, P. 1969. Cyclic nucleotide-dependent protein kinase. III. Purification and properties of adenosine 3′5′-monophosphate-dependent protein kinase from bovine brain. *Journal of Biological Chemistry* 244:6395–6402.

OLIVERIO, A. 1968. Neurohumoral systems and learning. In *Psychopharmacology. A Review of Progress 1957–1967*. U.S. Public Health Service Publication No. 1836. pp. 867–878.

PALMER, G. C., DAVENPORT, G. R., and WARD, J. W. 1970. The effect of neurohumoral drugs on the fixation of spinal reflexes and the incorporation of uridine into the spinal cord. *Psychopharmacologia (Berlin)* 17:59–69.

RANDT, C. T., QUARTERMAIN, D., GOLDSTEIN, M., and ANAGNOSTE, B. 1971. Norephinephrine biosynthesis inhibition: Effects on memory in mice. *Science* 172:498–499.

REIVICH, M., and GLOWINSKI, J. 1967. An autoradiographic study of the distribution of C¹⁴-norepinephrine in the brain of the rat. *Brain* 90:633–646.

ROSENZWEIG, M. R., and BENNETT, E L. 1969. Effects of differential environments on brain weights and enzyme activities in gerbils, rats and mice. *Developmental Psychobiology* 2:87–95.

SCHEIBEL, M. E., and SCHEIBEL, A. B. 1967. Structural organization of nonspecific thalamic nuclei and their projection toward cortex. *Brain Research* 6:60–94.

SHEARD, M. H., APPEL, J. B., and FREEDMAN, D. X. 1967. The effect of central nervous system lesions on brain monoamines and behavior. *Journal of Psychiatric Research* 5:237–242.

SIGGINS, G. R., HOFFER, B. J., and BLOOM, F. E. 1969. Cyclic adenosine monophosphate: Possible mediator for norepinephrine effects of cerebellar Purkinje cells. *Science* 165:1018–1020.

SNEDDON, J. M., and KEEN, P. 1970. The effect of noradrenaline on the incorporation of ³²P into brain phospholipids. *Biochemical Pharmacology* 19:1297–1306.

WIDROW, B., and ANGELL, J. B. 1962. Reliable trainable networks for computing and control. *Aerospace Engineering* 21:78–123.

Synaptogenesis,
Stressing Plasticity

22

Synaptogenesis: Effects of Synaptic Use

L. T. RUTLEDGE

ABSTRACT The question "What happens in the nervous system when learning occurs?" has been of special concern to neurobiologists for nearly one hundred years. The basic idea that the nervous system is modifiable is undoubtedly much older, for it has been commonly assumed that as a result of training and practice, nervous-system function improves and knowledge and memories are accumulated and stored. However, there have been few successful attempts to find specific electrical, chemical, or morphological neural changes associated with increased neuronal activity (use). A lack of good models continues to delay experimental work. The author and associates have devised a means of isolating for study the effects of activity on the neural systems linking the two cerebral hemispheres. Electrical responses in one system were seen to vary as an animal learned to use an electrical stimulation of the system as a signal to avoid a foreleg shock. Associated with the electrical change were alterations in certain structures of cortical neurons. Receptive fields (apical dendritic trees) of pyramidal cells increased in size and complexity, and at certain locations synaptic contacts (spines) appeared to become more numerous. Some of the observed changes seemed to appear only when the animal's behavior (learning) was involved, but others occurred with brain stimulation alone (no training). Results are interpreted to mean that neurons participating in circuits where an increase in interneuronal traffic (synaptic use) has occurred respond in part with morphological and functional alterations. Explanations and possible bases for the observations are discussed.

22.1 THE USE-DISUSE HYPOTHESIS

In our efforts to understand the neural basis for learning and memory in the mammalian nervous system, one rather old theory is still popular. This is the "growth theory," sometimes called the "use-disuse hypothesis." It postulates the modification of existing interneuronal connections, or the growth of new connections, as a result of their exercise or use, so that the subsequent passage of neural activity along these pathways is facilitated. Conversely, unused connections tend to regress and become nonfunctional. The origin of this basically commonsense idea is uncertain, but it seems to have been a consequence of the emergence of the "neuron theory" late in the nineteenth century. The acceptance of the existence of

specific interneuronal connections led to the idea that learning and memory are established as a result of the strengthening of these connections between neural cells.

Before the turn of the century a presynaptic basis for the development of better bonds or associations between neurons was proposed by Tanzi (1893). He thought that nerve impulses would increase the metabolic activity of a cell and that this would lead to an increase in cell volume. With more activity, the increase in volume would eventually move the ending ("presynaptic terminal" in present terminology) closer to the next neuron.

It may have been Foster and Sherrington in 1897 (see Gomulicki's excellent review of 1953) who proposed the "synapse as a connection," but it was probably Ramón y Cajal who first described a "use-disuse hypothesis." His original 1895 paper is not readily available. However, a later discussion (Ramón y Cajal, 1911) clearly sets forth his views and provides an appropriate orientation for our purposes. He believed that preexisting pathways in the nervous system (genetically determined, we would say) are reinforced by exercise and that new pathways are established as a result of the growth of dendritic and axonal arborizations. The initial connections present in infancy are modified by exercise throughout life. Neuronal elements extend, grow, multiply, and regress depending upon whether they are exercised (used) or not (disused). These mechanisms form the basis for the development of intellectual capacities, higher functions, memory, logic, etc. It was also Ramón y Cajal's contention that, following lesions of the nervous system, intact cells could restore connections and make new contacts as a result of axonal growths. Contacts between neurons were established by "chemotaxis."

Even without a solid scientific foundation, this hypothesis has provided a theoretical orientation for many workers, and it has been suggested as a basis for learning, memory, neural organization, etc. Konorski (1948) adopted an idea of "morphological plasticity of synaptic connections" to explain classical conditioning. Repetitive association of conditional and unconditional stimuli would transform potential connections in anatomical paths into actual connections. On the other hand, there

L. T. RUTLEDGE, Department of Physiology, University of Michigan Medical School, Ann Arbor, MI

would be a fading or atrophy of synaptic connections with disuse. Critical to Hebb's (1949) ideas on central organization was a synaptic growth process. He hypothesized that new functional groupings of neurons occur as a result of neural activity, lowered synaptic resistance, and synaptic knob growth. Among more recent proponents of the synaptic use theory have been Eccles (1966), Schmitt (1969), Barondes (1970), and Bloom (1970). Eccles (1972) has now modified his earlier viewpoint.

Virtually all of the experiments on the "use-disuse hypothesis" have used the spinal cord as a model. The results of these investigations have been less than definitive, leading Eccles (1966) to conclude that the experiments had failed to demonstrate a synaptic basis for learning. He felt that the spinal cord did not have pre-existing (genetically determined) structures with plastic properties. More recent experiments suggest that disuse may be associated with increased synaptic effectiveness, a point previously stressed by Sharpless (1964). April and Spencer (1969) investigated the monosynaptic response in the ascending spinocerebellar tract and found that chronic tenotomy and de-efferentation *increased* the amplitude of the Group I response. Robbins and Nelson (1970) obtained similar results on a monosynaptic reflex; however, they determined that the enhanced reflex (after the supposed disuse) was a presynaptic phenomenon, the probable cause being the availability of more transmitter. Higher in the nervous system, Burke and Hayhow (1968) achieved disuse by poisoning retinal receptors. Ganglion cells were not damaged, and thus there was no deafferentation. The experiments were therefore different from those of Eccles and others on the spinal cord. Repetitive stimulation of the optic nerve produced increased excitability when action potentials of the lateral geniculate body were recorded. Burke and Hayhow believed that their results could be explained by "hypersensitivity" or an increased accumulation of transmitter in terminals.

A common feature of most of the experiments on use and disuse has been an emphasis on electrophysiological signs of the effects of synaptic disuse. What is needed are good models for investigating possible effects of increased synaptic exercise or use. To this reviewer the abandonment of the use-disuse hypothesis, as implied by Sharpless (1964), would now seem to be unwise. With the reemergence of the Golgi method for selective quantitative study of neural elements, the improvement of long-term stimulating and recording techniques, the rapid advances in computers and related technology, and the use of the electron microscope for quantitative studies, a more concerted approach to the general problem of use and disuse now seems plausible.

22.2 INTERHEMISPHERIC SYSTEMS AS MODELS FOR EFFECTS OF INCREASED SYNAPTIC USE

22.2.1 Results from the study of electrophysiological responses

An acceptable model for the study of use and disuse in the central nervous system may be found in some of our experiments first described several years ago (Rutledge, 1965). In those studies changes in an electrical response, mediated by an extracallosal system, occurred only following training of a behavioral response. The experiments can be described with reference to Figure 22.1.

When the suprasylvian gyrus on one hemisphere is electrically stimulated, two major interhemispheric projection systems may be activated. One is a relatively straight-through, strongly monosynaptic system via the corpus callosum. At least in the rabbit (Globus and Scheibel, 1967), part of the contralateral projection of the corpus callosum is to oblique branches of pyramidal-cell apical dendrites. Recently, specific projection routes in the cat have been carefully defined by Heath and Jones (1971). The other system, which may be activated by the same stimulus, is extracallosal, and relays multisynaptically through the rostral mesencephalon to the contralateral cortex (Rutledge and Kennedy, 1961). The cortical electrical response of this system includes a large positive potential, which may be considered to represent underlying synchronous excitatory postsynaptic poten-

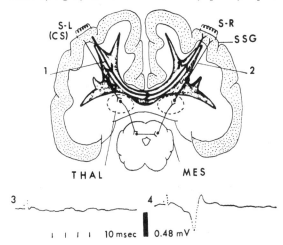

FIGURE 22.1 Callosal and extracallosal pathways and the conditioning experiments. S-L(CS): conditional electrical stimulation of left suprasylvian gyrus (SSG). 1: corpus callosum projection to contralateral cortex. 2: extracallosal system relaying through the rostral mesencephalon (MES) to contralateral cortex. THAL: thalamus. The computer-averaged response on the right gyrus to left stimulation (4) was found after training. No response appeared on the left gyrus (3) after comparable test stimulations to right gyrus.

tials (EPSPs) of apical dendrites. The projection in this system may be considered to be in part to the upper apical dendritic trees of pyramidal cells. This suggestion has no anatomical support, but postsynaptic potentials of apical dendrites following reticular-formation stimulation were described by Purpura (1958).

In the early experiments adult cats were trained with conditional electrical stimulation of the suprasylvian gyrus on one hemisphere (Figure 22.1; Rutledge, 1965). The unconditional stimulus was foreleg shock. Conditioned foreleg flexions were established, and the animals were overtrained. Each cat received 20 training trials per day for about 50 days. Tests for the electrical responses mediated by the callosal and extracallosal systems were made during training and/or in terminal acute experiments. Electrical potentials in the cortical projection of the extracallosal system were markedly enhanced contralateral to the conditoning (see the response labeled 4 in Figure 22.1). In the opposite direction responses were not present when comparable stimulation parameters were used. The electrical potential differences in the responses recorded from the two suprasylvian gyri lasted for at least several weeks, even in the absence of intervening training or brain stimulation. Foot flexions conditioned to brain stimulation in various loci may thus be relatively permanent once established. Cats retain the response ability for many months without periodic training. The results summarized in Figure 22.1 are offered as evidence that the facilitation of conduction in a multi-synaptic pathway occurred along with the training the animals received. In control cats, brain stimulation without foreleg shock did not produce similar results. The control experiments showed that exercise or use of an interhemispheric pathway was insufficient by itself to produce permanent electrical signs of facilitated transmission in the pathway.

The facilitation experiments (Rutledge, 1965) led to a consideration of the possible changes in cortical neuronal morphology which might also be found to occur as a result of the training (conditioning). Were there changes in apical dendritic spines as projection sites of the interhemispheric systems? Did apical dendritic fields change? Would pyramidal-cell axons participating in a chronically stimulated pathway change in any way? These important questions conceivably could be answered by careful quantitative study using the Golgi method and the light microscope.

Figure 22.2 depicts the projections of the callosal and extracallosal pathways and cortical elements, which seemed to be logical places for careful study. It was assumed that both systems project in part to various portions of pyramidal-cell apical dendrites. Attention was

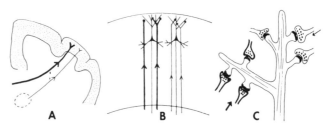

FIGURE 22.2 Contralateral projections of callosal (dark lines) and extracallosal (light lines) systems. A: both systems project contralaterally to homotopic cortex. B: both systems project strongly to apical dendrites of pyramidal cells in layers II and III. C: the corpus callosum projects in part to spines on oblique branches; the extracallosal projection is in part to spines on vertical portions of apical dendrites.

directed to pyramidal cells of the upper cortical layers and to dendritic spines on vertical, oblique, and terminal branches (Figure 22.2B,C). Basal dendrites were studied as controls since it is likely that neither system projects strongly to them. The pyramidal-cell apical dendritic tree was considered for possible changes in its branches, in the lengths or density of elements. Specifically, data were sought on the various measures described in Figure 22.3. Not shown are the measures made on numbers of

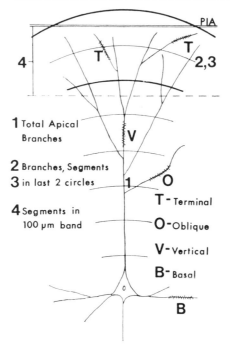

FIGURE 22.3 Areas measured on pyramidal-cell dendrites. Soma locations about 400μm from pia. Concentric circles are spaced at 50-μm intervals to pia. 1: total apical dendritic branches. 2,3: branches and segments found in last two areas of concentric circles. 4: segments in 100-μm band parallel to pia (this is a more consistent area for measurement because of the unpredictable spacing of the last circle area). Spinal counts were made in 10-μm portions at the locations indicated.

axon collaterals and their branches. Details of these experiments are available elsewhere (Rutledge, Wright, and Duncan, 1974).

In the present investigations adult cats were trained as in the "facilitation experiments" (Rutledge, 1965). No recordings of electrical responses were made. Electrodes were implanted on one side only, and they differed slightly from the earlier experiments in being 6–8 mm apart. Control animals were not trained: they received brain stimulation and foreleg shock, but separated by about 30 sec. No conditioned responses occurred in the untrained cats.

Brain tissues were removed from stimulated and homotopic cortex. The Golgi-Cox method as we have described it (Rutledge, Duncan, and Beatty, 1969) was used. All study of tissue sections was done blind, with the identity of brain side and treatment (trained or untrained) coded.

22.2.2 Results from the study of apical dendrites

For present purposes, only averaged data are given, and differences are shown as percentages (Table 22.1). All measures on apical dendrites, in both trained and untrained cats, were significantly greater in contralateral cortex. Greater percentage differences were seen in data from the trained cats than in data from controls. It seems reasonable to conclude that chronic brain stimulation produces morphological changes in apical dendritic branches and segments of the contralateral cortex.

TABLE 22.1
Apical dendritic measurements in stimulated (S) and contralateral (C) cortex

| | Means | | % increase | |
	S	C	(C−S)/S	p
Trained (126 measures each side)				
Total branches	11.05	12.69	15	<0.0001
Branches in last 2 circles	0.57	1.38	142	<0.0001
Segments in last 2 circles	4.17	8.94	114	<0.0001
Segments in 100-μm band	4.01	10.75	168	<0.0001
Untrained (66 measures each side)				
Total branches	12.11	13.46	11	∼0.05
Branches in last 2 circles	0.71	1.55	118	<0.003
Segments in last 2 circles	4.97	8.71	75	<0.001
Segments in 100-μm band	4.64	11.89	153	<0.0001

Four trained animals (126 measures) and two untrained animals (66 measures) were studied. Probability levels (p) were determined by t-test on the raw data.

TABLE 22.2
Dendritic-spine counts at four locations on pyramidal cells

	S	C	% increase (C−S)/S	p
Vertical				
Trained	7.64 (64)	8.46 (84)	10.7	∼0.001
Untrained	8.44 (62)	8.33 (64)	−1.3	0.73
Oblique				
Trained	6.32 (74)	7.54 (74)	19.3	<0.0001
Untrained	7.48 (81)	7.62 (85)	1.9	0.60
Terminal				
Trained	5.85 (73)	6.56 (73)	12.1	0.03
Untrained	6.54 (54)	7.51 (57)	14.8	0.01
Basal				
Trained	6.03 (74)	6.02 (64)	0.0	0.96
Untrained	6.14 (81)	5.80 (82)	−5.5	0.13

Counts were made in stimulated cortex (S) and contralateral cortex (C). The number of samples is given in parentheses. Probability levels (p) were determined from t-tests on raw data.

22.2.3 Results from the study of dendritic spines

Table 22.2 is a summary of the spine measures made at four locations on pyramidal cells in layers II and III. Counts made of spines on vertical and oblique branches were significantly greater in contralateral cortex, but only in trained animals. A reasonable conclusion is that training is necessary to produce spinal increases in the two locations. For terminal counts, brain stimulation alone seems to have been the only necessary procedure. There were significantly more spines contralaterally in both groups of animals. Spinal counts on basal branches were the same on both sides of the brain in both groups. The finding of no differences in these basal measures lends more importance to the other observed differences.

TABLE 22.3
Numbers of axon collaterals and branches in layer-II and layer-III pyramidal cells

	S	C	% increase (S−C)/C	p
Trained	(101)	(129)		
Collaterals	4.71	4.25	10.8	0.07
Branches	8.44	8.24	2.4	0.75
Untrained	(56)	(57)		
Collaterals	4.05	3.68	10.1	0.24
Branches	7.55	5.86	28.8	0.02

Counts were made in stimulated cortex (S) and contralateral cortex (C). The number of measurements is given in parentheses. Probability levels (p) were determined from t-tests on raw data.

As discussed above, no differences were expected on the basal dendrites since projections from the two interhemispheric systems to basal regions are supposedly sparse.

22.2.4 Results from axon measurements

Data on axon collaterals and their branches are summarized in Table 22.3. In contrast to the measures of Tables 22.1 and 22.2, counts here were greater on the stimulated than on the contralateral side. However, in only one instance (branches in untrained animals) were values statistically greater on the stimulated side. These data therefore offer only equivocal support for the hypothesis that pyramidal-cell axons in the stimulated gyrus reflect axonal changes as a result of the stimulation. Further discussion of these data does not seem warranted.

22.2.5 Microscopic qualitative observations

The low-power microscopic picture of the histological material showed apical dendrites, in cortex contralateral to the stimulated gyrus, packed rather closely to the pia. Figure 22.4 shows photomicrographs taken from both sides of the brain in an experimental cat and one from an experimentally naive cat. Pictures taken at one focal plane do not convey fully the marked patterns of bundle-like dendritic groupings in contralateral cortex. Groups were arranged in a drooping, weeping-willow, semicircular manner near the pia. Similar features are never as marked or as prominent in cortex on the stimulated gyrus or in the suprasylvian gyrus in naive animals. As visually assuring and esthetically pleasing as photomicrographs of Golgi-impregnated neocortex may be, the great density of branches and arches of apical dendrites (see also Scheibel and Scheibel, 1971) renders them unusable for comparative purposes. A method was therefore devised to describe the differences in dendritic terminals between the two sides. Upon closer study at higher magnification, it could be seen that apical dendritic terminals in many sections had unusual contortions, sharp angles, tips touching the pia, and other unusual features. Drawings were made to illustrate the various types. After the identifying code was broken, the examples were assigned to the correct brain sides, stimulated or contralateral. Some representative examples are assembled in Figure 22.5. Several types of terminals were found readily in contralateral cortex but infrequently in stimulated cortex. The most common type consisted of tips that reflected back from the pia at an acute angle or with a circular inclination (Figure 22.5, lower). Another frequently seen type in contralateral cortex consisted of tips that gave the impression of having firmly touched the pia (Figure 22.5, middle). Especially thin and/

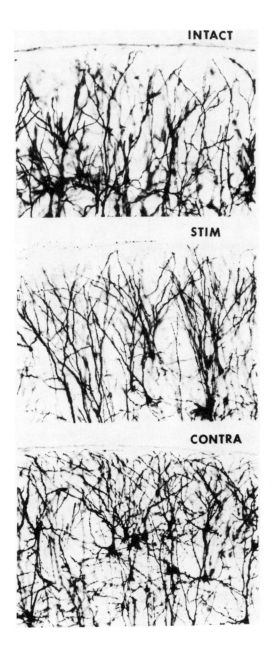

FIGURE 22.4 Photomicrographs of upper cortex in suprasylvian gyri stained by Golgi method. All taken at × 100. Tissue sections are 100 μm thick. INTACT: from nonexperimental adult cat. STIM: from cortex chronically stimulated. CONTRA: from cortex homotopic to that receiving conditional excitation. CONTRA and STIM are from same cat. Because of focal-plane differences in the microscope, only gross appearance can be illustrated. Both INTACT and STIM had some terminals closer to pia at other focal planes, but CONTRA showed terminals reaching pia in all focal planes. Notice the greater density of apical dendrites in CONTRA. In other tissues apical dendrites were more packed, and whorls or bundles appeared.

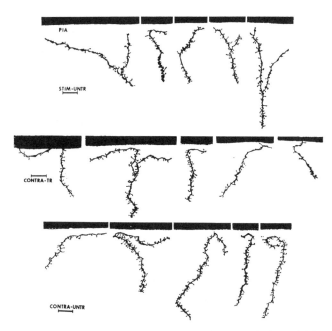

FIGURE 22.5 Accurate scale drawings of some apical dendritic terminal types. The bar represents 10 μm. The upper row comes from stimulated cortex, untrained cat; middle row from contralateral cortex, trained cat; lower from contralateral cortex, untrained cat. In two examples (middle) tips seemed to touch the pia even when the microscope focal plane was optimal for visualizing pia-terminal separation.

or long spines seemed to appear more frequently in contralateral cortex than they did in stimulated cortex. Note, for example, the two long spines at the tip of the second ending from the right in the middle row of Figure 22.5. Less frequently, similar spines were seen in stimulated cortex, such as the second one from the right in the upper row. Our distinct impression, then, was that the microscopic picture of layers I and II differed greatly between stimulated and contralateral cortex and between trained and untrained animals.

22.2.6 Possible limitations on observations

A criticism of these findings is that the histological procedure is unreliable for precise, adequately controlled quantitative work. The capriciousness of the Golgi method in its various modifications is well known. Sotelo and Palay (1968) have cautioned that Golgi methods do not give a true picture of dendritic tips. Very fine tips are probably not stained and thus are not seen. However, our laboratory has successfully used the Golgi method in previous quantitative work (Cant, 1973; Rutledge, 1969; Rutledge, Duncan, and Beatty, 1969; Rutledge, Duncan, and Cant, 1972). Furthermore, in the present experiments each animal was its own control since the two sides of the brain were compared; the tissue from both sides of a brain were treated alike and processed to-

gether; and in one important measure, basal dendritic spines, no difference between the two sides was found. Nevertheless, further studies of a similar nature, especially using the electron microscope, should be carried out. It would also be helpful to have comparative data from normal, nonexperimental adult cats. Ongoing work includes this feature.

Another criticism has to do with the question of whether the presence of electrodes in stimulated cortex has a detrimental effect upon nearby neuronal architecture. This possibility has not been absolutely ruled out. The precaution of using tissue only from the central 4 mm or so of electrode locations 6–8 mm apart would seem to be a partial answer to this criticism. Further, no signs of damage, gliosis, or loss of neurons were found beyond about 300–500 μm from the electrode locations. Current work includes a quantitative study of neuronal elements in cortex between indwelling electrodes in otherwise experimentally naive cats.

An important consideration in these observations is whether the results may have been simply an epiphenomenon resulting from better staining of those neurons that had been more active before death. More cells are stained by the Golgi method immediately following intensive sensory stimulation (Schapiro and Vukovich, 1970). However, this does not apply to the animals used here, since they were not killed until about 110 hours after the last brain stimulation. Moreover, whether cells had been used for short or long periods did not seem to make any difference in a report of staining with methylene blue (Edström, 1957). Another report has described a decrease in the cytoplasmic or nuclear volume of spinal motoneurons after exercise (Geinismann, Larina, and Mats, 1971). Our findings show increases in neuronal elements.

22.3 INTERPRETATIONS, SPECULATIONS, AND SYNTHESIS

22.3.1 Interpretations

Data reported in these experiments support the "synaptic exercise" or "use" theory. Increased use of neural systems produced changes in morphological growth in some of the participating components. Postsynaptic structures, apical dendrites and their spines, showed evidence of growth as a consequence of increased use. These changes were in pyramidal cells of layers II and III and apparently resulted from electrical stimulation of neurons in the opposite cortex projecting directly or indirectly to the other side of the brain. Evidence suggested that spines increased in two locations, on vertical and oblique branches, only as a result of training.

The essential features of the observations, plus some

extensions and assumptions, are summarized in the diagram of Figure 22.6. These, of course, are the changes seen contralaterally to the chronically stimulated cortex. Part 1 includes an increased length of terminal portions of apical dendrites and new spines appearing on new surfaces of vertical dendrites. In part 2 are new (immature?) small spines on new, thin, terminal twigs. No direct measurements were made of oblique apical dendrites, but it is supposed that new lengths would appear on these components along with an increase in number of spines (part 3). Part 4 represents how some of the new spines may form near established spines. This budding of secondary spines has been observed in the developing cerebellum by Hámori and Szentágothai (1964). Finally, it is suggested that as a consequence of increased synaptic activity, some established spines may increase their area of synaptic contact (part 5). If these interpretations of growth processes are even partly correct, it is important to consider whether there are any precedents of similar observations. One would suppose that at least certain aspects of the growth processes described here may not be unique to these experiments.

At birth there are few if any dendritic spines or fine dendritic terminals in cat neocortex (Voeller, Pappas, and Purpura, 1963; Adinolfi, 1971). Dendritic modifications leading to establishment of synaptic contacts thus occur to a great extent in the neonatal period. Investigators have observed relatively rapid growth and the appearance of many synapses by 14 days of age. "Growth cones" at the ends of immature dendrites were found by Morest (1969). However, although a search was made, no elements similar to "growth cones" have been found in any of the present work. Perhaps the very long and thin dendrites and spines seen in adult brains are the equivalents of dendritic terminal "growth cones" in the rapidly maturing neocortex.

I contend that the most plastic elements of neocortex

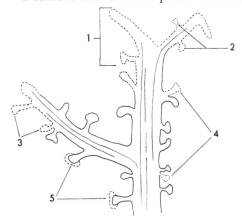

FIGURE 22.6 Specific loci and types of morphological changes observed or postulated in apical dendrites of contralateral cortex. Descriptions in text.

are postsynaptic. Small dendritic twigs, terminals, and spines may be capable of not so subtle changes if a strong synaptic drive is repeatedly directed toward them. This viewpoint has been discussed most recently by Hámori (1969) and Szentágothai (1971). Eccles (1973) has objected to a simple interpretation of the growth theory since it would imply a continued hypertrophy of "used" interconnections. It seems reasonable to assume, though, that "unused" connections might ordinarily regress, thus resulting in little if any net increase in total structural synaptic routes. The present findings would seem to be the result of a repetitive, synchronous synaptic drive produced by electrical stimulation of selected neuronal pathways. This excessive bombardment is, of course, a highly artificial situation. Whether similar results or more subtle changes can be produced by natural activation (such as primary sensory stimulation), remains for future study to determine. The channeling of functional load (Szentágothai, 1971) into neocortex would seem to be a reasonable basis for interpreting the observations made in "enriched-environment" studies. Increasing sensory input in these studies leads to more dendritic spines and dendritic branchings (Globus et al., 1973; Greenough and Volkmar, 1973). There are also increases in cortical weight (Rosenzweig, Bennett, and Krech, 1964; Rosenzweig, Love, and Bennett, 1968; Riege, 1971), increased depth (Walsh et al., 1972), larger synaptic contacts (Møllgaard et al., 1971; West and Greenough, 1972), and an increase in depth and number of glia (Diamond et al., 1966). The relative contribution of glial increases to cortical depth and weight has not been determined.

The emphasis in this discussion has been on postsynaptic structures, but presynaptic elements involved in the two pathways must also show growth changes. Our axonal measurements probably did not provide an adequate test for these. Mechanisms of regeneration and the likely formation of new synaptic contacts by growing and sprouting axons are discussed elsewhere in this volume. Assuming that some regenerating axons make new functional contacts (Raisman, 1969; Lynch, Deadwyler, and Cotman, 1973), it will be appropriate, when we have more definitive knowledge, to tie together mechanisms of pre- and postsynaptic alterations following increased synaptic use and axonal growth.

22.3.2 Speculations on mechanisms

It is suggested that the postsynaptic structural changes described here, and apparently dependent upon activity in interhemispheric neural routes, involve the following events:

1. increased presynaptic action potentials
2. increased release of transmitter at existing synapses

3. prolonged excitatory postsynaptic potentials (EP-SPs), with or without action potentials

4. formation of new postsynaptic membrane, with increased dendritic length

5. appearance of new synaptic elements, including specialized receptors

6. a response in presynaptic terminals marked by growth toward receptors.

Evidence in support of some of these suggestions has existed for some time, and more is now appearing. The first one seems to present no problem since it is assumed that action potentials are elicited in axons leaving the cortex on the stimulated side. On the second point, there is sufficient evidence to relate presynaptic activity to the density of synaptic vesicles, and in turn to the amount of transmitter released. In an important study of terminals in cat cerebral cortex, Fehér, Joó, and Halász (1972) showed that as little as 30 minutes of click stimulation could increase or decrease vesicle density, depending upon terminal size and probable type. Garey and Pettigrew (1974) found that visual stimulation after light deprivation in kittens produced an increase in the terminal-vesicle density of visual-cortex axons. From experiments on monkeys (Siegesmund, Sances, and Larson, 1969) it is not clear whether our type of electrical stimulation can be expected to produce an increase or a decrease in vesicle density. Certainly frequency and duration of stimulation, as well as time elapsed between stimulation and tissue death, are critical factors in the vesicle-density problem. The third point, prolonged EPSPs with or without soma action potentials, seems logical, assuming release of transmitter.

It is suggested that one adequate stimulus for post-synaptic cellular RNA and protein synthesis, the presumed basis for the fourth point, is related to membrane potential changes and action potentials in a critical time period. As these electrical events increase, synthesis increases. Direct evidence supporting this point is not as well established as might be desired. More indirect support is reasonably convincing. Booth (1973), after summarizing a number of experiments, concluded that RNA synthesis is specific to brain and occurs as a result of learning. In a nonmammalian system the rate of RNA synthesis increased with the number of action-potential spikes produced per hour (Berry, 1969). Hydén et al. (1974) have recently described a change in RNA base compositions in neocortex after visual-discrimination learning in the monkey. During a learning experiment in rats, incorporation of RNA precursors increased in neurons and glia (Pohle and Matthies, 1974). In the visual cortex, protein metabolism was found to be directly related to the amount of visual stimulation (Talwar et al., 1966). These studies, repre-sentative but not exhaustive, have certainly established a relationship between neuronal protein synthesis and various kinds of learning or, more simply, synaptic use. As has been pointed out by Rose (1973), and again at this conference, the direct relationship is not yet established. Protein synthesis may result from stress, motor activity, emotional disturbance, or increased sensory input.

If one accepts the possibility of an increase in RNA and protein synthesis in the postsynaptic neuron, then the appearance of new elements in the postsynaptic structure, including specialized receptors, may be inferred (fifth point). Further, presynaptic terminals may then respond with growth toward receptors (sixth point). I believe that it is now possible to study these two postulated events in the model that has been discussed here. Determination of specific protein changes in various neuronal elements would be exceedingly important. I feel strongly that the experiments of Raisman (1969) and Lynch (this volume; see also Lynch, Deadwyler, and Cotman, 1973), as well as those of others, already point to axonal terminal growth and the development of new synaptic connections. What distinguishes my model is that it supposes that changes in axons must occur in response to postsynaptic structural changes.

Finally, I would argue that there is already some support for ultrastructural changes at the synapse as a result of increased sensory input. The work of Cragg (1967, 1969, 1973), Møllgaard et al. (1971), and West and Greenough (1972) has shown that it is possible to do quantitative studies of the synapse using the electron microscope. Further work should be undertaken in order to establish firmly the nature of changes in synaptic contacts as a consequence of increased synaptic use or increased sensory input.

22.3.3 Synthesis and applications

The experimental results discussed here have been interpreted as suggesting that certain structures and related functions are modifiable in the adult nervous system by increased synaptic exercise or use. An associated learned behavior (foot flexion) may have been related causally to certain specific structural changes. These findings, supporting a growth theory of neuronal interconnections, help to extend our thinking about plasticity to include the adult nervous system. We cannot even begin to imagine what limitations there may be to pre- and postsynaptic plasticity and functional change in the mature brain. However, I suspect that, practically speaking, synaptogenesis is mostly under genetic control (see Crain, 1974; Berry, 1974). I agree with Sperry's (1965) clearly stated viewpoint that most of the circuitry in the nervous system is genetically determined and is established without much influence of functional demands during growth and differentiation. Neural changes associated with learning, he thinks, may be micro or molecular and may affect such things as excitability, conductance, and endogenous discharges. Another discussion, by Kandel et al. (1970), summarizes a similar belief and places heavy emphasis upon interneuronal connections that have been genetically determined.

Understanding synaptogenesis as related to learning and memory becomes an especially difficult problem when one tries to identify the more subtle plastic changes. It would seem that the careful electron microscopic studies by Sotelo and Palay (1968, 1971) on the vestibular nucleus may have elucidated some of the possible subtlety. Their work leads one to believe that in the intact adult rat nervous system, there may be continual, ongoing plastic changes. Certain signs indicate likely growth mechanisms in both axons and dendrites. Other nuclei or areas should be intently studied for possible similar evidence.

The data I have reported are the results of a special case of trying to overload neural systems with intense activity in an effort to see if, in the extreme, morphological changes can be provoked. Such changes, as observed, clearly do not establish a neural basis for learning and memory. As a first step in this direction, though, some of the basic neural effects of intensive synaptic use may have been defined. At the very least, an area of research has been opened by utilizing a new model for the study of synaptic plasticity and synaptogenesis. An important design element in our experiments was that the amount of stimulation or training necessary to produce the effects was actually very little each day. Total daily stimulation was only 40 seconds. Even less may be just as efficient. What is thought to be critical is the 24 hours between stimulation periods. A considerable amount of "consolidation time" is probably necessary to produce the changes we found. If synthesis of RNA and protein forms the basis for the effects described, this must occur between the training periods. Further work should consider some means of interfering with protein synthesis in order to observe possible effects upon the developed functional and structural changes.

ACKNOWLEDGMENT

Much of the data collection and analysis for the study of cortical neuronal morphology was done with the collaboration of Joyce Duncan and Cheryl Wright. The work was supported in part by NIH Grant 04119.

REFERENCES

ADINOLFI, A. M. 1971. The postnatal development of synaptic contacts in the cerebral cortex. In M. B. Sterman, D. J. McGinty, and A. M. Adinolfi, eds., *Brain Development and Behavior*. New York: Academic Press, pp. 73–89.

APRIL, R. S., and SPENCER, W. A. 1969. Enhanced synaptic effectiveness following prolonged changes in synaptic use. *Experientia* 25: 1272–1273.

BARONDES, S. H. 1970. Relationship of biological regulatory mechanisms to learning and memory. *Nature* 205: 18–21.

BERRY, M. 1974. Development of the cerebral neocortex of the rat. In G. Gottlieb, ed., *Aspects of Neurogenesis*. New York: Academic Press, pp. 7–67.

BERRY, R. W. 1969. Ribonucleic acid metabolism of a single neuron: Correlation with electrical activity. *Science* 166: 1021–1023.

BLOOM, F. E. 1970. Correlating structure and function of synaptic ultrastructure. In F. O. Schmitt, ed., *The Neurosciences: Second Study Program*. New York: Rockefeller University Press, pp. 729–746.

BOOTH, D. A. 1973. Protein synthesis and memory. In J. A. Deutsch, ed., *The Physiological Basis of Memory*. New York: Academic Press, pp. 27–58.

BURKE, W., and HAYHOW, W. R. 1968. Disuse in the lateral geniculate nucleus of cats. *Journal of Physiology* 194: 495–519.

CANT, N. W. B. 1973. Alterations in structure and function of the visual system after eye enucleation in adult cats. Unpublished Ph.D. dissertation, University of Michigan.

CRAGG, B. G. 1967. Changes in visual cortex on first exposure of rats to light. *Nature* 215: 251–253.

CRAGG, B. G. 1969. The effects of vision and dark-rearing on the size and density of synapses in the lateral geniculate nucleus measured by electron microscopy. *Brain Research* 13: 53–67.

CRAGG, B. G. 1973. Plasticity of synapses. In G. H. Bourne, ed., *The Structure and Function of Nervous Tissue*. New York: Academic Press, pp. 1–60.

CRAIN, S. 1974. Tissue culture models of developing brain functions. In G. Gottlieb, ed., *Aspects of Neurogenesis*. New York: Academic Press, pp. 69–114.

DIAMOND, M. C., LAW, F., RHODES, H., LINDNER, B., ROSENZWEIG, M. R., KRECH, D., and BENNETT, E. L. 1966. Increases in cortical depth and glia numbers in rats subjected to enriched environments. *Journal of Comparative Neurology* 128: 117–126.

ECCLES, J. C. 1953. *The Neurophysiological Basis of Mind*. London: Oxford University Press, pp. 203–327.

ECCLES, J. C. 1966. Conscious experience and memory. In J. C. Eccles, ed., *Brain and Conscious Experience*. New York: Springer-Verlag, pp. 314–344.

ECCLES, J. C. 1972. Possible synaptic mechanisms subserving learning. In A. G. Karczmar and J. C. Eccles, eds., *Brain and Human Behavior*. New York: Springer-Verlag, pp. 39–61.

ECCLES, J. C. 1973. *The Understanding of the Brain*. New York: McGraw-Hill, pp. 175–186.

EDSTRÖM, J. 1957. Effects of increased motor activity on the dimensions and the staining properties of the neuron soma. *Journal of Comparative Neurology* 107: 295–304.

FEHÉR, O., JOÓ, F., and HALÁSZ, N. 1972. Effect of stimulation on the number of synaptic vesicles in nerve fibers and terminals of the cerebral cortex of the cat. *Brain Research* 47: 37–48.

GAREY, L. J., and PETTIGREW, J. D. 1974. Ultrastructural changes in kitten visual cortex after environmental modification. *Brain Research* 66: 165–172.

GEINISMANN, YU. YA., LARINA, V. N., and MATS, V. N. 1971. Changes of neurones' dimensions as a possible morphological correlate of their increased functional activity. *Brain Research* 26: 247–257.

GLOBUS, A., ROSENZWEIG, M. R., BENNETT, E. L., and DIAMOND, M. C. 1973. Effects of differential experience on dendritic spine counts in rat cerebral cortex. *Journal of Comparative and Physiological Psychology* 82:175–181.

GLOBUS, A., and SCHEIBEL, A. B. 1967. Synaptic loci on visual cortical neurons of the rabbit: The specific afferent radiation. *Experimental Neurology* 18: 116–131.

GOMULICKI, B. R. 1953. The development and present status of the trace theory of memory. *British Journal of Psychology Monograph, Supplement* 29: 1–94.

GREENOUGH, W. T., and VOLKMAR, F. R. 1973. Pattern of dendritic branching in occipital cortex of rats reared in complex environments. *Experimental Neurology* 40: 491–504.

HÁMORI, J. 1969. Development of synaptic organization in the partially agranular and in the transneuronally atrophied cerebellar cortex. In R. Llinas, ed., *Neurobiology of Cerebellar Evolution and Development*. Chicago: AMA Education and Research Foundation, pp. 845–858.

HÁMORI, J., and SZENTÁGOTHAI, J. 1964. The "crossing over" synapse. An electron microscope study of the molecular layer in the cerebellar cortex. *Acta Biologica Academiae Scientiarum Hungaricae* 15: 95–117.

HEATH, C. J., and JONES, E. G. 1971. The anatomical organization of the suprasylvian gyrus of the cat. *Ergebnisse der Anatomie und Entwicklungsgeschichte* 45-3: 1–64.

HEBB, D. O. 1949. *The Organization of Behavior*. New York: John Wiley & Sons, pp. 60–66.

HYDÉN, H., LANGE, P. W., MIHAILOVIĆ, L. J., and PETROVIC-MINIĆ, B. 1974. Changes of RNA base composition in nerve cells of monkeys subjected to visual discrimination and delayed alternation performance. *Brain Research* 65: 215–230.

KANDEL, E., CASTELLUCCI, V., PINSKER, H., and KUPFERMAN, I. 1970. The role of synaptic plasticity in the short-term modification of behavior. In G. Horn and R. A. Hinde, eds., *Short-Term Changes in Neural Activity and Behaviour*. London: Cambridge University Press, pp. 281–322.

KONORSKI, J. 1948. *Conditioned Reflexes and Neuron Organization*. London: Cambridge University Press, pp. 87–90.

LYNCH, G., DEADWYLER, S., and COTMAN, C. 1973. Postlesion axonal growth produces permanent functional connections. *Science* 180: 1364–1366.

MØLLGAARD, K., DIAMOND, M. C., BENNETT., E. L., ROSENZWEIG, M. R., and LINDNER, B. 1971. Quantitative synaptic changes with differential experience in rat brain. *International Journal of Neuroscience* 2: 113–128.

MOREST, D. K. 1969. The growth of dendrites in the mammalian brain. *Zeitschrift fuer Anatomie und Entwicklungsgeschichte* 128: 290–317.

POHLE, W., and MATTHIES, H. 1974. Incorporation of RNA precursors into neuronal and glial cells of rat brain during a learning experiment. *Brain Research* 65: 231–237.

PURPURA, D. P. 1958. Organization of excitatory and inhibitory synaptic electrogenesis in the cerebral cortex. In H. H. Jasper et al., eds., *Reticular Formation of the Brain*. Boston: Little, Brown, pp. 435–457.

RAISMAN, G. 1969. Neuronal plasticity in the septal nuclei of the adult rat. *Brain Research* 14: 25–48.

RAMÓN Y CAJAL, S. 1911. *Histologie du Système Nerveux de L'Homme et des Vertébrés*, Vol. 2. Paris: Maloine, pp. 887–890.

RIEGE, W. H. 1971. Environmental influences on brain and behavior of year old rats. *Developmental Psychobiology* 4: 175–167.

ROBBINS, N., and NELSON, P. G. 1970. Tenotomy and the monosynaptic reflex. *Experimental Neurology* 27: 66–75.

ROSE, S. 1973. *The Conscious Brain*. New York: Alfred A. Knopf, pp. 196–199.

ROSENZWEIG, M. R., BENNETT, E. L., and KRECH, D. 1964. Cerebral effects of environmental complexity and training among adult rats. *Journal of Comparative and Physiological Psychology* 57: 438–439.

ROSENZWEIG, M. R., LOVE, W., and BENNETT, E. L. 1968. Effects of a few hours a day of enriched experience on brain chemistry and brain weights. *Physiology and Behavior* 3: 819–825.

RUTLEDGE, L. T. 1965. Facilitation: Electrical response enhanced by conditional excitation of cerebral cortex. *Science* 148: 1246–1248.

RUTLEDGE, L. T. 1969. Effect of stimulation on isolated cortex. In H. H. Jasper, A. A. Ward, Jr., and A. Pope, eds., *Basic Mechanisms of the Epilepsies*. Boston: Little, Brown, pp, 349–355.

RUTLEDGE, L. T., DUNCAN, J., and BEATTY, N. 1969. A study of pyramidal cell axon collaterals in intact and partially isolated adult cerebral cortex. *Brain Research* 16: 15–22.

RUTLEDGE, L. T., DUNCAN, J., and CANT, N. 1972. Long-term status of pyramidal cell axon collaterals and apical dendritic spines in denervated cortex. *Brain Research* 41: 249–262.

RUTLEDGE, L. T., and KENNEDY, T. T. 1961. Brain-stem and cortical interactions in the interhemispheric delayed response. *Experimental Neurology* 4:470–483.

RUTLEDGE, L. T., WRIGHT, C., and DUNCAN, J. 1974. Morphological changes in pyramidal cells of mammalian neocortex associated with increased use. *Experimental Neurology* 44:209–228.

SCHAPIRO, S., and VUKOVICH, K. R. 1970. Early experience effects upon cortical dendrites: A proposed model for development. *Science* 167: 292–294.

SCHEIBEL, M. E., and SCHEIBEL, A. B. 1971. Selected structural-functional correlations in postnatal brain. In M. B. Sterman, D. J. McGinty, and A. M. Adinolfi, eds., *Brain Development and Behavior*. New York: Academic Press, pp. 1–21.

SCHMITT, F. O. 1969. Brain cell membranes and their microenvironment. *Neurosciences Research Program Bulletin* 7: 281–417.

SHARPLESS, S. K. 1964. Reorganization of function—Use and disuse. *Annual Review of Physiology* 26: 357–388.

SIEGESMUND, K. A., SANCES, JR., A., and LARSON, S. J. 1969. Effects of electroanesthesia on synaptic ultrastructure. *Journal of Neurological Sciences* 9: 89–96.

SOTELO, C., and PALAY, S. L. 1968. The fine structure of the lateral vestibular nucleus of the rat. I. Neurons and neuroglial cells. *Journal of Cell Biology* 36: 151–179.

SOTELO, C., and PALAY, S. L. 1971. Altered axons and axon terminals in the lateral vestibular nucleus of the rat. *Laboratory Investigation* 25: 653–671.

SPERRY, R. W. 1965. Embryogenesis of behavioral nerve nets. In R. L. DeHaan and H. Ursprung, eds., *Organogenesis*. New York: Holt, Rinehart and Winston, pp. 161–186.

SZENTÁGOTHAI, J. 1971. Memory functions and the structural organization of the brain. *Symposia Biologica Hungarica* 10: 21–35.

TALWAR, G. P., CHOPRA, S. P., GOEL, B. K., and D'MONTE,

B. 1966. Correlation of the functional activity of the brain with metabolic parameters. III. Protein metabolism of the occipital cortex in relation to light stimulus. *Journal of Neurochemistry* 13: 109–116.

Tanzi, E. 1893. I fatti e le induzioni nell'odierna istologia del sistema nervosa. *Revista Sperimentale di Freniatria* 19: 419–472.

Voeller, K., Pappas, G. D., and Purpura, D.P. 1963. Electron microscope study of development of cat superficial neocortex. *Experimental Neurology* 7:107–130.

Walsh, R. N., Cummins, R. A., Budtz-Olsen, O. E., and Torok, A. 1972. Effects of environmental enrichment and deprivation on frontal cortex. *International Journal of Neuroscience* 4: 239–242.

West, R. W., and Greenough, W. T. 1972. Effect of environmental complexity on cortical synapses of rats: Preliminary results. *Behavioral Biology* 7: 279–284.

23

Synaptogenesis and the Morphology of Learning and Memory

ROBERT Y. MOORE

ABSTRACT The purpose of this contribution is to review morphological aspects of central-nervous-system plasticity which may be relevant to the events of learning and memory. In particular, the role that growth and synaptogenesis might play in these events is examined. A number of studies have demonstrated a remarkable neuronal plasticity in the developing nervous system in the formation of connections. Similarly, neurons in the adult nervous system are capable of growth and formation of new synapses following axonal section. Noninjured central neurons have been shown to increase their terminal axonal plexus by sprouting collateral branches from intact axons in response to the removal of other axonal input into the area innervated. These observations indicate that both the developing and the adult nervous systems are capable of growth and synaptogenesis and that there is significant plasticity in the process, involving both pre- and postsynaptic neural elements. The mechanisms by which such events might participate in learning and memory are discussed.

The phenomena of learning and memory imply that there is modifiability, or plasticity, in the organization of the central nervous system (CNS). It has been a basic tenet of neurobiology that CNS organization at any point in time is a function of both genetic and environmental influences. Our knowledge of the gross, genetically determined patterns of brain organization is well advanced, but we have little understanding of those aspects determined by the interplay of genetic and environmental factors, particularly as these are expressed at the cellular, or synaptic, level. The purpose of this review is to examine the role that synaptogenesis might play in neural mechanisms of learning and memory. The term "synaptogenesis" implies growth, and because of this I shall review some aspects of axonal growth as these occur both in the developmental period and in the adult organism as a basis for some speculation concerning the the role that synaptogenesis might play in learning and memory.

23.1 SYNAPTOGENESIS: SOME ASPECTS IN THE DEVELOPING AND ADULT CNS

An emerging exception to our ignorance concerning en-

ROBERT Y. MOORE, Department of Neurosciences, School of Medicine, University of California, San Diego, La Jolla, CA

vironmental influences on CNS organization lies in the many studies which have shown the effects of early sensory stimulation or deprivation on brain development (see, e.g., Greenough, Bennett, Rose, and Chapter 18, this volume). These highlight the plasticity of CNS organization in the developing organism, and I would like to amplify this point with two further examples. The first of these comes from the studies of Schneider (1973), who has examined responses to injury in the developing visual system. Schneider's work demonstrates that ablation of the superior colliculus in the newborn hamster results in a significant reorganization of the retinal input to the brain. In the normal animal, axons arising from retinal ganglion cells terminate in the thalamus in the dorsal and ventral divisions of the lateral geniculate nucleus and in the tectum in the superficial layers of the superior colliculus. Axons arising from neurons in the

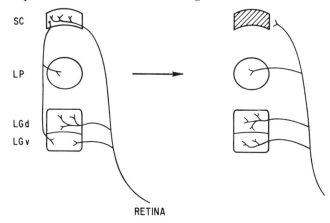

FIGURE 23.1 Effect of neonatal ablation of the superior colliculus on the development of retinal projections in the hamster. On the left is shown the organization of retinal projections to the thalamus and superior colliculus and the organization of superior-colliculus projections to the thalamus in the normal hamster brain (SC, superior colliculus; LP, lateral posterior nucleus of the thalamus; LGd, dorsal lateral geniculate nucleus; LGv, ventral lateral geniculate nucleus). The right part of the figure depicts the organization of retinal projections after neonatal superior-colliculus ablation. In this situation there is anomalous innervation to the lateral posterior nucleus and increased innervation from the retina to the ventral lateral geniculate nucleus. Redrawn from Schneider (1973).

superior colliculus terminate in the lateral posterior nucleus of the thalamus and the ventral lateral geniculate nucleus (Figure 23.1). When the superior colliculus is completely removed in the newborn hamster, there is increased retinal input to the ventral division of the lateral geniculate, and an anomalous retinal projection is formed into the lateral posterior nucleus of the thalamus. The lateral posterior nucleus normally receives input from the superior colliculus, as does the ventral lateral geniculate, but it does not receive retinal input in the normal animal (Figure 23.1).

Schneider has employed two concepts to explain these observations. The first concerns the availability of terminal space in innervated structures. Normally, in the adult nervous system, the postsynaptic sites are completely filled by presynaptic elements. In any given terminal area the normal organization of presynaptic elements occurs through a competition during development for the available terminal space. Following ablation of the superior colliculus in the neonatal hamster, there is a failure in the development of input from the colliculus to the lateral posterior nucleus of the thalamus and to the ventral nucleus of the lateral geniculate body. In both of these structures, then, there is available terminal space which will not be occupied by developing axons growing in from the neurons of the superior colliculus. Since there is ample evidence that dendritic growth is not dependent upon innervation by axons (e.g., Sotelo, 1973; Rakic and Sidman, 1973), this terminal space would still form and be available for occupation by axons arising from the retina (Figure 23.2), and these axons would be able to expand into the terminal space without competition.

The second concept relates to the formation of an axonal plexus of a specific size by a given neuron. When the superior colliculus is ablated, a major site of optic-tract terminal aborization is removed. This results in less available terminal space for optic-tract axons than in the normal state, and it is Schneider's view that these neurons attempt to preserve a minimum quantity of terminal axonal arborization (Figure 23.3). To do this the growing axons of retinal ganglion cells produce increased innervation to the ventral nucleus of the lateral

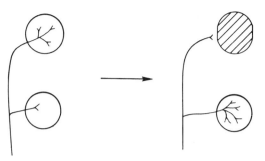

FIGURE 23.3 Conservation of a minimal terminal axonal plexus. The axon on the left normally innervates two areas. When one area is removed during development (as on the right), the axon produces its usual complement of terminal plexus. Redrawn from Schneider (1973).

geniculate body and to the lateral posterior nucleus, filling the terminal space made available by loss of the superior-colliculus input. The input to the lateral posterior nucleus is anomalous in the sense that the nucleus is not normally innervated by the retina, but it can be considered part of the visual system since it is normally innervated by superior colliculus and visual cortex. The anomalous growth of axons is not restricted to the visual system, however. In many of Schneider's experiments the brachium of the inferior colliculus was transected to produce a partial denervation of the thalamic auditory-relay nucleus, the medial geniculate. In these brains there was anomalous growth of optic-tract axons into the medial geniculate nucleus as well as into visual-system structures. Schneider has provided substantive evidence that some of the anomalous visual projections are functional, and he has studies underway to demonstrate whether the input to the medial geniculate body also forms functional synapses.

These observations do not fully establish the concept of conservation of a minimum terminal arborization, since nearly all of the axonal growth occurred in at least partially denervated areas and denervated sites may stimulate growth. Further evidence to support the concept comes from recent work by Singh and de Champlain (1972) and Jonsson et al. (1974). In these studies a neurotoxic compound, 6-hydroxydopamine (6-HDA), was administered parenterally to newborn rats. 6-HDA does not pass the blood-brain barrier significantly in the adult animal but does do so in the neonate (Sachs, 1973). The principal effect of 6-HDA appears to be a selective neurotoxicity for adrenergic neurons. When 6-HDA was administered to the newborn animal, the normal adrenergic innervation of the telencephalon did not develop. In the brainstem, however, there was a marked increase in adrenergic innervation in structures that normally contain such innervation. The brainstem and telencephalic innervations arise from the same neurons (Unger-

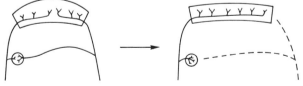

FIGURE 23.2 Competition for available terminal space. In the drawing on the left, two sources innervate the available terminal space. On the right, one of these has been removed during development, eliminating any competition for available terminal space, and the other innervation spreads to occupy that space. Redrawn from Schneider (1973).

stedt, 1971; Jonsson et al., 1974), and since the nonadrenergic innervation to the affected brainstem areas is not altered by 6-HDA effects, this would appear to be a clear demonstration of conservation of a minimum quantity of terminal arborization. That is, the loss of the telencephalic terminals is compensated for by the marked increase in brainstem adrenergic innervation to otherwise intact nuclei. Another facet of the increase in brainstem innervation is that it must occur at the expense of other innervation to the relevant nuclei, suggesting that the adrenergic innervation is in this circumstance more capable of competing for terminal space than are other types of input. This observation obviously requires further study, but it does have intriguing functional implications.

Both of these examples have dealt with manipulations that either remove part of the terminal area of developing neurons or partially alter axonal growth. They have demonstrated a marked plasticity in developing systems in response to experimental manipulation. In all likelihood there is a disparity among neurons in the degree of plasticity which may be shown and the time course over which this plasticity may be induced. This concept has been formalized by Jacobson (1970), who proposes that some neurons are specified early in development and are not readily modified, whereas others are specified late in development or may not be specified until well into the postnatal period. There is also the possibility that some neurons cannot become rigidly specified and may have an inherent plasticity greater than that of other neurons. If this is continued into the adult life of an animal, it has obvious implications for learning and memory.

Adrenergic neurons are certainly among those which may be endowed with a greater plasticity. In addition to the studies on developmental plasticity, there are a number of additional pieces of evidence to indicate that adrenergic neurons are capable of exhibiting remarkable plasticity during the adult life of animals. These studies have investigated the capacity of adrenergic neurons to make regenerative responses to injury (see Moore, Björklund, and Stenevi, 1974, for review). Within the central nervous system, the cell bodies of adrenergic neurons are found primarily in the brainstem (Ungerstedt, 1971). Some of their axons ascend in the brainstem reticular formation and enter the diencephalon, largely within the medial-forebrain-bundle complex, to innervate widespread areas of diencephalon and telencephalon (Ungerstedt, 1971). When the adrenergic axons ascending in the medial forebrain bundle are severed, there is vigorous regenerative sprouting from the proximal stumps, and the severed axons form a vast plexus of anomalously distributed terminals in the vicinity of the lesion (Katzman et al., 1971). This axonal growth is extremely vigorous in the first two weeks after a lesion, but the new axonal plexus then stabilizes. This axonal growth appears to represent an instance, in the adult nervous system, of the principle noted above: conservation of a minimum quantity of terminal axonal arborization. There is no evidence to indicate that the anomalous axon terminals formed in vast profusion in the vicinity of the lesion represent a functional plexus, so that the growth cannot be taken to represent regeneration in any strict sense. It does, however, represent evidence that central adrenergic axons are capable of substantial growth in the adult organism.

Further studies (Björklund and Stenevi, 1971; Björklund et al., 1971) have established that severed axons of adrenergic neurons will grow to innervate transplants of peripheral tissues that normally receive peripheral adrenergic innervation. The best example of this growth is into a transplanted iris (Figure 23.4). When an iris is removed from the anterior chamber of the eye and transplanted into the medial forebrain bundle, it severs the ascending axons within that tract, and they then undergo vigorous regenerative sprouting of the type noted above. The iris, which is denervated in the process of being transplanted, survives well in the brain, and the growing axons arising from noradrenaline cells of the pontine-nucleus locus ceruleus grow across the zone of transection and into the transplant. In the transplanted iris they form a pattern of innervation which does not differ

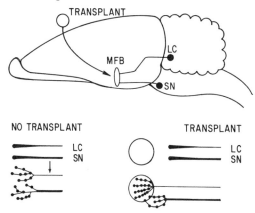

FIGURE 23.4 Regenerative growth of adrenergic axons in the mammalian central nervous system. The axons of adrenergic neurons arising from the locus ceruleus (LC) and substantia nigra (SN) ascend in the medial forebrain bundle (MFB). If they are transected in the MFB, the axons will grow to form a new, but anomalous, terminal plexus in the area of the transection (bottom left of figure). If a transplant of peripheral tissue, such as iris, is placed in the MFB, the axons of ascending adrenergic neurons are transected by the mechanical act of placing the transplant. In this situation both the LC and SN axons sprout, but the iris is reinnervated chiefly by LC axons, which produce the same neurotransmitter, noradrenaline as the axons that normally innervate the iris in the periphery. Redrawn from Moore, Björklund, and Stenevi (1974).

significantly from that in the normal iris. If another tissue, such as a mitral valve, which is normally innervated by peripheral sympathetic neurons, is transplanted into the central nervous system, it is also reinnervated by central noradrenergic neurons, and in this case the pattern of innervation is typical of the innervation of a normal mitral valve. Tissues that are not normally innervated by adrenergic neurons—for example, diaphragm or uterus—are not innervated by central axons. In addition, the axons of other central monoamine neuron systems, such as dopamine or serotonin neuron systems, do not innervate any of the transplants. These observations indicate that the axons of severed central adrenergic neurons are not only able to grow, but are capable of forming a terminal innervation plexus. It has not yet been established that these new terminal arborizations are functional, but the pattern of innervation certainly suggests that they are.

Nearly all studies of growth in the adult mammalian nervous system have examined the regenerative capacity of injured axons. There is another form of axonal growth in the adult nervous system which has been observed on only a few occasions. This is the phenomenon of collateral sprouting from intact axons. The most extensive examination of this phenomenon in the central nervous system has been carried out by Raisman (1969) and Raisman and Field (1973) on the innervation of the septal nuclear complex of the rat. This has been reviewed extensively by Raisman (this volume) and will not be further commented upon here. In these sudies, and in those of others, the basic paradigm has been to produce a distant lesion which results in degeneration of axons innervating the area under investigation. Following degeneration of the axons, there are vacated synaptic sites on dendrites or dendritic spines, and these are then filled by collateral axonal sprouts from the remaining, intact innervation to the partially denervated area.

The septal area receives a dense adrenergic innervation (Moore, Björklund, and Stenevi, 1971) from the medial forebrain bundle. Because of the marked growth capacity of adrenergic axons shown in the studies of regenerative sprouting, it appeared worthwhile to determine if these neurons participated in the phenomena described by Raisman (1969) and Raisman and Field (1973). Moore, Björklund, and Stenevi (1971) subjected rats to unilateral section of the fornix. Since the fornix projects nearly exclusively on the ipsilateral septal nuclei, the neurons of those nuclei were denervated and the contralateral septal nuclei served as a control. Following unilateral fornix section, a marked increase in adrenergic axons developed on the denervated side of the septum in comparison to the control side; this is shown diagrammatically in Figure 23.5. These observa-

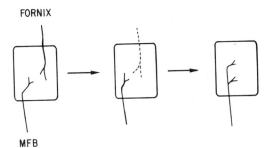

FORNIX

MFB

FIGURE 23.5 Collateral sprouting of central adrenergic axons. The septal area (designated by the rectangle in the figure) is innervated by two sets of axons, one from the hippocampus via the fornix and the other from the brainstem via the medial forebrain bundle (MFB). The latter group includes adrenergic axons arising in the locus ceruleus. When the fornix innervation is removed (center figure), the intact MFB innervation undergoes collateral sprouting to form new axon terminals.

tions indicate that the adrenergic innervation of the septum undergoes collateral sprouting in response to denervation, and this has been confirmed by other methods (Moore, 1974). Additional studies have shown that, under appropriate conditions, adrenergic axons in the mammalian central nervous system are capable of demonstrating collateral sprouting in a number of different areas (Moore, Björklund, and Stenevi, 1974), so that this phenomenon is not restricted to the innervation of the septum.

There are several aspects of this that warrant further comment. First, despite the remarkable instances of collateral sprouting observed in adrenergic neurons, this phenomenon is not restricted to the adrenergic neuron; it has been observed in the axons of a number of different types of neurons in a number of different areas (see Sidman and LaVail, 1975, for review). It is not established that one group of neurons is more capable than others of demonstrating this sort of phenomenon, but it is clear that collateral sprouting is not seen in certain experimental situations where it might be expected (Kerr, 1972; Guillery, 1972; Moore, Björklund, and Stenevi, 1974).

Second, the occurrence of collateral sprouting implies that certain central axons are capable of expanding their terminal plexus when available postsynaptic sites are present, and it further indicates that there is considerable plasticity in the membranes of the postsynaptic elements in the production of new receptor sites for the appropriate neurotransmitter substances. The latter is not surprising in that the postsynaptic neuron is simply producing new receptor sites that would be appropriate for transmitters with which it is already familiar. The only difference is that the location of the receptor sites is altered. This would be even further understandable if one accepted the hypothesis that there is a continuing turnover of terminals within a given area of neuropil. That is, if a continuing change occurred in the neuropil, with degeneration of some axon terminals and their replacement by newly formed terminals, a normal balance among afferent inputs to the area would be maintained by a competition for the available synaptic space. In such a dynamic situation, however, an advantage in the competition might occur with increased use of one input so that an alteration in the normal balance would result. This alteration in the synaptic organization of the neuropil could have important consequences in functional phenomena such as learning and memory. There are substantial data to indicate that synaptic proteins are constantly replaced (Droz, 1973), and some evidence exists for a continuing turnover of terminals in the mammalian CNS. The concept of continuing growth of axon terminals and reorganization of synaptic architecture in the adult nervous system has been reviewed on several occasions (Rose et al., 1960; Cohen and Pappas, 1969; Moore, Björklund, and Stenevi, 1971; Sotelo and Palay, 1971; Chan-Palay, 1973) and will not be elaborated further. Such a concept is obviously useful in considering synaptogenesis as a basis for learning and memory.

There is one further example of collateral sprouting of adrenergic axons that is of interest in this regard. Pickel and co-workers have recently demonstrated a remarkable collateral sprouting from adrenergic axons innervating the rat cerebellum (Pickel, Krebs, and Bloom, 1973; Pickel, Segal, and Bloom, 1974). It appears that severing one collateral of an adrenergic axon results in a marked sprouting of the remaining collaterals of the same axon. In this case, however, the phenomenon appears to be self-limited, and the newly formed collaterals are present only for a period of approximately six weeks. This contrasts, for example, with the collateral sprouting of adrenergic axons in the septum, where the effect appears to be permanent (Moore, Björklund, and Stenevi, 1971). One interpretation of Pickel's observations would be that the adrenergic neuron is maintaining its minimum quantity of terminal arborization by collateral sprouting, and as regenerative sprouting and new terminals occur at the proximal stump of the severed axon, the collaterals are resorbed. An interesting aspect of these observations is that the adrenergic axon in this situation, as in the developing brainstem (Jonsson et al., 1974), appears capable of competing advantageously with other intact axons for terminal space, in the areas in which its terminals are present, during the period of collateral sprouting. The fact that they are capable of doing so in response to injury raises the issue of whether functional influences alone are sufficient to induce such changes. This would be critical, of course, to any proposal sug-

gesting collateral sprouting as a mechanism for synaptic change in learning and memory.

In summary, all of the studies outlined above have demonstrated that neurons in the adult nervous system are capable of growth. This is the obvious foundation for the hypothesis that growth and reorganization of neural connections occur as the result of a functional state rather than in response to injury. This will now be considered in further detail.

23.2 SYNAPTOGENESIS AS A MECHANISM OF LEARNING AND MEMORY

There would appear to be at least three principal types of synaptic change that might occur during learning and memory. These are shown diagrammatically in Figure 23.6, and obviously, in a given area or circumstance, either one or a combination of them might be operative. The first of these (Figure 23.6A) is a form of growth in which there is a change in the length of synaptic contact. That is, with increased use of a specific input, growth would occur in the region of synaptic contacts, so that the area of axonal and dendritic, or somatic, contacts would be longer. This would necessitate the development of new receptor molecules by the postsynaptic components of the contact, and would further imply a loss or modification of adjacent axonal elements. It is known (Larramendi, 1969) that changes in length of axonal contacts occur during development, and such changes have been demonstrated as a consequence of

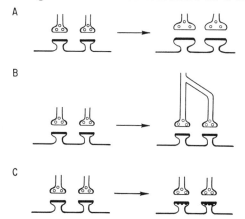

FIGURE 23.6 Three proposals of possible synaptic changes in learning and memory. In A, two axon terminals are diagrammatically represented as making contact with dendritic spines. The change would involve the growth of both pre- and postsynaptic membranes to form a more extensive synaptic contact. In B, two axons are again shown making contact with dendritic spines. The change is for one axon to undergo collateral sprouting, replacing the other axon terminal in order to increase the density of innervation from one source in the innervated area. In C, the change is a modification of receptor organization at the postsynaptic membrane.

344   ROBERT Y. MOORE

environmental input (Greenough, this volume; Bennett, this volume). The work of Rutledge and his collaborators has demonstrated changes in dendritic arborizations as a consequence of functional input (Rutledge, this volume), and this certainly implies that there has been some change in axonal morphology as well. It is extremely difficult to provide accurate quantitation of the lengths of synaptic contacts in given nuclei, and to accurately assess changes in this parameter of synaptic morphology would provide even greater technical obstacles. Consequently, it is unlikely that this type of change in synaptic morphology could be identified at the present time, but a theoretical molecular basis for expansion of synaptic contacts during learning has been put forth by Kosower (1972).

A second type of change in synaptic organization would occur as a result of collateral sprouting (Figure 23.6 B). In this situation, alteration in the functional state of a terminal area would lead to a loss of terminals from one source of innervation to the area, with replacement by collateral sprouting from other, intact, innervation. As noted above (see also Cohen and Pappas, 1969; Sotelo and Palay, 1971; Chan-Palay, 1973), degenerating axon terminals can be shown electron microscopically in the normal brain. Whether this results from altered input to the areas or from an event unrelated to functional state is unknown. It is certainly tempting to speculate that there is a normal turnover of synaptic terminals which can be altered by functional input, but this cannot be demonstrated at the present time.

The third type of synaptic modification that might underlie learning and memory would be a modification of receptor mechanisms (Figure 23.6 C). For example, an alteration in either receptor density or receptor configuration at the postsynaptic site could result from alterations in functional input. Since there is very little known about the distribution and organization of receptor molecules, this can only be stated in a general way. Two possible mechanisms for receptor modification are evident. One is a change in receptors in response to either increased or decreased neurotransmitter input. The other, which has not been extensively investigated and requires further attention, reflects the role of nontransmitter mechanisms in neuronal interaction. The existence of "trophic" factors has been a subject of discussion for many years. The mechanism by which these factors participate in neuronal interactions is not well known, but trophic influences do appear to be separate from transmitter functions. An elegant example of such an interaction has been demonstrated by the recent work of Aguilar et al. (1973). In their studies, dealing with innervation of amphibian limbs, blockade of rapid axonal transport by application of colchicine to

a peripheral nerve has been shown to be equivalent to nerve section in that nerves adjacent to the one in which axonal transport is blocked undergo collateral sprouting to innervate the area that is innervated by the colchicine-blocked nerve, even though that nerve is morphologically intact and conducting impulses. This suggests that a protein, or some other material carried in the rapid phase of axonal transport, is required to maintain a trophic interaction between the nerve and innervated tissue. There are no such examples from the central nervous system, but there is one interesting observation which suggests that such interactions might occur there as well. Grafstein and Laureno (1973) have shown that tritiated proline injected into the eye is incorporated into protein in retinal ganglion cells and transported to the lateral geniculate body by rapid axonal transport. Five hours after the appearance of labeled protein in the lateral geniculate body, it also appears in the visual cortex, and the amount in cortex is proportional to that transported to the lateral geniculate nucleus. Although alternative interpretations are possible, these observations suggest that there is a constant transfer of protein from labeled optic-nerve axon terminals to the postsynaptic elements in the lateral geniculate. If transsynaptic transfer of protein could be shown to be a general phenomenon in the nervous system, it would have significant functional consequences, for it is apparent that protein transfer from one nerve cell to another provides a mechanism for the exchange of information between neurons that is different from the conventional neurotransmitter function. A transfer of information of this type could be extremely important in long-term effects of synaptic use—for example, in the modification of receptor protein molecules at the synaptic surface.

Another example of a potential nontransmitter mechanism for altering neuronal function, and possibly morphology, is demonstrated by the work of McEwen et al. (1974) on the binding of adrenal steroids to the brain. These investigators have shown that the adrenal corticoid, corticosterone, is bound to neurons in two principal areas in the rat brain, the hypothalamus-preoptic region and the hippocampus. The binding to hypothalamic neurons is easily understandable in terms of feedback regulation to the hypothalamus-pituitary-adrenal system, but that to the hippocampal neurons is less explicable in that context and is of particular interest because of the well-known role of the hippocampus in memory function. It is known from the work of McEwen et al. (1974) that the hormone probably results in altered protein metabolism within the neurons to which it is bound. Thus one can visualize a situation in which there would be increased adrenal corticosterone output during the stress of a learning situation, and the effect of this hormone upon hippocampal neurons would interact with the effect of direct neuronal input to produce alterations, at least at the biochemical level, which might participate in the phenomena of learning and memory. These changes obviously would not be essential to learning or memory since these phenomena do occur in an adrenalectomized or hypophysectomized animal.

The speculations outlined in this review are meant only to be preliminary and tentative. Their intent is to point out directions which might be profitable in increasing our understanding of the neural mechanisms of learning and memory. To further this understanding will require great technical innovation in order to provide a basis for elucidating chemical and morphological quantitation of events occurring at synaptic contacts during the learning process. All of the data currently available indicate that the synapse is the site at which the critical events of learning and memory occur. The problem remaining is to identify and characterize these events. The purpose of this review has been to note some aspects of the morphological plasticity of the mammalian central nervous system in order to suggest that the events occurring in learning and memory may include growth, or synaptogenesis.

ACKNOWLEDGMENT

The preparation of this review and some of the work discussed in it was supported in part by grants NS-12080 and HD-04583 from the National Institutes of Health, USPHS.

REFERENCES

AGUILAR, E. C., BISBY, M. A., COOPER, E., and DIAMOND, J. 1973. Evidence that axoplasmic transport of trophic factors is involved in the regulation of peripheral nerve fields in salamanders. *Journal of Physiology* 234: 449–464.

BJÖRKLUND, A., KATZMAN, R., STENEVI, U., and WEST, K. 1971. Development and growth of axonal sprouts from noradrenaline and 5-hydroxytryptamine neurons in the rat spinal cord. *Brain Research* 31: 21–33.

BJÖRKLUND, A., and STENEVI, U. 1971. Growth of central catecholamine neurons into smooth muscle grafts in the rat mesencephalon. *Brain Research* 31: 1–20.

CHAN-PALAY, V. 1973. Neuronal plasticity in the cerebellar cortex and lateral nucleus. *Zeitschrift für Anatomie und Entwicklungsgeschichte* 142: 23–35.

COHEN, E. B., and PAPPAS, G. D. 1969. Dark profiles in the apparently normal nervous system: A problem in the electron microscopic identification of early anterograde degeneration. *Journal of Comparative Neurology* 136: 375–396.

DROZ, B. 1973. Renewal of synaptic proteins. *Brain Research* 62: 383–394.

GRAFSTEIN, B. and LAUREMO, R. 1973. Transport of radioactivity from eye to visual cortex in the mouse. *Experimental Neurology* 39: 44–57.

GUILLERY, R. W. 1972. Experiments to determine whether retinogeniculate axons can form translaminar collateral sprouts in the dorsal lateral geniculate nucleus of the cat. *Journal of Comparative Neurology* 146: 407–420.

JACOBSON, M. 1970. *Developmental Neurobiology*. New York: Holt, Rinehart and Winston.

JONSSON, G., PYCOCK, C., FUXE, K., and SACHS, C. 1974. Changes in the development of central noradrenaline neurons following neonatal administration of 6-hydroxydopamine. *Journal of Neurochemistry* 22: 419–426.

KATZMAN, R., BJÖRKLUND, A., OWMAN, CH., STENEVI, U., and WEST, K. A. 1971. Evidence for regenerative axon sprouting of central catecholamine neurons in the rat mesencephalon following electrolytic lesions. *Brain Research* 25: 579–596.

KERR, F. W. 1972. The potential of cervical primary afferents to sprout in the spinal nucleus of V following long-term trigeminal denervation. *Brain Research* 43: 547–560.

KOSOWER, E. M. 1972. A molecular basis for learning and memory. *Proceedings of the National Academy of Sciences* 69: 3292–3296.

LARRAMENDI, L. M. H. 1969. Analysis of synaptogenesis in the cerebellum of the mouse. In R. Llinás, ed., *Neurobiology of Cerebellar Evolution and Development*. Chicago: American Medical Association, pp. 803–843.

McEWEN, B. S., DENEF, C. J., GERLACH, J. L., and PLAPINGER, L. 1974. Chemical studies of the brain as a steroid hormone target tissue. In F. O. Schmitt and F. G. Worden, eds., *The Neurosciences: Third Study Program*. Cambridge, Mass.: MIT Press, pp. 599–620.

MOORE, R. Y. 1974. Growth of adrenergic neurons in the adult mammalian nervous system. In K. Fuxe, Y. Zotterman, and L. Olson, eds., *Dynamics of Degeneration and Growth in Neurons*. New York: Pergamon Press, pp. 379–388.

MOORE, R. Y., BJÖRKLUND, A., and STENEVI, U. 1971. Plastic changes in the adrenergic innervation of the rat septal area in response to denervation. *Brain Research* 33: 13–35.

MOORE, R. Y., BJÖRKLUND, A., and STENEVI, U. 1974. Growth and plasticity of adrenergic neurons. In F. O. Schmitt and F. G. Worden, eds., *The Neurosciences: Third Study Program*. Cambridge, Mass.: MIT Press, pp. 961–977.

PICKEL, V. M., KREBS, H., and BLOOM, F. E. 1973. Proliferation of norepinephrine-containing axons in rat cerebellar cortex after peduncle lesions. *Brain Research* 59: 169–178.

PICKEL, V. M., SEGAL, M., and BLOOM, F. E. 1974. Axonal proliferation following lesions of cerebellar peduncles. A combined fluorescence microscopic and autoradiographic study. *Journal of Comparative Neurology*. 155: 43–60.

RAISMAN, G. 1969. Neuronal plasticity in the septal nuclei of the adult rat. *Brain Research* 14: 25–48.

RAISMAN, G., and FIELD, P. M. 1973. A quantitative investigation of the development of collateral reinnervation after partial deafferentation of the septal nuclei. *Brain Research* 50: 241–264.

RAKIC, P., and SIDMAN, R. L. 1973. Organization of cerebellar cortex secondary to deficits of granule cells in weaver mutant mice. *Journal of Comparative Neurology* 152: 133–162.

ROSE, J. E., MALIS, L. I., KRUGER, L., and BAKER, C. P. 1960. Effects of heavy, ionizing, monoenergetic particles on the cerebral cortex. II. Histological appearance of laminar lesions and growth of nerve fibers after laminar destructions. *Journal of Comparative Neurology* 115: 243–296.

SACHS, C. 1973. Development of the blood-brain barrier for

6-hydroxydopamine. *Journal of Neurochemistry* 20: 1753–1760.

SCHNEIDER, G. E. 1973. Early lesions of the superior colliculus: Factors affecting the formation of abnormal retinal connections. *Brain, Behavior and Evolution* 8: 73–109.

SIDMAN, R. L., and LaVAIL, J. 1975. Biology of the regenerating neuron. *Neurosciences Research Program Bulletin* (in press).

SINGH, B., and DE CHAMPLAIN, J. 1972. Altered ontogenesis of central noradrenergic neurons following neonatal treatment with 6-hydroxydopamine. *Brain Research* 48: 432–437.

SOTELO, C. 1973. Permanence and rate of paramembranous synaptic specializations in "mutant" and experimental animals. *Brain Research* 62: 345–351.

SOTELO, C., and PALAY, S. L. 1971. Altered axons and axon terminals in the lateral vestibular nucleus of the rat. Possible example of axonal remodeling. *Laboratory Investigation* 25: 653–672.

UNGERSTEDT, U. 1971. Stereotaxic mapping of the monoamine pathways in the rat brain. *Acta Physiologica Scandinavica* Supplement 367: 1–48.

24

The Reaction of Synaptogenesis in the Central and Peripheral Nervous Systems of the Adult Rat

GEOFFREY RAISMAN

ABSTRACT It is generally assumed that the functions of learning and memory depend upon the presence of synaptic connections in appropriate parts of the nervous system. There is, however, very little evidence as to whether synapses can undergo structural modification in the brains of adult mammals. The present experimental approach has been to make selective lesions of axons running into specific areas. As a result of such lesions, axon terminals degenerate and synapses are lost. By making quantitative ultrastructural studies of the numbers and types of synapses remaining, it is possible to estimate the degree of deafferentation and to follow the time course of subsequent events.

It is found that in a specific site in the central nervous system—the septal nuclei—and also in a peripheral site—the superior cervical sympathetic ganglion—deafferenting lesions are followed by a major reaction of synaptogenesis. In both cases the newly formed synapses appear in sufficient numbers to reinnervate all the denervated sites and thus restore the total number of synapses in the denervated tissue to its normal, preoperative level. In the septal nuclei these new synapses are created by adjacent undamaged axons which form additional synaptic contacts. In the sympathetic ganglion the new synapses are formed by regenerating sprouts from the originally cut axons.

These observations support the idea that new synapses can be rapidly formed in both the central and the peripheral nervous systems of the adult rat after deafferenting injuries; they also suggest an experimental approach which might be useful for investigating the possibility of synaptogenesis under other experimental conditions.

24.1 INTRODUCTION

When an axon is cut, the part of the neuron that is detached from the nucleus—the distal portion—undergoes degeneration. In the peripheral nervous system of mammals, the proximal end of the cut axon emits large numbers of tiny, rapidly growing, highly mobile sprouts. These sprouts advance in an exploratory fashion through the environment and can travel for considerable distances to reach the denervated target tissue. They are capable of regenerating a new terminal apparatus and

GEOFFREY RAISMAN, Laboratory of Neurobiology, National Institute for Medical Research, London, England

reestablishing functional contacts (Guth, 1956). Such a process is aptly called "true regeneration" because the original connections are restored both anatomically and functionally. In this sense, the term "regeneration" implies a restitution of the status quo.

It is a long-established but still curious fact that while regeneration can occur in the peripheral nervous system, it does not occur after lesions in most parts of the central nervous system of adult warm-blooded vertebrates (Guth and Windle, 1970). Although cut central axons do show a regenerative type of sprouting, this reaction is abortive (Ramón y Cajal, 1928) in all but a few specialized cases (see, e.g., Katzman et al., 1971; Raisman, 1973). This failure of regeneration is frequently taken to imply that there is some radical difference either between the neurons in the two sites or between the environments in which the axon sprouts find themselves. In the present series of studies we have compared the mode of reinnervation of a peripheral nervous site (the superior cervical ganglion of the rat; see Raisman et al., 1974) with the reactions seen in a partially denervated central nervous area (the septal nuclei after section of the ipsilateral fimbria; see Raisman, 1969, and Raisman and Field, 1973). This led us to the conclusion that central and peripheral nervous reactions in fact have several similarities.

24.2 RESULTS

24.2.1 Superior cervical ganglion

The simplest experimental situation that we have studied is the superior cervical ganglion of the sympathetic nervous system in the rat. In a preliminary series of quantitative ultrastructural observations, samples of neuropil were examined from sections through the ganglion, and all synapses related to the principal ganglionic neurons were counted. Axon terminals in this ganglion establish contacts with dendrites or with irregularly shaped dendritic protuberances, which we have loosely designated "spinelike" in order to distinguish them from the synapses on the dendritic shafts. Axon terminals do not make synaptic contacts directly onto cell bodies. The majority of axon terminals contain small, clear-centered synaptic vesicles of around 50 nm diameter and an appreciable number of larger, dense-cored vesicles of around 100 nm diameter. These dense-cored vesicles are characteristic of the preganglionic (cholinergic) axon terminals. In the normal superior cervical ganglion there are, on the average, about 30 synapses in a tissue area of 1.8×10^4 sq. μm. Many of the synapses are marked on the postsynaptic side by a membrane-associated density.

In a further series of animals the preganglionic chain was completely sectioned at a point some 2 mm below the inferior pole of the ganglion. This led to rapid degeneration of the preganglionic axons and their terminals. Within 24 hours there was a dramatic fall in the number of synapses left in the ganglion. The synaptic density fell from about 30 to 3 per 1.8×10^4 sq. μm. (We do not know the source of these few remaining axon terminals. They may belong to preganglionic axons that take a course outside the main preganglionic trunk, or they may represent intrinsic synapses made by axons originating within the ganglion itself.) While the axon terminals disappear, the postsynaptic membrane thickenings persist in a recognizable form, but apposed now not by an axonal structure but by satellite cell processes. These configurations appear at the same time as the axon terminals disappear; their relative distribution on dendritic shafts as compared to dendritic spines is the same as that of the synapses in the normal ganglia. We therefore interpret them as synaptic thickenings vacated by removal of the presynaptic elements. In a study of the response to denervation at progressively longer postoperative survival times, it was found that if the preganglionic chain is prevented from regenerating back into the ganglion (by suturing it to the thoracic musculature), the number of ganglionic synapses remains low and the number of vacated synaptic thickenings remains high. This situation still holds as long as thirteen months after operation.

Quite a different situation occurs if the preganglionic fibers are allowed to regenerate back into the ganglia. To show this, the preganglionic chain was frozen with a small fragment of dry ice. This destroys all the constituent axons but leaves the sheath of the nerve in continuity. Under these circumstances, rapid, consistent, and efficient regeneration was observed. For the first month after operation the results were indistinguishable from that of sectioning and tying down the preganglionic chain. This proves that the freeze lesion destroys all the axons in the preganglionic chain. During the second month after the freeze lesion, however, the number of

normal synapses began to rise again. It rose progressively until it reached normal levels by the beginning of the third month after the operation. From this time onwards there was no further increase. The newly reappeared synapses were distributed on dendritic shafts and spines in exactly the same ratio as the synapses in normal ganglia, or as the vacated synaptic thickenings in the denervated ganglia. In addition, as the number of synapses increased, the number of vacated synaptic thickenings decreased. By three months after the operation the numbers of synapses and vacated thickenings were back to normal levels. In four such animals we then sectioned the preganglionic chain surgically and observed exactly the same response to denervation as occurred when we cut the chain in the normal animals. This proves that the newly formed synapses do have their parent axons in the preganglionic trunk.

On the basis of these observations, we suggested the following conclusions:

1. When denervated, postsynaptic sites persist for at least several months; i.e., synaptic sites are not lost.

2. The original cut axons regenerate back into the ganglion, and when they reach the ganglion, they reoccupy the sites that were left vacant.

3. Hyperinnervation does not occur, indicating that no new synaptic sites are formed.

This reaction is one of true regeneration in the sense that preganglionic fibers reoccupy denervated sites previously occupied by preganglionic fibers. As yet we do not know to what extent a given pattern of connections may be reestablished by this type of regeneration, nor the full extent of the functional restitution. (For studies of trans-synaptic enzyme regulation in this situation, see Raisman et al., 1974.)

24.2.2 Septal nuclei

We have used a similar methodology to study the effects of selective partial denervation of a site in the central nervous system (Raisman, 1969; Raisman and Field 1973). The septal nuclei receive a massive input from the hippocampus of the same side. The majority of these fibers pass through the ipsilateral fimbria, a tract which can conveniently be destroyed completely by a lesion placed a few millimeters behind the caudal pole of the septum.

In the present study we have selected the neuropil of the lateral septal nucleus. In this region synapses are much more frequent than in the sympathetic ganglion. As opposed to the ganglion, which has 30 synapses per 1.8×10^4 sq. μm, the septal neuropil has 900 synapses in the same area. These synapses are distributed roughly as follows: 64 percent on dendritic spines; 32 percent on dendritic shafts; and 4 percent on cell somata. A majority of the synapses have recognizable postsynaptic thickenings, and there are no vacated synaptic thickenings in the normal septal neuropil.

After section of the ipsilateral fimbria, the axon terminals undergo orthograde degeneration, and they are ultimately removed by phagocytosis by nonneuronal cells in the same way as are those in the sympathetic ganglion. However, the time course of the reaction in the septum is entirely different from that in the ganglion. The fimbrial fiber terminals do not begin to show degeneration for at least 24 hours after the operation. They then undergo shrinkage, an increase in electron density, and degradation of their contents. Although showing these obvious signs of degeneration, the terminals remain in contact with the postsynaptic sites for up to a week in the majority of cases (some for longer). Subsequently they are removed by astroglial phagocytosis. Compared with the ganglion, this slower process of removal of degenerating terminals means that synaptic sites are only gradually vacated. After section of the fimbria, about half of the synapses on dendritic spines undergo degeneration; by contrast, only about 10 percent of those on dendritic shafts degenerate. Thus, during the first week after operation the number of nondegenerating synapses remaining on dendritic spines is reduced to about half that found in normal animals.

At survival times longer than one week, the degenerating synapses are removed, and by one month after operation there are practically no degenerating terminals left in contact with the synaptic thickenings. Although a few vacated synaptic thickenings are seen, they are never numerous. What has happened to the denervated sites becomes obvious when we study the incidence of nondegenerating synapses on dendritic spines. For the first postoperative week, while the degeneration is at its maximum, the number of nondegenerating synapses is reduced by half. This is not surprising—half the synapses degenerate, so only half remain. Over the next three weeks, however, as the number of degenerating terminals falls, the number of nondegenerating terminals on dendritic spines rises. It continues to rise until it reaches normal levels, at which time there is no further increase. The time course of reappearance of normal spinal synapses is exactly in phase with the time course of the disappearance of the degenerating synapses.

On the basis of these observations, we suggest the following conclusions:

1. When axon terminals are lost as a result of degeneration, the postsynaptic sites persist; i.e., there is no loss of synaptic sites.

2. Unlike the ganglion, the postsynaptic sites do not appear in large numbers as vacated thickenings.

3. Instead, the vacated postsynaptic sites are occupied rapidly (upon removal of the degeneration) by adjacent normal axonal terminals that have survived.

4. The process of reinnervation is efficient in reclaiming almost all the vacated synaptic sites, and it therefore restores exactly the previous ratio of spine to shaft synapses.

5. There is no hyperinnervation.

This postulated process of reinnervation involves the formation of connections by axons already present in the region, and it has therefore been called "collateral reinnervation" (by analogy with a similar reaction in the peripheral nervous system; see below). The process of collateral reinnervation in the septum is extremely rapid; it follows directly upon the removal of the degenerating terminals, without an intervening phase of vacated thickenings. It is also highly efficient, since it results in a reclamation of all the vacated sites. It is by no means a random reaction. However, it differs from the reaction seen in the ganglion in that the sites are reinnervated by undamaged fibers from the surrounding region. These are adventitious contacts which the normal septum does not have. The original, cut fimbrial axons do not grow back into the septum. Thus the process is not one of regeneration in the true sense—it does not result in a restoration of the original hippocamposeptal projection. Functionally, therefore, it cannot restore the interrupted hippocamposeptal relationship.

24.3 DISCUSSION

In considering why the ganglionic reaction differs from that of the septum, one fact is clear. The normal septal neuropil has 900 synapses per 1.8×10^4 sq. μm, whereas the ganglionic neuropil has only 30 in the same area. After preganglionic section the ganglionic neuropil is almost totally denervated—only 3 synapses per 1.8×10 sq. μm remain—whereas in the fimbrially denervated septum 650 synapses remain. Thus, even if the ganglion were able to mount a reaction of collateral reinnervation comparable to that seen in the septum, there would simply not be enough synapses left to provide a reaction of sufficient magnitude to reclaim a significant proportion of the vacated sites. This seems a reasonable explanation of why large numbers of vacated thickenings appear in the ganglion and only a very few in the septum.

On the other hand, this explanation cannot resolve all the differences between the ganglion and the septum. In reported experiments where the ganglion has been partially denervated by section of selected preganglionic nerve roots (Guth and Bernstein, 1961), physiological data suggest that the remaining fibers in the ganglion acquired additional functional connections with the cells denervated by the partial deafferentation. Nonetheless, in these animals the cut preganglionic roots did commence regeneration and grew steadily back to the ganglion. When they arrived there, they reestablished contact with the originally denervated cells and at the same time abolished the effectiveness of the abnormal (collateral) innervation (see also Mark and Marotte, 1972). Thus, although the partially denervated ganglion shows an initial reaction of collateral reinnervation, this process is superseded by true regeneration. In the septum, the fimbrial axons do not regenerate back into the septal region, although as Ramón y Cajal (1928) described, cut central axons do make abortive attempts at regeneration. Thus the septal neuropil does not appear to be capable of progressing from collateral reinnervation to true regeneration.

The present observations do make some inroads into the established idea that the neurons of the central nervous system are incapable of a positive reaction to injury: they show that central neurons are capable of rapid and efficient synaptogenesis in the adult. Unfortunately, they still leave open the intriguing question of why these neurons cannot exploit this reaction so as to produce true regeneration. Be that as it may, we feel that one frontier has been crossed: synaptogenesis is not the sole prerogative of peripheral neurons.

Investigations exploiting this similarity between the reactions to axonal injury in the central and peripheral nervous systems could eventually give rise to a more hopeful approach to the treatment of patients with central nervous trauma. Furthermore, this similarity may go some way toward explaining the apparent paradox that the mammalian central nervous system, which is regarded as specialized for maximum behavioral plasticity and adaptability, should be so much less plastic anatomically than either the peripheral nervous system (Guth, 1956) or even the central nervous system of cold-blooded vertebrates (Gaze, 1970). The present results cannot, of course, have a direct bearing on this problem, but they do suggest that in the regions where the greatest functional adaptability is present, the neuropil shows the greatest degree of collateral reinnervation. Conversely, where collateral reinnervation is a less prominent feature of the reaction to injury, true regeneration can take place; these are the parts of the nervous system where functional adaptability is at its least—i.e., the peripheral nervous system, and the central nervous system of lower vertebrates, both of which show much more stereotyped patterns of behavior. One could argue speculatively that the ability to regenerate nervous connections requires a specificity of synaptic matching which favors regeneration of the originally cut fibers and precludes collateral reinnervation by heterotypic fibers. By contrast, in the central nervous system of higher vertebrates, the nerve cells have a greater degree of freedom. As a result, when fibers are cut, collateral reinnervation develops readily and the denervated synaptic sites are reoccupied. This collateral competition for the postsynaptic sites might in some way militate against true regeneration.

This, however, is to look only at the narrow field of the response of the nervous system to axonal injury. A loss of the ability to regenerate after injury would seem to be an evolutionary disadvantage. What positive advantage could such a step confer upon an animal? Possibly the freedom from rigid synaptic specificity has quite another function—namely, to allow new connections to be readily formed during adult life. Our results clearly establish that rapid, efficient synaptogenesis is indeed a property of at least some neurons in the adult central nervous system. Can the occurrence of this sort of synaptogenesis explain some of the reactions involved in memory or learning?

REFERENCES

GAZE, R. M. 1970. *The Formation of Nerve Connections*. New York: Academic Press.

GUTH, L. 1956. Regeneration in the mammalian peripheral nervous system. *Physiological Review* 36:441–478.

GUTH, L., and BERNSTEIN, J. J. 1961. Selectivity in the reestablishment of synapses in the superior cervical sympathetic ganglion of the cat. *Experimental Neurology* 4:59–69.

GUTH, L., and WINDLE, W. F. 1970. The enigma of central nervous regeneration. *Experimental Neurology* Supplement 5:1–43.

KATZMAN, R., BJÖRKLUND, A., OWMAN, C., STENEVI, U., and WEST, K. A. 1971. Evidence for regenerative axon sprouting of central catecholamine neurons in the rat mesencephalon following electrolytic lesions. *Brain Research* 25:579–596.

MARK, R. F., and MAROTTE, L. R. 1972. The mechanisms of selective reinnervation of fish eye muscles. III. Functional, electrophysiological and anatomical analysis of recovery from section of the IIIrd and IVth nerves. *Brain Research* 46:131–148.

RAISMAN, G. 1969. Neuronal plasticity in the septal nuclei of the adult rat. *Brain Research* 14: 25–48.

RAISMAN, G. 1973. Electron microscopic studies of the development of new neurohaemal contacts in the median eminence of the rat after hypophysectomy. *Brain Research* 55:245–261.

RAISMAN, G., and FIELD, P. M. 1973. A quantitative investigation of the development of collateral reinnervation after partial deafferentation of the septal nuclei. *Brain Research* 50:241–264.

RAISMAN, G., FIELD, P. M., OSTBERG, A. J. C., IVERSEN, L. L., and ZIGMOND, R. E. 1974. A quantitative ultrastructural and biochemical analysis of the process of reinnervation of the superior cervical ganglion in the adult rat. *Brain Research* 71:1–16.

RAMÓN y CAJAL, S. 1928. *Degeneration and Regeneration of the Nervous System*. London: Oxford University Press. (Reprint, New York: Hafner Publishing Company, 1968).

Simple Systems in the
Study of Memory:
Tissue-Culture Approaches

25

Neuronal Cell Cultures and Their Application to the Problem of Plasticity

PHILLIP G. NELSON AND
CLIFFORD N. CHRISTIAN

ABSTRACT Neurons from the vertebrate central nervous system can be grown in surface cultures at densities allowing considerable experimental resolution of cell properties. Small circuits of neurons can be characterized physiologically as to electrical activity, chemosensitivity, and synaptic connectivity. Subsequent morphological analysis of these same neurons might include silver staining or electron microscopy. Biochemical studies of entire cultures are readily made, and currently feasible technologies allow enzymatic and protein-synthesis studies to be done on a single cell or small groups of cells. Chronic long-term control of the electrical activity of entire cultures or of smaller neuronal networks is feasible. The simplification, accessibility, and manipulability of cultured neurons offer a number of unique opportunities for the study of the cellular mechanisms of plasticity.

The cellular-connectionistic theory of brain function, which explains the storage of information in terms of the formation or modulation of synapses (Kandel and Spencer, 1967) has attained a nearly universal acceptance, at least as a methodological approach to the study of learning and memory. We shall argue that tissue and cell cultures of the central nervous system offer unique opportunities to study intercellular connections and their plasticity. After making a general case for in vitro studies of neuronal interactions, we shall describe some findings relevant to the electrophysiological, morphological, and biochemical approaches to plasticity.

25.1 THE ANALYSIS OF SYNAPTIC FUNCTION

25.1.1 In vitro techniques employing peripheral organs

Much of our present knowledge of synaptic transmission derives from work on short-term organ cultures of the vertebrate peripheral nervous system. Its hardiness and accessibility to experimental manipulation have made the vertebrate neuromuscular junction a preeminent in vitro preparation. The quantal packaging of transmitter, the temporally random release of quanta, the increased probability of quantal release with depolariza-

tion of the presynaptic terminal, the change in the permeability of the postsynaptic membrane, the enzymatic deactivation of transmitter, the localization of postsynaptic transmitter sensitivity, the increased postsynaptic sensitivity with denervation—in short, most of our current concepts of synaptic transmission—are derived from studies on this preparation (Katz, 1969). If one is ever to understand learning in vertebrates as the modulation of synaptic transmission, then it will be necessary to have preparations of CNS neurons that are at least as accessible to experimental manipulation and long-term study as the in vitro neuromuscular junction.

The adult sympathetic ganglion, which can be maintained for at least a day in a chemically defined medium, is another useful preparation. In addition to a fast excitatory postsynaptic potential (EPSP) and inhibitory postsynaptic potential (IPSP), cells in this ganglion exhibit a slow EPSP and IPSP, lasting many seconds, produced by decreases in ionic conductance (Weight, 1973). Libet and Tosaka (1970) report that a short exposure to dopamine potentiates the slow EPSP for a period of hours. It has been proposed that acetylcholine (ACh) produces a similar slow EPSP in many CNS neurons (Krnjević, 1974). This type of EPSP, by increasing the input resistance of a neuron, would tend to make it more responsive to any additional synaptic input, and hence is one model of heterosynaptic facilitation. Its time course makes it a candidate, along with reverberating circuits, for the short-term storage of information.

25.1.2 Tissue-slice preparations

The use of tissue slices from the adult CNS improves accessibility and manipulation, and a wide range of biochemical and pharmacological studies have been carried out (McIlwain, 1971). Although tissue slicing subjects the neurons studied to gross damage from which they have little time to recover, intracellularly recorded neuronal activity has been elicited by stimulating the tracts attached to a slice of mammalian cortex (Richards and Sercombe, 1968; Yamamoto, 1972). Direct electrical stimulation of a slice lowers its incorporation of

PHILLIP G. NELSON and CLIFFORD N. CHRISTIAN, Behavioral Biology Branch, National Institute of Child Health and Human Development, Bethesda, MD

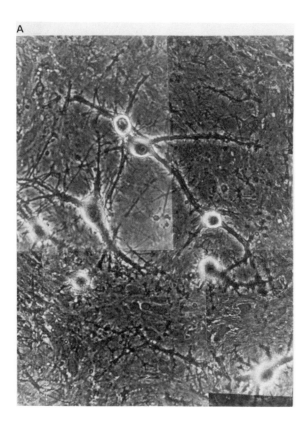

FIGURE 25.1(a) A composite phase-contrast photomicrograph of dissociated neuronal tissue. Ten-week-old spinal-cord cultures, with a group of large multipolar neurons.

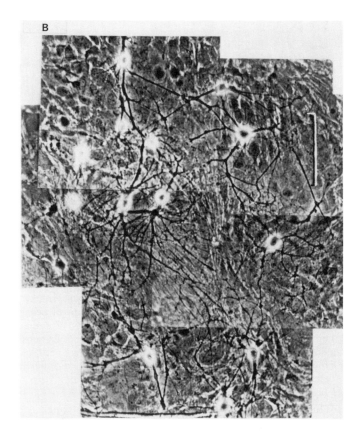

FIGURE 25.1(b) Five-week-old fetal rat cerebral cortex. The bar is 50 μm and applies to both montages.

radioactive precursors into both protein (Orrego and Lipmann, 1967) and RNA (Prives and Quastel, 1969). The decrease in RNA incorporation is prevented when electrical activity is blocked by tetrodotoxin. Schultz and Daly (1973) have demonstrated that adenosine and norepinephrine combine to elevate cyclic AMP levels in brain slices by over 100-fold. This is relevant to the theory that adrenergic activation of forebrain structures produces consolidation in recently activated synapses (Kety, 1970, and this volume).

Unfortunately, tissue slices of adult brain are not stable for any length of time in vitro. We shall therefore turn our attention to cell and tissue cultures, the properties of which have a more constant baseline against which long-term modulation can be examined.

25.1.3 Advantages of tissue and cell culture

One attractive feature of present-day culture technology is that, to a certain extent, an investigator can select a system of neurons (we refrain from saying a nervous system) with the types of cell density, connections, and organization most suited to his experimental needs. Organ or tissue explants retain a high degree of topo-

graphic specificity and are similar in anatomical organization to the tissue of origin (Seil and Leiman, this volume). Reaggregates of single cells display neuronal enzyme activities as high as those of the adult CNS (Seeds, 1973) and even show a geometry that is apparently specified by the cells composing them (DeLong, 1970). Cell cultures or surface cultures of dissociated cells develop neuronal networks of moderate complexity and exhibit a number of highly differentiated neuronal characteristics. Surface cultures are also amenable to analysis at the cellular level, because living preparations can be analyzed electrophysiologically and morphologically with considerable cellular detail (Figure 25.1). The growing literature describing methods and techniques (for reviews see Murray and Kopech, 1953; Murray, 1965, 1971; Lumsden, 1968; Nelson, 1975) indicates that it may become easier to grow systems of neurons for a given experimental application than to search out appropriate species having the required properties.

In addition to the obvious simplification and accessibility that culture techniques offer, they provide a number of other unique and useful features. For example, long-term treatments with pharmacologically active compounds, such as toxins and anesthetics, can be done most readily and under the most controlled conditions in vitro.

Another feature reflects the techniques by which cultures can be enriched with the cell type of interest. Differential cell plating has been used to increase the ratio of neuronal to nonneuronal cells in cultures of dorsal-root ganglion and sympathetic ganglion (Okun, Ontkean, and Thomas, 1972; Varon and Raiborn, 1972; Mains and Patterson, 1973a), and also in chick cerebral hemispheres (Varon and Raiborn, 1969). This ratio may also be altered by various pharmacological treatments (Shapiro, 1973) or by plating cells from embryos of different ages. Although it is not presently possible to isolate a pure population of neurons, one can expect some success with the techniques of differential sedimentation, electrophoresis, selective absorption, and affinity chromatography.

Small internuncial neurons, because they are among the last cells to develop ontogenetically (Altman, 1967) and phylogenetically, are correlated with behavioral plasticity (Young, 1966), and they may play important roles in learning and memory. However, they are too small for electrophysiological analysis even in invertebrates (Cohen, 1970). There is a growing corpus of techniques by which the size of neurons may be influenced in vitro, by special media (Mains and Patterson, 1973a,b), treatments with cyclic AMP (Shapiro, 1973; Schrier and Shapiro, 1973), antimitotic agents (Peacock et al., 1972), or x-irradiation (Prasad, 1971). Some cell types not amenable to study in vivo may possibly be studied in vitro.

The use of surface cultures of neurons permits electrodes to be readily positioned near the cells in relatively complex configurations involving several recording and stimulating electrodes. In addition to the electrodes, perfusion cannulas can be used to manipulate the cell's environment.

25.1.4 Assumptions and problems in cell and tissue culture

There is no doubt that many features of nervous-system function are permanently obliterated by the dissociation and culturing procedure. Many differentiated neurobiological features do persist, however, and it is our working hypothesis that these cultures exhibit enough of the properties of normal tissue to make their study relevant to the elucidation of neuronal mechanisms important to the intact organism.

In particular, we suppose that, in culture, cells mature and differentiate to have the same constellation of morphological and functional properties as cells in organisms.

This is difficult to validate, but there is some evidence that specific properties of cell type are determined at a relatively early stage of neurodifferentiation and may not be substantially altered by conditions of growth. As pictured in Figure 25.2, cells derived from spinal cord and dorsal-root ganglion maintain their characteristic appearances and electrophysiological properties when grown in culture. Reidentifiable cells (having unique and constant properties in each example of a species) are an unavailable luxury in vertebrate culture preparations, but they may be possible in long-term cultures of invertebrate ganglia (Levi-Montalcini and Seshan, 1973).

That neurons in vitro do maintain characteristic neuronal properties has occupied the bulk of the literature of neuronal cultures (Nelson, 1975). This often produces a feeling of in vitro déjà vu: yet another paper demonstrates that some phenomenon already known to exist in vivo can exist with something less than a traditional life-support system. Such studies are necessary, however, to establish in these fledgling systems replicable baseline parameters against which modulation and plasticity can be studied. As in any system, invariant properties must first be found before functional modifica-

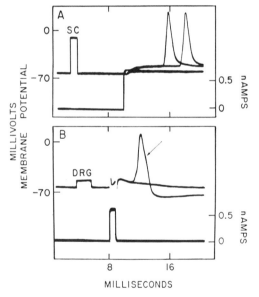

FIGURE 25.2 Characteristic properties of cells of spinal cord (SC) and dorsal-root ganglion (DRG) in monolayer cultures. (A) Action potentials from an SC cell are shown in the upper trace during sequential sweeps of an oscilloscope. Voltage calibration pulse is 50 mV by 1 msec long. The lower trace shows the stimulating current pulse. (B) An action potential from a DRG cell showing change from an initally slow phase (arrow) to a faster repolarization phase and then a more negative afterpotential than the SC cell. One of the two superimposed stimuli (lower trace) failed to elicit an action potential. Voltage calibration pulse is 10 mV by 2 msec. From Peacock, Nelson, and Goldstone (1973).

C

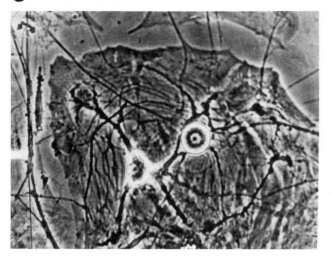

FIGURE 25.2(C) Morphologies of the two cell types, grown together in dissociated cultures. A multipolar SC cell on the left can be distinguished from the more spheroid DRG cell on the right, the latter having fewer processes.

tions can be analyzed, or even recognized as something other than experimental variation.

Behavior is conspicuously absent from a tissue-culture plate. Hence, modifiable cellular mechanisms analyzed in this milieu can be offered at the present time only as possible mechanisms to account for the changes in behavior that result from experience. Moreover, lacking any example of learning to pursue to its cellular substrate, experimenters using culture techniques are dependent on analyses of whole organisms for their choice of materials and experimental orientation. It is in this light that we shall review areas of research in the neurobiology of learning and memory and relate them to parallel work now underway with cell and tissue cultures. Not having to bear the weight of a behavioral analysis, and possessing a number of unique experimental advantages, cell and tissue culture approaches will perhaps make some substantial strides in analyzing cellular mechanisms of information storage.

D

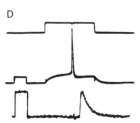

Figure 25.2(D) Synaptic interaction in an SC–SC pair. Current passed into one SC cell produced an action potential (upper two traces), which elicited an EPSP in the second SC cell (lower trace). Both calibration pulses are 10 mV by 5 msec.

25.2 ELECTROPHYSIOLOGICAL ANALYSIS OF PLASTICITY IN INTACT SYSTEMS

25.2.1 Habituation

The habituation of the flexion reflex in the spinal cat has many of the same behavioral parameters as various types of habituation in the intact organism (Thompson and Spencer, 1966). The plasticity of this reflex could result from desensitization (Sharpless, 1964), posttetanic potentiation of inhibitory synapses (Wickelgren, 1967a, b; Wall, 1970), or self-generated depression at an excitatory synapse (Horn, 1967). Intracellular recordings from spinal motoneurons during the habituation of the flexion reflex show an attenuation in both depolarizing and hyperpolarizing synaptic potentials. Such responses, reflecting the sum of many simultaneous synaptic inputs, do not rule out any proposed mechanism.

In a review of the behavioral literature, Groves and Thompson (1970) argued that repetitive stimulus presentations first produce a period of incremental responding (sensitization), and then habituation; this is also true in the spinal cat. Using extracellular electrodes, they found two types of spinal-cord interneurons that display plasticity during repetitive stimulation of the skin or cutaneous nerves. One set, located primarily in the dorsal grey matter, responds with a short-latency, high-frequency activity which progressively decreases with repetition. A second set, located more ventrally, responds with a longer latency, has a longer period of firing, and shows an initial increase in responsiveness with repetition, followed by maintained or decreased activity. They argued, therefore, that the two components of the behavioral responsiveness to repetitive stimuli are produced by separate plastic circuits. They have reviewed a number of models for habituation (Groves and Thompson, 1970, 1973), and have argued on indirect grounds that during stimulus repetition, intrinsic synaptic mechanisms in the excitatory pathway of the flexion reflex produce either decremental or initially incremental transmission.

Single units in many areas rostral to the spinal cord show response attenuation to repetitive stimuli (Segundo and Bell, 1970). Interestingly, about 75 percent of recorded units in the superior colliculus and brainstem reticular formation show such attenuation (Bell et al., 1964; Groves, Miller, and Parker, 1972; Horn and Hill, 1966a; Scheibel and Scheibel, 1965). Because habituating units have been observed in the mesencephalon of decorticate animals (Horn and Hill, 1966b), and in the sectioned spinal cord (Spencer, Thompson, and Neilson, 1966a,b,c), many forms of habituation are probably not due to inhibitory control by higher brain centers but are, rather, localized in each area of the brain.

25.2.2 Electrophysiological studies of associative learning in vertebrates

Extracellularly recorded neuronal activity has been sampled in an attempt to analyze the changes in the interconnection of neurons taking place during associative learning and to localize this plasticity. The classical or sensory conditioning of restrained or curarized animals has been shown to change the response of many single units to a conditioned stimulus. With intertrial intervals of from 3 to 30 seconds, modifiable units have been found in the brainstem reticular formation (Burešová and Bureš, 1965; Lindsley et al., 1973; Yoshii and Ogura, 1960), the thalamus (Chow, Lindsley, and Gollender, 1968; Kamikawa, McIlwain, and Adey, 1964), the sensory cortex (Adam, Adey, and Porter, 1966) and the motor cortex (O'Brien and Fox, 1969a,b). Generally, more caudal areas contain a greater percentage of modifiable units and exhibit conditioned responses after fewer trials. By this criterion, reticular systems are the most modifiable, with 50 percent of all recorded units demonstrating some plasticity, often within 25 trials. A more rapid conditionability of lower brain structures was also found with multiunit recording techniques (Buchwald, Halas, and Schramm, 1966; Halas, Beardsley, and Sandlie, 1970). Such results do not demonstrate that the recorded cells have undergone modification themselves, rather than following the altered output of a plastic circuit located elsewhere in the brain. They do suggest that brainstem reticular structures may be useful tissue to employ in testing cellular models of associational mechanisms.

One of the most ambitious electrophysiological studies of learning has partially mapped the entire brain during the classical conditioning of unrestrained rats (Olds et al., 1972). Single or multiunit responses elicited by a tone are recorded with chronic electrodes during pseudoconditioning and during the pairing of the tone with the delivery of food. If previously unused circuits are switched in to produce the conditioned response of approaching the food dispenser during the positive conditioned stimulus (CS), then the area in which this switching occurs will exhibit an altered responsiveness to the CS. Of course, many units will be driven by the altered output of other areas as well as by feedback from the learned response. Hence, the area with the shortest latency of CS-elicited activity that is altered by conditioning has the highest probability of containing the neurons undergoing switching. Furthermore, the plastic area must "learn" the response at least as fast as the behavior is acquired. Therefore, this experimental approach has measured both the latency of detectable changes in CS-elicited activity and the number of trials required for this change to take place. A preliminary inspection of the brain has been made to find the "earliest new response" in various neuronal systems.

Of the hindbrain and midbrain areas sampled, short-latency activity specific to the positive CS was found in the midlateral region of the ventral brainstem (Kornblith and Olds, 1973) and the ventral tegmentum (Olds et al., 1972), but not in the tectum or the adjacent dorsal midbrain reticular formation. The posterior thalamic nucleus contained the highest proportion of units exhibiting modified responses to the CS during conditioning (Olds et al., 1972). In general, the hypothalamus had no early responses that were modified by training (Olds, 1973), with the exception of the preoptic boundary with the striatum, where short-latency responses were learned very quickly (Linseman and Olds, 1973). Learning points were found in all parts of the neocortex, and many of them were specific to the positive CS (Disterhoft and Olds, 1972).

The method of studying CS-elicited latencies and single-unit learning curves has been applied most thoroughly to a study of the plasticity of sensory processing in the hippocampus, where latencies are the shortest of any region in the forebrain (Segal, 1973; Segal and Olds, 1972). Because area CA3 has shorter-latency responses and demonstrates faster learning than units in CA1, it has been proposed that CA3 passes learned information to area CA1. Although both the dentate and the entorhinal cortex are afferent to CA3, they have longer CS latencies than CA3, and thus cannot explain CA3 plasticity.

All single-unit studies during classical conditioning suggest that lower brain structures may possess a great deal of plasticity. In addition, they affirm a general caudal-to-rostral gradient in the number of trials necessary to produce detectable changes in CS-elicited neuronal activity during conditioning.

Instead of systematically mapping the brain, Woody and his collaborators have used a paradigm with a discrete behavioral response of short latency, which hopefully involves a restricted area of the brain. In a steady-state analysis, they compared populations of cells from naive animals, animals thoroughly conditioned by the pairing of a click with glabellar tap, and animals extinguished by reversing the order of CS and US presentation. The conditioned response, an eyeblink, was monitored by electromyography of the orbicularis oculi muscles. After the activity of a single unit was studied, its projection to the orbicularis oculi was affirmed by checking whether a low stimulating current passed from the recording electrode elicited an electromyographic response.

The coronal-pericruciate area probably contains, or is directly connected to, a region in which the registration of a conditioned response occurs (Woody, Vassilersky, and Engel, 1970; Woody et al., 1974). The readout of this conditioned response has been investigated with intracellular electrode techniques (Woody and Black-Cleworth, 1973). After conditioning, no change in the spontaneous discharge rate or the rate of PSPs in relevant neurons was noted. However, in units projecting to the target muscles of the conditioned response, current thresholds for spike initiation were lowered. Such a postsynaptic effect, which suggests an increase in neuronal input resistance, can account for both the motor specificity and the nonspecific effects of conditioning, such as increases in spontaneous blinking and responsiveness to glabellar tap. There may, however, be other cellular mechanisms that account for the sensory specificity of conditioned animals.

25.2.2 Cellular theories of associative learning

Despite a paucity of data, many theorists of the neurophysiology of learning, following Hebb (1949), have been convinced that learning cannot be accounted for by the long-term modulation with use of a single synapse. Rather, the associative nature of learning, a major notion in psychology since the time of Locke and Hume, apparently calls for a mechanism of plasticity initiated by the temporal association of two events in one neuron. In some forms of classical conditioning the unconditioned stimulus must follow shortly after the conditioned stimulus, and in some forms of operant conditioning a reward must closely follow the response that is to be reinforced. The temporal properties of these behavioral paradigms have been explained by plastic mechanisms at the cellular level which are triggered by the simultaneous occurrence of two events (Leiman and Christian, 1973). Possible plastic synapses that could account for classical conditioning have been described by Brindley (1967, 1969) and extended to operant conditioning by Kupfermann and Pinsker (1969).

Krasne (this volume) points out the present inadequacy of the argument for the parametric similarity of cellular and behavioral events. Certainly, important types of associative learning may have temporal properties far removed from those characterizing classical conditioning (Garcia and Levine, this volume). Further, the temporal specificity of a circuit ocan be btained by presently known mechanisms plus appropriately wired interneurons, and thus need not require that a single neuron recognize the simultaneous occurrence of two events (Kupfermann and Pinsker, 1969). In the few cases of heterosynaptic facilitation in invertebrates that require the specific pairing of two stimuli, the presence of interneurons has not been ruled out, and hence it has not been proved that a specific associative cellular mechanism exists. Despite this lack of confirming behavioral or neurophysiological data, interest in associative cellular mechanisms remains high, perhaps due to their elegant simplicity, or to the difficulty in imagining how the change with use of a single synapse could account for all examples of learning and memory.

In our treatment we shall classify associative cellular mechanisms in a methodological rather than a conceptual manner. We shall thus classify plastic cell interactions not in terms of what function they may perform in a circuit to produce behavior, but in terms of how their presence can be verified. Homosynaptic mechanisms can be discovered by placing two electrodes in the somata of the pre- and postsynaptic cells of a single synapse. The testing of heterosynaptic mechanisms requires at least one additional electrode in a neuron that modulates the efficiency of the tested synapse.

In Table 25.1A we have described four homosynaptic tests of temporal specificity. It is hypothesized that a repetitive pairing of an elicited PSP with either an action potential or a hyperpolarization in the postsynaptic neuron will modify the subsequent size of that PSP. Since the resulting modulation could be either an increase or a decrease in the size of the PSP, there are eight possible outcomes. To demonstrate temporal specificity, unpaired controls are required, as well as tests to demonstrate the effect of postsynaptic membrane manipulation alone.

This scheme is a generalization of the Brindley-Hebb and perceptron synapses (Hebb, 1949; Brindley, 1967; Rosenblatt, 1962). Arbib, Kilmer and Spinelli (this volume) have described how these plastic elements might function in circuits to perform definite learning tasks.

Another associative mechanism may be testable by a monosynaptic paradigm. Kety (1970) has hypothesized that aminergic pathways, originating in the brainstem, fan out through all parts of the brain and, when active, modulate the efficiency of simultaneously active synapses. A formal treatment of this notion has been elaborated for the climbing fibers of the cerebrum (Blomfield and Marr, 1970) and cerebellum (Marr, 1970). In cultures of cerebrum lacking brainstem neurons, the effects of climbing-fiber activity can be mimicked by perfusion with biogenic amines or brainstem extracts.

In addition to the modulation of synaptic transmission, these paradigms might produce other effects (von Baumgarten, 1970), including a slow polarization due to an ionic pump, the initiation of pacemaker activity, and a change in membrane properties that alters the firing level.

There is evidence that synaptic input, rather than depolarization alone, is required for the initiation of metabolic changes (Geinismann, 1972; Peterson and

TABLE 25.1
Results of various experimental manipulations for testing the specificity of two cellular events

	A. Homosynaptic mechanisms. Current passed into B produces:		B. Heterosynaptic mechanisms with target interaction. Stimulation of C produces in B:		C. Heterosynaptic mechanisms with afferent interaction. Stimulation of C produces as presynaptic modulation of A:	
	Action potential	Hyperpolarization	EPSP	IPSP	Facilitation	Inhibition
Stimulation of A produces in B:						
EPSP	Successful use	Unsuccessful use	Augmentation	Reduction	Increase of excitation	Decrease of excitation
IPSP	Unsuccessful use	Successful use	Reduction	Augmentation	Decrease of excitation	Increase of excitation

Experimental paradigms for testing the effect of the association of two events on long-term synaptic efficiency. In each paradigm a postsynaptic potential (PSP) in the test pathway is paired with another event during conditioning (see Figure 25.3). It is postulated that the pairing produces a long-term change in the size of the test PSP. In the homosynaptic paradigm (A) the test PSP is paired with current injection into the target cell. In the two simplest cases of heterosynaptic associative interactions, the test PSP is paired with the elicited activity of the modulator cell. The interactions of these two events can take place in the target cell (B) or in the synaptic terminals of the test pathway (C).

Loh, 1973). In the giant neuron R_2 of the *Aplysia* abdominal ganglion, synaptic input that elicited action potentials increased the incorporation of a radioactive RNA precursor. However, intracellular depolarization producing an equivalent number of spikes failed to increase incorporation (Peterson and Kernell, 1970; Kernell and Peterson, 1970). This alteration in RNA metabolism may be due to an alteration in the size of the precursor pool rather than a direct action on RNA synthesis (Berry and Cohen, 1972). These data suggest that synaptic inputs, rather than spike activity per se, are important events in altering metabolic activity. Associative mechanisms may therefore depend on the temporal interaction of two or more synaptic events (see Figure 25.3). We shall define heterosynaptic associational mechanisms to be those in which the simultaneous activation of two afferents to one cell subsequently modifies the efficiency of one of the afferents.

In heterosynaptic associative mechanisms with target or postsynaptic interaction, both inputs produce PSPs in

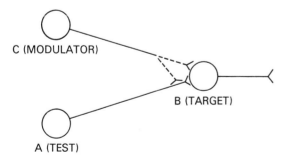

FIGURE 25.3 Possible sites for the interaction of activity in a test pathway with simultaneous activity in a target or modulator cell.

the postsynaptic cell. The possibilities of associative interaction between a test and a modulator input to a target cell are detailed in Table 25.1B. Mark (1970) has proposed one of these possibilities on the basis of studies of the competitive reinnervation of muscle. An inappropriate motor nerve will innervate denervated muscle, but its synaptic transmission will be quickly switched off if an appropriate motor nerve subsequently innervates the muscle (Mark, Marotte, and Mart, 1972). This suggests that activity of one synapse on a neuron may decrease the efficiency of other synapses on that cell, and one might postulate a postsynaptic mechanism as the basis for this decrease.

Heterosynaptic associative mechanisms might also be based on afferent interactions (Table 25.1C), and the known phenomena of presynaptic facilitation and inhibition (Eccles, 1964; Tauc, 1965) could serve as the mechanism underlying such effects. In afferent interactions the modulator neuron contacts the test pathway at a point presynaptic to the target cell. It is well known that presynaptic interactions between afferent fibers occur, and the mechanisms underlying presynaptic facilitation and inhibition have received much study. If these mechanisms are to be related to heterosynaptic associative phenomena, however, some temporal relationship between the activation of the two pathways is crucial to the long-term efficiency of one pathway. Researchers have attempted to show that some cases of heterosynaptic facilitation do have a temporally specific component (Kandel and Tauc, 1965a,b; Tauc and Epstein, 1967; Epstein and Tauc, 1970). They have established that the effect is due to presynaptic interactions, but they have not conclusively ruled out a role for interneurons in securing temporal specificity, and hence have not implicated a mechanism with more specificity than presynaptic facilitation.

25.3 IN VITRO STUDIES

There are now sufficient examples in the literature to justify the generalization that any given area of the CNS can be grown and will differentiate in vitro to possess a degree of synaptic activity that will warrant using this preparation to study intercellular plasticity. We shall emphasize the analytical advantages of such preparations: the morphological identification of cell type and connection, the possibility of recording intracellularly from both the presynaptic and postsynaptic neurons of a connection, and the testing of neuronal membrane properties by perfusion and microiontophoretic application of drugs. These techniques permit an advanced analysis of the neuronal plasticity observed during animal training and allow the direct testing of certain hypothesized cellular mechanisms of learning and memory.

25.3.1 In vitro neuronal models
Because of its relative simplicity and known pharmacology, the sympathetic ganglion is an excellent system for a range of problems in neurobiology. Explants of sympathetic ganglion have been used to study the action of nerve growth factor (NGF) (Levi-Montalcini and Angeletti, 1968) and the migration of cell types (Chamley et al., 1972). Dissociated cells can be readily cultured, form extensive processes (Bunge, 1973), bind α-bungarotoxin (Greene et al., 1973), and have neuronal electrical properties.

A method has been found to culture dissociated neurons in the virtual absence of nonneuronal cells (Mains and Patterson, 1973a,b,c). With time, such cultures develop the capacity to accumulate and synthesize catecholamines and resemble the norepinephrine cells of the in vivo ganglion. The uniformity and purity of this cell type in culture should facilitate studies of the modulation of receptor and enzyme concentrations by treatments with ACh, NGF, and coculturing with spinal-cord or sympathetic target tissues. Hence, various models of "change with use" can be investigated with sympathetic-ganglion neurons (Thoenen, 1974).

A number of laboratories are producing cultures of spinal cord and dorsal-root ganglion which possess differentiated neuronal properties characteristic of the tissue of origin. They should be good preparations for analyzing the possible mechanisms of habituation, sensitization, and posttetanic potentiation which are exhibited by the spinal cord in vivo. Spinal-cord explants develop connections and become myelinated in vitro (Peterson, Crain, and Murray, 1965), and they maintain characteristic spinal-cord structures (Guillery, Sobkowicz, and Scott, 1968, 1970).

Dissociated cell cultures, although they lack myelination, are also highly differentiated (Meller et al., 1969) and are optimal for concurrent morphological and electrophysiological analyses (see Figure 25.2). The neuronal form expressed in cell cultures of spinal cord (SC) and dorsal-root ganglion (DRG) is reminiscent of the form that develops normally in vivo. DRG cells have a highly characteristic round cell body, with a central nucleus, a prominent nucleolus, and one or two sparsely branched, thin processes which taper very little. These contrast very strongly with another identifiable group of cells, the large multipolar SC cells, which have several processes with rapid tapers and rich branching patterns. Silver stains usually reveal one very long process with less taper and fewer branches, which presumably represents an axon. A number of factors are involved in the development of cell processes—for example, the nature of the surface to which the processes attach. However, the difference between SC and DRG cells cannot be ascribed to such features of the cell microenvironment. It represents, to a significant degree, a feature of the differentiation of these cells which, once initiated, is controlled largely by the cells themselves. Thus cellular control mechanisms must exist which will account for such morphological specialization more or less independently of the environment.

The differentiation of electrophysiological properties has been shown to parallel the morphological differentiation of SC and DRG cells from the mouse (Peacock, Nelson, and Goldstone, 1973) and the chick (Fischbach and Dichter, 1974). The action-potential configuration is different in the cell types; the DRG action potential has an initial relatively slow phase of repolarization followed by a more rapid phase, while the SC action potential has a smooth uninflected falling phase (Figure 25.2a,b). A more pronounced hyperpolarizing afterpotential follows the action potential in DRG than in SC cells. Fischbach and Dichter have shown that the ionic mechanisms involved in generation of the two cell types are different. Both Ca^{++} and Na^+ ions participate in the depolarizing phase of the action potential generated in DRG cell somata, while only Na^+ ions are involved in SC-cell action-potential generation. Ca^{++} ions do not appear to be involved in action potentials propagated along the axons of the DRG or SC cells. The functional implications of these properties are not clear, but they certainly represent maintained and differentiated physiological properties that correlate precisely with cell morphology.

Extensive synaptic connections occur in these cultures,

and networks of some complexity develop as they mature; both excitatory and inhibitory postsynaptic potentials occur. Morphologically identified pairs of SC and DRG cells have been studied with intracellular electrodes (Figure 25.2d). In many cases a single action potential, elicited in the DRG by direct stimulation, produced an EPSP in the SC neuron. No postsynaptic activity in DRG neurons followed SC-cell action potentials, even though a few DRG neurons displayed some apparently spontaneous synaptic input (Fischbach and Dichter, 1974). Synaptic coupling was also readily demonstrated between pairs of SC neurons.

Dissociated brain cells have also been successfully cultured, and they have exhibited synapse formation, myelinated fibers (Bornstein and Model, 1972), and complex electrical activity (Crain and Bornstein, 1972). Various morphological cell types have been observed (Grosse and Lindner, 1970), but their correspondence to in vivo cell types is not known. The identification of cells that have active uptake systems for various neurotransmitters may be quite useful in identifying cell types in vitro. For example, cerebellar cultures contain neurons that concentrate extracellular γ-aminobutyric acid (GABA) (Lasher and Zagon, 1972). Intracellular recordings from cerebellar neurons have disclosed hyperpolarizing IPSPs and EPSPs, and have demonstrated the feasibility of analyzing small networks of neurons (Nelson and Peacock, 1973). Rat brain cell cultures have been produced that are optimal for concurrent morphological and electrophysiological studies (Godfrey et al., 1975).

25.3.2 Receptor-surface mapping

A striking property of cell cultures is the accessibility of the entire dendritic tree of a neuron, in contradistinction to the hermetic neuropil of the vertebrate CNS or the invertebrate ganglion. In many cases a drug pipette can be positioned under direct visual guidance, which allows topographic mapping of the receptor surface of a cell (Figure 25.4). The tip of the pipette can be brought close to the membrane surface, thereby producing a high degree of spatial resolution with low iontophoretic currents and minimizing artifacts.

With this method it was found that in rat brain cell cultures the reversal potentials of IPSPs for GABA and glycine are very similar if not identical (Godfrey et al., 1975). The effect of these compounds is therefore compatible with their suggested role as neurotransmitters.

In some of the cultured SC cells where a glutamate response and an EPSP were tested concurrently, there were clear differences in the reversal potentials. Both somatic and distal dendritic regions could be tested with glutamate, and the results appeared to be incompatible

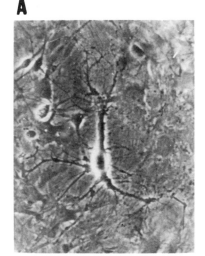

A

$\underline{50\,\mu}$

FIGURE 25.4(A) Topographic mapping of the responsiveness of a spinal-cord cell 4 weeks in culture, as it appeared in phase contrast during mapping.

with the hypothesis that glutamate functions as the excitatory transmitter (Ransom and Nelson, 1975). Topographic mapping revealed large differences in receptor-surface sensitivity. Some SC cells were also sensitive to glycine but were desensitized by concentrations of glycine at which GABA responses could still be elicited. Thus the glycine receptor of SC cells differs from that found in brain, and the glycine and GABA receptors of SC cells can be unequivocally differentiated. Even when cells were chronically exposed to glycine, glycine responses could be elicited as soon as the cells were placed in a glycine-free medium. In such cultures, however, preliminary results indicate that the incidence of IPSPs

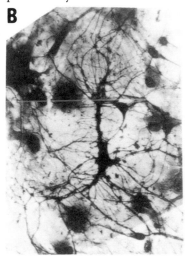

B

FIGURE 25.4(B) Same cell culture after fixation and silver staining.

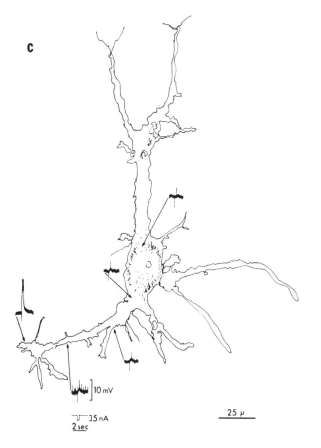

c

10 mV

5 nA

2 sec

25 μ

FIGURE 25.4(C) The depolarizing responses of the cell, recorded with a microelectrode in the soma, to the microiontophoretic application of glutamate. The arrows indicate the position of the electrode filled with 0.5 M glutamate, through which current was passed to release the ion (lower-left current trace). Different locations on the cell surface were not equally responsive.

is greatly reduced (three- to fivefold reduction) in comparison to cultures grown in the absence of glycine. This work indicates that the regulation of extracellular levels of amino acids and other transmitters may control the overall behavior of neuronal circuits.

Microiontophoretic application of acetylcholine (ACh) has been used to map the surface of cultured muscle cells. In rat muscle organ cultures, Fambrough (1970) demonstrated that the spread in ACh sensitivity with denervation was dependent on RNA and protein synthesis. Cohen and Fischbach (1973) demonstrated that this muscle-fiber sensitivity was related to the electrical activity of the muscle. In both innervated and uninnervated muscle, when the muscle action potential was blocked by lidocaine or tetrodotoxin, ACh sensitivity increased. Direct electrical stimulation, on the other hand, decreased sensitivity. If such work can be extended to CNS neurons, it will have important consequences for our understanding of how a neuron modu-

lates its receptor surface to maintain a given level of tonic activity. Such a mechanism could explain how chronic activity at one excitatory synapse can, by lowering the general sensitivity of a cell, decrease the efficiency of other excitatory synapses on that cell.

The feasibility of cellular topographic mapping and of the morphological methods to be discussed in the next section, allows a further refinement of the questions that have been asked concerning associative cellular mechanisms. If the simultaneous occurrence of two inputs modulates synaptic efficiency, it can be determined whether the two inputs need to be on the same neuron, or on the same dendrite, or even on contiguous patches of membrane.

25.3.3 Long-term extracellular studies

Even under favorable conditions, intracellular records can be obtained from a neuron for no more than a few hours. Thus, for long-term studies and for studies of explants, where intracellular recording is difficult, extracellular recording has been employed (Crain, 1973). Seil and Leiman (this volume) describe both the organotypic morphology and stereotyped electrical activity of cerebellar and cerebral explants. Methods of signal analysis, probably necessary for the success of a circuit approach to plasticity, have been applied to in vitro extracellular recordings (Calvet, 1974; Corner and Crain, 1972; Gahwiler, Mamoon, and Tobias, 1973; Schlapfer, Mamoon, and Tobias, 1972).

25.4 STUDIES OF MORPHOLOGICAL DYNAMICS

25.4.1 In vivo studies

A recurrent theme in this volume is the impact of experience on brain morphology. Various types of differential experience produce detectable changes in brain weight and size, cell numbers, the size and shape of dendrites, the number of dendritic spines, the size of synaptic profiles, and the number of presynaptic vesicles (Greenough, Bennett, Rutledge, and Chapter 18, this volume). It is assumed that these morphological effects are due, at least in part, to altered activity in brain circuits. Some support for this assumption has been provided by ruling out systemic effects in certain cases. The effects are pronounced if input is restricted to one half of a brain and comparisons are made across the midline (Rutledge, this volume), or if systemic variables are directly manipulated (Rosenzweig, Bennett, and Diamond, 1972).

The morphological alterations that result from experience have often been seen as a subset of the changes comprising development. From this point of view, learning involves modulation of the basic cellular mechanisms of neural ontogeny (Szentágothai, 1971). Cellular interactions during development have been studied by ablation and surgical transposition (Jacobson, 1970), and interesting genetic models are now receiving attention (Rakic and Sidman, 1973).

The presentation of Greenough in this volume suggests that there is a class of neuronal structures, determined by developmental history, that can be quickly modulated by experience (see also Chapter 18, this volume). Short-term sensory stimulation produces in relevant sensory pathways detectable changes in the synaptic ultrastructure of neurons (Cragg, 1968; Fehér, Joó, and Halázs, 1972). These changes are presumably due to the altered activity in these pathways that is elicited by stimulation. Pettigrew has shown that in the visual cortex, the responsiveness of single cells to visual input changes during visual stimulation, which produces changes in the ultrastructure of terminals. However, because the morphological studies have employed statistical methods on large volumes of tissue, it has not been directly shown that structures are altered by their previous activity, or that their function has been changed. With in vitro preparations it is possible to stimulate a known synapse accurately and to study its morphology. For example, Heuser and Reese (1973) have shown that five minutes' stimulation of the frog neuromuscular junction modifies the ultrastructure of that synapse.

25.4.2 In vitro approaches

Phase-contrast microscopes have for years permitted the resolution of somata, fibers, and growth cones of living neurons (Pomerat et al., 1967; Nakai, 1964). The introduction of differential-interference-contrast optical systems (e.g., Nomarski optics) makes possible the visualization of some synaptic connections, as well as larger intracellular organelles (Figure 25.5). In favorable preparations, nerve terminals have been visually identified on ganglion cells of the heart (McMahan and Kuffler, 1971) and on striate muscle (McMahan, Spitzer, and Peper, 1972).

Because cell cultures are monitored visually, a studied cell can be easily relocated after fixation and embedding, and its position can be marked for thin sectioning. Thus, after morphological and electrophysiological studies, one can obtain an ultrastructural classification and analysis of structures whose behavior is known (Breuer et al., 1975). Such methods permit a direct test of the "change-with-use" hypothesis of synaptic activity.

SYNAPTOGENESIS AND TROPHIC FUNCTION. Up to the present, attempts to modulate synaptogenesis in vitro

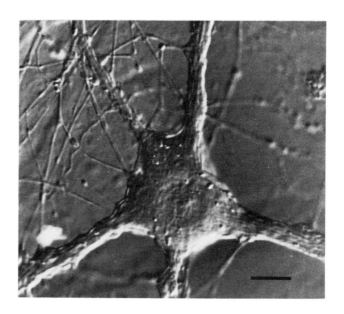

FIGURE 25.5 A Nomarski interference-contrast photomicrograph of a living fetal rat brain cell, 41 days in culture. Some of the organelles were seen to translocate within the soma and along the processes. A number of possible synaptic connections can be seen. The bar is 10 μm.

have been largely negative. Because functional synapses form in cultures of isolated spinal cord, input or neurotrophic influences from rostral or peripheral structures are not obligatory for synaptogenesis. Moreover, the electrical activity of a fetal tissue can be completely suppressed by chronic treatment with xylocaine, while synaptic activity can be prevented by high Mg^{++} concentrations. When these agents are removed after several days or weeks, a normal pattern of complex bioelectric activity immediately begins (Crain, Bornstein, and Peterson, 1968; Model et al., 1971). Thus synaptogenesis can occur in the absence of normal ongoing electrical activity. A similar negative result was found in nerve-muscle cultures. When neuromuscular transmission is blocked with hemicholinium or curariform agents, formation of neuromuscular connections proceeds normally (Crain and Peterson, 1971; Cohen, 1972).

"Trophic" interactions are of great interest and have been studied extensively in vitro, where it has been shown that the neuron exerts a sustaining effect on the target cell. This process has been observed in interactions between spinal-cord and muscle cells. Dissociated or explanted muscle in culture eventually atrophies. If nerve explants are added, innervation occurs, with subsequent reversal of muscle atrophy (Robbins and Yonezawa, 1971; Lentz, 1972). A similar effect on end-organ differentiation has been seen in the innervation of taste buds (Farbman, 1972; Zalewski, 1972, 1973). It is not clear whether this reversal of atrophy is due to the neurogenic activation of the end organ or to some direct metabolic interaction. Spinal-cord cultures develop many morphologically defined synapses in vitro, but after some two to three weeks these undergo considerable atrophy or degeneration. If muscle cells are included in the cultures, this degeneration is substantially reduced. This sustaining effect of the muscle is clearly seen on synapses between nerve cells; it is not restricted to the maintenance of synapses that are established on muscle cells (Meller et al., 1969).

The specificity of neuronal connections during fiber outgrowth has been studied by coculturing explants. More fibers grow between topographically related than between unrelated explants of cerebellum (Allerand and Murray, 1968). Cocultured explants of superior cervical ganglion, spinal cord, and cerebral cortex all show cross-innervation, but more synapses form when the ganglion is grown with spinal cord (Olson and Bunge, 1973). Sympathetic-ganglion outgrowth has an affinity for cultured autonomic target tissues (Mark, Chamley, and Burnstock, 1973). Hunt and Jacobson (1972) have demonstrated that after retinal specification, the retina can be maintained in vitro and, when reimplanted, it retains the retinotectal specificity of the donor animal.

NEURITE MOTILITY. The experiential modulation of the number of synapses in certain areas of the cortex, and the stimulation of dendritic growth (see Greenough, Rutledge, this volume), suggests that neurite motility can be switched on and off in the adult as well as the developing animal. Although switchboard theories of behavioral plasticity, and concomitant cellular mechanisms such as neurobiotaxis (Kappers, 1917), have been out of favor, the cellular-connectionistic orientation of current neurobiologists and the data of morphological plasticity may well revivify these theories in a more detailed and sophisticated form.

The study of neurite outgrowth from explants or single cells, perhaps the most dramatic feature of neuronal culture systems, has been studied as long as neurons have been cultured. Cinematography vividly reveals the dynamic nature of neurite outgrowth (Hughes, 1953) and the ceaseless motion of the neurite growth cone (Nakai and Kawasaki, 1959; Nakai, 1964). More recently, electron microscopy has shown the organized structure of organelles and microfilaments in growth cones' (Bray, 1973; Yamada, Spooner, and Wessells, 1970, 1971).

The modulation of neurite elongation has been best analyzed in cultures of DRG and sympathetic ganglion which are responsive to nerve growth factor (NGF) (for review see Levi-Montalcini and Angeletti, 1968). In producing neurite outgrowth, NGF enhances micro-

tubule assembly (Roisen, Murphy, and Braden, 1972; Roisen and Murphy, 1973). Both NGF and dibutyryl cyclic AMP stimulate the neurite outgrowth of DRG cells, apparently by different mechanisms (Frazier et al., 1973). Interestingly, dibutyryl cyclic AMP in vivo also promotes the reinnervation of denervated muscle (Pichichero, 1973), although this system is not responsive to NGF. Tissue culture offers a convenient bioassay system for testing growth factors (see Mandel, this volume) and permits the assessment of the short-term effects of putative neurotransmitters on growth-cone mobility.

MORPHOLOGICAL STUDIES OF AXOPLASMIC TRANSPORT. If the synthetic machinery of the neuronal soma is involved in plasticity, then the axoplasmic transport of materials to dendrites and presynaptic terminals may play a role in the "consolidation" of morphological and functional alterations (Barondes, 1967). Colchicine, which disaggregates microtubules and blocks fast axoplasmic transport (100–500 mm/day), when given immediately after training eliminates the subsequent savings in shock-avoidance learning of goldfish (Cronly-Dillon, 1973). The effect is apparently not due to alterations in neuronal activity or protein synthesis.

The motion of organelles, visualized by Nomarski optics, probably mediates some of the axoplasmic transport measured by biochemical methods (Kirkpatrick, Bray, and Palmer, 1972; Breuer et al., 1975). By such optical methods, it is possible to estimate the rate and direction of axoplasmic transport in individual neurons. Particles exhibiting fast transport (50–100 mm/day) have been observed in the neurites of cultured cells from the DRG, SC, brain, and a variety of continuous cell lines. In many neurites there are as many particles moving toward as moving away from the neuronal soma, which suggests that axoplasmic transport may be important in delivering materials to the soma.

Such studies may demonstrate which normal structures can intercommunicate by means of fast transport. For example, in the primary bifurcation of a cultured DRG neuron, particles move to and from the soma and each neurite branch, but do not move between branches. This traffic corresponds to the distribution of microtubules, which are plentiful in the DRG neuron processes but do not connect the branches at the primary bifurcation (Ha, 1970). If it could be established that fast axoplasmic transport reflects the distribution of microtubules, then the avenues of fast communication within a cell type could be mapped by electron microscopy. If it were established, for example, that two dendrites of the same cell cannot communicate by fast axoplasmic transport, except via the soma, this would set constraints on theories of dendritic interaction and the time course of consolidation. In cell cultures the predicted traffic can be verified directly in single cells of any geometry and size.

25.5 BIOCHEMICAL APPROACHES

Studies on the biochemistry of learning have primarily focused on changes in the rates of protein and RNA synthesis associated with a learning experience (Rose, Dunn, this volume). In addition, an active field of research using drugs that affect synthetic activity has attempted to determine whether protein or RNA synthesis is in fact necessary for the long-term retention of learning (Jarvik and Flood, this volume). On the other hand, biochemical studies of cultured neuronal tissue have concentrated on changes in enzyme activity with development and cell interaction in vitro (Nelson, 1975). Continuous cell lines have been exploited in a genetic analysis of neuronal characteristics and in studies of biochemical regulation (Mandel, this volume; McMorris, Nelson and Ruddle, 1973).

25.5.1 Enzyme induction
The time course of the development of a variety of neuron-specific enzymes has been studied in cell cultures of brain, spinal cord, and sympathetic ganglion (Kim, Oh, and Johnson, 1972; Mains and Patterson, 1973a, b,c; Schrier, 1973). It is assumed that the activity of an enzyme such as choline acetyltransferase (CAT) reflects the state of development of a specific class of neurons. Thus, in contrast to the situation of individual cell analyses by morphological and electrophysiological techniques, single-gene products can be examined using biochemical techniques. Characteristic developmental time courses for the different enzymes indicate that they are under separate regulatory influence, and one reasonable hypothesis is that this represents differential maturation of different cell types.

The presence of muscle cells in cocultures with spinal-cord cells results in an approximately tenfold increase in CAT activity (Giller et al., 1973). CAT activity is changed in a relatively specific manner, since a number of other enzymes show little or no alteration in the combined cultures. This effect is at least partly mediated by a diffusible substance, since a conditioned medium from muscle cultures produces a substantial increase in CAT activity when added to spinal-cord cultures. The substance involved is not dialyzable.

It can also be shown that the increases in CAT activity due to muscle and conditioned medium are additive. It may well be that a diffusible substance and a synaptically mediated inductive effect are both operative. Both skeletal muscle and heart muscle are much more effective than fibroblasts in eliciting the increased enzyme activity. Because spinal-cord motoneurons are cholinergic, this inductive effect may represent the modulation of neurons by target cells to increase the efficiency of their synaptic connections. It remains to be seen whether the synthesis of the inducing substance can itself be regulated by treatment of the target cells.

25.5.2 Neurotoxin binding and the modulation of receptor density
As mentioned above, myotubes, formed in vitro by the fusion of dissociated myoblasts, are responsive to locally applied ACh (Fambrough and Rash, 1971). This effect can be monitored biochemically with radioactive α-bungarotoxin (BNT), which binds irreversibly and specifically to the ACh receptors of myotubes (Vogel, Sytkowski, and Nirenberg, 1972) and has the same distribution of binding as the distribution of responsiveness to ACh (Fischbach and Cohen, 1973). Fischbach and Cohen also found that noninnervated as well as innervated chick myotubes have localized areas of high BNT binding.

One day of treatment with tetrodotoxin (TTX), which blocks the active sodium channel, prevents spontaneous muscle contractions, and increases BNT binding five-to tenfold. This is probably due both to an increase in binding to receptor clusters and an increase in the diffuse labeling of the myotubes. Preliminary data indicate that incubation with ACh, followed by extensive washing to reverse desensitization, decreased BNT binding fivefold. ACh does not prevent the TTX increase in BNT binding.

It is not clear how the receptor density of myotubes is regulated. The influx of Na^+, the release of sequestered Ca^{++}, or some metabolic consequence of the twitch itself, are all possible mechanisms. Myotube cultures provide a useful model for postsynaptic plasticity in the central nervous system, and they can be used to test a number of current theories.

Guided by the finding that direct electrical stimulation of muscle prevents denervation supersensitivity (Lømo and Rosenthal, 1972), Stent (1973) proposed that the reversal of membrane potential during an action potential destabilizes muscle ACh receptors. If a neuromuscular junction is active during the action potential, the resulting EPSP, by increasing nonspecific ionic conductance, clamps the membrane and prevents an overshoot in the region of the synapse. Hence, postsynaptic receptors are protected from degradation, and the efficiency of that synapse is increased.

The theory does not explain the focal BNT binding observed in pure myotube cultures. Contrary to our observations, Stent's theory predicts that these myotubes should exhibit uniform BNT binding unless innervated. The theory also predicts that long-term treatment of muscle with ACh should either increase ACh receptors or, if desensitization occurs, have no effect. In fact, ACh treatment significantly decreases BNT binding.

25.6 CONTINUOUS CELL LINES

A number of continuously dividing lines of tumor cells derived from the nervous system demonstrate interesting neuronal or glial properties. Procedures are available for inducing rapid differentiation of the neurobiological characteristics of these cell lines, and quite homogenous populations of cells can be easily grown. They are particularly convenient for biochemical studies, and it is clear that for a wide range of neurobiological properties the neuroblastoma and glial lines represent attractive model systems.

The mouse C-1300 neuroblastoma arose spontaneously in a mouse in the Jackson Laboratories several decades ago. The cells have been adapted to tissue culture, and a large number of cell lines have been established by cloning techniques. In general, the clones exhibit some degree of chromosomal heterogeneity, so that, despite the fact that a clone may consist exclusively of daughter cells from a single parent cell, the genetic makeup of all cells is not identical. Particular clones have characteristic biochemical, morphological, and electrophysiological characteristics. In a variety of clones the transmitter-related enzymes CAT, tyrosine hydroxylase (TH), and acetylcholinesterase (AChE) were independently expressed. High levels of AChE activity could be found in clones with high levels of either CAT or TH. No clones were found, however, with high levels of both CAT and TH. The mutual exclusivity of TH and CAT indicates an interrelated regulation of these enzymes, as would be required to ensure that a given neuron would be either cholinergic or adrenergic but not both (Amano, Richelson, and Nirenberg, 1972). Clones synthesizing tyramine, octopamine, serotonin, or histamine have also been found.

Electrophysiological study of neuroblastoma cells has demonstrated their electrical and chemical excitability. Both Na^+ and Ca^{++} ions are involved in the generation of action potentials, and cells generate both depolarizing and hyperpolarizing responses to applied neurohormones such as ACh. The cells develop long, branching processes, and both electrical and chemically responsive regions occur in both cell bodies and processes. Although original attempts to induce synaptogenesis in clonal cell lines were unsuccessful (Giller et al., 1975), we have recently found cholinergic synapses between neuroblastoma-glioma hybrid cells and cultured striate muscle.

Glial tumor cells have been grown in culture, cloned, and studied biochemically. Treatment with norepinephrine and some other putative neurotransmitters causes a very large increase in the intracellular concentration of cyclic AMP in glial clones (Clark and Perkins, 1971; Gilman and Minna, 1973). These cells can take up, metabolize, or secrete a number of neuroactive compounds, such as glutamate, GABA, and taurine (Schrier and Thompson, 1974). The glial cells of dorsal-root ganglia respond to depolarizing levels of potassium with a calcium-dependent efflux of GABA (Minchin and Iversen, 1974). This suggests that glia may play a significant role in regulating the extracellular concentration of a number of amino acids and other molecules that strongly affect neuronal excitability. Because glial metabolism itself is strikingly responsive to norepinephrine, mechanisms may exist for powerful interactions between nerve and glial cells.

Glial clones also synthesize S-100 protein, which is specific to nervous tissue and thought to be produced by normal glia in vivo. It has been shown that during transfer-of-handedness training in rats, the synthesis of S-100 protein increases in area CA3 of the hippocampus. Antiserum to S-100 protein prevents the normal acquisition of this task (Hydén and Lange, 1970). Training also produces apparent conformational changes in S-100 protein that are related to intracellular Ca^{++} concentrations in the hippocampus (Haljamäe and Lange, 1972). Although it is unclear how these effects are related to learning, the glial-neuron unit may be important in neuronal activity and may have a role in the storage of information (Galambos, 1961). The responsiveness of glial cell lines to neuroactive substances, and the fact that glial cells constitute half the volume of the brain, suggest important functions, with a cellular specificity perhaps equal to that of neurons. Clonal cell lines at the present time offer good model systems for studying the possible interactions of glia and neurons.

25.7 A TISSUE-CULTURE PROSPECTUS

It is clear from the foregoing that tissue culture has as yet made little substantive contribution to our understanding of the cellular mechanisms that might underlie behavioral plasticity. It seems equally clear to us, however, that hypotheses regarding these mechanisms can be tested by tissue-culture methods now technically feasible. We shall suggest experiments that summarize some of these possibilities.

The attenuation or augmentation of responses to iterated stimuli is ubiquitous in the CNS, which suggests that habituation and sensitization paradigms can be studied in cultures of various nervous-system regions, including the spinal cord. Low-density cocultures of spinal cord and dorsal-root ganglion would provide favorable conditions for analyzing these phenomena.

Electrodes can be placed in synaptically coupled DRG-SC pairs, so that electrical stimulation of the DRG cell elicits a monosynaptic EPSP in the SC cell. The effect of slow, repetitive stimuli or posttetanic potentiation can be studied, and similar experiments can be done on two SC cells synaptically coupled with excitatory or inhibitory connections. Low noise levels would permit a quantitative analysis of the transmission process at these synapses, and the responsiveness of the postsynaptic membrane would be determined by direct iontophoretic application of putative neurotransmitters. The role of Ca^{++} can be studied either by altering the level of the cation in the medium or by injecting Ca^{++} into the pre- or postsynaptic cell. Fine structural studies of the cells can be attained by fixation during the habituation paradigm, with the cells marked by intracellular tracers such as peroxidase.

Regions other than the spinal cord may show particularly marked degrees of alteration in connectivity with stimulation. For instance, a frequency potentiation of the perforant-pathway endings on hippocampal cells lasts for a period of hours (Bliss, Gardner-Medwin, and Lømo, 1973). The increased transmission in this pathway is probably due both to the increased synaptic coupling between the presynaptic endings and hippocampal granule cells, and to the increased excitability of the granule cells. By coculturing pre- and postsynaptic tissues, it is possible to stimulate and record from both elements of a synapse and to determine if the facilitative effect is monosynaptic. Such a system may reveal long-term posttetanic potentiation in the central nervous system.

The associational paradigms described above can, with varying degrees of difficulty, be applied to cultured cells (see Table 25.1). In cell monolayers from brain or spinal cord, neurons can be visually located which have a high probability of making direct synaptic contact, and the role of interneurons can be determined by physiological and anatomical methods. Stimulating and recording can be carried out simultaneously in a number of cells for periods of an hour or more. Noise caused by extraneous spontaneous synaptic potentials can be reduced by using sparsely plated cells, or by breaking the neurites of all neurons except those being studied. Various temporal contingencies can be arranged and the consequences determined. For instance, two cells, each of which is synaptically linked to a third cell, can be activated in a variety of sequences with and without postsynaptic spike generation. If positive effects are found, a variety of ionic agents (Ca^{++}, TEA, D-600, ouabain) or metabolic agents (DNP, protein-synthesis inhibitors) can be used to get at possible mechanisms.

Cultures of single neurons responsive to a number of iontophoretically applied putative neurotransmitters make it possible to test the interaction of postsynaptic receptor mechanisms. It has generally been held that PSPs sum spatially and temporally in the initiation of an action potential. It is useful to test this assumption in vitro, with various neuronal types, and to look for non-linearities or long-term effects of the interaction of different neurotransmitters on a single neuron. One can directly test postsynaptic models of heterosynaptic facilitation by pairing iontophoretic drug applications with the synaptic activation of neurons.

The fast changes in synaptic morphology caused by the short-term experiential manipulation of animals suggest that, in culture, precisely controlled electrical stimulation of an identified neuron might produce a noticeable effect on its morphology and biochemistry. The size and shape of individual synaptic endings, as well as neurite movements, can be followed visually during a regimen of stimulation or drug application. The ultrastructure of neurons with a known history of activity or synaptic input can be determined. Because neurons often grow upon a layer of supporting cells, single neurons, uncontaminated by other cells, can be picked from a culture plate for enzyme assays or microgel electrophoresis.

Biochemical alteration in neurons as a consequence of altered electrical activity can be readily examined. Single-cell studies are probably feasible, and long-term alteration in culture activity by chronic administration of anesthetics, epileptogenic agents, or magnesium (to block synaptic activity) can certainly be accomplished. Despite experiments cited earlier indicating that neuro-electric activity does not influence synaptogenesis, this important issue needs further investigation. It is crucial to have high-resolution methods for examining the physiological, pharmacological, morphological, and biochemical consequences of a variety of manipulations. We feel that these methods are at hand and should yield much valuable information about the mechanisms of plasticity.

REFERENCES

ADAM, G., ADEY, W. R., and PORTER, R. W. 1966. Interoceptive conditional responses in cortical neurones. *Nature* 209: 920–921.

ALLERAND, C. D., and MURRAY, M. R. 1968. Myelin formation *in vitro*. Endogenous influences on cultures of newborn mouse cerebellum. *Archives of Neurology* 19: 292–301.

ALTMAN, J. 1967. Postnatal growth and differentiation of the mammalian brain, with implications for a morphological theory of memory. In G. C. Quarton, T. Melnechuk, and

F. O. Schmitt, eds., *The Neurosciences: A Study Program*. New York: Rockefeller University Press, pp. 723–743.

AMANO, T., RICHELSON, E., and NIRENBERG, M. 1972. Neurotransmitter synthesis by neuroblastoma clones. *Proceedings of the National Academy of Sciences* 69: 258–263.

BARONDES, S. H. 1967. Axoplasmic transport. *Neurosciences Research Program Bulletin* 5: 307–419.

BELL, C., SIERRA, B., BUENDIA, N., and SEGUNDO, J. P. 1964. Sensory properties of neurons in the mesencephalic reticular formation. *Journal of Neurophysiology* 27: 961–987.

BERRY, R. W., and COHEN, M. J. 1972. Synaptic stimulation of RNA metabolism in the giant neuron of *Aplysia californica*. *Journal of Neurobiology* 3: 209–222.

BLISS, T. V. P., GARDNER-MEDWIN, A. R., and LØMO, T. 1973. Synaptic plasticity in the hippocampal formation. In G. B. ANSELL and P. B. BRADLEY, eds., *Macromolecules and Behavior*. New York: Macmillan, pp. 193–203.

BLOMFIELD, S., and MARR, D. 1970. How the cerebellum may be used. *Nature* 227: 1224–1228.

BORNSTEIN, M. B., and MODEL, P. G. 1972. Development of synapses and myelin in cultures of dissociated embryonic mouse spinal cord, medulla and cerebrum. *Brain Research* 37: 287–293.

BRAY, D. 1973. Model for membrane movements in the neural growth cone. *Nature* 244: 93–95.

BREUER, A. C., CHRISTIAN, C. N., HENKART, M., and NELSON, P. G. 1975. Computer analysis of organelle translocation in primary neuronal cultures and continuous cell lines. *Journal of Cell Biology* 65: 562–576.

BRINDLEY, G. S. 1967. The classification of modifiable synapses and their use in models for conditioning. *Proceedings of the Royal Society (London)* B 168: 361–376.

BRINDLEY, G. S. 1969. Nerve net models of plausible size that perform many simple learning tasks. *Proceedings of the Royal Society (London)* B 174: 173–191.

BUCHWALD, J. S., HALAS, E. S., and SCHRAMM, S. 1966. Changes in cortical and subcortical unit activity during behavioral conditioning. *Physiology and Behavior* 1: 11–22.

BUNGE, M. B. 1973. Fine structure of nerve fibers and growth cones of isolated sympathetic neurons in culture. *Journal of Cell Biology* 56: 713–735.

BUREŠOVÁ, O., and BUREŠ, J. 1965. Classical conditioning and reticular units. *Acta Physiologica Academiae Scientiarum Hungaricae* 26: 53–57.

CALVET, M. 1974. Patterns of spontaneous electrical activity in tissue cultures of mammalian cerebral cortex vs. cerebellum. *Brain Research* 69: 281–295.

CHAMLEY, J. H., MARK, G. E., CAMPBELL, G. R., and Burnstock, G. 1972. Sympathetic ganglia in culture. I. Neurons. *Zeitschrift fuer Zellforschung und Mikroskopische Anatomie* 135: 287–314.

CHOW, K. L., LINDSLEY, D. F., and GOLLENDER, M. 1968. Modification of response patterns of lateral geniculate neurons after paired stimulation of contralateral and ipsilateral eyes. *Journal of Neurophysiology* 31: 729–739.

CLARK, R. B., and PERKINS, J. P. 1971. Regulation of adenosine 3′,5′-cyclic monophosphate concentration in cultured human astrocytoma cells by catecholamines and histamine. *Proceedings of the National Academy of Sciences* 68: 2757–2760.

COHEN, M. J. 1970. A comparison of invertebrate and vertebrate central neurons. In F. O. Schmitt, ed., *The Neurosciences: Second Study Program*. New York: Rockefeller University Press, pp. 798–812.

COHEN, M. W. 1972. The development of neuromuscular connexions in the presence of D-tubocurarine. *Brain Research* 41: 457–463.

COHEN, S. A., and FISCHBACH, G. D. 1973. Regulation of muscle acetylcholine sensitivity by muscle activity in cell cultures. *Science* 181: 76–78.

CORNER, M. A., and CRAIN, S. M. 1972. Patterns of spontaneous bioelectric activity during maturation in culture of fetal rodent medulla and spinal cord tissues. *Journal of Neurobiology* 3: 25–45.

CRAGG, B. G. 1968. Are there structural alterations in synapses related to functioning? *Proceedings of the Royal Society* B 171: 319–323.

CRAIN, S. M. 1973. Microelectrode recording in brain tissue cultures. In R. F. Thompson and M. M. Patterson, eds., *Bioelectric Recording Techniques*. Part A: *Cellular Processes and Brain Potentials*. New York: Academic Press, pp. 39–75.

CRAIN, S. M., and BORNSTEIN, M. B. 1972. Organotypic bioelectric activity in cultured reaggregates of dissociated rodent brain cells. *Science* 176: 182–184.

CRAIN, S. M., BORNSTEIN, M. B., and PETERSON, E. R. 1968. Maturation of cultured embryonic CNS tissue during chronic exposure to agents which prevent bioelectric activity. *Brain Research* 8: 363–372.

CRAIN, S. M., and PETERSON, E. R. 1971. Development of paired explants of fetal spinal cord and adult skeletal muscle during chronic exposure to curare and hemicholinium. *In Vitro* 6: 373.

CRONLY-DILLON, J. 1973. The effect of colchicine on memory. *Journal of Physiology* 234: 104 p.

DeLONG, G. R. 1970. Histogenesis of fetal mouse isocortex and hippocampus in reaggregating cell cultures. *Developmental Biology* 22: 563–583.

DISTERHOFT, J. F., and OLDS, J. 1972. Differential development of conditioned unit changes in thalamus and cortex of rat. *Journal of Neurophysiology* 35: 665–679.

ECCLES, J. C. 1964. *The Physiology of Synapses*. Berlin: Springer-Verlag.

EPSTEIN, R., and TAUC, L. 1970. Heterosynaptic facilitation and post-tetanic potentiation in *Aplysia* nervous system. *Journal of Physiology* 209: 1–23.

FAMBROUGH, D. M. 1970. Acetylcholine sensitivity of muscle fiber membranes. Mechanism of regulation by motoneurons. *Science* 168: 372–373.

FAMBROUGH, D., and RASH, J. E. 1971. Development of acetylcholine sensitivity during myogenesis. *Developmental Biology* 26: 55–68.

FARBMAN, A. I. 1972. Differentiation of taste buds in organ culture. *Journal of Cell Biology* 52: 489–493.

FEHÉR, O., JOÓ, F., and HALÁZS, N. 1972. Effects of stimulation on the number of synaptic vesicles in nerve fibres and terminals of the cerebral cortex in the cat. *Brain Research* 47: 37–48.

FISCHBACH, G. D., and COHEN, S. A. 1973. The distribution of acetylcholine sensitivity over uninnervated and innervated muscle fibers grown in cell culture. *Developmental Biology* 31: 147–162.

FISCHBACH, G. D., and DICHTER, M. A. 1974. Electrophysiologic and morphologic properties of neurons in dissociated chick spinal cord cell cultures. *Developmental Biology* 37: 100–116.

FRAZIER, W. A., OHLENDORF, C. E., BOYD, L. F., ALOE, L., JOHNSON, E. M., FERRENDELLI, J. A., and BRADSHAW, R. A.

1973. Mechanism of action of nerve growth factor and cyclic AMP on neurite outgrowth in embryonic chick sensory ganglia: Demonstration of independent pathways of stimulation. *Proceedings of the National Academy of Sciences* 70: 2448–2452.

GAHWILER, B. H., MAMOON, A. M., and TOBIAS, C. A. 1973. Spontaneous bioelectric activity of cultured cerebellar Purkinje cells during exposure to agents which prevent synaptic transmission. *Brain Research* 53: 71–79.

GALAMBOS, R. 1961. A glia-neural theory of brain function. *Proceedings of the National Academy of Sciences* 47: 129–136.

GEINISMANN, Yu. Ya. 1972. Effects of excitatory and inhibitory synaptic actions on RNA content of spinal motoneurones. *Brain Research* 44: 221–229.

GILLER, E. L., BREAKEFIELD, X. O., CHRISTIAN, C. N., NEALE, E. A., and NELSON, P. G. 1975. Expression of neuronal characteristics in culture: Some pros and cons of primary cultures and continuous cell lines. In M. Santini, ed., *Golgi Centennial Symposium*. New York: Raven Press, pp. 603–623.

GILLER, E. L., SCHRIER, B. K., SHAINBERG, A., FISK, H. R., and NELSON, P. G. 1973. Increased choline acetyltransferase activity in combined cultures of spinal cord and muscle cells from the mouse. *Science* 182: 588–589.

GILMAN, A. G., and MINNA, J. D. 1973. Expression of genes for metabolism of cyclic adenosine 3′,5′-monophosphate in somatic cells. I. Responses to catecholamines in parental and hybrid cells. *Journal of Biological Chemistry* 248: 6610–6617.

GODFREY, E. W., NELSON, P. G., SCHRIER, B. K., BREUER, A. C., and RANSOM, B. R. 1975. Neurons from fetal rat brain in a new cell culture system: A multidisciplinary approach. *Brain Research* 90: 1–21.

GREENE, L. A., SYTKOWSKI, A. J., VOGEL, Z., and NIRENBERG, M. W. 1973. α-bungarotoxin used as a probe for acetylcholine receptors of cultured neurones. *Nature* 243: 163–166.

GROSSE, G., and LINDNER, G. 1970. Untersuchungen zur Differenzierung isolierter Nerven und Gliazellen des zentralnervasen Gewebes von Hühnerembryonen in der Zellkultur. *Journal für Hirnforschung* 12: 207–215.

GROVES, P. M., MILLER, S. W., and PARKER, M. V. 1972. Habituation and sensitization of neuronal activity in the reticular formation of the rat. *Physiology and Behavior* 8: 589–594.

GROVES, P. M., and THOMPSON, R. F. 1970. Habituation: A dual-process theory. *Psychological Review* 77: 419–450.

GROVES, P. M., and THOMPSON, R. F. 1973. A dual-process theory of habituation: Neural mechanisms. In H. V. S. Peeke and M. J. Herz, eds., *Habituation*, Vol. 2. New York: Academic Press, pp. 175–205.

GUILLERY, R. W., SOBKOWICZ, H. M., and SCOTT, G. L. 1968. Light and electron microscopical observation of the ventral horn and ventral root in long-term cultures of the spinal cord of the fetal mouse. *Journal of Comparative Neurology* 134: 433–476.

GUILLERY, R. W., SOBKOWICZ, H. M., and SCOTT, G. L. 1970. Relationships between glial and neuronal elements in the development of long-term cultures of the spinal cord of the fetal mouse. *Journal of Comparative Neurology* 140: 1–34.

HA, H. 1970. Axonal bifurcation in the dorsal root ganglion of the cat: A light and electron microscopic study. *Journal of Comparative Neurology* 140: 227–240.

HALAS, E. S., BEARDSLEY, J. V., and SANDLIE, M. E. 1970. Conditioned neuronal responses at various levels in conditioning paradigms. *Electroencephalography and Clinical Neurophysiology* 28: 468–477.

HALJAMÄE, H., and LANGE, P. W. 1972. Calcium content and conformational changes of S-100 protein in the hippocampus during training. *Brain Research* 38: 131–142.

HEBB, D. O. 1949. *The Organization of Behavior*. New York: John Wiley &. Sons.

HEUSER, J. E., and REESE, T. S. 1973. Evidence for recycling of synaptic vesicle membrane during transmitter release at the frog neuromuscular junction. *Journal of Cell Biology* 57: 315–344.

HORN, G. 1967. Neuronal mechanisms of habituation. *Nature* 215: 707–711.

HORN, G., and HILL, R. M. 1966a. Responsiveness to sensory stimulation of units in the superior colliculus and subjacent tectotegmental regions of the rabbit. *Experimental Neurology* 14: 199–224.

HORN, G., and HILL, R. M. 1966b. Effect of removing the neocortex on the response to repeated sensory stimulation of neurons in the mid-brain. *Nature* 202: 296–298.

HUGHES, A. 1953. The growth of embryonic neurites. A study on cultures of chick neural tissues. *Journal of Anatomy* 87: 150–162.

HUNT, R. K., and JACOBSON, M. 1972. Specificaton of positional information in retinal ganglion cells of Xenopus: Stability of the specified state. *Proceedings of the National Academy of Sciences* 69: 2860–2864.

HYDÉN, H., and LANGE, P. W. 1970. Protein changes in nerve cells related to learning and conditioning. In F. O. Schmitt, ed., *The Neurosciences: Second Study Program*. New York: Rockefeller University Press, pp. 278–289.

JACOBSON, M., ed. 1970. *Developmental Neurobiology*. New York: Holt, Rinehart and Winston.

KAMIKAWA, K., McILWAIN, T., and ADEY, W. R. 1964. Response patterns of thalamic neurons during classical conditioning. *Electroencephalography and Clinical Neurophysiology* 17: 485–496.

KANDEL, E. R., and SPENCER, W. A. 1968. Cellular neurophysiological approaches in the study of learning. *Physiological Reviews* 48: 65–134.

KANDEL, E. R., and TAUC, L. 1965a. Heterosynaptic facilitation in neurones of the abdominal ganglion of *Aplysia depilans*. *Journal of Physiology* 181: 1–27.

KANDEL, E. R., and TAUC, L. 1965b. Mechanism of heterosynaptic facilitation in the giant cell of the abdominal ganglion of *Aplysia depilans*. *Journal of Physiology* 181: 28–47.

KAPPERS, C. U. A. 1917. Further contributions on neurobiotaxis. IX. *Journal of Comparative Neurology* 27: 261–298.

KATZ, B., ed. 1969. *The Release of Neural Transmitter Substances*. Liverpool: Liverpool University Press.

KERNELL, D., and PETERSON, R. P. 1970. The effect of spike activity versus synaptic activation on the metabolism of ribonucleic acid in a molluscan giant neuron. *Journal of Neurochemistry* 17: 1087–1094.

KETY, S. S. 1970. The biogenic amines in the central nervous system. Their possible roles in arousal, emotion and learning. In F. O. Schmitt, ed., *The Neurosciences: Second Study Program*. New York: Rockefeller University Press, pp. 324–336.

KIM, S. U., OH, T. H., and JOHNSON, D. D. 1972. Developmental changes of acetylcholinesterase and pseudocholinesterase in organotypic cultures of spinal cord. *Experimental Neurology* 35: 274–281.

KIRKPATRICK, J. B., BRAY, J. J., and PALMER, S. M. 1972.

Visualization of axoplasmic flow *in vitro* by Nomarski microscopy. Comparison to rapid flow of radioactive proteins. *Brain Research* 43: 1–10.

KORNBLITH, C., and OLDS, J. 1973. Unit activity in the brain stem reticular formation of the rat during learning. *Journal of Neurophysiology* 36: 489–501.

KRNJEVIĆ, K. 1974. Chemical nature of synaptic transmission in vertebrates. *Physiological Reviews* 54: 418–540.

KUPFERMANN, I., and PINSKER, H. 1969. Plasticity in *Aplysia* neurons and some simple neuronal models of learning. In J. T. Tapp, ed., *Reinforcement and Behavior*. New York: Academic Press, pp. 356–386.

LASHER, R. S., and ZAGON, I. S. 1972. The effect of potassium on neuronal differentiation in cultures of dissociated newborn rat cerebellum. *Brain Research* 41: 482–488.

LEIMAN, A. L., and CHRISTIAN, C. N. 1973. Electrophysiological analyses of learning and memory. In J. A. Deutsch, ed., *The Physiological Basis of Memory*. New York: Academic Press, pp. 125–165.

LENTZ, T. L. 1972. Development of the neuromuscular junction. III. Degeneration of motor endplates after denervation and maintenance *in vitro* by nerve explants. *Journal of Cell Biology* 55: 93–103.

LEVI-MONTALCINI, R., and ANGELETTI, P. U. 1968. Nerve growth factor. *Physiological Reviews* 48: 534–569.

LEVI-MONTALCINI, R., and SESHAN, K. R. 1973. Long-term cultures of embryonic and mature insect nervous and neuroendocrine systems. In G. Sato, ed., *Tissue Culture of the Nervous System*. New York: Plenum Press, pp. 1–33.

LIBET, B., and TOSAKA, T. 1970. Dopamine as a synaptic transmitter modulator in sympathetic ganglia: A different type of synaptic action. *Proceedings of the National Academy of Sciences* 67: 667–673.

LINDSLEY, D. F., RANF, S. K., SHERWOOD, M. J., and PRESTON, W. G. 1973. Habituation and modification of reticular formation neuron responses to peripheral stimulation in cats. *Experimental Neurology* 41: 174–189.

LINSEMAN, M. A., and OLDS, J. 1973. Activity changes in rat hypothalamus, preoptic area and striatum associated with Pavlovian conditioning. *Journal of Neurophysiology* 36: 1038–1050.

LØMO, T., and ROSENTHAL, J. 1972. Control of ACh sensitivity by muscle activity in the rat. *Journal of Physiology* 221: 493–513.

LUMSDEN, C. E. 1968. Nervous tissue in culture. In G. H. Bourne, ed., *The Structure and Function of Nervous Tissue*. New York: Academic Press, pp. 67–140.

MAINS, R. E., and PATTERSON, P. H. 1973a. Primary cultures of dissociated sympathetic neurons. I. Establishment of long-term growth in culture and studies of differentiated properties. *Journal of Cell Biology* 59: 329–345.

MAINS, R. E., and PATTERSON, P. H. 1973b. Primary cultures of dissociated sympathetic neurons. II. Initial studies of catecholamine metabolism. *Journal of Cell Biology* 59: 346–360.

MAINS, R. E., and PATTERSON, P. H. 1973c. Primary cultures of dissociated sympathetic neurons. III. Changes in metabolism with age in culture. *Journal of Cell Biology* 59: 361–366.

MARK, G. E., CHAMLEY, J. H., and BURNSTOCK, G. 1973. Interactions between autonomic nerves and smooth and cardiac muscle cells in culture. *Developmental Biology* 32: 194–200.

MARK, R. F. 1970. Chemospecific synaptic repression as a possible memory store. *Nature* 225: 178–179.

MARK, R. F., MAROTTE, L. R., and MART, P. E. 1972. The mechanism of selective reinnervation of fish eye muscles. IV. Identification of repressed synapses. *Brain Research* 46: 149–157.

MARR, D. 1970. A theory for cerebral neocortex. *Proceedings of the Royal Society* (*London*) B 176: 161–234.

MCILWAIN, H., ed. 1971. *Biochemistry and the Central Nervous System*, 4th ed. Baltimore: Williams & Wilkins.

MCMAHAN, U. J., and KUFFLER, S. W. 1971. Visual identification of synaptic boutons on living ganglion cells and of varicosities in postganglionic axons in the heart of the frog. *Proceedings of the Royal Society* (*London*) B 177: 485–508.

MCMAHAN, U. J., SPITZER, N. C., and PEPER, K. 1972. Visual identification of nerve terminals in living isolated skeletal muscle. *Proceedings of the Royal Society* (*London*) B 181: 421–430.

MCMORRIS, F. A., NELSON, P. G., and RUDDLE, F. H. 1973. Clonal systems in neurobiology. *Neurosciences Research Program Bulletin* 11: 411–536.

MELLER, K., BREIPOHL, W., WAGNER, H. H., and KNUTH, A. 1969. Die Differenzierung isolierter Nerven und Gliazellen aus trypsinierten Ruckenmark von Hühnerembryonen in Gewebekulturen. *Zeitschrift fuer Zellforschung und Mikroskopische Anatomie* 101: 135–151.

MINCHIN, M. C. W., and IVERSEN, L. L. 1974. Release of [³H]gamma-aminobutyric acid from glial cells in rat dorsal root ganglion. *Joural of Neurochemistry* 23: 533–540.

MODEL, P. G., BORNSTEIN, M. B., CRAIN, S. M., and PAPPAS, G. D. 1971. An electron microscopic study of the development of synapses in cultured fetal mouse cerebrum continuously exposed to xylocaine. *Journal of Cell Biology* 49: 362–371.

MURRAY, M. R. 1965. Nervous tissue *in vitro*. In E. N. Wilmer, ed., *Cells and Tissues in Culture*, Vol. 2. New York: Academic Press, pp. 373–455.

MURRAY, M. R. 1971. Nervous tissues isolated in culture. In A. Lajtha, ed., *Handbook of Neurochemistry*, Vol. 5A. New York: Plenum Press, pp. 373–438.

MURRAY, M. R., and KOPECH, G., eds. 1953. *A Bibliography of the Research in Tissue Culture*, 2 vols. New York: Academic Press.

NAKAI, J. 1964. The movements of neurons in tissue culture. In R. D. Allen and N. Kamiya, eds., *Primitive Motile Systems in Cell Biology*. New York: Academic Press, pp. 377–385.

NAKAI, J., and KAWASAKI, Y. 1959. Studies on the mechanism determining the course of nerve fibers in tissue culture. I. The reaction of the growth cone to various obstructions. *Zeitschrift fuer Zellforschung und Mikroskopische Anatomie* 51: 108–122.

NELSON, P. G. 1975. Nerve and muscle cells in culture. *Physiological Reviews* 55: 1–61.

NELSON, P. G., and PEACOCK, J. H. 1973. Electrical activity in dissociated cell cultures from fetal mouse cerebellum. *Brain Research* 61: 163–174.

O'BRIEN, J. H., and FOX, S. S. 1969a. Single-cell activity in cat motor cortex. I. Modifications during classical conditioning procedures. *Journal of Neurophysiology* 32: 267–284.

O'BRIEN, J. H., and FOX, S. S. 1969b. Single-cell activity in cat motor cortex. II. Functional characteristics of the cell related to conditioning changes. *Journal of Neurophysiology* 32: 285–296.

OKUN, L. M., ONTKEAN, F. K., and THOMAS, JR., C. A. 1972.

Removal of non-neuronal cells from suspensions of dissociated embryonic dorsal root ganglia. *Experimental Cell Research* 73: 226–229.

OLDS, J., DISTERHOFT, J. F., SEGAL, M., KORNBLITH, C. L., and HIRSH, R. 1972. Learning centers of rat brain mapped by measuring latencies of conditioned unit responses. *Journal of Neurophysiology* 35: 202–219.

OLDS, M. E. 1973. Short-term changes in the firing pattern of hypothalamic neurons during Pavlovian conditioning. *Brain Research* 58: 95–116.

OLSON, M. I., and BUNGE, R. P. 1973. Anatomical observations on the specificity of synapse formation in tissue culture. *Brain Research* 59: 19–33.

ORREGO, F., and LIPMANN, F. 1967. Protein synthesis in brain slices: Effects of electrical stimulation and acidic amino acids. *Journal of Biological Chemistry* 242: 665–671.

PEACOCK, J., MINNA, J., NELSON, P., and NIRENBERG, M. 1972. Use of aminopterin in selecting electrically active neuroblastoma cells. *Experimental Cell Research* 73: 367–377.

PEACOCK, J. H., NELSON, P. G., and GOLDSTONE, M. W. 1973. Electrophysiologic study of cultured neurons dissociated from spinal cords and dorsal root ganglia of fetal mice. *Developmental Biology* 30: 137–152.

PETERSON, E. R., CRAIN, S. M., and MURRAY, M. R. 1965. Differentiation and prolonged maintenance of bioelectrically active spinal cord cultures (rat, chick and human). *Zeitschrift fuer Zellforschung und Mikroskopische Anatomie* 66: 130–154.

PETERSON, R. P., and KERNELL, D. 1970. Effects of nerve stimulation on the metabolism of ribonucleic acid in a molluscan giant neuron. *Journal of Neurochemistry* 17: 1075–1085.

PETERSON, R. P., and LOH, Y. P. 1973. The role of macromolecules in neuronal function in *Aplysia*. In G. A. Kerkut and J. W. Phillis, eds., *Progress in Neurobiology*, Vol. 2, Part 2. New York: Pergamon Press, pp. 179–203.

PICHICHERO, M. 1973. Effects of dibutyryl cyclic AMP on restoration of function of damaged sciatic nerve in rats. *Science* 182: 724–725.

POMERAT, C. M., HENDLEMAN, W. J., RAIBORN, Jr., C. W., and MASSEY, J. F. 1967. Dynamic activities of nervous tissues *in vitro*. In H. Hydén, ed., *The Neuron*. New York: American Elsevier, pp. 119–178.

PRASAD, K. N. 1971. X-ray-induced morphological differentiation of mouse neuroblastoma cells *in vitro*. *Nature* 234: 471–473.

PRIVES, C., and QUASTEL, J. H. 1969. Effects of cerebral stimulation in the biosynthesis *in vitro* of nucleotides and RNA in brain. *Nature* 221: 1053.

RAKIC, P., and SIDMAN, R. L. 1973. Weaver mutant mouse cerebellum: Defective neuronal migration secondary to abnormality of Bergmann glia. *Proceedings of the National Academy of Sciences* 70: 240–244.

RANSOM, B. R., and NELSON, P. G. 1975. Neuropharmacological responses from nerve cells in tissue culture. In L. L. Iversen, S. D. Iversen, and S. H. Snyder, eds., *Handbook of Psychopharmacology*, Vol. 2. New York: Plenum Press, pp. 101–127.

RICHARDS, C. D., and SERCOMBE, R. 1968. Electrical activity observed in guinea pig olfactory cortex maintained *in vitro*. *Journal of Physiology* 197: 667–683.

ROBBINS, N., and YONEZAWA, T. 1971. Physiological studies during formation and development of rat neuromuscular junctions in tissue culture. *Journal of General Physiology* 58: 467–481.

ROISEN, F. J., and MURPHY, R. A. 1973. Neurite development *in vitro*. II. The role of microfilaments and microtubules in dibutyryl adenosine 3′,5′-cyclic monophosphate and nerve growth factor stimulated maturation. *Journal of Neurobiology* 4: 397–412.

ROISEN, F. J., MURPHY, R. A., and BRADEN, W. G. 1972. Neurite development *in vitro*. I. The effects of adenosine 3′5′-cyclic monophosphate (cyclic AMP). *Journal of Neurobiology* 3: 347–368.

ROSENBLATT, F. 1962. *Principles of Neurodynamics: Perceptrons and the Theory of Brain Mechanisms*. Washington, D. C.: Spartan Books.

ROSENZWEIG, M. R., BENNETT, E. L., and DIAMOND, M. C. 1972. Chemical and anatomical plasticity of brain: Replications and extensions. In J. Gaito, ed., *Macromolecules and Behavior*, 2nd ed. New York: Appleton-Century-Crofts, pp. 205–277.

SCHEIBEL, M. E., and SCHEIBEL, A. B. 1965. The response of reticular units to repetitive stimuli. *Archives Italiennes de Biologie* 103: 279–299.

SCHLAPFER, W. T., MAMOON, A.-M., and TOBIAS, C. A. 1972. Spontaneous bioelectric activity of neurons in cerebellar cultures: Evidence for synaptic interaction. *Brain Research* 45: 345–363.

SCHRIER, B. K. 1973. Surface culture of fetal mammalian brain cells: Effect of subculture on morphology and choline acetyltransferase activity. *Journal of Neurobiology* 4: 117–124.

SCHRIER, B. K., and SHAPIRO, D. L. 1973. Effects of N^6-monobutyryl cyclic AMP on glutamate decarboxylase activity in fetal rat brain cells and glial tumor cells in culture. *Experimental Cell Research* 80: 459–462.

SCHRIER, B. K., and Thompson, E. 1974. On the role of glial cells in the mammalian nervous system: Uptake, excretion and metabolism of putative neurotransmitters by cultured glial tumor cells. *Journal of Biological Chemistry* 249: 1769–1780.

SCHULTZ, J., and DALY, J. W. 1973. Adenosine 3′,5′-monophosphate in guinea pig cerebral cortical slices: Effects of α and β-adrenergic agents, histamine, serotonin and adenosine. *Journal of Neurochemistry* 21: 573–579.

SEEDS, N. W. 1973. Differentiation of aggregating brain cell cultures. In G. Sato, ed., *Tissue Culture of the Nervous System*. New York: Plenum Press, pp. 35–53.

SEGAL, M. 1973. Flow of conditioned responses in limbic telencephalic system of the rat. *Journal of Neurophysiology* 36: 840–854.

SEGAL, M. and OLDS, J. 1972. Behavior of units in hippocampal circuit of the rat during learning. *Journal of Neurophysiology* 35: 680–690.

SEGUNDO, J. P., and BELL, C. C. 1970. Habituation of single nerve cells in the vertebrate nervous system. In G. Horn and R. A. Hinde, eds., *Short-term Changes in Neural Activity and Behaviour*. London: Cambridge University Press, pp. 77–94.

SHAPIRO, D. L. 1973. Morphological and biochemical alterations in foetal rat brain cells cultured in the presence of monobutyryl cyclic AMP. *Nature* 241: 203–204.

SHARPLESS, S. K. 1964. Reorganization of function in the nervous system—Use and disuse. *Annual Review of Physiology* 26: 357–388.

SPENCER, W. A., THOMPSON, R. F., and NEILSON, JR., D. R. 1966a. Response decrement of flexion reflex in acute spinal cat and transient restoration by strong stimuli. *Journal of Neurophysiology* 29: 221–239.

SPENCER, W. A., THOMPSON, R. F., and NEILSON, JR., D. R.

1966b. Alterations in responsiveness of ascending and reflex pathways activated by iterated cutaneous afferent volleys. *Journal of Neurophysiology* 29: 240–252.

SPENCER, W. A., THOMPSON, R. F., and NEILSON, JR., D. R. 1966c. Decrement of ventral root electrotonus and intracellularly recorded post-synaptic potentials produced by iterated cutaneous afferent volleys. *Journal of Neurophysiology* 29: 253–274.

STENT, G. S. 1973. A physiological mechanism for Hebb's postulate of learning. *Proceedings of the National Academy of Sciences* 70: 997–1001.

SZENTÁGOTHAI, J. 1971. Memory functions and the structural organization of the brain. In G. ÁDÁM, ed., *Biology of Memory*. New York: Plenum Press, pp. 21–35.

TAUC, L. 1965. Presynaptic inhibition in the abdominal ganglion of *Aplysia*. *Journal of Physiology* 181: 282–307.

TAUC, L., and EPSTEIN, R. 1967. Heterosynaptic facilitation as a distinct mechanism in *Aplysia*. *Nature* 214: 724–725.

THOENEN, H. 1974. Trans-synaptic enzyme-induction. *Life Science* 14: 223–235.

THOMPSON, R. F., and SPENCER, W. A. 1966. Habituation: A model phenomenon for the study of neuronal substrates of behavior. *Psychological Review* 73: 16–43.

VARON, S., and RAIBORN, JR., C. W. 1969. Dissociation, fractionation, and culture of embryonic brain cells. *Brain Research* 12: 180–199.

VARON, S., and RAIBORN, JR., C. W. 1972. Dissociation, fractionation and culture of chick embryo sympathetic ganglia cells. *Journal of Neurocytology* 1: 211–221.

VOGEL, Z., SYTKOWSKI, A. F., and NIRENBERG, M. W. 1972. Acetylcholine receptors of muscle grown *in vitro*. *Proceedings of the National Academy of Sciences* 69: 3180–3184.

VON BAUMGARTEN, R. J. 1970. Plasticity in the nervous system at the unitary level. In F. O., Schmitt, ed., *The Neurosciences: Second Study Program*. New York: Rockefeller University Press, pp. 260–271.

WALL, P. D. 1970. Habituation and post-tetanic potentiation in the spinal cord. In G. Horn and R. A. Hinde, eds., *Short-Term Changes in Neural Activity and Behaviour*. London: Cambridge University Press, pp. 181–210.

WEIGHT, F. F. 1973. Physiological mechanisms of synaptic modulation. In F. O. Schmitt and F. G. Worden, eds., *The Neurosciences: Third Study Program*. Cambridge, Mass.: MIT Press, pp. 929–941.

WICKELGREN, B. G. 1967a. Habituation of spinal motoneurons. *Journal of Neurophysiology* 30: 1404–1423.

WICKELGREN, B. G. 1967b. Habituation of spinal interneurons. *Journal of Neurophysiology* 30: 1424–1438.

WOODY, C. D., and BLACK-CLEWORTH, P. 1973. Differences in excitability of cortical neurons as a function of motor projection in conditioned cats. *Journal of Neurophysiology* 36: 1104–1116.

WOODY, C. D., Vassilersky, N. N., and ENGEL, J. 1970. Conditioned eye blink: Unit activity at coronal-precruciate cortex of the cat. *Journal of Neurophysiology* 33: 851–864.

WOODY, C. D., YAROWSKY, P., OWENS, J., BLACK-CLEWORTH, P., and CROW, T. 1974. Effect of lesions of cortical motor axons on acquisition of conditioned eye blink in the cat. *Journal of Neurophysiology* 37: 385–394.

YAMADA, K. M., SPOONER, B. S., and WESSELLS, N. K. 1970. Axon growth: Roles of microfilaments and microtubules. *Proceedings of the National Academy of Sciences* 66: 1206–1212.

YAMADA, K. M., SPOONER, B. S., and WESSELLS, N. K. 1971. Ultrastructure and function of growth cones and axons of cultured nerve cells. *Journal of Cell Biology* 49: 614–635.

YAMAMOTO, C. 1972. Activation of hippocampal neurons by mossy fiber stimulation in thin brain sections *in vitro*. *Experimental Brain Research* 14: 423–535.

YOSHII, N., and OGURA, H. 1960. Studies of the unit discharge of brainstem reticular formation in the cat. I. Changes of recticular unit discharge following conditioning procedure. *Medical Journal of Osaka University* 11: 1–17.

YOUNG, J. Z. 1966. *The Memory System of the Brain*. Berkeley: University of California Press.

ZALEWSKI, A. A. 1972. Regeneration of taste buds after transplantation of tongue and ganglia grafts to the anterior chamber of the eye. *Experimental Neurology* 35: 519–528.

ZALEWSKI, A. A. 1973. Regeneration of taste buds in tongue grafts after reinnervation by neurons in transplanted lumbar sensory ganglia. *Experimental Neurology* 40: 161–169.

26

Nerve Cell Cultures as a Tool for Investigating Basic Cellular Mechanisms of Learning and Memory

PAUL MANDEL

ABSTRACT There is good evidence for a chemical basis of learning and memory. However, it is very difficult to study the molecular mechanisms involved in this phenomenon because of the great diversity of nerve cells, the variety of their functions, the multiple interactions between individual nerve cells, and finally because of the influence of the whole organism on the central nervous system. A novel approach to basic molecular studies of nervous activity is the use of various types of cell cultures. The advantage of cell culture is that the cells are isolated from the rest of the organism in a well-defined medium, thereby avoiding the ambiguities of experiments in vivo. Thus investigations of the molecular basis of nerve cell differentiation and its specificity and function are easier in cell cultures. Also, studies of the effects of biologically active substances, including hormones, transmitters, and drugs, are facilitated in cell cultures.

There are different types of cell cultures: explants (i.e., tissue fragments), whole ganglia, and dissociated cells from ganglia or cerebral and cerebellar hemispheres. All of these cells have a very limited life span, and they can be obtained only in small amounts. In contrast, clonal cell lines, derived from a single cell of tumoral origin or transformed by a virus, may proliferate, producing enough cells for a wide range of biochemical investigations. Moreover, some of these clones undergo neuronlike differentiation under the influence of compounds such as cyclic nucleotides, bromodeoxyuridine, nerve growth factor, or insulin. In this way the acquisition of specific structures, the modulation of energy production through oxygen consumption, the biosynthesis and degradation of transmitters (acetylcholine, catecholamines, etc.), cell-cell interaction and communication, the effects of drugs, and even the mechanism of drug tolerance and dependence can be investigated.

Thus studies on nerve cell cultures of various types seem to offer an interesting approach to the study of the basic cellular phenomena which may be involved in the regulation of behavioral states. The findings concerning the plasticity of neuronal and glial cells, and the effects of the molecular environment (in particular, of trophic factors), may be of great importance in understanding behavioral mechanisms.

Interesting developments may be expected through the mapping of genes involved in the control of the biosynthesis of transmitters or other biologically active molecules. Development of new clonal lines and new biochemical, immunological, and electrophysiological methods are necessary in order to

PAUL MANDEL, Centre de Neurochimie du CNRS, and Institut de Chimie Biologique, Faculté de Médecine, Strasbourg, France

allow our knowledge of nervous tissue in culture and basic cellular mechanisms to progress. We should keep in mind, however, the extraordinary complexity of molecular events when the number of cells interacting increases up to the cell population involved in the simplest of learning tasks. Moreover, the limitations of some investigations on clonal lines have to be considered.

26.1 INTRODUCTION

Ultimately, like all biological phenomena, learning and memory must be explained at the molecular and cellular levels, as well as at the level of the whole animal. In fact, we know that manipulation of these three levels—by using pharmacological agents, by making lesions, or by varying the psychosocial environment—can lead to behavioral changes.

It is evident that a given individual is the result of a genetically determined program expressed at the molecular and cellular levels, but the expression of this program may be modulated by the molecular environment. All of these phenomena will be controlled by the repression and derepression of certain genes, leading to changes in the macromolecular composition (proteins, nucleic acids, and membranes) of the cell. In the central nervous system there is a contribution from each individual cell, but there is also, and perhaps more importantly, an organization of cells into specific pathways. It is thus necessary to study the biochemistry of the brain at this level as well.

The advantage of tissue cultures is that they are isolated from the rest of the organism in a well-defined medium. In particular, the effects of growth factors, differentiation factors, hormones, and pharmacological agents can be defined in a tissue culture, so that the ambiguities arising in experiments carried out in vivo from effects exerted on other organs are avoided.

The first experiment using tissue culture of the nervous system was performed by Harrisson (1907); it confirmed the neuron doctrine that had been proposed by Cajal and His, since neurons and nerve fibers could be observed directly. This concept now forms the basis of our understanding of nervous function. But there are many problems involved in the use of tissue cultures of the nervous system. It was once thought that, under appropriate conditions, mammalian cells could grow in culture indefinitely, as do microorganisms. If, in certain cases, this has proved to be possible, the extreme fragility of cells taken from their natural environment and placed in an artificial medium must nevertheless be borne in mind. The natural environment is the result of a long process of development, relative to which the time cells have to adapt to an artificial medium is extremely short. Cells often take on different forms and functions in response to their environment, and to the methodology used. Thus rigorous morphological (including karyotypical) and biochemical controls are necessary to assure that the original cell type has been maintained in culture. It must also be borne in mind that cells divide less rapidly after a certain time in culture, and frequent renewal of the medium is often necessary for their survival.

26.2 THE TYPES OF TISSUE CULTURE

Tissue culture of the nervous system has been performed on explants (i.e., on tissue fragments), on primary cultures of dissociated or reaggregated cells, and on clonal lines of neuroblastoma, glioblastoma, and glial cells.

26.2.1 Explant cultures

After the initial experiments of Harrisson (1907), the use of tissue culture of the nervous system developed very slowly, but interest in the field has quickened over the past twenty years (for review see Murray, 1971). The techniques used have been gradually improved, and cells survive longer and longer in culture, which extends the range of experimentation possible. Most of the earlier experiments reported have dealt with explant cultures and their morphological characterization. In particular, cell migration, the formation of nerve fibers, synaptogenesis, and myelinization have been studied.

The stimulatory effect of nerve growth factor on the formation of nerve fibers and cell differentiation in explants of embryonic sympathetic and sensory ganglia shown by Levi-Montalcini, Meyer, and Hamburger (1954) is now classic. We have observed that an extract of embryonic chick cerebral cortex stimulates the growth of neurites in cerebral-cortex explants (Treska et al., 1968; see Figure 26.1).

Demyelinization has been induced by adding to the culture medium serum or lymphocytes taken from patients with multiple sclerosis or the Guillain-Barré syndrome, or from animals with experimental allergic

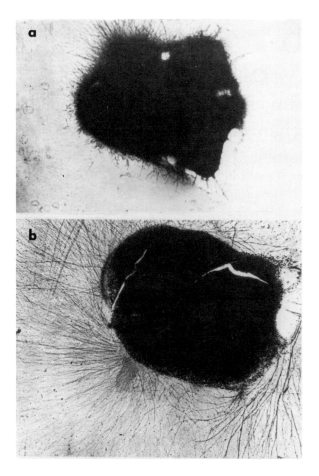

FIGURE 26.1 The effect of brain extract on the morphological differentiation of nerve cells in culture. Cerebral-hemisphere explants from 7-day-old chick embryos are shown after 24 days of culture (Bodian stain) (a) with total embryo extract (Obj. × 10), and (b) with embryonic brain extract (Obj. × 10).

encephalomyelitis (Bornstein and Appel, 1961; Berg and Kallen, 1964; Yonezawa, Ishihara, and Matsuyama, 1968). Demyelinization has also been induced by Silberberg (1967, 1969) in a medium containing metabolites from patients suffering from mental retardation due to genetic maladies such as phenylketonuria and maple-syrup disease.

Disturbed electrical activity has been observed in demyelinizing cultures by Bornstein and Crain (1965, 1971) (see reviews by Crain, 1966, and Murray, 1971).

Myelinization is stimulated by added thyroxine, in agreement with observations in vivo. Recently myelinization has been studied biochemically, particularly the synthesis of sulphatides (Silberberg et al., 1972; Fry, Lehrer, and Bornstein, 1972) and the accumulation of 2′, 3′-cyclic AMP 3′-phosphohydrolase.

One of the problems in explant cultures is that the development of the different cells of an explant is not necessarily synchronous, as is suggested by the work of

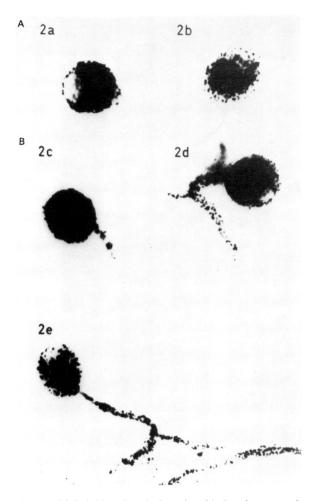

Allerand and Murray (1968), where myelinization was shown to extend over a long period. However, cultures of contiguous cerebellar explants myelinate within much narrower time limits. Synaptogenesis has been studied electron microscopically (Bunge, Bunge, and Peterson, 1967) and electrophysiologically (Crain, 1966); this topic is reviewed in detail by Nelson and Christian (this volume).

It is clear that detailed biochemical studies are needed in order to obtain the maximum amount of data from these cultures. Yet such cultures are difficult to study because they generally maintain the cellular heterogeneity of the tissue from which they are derived. Thus it is extremely difficult to decide which cells are responsible for the changes observed, and to elucidate the role of cellular interactions. It is therefore generally necessary to study processes for which there are well-defined markers, as is the case for myelinization, the development of enzymes involved in transmitter synthesis, and the formation of synapses. Moreover, in view of the limited amounts of material available, biochemical, immunological, and pharmacological techniques must often be adapted to a microanalytical level for use on these cultures.

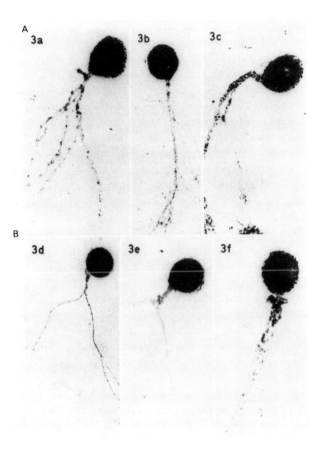

FIGURE 26.2 A histochemical study of isolated neurons in culture from chick embryo spinal ganglia. *Above*: Succinate dehydrogenase (SDH) activity in a medium (A) with total embryonic extract (2a: 1-day culture; 2b: 2-day culture); (B) with total embryonic extract and nerve growth factor (2c: 1-day culture; 2d: 2-day culture; 2e: 3-day culture). *Right*: Mitochondrial enzymatic activity in a 4-day culture in a medium of cultivation (A) with total embryonic extract and nerve growth factor (3a: succinate dehydrogenase; 3b: monoamine oxidase; 3c: glutamate dehydrogenase); (B) with embryonic spinal-cord extract (3d: succinate dehydrogenase; 3e: monoamine oxidase; 3f: glutamate dehydrogenase). (Obj. × 30, except 3d, which is Obj. × 19)

26.2.2 Cultures of dissociated cells

METHODOLOGY AND GENERAL CHARACTERISTICS. Cultures of dissociated cells overcome certain of the objections to explants. Initially developed by Moscona (1952) and extended by Cavanaugh (1955), Nakai (1956), Cohen, Nicol, and Richter (1964), Shimizu (1965), Utakoji and Hsu (1965), Scott, Engelbert, and Fisher (1969), Sensenbrenner et al. (1969, 1971), and Varon and Raiborn (1971), cultures are usually made from spinal or sympathetic ganglia or from chick, mouse, or rat cerebral cortex, either treated with trypsin or dissociated mechanically in such a way that the individual cells can be observed. Generally the cells are cultured in Maximow chambers (Maximow, 1925), Rose chambers (Rose, 1954), or Falcon flasks. The techniques are constantly being improved (Booher and Sensenbrenner, 1972; Sensenbrenner et al., 1972; Miller et al., 1970; Scott and Fisher, 1970, 1971). Recently methods for enriching the suspension in neurons before culture have been reported (di-Zerega et al., 1970; Okun, Ontkean, and Thomas, 1972).

We have observed that neurons derived from either sympathetic or spinal ganglia, or cerebral cortex, and cultivated in this way, can start to differentiate and grow neurites even in the absence of glial cells, but they degenerate rapidly. In the case of sympathetic-ganglion neurons, nerve growth factor prolongs survival, and similar effects can be obtained with nerve growth factor or spinal-cord extract on spinal-ganglion neurons, and with embryonic cerebral-cortex extract on cerebral-cortex neurons. The neurons can survive for several weeks and can differentiate, as can be seen by the appearance of enzymes involved in transmitter metabolism (Ciesielski-Treska, Hermetet, and Mandel, 1970; see Figures 26.2 and 26.3). The stimulations observed with nerve growth factor, spinal-cord or cerebral-cortex extracts (Sensenbrenner et al., 1969), and even with insulin (see Section 26.3), pose the problem of the structural relationships between and the phylogenesis of these various factors.

Dissociated neurons from dorsal-root ganglia of 8- to 12-day-old chick embryos have been cultivated in Rose chambers for up to five weeks. Newly formed fibers appeared either singly or grouped in bundles. The diameters of the fibers increased progressively, and a number of varicosities appeared. During the second week in culture, Schwann cells were easily recognized (Lodin et al., 1973). Mitochondrial enzymes such as succinate dehydrogenase, glutamate dehydrogenase, and monoamine oxidase could be detected in the cells and in the fibers (Ciesielski-Treska, Hermetet, and Mandel, 1970). RNA synthesis in short-term cultures of chick embryo spinal ganglia was higher in the presence of nerve growth factor.

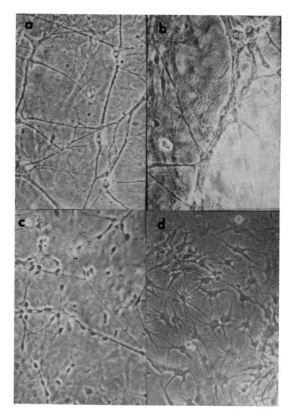

FIGURE 26.3 Stimulation of the differentiation of nerve and glial cells by a brain extract. Cultures of dissociated cells from 5-day-old chick embryo cerebral hemisphere are shown in the presence of brain extract from 8-day-old embryo: (a, b) after 15 days (multipolar neurons), (c) after 15 days (oligodendrocytelike cells along the fibers), (d) after 30 days (typical astrocytes). (Obj. × 25)

Other factors, such as concanavalin A, can stimulate the development of neurites in cultures of chick embryo spinal ganglia. α-Methylmannoside inhibits this effect, which suggests that it is concanavalin A bound to terminal mannose residues of plasma membrane glycoproteins which exerts the effect observed (Ciesielski-Treska, Gombos, and Morgan, 1971). Certain glycopeptides can produce similar effects (Gombos et al., 1972). Thus new possibilities for influencing cell plasticity are becoming available.

Dissociated sympathetic neurons maintained in culture without direct contact with glial cells still show characteristic catecholamine fluorescence; they also maintain enzyme activities such as those of the carboxylic esterases, succinate dehydrogenase, glutamate dehydrogenase, monoamine oxidase, lactate dehydrogenase, and alcohol dehydrogenase for short periods of time. Nerve growth factor maintains mitochondrial enzymes, acetylcholinesterase and nonspecific cholinesterases, and lactate dehydrogenase in sympathetic neurons for several weeks. In the absence of nerve growth factor, the more primitive enzymes, such as alcohol dehydrogenase, or the less specific, such as α-naphthol esterases, are retained for some time, whereas the mitochondrial and cholinesterase activities are lost rapidly.

Eight-day-old chick embryo brain extract stimulated the differentiation of dissociated cells of chick embryo cerebral hemispheres to large multipolar and pyramidal neurons, whereas 12-day-old chick embryo brain extract influenced the maturation of bipolar neurons of 5- and 7-day-old chick embryo cerebral-hemisphere cultures. Both extracts stimulated the differentiation of oligodendrocytes and of astrocytes, but the brain extracts from older embryos seemed to be more favorable for the maturation of astrocytes. The development of Nissl substance and the increase in acetylcholinesterase activity were stimulated by these extracts during the differentiation of the neurons (Sensenbrenner et al., 1972). This observation suggests that differentiation factors, which could play a fundamental role at a precise time, appear sequentially in the nervous system. Can this program or its expression be influenced by the environment, or is there a possibility of production of similar substances in later stages of development or in the adult? The existence of trophic or stimulatory factors is of obvious importance for research on cell plasticity. Perhaps such factors appear in vivo under certain conditions of afferent input or environment. In these investigations tissue cultures may be extremely useful.

Dissociated cerebral-hemisphere neurons and glial cells from chick, rat, and human embryos have been cultivated in Falcon plastic flasks. Neuronal elements from 5- to 13-day-old embryonic chick, 7- to 9-day-old embryonic rat, and 13- to 19-week-old human fetal brain have been established and maintained for varying periods of time in culture. Thus enough material for biochemical investigation may be available (Booher and Sensenbrenner, 1972).

Attempts to cultivate dissociated brain cells from older chick and rat embryonic material have been unsuccessful in producing a neuronal population; instead, layers of glial-cells tend to be produced.

We have observed that neuroblasts may develop into neurons without direct contact with glial cells. However, in the case of the dissociated cultures of chick embryo cortex which we have studied in some detail, underlying glial-cell layers considerably stimulate the differentiation of dissociated neuroblasts.

The first stages of myelin formation are observed in cultures to which embryonic brain extract has been added. Typical oligodendrocytes are observed to accumulate about thick fibers in these preparations.

Synapses also appear in these cultures but degenerate rapidly. The noradrenergic synapses appear to be the most resistant.

As in the case of explants, a number of specialized techniques need to be applied in order to obtain the maximum amount of information from these cultures. Morphological data give a measure of differentiation and cell integrity. Histochemical techniques can detect certain molecules (catecholamines, serotonin) or certain enzymes, but above all, quantitative and qualitative microanalysis will be necessary.

One important point is to determine to what extent the development of the culture parallels that of the tissue in vivo. We have attempted to analyze this problem in three areas: energy metabolism (Dittmann et al., 1973b), the cholinergic system (Ebel et al., 1974), and free nucleotides (Dittmann et al., 1973a).

OXYGEN UPTAKE. Oxygen uptake, lactate production, and the content of ATP per neuronal cell were measured at different times of cultivation and compared with the same parameters in cells obtained from the brains of living embryos.

The rate of oxygen consumption increased with the age of the culture, in parallel with the increase in the rate of oxygen uptake observed in the embryo. Neuronal oxygen uptake was about four times higher than that of glial cells. The rate of anaerobic lactate production increased as a function of the age of the culture (as known from other in vitro systems), whereas the glycolytic rate in the embryo decreased with development. The ATP content remained approximately constant (Schousboe, Booher, and Hertz, 1970).

No stimulatory effect of potassium on neuroblast cell respiration was observed. This supports the idea (Hertz, 1966; Haljamäe and Hamberger, 1971) that neurons are not affected by excess potassium, and that the stimulation of oxygen uptake in slices of brain cortex is a glial phenomenon.

These observations suggest that cultures of dissociated brain cells may undergo a considerable degree of metabolic differentiation and thus be well suited for studies of metabolic events in the nervous system. But some limitations have to be taken into consideration (Dittmann et al., 1973a,b).

CHOLINE UPTAKE. Cultures of dissociated nerve cells from chick embryo cerebral hemispheres can be manipulated to give cell populations with different proportions of neurons and glial cells. Ten-day cultures of 8-day-old embryos contain a high proportion of neurons. When a biphasic curve for choline uptake was expressed as a

Lineweaver-Burk plot, it demonstrated the presence of high- and low-affinity choline uptake systems. In contrast, in a 21-day culture of 14-day-old embryos, where all neurons had degenerated and an exclusively glial culture was obtained, only low-affinity uptake could be detected. These data show again that neuron differentiation characteristics such as choline uptake can be investigated in dissociated cell cultures (Massarelli et al., 1973b, 1974).

CHOLINE ACETYLTRANSFERASE AND ACETYLCHOLINESTERASE. The development of the enzymes involved in acetylcholine metabolism (choline acetyltransferase, acetylcholinesterase) was investigated in cell cultures from cerebral hemispheres of 7- and 12-day-old chick embryos and in vivo. A major difficulty encountered in this study was that such cultures give rise to both neuronal and glial cells, with an increase of total protein that makes the interpretation of specific enzymatic activities difficult. To avoid this inconvenience we have calculated the choline acetyltransferase/acetylcholinesterase ratio. It is noteworthy that, at the period corresponding to hatching time, cultures from 7- and 12-day-old chick embryos showed values very similar to those of hatching embryos. Thus primary cultures of embryonic cortical brain cells may provide a tool for pharmacological studies (Ebel et al., 1974).

GUANYL CYCLASE. In a 10-day culture of cerebral hemispheres of an 8-day-old chick embryo, where the proportion of neurons is rather high, guanyl cyclase activity is also high. In contrast, in a 21-day culture from cerebral hemispheres of a 14-day-old chick embryo, where only glial cells can be found, guanyl cyclase activity could not be detected. These data suggest that guanyl cyclase is mainly concentrated in neurons, as was first indicated by subcellular fractionation (Goridis and Morgan, 1973). A role for cyclic GMP in neuronal activity or in behavioral states may thus be expected (Goridis et al., 1974).

REAGGREGATION OF DISSOCIATED CELLS. We have observed that dissociated 5- or 7-day-old chick embryo cells tend to reaggregate, and that reaggregation favors the survival and differentiation of cells in culture. Isolated cells differentiate more slowly, particularly in low-density cultures, and in the absence of growth factors, they degenerate more rapidly (Sensenbrenner et al., 1972).

Moreover, cells dissociated in tissue culture reaggregate to form clumps, and in certain cases they form cellular aggregates which resemble histologically the original tissue. The reaggregation technique (Moscona,

1965) has recently been applied to the nervous system (Ishii, 1966; Stefanelli et al., 1967). Dissociated fetal isocortex and hippocampal cells reaggregate in layers which are organized histologically as in vivo (DeLong, 1970). This indicates that the intercellular signals and recognition phenomena are quite well conserved. It is also interesting that reaggregation favors the expression of certain specific enzymes (Seeds, 1971). The importance of intercellular contact and interaction (for the cellular functioning which is the basis of psychophysiological activity) is thus evident. The use of appropriate histochemical, chemical, and immunological techniques may enable us to determine the role of the different cell types in the formation of organized aggregates and in the expression of neural functioning.

Reaggregation is in part regulated by specific factors (Garber and Moscona, 1972a,b) whose activity depends upon the age of the culture from which they are extracted. The maximum effect was observed in cultures of 14-day-old mouse embryo brain with extracts from similar cultures. These factors seem to have a marked regional specificity. The elucidation of the nature and structure of these factors is obviously of great interest, particularly if they can be used to promote certain interactions and integrations of cellular physiological and psychic activities.

The fact that cells in culture produce substances which promote their differentiation and that of other cells is extremely important. These substances probably have a role in the maintenance and stimulation of nerve cells in vivo.

26.3 CLONAL CULTURES: NEUROBLASTOMA CELL CULTURES

Primary cultures of dissociated nervous-tissue cells are still mixtures of cell types, although they may be simpler than explants. It is obviously preferable to have homogeneous cultures that divide synchronously, maintain certain differentiated properties, and can thus be used to analyze the effects of environment on the inherited characteristics. Unfortunately, it has not been possible to obtain such cultures for neurons, and only rarely have they been obtained for glial cells. However, human and mouse neuroblastoma cells have been cultured, and a number of clones are now available (Klebe and Ruddle, 1969; Schubert et al., 1969; Augusti-Tocco and Sato, 1969). Similarly, the C_6 clone astrocytoma cells (Benda et al., 1968) and the NN strain of hamster astroblasts (Shein et al., 1970) are available. Clones of neurons could perhaps be produced by chemical or viral transformation of embryonic cells.

Continuous clonal cell lines which undergo neuronlike

differentiation can be obtained from the mouse neuroblastoma C1300 (Klebe and Ruddle, 1969; Schubert et al., 1969; Augusti-Tocco and Sato, 1969). The primary cultures of the cloned cells divide rapidly in suspension in a medium supplemented with fetal calf serum and retain their round cell morphology (Schubert et al., 1969). The average cell doubling time is about 18–24 hours. Some of the cells classified as "active" maintain the ability to produce the following enzymes involved in the synthesis and degradation of transmitters, as measured by biochemical methods: choline acetyltransferase (Rosenberg et al., 1971; Amano, Richelson, and Nirenberg, 1972); acetylcholinesterase (Blume et al., 1970; Schubert et al., 1971; Minna, Glazer, and Nirenberg, 1972; Amano, Richelson, and Nirenberg, 1972;) tyrosine hydroxylase (Schubert et al., 1969; Richelson, 1972; Waymire, Weiner, and Prasad, 1972; Amano, Richelson, and Nirenberg, 1972; Prasad et al., 1973); DOPA decarboxylase (Mack, Zwiller, and Mandel, unpublished data); dopamine-β-hydroxylase (Anagnoste et al., 1972); and monoamine oxidase (Goridis, Ciesielski-Treska, Hermetet, and Mandel, in preparation). We have also found evidence suggesting the presence of enzyme inhibitors of DOPA decarboxylase and dopamine-β-hydroxylase.

Microtubule proteins and the 14–3–2 protein are also present in neuroblastoma cell cultures (Herschman and Lerner, 1973). The presence of all these molecular species together with the electrophysiological properties of these cultures (see Nelson and Christian, this volume) indicates a high degree of neuronal differentiation.

26.3.1 Differentiation of neuroblastoma cells

Several investigators have reported on the morphological, biochemical, and neurophysiological differences among neuroblastoma cells grown under different conditions.

An increase in cellular and nuclear size and the formation of cytoplasmic processes longer than 50 μm as well as a production of a molecular phenotype resembling that of neurons have been obtained under the following conditions: (1) transfer of the cell suspension in a medium containing either 10 or 0.2 percent serum to a surface to which cells could attach, such as glass, collagen, or commercially treated tissue-culture dishes (Blume et al., 1970); (2) removal of the calf serum from the culture medium (Seeds et al., 1970); (3) addition of butyryl cyclic AMP or cyclic AMP phosphodiesterase inhibitors (Furmanski, Silverman, and Lubin, 1971; Prasad and Hsie, 1971; Kirkland and Burton, 1972; Richelson, 1972; Prasad and Sheppard, 1972; Prasad et al., 1973; Waymire, Weiner, and Prasad, 1972); (4) addition of bromodeoxyuridine (an inhibitor of DNA synthesis) (Schubert and Jacob, 1970; Kates, Winterton,

and Schlessinger, 1971); (5) addition of prostaglandin E1 (Prasad, 1972; Prasad et al., 1973); (6) x-irradiation (Prasad, Waymire, and Weiner, 1972). We have also shown that the nerve growth factor of Levi-Montalcini (Hermetet, Ciesielski-Treska, and Mandel, 1972a,b) and insulin (Hermetet et al., 1973) may have similar effects. In general, the induction of the growth of axonlike processes parallels the inhibition of cellular DNA synthesis. But dopamine, 6-hydroxydopamine, and DL-glyceraldehyde, which inhibit cell division, do not induce morphological differentiation (Prasad, 1971a,b).

Neuroblastoma cells vary in their sensitivity to induced differentiation by dibutyryl cyclic AMP, bromodeoxyuridine, and removal of serum, as has been shown chemically and by investigations of enzyme activities and of cell morphology.

26.3.2 Clonal and intraclonal heterogeneity of neuroblastoma cells

It should be pointed out that a great heterogeneity exists among the neuroblastoma clones and within cells of the same culture, as has been demonstrated by biochemical enzyme assays, by traditional histochemistry, by histofluorescence, and by karyotype analysis. Thus, in clones containing the enzymes involved in the metabolism of catecholamines, cells possessing serotonin or histamine can be found (Mandel et al., 1973a). In addition, process-poor clones may contain choline acetyltransferase and tyrosine hydroxylase in higher amounts than related process-rich clones.

Using histochemical methods, we found that the relative number of cells having processes is similar in a given clone after removal of serum and after addition of bromodeoxyuridine, butyryl cyclic AMP, nerve growth factor, or insulin. However, in clones in which 30–40 percent of the cells have extended processes during the stationary phase, only 15 percent show acetylcholinesterase activity. Similarly, in several adrenergic clones catecholamine-specific histofluorescence can be detected in only 30–40 percent of cells. The percentage of processes containing acetylcholinesterase was significantly higher after addition of the inducer substances than after removal of the serum. Nerve-growth-factor antiserum did not prevent the growth of processes. However, cellular alterations developed progressively (vacuolation, pyknosis), and the specific catecholamine fluorescence disappeared in all cell lines. The acetylcholinesterase activity of the cells was variably affected (Mandel et al., 1973a,b).

Neuroblastoma cells are often aneuploid. In most clones tetraploid as well as octaploid cells can be found. This intraclonal as well as interclonal heterogeneity with respect to chromosome number is not necessarily correlated with loss of differentiated function. Conversely, diploidy is not necessarily correlated with retention of differentiated characteristics. In principle, is it useful to isolate less aneuploid cell lines, although their karyotypic stability cannot be guaranteed. These karyotypic abnormalities show that neuroblastoma cells are not normal neurons. They exhibit, however, many of the properties of the neurons, and they may be used as a valuable model system for neurobiology and developmental biology.

The specific activity of some enzymes is modulated during the culture cycle, while that of others is not. Modulation as a function of culture conditions has been reported for acetylcholinesterase (Blume et al., 1970; Schubert et al., 1971) and for choline acetyltransferase (Amano, Richelson, and Nirenberg, 1972; Rosenberg et al., 1971). In contrast, no changes during the growth cycle were observed for catechol-O-methyltransferase (Blume et al., 1970) or for 14–3–2 specific protein in the human neuroblastoma (Herschman and Lerner, 1973). These phenomena, if they exist in vivo, may play a role in brain development and perhaps in early behavioral development. Synapse formation using clonal cell lines has not been reported.

26.3.3 Metabolic and molecular changes during differentiation and under the action of inducers

OXYGEN CONSUMPTION AND GLUCOSE METABOLISM. Neuroblastoma cell differentiation offers a good model for investigating the plasticity of neuronal type cells in the acquisition of high-energy production patterns.

Removal of serum from neuroblastoma cultures (Nissen et al., 1972), or addition of butyryl cyclic AMP (Furmanski, Silverman, and Lubin, 1971; Prasad and Hsie, 1971; Kirkland and Burton, 1972; Prasad et al., 1973) or of bromodeoxyuridine (Schubert and Jacob, 1970; Kates, Winterton, and Schlessinger, 1971) produces, in parallel with other differentiation phenomena, a striking increase in the oxygen uptake. However, the change in oxygen uptake differs from one clone to another and from one inducer to another, showing the great plasticity of basic neural functions.

In parallel with the increase in oxygen uptake, we have observed changes in the activities of some of the enzymes of intermediary metabolism: decreased lactate dehydrogenase activity and increased activities of the enzymes involved in oxidative metabolism of glucose, glutamate dehydrogenase, mitochondrial malate dehydrogenase, and isocitrate dehydrogenase (Ciesielski-Treska et al., 1972; Tholey et al., 1972). There are striking changes in the distribution of enzymes involved in glucose metabolism and their isoenzymes. This is particularly the case

for lactate dehydrogenase (Tholey, Ciesielski-Treska, and Mandel, unpublished data).

It seems likely that, in vivo, changes in the energy metabolism of nerve cells may parallel higher functional activity and that these changes may influence behavioral patterns.

TRANSMITTERS AND ENZYMES INVOLVED IN NEUROTRANSMITTER BIOSYNTHESIS. The distribution of catecholamines, serotonin, and histamine in neuroblastoma clones has been determined by a dansylation method (Table 26.1). Marked differences in the proportion and in the absolute quantities of different amines were observed. Chemical findings indicate that some neuroblastoma cells in culture contain both catecholamines and acetylcholinesterase (Hermetet, Ciesielski-Treska, and Mandel, 1972c). The presence of serotonin or histamine in the same cultures as catecholamines has been demonstrated in certain cells by coupling histochemical, histofluorescence, and biochemical methods (Mandel, 1973; Mandel et al., 1973a).

During the stationary phase of growth, or during induced differentiation, there is an increase in the specific activity of acetylcholinesterase in some clones (Blume et al., 1970; Schubert et al., 1971; Minna, Glazer, and Nirenberg, 1972; Amano, Richelson, and Nirenberg, 1972), of choline acetyltransferase in cholinergic clones (Rosenberg et al., 1971; Amano, Richelson, and Nirenberg, 1972), and of tyrosine hydroxylase in adrenergic clones (Schubert et al., 1969; Richelson, 1972; Waymire, Weiner, and Prasad, 1972; Prasad et al., 1973). However, the rate of the increase varies from one clone to another and during transfers of the clones.

It has been reported that simultaneous treatment of neuroblastoma cells in monolayers with cortisol, growth hormone, and thyroxine results in an increase in protein synthesis, neurite number, and neurite branching (De Vellis et al., 1971; De Vellis, Inglish, and Galey, 1971). Treatment with each hormone separately had no discernible effect. It would be interesting to confirm these

TABLE 26.1
Distribution of catecholamines in two adrenergic clones

	N1E-115	M1
Dopamine	0.2 ±0.1	2.0 ±0.7
Norepinephrine	1.8 ±0.7	13.6 ±1.4
Normetanephrine	0.9 ±0.4	21.1 ±1.2
Epinephrine	0.4 ±0.2	0.3 ±0.1
Serotonin	0.2 ±0.1	
Histamine	0.2 ±0.1	

Each value is the mean ±S.D. of 5 determinations expressed in 10^{-12} mol/mg proteins (Zwiller et al., 1973).

data on other models, in view of the cellular basis of the hormonal effects on behavior.

Antibodies against acetylcholinesterase were used to select neuroblastoma clones with a low acetylcholinesterase activity. The decrease of the enzyme activity was not associated with a decrease of choline acetyltransferase (Siman-Tov and Sachs, 1972, 1973). The independent control of these two enzymes was further shown under other experimental conditions (Blume et al., 1970; Prasad and Hsie, 1971; Rosenberg et al., 1971; Schubert et al., 1971; Amano, Richelson, and Nirenberg 1972; Minna, Glazer, and Nirenberg, 1972). We also found that cytidine diphosphate choline produces an increase of acetylcholinesterase, while phosphatidyl choline and insulin produce an increase of choline acetyltransferase activity (Mandel, Ayad, and Ebel, unpublished data).

Striking changes in neurotransmitter synthesis can occur in nutritional mutants of clonal lines of neuroblastoma. Thus, in an azaguanine-resistant cholinergic clone there is a twentyfold increase in choline acetyltransferase activity (Ebel, Ayad, Ciesielski-Treska, and Mandel, unpublished data). Changes in neurotransmitter equilibrium under mitogenic conditions may therefore occur, producing secondary behavioral changes.

UPTAKE OF CHOLINE. The uptake of choline in a cloned cell line derived from mouse neuroblastoma was higher in the so-called differentiating than in proliferating cells (Massarelli, Ciesielski-Treska, Ebel, and Mandel, unpublished data). The uptake was strongly inhibited if cesium or lithium ions or sucrose was substituted for sodium ions. Substitution of sodium for potassium also inhibited the uptake of choline. Incubation with potassium ferricyanide or at low temperature inhibited the incorporation of choline in both proliferating and differentiating cells. Thus it can be concluded that there is a strict relationship between choline uptake and the sodium pump, and that an active, energy-dependent component is involved in choline transport in neuroblastoma cells (Massarelli et al., 1973a). Furthermore, the presence of carriers necessary for choline transport in neuroblastoma cultures has been demonstrated by an analysis of the kinetics of choline uptake.

Thus, in respect to choline uptake, which undoubtedly plays an important role in cholinergic neurons, some neuroblastoma clones may behave like neurons.

ATPASE ACTIVITY. ATPase is inherently linked with the transport of cations across the neuronal membrane. An increase of ATPase activity during neuroblastoma cell differentiation has been observed (Ledig, Cam, and Ciesielski-Treska, 1972). In addition, an active "ecto"-ATPase has been demonstrated in neuroblastoma cells (Stefanovic et al., 1974).

GANGLIOSIDES OF NEUROBLASTOMA CELLS. Dawson et al. (1971) and Yogeeswaran et al. (1973) have recently reported marked differences in ganglioside patterns of neuroblastoma cell clones. Similar differences have been observed in our laboratory. We expected during differentiation a shift toward a preponderance of polysialic gangliosides, as is observed during ontogenesis of the nervous system. Although an increase in total ganglioside and in the G_{D3} content was observed in differentiated neuroblastoma cells, G_{D1b}, G_{T1}, and G_{Q1} gangliosides could not be detected (Rebel, Ciesielski-Treska, and Mandel, 1973). Thus the "neuronal" distribution was not observed. Since gangliosides are mainly localized in neuronal membranes, and particularly in synaptic membranes, the lack of production of synaptic contacts may be related to the inability to produce the polysialic gangliosides.

NEUROBLASTOMA CELL HYBRIDIZATION. Hybridization of somatic cells is particularly useful for investigation of the regulation of cell differentiation and for chromosomal mapping. The expression of different phenotypes makes it possible to determine whether different patterns are regulated individually or en bloc. When neuroblastoma cells are fused with human fibroblasts, a reexpression of a neuronal phenotype in the hybrid clone which correlates with a loss of a particular human chromosome may suggest the presence of a regulatory gene on this chromosome. Moreover, if, for example, mouse neuroblastoma cells are hybridized with human neuroblastoma and the hybrids continue to express neuronal phenotypes, one should thereby be able to correlate a particular enzyme —acetylcholinesterase, or tyrosine hydroxylase—with the loss of a specific human chromosome from hybrid clones. Mapping of structural and regulatory genes for differentiated phenotypes can be developed in this way.

By hybridization of neuroblastoma and L cells (a stable line derived from mouse fibroblasts), Minna, Glazer, and Nirenberg (1972) found a correlation between acetylcholinesterase activity and total chromosome number. Those clones with the lowest acetylcholinesterease activity had a lower average chromosome number; almost all acetylcholinesterase-positive clones had neurites.

The neutral glycosphingolipid patterns in neuroblastoma/L-cell hybrids are essentially the sum of the parental patterns (Yogeeswaran et al., 1973). In hybrid clones that exhibit widely different degrees of neuronal differentiation, no large differences are found among the glycosphingolipids, suggesting that the different metabolic patterns are independently controlled.

26.4 CLONAL CULTURES: GLIAL CELL CULTURES

Glial cell cultures may be of a great interest for investigation of the specific patterns of growth of glial cells and their interaction with neurons. Several lines of glial material are available: a clone of cells isolated from a rat glioma induced by injections of N-nitrosomethylurea (Benda et al., 1968), a clonal line developed from a human astrocytoma (CHB), and an astrocyte line derived from hamster (NN). The acidic protein S-100 described by Moore and co-workers (Moore, 1965; Moore and McGregor, 1965) can be used as a chemical marker of glial cell differentiation, as can 2′,3′-cyclic nucleotide 3′-phosphohydrolase. It is interesting to note that S-100 accumulation in C_6 glial cells depends on the pH of the medium: the synthesis and the proliferation proceed somewhat more rapidly at alkaline pH, and accumulation occurs more rapidly at slightly acidic pH. Cortisol induction of glucose-6-phosphate dehydrogenase was observed in C_6 glioma cells (De Vellis and Inglish, 1969; De Vellis et al., 1971; De Vellis, Inglish, and Galey, 1971). Lactate dehydrogenase was also found to be inducible in C_6 glioma cells (De Vellis and Inglish, 1969: De Vellis et al., 1971; De Vellis, Inglish, and Galey, 1971; De Vellis and Brooker, 1972). It should, however, be pointed out that the ganglioside pattern is extremely simple in C_6 cells and resembles that of nonneural tissue. Only G_{M3} was found in these cells. In contrast, a much greater variety of gangliosides was detected in the NN astroblast line (Rebel, Robert, and Mandel, unpublished data).

Several findings (Davidson and Benda, 1970; Benda and Davidson, 1971) on glial-cell/mouse-fibroblast hybrids suggest strongly that the synthesis of glial-cell-specific protein may be controlled by soluble diffusible regulators. In a mixed culture of a neuroblastoma adrenergic clone and NN cells, cells resembling the NN parents but with markedly increased ATPase activity appear (Stefanovic, Ciesielski-Treska, Ebel, and Mandel, unpublished data). The mechanism of this phenomenon is under investigation. All these data show the complexity of regulatory mechanisms and demonstrate that the genetically determined patterns may be modulated under different conditions. New aspects of neural plasticity have thus been discovered.

26.5 THE AGING OF CLONES OF MAMMALIAN CELLS

Hayflick and Moorehead (1961) and Hayflick (1965)

have emphasized a possible connection between aging changes observed in whole animals and the senescence of clones and cultures. Hayflick's experiments on fibroblast cultures can, however, be criticized on a number of grounds: the dependence of the longevity of the cell lines on the donor species, especially on the age of the donor; the cell type studied; and the culture conditions employed.

Supplementing a medium with hydrocortisone or tyrosine leads to a substantial increase in the number of divisions in the period when the growth capacity normally declines (Maciero-Coelho, 1966; Cristofalo, 1970; Litwin, 1972). Numerous proteins that differ from the standard proteins have been detected in aged cell lines (Holliday and Tarrant, 1972). Thus glucose-6-phosphate dehydrogenase mutants are more common in old than in young human fibroblasts (S. Fulder, quoted in Orgel, 1973). On the basis of the experiments available, it cannot be asserted that intracellular errors of macromolecular synthesis are responsible for in vivo aging. However, it seems likely that the investigation of cell cultures will be useful in the study of the aging of nerve cells and, in fact, of all cells.

26.6 EFFECTS OF DRUGS

Neuroblastoma cells can be used to test inhibitors of monoamine oxidase. The addition of different MAO inhibitors to a culture of an adrenergic clone increased the fluorescence without changing the number of catecholamine-containing neuroblasts. Addition of reserpine to the cultivation medium decreased the specific catecholamine fluorescence. Incubation with reserpine decreased acetylcholinesterase, especially in one clone, where acetylcholinesterase-positive varicosities completely disappeared. 6-Hydroxydopamine induced rapid degeneration of differentiated neuroblasts, characterized by morphological alterations (vacuolation, pyknosis) and the disappearance of catecholamine fluorescence and acetylcholinesterase. These effects were observed for all the cells of every adrenergic clone tested (Mandel, 1973; Mandel et al., 1973b).

As with other drugs, the biochemistry of morphine tolerance and dependence has primarily been studied on whole animals or on tissues taken from tolerant animals. Therefore, some of the phenomena observed may result from secondary effects rather than the primary action of morphine. Here again, the problem arises of whether it is possible to use tissue cultures to investigate the mechanism of action of a drug that produces striking behavioral changes. What we would like to find is the molecular mechanism of action of morphine on the cellular level, which is the first part of the behavioral change; the development of tolerance to and dependence on morphine has therefore been investigated in a variety of cultured cells (Semura, 1933; Sasaki, 1938; Corssen and Skora, 1964; Ghadirian, 1969). Several investigators concluded that cholinergic mechanisms are significantly affected by morphine (Hano et al., 1964; Beleslin and Polak, 1965; Jhamandas, Pinsky, and Phillis, 1970; Datta, Thal, and Wajda, 1971; Large and Milton, 1971). Recently the effect of morphine on the survival, cell proliferation rate, and choline acetyltransferase and acetylcholinesterase activities has been investigated in the human neuroblastoma IMR-32 line (Manner et al., 1974) and in a cloned mouse neuroblastoma line. It appears that cells exposed to morphine for thirty generations tolerate a previously lethal morphine concentration. Also, cell proliferation slows down in such cultures when morphine is completely withdrawn. However, normal morphology and proliferation are regained within a few days. Long-term exposure to morphine causes a striking increase in cholinesterase and a decrease in choline acetyltransferase. These changes persist in cultures habituated to morphine for at least two weeks after the withdrawal of the drug. It has also been shown that neuroblastoma cells exposed to the drug in vivo by propagation in morphine-tolerant mice are "dependent" on morphine when transferred to a culture. This is reflected in low levels of choline acetyltransferase and acetylcholinesterase when the cultures are grown without the drug (Peterson and Shuster, 1973).

Obviously, observations made on cells of an established line do not necessarily reflect the mechanisms of morphine habituation in the normally nondividing cells of the nervous system in the intact animals. Moreover, the morphine concentration applied in the experiments was higher than those reported in the brains of narcotized animals. Nevertheless, the results show that morphine tolerance can be induced in neuronlike cells without the mediation of other organs and tissues.

Changes do occur in the activities of enzymes involved in cholinergic neurotransmission. How these changes, which compensate for the effects of morphine, are brought about—whether by selective enzyme repression or induction—remains unknown.

Experiments have obviously to be done to extend the interpretation of the tissue-culture data. However, the fact that neuroblastoma cells in culture respond to added morphine suggests that this system holds much potential for the investigation of narcotic-related phenomena.

26.7 CONCLUSIONS

Investigations on nerve cell cultures seem to offer an interesting approach to the study of the basic cellular phenomena that may be involved in the regulation of behavioral states. Findings concerning the plasticity of neuronal and glial cells, their interactions, and the effects of the molecular environment, in particular of trophic factors, may be of great importance in understanding behavioral mechanisms.

Interesting developments may be expected through mapping of genes involved in the biosynthesis of transmitters or other biologically active molecules. Development of new clonal lines and new biochemical, immunological, and electrophysiological methods are necessary in order to allow our knowledge on nervous-tissue culture and basic cellular mechanisms to progress. However, we must keep in mind the extraordinary complexity of molecular events that results when the number of interacting cells increases up to the cell population involved in the simplest of learning tasks.

REFERENCES

ALLERAND, C. D., and MURRAY, M. R. 1968. Myelin formation in vitro. Endogenous influences on cultures of newborn mouse cerebellum. Archives of Neurology 19: 292–301.

AMANO, T., RICHELSON, E., and NIRENBERG, M. 1972. Neurotransmitter synthesis by neuroblastoma clones. Proceedings of the National Academy of Sciences (USA) 69: 258–263.

ANAGNOSTE, B., FREEDMAN, L. S., GOLDSTEIN, M., BROOME, J., and FUXE, K. 1972. Dopamine-β-hydroxylase activity in mouse neuroblastoma tumors and in cell cultures. Proceedings of the National Academy of Sciences (USA) 69: 1883–1886.

AUGUSTI-TOCCO, G., and SATO, G. 1969. Establishment of functional clonal lines of neurons from mouse neuroblastoma. Proceedings of the National Academy of Sciences (USA) 64: 311–315.

BELESLIN, D., and POLAK, R. L. 1965. Depression by morphine and chloralose of acetylcholine release from the cat's brain. Journal of Physiology 177: 411–419.

BENDA, P., and DAVIDSON, R. L. 1971. Regulation of specific functions of glial cells in somatic hybrids. I. Control of S100 protein. Journal of Cell Physiology 78: 209–216.

BENDA, P., LIGHTBODY, J., SATO, G., LEVINE, L., and SWEET, W. 1968. Differentiated rat glial cell strain in tissue culture. Science 161: 370–371.

BERG, O., and KALLEN, B. 1964. Effect of mononuclear blood cells from multiple sclerosis patients on neuroglia in tissue culture. Journal of Neuropathology and Experimental Neurology 23: 550–559.

BLUME, A., GILBERT, F., WILSON, S., FARBER, J., ROSENBERG, R. and NIRENBERG, M. 1970. Regulation of acetylcholinesterase in neuroblastoma cells. Proceedings of the National Academy of Sciences (USA) 67: 786–792.

BOOHER, J., and SENSENBRENNER, M. 1972. Growth and cultivation of dissociated neurons and glial cells from embryonic chick, rat and human brain in flask cultures. Neurobiology 2: 97–105.

BORNSTEIN, M. B., and APPEL, S. H. 1961. The application of tissue culture to the study of experimental "allergic" encephalomyelitis. I. Patterns of demyelination. Journal of Neuropathology and Experimental Neurology 20: 141–157.

BORNSTEIN, M. B., and CRAIN, S. M. 1965. Functional studies of cultured brain tissues as related to "demyelinative disorders." *Science* 148: 1242–1244.

BORNSTEIN, M. B., and CRAIN, S. M. 1971. Lack of correlation between changes in bioelectric functions and myelin in cultured CNS tissues chronically exposed to sera from animals with EAE. *Journal of Neuropathology and Experimental Neurology* 30: 129.

BUNGE, M. B., BUNGE, R. P., and PETERSON, E. R. 1967. The onset of synapse formation in spinal cord cultures as studied by electron microscopy. *Brain Research* 6: 728–749.

CAVANAUGH, M. W. 1955. Neuron development from trypsin-dissociated cells of differentiated spinal cord of the chick embryo. *Experimental Cell Research* 9: 42–48.

CIESIELSKI-TRESKA, J., GOMBOS, G., and MORGAN, I. G. 1971. Effet de la concanavaline A sur les neurones de ganglions spinaux d'embryons de poulet en culture. *Comptes Rendus (Paris)* série D 273: 1041–1043.

CIESIELSKI-TRESKA, J., HERMETET, J. C., and MANDEL, P. 1970. Histochemical study of isolated neurons in culture from chick embryo spinal ganglia. *Histochemie* 23: 36–43.

CIESIELSKI-TRESKA, J., MANDEL, P., THOLEY, G., and WURTZ, B. 1972. Enzymatic activities modified during multiplication and differentiation of neuroblastoma cells. *Nature* 239: 180–181.

COHEN, A. I., NICOL, E. C., and RICHTER, W. 1964. Nerve growth factor requirement for development of dissociated embryonic sensory and sympathetic ganglia in culture. *Proceedings of the Society for Experimental Biology* 116: 784–789.

CORSSEN, G., and SKORA, I. A. 1964. "Addiction" reactions on cultured human cells. *Journal of the American Medical Association* 187: 328–332.

CRAIN, S. M. 1966. Development of "organotypic" bioelectric activities in central nervous tissues during maturation in culture. *International Review of Neurobiology* 9: 1–43.

CRISTOFALO, V. J. 1970. Metabolic aspects of aging in diploid human cells. In E. Holeckova and V. J. Cristofalo, eds., *Aging in Cell and Tissue Culture*. New York: Plenum Press, pp. 83–119.

DATTA, K., THAL, L., and WAJDA, I. 1971. Effects of morphine on choline acetyltransferase levels in the caudate nucleus of the rat. *British Journal of Pharmacology* 41: 84–93.

DAVIDSON, R. L., and BENDA, P. 1970. Regulation of specific functions of glial cells in somatic hybrids. II. Control of inducibility of glycerol-3-phosphate dehydrogenase. *Proceedings of the National Academy of Sciences (USA)* 67: 1870–1877.

DAWSON, G., KEMPF, S. F., STOOLMILLER, A. C., and DORFMAN, A. 1971. Biosynthesis of glycosphingolipids by mouse neuroblastoma (NB41A), rat glia (RGC-6) and human glia (CHB-14) in cell culture. *Biochemical and Biophysical Research Communications* 44: 687–694.

DELONG, G. R. 1970. Histogenesis of fetal mouse isocortex and hippocampus in reaggregating cell cultures. *Developmental Biology* 22: 563–583.

DE VELLIS, J., and BROOKER, G. 1972. Effect of catecholamines on cultured glial cells: correlation between cyclic AMP levels and lactic dehydrogenase induction. *Federation Proceedings* 31: 513a.

DE VELLIS, J., and INGLISH, D. 1969. Effect of cortisol and epinephrine on the biochemical differentiation of cloned glial cells in culture and of the developing rat brain. In R. Paoletti, R. Fumagalli, and C. Galli-Tamburini, eds. *Second Meeting of the International Society for Neurochemistry*, Milan, pp. 151–152.

DE VELLIS, J., INGLISH, D., COLE, R., and MOLSON, J. 1971. Effects of hormones on the differentiation of cloned lines of neurons and glial cells. In *Influence of Hormones on the Nervous System* (Proceedings of the International Society of Psychoendocrinology). Basel: S. Karger AG. pp. 25–39.

DE VELLIS, J., INGLISH, D., and GALEY, F., 1971. Effects of cortisol and epinephrine on glial cells in culture. In D. C. Pearse, ed., *Cellular Aspects of Neural Growth and Differentiation*. Berkeley: University of California Press, pp. 23–32.

DITTMANN, L., HERTZ, L., SCHOUSBOE, A., FOSMARK H., SENSENBRENNER, M., and MANDEL, P. 1973a. Energy metabolism of nerve cells during differentiation. *Experimental Cell Research* 80: 425–431.

DITTMANN, L., SENSENBRENNER, M., HERTZ, L., and MANDEL, P. 1973b. Respiration by cultivated astrocytes and neurons from the cerebral hemispheres. *Journal of Neurochemistry* 21: 191–198.

diZEREGA, G., JOHNSON, L., MORROW, J., and KASTEN, F. H. 1970. Isolation of viable neurons from embryonic spinal ganglia by centrifugation through albumin gradients. *Experimental Cell Research* 63: 189–192.

EBEL, A., MASSARELLI, R., SENSENBRENNER, M., and MANDEL, P. 1974. Choline acetyltransferase and acetylcholinesterase activities in chicken brain hemispheres *in vivo* and in cell culture. *Brain Research* 76: 461–472.

FRY, J. M., LEHRER, G. M., and BORNSTEIN, M. B. 1972. Sulfatide synthesis: Inhibition by experimental allergic encephalomyelitis serum. *Science* 175: 192–194.

FURMANSKI, P., SILVERMAN, D. J., and LUBIN, M. 1971. Expression of differentiated functions in mouse neuroblastoma mediated by dibutyryl-cyclic adenosine monophosphate. *Nature* 233: 413–415.

GARBER, B. B., and MOSCONA, A. A. 1972a. Reconstruction of brain tissue from cell suspensions. I. Aggregation patterns of cells dissociated from different regions of the developing brain. *Developmental Biology* 27: 217–234.

GARBER, B. B., and MOSCONA, A. A. 1972b. Reconstruction of brain tissue from cell suspensions. II. Specific enhancement of aggregation of embryonic cerebral cells by supernatant from homologous cell cultures. *Developmental Biology* 27: 235–243.

GHADIRIAN, A. 1969. A tissue culture study of morphine dependence on the mammalian CNS. *Canadian Psychiatric Association Journal* 14: 607–615.

GOMBOS, G., HERMETET, J. C., REEBER, A., ZANETTA, J. P., and CIESIELSKI-TRESKA, J. 1972. The composition of glycopeptides, derived from neural membranes, which affect neurite growth *in vitro*. *FEBS Letters* 24: 247–250.

GORIDIS, C., MASSARELLI, R. SENSENBRENNER, M., and MANDEL, P. 1974. Guanyl cyclase in chick embryo brain cell cultures: Evidence of neuronal localization. *Journal of Neurochemistry* 23: 135–138.

GORIDIS, C., and MORGAN, I. G. 1973. Guanyl cyclase in rat brain subcellular fractions. *FEBS Letters* 34: 71–73.

HALJAMÄE, H., and HAMBERGER, A. 1971. Potassium accumulation by bulk prepared neuronal and glial cells. *Journal of Neurochemistry* 18: 1903–1912.

HANO, K., KANETO, H., KAKUNAGA, T., and MORIBAYASHI, N. 1964. Pharmacological studies of analegesics. VI. The administration of morphine and changes in acetylcholine

386   PAUL MANDEL

metabolism in mouse brain. *Biochemical Pharmacology* 13: 441–447.

HARRISSON, R. G. 1907. Observation on the living developing nerve fiber *Anatomical Record* 1: 116–118.

HAYFLICK, L. 1965. The limited *in vitro* lifetime of human diploid cell strains. *Experimental Cell Research* 37: 614–636.

HAYFLICK, L., and MOOREHEAD, P. S. 1961. The serial cultivation of human diploid cell strains. *Experimental Cell Research* 25: 585–621.

HERMETET, J. C., CIESIELSKI-TRESKA, J., and MANDEL, P. 1972a. Effets du NGF sur des cultures de neuroblastes du neuroblastome C1300. *Comptes Rendus de Société de Biologie* 166: 1120–1125.

HERMETET, J. C., CIESIELSKI-TRESKA, J., and MANDEL, P. 1972b. Effets du NGF sur un neuroblastome murin. *Comptes Rendus de Société de Biologie* 166: 708–711.

HERMETET, J. C., CIESIELSKI-TRESKA, J., and MANDEL, P. 1972c. Cytochemical demonstration of catecholamines and acetylcholinesterase activity in neuroblastoma cells in culture. *Journal of Histochemistry and Cytochemistry* 20: 137–138.

HERMETET, J. C., CIESIELSKI-TRESKA, J., WARTER, S., and MANDEL, P. 1973. Effets différentiels de l'insuline sur divers clones du neuroblastome C1300 de la souris. *Journal de Physiologie* 67: 280.

HERSCHMAN, H. R., and LERNER, M. P. 1973. Production of a nervous-system-specific protein (14-3-2) by human neuroblastoma cells in culture. *Nature; New Biology* 241: 242–244.

HERTZ, L. 1966. Neuroglial localization of potassium and sodium effects on respiration in brain. *Journal of Neurochemistry* 13: 1373–1387.

HOLLIDAY, R., and TARRANT, G. M. 1972. Altered enzymes in ageing human fibroblasts. *Nature* 238: 26–30.

ISHII, K. 1966. Reconstruction of dissociated chick brain cells in rotation mediated culture. *Cytologica* 31: 89–98.

JHAMANDAS, K., PINSKY, C., and PHILLIS, J. W. 1970. Effects of morphine and its antagonists on release of cerebral cortical acetylcholine. *Nature* 228: 176–177.

KATES, J. R., WINTERTON, R., and SCHLESSINGER, K. 1971. Induction of acetylcholinesterase activity in mouse neuroblastoma tissue culture cells. *Nature* 229: 345–347.

KIRKLAND, W. L., and BURTON, P. R. 1972. Cyclic adenosine monophosphate-mediated stabilization of mouse neuroblastoma cell neurite microtubules exposed to low temperature. *Nature; New Biology* 240: 205–217.

KLEBE, R. J., and RUDDLE, F. H. 1969. Neuroblastoma: Cell culture analysis of a differentiating stem cell system. *Journal of Cell Biology* 43: 69A.

LARGE, W. A., and MILTON, A. S. 1971. Effects of morphine, levorphanol, nalorphine and naloxone on the release of acetylcholine from slices of rat cerebral cortex and hippocampus. *British Journal of Pharmacology* 41: 398P +.

LEDIG, M., CAM, Y., and CIESIELSKI-TRESKA, J. 1972. Etude de l'activité ATPasique (Na$^+$- K$^+$) dans les cellules de neuroblastome en culture. *Journal de Physiologie* 65: 137A.

LEVI-MONTALCINI, R., MEYER, H., and HAMBURGER, V. 1954. *In vitro* experiments on the effects of mouse sarcoma 180 and 37 on the spinal and sympathetic ganglia of the chick embryo. *Cancer Research* 14: 49–57.

LITWIN, J. 1972. Human diploid cell response to variations in relative amino acid concentrations in Eagle medium. *Experimental Cell Research* 72: 566–568.

LODIN, Z., FALTIN, J., BOOHER, J., HARTMAN, J., and SENSEN-

BRENNER, M. 1973. Fiber formation and myelinization of cultivated dissociated neurons from chicken dorsal root ganglia. *Neurobiology* 3: 66–87.

MACIERO-COELHO, A. 1966. Action of cortisone on human fibroblasts *in vitro*. *Experientia* 22: 390–391.

MANDEL, P. 1973. Intérêt de la culture de neurones isolés, en neurochimie et en neuropharmacologie. In *Actualités Pharmacologiques*, 26ème série, Paris: Masson et Cie., pp. 1–25.

MANDEL, P., CIESIELSKI-TRESKA, J., HERMETET, J. C., ZWILLER, J., MACK, G., and GORIDIS, C. 1973a. Neuroblastoma cells as a tool for neuronal molecular biology. In E. Usdin and S. Snyder, eds., *Frontiers in Catecholamine Research*. Oxford: Pergamon Press, pp. 277–283.

MANDEL, P., CIESIELSKI-TRESKA, J., HERMETET, J. C., HERTZ, L., NISSEN, C. THOLEY, G., and WARTER, F. 1973b. Some histochemical, biochemical, and pharmacological aspects of differentiation of neuroblastoma cells of mouse. In E. Genazzani and H. Herken, eds., *Central Nervous System. Studies on Metabolic Regulation and Function*. Heidelberg: Springer-Verlag, pp. 223–230.

MANNER, G., FOLDES, F. F., KULEBA, M., and DEERY, A. M. 1974. Morphine tolerance in a human neuroblastoma line: Changes in choline acetylase and cholinesterase activities. *Experientia* 30: 137–138.

MASSARELLI, R., CIESIELSKI-TRESKA, J., EBEL, A. and MANDEL, P. 1973a. Choline uptake in neuroblastoma cell cultures: Influence of ionic environment. *Pharmacological Research Communications* 5: 397–406.

MASSARELLI, R., SENSENBRENNER, M., EBEL, A., and MANDEL, P. 1973b. Choline uptake in culture of dissociated cerebral cells from chick embryos. In *Proceedings of the 4th Meeting of the International Society for Neurochemistry*, Tokyo, p. 296 (Abstract).

MASSARELLI, R., SENSENBRENNER, M., EBEL, A. and MANDEL, P. 1974. Choline uptake in nerve cell cultures. I. Uptake in neuron-glial and glial cell population. *Neurobiology* 4:293–300.

MAXIMOW, A., 1925. Tissue cultures of young mammalian embryos. *Contributions to Embryology* (Carnegie Institute) 16: 47–113.

MILLER, R., VARON, S., KRUGER, L., COATES, P. W., and ORKAND, P. M. 1970. Formation of synaptic contacts on dissociated chick embryo sensory ganglion cells *in vitro*. *Brain Research* 24: 356–358.

MINNA, J., GLAZER, D., and NIRENBERG, M. 1972. Genetic dissection of neural properties using somatic cell hybrids. *Nature; New Biology* 235: 225–231.

MOORE, B. W. 1965. A soluble protein characteristic of the nervous system. *Biochemical and Biophysical Research Communications* 19: 739–744.

MOORE, B. W., and MCGREGOR, D. 1965. Chromatographic and electrophoretic fractionation of soluble proteins of brain and liver. *Journal of Biological Chemistry* 240: 1647–1653.

MOSCONA, A. A. 1952. Cell suspensions from organ rudiments of chick embryo. *Experimental Cell Research* 3: 535–539.

MOSCONA, A. A, 1965. Recombination of dissociated cells and the development of cell aggregates. In E. N. Willmer, ed., *Cells and Tissues in Culture*, Vol. 1. London: Academic Press, pp. 489–529.

MURRAY, M. R. 1971. Nervous tissues isolated in cultures. In A. Lajtha, ed., *Handbook of Neurochemistry*, Vol. 5, Part A. New York: Plenum Press, pp. 373–438.

NAKAI, J. 1956. Dissociated dorsal root ganglia in tissue culture. *American Journal of Anatomy* 99: 81–103.

NISSEN, C., CIESIELSKI-TRESKA, J., HERTZ, L., and MANDEL, P. 1972. Rates of oxygen uptake in proliferating and differentiating neuroblastoma. *Brain Research* 39: 264–267.

OKUN, L. M., ONTKEAN, F. K., and THOMAS, C. A. 1972. Removal of non-neuronal cells from suspensions of dissociated embryonic dorsal root ganglia. *Experimental Cell Research* 73: 226–229.

ORGEL, L. E. 1973. Ageing of clones of mammalian cells. *Nature* 243: 441–445.

PETERSON, G. R., and SHUSTER, L. 1973. Effects of morphine on choline acetyltransferase and acetylcholinesterase in cultured mouse neuroblastoma. *Proceedings of the Western Pharmacological Society* 16: 129–133.

PRASAD, K. N. 1971a. X-Ray induced morphological differentiation of mouse neuroblastoma cells *in vitro*. *Nature* 234: 471–473.

PRASAD, K. N. 1971b. Effect of dopamine and 6-hydroxydopamine on mouse neuroblastoma cells *in vitro*. *Cancer Research* 31: 1457–1460.

PRASAD, K. N. 1972. Morphological differentiation induced by prostaglandin in mouse neuroblastoma cells in culture. *Nature; New Biology* 236: 49–52.

PRASAD, K. N., and HSIE, A. W. 1971. Morphological differentiation of mouse neuroblastoma cells induced *in vitro* by dibutyryl adenosine 3′:5′-cyclic monophosphate. *Nature; New Biology* 233: 141–142.

PRASAD, K. N., MANDAL, B., WAYMIRE, J. C., LEES, G. J., VERNADAKIS, A., and WEINER, N. 1973. Basal level of neurotransmitter synthesizing enzymes and effect of cyclic AMP agents on the morphological differentiation of isolated neuroblastoma clones. *Nature; New Biology* 241: 117–119.

PRASAD, K. N., and SHEPPARD, J. R. 1972. Inhibitors of cyclic-nucleotide phosphodiesterase induce morphological differentiation of mouse neuroblastoma cell culture. *Experimental Cell Research* 73: 436–440.

PRASAD, K. N., WAYMIRE, J. C., and WEINER, N. 1972. A further study on the morphology and biochemistry of X-ray and dibutyryl cyclic AMP-induced differentiated neuroblastoma cells in culture. *Experimental Cell Research* 74: 110–114.

REBEL, G., CIESIELSKI-TRESKA, J., and MANDEL, P. 1973. Etude des gangliosides d'un clone de cellules de neuroblastome. *Comptes Rendus (Paris)* série D 277: 1193–1195.

RICHELSON, E. 1972. Stimulation of tyrosine hydroxylase activity in an adrenergic clone of mouse neuroblastoma by dibutyryl cyclic-AMP. *Nature; New Biology* 242: 175–177.

ROSE, G. G. 1954. A separable and multipurpose tissue culture chamber. *Texas Reports on Biology and Medicine* 12: 1074–1083.

ROSENBERG, R. N., VANDEVENTER, L., DE FRANCESCO, L., and FRIEDKIN, A. E. 1971. Regulation of the synthesis of choline-O-acetyltransferase and thymidylate synthetase in mouse neuroblastoma in cell culture. *Proceedings of the National Academy of Sciences (USA)* 68: 1436–1440.

SASAKI, M. 1938. Studies on phenomena of morphine abstinence of cultures *in vitro* of fibroblasts, and on curative effect of morphine and its derivatives on them. *Archive fuer Experimentelle Zellforschung* 21: 289–307.

SCHOUSBOE, A., BOOHER, J., and HERTZ, L. 1970. Content of ATP in cultivated neurons and astrocytes exposed to balanced and potassium-rich media. *Journal of Neurochemistry* 17: 1501–1504.

SCHUBERT, D., HUMPHREYS, S., BARONI, C., and COHN, M. 1969. *In vitro* differentiation of a mouse neuroblastoma. *Proceedings of the National Academy of Sciences (USA)* 64: 316–323.

SCHUBERT, D., and JACOB, F. 1970. 5-Bromodeoxyuridine-induced differentiation of a neuroblastoma. *Proceedings of the National Academy of Sciences (USA)* 67: 247–254.

SCHUBERT, D., TARIKAS, H., HARRIS, A. J., and HEINEMANN, S. 1971. Induction of acetylcholine esterase activity in a mouse neuroblastoma. *Nature; New Biology* 233: 79–80.

SCOTT, B. S. 1971. Effect of potassium on neuron survival in cultures of dissociated human nervous tissue. *Experimental Neurology* 30: 297–308.

SCOTT, B. S., ENGELBERT, V. E., and FISHER, K. C. 1969. Morphological and electrophysiological characteristics of dissociated chick embryonic spinal ganglion cells in culture. *Experimental Neurology* 23: 230–248.

SCOTT, B. S., and FISHER, K. C. 1970. Potassium concentration and number of neurons in cultures of dissociated ganglia. *Experimental Neurology* 27: 16–22.

SCOTT, B. S., and FISHER, K. C. 1971. Effect of choline, high potassium and low sodium on the number of neurons in cultures of dissociated chick ganglia. *Experimental Neurology* 31: 183–188.

SEEDS, N. W. 1971. Biochemical differentiation in reaggregating brain cell culture. *Proceedings of the National Academy of Sciences (USA)* 68: 1858–1861.

SEEDS, N. W., GILMAN, A. G., AMANO, T., and NIRENBERG, M. 1970. Regulation of axon formation by clonal lines of a neural tumor. *Proceedings of the National Academy of Sciences (USA)* 66: 160–167.

SEMURA, S. 1933. Experimentelle studien über die Morphingewöhrung mittels gezüchteter gewebe. *Folia Pharmacologica Japonica* 17: 3–4; 4–5.

SENSENBRENNER, M., BOOHER, J., and MANDEL, P. 1971. Cultivation and growth of dissociated neurons from chick embryo cerebral cortex in the presence of different substrates. *Zeitschrift für Zellforschung* 117: 559–569.

SENSENBRENNER, M., LODIN, Z., TRESKA, J., JACOB, M., KAGE, M. P., and MANDEL, P. 1969. The cultivation of isolated neurons from spinal ganglia of chick embryo. *Zeitschrift für Zellforschung* 98: 538–549.

SENSENBRENNER, M., SPRINGER, N., BOOHER, J., and MANDEL, P. 1972. Histochemical studies during the differentiation of dissociated nerve cells cultivated in the presence of brain extracts. *Neurobiology* 2: 49–60.

SHEIN, H. M., BRITVA, A., HESS, H. H., and SELKOE, D. J. 1970. Isolation of hamster brain astroglia by *in vitro* cultivation and subcutaneous growth, and content of cerebroside, ganglioside, RNA and DNA. *Brain Research* 19: 497–501.

SHIMIZU, Y. 1965. The satellite cells in cultures of dissociated spinal ganglia. *Zeitschrift für Zellforschung* 67: 185–195.

SILBERBERG, D. H. 1967. Phenylketonurea metabolism in cerebellum culture morphology. *Archives of Neurology* 17: 524–529.

SILBERBERG, D. H. 1969. Maple syrup urine disease metabolites studied in cerebellum cultures. *Journal of Neurochemistry* 16: 1141–1146.

SILBERBERG, D. H., BENJAMINS, J., HERSCHKOWITZ, N., and McKHANN, G. M. 1972. Incorporation of radioactive sulphate into sulfatide during myelination in cultures of rat cerebellum. *Journal of Neurochemistry* 19: 11–18.

SIMAN-TOV, R., and SACHS, L. 1972. Enzyme regulation in neuroblastoma cells. *European Journal of Biochemistry* 30: 123–129.

SIMAN-TOV, R., and SACHS, L. 1973. Regulation of acetylcholine receptors in relation to acetylcholinesterase in neuroblastoma cells. *Proceedings of the National Academy of Sciences (USA)* 70: 2902–2905.

STEFANELLI, A., ZACCHEI, A. M., CARAVITA, S., CATALDI, A., and IERADI, L. A. 1967. New-forming retinal synapses *in vitro*. *Experientia* 23: 199–200.

STEFANOVIC, V., CIESIELSKI-TRESKA, J., EBEL, A., and MANDEL, P. 1974. Mise en évidence d'une ATPase sensible à l'ouabaine à la surface externe des cellules de neuroblastome et de cellules gliales en culture. *Comptes Rendus (Paris)* série D 278: 2041–2044.

THOLEY, G., CIESIELSKI-TRESKA, J., WURTZ, B., and MANDEL, P. 1972. Variations de diverses activités enzymatiques liées au métabolisme glucidique dans des cellules de neuroblastome en prolifération et en différenciation. *Comptes Rendus (Paris)* série D 275: 1715–1718.

TRESKA, J., SENSENBRENNER, M., LODIN, Z., JACOB, M., and MANDEL, P. 1968. Action d'extraits embryonnaires de cerveau sur la différenciation morphologique de cellules nerveuses en culture *in vitro*. *Comptes Rendus (Paris)* série D 267: 2034–2036.

UTAKOJI, T., and HSU, T. E. 1965. Nucleic acids and protein synthesis of isolated cells from chick embryonic spinal ganglia in culture. *Journal of Experimental Zoology* 158: 181–202.

VARON, S., and RAIBORN, JR., C. 1971. Excitability and conduction in neurons of dissociated ganglionic cell cultures. *Brain Research* 30: 83–98.

WAYMIRE, J. C., WEINER, N., and PRASAD, K. N. 1972. Regulation of tyrosine hydroxylase activity in cultured mouse neuroblastoma cells: Elevation induced by analogs of adenosine $3':5'$-cyclic monophosphate. *Proceedings of the National Academy of Sciences (USA)* 69: 2241–2245.

YOGEESWARAN, G., MURRAY, R. K., PEARSON, M. L., SANWAL, B. D., McMORRIS, F. A., and RUDDLE, F. H. 1973. Glycosphingolipids of clonal lines of mouse neuroblastoma and neuroblastoma X L hybrids. *Journal of Biological Chemistry* 248: 1231–1239.

YONEZAWA, T., ISHIHARA, Y., and MATSUYAMA, H. 1968. Studies on experimental allergic peripheral neuritis. Demyelinating patterns studies *in vitro*. *Journal of Neuropathology and Experimental Neurology* 27: 453–463.

ZWILLER, J., CIESIELSKI-TRESKA, J., MACK, G., and MANDEL, P. 1973. Amines biogènes des cellules de neuroblastome en culture. *Journal de Physiologie* 67: 225 A.

27

Neural Subsystems and Learning: Tissue-Culture Approaches

FREDRICK J. SEIL AND ARNOLD L. LEIMAN

ABSTRACT Portions of the nervous system removed either around the time of birth or during a prenatal period can be maintained in isolation from the rest of the brain. Such tissue cultures of the central nervous system show the development in isolation of connections and organizational patterns characteristic of the region from which the tissue culture is derived. Examples of tissue cultures of cerebral and cerebellar neocortex suggest that many aspects of anatomical relations in these regions are pre-programmed by genetic mechanisms. Characteristic forms of electrical activity are evident in tissue cultures derived from these regions. The use of neural tissue cultures in learning and memory experiments may enable a closer look at the distinctive memory operations or devices of particular brain regions removed from systemic and other brain influences.

The study of the biology of learning and memory has been rich in theories about ways in which nervous systems might store information, but it has been somewhat less fortunate in the elaboration of suitable experimental strategies and tactics. The disparity between conjecture and the attainments of research has contributed to an emphasis on the analytic advantages of nervous-system organizations simpler than that of the intact mammalian brain with its billions of neurons (e.g., Kandel and Spencer, 1968; Leiman and Christian, 1973). The quest for simplicity has led some experimenters to concentrate on the study of invertebrates, and this perspective is offered in other chapters in this volume.

Another approach to the problem at a somewhat different organizational level is provided by vertebrate cell- and tissue-culture techniques. The method of cell culture is based on the dissociation of cells from each other by enzymatic, chemical, or mechanical means. The method of tissue culture is based on the explantation of isolated but intact fragments of nervous tissue, enabling the maintenance of those interneuronal relationships that already exist and allowing the development of further intercellular relationships. With this technique an organizational level is achieved in isolated and easily observable bits of nervous tissue which incorporates some of the complexity of particular central-nervous-system (CNS) regions.

FREDRICK J. SEIL, Department of Neurology, Veterans Administration Hospital, Palo Alto, CA, and ARNOLD L. LEIMAN, Department of Psychology, University of California, Berkeley

27.1 TISSUE-CULTURE METHODS

A variety of tissue-culture methods have been used for both central and peripheral nervous system (for reviews see Murray, 1965, 1971). Major differences in technique include:

1. the types of chambers employed, such as roller tubes, or Rose or Maximow chambers (some chambers involve immersion of the tissues in a fluid medium, while others emphasize a thin layer of medium overlying the cultures to allow a freer exchange of gases);

2. the choice of substrates, ranging from two-dimensional systems such as glass or plastics, with or without a coating of collagen gel, to quasi-three-dimensional systems such as plasma clots, to fully three-dimensional systems such as gelatin foam;

3. the compositon of feeding media, with fully synthetic media at one end of the spectrum and so-called natural media, a major component of which is serum of animal or human origin, at the other end.

Generally, single fragments of nervous system tissue are explanted, but most culture systems are adaptable to explantation of several adjoining fragments of tissue, provided the total tissue mass is kept small enough that its nutritive and oxygen requirements can be met. The explantation of multiple fragments of nervous-system tissue has been used to advantage by Crain, Peterson, and Bornstein (1968), who demonstrated that functional interconnections develop between such explants.

The specific tissue-culture method we employ is the Maximow-chamber method (Murray, 1965, 1971). In this system an explant is placed on a round glass coverslip previously coated with rat-tail collagen and covered with a drop of nutrient medium. The round glass coverslip is attached with a drop of fluid to a square glass coverslip, which is inverted over a Maximow depression slide and sealed with paraffin. The cultures are incubated at 35.5–36°C in the lying-drop position. The nutrient medium is changed twice weekly under aseptic conditions. The composition of the nutrient medium currently employed in our laboratory for cerebellar and cerebral neocortex cultures is as follows: 2 parts of 3 units/ml low-zinc insulin (from Squibb Institute for Medical

Research); 1 part of 20 percent dextrose; 4 parts of bovine serum ultrafiltrate; 4 parts of Eagle's minimum essential medium with Hanks's base and added L-glutamine; 7 parts of Simms's X-7 balanced salt solution (BSS) with sufficient added N-2-hydroxyethylpiperazine-N′-2-ethanesulfonic acid (HEPES) to make its concentration 0.01 M in the fully constituted nutrient medium; and 12 parts of human placental serum. During electrophysiological recording procedures this medium is replaced by BSS additionally buffered with 0.015 M HEPES. Our reasons for choosing the Maximow-chamber method include the ease of microscopic observation which the system allows and the fact that CNS explants appear to achieve a greater degree of anatomical organization and functional integrity with this system than with other methods (Seil, 1972; Leiman and Seil, 1973).

27.2 STRUCTURAL ORGANIZATION OF CNS EXPLANTS

Cultures of spinal cord, cerebellum, hippocampus, and cerebral neocortex attain, after several weeks in vitro, organizational characteristics that suggest their tissue of origin, and that allow them to be readily distinguished from each other (Sobkowicz, Guillery, and Bornstein, 1968; Kim, 1972; Seil, 1972; LaVail and Wolf, 1973; Seil, Kelly, and Leiman, 1974). This point will be

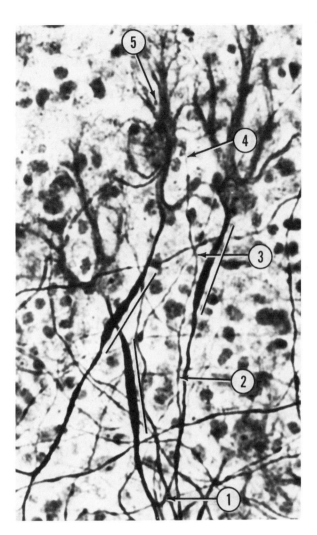

FIGURE 27.2 Purkinje cells from a cerebellar culture, 28 days in vitro. Axons are easily identified by their enlarged proximal segments (indicated by adjacent straight lines). Arrows (successively numbered) trace a collateral originating (No. 1) from the axon of the Purkinje neuron whose cell body is on the left to its termination (No. 5) as a club-shaped ending near a dendritic branch of the cell in the center. Holmes stain, × 615. Modified from Seil (1972). Reproduced with the permission of ASP Biological and Medical Press (Elsevier division).

illustrated by a description of two levels of the CNS that we have studied in some detail, namely, cerebellum and cerebral neocortex.

27.2.1 Cerebellar tissue cultures

Parasagittally cut explants of newborn mouse cerebellum present a complex organization after 3–4 weeks in vitro (Seil and Herndon, 1970; Seil, 1972). Figure 27.1 illustrates such an explant after one month in culture; a cortical area and subcortical (intracerebellar and vestibular) nuclei are readily apparent. Purkinje-cell axons can be seen to converge upon an intracerebellar

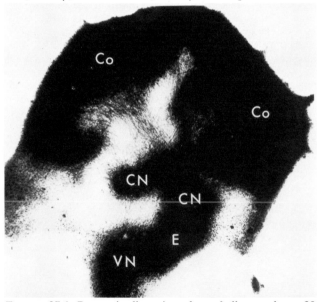

FIGURE 27.1 Parasagittally oriented cerebellar explant, 29 days in vitro, with cortical (Co), intracerebellar nuclear (CN), and vestibular nuclear (VN) zones. An ependymal (E) zone is also indicated, as the ependyma distinguishes the caudal from the rostral end of the explant. Fibers originating from Purkinje cells in the cortex converge upon the intracerebellar nucleus. Holmes stain, × 40.

nucleus. Characteristic neuronal types are found in each of the cortical and subcortical nuclear areas. Details of the neuronal types in the subcortical nuclei can be found in the original publication (Seil, 1972). There is some evidence for the presence of each of the five expected cell types in the cortical zones of these cultures. For purposes of the present discussion, we shall concentrate on the two major classes of cerebellar cortical neurons, the Purkinje and granule cells.

Purkinje cells are abundantly present in cerebellar cultures. They are easily recognized in the living state by their cortical location and their large, prominent nuclei. Figure 27.2 illustrates three such cells which have been impregnated with silver. While their dendritic trees do not achieve the full adult elaboration in vitro, their morphology is nevertheless consistent with that of Purkinje cells in situ (Meller and Glees, 1969). Also illustrated in this photomicrograph is a common finding in cerebellar cultures, namely, the presence of Purkinje-cell axon collaterals. An axon collateral can be traced (arrows) from its origin on the axon of the cell on the left to its termination as a club-shaped ending near one of the dendritic branches of the cell in the center.

Granule cells are also abundant in cerebellar cultures, and some of these neurons are illustrated in Figure 27.3. The cells in this figure have been impregnated by the Golgi-Cox method (Wolf and Dubois-Dalcq, 1970), and a typical "claw-shaped" dendrite is seen emanating from one of them. Although mossy fibers are absent or occur infrequently in culture preparations because they are severed during explantation, ultrastructural studies have demonstrated that the granule-cell dendrites do receive Golgi axon terminals (Seil and Herndon, 1970). Granule-cell axons appear as bundles of parallel fibers, as shown by electron microscopy (Figure 27.4, top), and

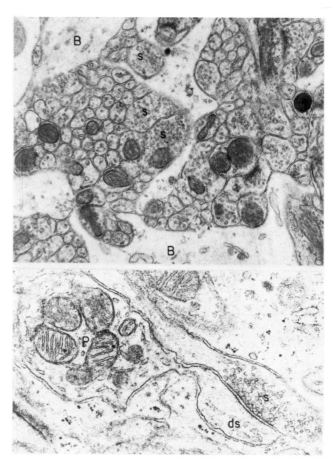

FIGURE 27.4 *Top*: Electron micrograph from a cerebellar culture, 26 days in vitro. Bundles of parallel fibers are seen, separated by processes of Bergmann astrocytes (B). A number of enlargements (s) containing synaptic vesicles are seen, but points of synaptic contact are not demonstrated in this field. × 18,200.

Bottom: Electron micrograph from a cerebellar culture, 33 days in vitro. Demonstrated is a Purkinje-cell dendrite (P) with a dendritic branchlet spine (ds) in synaptic contact with the terminal enlargement of a parallel fiber (s). × 23,100. From Seil and Herndon (1970). Reproduced with the permission of The Rockefeller University Press.

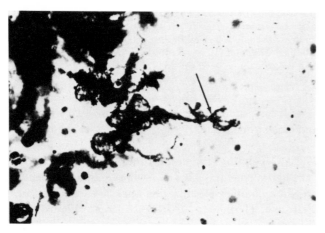

FIGURE 27.3 Granule cells from a cerebellar culture, 32 days in vitro. The arrow points to a "claw-shaped" dendrite emanating from one of a cluster of three granule cells. Golgi-Cox stain, × 690.

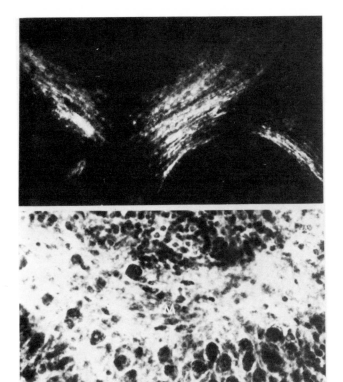

FIGURE 27.5 *Top*: Bundles of myelinated Purkinje-cell axons from a cerebellar culture, 15 days in vitro. The preparation was photographed with polarized light in the living state. × 140. *Bottom*: Lamination in the cortex of a cerebellar explant, 25 days in vitro. Below the molecular layer (M) is a layer several cells thick of large Purkinje cells. A relatively thin layer of small granule cells, the internal granular layer, is evident below the Purkinje cells. A thicker outer granular layer is seen above the molecular layer. Thionine stain, photographed with phase-contrast optics, × 300.

the parallel fibers form appropriate synapses with Purkinje-cell dendritic spines (Figure 27.4, bottom). Such synapses are commonly found after several weeks in vitro, suggesting that a pathway for excitation of Purkinje cells is readily available in these cultures.

The development of the parallel-fiber/Purkinje-cell synapses must be a postexplantation phenomenon, since mouse cerebellar granule cells at birth, which is when the explants are prepared, are dividing neuroblasts that have not yet formed synapses (Miale and Sidman, 1961). The subsequent formation of such synapses in the complete isolation of the culture chamber indicates that input such as that provided by limb movements after birth is not necessary for their development.

Another postexplantation phenomenon is myelin formation. The mouse cerebellum is unmyelinated at birth. Myelin generally appears in cerebellar explants after 9–12 days in vitro. The first appearance of myelin is usually in the ventral portion of the cultures, with the axons of subcortical nuclear neurons and the axons of Purkinje cells in the rostral half of the culture myelinating first. The distal portions of Purkinje-cell axons appear to myelinate before proximal portions, and Purkinje-cell axon myelination precedes myelination of axon collaterals. Figure 27.5 (top) demonstrates myelinated bundles of Purkinje-cell axons in a cerebellar culture after 15 days in vitro. These fibers were photographed in the living state with polarized light.

The overall organization of the cerebellar cortex is a laminar one. This is illustrated in Figure 27.5 (bottom), in which granule and Purkinje cells appear as distinct layers and a molecular layer is also evident. The Purkinje-cell layer is several cells deep since the monolayer that is typical of the adult does not usually develop in vitro. There are also both outer and internal granular layers, the former appearing dorsal to the molecular layer in Figure 27.5 (bottom) and the latter appearing ventral to the Purkinje cells. The persistence of an outer granular layer in tissue culture could represent a premature arrest of granule-cell migration (Seil, 1972). It has also been postulated (Wolf, 1970) that a double granular layer is formed in vitro because of granule-cell migration in two directions, rather than in one as in vivo.

27.2.2 Cerebral neocortex tissue cultures

Parasagittally oriented explants of cerebral neocortex derived from frontal and parietal cortex of 2- to 3-day-old mice present an organization different from that of cerebellar cultures (Seil, Kelly, and Leiman, 1974). As shown in Figure 27.6, the original cortical surface remains easily recognizable in crescent-shaped cerebral neocortical explants after several weeks in vitro. A horizontal laminar organization is the major structural

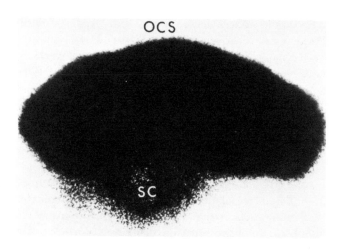

FIGURE 27.6 Parasagittally oriented cerebral neocortex explant, 18 days in vitro. The original cortical surface (OCS) of the explant remains identifiable by its curvature. A subcortical (SC) zone of tissue is also illustrated, Holmes stain, × 45.

feature of these cultures, and the outstanding elements of this organization are four bundles of horizontally coursing neurites (Figure 27.7). We have designated these bundles, beginning dorsally, as the tangential, submarginal, intermediate, and deep bands.

The tangential band appears at the cortical surface and courses along the entire dorsal margin of the explant. It is composed, in part, of both dendrites and axons of superficial cortical neurons. Running parallel to the tangential band, but separated from it by a layer of closely packed neurons, is the submarginal band. This band also appears to be composed, at least in part, of axons originating from superficial cortical neurons.

The layer of neurons separating the dorsally located bands, designated the external granular layer in Figure 27.7, is composed of predominantly multipolar cells (Figure 27.8, upper left), which may represent stellate or modified pyramidal cells. This layer probably corresponds to the second cortical layer in situ (Meller, Breipohl, and Glees, 1968). Axons from the neurons of the external granular layer appear in cerebral neocortical cultures in both the tangential and submarginal bands, where they have been traced from one end of the culture to the other, possibly acting as association fibers connecting rostral with caudal portions of the explant.

The dominant neuronal types ventral to the submarginal band are pyramidal cells. Their vertically oriented apical dendrites stand out from background fibers in silver-stained preparations (Figure 27.8, upper right). Both large and small pyramidal neurons are present. Most demonstrate the classic morphology, with apical dendrites having oblique branches and with horizontally or obliquely oriented basilar dendrites (Figure 27.8, lower left). The basilar dendrites achieve a considerable

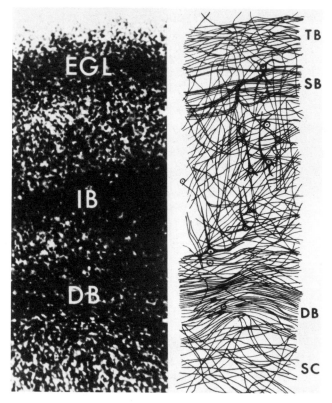

FIGURE 27.7 *Left*: A horizontal laminar organization is evident in a cerebral neocortical explant, 19 days in vitro. The cortical surface of the explant is at the top of the figure. Distinguishable as relatively dense structures are an external granular layer of neurons (EGL) and intermediate (IB) and deep (DB) bands of horizontally coursing fibers. The deep band is at the ventral margin of the cortical region of the explant, and the tissue that appears ventral to the deep band is subcortical tissue. Holmes stain, × 95.

Right: Drawing based on a camera lucida tracing of a Holmes-stained preparation of a cerebral neocortex culture, 21 days in vitro. The drawing is of an area of the explant comparable to that on the left. Shown are the tangential (TB), submarginal (SB), and deep (DB) bands of fibers, as well as some subcortical neurites (SC). This culture does not have an intermediate band of fibers, as is true for more than half of the cerebral neocortex cultures. Also demonstrated are some neurites between the major fiber bands and some silver-impregnated neurons. × 125. From Seil, Kelly, and Leiman (1974). Reproduced with the permission of Academic Press, Inc.

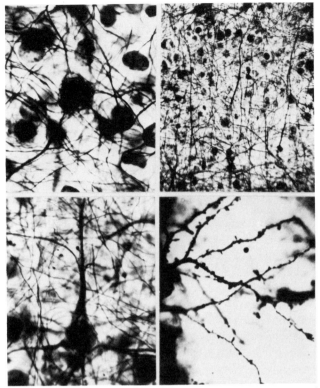

FIGURE 27.8 *Upper Left*: Multipolar neuron from the external granular layer of a cerebral neocortex culture, 21 days in vitro. Holmes stain, × 810. *Upper Right*: Pyramidal-cell apical dendrites stand out as thick vertically oriented elements from the background fibers in a cerebral neocortex culture, 21 days in vitro. Holmes stain, × 250. *Lower Left*: Classical pyramidal neuron from a cerebral neocortical culture, 21 days in vitro. Oblique branches emanate from the stout apical dendrite. Horizontally oriented basilar dendrites originate from the neuronal cell body near the bottom of the figure. An axon is directed straight downward. Holmes stain, × 725. *Lower Right*: Pyramidal-cell basilar dendrites from a cerebral neocortex explant, 21 days in vitro. A considerable degree of branching and dendritic spine formation is evident. Golgi-Cox stain, × 890. From Seil, Kelly, and Leiman (1974). Reproduced with the permission of Academic Press, Inc.

degree of branching and spine formation after several weeks in vitro (Figure 27.8, lower right). This too is a postexplantation phenomenon, as the degree of pyramidal-cell basilar dendritic complexity illustrated in Figure 27.8 (lower right) is not present in the mouse at the time of explantation (Ramón y Cajal, 1960).

The intermediate band of fibers is present in less than one-half of the explants. This possibly relates to the fact that the explants are variously derived from frontal or parietal cortex. When the intermediate band is present, it intersects a dense layer of interwoven pyramidal-cell basilar dendrites, rather reminiscent of the basilar dendritic bundles described by Scheibel et al. (1974). While it has not been possible to trace the origin of the intermediate band of fibers with certainty, we have, because of their close association with basilar dendrites, postulated that these fibers might represent pyramidal-cell axon collaterals, which are otherwise abundantly present.

The deep band of fibers is located at the ventral margin of the explant. It contains many thick neurites, at least some of which are pyramidal-cell axons, as determined by fiber tracing. A similar deep tangential band of fibers has been described in situ in the rat, in which species the neurites appear to be association fibers (Krieg, 1946). Myelin initially appears in the deep band of fibers and in the more ventrally located subcortical fibers in cerebral neocortex cultures, generally after 10–14 days in vitro (Seil, Kelly, and Leiman, 1974).

Lamination is poorly developed in neonatal mouse or rat cerebral neocortex, and few axons are present at birth or during early postnatal stages in the rat (Eayrs and Goodhead, 1959; Kobayashi et al., 1964). The degree of laminar formation and fiber organization present in cerebral neocortex cultures after 2–4 weeks in vitro therefore represents developments which have occurred in the tissues after explantation.

These anatomical studies demonstrate that structurally different levels of the central nervous system retain their differences when maintained in a tissue-culture system. The studies also demonstrate that a high degree of organizational complexity can be attained in such cultures in the absence of the usual afferent components. Cultures of cerebellum and cerebral neocortex show typical cell types, neuronal groupings, and internal network relations. These observations suggest that the organizational development of nervous systems is largely guided by intrinsic instructional mechanisms. Although indicants of functional plasticity of the nervous system have been frequently noted (Cragg, 1972), observations from tissue-culture studies suggest that the range of possibilities for structural plasticity is considerably narrower.

27.3 ELECTROPHYSIOLOGICAL PROPERTIES OF CNS EXPLANTS

The functional properties of CNS tissue cultures have been explored in many neurophysiological studies using both extracellular and intracellular recording techniques. In reviewing these studies it is useful to consider extant data from the perspective of the kind of problems and questions to which these studies have been addressed.

Since the earliest demonstrations of Crain (1956), there have been many experiments showing that the forms of electrical activity recorded in various explants are similar to those observed in vivo. Thus properties of electrogenesis are maintained in the "dish-grown" nervous system whether it is cerebral or cerebellar cortex, brainstem, or spinal cord (Crain and Bornstein, 1964; Crain and Peterson, 1964; Crain, Peterson, and Bornstein, 1968; Leiman and Seil 1973).

The functional concomitants of in vitro growth and differentiation have not been examined in an exhaustive manner, particularly in a way that can be readily related to developmental events such as neurite organization, myelin formation, and synapse elaboration. Crain (1974) has emphasized a similarity in the functional development of diverse tissue cultures, particularly those of spinal cord and cerebral neocortex. He has suggested that the sequence of electrical responsiveness starts with simple "spike" responses, which in the spinal cord seem correlated with the appearance of axodendritic synapses. The maturation of electrical activity with increasing age in vitro includes, according to Crain, a succession of events leading to more tonic barrages of stimulus-elicited activity. Prolonged periods of afterdischarge appear to characterize the most mature cultures. The underlying structural developments have not been examined.

27.3.1 Cerebellar tissue cultures

The functional correlates of anatomical arrangements in cerebellar tissue cultures have been examined in extracellular microelectrode studies (Leiman and Seil, 1973). These cultures have been recorded from at various ages following explantation ranging from 19 to 27 days in vitro. In these explants a high level of spontaneous activity is present just below the cortical surface. The patterns of such activity are displayed in Figure 27.9. This high level of endogenous activity persists across a wide range of temperature, and some investigators of cerebellar tissue cultures have attributed this response to an internal pacemaker as opposed to a synaptically driven system (Schlapfer, Mamoon, and Tobias, 1972; Calvet, 1974).

Activity elicited by dorsal-surface stimulation includes both short and long-latency spike activity restricted to a

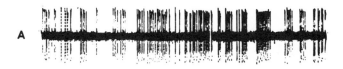
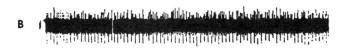

FIGURE 27.9 Spontaneous activity recorded extracellularly from cerebellar cultures, 22 days in vitro. In A, neuronal discharges occur in a burst pattern. In B, recorded from another culture, more regularly occurring discharges are seen. The time base indicator equals 1 sec. From Leiman and Seil (1973). Reproduced with the permission of Academic Press, Inc.

rather limited cortical sector. A marked sensitivity of stimulus-elicited firing to repetition rate is particularly evident. Figure 27.10 displays a marked diminution over successive responses whenever stimuli are repeated at a rate of one every two seconds. This phenomenon has been commonly noted in studies of intact immature cortex (Purpura and Shofer, 1972), although in tissue cultures this may also be a reflection of afferent deprivation.

27.3.2 Cerebral neocortex tissue cultures

Tissue cultures of cerebral neocortex exhibit electrical properties which are dissimilar from those displayed by cerebellar cultures. Endogenous activity is much less evident in our neurophysiological observations of cerebral neocortex cultures ranging in age from 1 to 33 days in vitro (Leiman, Seil, and Kelly, 1975). Activity elicited

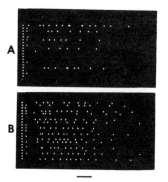

FIGURE 27.10 Extracellular responses elicited by cortical-surface stimulation in a cerebellar culture, 20 days in vitro, displayed as dots. The initial dot in each horizontal row marks the stimulus artifact, and succeeding dots indicate responses. This figure demonstrates the effects of stimulus repetition rate. In A, the stimulus was presented once every 2 sec; in B, once every 10 sec. An attenuation of responsiveness is evident at the faster rate. The time base marker equals 50 msec. From Leiman and Seil (1973). Reproduced with the permission of Academic Press, Inc.

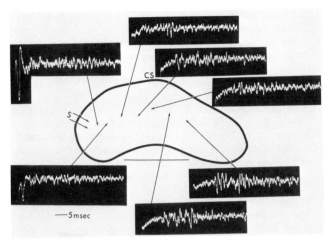

FIGURE 27.11 Spatial distribution of extracellularly recorded activity evoked by stimulation near the cortical surface (CS) in a cerebral neocortex culture, 19 days in vitro. Wide propagation of stimulus-elicited activity is evident. Small-amplitude spike responses and large-amplitude positive-negative wave sequences are illustrated. The outline of the explant is indicated. The site of the stimulating electrodes (S) is designated by two arrows, while the other arrows indicate the location of the varying responses. The bar adjacent to the ventral surface of the culture represents 1 mm. The given time base applies to all responses.

by cortical-surface stimulation is widely propagated (Figure 27.11) and not restricted, as it is in cerebellar explants.

Various forms of stimulus-provoked activity have been evident in cultures of cerebral neocortex. Crain and Bornstein (1964) observed "complex bioelectric responses" which consisted of large-amplitude slow-wave activity frequently characterized by a prolonged oscillatory afterdischarge. Long-duration activity, which is sensitive to repetition rate, can also be observed (Figure 27.12). Detailed topographic analysis of these cultures

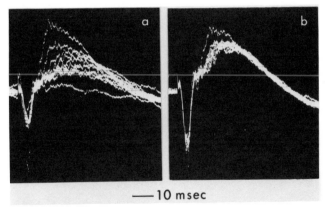

FIGURE 27.12 Stimulus-repetition-rate effects in a cerebral neocortex culture, 20 days in vitro. In a, the stimulus was presented once per sec; in b, once every 10 sec. Decremental responsiveness of slow-wave activity is evident at the more rapid rate.

suggests that many characteristics of evoked activity are closely related to the dendritic fields of pyramidal cells, although phase reversal of these responses with increasing depth of recording occurs infrequently in our observations (Leiman, Seil, and Kelly, 1975).

These electrophysiological studies demonstrate that differing functional characteristics of two levels of the CNS are retained in vitro. Thus functional as well as structural signatures of particular CNS regions may be preserved in tissue-culture systems.

27.4 RELATIONSHIP OF TISSUE CULTURE TO PROBLEMS OF LEARNING AND MEMORY

What is the potential relevance of tissue-culture studies to inquiries about the biology of learning and memory? An obvious answer is usually posed in the form of the simplicity of this system in comparison with the in vivo state. Fewer nerve cells, relieved of a wide variety of customary neural and humoral influences, should provide a more stable and, almost by definition, a less complex organization. The consideration of simplification per se does not complete the rationale for the exploitation of in vitro systems in experimental efforts related to the phenomena of learning and memory. From our vantage point, tissue culture provides a useful system in which to explore the relations of characteristic intrinsic forms of neural organization to learning and memory. Consider the possibility that a mammalian brain includes a variety of learning or memory devices, each represented structurally by a distinctive circuitry arrangement of some small assembly of elements. From this perspective information storage (e.g., by a cerebellar cortical organization) may embody a rule for storage that is discriminably different from rules posed by other forms of neural arrangements. The techniques of cell and tissue culture provide unique opportunities for examining the learning and memory capabilities of prototypic neural arrangements disengaged from the complexity of modulating influences encountered in vivo.

REFERENCES

CALVET, M. C. 1974. Patterns of spontaneous electrical activity in tissue cultures of mammalian cerebral cortex vs. cerebellum. *Brain Research* 69: 281–295.

CRAGG, B. G. 1972. Plasticity of synapses. In G. H. Bourne, ed., *The Structure and Function of Nervous Tissue*, Vol. 4. New York: Academic Press, pp. 1–60.

CRAIN, S. M. 1956. Resting and action potentials of cultured chick embryo spinal ganglion cells. *Journal of Comparative Neurology* 104: 285–330.

CRAIN, S. M. 1974. Tissue culture models of developing brain functions. In G. Gottlieb, ed., *Studies on the Development and Behavior of the Nervous System*. Vol. 2: *Aspects of Neurogenesis*. New York: Academic Press, pp. 69–114.

CRAIN, S. M., and BORNSTEIN, M. B. 1964. Bioelectric activity of neonatal mouse cerebral cortex during growth and differentiation in tissue culture. *Experimental Neurology* 10: 425–450.

CRAIN, S. M., and PETERSON, E. R. 1964. Complex bioelectric activity in organized tissue cultures of spinal cord (human, rat and chick). *Journal of Cellular and Comparative Physiology* 64: 1–15.

CRAIN S. M., PETERSON, E. R., and BORNSTEIN, M. B. 1968. Formation of functional interneuronal connections between explants of various mammalian central nervous tissues during development *in vitro*. In G. E. W. Wolstenholme and M. O'Connor, eds., *Ciba Foundation Symposium: Growth of the Nervous System*. Boston: Little, Brown, pp. 13–31.

EAYRS, J. T., and GOODHEAD, B. 1959. Postnatal development of the cerebral cortex in the rat. *Journal of Anatomy* 93: 385–402.

KANDEL, E. R., and SPENCER, W. A. 1968. Cellular neurophysiological approaches in the study of learning. *Physiological Review* 48: 65–134.

KIM, S. U. 1972. Light and electron microscopic study of mouse cerebral neocortex in tissue culture. *Experimental Neurology* 35: 305–321.

KOBAYASHI, T., INMAN, O. R., BUNO, W., and HIMWICH, H. E. 1964. Neurohistological studies of developing mouse brain. In W. A. Himwich and H. E. Himwich, eds., *Progress in Brain Research*, Vol. 9. Amsterdam: Elsevier, pp. 87–88.

KRIEG, W. J. S. 1946. Connections of the cerebral cortex. I. The albino rat. B. Structure of the cortical areas. *Journal of Comparative Neurology* 84: 277–324.

LaVAIL, J. H., and WOLF, M. K 1973. Postnatal development of the mouse dentate gyrus in organotypic cultures of hippocampal formation. *American Journal of Anatomy* 137: 47–66.

LEIMAN, A. L., and CHRISTIAN, C. N. 1973. Electrophysiological analyses of learning and memory. In J. A. Deutsch, ed., *The Physiological Basis of Memory*. New York: Academic Press, pp. 125–173.

LEIMAN, A. L., and SEIL, F. J. 1973. Spontaneous and evoked bioelectric activity in organized cerebellar tissue cultures. *Experimental Neurology* 40: 748–758.

LEIMAN, A. L., SEIL, F. J., and KELLY, J. M. 1975. Maturation of electrical activity of cerebral neocortex in tissue culture. *Experimental Neurology* 48:275–291.

MELLER, K., BREIPOHL, W., and GLEES, P. 1968. Synaptic organization of the molecular and the outer granular layer in the motor cortex in the white mouse during postnatal development. A Golgi and electron microscopic study. *Zeitschrift für Zellforschung und Mikroskopische Anatomie* 92: 217–231.

MELLER, K., and GLEES, P. 1969. The development of the mouse cerebellum. A Golgi and electron microscopic study. In R. Llinás, ed., *Neurobiology of Cerebellar Evolution and Development. Proceedings of the First International Symposium of the Institute for Biomedical Research*. Chicago: American Medical Association, pp. 783–801.

MIALE, I. L., and SIDMAN, R. L. 1961. An autoradiographic analysis of histogenesis in the mouse cerebellum. *Experimental Neurology* 4: 277–296.

MURRAY, M. R. 1965. Nervous tissues *in vitro*. In E. N. Willmer, ed., *Cells and Tissues in Culture*, Vol 2. New York: Academic Press, pp. 373–455.

MURRAY, M. R. 1971. Nervous tissues isolated in culture. In A. Lajtha, ed., *Handbook of Neurochemistry*, Vol. 5. New York: Plenum Press, pp. 373–438.

PURPURA, D. P., and SHOFER, R. A. 1972. Principles of synaptogenesis and their application to ontogenetic studies of mammalian cerebral cortex. In C. D. Clemente, D. P. Purpura, and F. E. Mayer, eds., *Sleep and the Maturing Nervous System*. New York: Academic Press, pp. 3–22.

RAMÓN y CAJAL, S. 1960. *Studies on Vertebrate Neurogenesis*. Translated by L. Guth. Springfield: Charles C Thomas.

SCHEIBEL, M. E., DAVIES, T. L., LINDSAY, R. D., and SCHEIBEL, A. B. 1974. Basilar dendritic bundles of giant pyramidal cells. *Experimental Neurology* 42: 307–319.

SCHLAPFER, W. T., MAMOON, A. M., and TOBIAS, C. A. 1972. Spontaneous bioelectric activity of neurons in cerebellar cultures: Evidence for synaptic interactions. *Brain Research* 45: 345–364.

SEIL, F. J. 1972. Neuronal groups and fiber patterns in cerebellar tissue cultures. *Brain Research* 42: 33–51.

SEIL, F. J., and HERNDON, R. M. 1970. Cerebellar granule cells *in vitro*. A light and electron microscopic study. *Journal of Cell Biology* 45: 212–220.

SEIL, F. J., KELLY, J. M., and LEIMAN, A. L. 1974. Antomical organization of cerebral neocortex in tissue culture. *Experimental Neurology* 45: 435–450.

SOBKOWICZ, H. M., GUILLERY, R. W., and BORNSTEIN, M. B. 1968. Neuronal organization in long term cultures of the spinal cord of the fetal mouse. *Journal of Comparative Neurology* 132: 365–395.

WOLF, M. K. 1970. Anatomy of cultured mouse cerebellum. II. Organtypic migration of granule cells demonstrated by silver impregnation of normal and mutant cultures. *Journal of Comparative Neurology* 140: 281–297.

WOLF, M. K., and DUBOIS-DALCQ, M. 1970. Anatomy of cultured mouse cerebellum. I. Golgi and electron microscopic demonstration of granule cells, their afferent and efferent synapses. *Journal of Comparative Neurology* 140: 261–280.

Plasticity in Invertebrates

28

Invertebrate Systems as a Means of Gaining Insight into the Nature of Learning and Memory

FRANKLIN B. KRASNE

ABSTRACT Many invertebrates are capable of good learning and memory in appropriate situations. Some invertebrates also have neural subsystems with special features which make them particularly amenable to physiological analysis. In a few cases very simple kinds of short-term learning have been found to be mediated by such analyzable subsystems, and there is reason to believe that more complex and more permanent learning will also soon be found.

So far, however, *detailed* analyses have been possible only for short-term, nonassociative learning processes, such as habituation. Data on these simple processes indicate that they are due to intrinsic changes of transmission efficacy at specific, specially designed synapses, that the changes are on the presynaptic side of those synapses, and that the development, expression, and retention of the changes can be controlled by other parts of the nervous system. Reasons are given for believing that long-term learning will soon be subjected to similar analyses and for suspecting that for any given kind of learning, short- and long-term changes may be very similar in nature while different *kinds* of learning may have different physiological bases at the cellular level.

28.1 INVERTEBRATES DO LEARN

The purpose of this review is to argue for and illustrate the usefulness of certain invertebrate animals for gaining insight into the physiological mechanisms of learning phenomena.

Long-term, associative-learning abilities are by no means a monopoly of the vertebrates. The lowliest invertebrates in which associative learning has been unequivocally demonstrated are the planarian flatworms. In the best experiments available (Jacobson, Fried, and Horowitz, 1967) subjects were presented with a random schedule of mild visual and vibratory stimuli, one or the other of which was consistently followed by an electrical shock that caused an unconditioned contraction response. When tested during experimental extinction, the animals reacted by contracting to the stimulus that preceded shock during training but not to the one that did not (Table 28.1). Such clear-cut experimental demonstrations on platyhelminths, annelids, and noncephalopod molluscs are relatively few and far between,

FRANKLIN. B. KRASNE, Department of Psychology, University of California, Los Angeles

perhaps as much because of deficiencies in experimental design as because of the tenuousness of the animals' learning abilities. However, by the time one comes to the arthropods, which in fact provide some of the most promising nervous systems for analytic attack, a capacity for associative learning not only becomes readily demonstrable, but in some cases is well known to play a clear and useful role in the animals' day-to-day lives. Members of this phylum utilize their learning abilities to aid in activities such as foraging, homing, and the establishment of stable dominance orders in much the same way that mammals do (see Krasne, 1973; a thorough three-volume review of invertebrate learning has recently been edited by Corning, Dyal, and Willows, 1973). Furthermore, mastery of traditional maze-learning and instrumental-discrimination tasks has been demonstrated many times. For example, if shrimps (*Leander*) or hermit crabs (*Pagurus striatus*) are repeatedly allowed to

TABLE 28.1
Number of responses to light and vibration during an extinction test series for a light-positive group and a vibration-positive group of flatworms*

Subject	Vibration	Light	Subject	Light	Vibration
V1	8	0	L1	7	2
V2	8	1	L2	6	2
V3	8	2	L3	6	4
V4	5	0	L4	5	3
V5	4	0	L5	4	2
V6	4	0	L6	3	1
V7	4	1	L7	5	4
V8	3	0	L8	4	3
V9	5	3	L9	4	3
V10	4	2	L10	3	2
V11	3	1	L11	4	4
V12	6	5	L12	1	1
V13	2	1	L13	5	6
V14	3	3	L14	5	6

*The extinction series consisted of 30 trials in a prearranged sequence of 15 presentations of vibration and 15 of light.
Source: Jacobson, Fried, and Horowitz (1967).

find food on a hook within a cylinder of one color, while a similar hook in a cylinder of a different color is never baited, they will, after about a week of training, enter a cylinder similar to the one in which they have found food to search for food, while the cylinder of the other color will not attract them (Mikhailoff, 1923). They do this even though the actual cylinders used in the tests have never been touched by food. Extinction in this case requires about a week of unreinforced training trials, indicating that memory is apparently quite stable. Honeybees learn such simple discriminations within a few trials and show no signs of forgetting over a fortnight (Figure 28.1), but once experimental extinction is instituted, they extinguish rapidly, showing some spontaneous recovery on the next day in much the same way that a rat would. Bees even learn conditional discriminations of the form "turn left when presented with a green signal and right with a blue one" (see Wells, 1973).

Effects which in mammals are sometimes thought to be mediated by internal, self-produced cues or to be signs of "higher mental processes" have also been reported on occasion. Thus slower extinction after partial (intermittent) reinforcement has been reported in earthworms (Wyers, Peeke, and Herz, 1964), while higher-order, Pavlovian conditioning appears to have been demonstrated in hermit crabs (Mikhailoff, 1923).

These examples of associative learning in invertebrates are offered to demonstrate that these "lowly" animals possess the neurological machinery required for the sort of learning that most challenges our understanding, and hence to indicate that they in principle have the potential for disclosing the mechanisms of that sort of learning.

However, I believe that it is useful and proper to *define* learning, more inclusively, as *any* fairly persistent change in behavioral attributes produced by the action of experi-

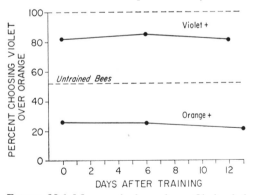

FIGURE 28.1 Memory in honeybees. Choice behavior of bees that have been given three opportunities to find food either on a violet plaque but not an orange one (upper curve), or conversely (lower curve), on day zero. After this training separate batches of bees were tested at various times for memory. Data from Menzel (1968).

ence on the central nervous system. Transient, "permanent," nonassociative, and associative behavioral changes are all encompassed by this definition; and specifically, sensitization and habituation phenomena as well as classical and instrumental conditioning are included. Also included are "hidden" learning phenomena, such as optokinetic memory (Horridge, 1968; York, Wiersma, and Yanagisawa, 1972; York, Yanagisawa, and Wiersma, 1972; see also Krasne, 1973), which are integral parts of some complex perceptual and motor achievements but do not fit into any of the usual paradigms of experimental psychology.

We shall turn below to attempts to take advantage of certain special features of invertebrate nervous systems to ease the difficult task of understanding how nervous systems produce learned behavioral change. As partially successful analyses are described, it will become apparent that whereas it would obviously be inadvisable to try using an animal that is not known to be capable of learning for such an analysis, the mere discovery of an invertebrate that is a facile learner in some domain in no way guarantees that a successful analytical attack on the learning phenomenon can be mounted. The strict requirement for progress, as will become clear below, is that the neural circuitry mediating the modifiable response be understandable in terms of individual neurons and their interconnections. And while this is a very stringent requirement, it is by no means a hopeless one in dealing with invertebrate behavior patterns.

28.2 CURRENTLY PROMISING PREPARATIONS

28.2.1 First attempts at defining neural correlates of invertebrate learning

Published attempts to use well-circumscribed invertebrate reflexes for the purpose of localizing and isolating neuronal entities that change during learning are largely of quite recent origin. The first explicit attempts of which I am aware were carried out by Adrian Horridge on the giant-fiber withdrawal reflexes of annelid worms. When well-rested individuals of many annelid species are disturbed by tactile, vibratory, or visual stimuli, they execute rapid shortening responses which tend to get them promptly away from the immediate point of stimulation. Such reflexes are almost always mediated in part by nerve cells whose axons are much larger than any other elements of the animals' nervous systems, and this of course makes them very convenient for physiological analysis. Their potential interest to students of behavior was introduced in the following way by Horridge: "A superficial examination . . . of . . . startle reflex responses . . . at once shows that the animal rapidly habituates to stimulation . . . . However, not only is the site of this habituation unknown, but the whole pathway of transmission of excitation from sensory cells via internuncial neurons to motor neurons and finally to muscle fibers is unexplored" (Horridge, 1959, p. 246).

Horridge proceeded to utilize the accessibility of the giant neurons, whose spike activity stands out boldly from all other nerve-cord activity and whose thresholds for direct electrical stimulation are lower than those of any other axons, to determine that the habituation in the species he studied occurred primarily between afferents and giant fibers, while transmission between giants and motoneurons was a relatively reliable process.

28.2.2 A catalogue of presently available preparations

Since Horridge's work, though not necessarily flowing from it, a number of investigators have attempted to elucidate neuron circuitry while searching for long-lasting behavioral modifications of various invertebrate behavior patterns. The result has been the development of about a dozen preparations which either have begun to yield insights into the nature of some simple learning phenomena or seem very likely to do so soon. These are listed as Table 28.2 along with brief characterizations of the types of learning so far discovered and the present status of efforts toward complete circuit analysis.

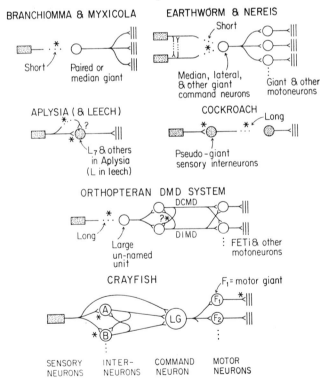

FIGURE 28.2 Circuit diagrams for some invertebrate escape reflexes. The reflexes and relevant references are specified in Table 28.2. Asterisks indicate labile synapses. Stippling indicates that a *population* of (parallel) neurons is involved.

It will be noticed that most of the response patterns listed in this table are evasive responses of some kind. There are good reasons why this is so. Escape behavior, which in large measure evolved to thwart capture by predators, is under powerful selection pressures for rapidity. As a result, many of the neurons that compose the escape-reflex circuitry have expanded to great size in order to speed rates of signal propagation, while the number of synapses in series between receptors and muscles has presumably been kept at the absolute minimum consistent with adequately integrated performance. The resultant circuitry, which is comprised of neurons with many large processes and has minimal organizational complexity, is ideal for physiological analysis.

Figure 28.2 illustrates schematically the neuronal circuits of a number of the escape reflexes of Table 28.2. The crayfish reflex shown at the bottom of the figure is one of the best worked out of these pathways and one to which we shall have frequent reference here. Working backward from the efferent side, the many motoneurons that are involved in the escape maneuver, which is a powerful flexion of the abdominal musculature, are all fed by a single interconnected pair of command elements (one on each side of the body), the lateral giant fibers (LGs). These command neurons in turn receive input from tactile receptors of the animal's abdomen, both monosynaptically and via a set of first-order interneurons, a number of which have been identified. The interneurons also tend to reinforce one another in excitatory fashion. Only the disynaptic pathway is effective enough to fire the lateral giants and so produce behavior. An indication of the physical appearance of some of the elements in this schematic diagram and some typical intracellular responses produced in the command neuron by afferent stimulation are shown in Figure 28.3.

Despite natural selection for simplicity, plasticity—the feature of our particular interest—has not been bred out of these reflexes. Escape must be rapid, but it is also highly adaptive for it to be subject to some measure of control by the past. The escape responses are generally such that they interfere massively with other ongoing activities and are metabolically expensive. Furthermore, the nature of the stimuli to which it is worthwhile reacting can change drastically from time to time and from microenvironment to microenvironment. The effects of the selection pressure thus produced are evident in several forms of plasticity among the escape reflexes.

Habituation to recurrent startling, but basically innocuous, stimuli is a feature of virtually all known escape reflexes and is well represented in Table 28.2. Figure 28.4 illustrates typical effects. In each of these cases the repetition of mild stimuli leads to a relatively rapid

TABLE 28.2
Catalogue of important preparations

Preparation	Description of relevant behavior	Retention*	Status of circuit analysis**	References***
Sabellid withdrawal reflex	*Habituation* of rapid withdrawal into tube in response to visual, tactile, or vibratory stimuli.	Moderate (or long?)	Partial	Nichol (1950, 1951) Roberts (1962a, b) Krasne (1965)
Nereid withdrawal reflex	*Habituation* of rapid withdrawal into burrow in response to visual, tactile, or vibratory stimuli.	Short	Partial	Horridge (1959, 1963) Clark (1960a, b) Evans (1966, 1969)
	Sensitization of rapid withdrawal into burrow. Visual stimuli become more effective in eliciting reaction when electric shocks and visual stimuli are presented randomly.	Short		
Earthworm withdrawal reflex	*Habituation* of rapid withdrawal into burrow in response to visual, tactile, or vibratory stimuli.	Short and long	Partial	Bullock (1945) Rushton (1946) Kuenzer (1958) Roberts (1962a, b, 1966) Gunther (1971, 1972) Gunther and Walther (1971)
Leech segmental shortening reactions	*Stimulation* of identified sensory neurons causes primarily segmental shortening reaction. As yet no studies of behavioral learning phenomena, but the preparation is very promising, and positive results of some kind seem likely.		Pathway closed	Nichols and Purves (1970) Stuart (1970)
Aplysia gill- and siphon-retraction reflex	*Habituation* of gill (and siphon) retraction to tactile stimulation of the siphon.	Short and long	Pathway closed	Kupfermann et al. (1969). Castellucci et al. (1970) Kupfermann et al. (1970) Pinsker et al. (1970) Carew, Pinsker, and Kandel (1972) Carew and Kandel (1973) Kandel (1973) Pinsker et al. (1973)
	Sensitization of siphon (and presumably gill) retraction to weak tactile stimulation of the siphon as a result of traumatic stimulation in the experimental situation.	Short and long		
Pleurobranchaea feeding and defensive reflexes	*Conditioned*† feeding response. If tactile stimulus which by itself would evoke withdrawal is repeatedly presented simultaneously with food, it will come to evoke feeding movements rather than withdrawal. Tactile stimuli repeatedly presented alone continue to evoke defense.	Long	Partial	Mpitsos and Davis (1973) Davis (this volume)
	Conditioned defensive response. Shocking animals trained as above when they give feeding responses to tactile stimuli causes return of defensive behavior. Controls given touch and yoked shocks continue to make feeding reaction.	Long		

TABLE 28.2 (*Continued*)

Preparation	Description of relevant behavior	Retention*	Status of circuit analysis**	References***
Tritonia escape swimming	*Habituation* of duration of swimming escape from model of natural predator. *Sensitization* of swimming response. Random or paired presentation of neutral S and UCS for swimming slightly raises probability of swimming response to neutral stimulus.	Moderate Moderate to long	Partial	Willows and Hoyle (1969) Abraham and Willows (1972) Dorsett, Willows, and Hoyle (1973) Willows (1973) Willows, Dorsett, and Hoyle (1973a,c)
Crayfish "lateral-giant" escape reflex	*Habituation* of tail-flip response to phasic tactile stimulation of abdomen.	Short and long	Pathway closed	Krasne (1969) Krasne and Woodsmall (1969) Wine and Krasne (1969) Zucker (1972)
Orthopteran descending movement-detector system	*Habituation* of excitatory input to jump motor neurons in response to small, dark moving objects in the visual field.	Short to moderate	Partial	Horn and Rowell (1968) Rowell (1971a–c) Burrows and Rowell (1973) O'Shea, Rowell, and Williams (1974) Rowell (this volume)
Cockroach evasion response	*Habituation* of forward running in response to stimulation of anal circi by air puffs.	Short to moderate	Rudimentary	Roeder (1948) Hughes (1965) Dagan and Parnas (1970) Zilber-Gachelin and Chartier (1973a,b)
Cockroach "antennal" cleaning response	*Learned change* (type not characterized) in posture permitting cleaning of antennae with one mesothoracic leg and mouthparts after removal of prothoracic legs.	Long	Rudimentary	Luco and Aranda (1964a, b, 1966) Aranda and Luco (1969)
Cockroach and locust "leg-lift" response	Instrumentally learned alteration of leg position to avoid electrical shock.	Long	Rudimentary	Horridge (1962) Eisenstein and Cohen (1965) Hoyle (1965) Eisenstein (1971) Burrows and Hoyle (1973) Hoyle (1973) Hoyle and Burrows (1973 a, b)

*Short: recovery in less than one hour. Moderate: recovery in 1–24 hr. Long: recovery substantially incomplete over days and possibly asymptotic at incomplete levels.

**Complete: all neurons of full excitatory pathway identified. Pathway closed: representatives of all classes of neurons in an effective conduction pathway between sensory and motor neurons identified. Partial: major segments of pathway closed. Rudimentary: some important elements have been identified.

***To save space these references have not been made exhaustive, but consultation of the papers cited will allow the construction of comprehensive bibliographies.

†Because sensitization controls in this experiment did not receive the same temporal pattern of UCS application as experimentals, there remains a possibility that long-term sensitization occurred rather than associative conditioning.

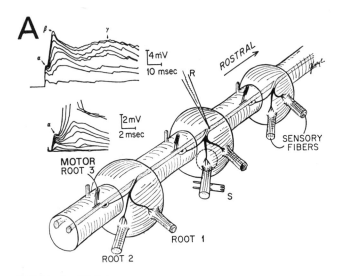

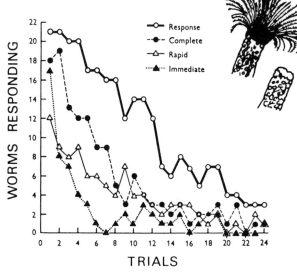

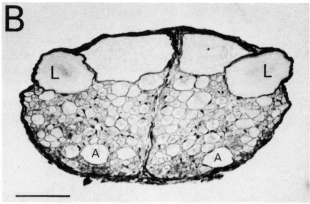

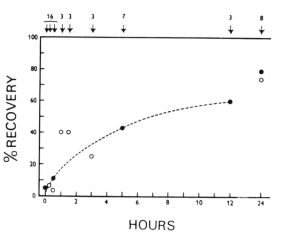

FIGURE 28.3 The LG escape-reflex system of the crayfish. A. *Lower right:* A schematic diagram of the middle portion of crayfish abdominal nerve cord to show the general organization of the reflex. The lateral giants are stippled; only that of the right side is shown in its entirety. The lateral giants are in fact a chain of neurons interconnected by unpolarized, reliable, electrical synapses. *Upper left:* Intracellular recordings from a lateral giant during shocks to a sensory root in two preparations (typical positions of stimulating and recording electrodes are shown below). Traces for a series of stimulus intensities are superimposed. Alpha and beta are the excitatory postsynaptic potentials produced by the monosynaptic and disynaptic pathways (Figure 28.2), respectively. From Krasne (1973). B. Transverse section through a connective between abdominal ganglia. Lateral giants (L) and interneuron A are labeled. Scale: 100 μm.

FIGURE 28.4(a) Habituation of moderate duration in *Branchiomma. Top:* The number of worms withdrawing into their tubes in response to successive brushings of the branchial crown at approximately 50-sec intervals. *Bottom:* Recovery of responses after failure. The number of responses made before the occurrence of 3 failures to respond was measured when each worm was fresh and again after a recovery period. The ratio of the two measurements (× 100) is the definition of percentage recovery. The numbers of worms tested are noted at the top of the graph. From Krasne (1965).

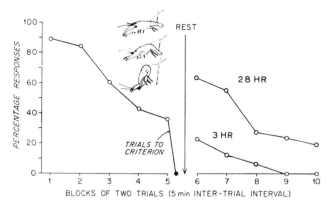

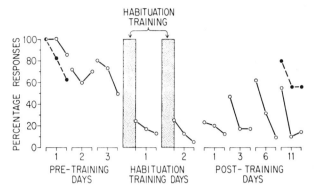

FIGURE 28.4(b) Habituation of moderate duration in the crayfish. *Left:* Mean percentage of trials on which tail flips (and also LG action potentials) occurred in rested animals in response to just-suprathreshold taps to the side of the abdomen. Trials to criterion consisted of taps at 1 per min in blocks of 10 separated by 10-min rests until completion of a block without any responses (mean trials to criterion was 20). *Right:* Responses after rests of the stated duration. Data from Wine and Krasne (1969).

FIGURE 28.5 Long-term habituation in crayfish LG reflex. Thirty just-suprathreshold tap stimuli per day were given at random points on the side of the abdomen of free animals at 15-sec intervals; percentage responses are calculated over 10-trial blocks. There is a significant drop of daily responses over the first 3 days of testing ($p < 0.01$, two tails). On the next two days animals were given 5-min bouts of 2 taps per sec at random all over the abdomen at 2, 4, and 6 hr before testing, in order to depress the reflex thoroughly. Subsequent tests given after rests of up to 5 days show an initial recovery (up to day 3 or 6) with little further recovery. Control animals given tests only on the first and last days of the experiment are significantly more responsive than experimental animals on the last day ($p < 0.01$, two tails). Unpublished data.

reduction of response probability. During rest both response probability and the number of trials required to rehabituate the animal to a specified criterion of nonresponsiveness recover over a period of hours: in the experiments illustrated, there was very little recovery during the first two hours, but substantial though not always complete recovery within twenty-four.

It is behavioral effects such as these which have already been pursued in some measure of depth to the physiological level; we shall therefore necessarily be confined to them in much of what follows.

The behaviors mediated by some of these simple escape-reflex pathways, as well as several other behavior patterns entered in Table 28.2, are also subject to long-term changes due to training. Habituation of long duration has been demonstrated in both *Aplysia* and crayfish escape reflexes. Long-term habituation in *Aplysia*, which is discussed extensively in the chapter by Davis, is on the verge of being pursued to the physiological level. [Davis's chapter will emphasize work on gastropod molluscs, while this chapter will emphasize work on arthropods and annelids. These three groups seem at present to hold the greatest promise for physiological analysis.]

The effect in crayfish, which has only recently been discovered, is illustrated in Figure 28.5. In each case retention is measured at least in weeks, but the upper limits have not been accurately probed. Long-lasting *augmentations* of withdrawal-reflex excitability have been produced in *Aplysia* by traumatic stimulation over a number of days, and work in progress indicates that a comparable effect can probably be obtained in the crayfish. Physiological analyses of these long-term effects are

almost certain to yield important insights into the nature of long-term behavioral modifications within the next few years.

Also included in Table 28.2 are several preparations that I believe hold great promise for the physiological analysis of long-term associative processes, but that still require more circuit analysis before they bear fruit. An essential feature of any analytically useful training procedure is that the learned behavior, or neuronal correlates of it, should be obtainable from nervous systems prepared for physiological analysis. This requirement seems to be met by conditioned feeding behavior in *Pleurobranchaea*, and for both shock-avoidance learning and postural learning in the insect preparations of Table 28.2.

Finally, I have included the leech segmental shortening reaction because it seems to provide exceptionally promising, but as yet untapped, material for behavioral study.

28.3 FINDINGS AND THEIR POSSIBLE IMPLICATIONS

Although a reasonable range of behavioral learning phenomena is included within the purview of Table 28.2, serious progress in getting at mechanisms has so far been confined mainly to habituation of short-to-moderate duration. The discoveries that have been made of course tell us a good deal about the mechanisms of this specific behavioral phenomenon, but they also provide some of the first answers that have become available—admittedly tentative and restricted ones—to certain general questions about mechanisms of learning. I shall use a discussion of some of these general concerns to focus and give meaning to my exposition of empirical findings. This will highlight the possible significance of the material, but the reader will have to keep in mind that, for the most part, the learning I am discussing is nonassociative, while the "engrams" I discuss are ones which may last for only a matter of hours.

28.3.1 The relationship between central and behavioral change

Learning, as I have defined it, encompasses many specific behavioral phenomena. These include habituation and sensitization of reflexive or instinctive responses due to stimulus repetition, increases or decreases in rates of emission of spontaneous behaviors and alterations of tonic postures or internal sets due to reward or punishment, development of apparently new stimulus-response relationships due to Pavlovian training procedures or to reward, and so on. I shall be concerned in this chapter with what we know or can guess about the sorts of *functional* changes in neurons that bring about these phenomena. I shall consider only lightly the question of the means nerve cells may use to produce and stabilize such expressed changes, because relatively little useful work has been done on this matter in the invertebrates.

Isomorphism? Neurophysiologists do know of physiological phenomena which, naively viewed, could easily be the basis of at least some of the shorter-term forms of certain learning phenomena. For instance, habituation could easily be due to depression of synapses in the innate reflex arcs that mediate behaviors that can be habituated (which we shall refer to as "habituable"), while sensitization could similarly be due to posttetanic potentiation or long-lasting interneuronal facilitation of those same synapses. That is, the neuronal changes responsible for these behavioral changes might be analogous or *isomorphic* to them in form. The idea that such isomorphism might be a general or very common feature of the neural substrates of behavioral change seems to me to be an implicit hypothesis of many investigators who search for neuronal analogues of this or that type of learning phenomenon (e.g., Bureš and Burešová, 1967; Kandel and Tauc, 1965).

Neuronal phenomena that are truly isomorphic to *associative* learning are largely unknown. Some highly suggestive phenomena have been discovered during mammalian visual-system development, and some fascinating theories have been put forward to explain how the synapses of neuron A on neuron B can be selectively "strengthened" by the contiguous firing of A and B (Stent, 1973; Griffith, 1966; Elul, 1967). But whether neurons really do possess internal mechanisms and lines of intercellular communication that can produce such an effect is as yet uncertain. The search for cellular analogues of behavioral learning phenomena is a worthwhile enterprise, but it is important to recognize that such analogues may not exist, and that even in those cases where analogous neuronal phenomena do exist, they might not actually be used in the way one might presume.

Parsimony? Indeed, it is entirely possible that the nervous system is highly parsimonious in its use of plastic processes and that but a single kind of persistent and input-inducible functional change in nerve cells underlies all types of learning. Logically speaking, a change in virtually any functional property of a neuron, when taken in conjunction with the various well-known properties of neurons, can yield any kind of learning.

To emphasize the point by an unlikely example, synaptic depression—the decrease of synaptic efficacy seen at certain synapses when they are used with more than some critical frequency—could produce not only habituation but also augmentations of behavior, as in sensitization, or specific associations of the sort seen in classical conditioning. One arrangement which would produce classical conditioning is illustrated in Figure 28.6. This scheme may seem absurd because it would require prewired circuits (of the sort provided by neurons

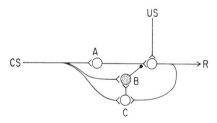

Figure 28.6 Synaptic depression *could* be the basis of classical conditioning. In this hypothetical system CS fires R only after CS and US have been paired. In the "naive" circuit US alone fires R reliably, while CS alone fires A but also fires the inhibitory neuron B which in turn prevents A from releasing enough transmitter to fire R. Neuron C's threshold is such that neither CS alone nor R alone can fire it; however, when US and CS fire *together*, they fire C, which in turn releases a large dose of slowly inactivated transmitter which causes B to fire at high frequency and thereby produces a long-lasting depression of inhibitory-transmitter output from B. Therefore, on subsequent trials B no longer prevents A from firing R; hence, CS now fires R.

A, B, and C in the figure for each association that an animal is capable of learning, but this requirement is not so preposterous as it may seem.

Honeybees efficiently learn associations between some kinds of odors and nectar, while other sorts of smells to which they are sensitive but which are not ordinarily encountered during foraging cannot become learned cues for feeding at all (von Frisch, 1953). Such limitations on learning ability are common in invertebrates and even seem to be present in mammals, in whom it used to be thought that learned associability was entirely arbitrary (Manning, this volume; Garcia and Levine, this volume). Perhaps even aspects of language learning in man are under such constraints (Lennenberg, 1967). Such considerations make it impossible to reject schemes like those of Figure 28.6 out of hand.

SOME DATA. Information on the sorts of neuronal changes that in fact mediate learned behavioral modifications in *any* kind of animal are very scanty.

For many years it was believed, largely on the basis of the behavioral phenomenon of "disinhibition" (Pavlov, 1927; Humphrey, 1930), that habituation is due to augmented inhibition of the excitatory pathways mediating the habituable responses. Some physiological studies supported this belief by the observation that the time course of spinally mediated habituation in cats is similar to that of posttetanic potentiation in the spinal cord, and it was thus suggested that the habituation was due to posttetanic potentiation of inhibitory pathways that play upon the habituable reflexes (Wickelgren, 1967a,b). However, when the crayfish and *Aplysia* withdrawal-reflex preparations made it possible to study habituation more critically, it became clear that, as had been suggested by some previous investigators (particularly Spencer, Thompson, and Neilson, 1966), habituation—at least in presently analyzable cases—is due to an intrinsic decline of the excitatory events that mediate habituating responses (see Section 28.3.3). Thus the neuronal events responsible for habituation seem to be analogous or isomorphic to the habituation itself.

Long-term sensitization has been demonstrated in *Aylysia*, a preparation that seems ready for analysis but has not yet been subjected to that analysis. Transient sensitization produced by single applications of stimuli similar to those that, when repeated over days, lead to long-term effects, has been analyzed and found probably to result from augmentations of transmitter release at excitatory synapses in the escape-reflex arc produced by activity in a presynaptic facilitative pathway (Castellucci et al., 1970; Carew, Castellucci, and Kandel, 1971). Once initiated, this augmentation may persist for some

minutes, but the cause of the persistence is as yet unknown, as is the entire basis of the long-term effects.

Ironically, posttetanic potentiation, which is one of the most intensively studied forms of synaptic plasticity, has not been definitively shown to be involved in any sort of learning phenomenon. However, there is suggestive evidence that it might be. When cockroaches are deprived of their forelegs, they "learn" over a period of some days to support their weight on the legs that remain. Until this postural readjustment is well advanced, the animals cannot use a middle leg to bring their antennae to their mouths for cleaning without toppling over, and this provides a useful test for the postural readjustment. Correlated with the development of a sufficient degree of readjustment to pass this test is a presumably intrinsic augmentation of probably monosynaptic excitatory transmission between certain unidentified interneurons descending from rostral ganglia and unidentified motoneurons to the hind legs (Figure 28.7). Since a very similar augmentation can be produced by tetanization of the presynaptic pathway of naive animals, Luco and Aranda (1964b) believe that the effect produced during the "learning" is probably also a result of repeated use. However, whereas the posttetanic potentiation that is produced acutely dissipates relatively rapidly, that produced by "training" seems to last for at least 20 days: even 20 days after an animal's forelegs have been allowed to grow back, the synaptic alteration persists to some degree, as does a savings in relearning the postural shift (Figure 28.7; Luco and Aranda, 1966). These data are clearly very suggestive. However, there is no actual evidence that the augmentation is intrinsic to the descending-interneuron/motoneuron synapses. Nor has it really been shown that "learning" did not induce a cerebrally directed postural change that maintained bombardment of the test synapse during the 20 days that the animal supposedly went without practice or reinforcement.

A variety of physiological studies have provided evidence that the endogenous spontaneous firing rates of some neurons can be altered for periods of minutes or hours by synaptic input (e.g., Parnas, Armstrong, and Strumwasser, 1974; Parnas and Strumwasser, 1974; see also Davis, this volume), but again there is as yet no clear-cut evidence that such a phenomenon is ever involved in learning. There is evidence, however, which may be considered suggestive, that such a change could be involved in a form of operant conditioning. If a cockroach, locust, or crab is shocked whenever it extends a particular leg, that leg will become tonically flexed (Table 28.2; see Krasne, 1973). Instead of training an animal behaviorally, reinforcement contingencies

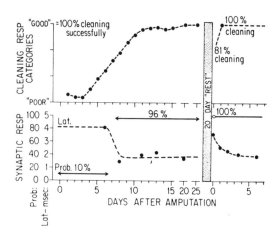

FIGURE 28.7 Successful antennal cleaning and successful synaptic transmission in the cockroach. *Upper*: The ability to clean the antennae without toppling over improves over some 5–10 days after amputation of forelegs in naive animals. After perfection of the response, forelegs were allowed to regenerate, and the animals were allowed 20 days with fully operative forelegs. When the legs were then reamputated, ability to clean without toppling over reappeared very rapidly. *Lower*: Probability and latency of transmission between an unidentified interneuron that descends from the brain and unidentified motoneurons to the hind legs. After amputation, efficient transmission becomes established after some 5–10 days. Over a 20-day rest transmission remains more efficient than in naive animals and returns to prerest levels within a few days of reamputation. Based on Luco and Aranda (1964b, 1966).

can be based directly upon selected motoneuron firing rates, which can thereby be arbitrarily raised or lowered (Hoyle, 1965, 1973). The slow anterior coxal adductor motoneuron (ACAd) of the locust has been especially studied in this regard. Intracellular analyses of the ACAd suggest that its firing rate is endogenously controlled; synaptic input can transiently alter the rate, but the rate seems to depend primarily on properties of the neuron itself, at least in the untrained preparation (Hoyle, 1973). This has led Hoyle to speculate that the changes of rate that can be produced in this neuron by training may be due to intrinsic alterations of the "trained" neuron's intrinsic rate of spontaneous firing. This is a fascinating possibility, but it must be emphasized that it is still in the realm of conjecture.

Most of the above is highly inconclusive. However, it is probably sufficient to motivate the hypothesis that all forms of behavioral change are not due to a single form of neuronal change. Moreover, the notion that there might be close parallels between behavioral changes and the neuronal changes that cause them remains viable.

However, Rescorla (personal communication) has pointed out that as a general rule isomorphism *cannot* be valid because of the arbitrariness with which responses

can be defined. For example, in a case where habituation of a response R is known to be due to synaptic depression, we might define a new response, not-R, which, operationally, would become *facilitated* because of (the same) depression. It seems to me that in many real situations where one is dealing with gross responses that occur against a behavioral background of relative quiescence, Rescorla's point becomes largely a logical quibble. However, it must be admitted that the fact that nervous systems are constructed in such a way that incompatible responses inhibit one another probably does (or will soon) lead to the invalidation of the isomorphism hypothesis as a completely general rule. For example, the same stimuli that elicit LG tail-flip behavior in crayfish can also evoke a backward thrust of the legs against the substrate that propels the animal rapidly forward. This ambulatory response, which is presumably inhibited by LG firing, replaces tail flips during the course of habituation (until it too habituates). We may quite properly say, therefore, that stimulus repetition leads to the *facilitation* of the ambulatory response as a result of the *depression* of synapses in an inhibitory pathway. If verified, this would seem to be a clear violation of the isomorphism principle.

28.3.2 Loci of change

The elucidation of nerve circuits that mediate modifiable responses and the location within those circuits of the points where transmission characteristics or spontaneity change so as to produce learned alterations of behavior are of course crucial intermediate steps in the search for the engram. Beyond this, however, they may also provide useful information in their own right.

We wish to know whether changes in transmission characteristics are distributed widely throughout plastic stimulus-response pathways or are confined to specific, specialized switch points. We need hard evidence to evaluate the old conception that the circuits for sensory analysis and motor elaboration are hard-wired and that learning occurs in the layer of association neurons interposed between these stable sensory and motor analyzers. We must discover whether learned behavioral change can occur in simple monosynaptic systems, or whether properties of polysynaptic pathways, such as repetitive interneuron firing, afterdischarge, or multiple foci of change, are crucial in establishing or maintaining altered firing characteristics. Elucidation of the circuitry of modifiable behavior patterns will lead rapidly to answers to such questions.

Habituation learning has yielded to circuit analysis before other forms of learning. This is because the mediating pathways are inborn, well defined, relatively stable, and not easily traumatized. The pathways of associatively learned reactions, by contrast, are not identifiable and may not even exist as localized pathways until learning has occurred. Furthermore, such pathways may fail to function in animals prepared for physiological analysis.

We may use the crayfish LG escape reflex to illustrate the analysis of habituable reflex pathways. It was known at the outset from work of Wiersma (1947) and Takeda and Kennedy (1964) that the motoneurons for the tail-flip response are fed by the LG command neurons (Figure 28.2). It was also known that the neuromuscular synapses between some of the motoneurons and the tail-flip muscles are extremely prone to depression, while the remainder are quite stable or actually tend to facilitate during repetitive activation (Takeda and Kennedy, 1964). Behavioral observations of responses to repetitive stimulation showed that while there is some waning in the vigor of responses during habituation, presumably ascribable in part to the depression-prone neuromuscular junctions, habituation is due to precipitous total failure to respond, not to a gradual reduction of response intensity to zero. This seemed to imply failure of command-neuron firing. Physiological experiments at once showed that saltatory failures of response are not seen when LGs are excited repetitively by direct shocks, and recordings from nerve cords of chronically prepared animals during habituation showed that the transmission failure responsible for habituation is indeed antecedent to the lateral giants (Figure 28.4; Krasne and Woodsmall, 1969; Wine and Krasne, 1969).

Intracellular recording from the lateral giants in acute

preparations then disclosed that sensory volleys reach them over both a monosynaptic (or alpha) route and a polysynaptic (or beta) route whose latency indicated that it is probably disynaptic (see Figure 28.3). Only the presumptive disynaptic route showed lability during stimulus repetition. The monosynaptic pathway was quite stable, but by itself never made a large enough contribution to fire the lateral giants (Figure 28.8). Details of the way in which failure occurs in the presumptive disynaptic pathway suggested that the failure was probably at the first synapse, but this inference could not be made solid (Krasne, 1969).

Several years later some of the interneurons between sensory neurons and lateral giants were identified (Zucker, Kennedy, and Selverston, 1971; Zucker, 1972); it was then easily shown that the pathway is disynaptic and that repetitive activation of sensory fibers results in cessation of interneuron firing, whereas direct activation of individual interneurons produces absolutely constant excitatory postsynaptic potentials (EPSPs) in the lateral giants even at very high interneuron firing frequencies (Figure 28.9). It was also discovered that there are excitatory cross-connections between the interneurons which tend to reinforce their synchrony and thereby their ultimate effect on the lateral giants; these cross-connecting synapses do not, however, seem to be prone to depression.

Of course, the interneurons analyzed in this way might have been in some way unusual; after all, it was the unusually large size of their axons in interganglionic connectives that led to their discovery. However, if there were a fairly general tendency for failure to

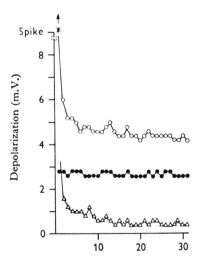

FIGURE 28.8(a) Intracellular recordings from crayfish lateral giant fibers during stimulus repitition. The experimental setup is shown in Figure 28.3 The effects on the alpha (monosynaptic) and beta (disynaptic) components of stimulation at approximately 3-sec intervals. Note the stability of alpha. Filled circles: alpha. Open circles: beta. Triangles: gamma.

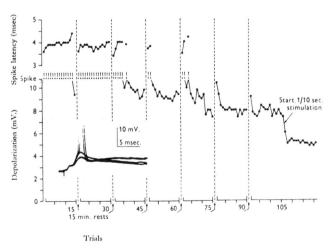

FIGURE 28.8(b) The effect of alternating blocks of 15 stimuli at 1 per min with 15-min periods of rest. The size of the beta (disynaptic) component is plotted on trials without a spike; spike latency is plotted on trials with a spike. The superimposed oscillograph traces from trials 61, 62, 63, and 75 have been inset at the lower left. Both parts from Krasne (1969).

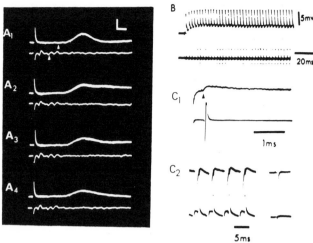

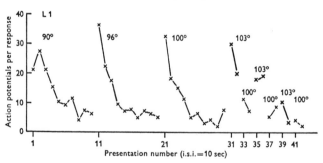

FIGURE 28.9 Properties of synapses in the crayfish LG reflex pathway. A. Sensory-neuron/interneuron synapse, showing the decline of a unitary EPSP in interneuron A (see Figures 28.2, 28.3). A_1–A_4 show responses on alternate trials at 1 per 2 sec (Upper traces show EPSPs; lower traces sensory-nerve activity.) Calibration: 2 mv and 2 msec. From Zucker, Kennedy, and Selverston (1971). Copyright 1971 by the American Association for the Advancement of Science. B. An interneuron/LG synapse. *Lower*: Spikes in interneuron A. *Upper*: EPSPs in the lateral giant. Note that there is no sign of decrement even at this very high frequency. From Zucker (1972). C. Interneuron/interneuron synapses. Lower traces show spikes in interneuron A; upper, EPSPs in interneuron C. C_1 shows a single trial at high sweep speed. C_2 shows that trials at 200 Hz produce no decline in the EPSP. From Zucker (1972).

develop between interneurons and the lateral giants or between one interneuron and another, there ought also to be some transfer (or generalization) of habituation between sensory inputs that converge on common first-order interneurons. But intensive efforts to find such effects have been essentially unsuccessful. Both Zucker and I have on occasion seen very marginal signs of generalization, but they are neither consistent nor strong enough to be taken very seriously in the present context (Zucker, 1972; Kramer, Krasne, and Lee, unpublished observations).

The picture emerging from this analysis is presented at the bottom of Figure 28.2, with the synapses at which transmission failure occurs indicated by asterisks. The results of similar analyses on a number of other preparations are given in the same figure.

From these analyses, taken together, several general points emerge. First, it is clear that adaptive degrees of behavioral change lasting from minutes to hours *can* be mediated by altered transmission at single synapses. There is no requirement for polysynaptic organization. This is clearest for the *Aplysia* and crayfish cases.

Second, those synapses at which transfer functions alter are not diffused throughout a reflex arc. The points at

which change occurs are specific and appear to be dictated by functional requirements. In the various reflexes that have been examined, the points utilized are all such as to promote strong stimulus specificity of habituation. This specificity is especially well illustrated by the descending-movement detector system studied by Rowell (Figure 28.10). In most of the systems the transmission failure responsible for habituation is thus at very early synapses prior to points of major sensory convergence. The only conspicuous exception to this rule is the cockroach evasion reflex (Figure 28.2; Zilber-Gachelin and Chartier, 1973a,b), but this may in fact be an exception that supports the rule: whereas habituation of the evasion response does involve alterations of transmission at points much beyond the first synapse, the sensory field of the reflex is itself so restricted (hairs on tiny anal circi) that further sensory specificity would presumably be of no adaptive value.

Third, while changeable transfer properties of *single* synapses probably govern behavioral habituation in *Aplysia*, crayfish, and perhaps other reflexes of Figure 28.2, unitary points of change are not an invariant rule. The cockroach evasion reflex provides a clear example of the cooperative interaction of altered transfer characteristics at several levels to produce profound behavioral lability (Zilber-Gachelin and Chartier, 1973a,b). The first synapse in the pathway becomes much less efficacious when airpuffs to anal circi are repeated at intervals on the order of twice per minute, and it shows a marginal decline at frequencies as low as once in five minutes. These effects are seen clearly only when natural stimuli (airpuffs to the anal circi), which produce repetitive, asynchronous bombardment of first-order synapses, are utilized; single shocks to afferent nerves produce only extremely marginal signs of depression. Volleys produced in first-order interneurons by airpuffs ascend to the

FIGURE 28.10 Stimulus-specific habituation of the locust descending-movement detector. Visual stimuli are presented serially to slightly different positions (indicated by visual angles) on the retina. Each point on the retina has to be independently habituated. Note from the manipulations at the right (e.g., 100° to 103° to 100°) that habituation at previously stimulated locations persists throughout a test of a fresh spot. From Rowell (1971c).

thoracic ganglia where, if sufficiently intense and prolonged, they release the evasion response. The requirement for a long, intense volley makes the evasion response
particularly sensitive to depression at the first synapse.
Furthermore, even when constant interneuron volleys
are repeated as infrequently as once in four minutes, their
ability to release evasion declines strongly. The net result is a behavioral response which is probably considerably more labile than either the first-level or second-
level labilities *alone* would lead us to expect.

Finally, I should like to return briefly to the failure-
prone neuromuscular junction in the crayfish LG reflex arc (the efferent synapses of F_1 in Figure 28.2).
Crustacean muscle fibers have attracted considerable
study because, like central neurons, synaptic transmission
to them is subject to both pre- and postsynaptic inhibition (Dudel and Kuffler, 1961). This has permitted
particularly detailed and informative analyses to be
made of these processes, which are normally found only
inside the central nervous system, where it is much more
difficult to study them. The reduced effectiveness of the
synapses between F_1 and the fast flexor muscles during
repeated LG firing may be thought of as another example of externalization of a normally central process.
There is little doubt that the alteration of transfer characteristics at these synapses must result in some, presumably adaptive, alterations in the intensity and form
of tail-flip behavior during repetitive stimulation (before
full habituation occurs). Thus, were it not for the peripheral locus of the synapses, we would not hesitate to
conclude that they participate critically in a kind of
habituation learning. It therefore may be particularly
justifiable to utilize these synapses in analytical work
aimed at understanding the physiological basis of the
alterations in synaptic transfer functions that are responsible for learning.

28.3.3 Extrinsically imposed versus intrinsic changes in circuitry mediating behavior as causes of learning

It is a persistent worry of neurophysiologists interested in
discovering the locus of the engram that they will locate
the points of altered transmission or rate of firing that
cause an alteration of behavior only to discover that
these local changes are, in turn, imposed from some
other, remote place in the nervous system. In fact, however, there is very little evidence to support such a pessimistic view. It is well known that one cannot produce
severe impairments of memory in the mammalian brain
without doing violence to the very perceptual and motor
circuitry that must directly mediate the learned behaviors, and this suggests that the engrams are localized
in the mediational circuitry itself. Moreover, it seems

unlikely on logical grounds that any region of the mammalian brain other than the classical input and output
"analyzers" themselves possess the articulate representation of sensory events and motor activities that would be
required to store highly stimulus- and response-specific
memories.

In invertebrate preparations we can, so far, address
this question of intrinsic versus extrinsic sites of fundamental change in detail only for the process of habituation. However, this process may be theoretically crucial
on this issue, because it is hard to imagine a sort of learning for which intrinsic change would seem *less* likely on
a priori grounds. The loss of the possibility of control
that is seemingly implied by depression intrinsic to the
excitatory pathway of a habituating response would
appear to be a very dangerous step, particularly in the
case of the survival-essential escape reactions that we
have available for study. It could be argued, therefore,
that if altered transmission during habituation in *these*
pathways is due to intrinsic depression processes, then
other forms of learning may, a fortiori, be due to intrinsic
change as well.

POTENTIAL SUBSTRATES FOR HABITUATION OF EXTRINSIC
ORIGIN IN THE CRAYFISH. The crayfish LG escape-reflex
system is a particularly interesting target for investigating the origin of the altered transmission characteristics
responsible for habituation, because a number of local
and higher-order modulatory control pathways which
could in principle mediate an extrinsically originating
effect are known to exist.

These are indicated in Figure 28.11; only inhibitory
controls have been included since it is presumably these
that would operate during habituation. We know of four
modes of inhibition in this pathway:
I.   presynaptic inhibition of afferent terminals (Krasne
and Bryan, 1973; Kennedy, Calabrese, and Wine, 1974);
II. postsynaptic inhibition of first-order interneurons
(Krasne and Bryan, 1973);
III. postsynaptic inhibition of the LG command neuron
(Roberts, 1968); and
IV. postsynaptic inhibition of some of the more important motoneurons of the tail-flip response (Hagiwara,
1958; Mittenthal and Wine, 1973).

These inhibitory effects are known to be produced in
various combinations by a variety of events:
1. The firing of the LG command neuron or of other
command neurons for escape (there are several of these
having different releasing stimuli and producing somewhat different trajectories or latencies of escape; see
Wine and Krasne, 1972) produces a virtually total shut-
down of the LG reflex pathways via input paths S, T,
and U; this inhibition starts right after the motoneurons

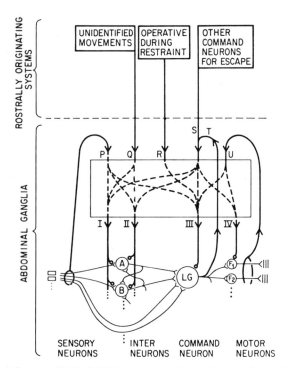

FIGURE 28.11 Inhibitory controls in the crayfish LG reflex pathway. The basic LG reflex circuit is drawn with thin lines. Known inhibitory pathways are drawn with bold lines. An explanation is given in the text.

for the escape pattern have fired and persists until the behavioral response is essentially complete. It presumably serves in part to prevent conflicting or confused response patterns (Roberts, 1968; Wine, 1971; Mittenthal and Wine, 1973; Krasne and Bryan, 1973).

2. Strong sensory input can lead via presumptive pathway P to widespread inhibition of the afferent limb of the LG reflex arc (Kennedy, Calabrese, and Wine, 1974; Krasne, unpublished observations). This inhibition normally starts late enough not to affect the probability that the eliciting stimulus will evoke LG responses, but it will drastically attenuate the effect of a slightly later stimulus. Its function is uncertain, but it could be involved in limiting the LG escape system to discrete phasic stimuli; other escape command systems specialize in setting up responses in the presence of persistent annoyances or gradually developing threat situations.

3. Restraining an animal so that it cannot escape effectively causes strong inhibition of transmission between interneurons and lateral giants via presumptive pathway R, which is of cephalad origin (Krasne and Wine, 1975).

4. Movements of the animal that have not yet been characterized are associated with a rostrally originating inhibition which, in distinction to that of pathway R, operates at the first synapse of the reflex pathway (route Q) (Kramer, Krasne, and Lee, unpublished observations) We do not know the function of this effect.

LACK OF EXTRINSIC EFFECTS. Route P obviously offers the possibility of some sort of augmentation of stimulus-produced inhibition as the mechanism of habituation. The existence of inhibitory pathways Q and R descending from higher centers suggests the possibility that habituation is in some measure due to tonic inhibition of the reflex by the brain. And since other escape commands, as well as unidentified movements, can inhibit the LG pathway, habituation could occur because some behavior other than and presumably incompatible with escape has become facilitated. Although these possibilities are all highly plausible, experiments designed to yield evidence in favor of them have given uniformly negative results.

Cutting the nerve cord between thorax and abdomen, so as to isolate the abdominal cord chronically and abolish the effects of inhibitory pathways descending from higher centers, produces an animal whose LG reflex is somewhat more excitable than that of a normal animal, but whose moderate-term habituation to repetitive stimuli seems entirely normal (Figure 28.12; Wine and Krasne, 1969; Wine, Krasne, and Chen, 1975).

Application of picrotoxin, which poisons known presynaptic and postsynaptic inhibitory actions in the crayfish nervous system, also produces an abnormally excitable LG reflex, but it does not abolish the failure of transmission that occurs when stimuli are repeated (Krasne and Roberts, 1967).

Intracellular recording from first-order interneurons during repetition-produced transmission failure provides no evidence of any postsynaptic inhibitory action. There are no emergent IPSPs, though hyperpolarizing IPSPs in the same neurons are seen when pathways S, T, or (sometimes) P are activated, nor is there any indication of any conductance increase in the interneurons. (Figure 28.13; Zucker, 1972).

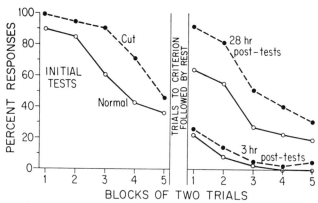

FIGURE 28.12 Habituation of moderate duration does not depend upon rostrally originating inhibition. "Cut" animals have had their cords sectioned between thorax and abdomen. The experimental procedure is identical to that described for crayfish in Figure 28.4. From Wine, Krasne, and Chen (1975).

414   FRANKLIN B. KRASNE

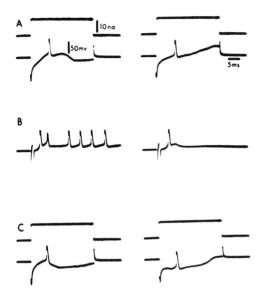

FIGURE 28.13 Tests for conductance or excitability changes in a first-order interneuron due to repeated direct or afferent bombardment. A. An electrode near the base of the dendritic tree of interneuron C was used simultaneously to pass a just suprarheobase current (upper trace) and to record the initiation of a spike (lower trace). The latency of the spike under such circumstances is a very sensitive measure of the cell's firing threshold. The left and right traces are the first and last of 10 current pulses at 1 per sec. Direct injection of current apparently produces no change of threshold. B. One sec after the above sequence a sensory-root feeding interneuron C was shocked 10 times at 1 per sec. The discharge in the neuron clearly declined. C. One sec later the procedure of A was repeated. Note that the repetitive afferent stimulation that resulted in a decline of firing in interneuron C produced no increase in its threshold. Modified from Zucker (1972).

The likelihood of *any* process external to sensory-neuron/interneuron synapses being necessarily involved in habituation is virtually nil, because even when individual tactile afferent fibers are stimulated to fire single spikes at moderate intervals, the resultant EPSPs in first-order interneurons diminish, while other synapses remain unaffected. In this situation it seems extremely unlikely that any neuron other than the activated sensory neuron would be driven to fire, and thus the nervous system as a whole should presumably not even be "aware" that anything has happened. Nevertheless, the decremental process occurs, and we therefore believe that it is intrinsic to the synapses that are recurrently stimulated (see Figure 28.20, below, and Zucker, 1972). One proviso must be made to this conclusion. There is some question as to whether the time course of recovery from habituation is the same in acute as in chronic preparations. It is thus possible that processes are operating in chronic preparations and intact animals that are not seen in acute experiments. See Wine, Krasne, and Chen (1975) for a discussion of relevant data.

Similar experiments have led to virtually identical conclusions for the withdrawal reflexes of *Aplysia* (Castellucci et al., 1970). Furthermore, a number of investigators have examined the effects of various ablations on habituation phenomena in many kinds of animals (see Groves and Lynch, 1972; Peretz and Howieson, 1973; Groves, Wilson, and Boyle, 1974; and references therein). While there have often been effects on extents or rates of habituation, it has never been possible to assess properly the baseline effects of the lesions on synaptic transmission through the reflex pathway. Without such information one cannot rule out the possibility that alterations in tonic levels of inhibition, excitation, or both drive some synaptic transfer functions to the extreme ends of their dynamic ranges, where changes that normally cause habituation can occur without being manifest. Furthermore, there is good reason for supposing that such alterations of tonic modulation have occurred in most studies reporting effects. Thus I believe it may be said that to date there has been no satisfactory demonstration of habituation being due to extrinsic inhibitory control in any animal.

SENSITIZATION IN *Aplysia*. An apparent exception to the hypothesis that engrams are generally intrinsic comes from experiments on sensitization in *Aplysia*. Strong or novel stimulation causes augmentation of the EPSPs produced by many or all of the synapses in the monosynaptic limb of the withdrawal-reflex pathway (Figure 28.2), and since no evidence for postsynaptic changes that could cause the augmentation has been found, it is believed that the effect is brought about by a pathway which presynaptically facilitates transmitter release from afferent neuron terminals (Carew, Castellucci, and Kandel, 1971; Castellucci et al., 1970). It therefore seems likely that the sensitization is established by an extrinsic route. The reason for classing this sensitization as a form of learning is that it outlasts by minutes or perhaps days the stimuli that initiate it (Kandel and Tauc, 1965; Carew, Castellucci, and Kandel, 1971; Pinsker et al., 1973). However, it is at present an open question whether the persistence is due to continuing activity in the presumptive facilitatory pathway or whether that pathway merely *establishes* an intrinsic change in the withdrawal-reflex pathway itself.

28.3.4 Superordinate control of plasticity
The notion that learning might be generally due to intrinsic synaptic changes in already formed transmission pathways does not mean that learning and performance are independent of the rest of the nervous system. This is particularly clear, for example, in the effects of hippocampal ablations in man, which massively disturb

learning ability while leaving many previously stored memories fully intact (see Rozin, this volume). In the invertebrates there are a number of known processes whereby extrinsic circuitry affects learning, performance, or retention of "engrams" which are themselves probably of intrinsic origin.

OVERRIDE OF LEARNED INTRINSIC CHANGES BY EXTRINSIC MODULATION. In his pioneering studies of the "intelligence" of lower animals, Yerkes (1912) performed maze-learning experiments on earthworms which suggested that these animals might be able to master a T maze. Performance was never very reliable; however, when the brain was removed from the trained animals, learned performance actually improved! When a new brain regenerated, performance again deteriorated. This experiment has been replicated several times (Heck, 1920; Zellner, 1966). It has similarly been found that although moderate-term habituation learning in cockroaches is independent of the brain (Zilber-Gachelin and Chartier, 1973a,b; but cf. Baxter, 1957), the brain does make the course of habituation much more variable. Results such as these indicate that neuronal pathways mediating learned behavior are subject to quite effective extrinsic control which can override or modulate learned performance.

Such override has been investigated in depth during studies of the habituation of withdrawal behavior in *Aplysia*. It is well established that habituation of this reflex is due to a depression of excitatory effectiveness that is intrinsic to those synapses between sensory and motor neurons of the reflex arc that have been repeti-

tively activated (see Section 28.3.3), When a habituated animal is given a strong or noxious stimulus, there is an apparent recovery from the habituated state. This makes adaptive sense, since the occurrence of the strong stimulus may mean that environmental conditions have changed in such a way that previously innocuous stimuli are now harbingers of danger. Careful investigations of this "dishabituation" have shown that it is caused by an augmented effectiveness of both depressed and undepressed (i.e., "unhabituated") synapses (Figure 28.14 A), which is probably due in turn to a widely generalized presynaptic facilitation of sensory-nerve terminals (Carew, Castellucci, and Kandel, 1971). In other words, it does not represent a recovery from habituation per se, but is rather a superimposed and highly generalized facilitation of synaptic transmission. In other preparations where these characteristics of dishabituation have been found, there is also a spontaneous reversion to the habituated state after the transient effect of the dishabituating stimulus wears off (Figure 28.14 B).

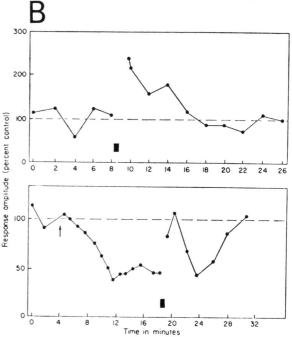

FIGURE 28.14(B) Effects of a strong stimulus (solid black rectangle) on the flexion reflex of a spinal cat. *Upper*: The strong stimulus transiently elevates flexion-reflex excitability in an unhabituated preparation. *Lower*: The same stimulus restores the responsiveness of a habituated preparation. After the presentation of the strong stimulus, the stimulus frequency for the flexion reflex was lowered to a rate which did not produce habituation (see above); testing of the reflex at this rate showed that after the effect of the strong stimulus wore off, reflex excitability returned spontaneously to the *habituated* level and then proceeded to undergo spontaneous recovery. From Thompson and Spencer (1966). Copyright 1966 by the American Psychological Association. Reproduced with permission.

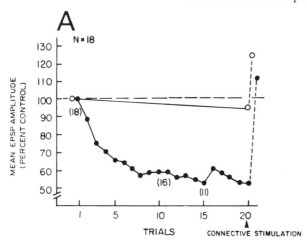

FIGURE 28.14(A) Apparent dishabituation due to transient facilitation. This part shows the effect of a "dishabituatory" stimulus (connective stimulation) on habituated (open circles) and unhabituated (filled circles) responses in *Aplysia*. EPSPs are in a withdrawal-reflex motoneuron. Note that connective stimulation increases responsiveness even in unhabituated preparations. From Carew and Kandel (1974).

416   FRANKLIN B. KRASNE

EXTRINSIC CONTROL OF ENGRAM FORMATION: PROMOTION OF CHANGE AND PROTECTION FROM CHANGE. Several lines of experimentation suggest that the extent to which synaptic change leading to learning will occur in a given situation may be subject to extrinsic regulatory control. The possibility that there might be natural mechanisms for preventing learning is manifest in the ease with which learning or consolidation can be disrupted by external agents, while the contrary possibility, that there might be natural mechanisms for promoting learning, is suggested by the existence of ablation and lesion maneuvers which prevent new learning while leaving old memories intact (see Flood and Jarvik, McGaugh and Gold, and Rozin, this volume). Experiments showing the facilitation of learning by certain pharmacological agents (McGaugh, 1973; Flood and Jarvik, this volume) might also be interpretable in this context.

The promotion of segmentally stored learning by cerebral machinery has also been shown in an invertebrate in an interesting experiment by Evans (1963) on the annelid worm *Nereis*. When placed headfirst into a glass tube, *Nereis* normally crawls promptly through the tube and exits from the other end; if given repeated trials its performance gradually improves. If, however, the worm is repeatedly shocked either before, during, or after its run through the tube, it becomes recalcitrant and refuses to crawl through. Furthermore, if the brain of an avoidance-trained worm is removed, its tube-crawling behavior remains largely indistinguishable from that of an unoperated control (Figure 28.15). This indicates that an "engram" for the "learned" avoidance response resides in the lower portions of the animal's nervous system. However, whereas the brain is apparently not needed for recall, it does seem to be required in some phase of the storage process, for if animals without brains are trained de novo, they learn in an almost normal fashion but do not retain this learning for even an hour (Figure 28.15).

Although it is thus clear that the integrity of function of one part of a nervous system can influence the laying down of engrams in other parts, this does not prove that modulation of engram formation is a *normal* activity of the nervous system. Recently, however, it has been shown that the labile synapses of the crayfish LG reflex are protected from depression, and hence the animal is protected from habituation during its own tail-flip movement (Figure 28.16). Were this not so, the water currents set up by the animal's own movements would discharge escape-reflex afferents and lead to self-produced habituation. This would be highly maladaptive, because crayfish utilize tail-flip responses under a variety of circumstances unrelated to escape from abdominal stimulation (Wine and Krasne, 1972); without a protective mechanism a bout of tail flips, no matter what its cause, would leave the animal unable to react to a subsequent threat. This protection from maladaptive synaptic change is brought about by a corollary discharge that originates with the firing of escape command neurons and acts by inhibiting the presynaptic terminals of depressible synapses (via Pathway I of Figure 28.11; see Krasne and Bryan, 1973). Whether this presynaptic inhibition prevents depression by sparing depletable transmitter stores or by some other means remains to be determined. However, it does demonstrate rather clearly that nervous systems (or at least this nervous system) possess control circuitry which functions to regulate the malleability of inherently plastic synapses and which thereby determines whether learning will occur.

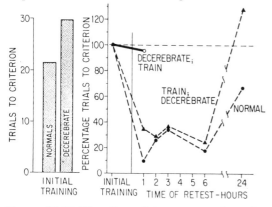

FIGURE 28.15 The effect of the supra-esophageal ganglion of *Nereis* on learning and retention. *Left*: "Decerebrates" readily "learn" not to crawl through a tube if they are shocked. Trials to criterion (3 successive failures to crawl to the end within 40 sec) are not greatly different for normals and decerebrates. *Right*: Both normals and worms decerebrated *after* being trained show large savings in retraining for at least 6 hr after the original sensitization learning. However, animals decerebrated and *then* trained for the first time show no savings even after only 1 hr of rest. Based on Evans (1963).

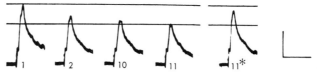

FIGURE 28.16 Protection from habituation in the crayfish LG escape reflex. Stimulation and recording are as in Figure 28.3A. 1, 2, 10, 11 are EPSPs in the lateral giant to the 1st, 2nd, 10th, and last of 11 stimulations at 1 per 5 sec. After a rest the same stimulus series was repeated, but each of the first 10 stimuli was preceded (by 20 msec) by activation of tail-flip motor circuitry (produced by stimulating non-LG escape command neuron); 11* is the EPSP on the last trial of this series. Note that preceding the stimuli by motor-circuit activation largely protected the reflex from becoming depressed. This effect is maximal at the time when the power stroke of the tail flip would be occurring if the animal were intact. Calibration: 4mv and 20 msec. From Krasne and Bryan (1973). Copyright 1973 by the American Association for the Advancement of Science.

"Erasure" of an engram—true dishabituation. The third possible way in which one part of a nervous system could exert control over the learning of other parts is through an active erasure process. In this era of analogies between computers and brains, it seems odd that we cannot point to memory-erasure processes in brains. However, there is some evidence from invertebrate systems that this sort of process might be a reality. In some preparations which show habituation, appropriate sorts of stimulation can cause an immediate recovery from habituation which looks as though it may involve a resetting of the depressed synapses rather than the sort of superimposed facilitative process discussed above (Rowell, 1971b).

Rowell's descending movement-detector system (Table 28.2; Figure 28.2) provides the most convincing evidence available for such an erasure or resetting process. The critical properties of dishabituation in this system are as follows: (1) Only responses to stimuli whose effectiveness is low due to *habituation* become enhanced. Responses that are low because stimulation was mild are unaffected by the dishabituating process (Figure 28.17A). (2) Recovery due to dishabituation is never to levels *above* those seen to the test stimulus in an unhabituated animal (cf. Figure 28.14). (3) The recovery produced by the dishabituation process appears to be permanent, despite the fact that the events initiating

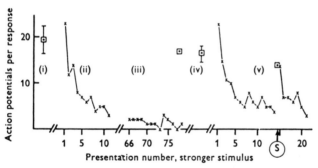

FIGURE 28.17(A) True dishabituation in the locust movement-detector system. Responses of the descending movement-detector neuron to a weak stimulus (square) and stronger stimulus (X) at two different loci on the retina. The weaker stimulus is presented at an interstimulus interval of 10 min throughout the experiment, at which frequency there is negligible decline of responsiveness; points (i) and (iv) are *means* for 11 and 5 successive stimuli, respectively. The stronger stimulus is presented as shown on the graph. At S, during a series of presentations of the stronger stimulus, an antenna was briefly shocked just before the scheduled presentations of both the stronger and weaker stimuli. The response to the stronger stimulus shows marked dishabituation, whereas that to the weaker stimulus is not affected. That the response to the weaker stimulus had not suffered decrement as a result of the repeated presentations of the strong stimulus per se is shown by the weak-stimulus presentation between strong-stimulus presentations number 77 and 78 of series (iii).

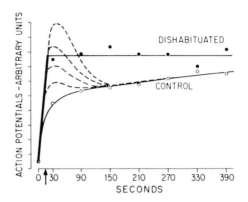

FIGURE 28.17(B) Recovery from habituation is shown for control runs by the open circles. On experimental runs a disturbing stimulus was given at the arrow; the result (filled circles) was an immediate and full recovery from habituation. The dashed lines indicate some of the sorts of recovery patterns that might have been expected on experimental runs if the effect of the disturbing stimulus had been to increase the excitability of the system transiently without actually abolishing the habituation. Both parts based on Rowell (1971b).

the recovery are presumably transient (Figure 28.17B; cf. Figure 28.14B).

Such data strongly suggest a process of resetting, but they are not absolutely compelling. Suppose that habituation were due to depression at synapses that are maximally effective, or "saturated," when fresh but that tend to run down *during* trains of arriving spikes when depressed (cf. "fresh" with "habituated" in Figure 28.18), while dishabituating stimuli facilitate transmitter release but cannot cause EPSPs to rise above their maximum possible size. Then dishabituating stimuli would not increase responses of fresh preparations (cf. fresh with fresh but also with facilitated cases for weak stimuli in Figure 28.18) but *would* cause recovery in habituated preparations (cf. habituated with habituated but also with facilitated cases for strong stimuli). The apparent permanence of dishabituation could merely indicate

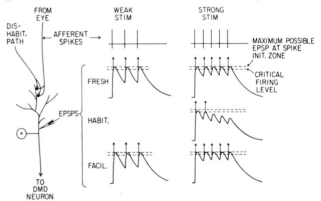

FIGURE 28.18 A scheme for explaining data such as that of Figure 28.17 without postulating "true" dishabituation. See text for explanation.

that the facilitative processes initiated by the dishabituating event outlast the depression produced by habituation training. Since habituation is not usually very long-lasting in the descending movement-detector system, this is not an implausible alternative.

If such an interpretation can be ruled out, the insect nervous system will have introduced us to a neuronal mechanism which one would expect to have become of major functional significance in animals that are heavily dependent upon learning.

28.3.5 On the nature of intrinsic change

In principle, changes in efficacy of transmission between one neuron and another could result from any of a host of pre- or postsynaptic alterations. The major known steps in synaptic transmission are indicated in Figure 28.19, along with some parameters that one might imagine could change so as to affect the transition from one step to the next. These parameters include resting potential levels, critical firing levels, membrane conductances, residual calcium-ion levels in terminals,

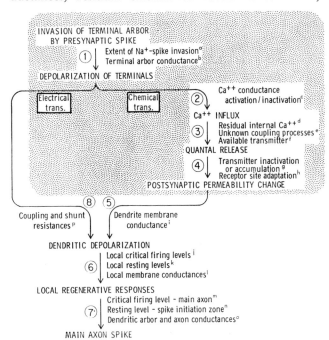

FIGURE 28.19 Major steps in synaptic transmission. The shaded region indicates those steps most likely to be involved in learned functional change. Some of the parameters that affect each step are listed. There is evidence that most of them are subject to at least brief changes as the result of usage. [References: Nastuk, 1967 (h); Katz and Miledi, 1968 (d); Betz, 1970 (e, f); Katz and Miledi, 1971 (b but *not* c); Sokolove and Cooke, 1971 (n); Wachtel and Kandel, 1971 (h); Brodwick and Junge, 1972 (i, k, l, n, o); Parnas, 1972 (a); Highstein and Bennett, 1973 (f); Jansen and Nicholls, 1973 (a, b); Stephens, 1973a,b (j or m); van Essen, 1973 (a); Woody and Black-Cleworth, 1973 (l, i); Zucker, 1973 (e or f); Spira and Bennett, 1971 (p).]

postsynaptic transmitter receptor site numbers and states of adaptation, and the condition of the unknown coupling processes between calcium-ion entry into terminals and the release of transmitter substance. Even this rather long list is surely not exhaustive. Furthermore, all of these parameters are, at least transiently, affected by prior activity.

The question, however, is whether variations in any of them are responsible for *learned* behavioral change.

Strictly speaking, we are in a position to comment only on habituation of moderate duration in *Aplysia* and crayfish. However, it will be useful to give some consideration as well to some other examples of use-produced depressions and potentiations of PSP size which are not necessarily responsible for learning.

STABILITY OF POSTSYNAPTIC ELECTRICAL EXCITABILITY. One of the most conspicuous ways in which synaptic transfer characteristics might be altered is by changes in the critical firing levels or resting potentials of postsynaptic cells. However, as soon as we were able to record intracellularly from the postsynaptic side of changing synapses in *Aplysia* and crayfish, it became immediately apparent that these parameters were not changing in any substantial way. Rather, EPSPs were altering drastically in size (Castellucci et al., 1970; Zucker, Kennedy, and Selverston, 1971). Furthermore, as could have been inferred from behavior, only the EPSPs of stimulated pathways changed, which ruled out any form of global change of the postsynaptic cell. These observations did not, however, rule out the possibility that altered EPSP sizes might be due to local changes in dendritic input impedance or to changes in the degree to which primary EPSPs are amplified by local, nonpropagated, regenerative responses in the dendritic tree.

In an attempt to evaluate such possibilities, careful comparisons of postsynaptic electrical properties and excitability before and after habituation have been made in *Aplysia* and crayfish. However, neither repetition of afferent input leading to synaptic depression nor repetition of injected current pulses sufficient to fire the postsynaptic cell have led to any demonstrable change in either postsynaptic conductance or the threshold current for producing regenerative responses (Figure 28.13; Castellucci et al., 1970; Zucker, 1972).

In *Aplysia* these experiments were done with electrodes in neuron somata; in crayfish the electrodes were probably located just at the base of the dendritic tree. The experiments are thus open to the criticism that they are relatively insensitive to conditions at substantial distances from these points of impalement. However, since some depressible EPSPs do seem to be of fairly proximal origin, this criticism is not devastating. Furthermore, the outcomes of these experiments conform to those of many kinds of experiments on nerve-muscle preparations which show that analogous, though shorter-lasting, forms of depression and also of poststimulation facilitation are invariably due to much earlier steps in the transmission process (see the discussion of presynaptic versus postsynaptic change, below).

The notion that the steps outside the shaded region of Figure 28.19 are not normally responsible for behaviorally significant degrees of synaptic lability is also bolstered by the observation that whereas chemical and electrical synapses traverse these steps in a similar way, only chemically operating synapses seem to be subject to significant degrees of lability.

The crayfish escape reflex is particularly interesting in this context, because in this one pathway those synaptic levels at which transmission is stable all seem to operate electrically, while the single level at which transmission is subject to failure operates chemically (Zucker, 1972). The synapses believed to be electrical are considered so because their EPSPs have vanishingly small synaptic delays, have rapid rise and fall times, and are not affected by mild polarizations of the membrane at the recording site. Those considered chemical have EPSPs with delays in excess of 0.5 msec, have relatively slow rise and fall times, and *are* readily affected by membrane polarization. These criteria are definitely not entirely satisfactory, but in other systems where more stringent criteria are also met, the rule that plastic synapses are chemical and not electrical continues to hold (Nicholls and Purves, 1972; Martin and Pilar, 1963, 1964). This suggests that changes occur only in the uniquely "chemical" steps 2–4 of Figure 28.19. But since another feature that distinguishes chemical from electrical synapses is a nonlinear, highly positively accelerating relation between terminal depolarization and transmitter release, transmission at chemical synapses would also be particularly sensitive to alterations in step 1.

DIFFERENCES BETWEEN CHEMICAL SYNAPSES. The way in which a given synapse reacts to repetitive activation seems to be a characteristic feature of that synapse. If one examines individual afferents synapsing on the largest first-order interneuron of the crayfish escape reflex, for example, one finds that some afferents produce constant EPSPs while others show either decrementing responses at relatively low frequencies or a degree of augmentation (Kennedy, 1971, and see the disussion of presynaptic versus postsynaptic change, below).

Such differences are not random or accidental. Motoneurons innervating crustacean muscle branch widely and multiterminally innervate each fiber of an entire muscle. The neuromuscular synapses thus formed by

single motoneurons differ from one another dramatically in the degree to which they tend to show augmentation of EPSPs during repetitive activation. However, all of the synapses on a *given* muscle fiber are uniform in the degree to which they show this tendency (Atwood and Bittner, 1971). Taken together, observations such as these indicate that both the synaptic contacts made by a single presynaptic neuron and those occurring on a single postsynaptic neuron may vary among themselves in their responses to repetitive activation, but that these patterns of response are nevertheless under fairly strict developmental or ongoing regulation. The nature of this control is unknown, but it is surely conceivable that changes in it in adult organisms are involved in learning phenomena.

The constancy of the individual synapse's mode of response to usage opens the possibility of undertaking morphological comparisons of differently behaving synapses. This has been done so far only for certain convenient crustacean neuromuscular synapses, and the comparisons have been largely qualitative (Atwood, 1967; Sherman and Atwood, 1972; Lang and Atwood, 1973). Comparisons between depression-prone and non-depression-prone synapses have shown the former to be poorer in mitochondria and synaptic vesicles and to have presynaptic processes of a relatively large diameter. The vesicle and mitochondria differences are plausible; the relatively large size of presynaptic processes may imply that presynaptic spikes fully invade the terminals and are not likely to be subject to conduction blockage. Comparisons between facilitation-prone and relatively stable synapses show the former to have fewer very large (and also fewer very small) presynaptic processes and more but smaller patches of specialized contact area. The relative absence of large presynaptic processes at the facilitative junctions has been viewed as consistent with physiological evidence suggesting that presynaptic spikes approaching such junctions are subject to propagation failures; in this view, facilitation is thought to be due to processes that improve the effectiveness with which these readily blockable spikes can lead to Ca^{++}-permeability increases in the terminals. So far such analyses have only been of heuristic value, but they seem to have considerable potential.

PRESYNAPTIC VERSUS POSTSYNAPTIC CHANGE. One of the major neurophysiological discoveries of the last few decades has been that transmitter release from presynaptic terminals is quantal and probabilistic. This discovery has, in turn, been of great use for determining the locus of responsibility for intrinsic depressions and augmentations of synaptic efficacy. Del Castillo and Katz (1954) showed in one of their early papers on quantal release that at frog neuromuscular junctions, quantal EPSP size of both depressed and facilitated junctions remained constant; it was the number of quanta released by the presynaptic terminals which varied. In other words, depression and facilitation, in this case at least, were presynaptic phenomena.

As other synapses showing plastic efficacy have been studied, the generality of this finding has not been successfully challenged (though see Highstein and Bennett, 1973). There is therefore every reason to suppose that it will continue to hold for the relatively persistent changes that mediate habituation in crayfish and *Aplysia*; however, the sorts of experiments required to test this hypothesis are fraught with difficulties when they are attempted at the relevant central synapses. Of several problems the greatest is that since quite a large number of quanta seem to be released by each presynaptic impulse, one never sees the effects of the release of a single quantum, identifiable as originating at the relevant synapse, in isolation. Drugs or cooling can in principle be used to lower quantal output, and such methods have been employed on *Aplysia* (Castellucci and Kandel, 1974), but one has little assurance that the synaptic depression seen under such circumstances has normal causality. It has therefore been necessary to make inferences about the sizes and numbers of quanta composing EPSPs on the basis of statistical variations in EPSP size (Hubbard, Llinás, and Quastel, 1969).

Because release is probabilistic, the precise number of quanta that compose an EPSP is a random variable. The mean (v) and standard deviation (σ_v) of observed EPSP size will reflect the mean (m) and standard deviation (σ_m) of the number of quanta released per trial. If the size of EPSP caused by a single quantal release is q, the so-called quantal efficiency, then $v = qm$ and $\sigma_v = q\sigma_m$, assuming that v remains far enough from its reversal potential so that summation remains "linear." Consequently, the coefficient of variation of observed EPSP size, $\sigma_v / v = \sigma_m / m$, is independent of q. If this statistic changes during alterations of synaptic efficacy, there must have been changes in the quantal release process on which the parameters m and σ_m depend. Conversely, if the coefficient of variation remains unaltered, the change in efficacy must have been due to a change in quantal efficiency (unless σ_m and m change proportionately, which is improbable); *this* sort of change could be of either pre- or postsynaptic origin.

In order to make realistic use of this approach, one must recognize that the quantal efficiency q is itself somewhat variable, presumably because of variations in such factors as the precise number of transmitter molecules per quantal packet and the precise distance between the recording electrode and the point on the postsynaptic membrane where a given dose of transmitter arrives. However, when this complication is taken into account it remains a reasonable conclusion that changes in the coefficient of variation reflect changes in presynaptic release mechanisms, while lack of such changes reflects alterations in quantal efficiency. [Assume that the variability of quantal efficiency is due to variation in the number of transmitter molecules per quantum and in the electrotonic distance from the recording electrode of arriving quanta (due in turn to differences in points of release), while postsynaptic sensitivity to transmitter is fairly uniform across the postsynaptic membrane and shows only negligible random fluctuations in time. Then we may write $\mathbf{q} = s\mathbf{ta}$ where $\mathbf{q}$, the quantal efficiency, is a random variable; s is local depolarization per transmitter molecule; $\mathbf{t}$, a random variable, is the number of transmitter molecules per quantum; and $\mathbf{a}$, a random variable, is the attenuation of the quantal depolarization between its point of origin and the recording electrode. The coefficient of variation then becomes

$$\sqrt{\left[\frac{\text{var}(\mathbf{ta})}{E^2(\mathbf{ta})}\frac{1}{m} + \frac{\sigma_m^2}{m^2}\right]},$$

where var and E are the variance and expected values, respectively (see Feller, 1950, for formulas for sums of random numbers of random variables). Since every quantity in this expression pertains to presynaptic events, a change in the coefficient of variation, under these assumptions, reflects presynaptic change.]

In a first attempt to utilize this approach on the crayfish escape-reflex synapses that participate in habituation, it was found that (after appropriate corrections on the data) a decrease in the mean EPSP from 4.13 to 3.17 mv was associated with a statistically reliable increase in the coefficient of variation from 0.049 to 0.068 (Zucker, 1972). On the face of it, this implied that habituation was at least partly due to changes in quantal release from presynaptic terminals. However, there were complications. In order to bring EPSP size sufficiently above noise level, it had been necessary to stimulate a number of afferents synchronously, a procedure which unfortunately leads to two problems.

First, differential changes in quantal efficiency among the activated synapses can alter the measured coefficient of variation even if quantal release statistics remain constant. [This stems from the fact that, for a given amount of variability in number of quanta released per impulse and a given size of EPSP at the recording electrode, there will (by the law of large numbers) be much less variability in EPSP magnitude if the EPSP is due to input from a large number of distant synapses (each making a small contribution) than if it is due to input from a small number of close synapses. Therefore, if an EPSP reduction were to result from a decline of synaptic efficacy at many very distal synapses, EPSP variance, which is mostly due to proximal synapses, would not change; hence, the coefficient of variation would rise. In the limiting case where all EPSP depression is due to postsynaptic desensitization of infinitely large numbers of infinitely distant (or otherwise ineffective) synapses, while no depression occurs at proximal synapses responsible for EPSP variability, $c_H / c_R = v_R / v_H$, where c_H and c_R are coefficients of variation in habituated and rested preparations, respectively, while v_H and v_R are the associated mean EPSP sizes. In the experiment described above, $c_H / c_R = 1.39$ and $v_R / v_H = 1.30$, which comes very close to corresponding to the limiting case. Since it is quite clear that different afferents on a given postsynaptic neuron are *not* uniformly depressible, the rise in c may have no implications for the mechanism of depression.]

Second, when, as was done in this experiment, a population of afferents is excited by a sensory-nerve shock that is near the threshold for some of the afferents, much of the variability in the EPSP can be due to the coming and going of precariously stimulated afferents. Attempts to monitor such a complex afferent volley accurately are usually unsatisfactory.

In order to try to remove some of these difficulties, we have attempted to repeat this analysis on an EPSP produced by a single afferent fiber. This is possible in interneuron A (Figure 28.2) because bending of some sensory hairs produces large and unitary EPSPs near the base of the dendritic tree (Kennedy, 1971). About 20 percent of the afferents we have tested evoke EPSPs that become depressed at moderate frequencies. In each of three successful experiments that we have so far carried out, stimulus repetition leading to depression has caused a decline in the coefficient of variation (Figure 28.20). While this again suggests that habituation is due at least in part to presynaptic changes, the occurrence of a decreased as opposed to an increased coefficient of variation is unexpected.

The two models of quantal release currently in vogue —Poisson and binomial (see, e.g., Zucker, 1973)— predict that decreased transmitter output should be associated with an increased coefficient of EPSPs variation. This prediction is inescapable for the Poisson model and highly *plausible* for the binomial model. There are several ways out of this dilemma. One, which seems to me implausible, is to assume that quantal release increases during depression, thus reducing the coefficient of variation, while quantal efficiency declines sufficiently to produce a decrease in mean EPSP size despite the rise in quantal release. A more likely way of explaining the observations is to assume that release of transmitter does

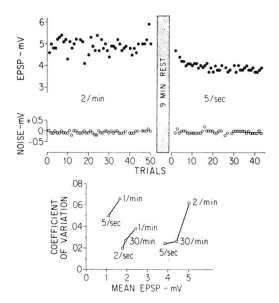

FIGURE 28.20 Changes in EPSP variability during depression at single synapses onto interneuron A of the crayfish LG escape reflex. *Upper*: Trial-by-trial data from a portion of one experiment. Noise measurements were (arbitrarily) taken at the moment the afferent fiber fired. Note the obvious decrease of EPSP variability during depression at 5 per sec. *Lower*: Coefficient of variation calculated for several experiments (noise variance subtracted out); the points for each experiment are joined by lines. As the mean EPSP decreases, the coefficient of variation falls. Unpublished data of Joan Bryan from the author's laboratory.

in fact fit a binomial model (i.e., each of a number of independent and specific release sites releases a quantum with probability p), but that the different release sites of a given presynaptic neuron do not all either have the same probability of release or react in the same way to repetitive activation. This model has the virtue of being able to account for either increases or decreases in the coefficient of variation (with decreasing total release). If some release sites have a very high and constant probability of release, while others have a low probability that decreases still further during repetitive activation, the coefficient of variation will fall. If all sites behave uniformly or if the initial probability of the labile sites is high, the coefficient of variation will rise. Clearly, such a model would require careful quantitative testing, but it could reconcile presently available observations.

It will be clear to anyone familiar with experiments on such "ideal" preparations as the neuromuscular junction that central synapses are a poor place to try to carry out analyses such as those just described, and it may be argued that we should use these more convenient preparations as models when dealing with phenomena such as depression, facilitation, and posttetanic potentiation which they do in fact display. However, though there is some merit in this argument, the greatest caution must attach to the assumption that depression, facilitation, etc., are unitary phenomena which will have identical explanations wherever they are found. Even at neuromuscular junctions in different species of animals, the mechanisms of apparently similar phenomena seem to be diverse.

For example, it has been hypothesized that synaptic depression at vertebrate neuromuscular junctions is due to depletion of the store of quanta available for release (Betz, 1970; Thies, 1965; Takeuchi, 1958). This hypothesis is based on several lines of evidence, one of which is that one can greatly diminish the extent to which depression will develop by altering Ca^{++}-Mg^{++} balance so as to reduce quantal output and thus "spare" transmitter. However, at the synapses between motor giant axons (F_1 of Figure 28.2) and fast flexor muscles in the crayfish abdomen, where depression not only occurs but has a time course long enough so that it really is a phenomenologically plausible model for the depressible synapses involved in habituation, reducing transmitter output by altering divalent cations has virtually no effect on the depression phenomenon. (In fact, there *is* a small effect on a mild depression which develops only with very prolonged stimulation; see Bruner and Kennedy, 1970.)

Again, at vertebrate neuromuscular junctions there is growing evidence that facilitation of transmitter release is due to the accumulation of Ca^{++} ions in nerve terminals during repetitive activation (Katz and Miledi, 1968). However, at several classes of crustacean neuromuscular synapses where the phenomenon of facilitation is extremely striking, this model seems unsatisfactory (see Lang and Atwood, 1973), though Zucker (1974) has made heroic and possibly successful efforts to save it. Furthermore, Sherman and Atwood (1971) have found a very long-term posttetanic augmentation at crab neuromuscular junctions which they believe is due to the accumulation of *sodium* ions in the nerve terminals.

If mechanisms of facilitation and depression differ even at different neuromuscular synapses, then clearly one must be very wary of generalizations from neuromuscular preparations to the central synapses responsible for learning. The neuromuscular preparations can provide hypotheses, but these must be tested at the actual synapses of interest.

28.3.6 Relationship between short- and long-term change

THE ROLE OF GENE TRANSCRIPTION OR TRANSLATION. A great deal of evidence from vertebrates encourages, though it does not demand, the view that long-term engram formation is a two-stage process: (1) Training initially establishes learned changes that are independent of protein synthesis and that are both temporary and susceptible to destruction by a variety of traumatic events. (2) Some time later, as the result of a "consolidation" process which seems to depend in some way on fresh genetic transcription or translation, the behavioral changes become resistant to both trauma and forgetting.

There is remarkably little information, given the technical ease of doing relevant experiments, on whether this general picture also holds for invertebrates.

Short-term habituation and sensitization learning in *Aplysia* have been shown to be quite unaffected by 95 percent inhibition of protein synthesis (Schwartz, Castellucci, and Kandel, 1971). There have been several attempts to investigate the effects of protein-synthesis inhibitors on learning in the cockroach "leg-lift" paradigm (Table 28.2), but the interpretation of results has been clouded by acute uncertainties as to whether the observed effects were in learning or in performance and whether short-term or consolidated learning was being studied (Brown and Noble, 1967; Glassman et al., 1970; Kerkut et al., 1970). Many of the difficulties of these experiments could probably be circumvented by using a learning phenomenon such as that illustrated in Figure 28.1 for honeybees.

There have also been a few attempts to measure the effect of leg-lift training on RNA base incorporation in both cockroaches and crabs (Kerkut et al., 1970; Kerkut, Emson, and Beesley, 1972; and unpublished experiments by D. Rafuse, quoted in Krasne, 1973), and these seem to have met with a measure of success. Trained animals have generally shown greater incorporation than either control animals receiving a comparable number of shocks or animals that have merely rested, and autoradiography has shown preferential incorporation in neurons that are probably involved in the task. More detailed work using further controls is definitely required, but the results to date are promising.

A unique approach to the question of what role genes may play in learning and memory is made possible in invertebrates by the fact that their gene-bearing neuron somata are set aside from the parts of the cell that are most obviously involved in information processing (Figure 28.21), and this suggests the possibility of examining the effects on plasticity of removing the cell body without totally disrupting the activities of the neuron. This is especially feasible because the neuron somata occur in relatively neat clusters at the periphery of the nervous system. Crustacean material seems to have special virtues for such experimentation; whereas the processes of most neurons begin to degenerate shortly after removal of their somata, there is growing evidence to suggest that both propagation and synaptic events in

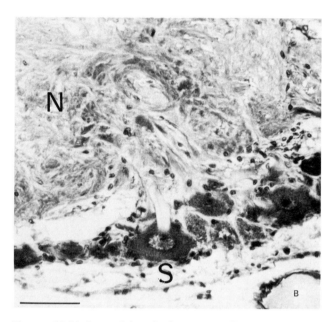

FIGURE 28.21 A crayfish unipolar neuron. Transverse section through a ventral portion of an abdominal ganglion. Neuropil (N) is above, and peripherally located cell bodies below. Just above the label S is a soma sending its unipolar process up into the neuropil. The ventral margin of the ganglion is just below S. The object at the lower right (B) is a medial artery lying just ventral to the nerve cord. Scale: 100 μm.

crustacean neurons remain normal for weeks or months after neurons have lost their gene-containing cell bodies.

As early as 1898 von Bethe removed all of the central cell bodies serving the neuropil of the second antenna of the crab, *Carcinus*. In the best of the several cases where he performed this difficult operation successfully, both reflex and spontaneous movements of the antenna continued normally for some three days after the operation; after that, thinking that he had perhaps missed some cell bodies or gotten his animals mixed up, von Bethe sacrificed the animal for histology, which confirmed that the somata were in fact all gone (Bethe, 1897). A variety of recent observations have successfully extended this sort of observation to various identified neurons and have shown that function remains normal for many weeks or even months (Hoy, Bittner, and Kennedy, 1967; Hoy, 1969; Wine, 1973).

The separation between somata and information processing in invertebrates also raises the interesting possibility that the consolidation of learning might have unusual attributes in invertebrates. If consolidation in any way requires interactions between information-processing parts of the neuron and the genome, one might expect greater consolidation time and greater susceptibility to manipulations affecting neuroplasmic flow than in vertebrates. A whole range of fascinating behavioral experiments suggests itself. There have in

fact been a few attempts to investigate the effects of temperature (Alloway, 1969, 1970), which affects the rate of axoplasmic flow, and of colchicine (Donoso and Fernandez, 1973) on learning and memory in insects, but no results of interest in the present context have yet emerged.

SHORT-TERM VERSUS LONG-TERM FUNCTIONAL CHANGES. At the functional level pursued in most of this chapter, the fundamental question to be asked in the present context is whether the functional changes of neurons that mediate the short- and long-term forms of a given behavioral change are one and the same. Does consolidation of an engram merely imply the stabilization of the specific central changes that have mediated freshly learned performance during training, or does it involve a restructuring of the neuronal basis of the new behavior? It seems to me highly unparsimonious to suppose that the functional neuronal basis for the short- and long-term versions of the same learned behavior will differ, but parsimony is a poor guide in biology.

We may expect to have some answers on this point very soon for the long-term habituation, and perhaps also the long-term sensitization, of gill and siphon withdrawal in *Aplysia* (see Table 28.2 and Davis, this volume), since the former effect, at least, seems to be obtainable in an abdominal ganglion maintained in organ culture (Carew and Kandel, 1973) and is therefore readily amenable to physiological analysis.

One of the particularly interesting features of long-term habituation in *Aplysia* is that, as in most forms of long-term learning in mammals, spaced trials are much more effective than massed ones for establishing a change that will last (Carew, Pinsker, and Kandel, 1972). The well-spaced occurrence of an environmental contingency of course provides some assurance that the contingency is not ephemeral, and this may provide an adaptive reason for the relative effectiveness of spaced learning trials. In any case, it will be interesting to see whether sensitivity to spacing is an intrinsic aspect of the intracellular mechanisms involved in consolidation. Particularly relevant in this context will be studies of the dynamics of synaptic stimulation-induced RNA synthesis in *Aplysia* neurons; there are already indications that such synthesis does not begin until about half an hour after transsynaptic stimulation is initiated (Peterson and Erulkar, 1973), which is commensurate with the observation that protein synthesis is not involved in short-term learning in *Aplysia*.

28.4 CONCLUSION

This essay has illustrated the use of invertebrate behavior

patterns that are mediated by definable neural circuitry for analyzing some simple learning phenomena. The power of the approach should be evident. However, the question of whether the sorts of long-term associative learning phenomena that interest us most will be found to occur in neural circuits that can be analyzed in this way remains open. Extrapolating from findings already on record, I believe that an affirmative answer is reasonably likely.

ACKNOWLEDGMENT

Preparation of this chapter was supported by USPHS Grant No. NS 8108. I wish to thank Joan Bryan, Andrew Kramer, Sun Hee Lee, and J. J. Wine for comments on the manuscript and access to unpublished data.

REFERENCES

ABRAHAM, F. D., and WILLOWS, A. O. D. 1972. Plasticity of a fixed action pattern in the sea slug *Tritonia diomedia*. *Communications in Behavioral Biology* A 6: 271–280.

ALLOWAY, T. M. 1969. Effects of low temperature upon acquisition and retention in the grain beetle, *Tenebrio molitor*. *Journal of Comparative and Physiological Psychology* 69: 1–8.

ALLOWAY, T. M. 1970. Methodological factors affecting the apparent effects of exposure to cold upon retention in the grain beetle, *Tenebrio molitor*. *Journal of Comparative and Physiological Psychology* 72: 311–317.

ATWOOD, H. L. 1967. Crustacean neuromuscular mechanisms. *American Zoologist* 7: 527–551.

ATWOOD, H. L., and BITTNER, G. D. 1971. Matching of excitatory and inhibitory inputs to crustacean muscle fibers. *Journal of Neurophysiology* 34: 157–170.

BAXTER, C. 1957. Habituation of the roach to puffs of air. *Anatomical Record* 128: 521.

BETHE, A. 1897. Vergleichende Untersuchungen über die Funktionen des Centralnerven Systems der Arthropoden. *Pfluegers Archiv für die Gesamte Physiologie des Menschen und der Tiere* 68: 449–545.

BETZ, W. J. 1970. Depression of transmitter release at the neuromuscular junction of the frog. *Journal of Physiology* 206: 629–644.

BRODWICK, M. S., and JUNGE, D. 1972. Post-stimulus hyperpolarization and slow potassium conductance increase in *Aplysia* giant neurone. *Journal of Physiology* 223: 549–570.

BROWN, B. M., and NOBLE, E. P. 1967. Cycloheximide and learning in the isolated cockroach ganglion. *Brain Research* 6: 363–366.

BRUNER, J., and KENNEDY, D. 1970. Habituation: Occurrence at a neuromuscular junction. *Science* 169: 92–94.

BULLOCK, T. H. 1945. Function of giant fibers in *Lumbricus*. *Journal of Neurophysiology* 8: 55–72.

BUREŠ, J., and BUREŠOVÁ, O. 1967. Plastic changes of unit activity based on reinforcing properties of extracellular stimulation of single neurons. *Journal of Neurophysiology* 30: 98–113.

BURROWS, M., and HOYLE, G. 1973. Neural mechanisms underlying behavior in the locust *Schistocera gregaria*. III. Topo-graphy of limb motoneurons in the metathoracic ganglion. *Journal of Neurobiology* 4: 167–186.

BURROWS, M., and ROWELL, C. H. F. 1973. Connections between descending visual interneurons and metathoracic motoneurons in the locust. *Journal of Comparative Physiology* 85: 221–234.

CAREW, T. J., CASTELLUCCI, V. F., and KANDEL, E. R. 1971. An analysis of dishabituation and sensitization of the gill-withdrawal reflex in *Aplysia*. *International Journal of Neuroscience* 2: 79–98.

CAREW, T. J., and KANDEL, E. R. 1973. Acquisition and retention of long-term habituation in *Aplysia*: Correlation of behavioral and cellular processes. *Science* 182: 1158–1160.

CAREW, T. J., and KANDEL, E. R. 1974. Synaptic analysis of the interrelationships between behavioral modifications in *Aplysia*. In M. V. L. Bennett, ed., *Synaptic Transmission and Neuronal Interaction*. New York: Raven Press, pp. 339–383.

CAREW, T. J., PINSKER, H. M., and KANDEL, E. R. 1972. Long-term habituation of a defensive withdrawal reflex in *Aplysia*. *Science* 175: 451–454.

CASTELLUCCI, V., and KANDEL, E. R. 1974. Further analysis of the synaptic decrement underlying habituation of the gill-withdrawal reflex in *Aplysia*. *Society for Neuroscience Fourth Annual Meeting*, Abstract no. 111.

CASTELLUCCI, V., KUPFERMANN, I., PINSKER, H., and KANDEL, E. R. 1970. Neuronal mechanisms of habituation and dishabituation of the gill withdrawal reflex in *Aplysia*. *Science* 167: 1445–1448.

CLARK, R. B. 1960a. Habituation of the polychaete *Neries* to sudden stimuli. I. General properties of the habituation process. *Animal Behaviour* 8: 82–91.

CLARK, R. B. 1960b. Habituation of the polychaete *Nereis* to sudden stimuli. II. The biological significance of habituation. *Animal Behaviour* 8: 92–103.

CORNING, W. C., DYAL, J. A., and WILLOWS, A. O. D., eds. 1973. *Invertebrate Learning*. Vol. 1: *Protozoans through Annelids*. Vol. 2: *Arthropods and Gastropod Mollusks*. Vol. 3: *Cephalopods and Echinoderms*. New York: Plenum Press.

DAGAN, D., and PARNAS, I. 1970. Giant fibre and small fibre pathways involved in the evasive response of the cockroach, *Periplaneta americana*. *Journal of Experimental Biology* 52: 313–324.

DEL CASTILLO, J., and KATZ, B. 1954. Statistical factors involved in neuromuscular facilitation and depression. *Journal of Physiology* 124: 574–585.

DONOSO, A. L., and FERNANDEZ, H. L. 1973. Effect of colchicine on long lasting synaptic modifications induced by hyperactivity. *Experientia* 29: 1089–1090.

DORSETT, D. A., WILLOWS, A. O. D., and HOYLE, G. 1973. The neuronal basis of behavior in *Tritonia*. IV. The central origin of a fixed action pattern in the isolated brain. *Journal of Neurobiology* 4: 287–300.

DUDEL, J., and KUFFLER, S. W. 1961. Presynaptic inhibition at the crayfish neuromuscular junction. *Journal of Physiology* 155: 543–562.

EISENSTEIN, E. M. 1972. Learning and memory in isolated insect ganglia. *Advances in Insect Physiology* 9: 111–181.

EISENSTEIN, E. M., and COHEN, M. J. 1965. Learning in an isolated insect ganglion. *Animal Behaviour* 13: 104–108.

ELUL, R. 1967. Fixed change in the cell membrane. *Journal of Physiology* 189: 351.

EVANS, S. M. 1963. The effect of brain extirpation on learning and retention in nereid polychaetes. *Animal Behaviour* 11: 172–178.

EVANS, S. M. 1966. Non-associative behavioral modifications in the polychaete *Nereis diversicolor*. *Animal Behaviour* 14: 107–112.

EVANS, S. M. 1969. Habituation of the withdrawal response in nereid polychaetes. 2. Rates of habituation in intact and decerebrate worms. *Biological Bulletin* 137: 105–117.

FELLER, W. 1950. *An Introduction to Probability Theory and its Applications*. New York: John Wiley & Sons.

GLASSMAN, E., HENDERSON, A., CORDLE, M., MOON, H. M., and WILSON, J. E. 1970. Effect of cycloheximide and actinomycin D on the behavior of the headless cockroach. *Nature* 225: 967–968.

GRIFFITH, J. S. 1966. A theory of the nature of memory. *Nature* 211: 1960.

GROVES, P. M., and LYNCH, G. S. 1972. Mechanisms of habituation of the brain stem. *Psychological Review* 79: 237–244.

GROVES, P. M., WILSON, C. J., and BOYLE, R. D. 1974. Brain stem pathways, cortical modulation, and habituation of the acoustic startle response. *Behavioral Biology* 10: 391–418.

GUNTHER, J. 1971. Microanatomy of the ventral cord of *Lumbricus terrestris* L. *Zeitschrift für Morphologie der Tiere* 70: 141–182.

GUNTHER, J. 1972. Giant motor neurons in the earthworm. *Comparative Biochemistry and Physiology* 42a: 967–973.

GUNTHER, J., and WALTHER, J. B. 1971. Functional anatomy of the dorsal giant fiber systems of *Lumbricus terrestris* L. *Zeitschrift für Morphologie der Tiere* 70: 254–280.

HAGIWARA, S. 1958. Synaptic potentials in the motor giant axon of the crayfish. *Journal of General Physiology* 41: 1119–1128.

HECK, L. 1920. Über die Bildung einer Assoziation biem Regenwurm auf Grund von Dressurversuchen. *Lotos* 68: 168–189.

HIGHSTEIN, S. M., and BENNETT, M. V. L. 1973. Fatigue of transmission at the Mauthner fiber–giant fiber synapses of the hatchet fish. *Society for Neurosciences 3rd Annual Meeting*, Abstract no. 47.7.

HORN, G., and ROWELL, C. H. F. 1968. Medium and long-term changes in the behavior of visual neurones in the tritocerebrum of locusts. *Journal of Experimental Biology* 49: 143–169.

HORRIDGE, G. A. 1959. Analysis of the rapid responses of *Nereis* and *Harmothoe* (Annelida). *Proceedings of the Royal Society (London)* B 150: 245–262.

HORRIDGE, G. A. 1962. Learning of leg position by the ventral nerve cord in headless insects. *Proceedings of the Royal Society (London)* B 157: 33–52.

HORRIDGE, G. A. 1963. Proprioceptors, bristle receptors, efferent sensory impulses, neurofibrils and number of axons in the parapodial nerve of the polychaete *Harmothoe*. *Proceedings of the Royal Society (London)* B 157: 199–222.

HORRIDGE, G. A. 1968. Five types of memory in crab eye responses. In F. Carlson, ed., *Physiological and Biochemical Aspects of Nervous Integration*. Englewood Cliffs, N. J.: Prentice Hall, pp. 245–265.

HOY, R. R. 1969. Degeneration and regeneration in abdominal flexor motor neurons in the crayfish. *Journal of Experimental Zoology* 172: 219–232.

HOY, R., BITTNER, G. D., and KENNEDY, D. 1967. Regeneration in crustacean motoneurons: Evidence for axonal fusion. *Science* 156: 251–252.

HOYLE, G. 1965. Neurophysiological studies on "learning" in headless insects. In J. E. Treherne and J. W. L. Beament, eds., *The Physiology of the Insect Central Nervous System*. New York: Academic Press, pp. 203–232.

HOYLE, G. 1973. Origin of behavioral rhythms in insect nervous systems. In J. Salanki, ed., *Neurobiology of Invertebrates. Mechanisms of Rhythm Regulation*. Budapest: Akademiai Kiado, pp. 233–247.

HOYLE, G., and BURROWS, M. 1973a. Neural mechanisms underlying behavior in the locust *Shistocerca gregaria*. I. Physiology of identified motoneurons in the metathoracic ganglion. *Journal of Neurobiology* 4: 3–41.

HOYLE, G., and BURROWS, M. 1973b. Neural mechanisms underlying behavior in the locust *Shistocerca gregaria*. II. Integrative activity in metathoracic neurons. *Journal of Neurobiology* 4: 43–67.

HOYLE, G., and WILLOWS, A. O. D. 1973. Neuronal basis of behavior in *Tritonia* II. Relationship of muscular contraction to nerve impulse pattern. *Journal of Neurobiology* 4: 239–254.

HUBBARD, J. I., LLINÁS, R., and QUASTEL, D. M. J. 1969. *Electrophysiological Analysis of Synaptic Transmission*. Baltimore: Williams & Wilkins.

HUGHES, G. M. 1965. Neuronal pathways in the insect central nervous system. In J. E. Treherne and J. W. L. Beament, eds., *The Physiology of the Insect Central Nervous System*. New York: Academic Press, pp. 79–112.

HUMPHREY, G. 1930. Extinction and negative adaption. *Psychological Review* 37: 361–363.

JACOBSON, A. L., FRIED, C., and HOROWITZ, S. D. 1967. Classical conditioning, pseudoconditioning, or sensitization in the planarian. *Journal of Comparative and Physiological Psychology* 64: 73–79.

JANSEN, J. K. S., and NICHOLLS, J. G. 1973. Conductance changes, an electrogenic pump and the hyperpolarization of leech neurones following impulses. *Journal of Physiology* 229: 635–655.

KANDEL, E. R. 1974. An invertebrate system for the cellular analysis of simple behaviors and their modifications. In F. O. Schmitt and F. G. Worden, eds., *The Neurosciences: Third Study Program*. Cambridge, Mass.: MIT Press, pp. 347–370.

KANDEL, E. R., CASTELLUCCI, V., PINSKER, H., and KUPFERMANN, I. 1970. The role of synaptic plasticity in the short-term modification of behavior. In G. Horn and R. A. Hinde, eds. *Short-term Changes in Neural Activity and Behaviour*. London: Cambridge University Press, pp. 281–322.

KANDEL, E. R., and TAUC, L. 1965. Heterosynaptic facilitation in neurons of the abdominal ganglion of *Aplysia depilans*. *Journal of Physiology* 181: 1–27.

KATZ, B., and MILEDI, R. 1968. The role of calcium in neuromuscular facilitation. *Journal of Physiology* 195: 481–492.

KATZ, B., and MILEDI, R. 1971. The effect of prolonged depolarization on synaptic transfer in the stellate ganglion of the squid. *Journal of Physiology* 216: 503–512.

KENNEDY, D. 1971. Crayfish interneurons. *Physiologist* 14: 5–30.

KENNEDY, D, CALABRESE, R., and WINE, J. 1974. Presynaptic inhibition: Primary afferent depolarization in crayfish neurons. *Science* 186: 451–454.

KERKUT, G. A., EMSON, P. C., and BEESLEY, P. W. 1972. Effect of leg-raising learning on protein synthesis and ChE activity in the cockroach CNS. *Comparative Biochemistry and Physiology* 41B: 635–645.

KERKUT, G. A., OLIVER, G. W. O., RICK, J. T., and WALKER, R. J. 1970. The effects of drugs on learning in a simple preparation. *Comparative General Pharmacology* 1: 437–483.

KRASNE, F. B. 1965. Escape from recurring tactile stimulation in *Branchiomma Vesiculosum*. *Journal of Experimental Biology* 42: 307–322.

KRASNE, F. B. 1969. Excitation and habituation of the crayfish escape reflex: The depolarizing response in lateral giant fibers of the isolated abdomen. *Journal of Experimental Biology* 50: 29–46.

KRASNE, F. B. 1973. Learning in Crustacea. In Corning, Dyal, and Willows (1973), Vol. 2, pp. 49–130.

KRASNE, F. B., and BRYAN, J. S. 1973. Habituation: Regulation through presynaptic inhibiton. *Science* 182: 590–592.

KRASNE, F. B., and ROBERTS, A. 1967. Habituation of crayfish escape response during release from inhibition induced by picrotoxin. *Nature* 215: 769–770.

KRASNE, F. B., and WINE, J. J. 1975. Extrinsic modulation of crayfish escape behavior. *Journal of Experimental Biology* (in press).

KRASNE, F. B., and WOODSMALL, K. S. 1969. Waning of the crayfish escape response as a result of repeated stimulation. *Animal Behaviour* 17: 416–424.

KUPFERMANN, I., CASTELLUCCI, V., PINSKER, H., and KANDEL, E. 1970. Neuronal correlates of habituation and dishabituation of the gill-withdrawal reflex in *Aplysia*. *Science* 167: 1743–1745.

KUPFERMANN, I., and KANDEL, E. R. 1969. Neural controls of a behavioral response mediated by the abdominal ganglion of *Aplysia*. *Science* 164: 847–850.

LANG, F., and ATWOOD, H. L. 1973. Crustacean neuromuscular mechanisms: Functional morphology of nerve terminals and the mechanism of facilitation. *American Zoologist* 13: 337–355.

LENNENBERG, E. H. 1967. *Biological Foundations of Language*. New York: John Wiley & Sons.

LUCO, J. V., and ARANDA, L. C. 1964a. An electrical correlate to the process of learning. Experiments in *Blatta orientialis*. *Nature* 201: 1330–1331.

LUCO, J. V., and ARANDA, L. C. 1964b. An electrical correlate to the process of learning. *Acta Physiologica Latino Americana* 14: 274–288.

LUCO, J. V., and ARANDA, J. C. 1966. Reversibility of an electrical correlate to the process of learning. *Nature* 209: 205–206.

MARTIN, A. R., and PILAR, G. 1963. Dual mode of synaptic transmission in the avian ciliary ganglion. *Journal of Physiology* 168: 443–463.

MARTIN, A. R., and PILAR, G. 1964. Presynaptic and postsynaptic events during post-tetanic potentiation and facilitation in the avian ciliary ganglion. *Journal of Physiology* 175: 17–30.

MCGAUGH, J. L. 1973. Drug facilitation of learning and memory. *Annual Review of Pharmacology* 13: 229–241.

MENZEL, R. 1968. On the honey bee's memory of spectral colours. I. Long-term and short-term retention. *Zeitschrift für Vergleichende Physiologie* 60: 82–102.

MIKHAILOFF, S. 1923. Expérience réflexologique: Expériences novelles sur *Pagurus striatus, Leander xiphiaas et treillianus*. Institute Océanographique, Monaco, *Bulletin*, no. 422.

MILNER, B. 1959. The memory defect in bilateral hippocampal lesions. *Psychiatric Research Reports* 11: 43–52.

MITTENTHAL, J. E., and WINE, J. J. 1973. Connectivity patterns of crayfish giant interneurons: Visualization of synaptic regions with cobalt dye. *Science* 179: 182–184.

MPITSOS, G. J., and DAVIS, W. J. 1973. Learning: Classical and avoidance conditioning in the mollusk *Pleurobranchaea*. *Science* 180: 317–321.

NASTUK, W. L. 1967. Activation and inactivation of muscle postjunctional receptors. *Federation Proceedings* 26: 1639–1646.

NICHOL, J. A. C. 1950. Responses of *Branchiomma vesiculosum* (Montagu) to photic stimulation. *Journal of the Marine Biological Association (United Kingdom)* 29: 303–320.

NICHOL, J. A. C. 1951. Giant axons and synergic contractions in *Branchiomma vesiculosum*. *Journal of Experimental Biology* 28: 22–31.

NICHOLLS, J. G., and PURVES, D. 1970. Monosynaptic chemical and electrical connexions between sensory and motor cells in the central nervous system of the leech. *Journal of Physiology* 209: 647–667.

NICHOLLS, J. G., and PURVES, D. 1972. A comparison of chemical and electrical synaptic transmission between single sensory cells and a motoneurone in the central nervous system of the leech. *Journal of Physiology* 225: 637–656.

O'SHEA, M., ROWELL, C. H. F., and WILLIAMS, J. L. D. 1974. The anatomy of a locust visual interneurone; the descending contralateral movement detector. *Journal of Experimental Biology* 60: 1–12.

PARNAS, I. 1972. Differential block at high frequency of branches of a single axon innervating two muscles. *Journal of Neurophysiology* 35: 903–914.

PARNAS, I., ARMSTRONG, D., and STRUMWASSER, F. 1974. Prolonged excitatory and inhibitory synaptic modulation of a bursting pacemaker neuron. *Journal of Neurophysiology* 37: 594–608.

PARNAS, I., and STRUMWASSER, F. 1974. Mechanisms of long-lasting inhibition of a bursting pacemaker neuron. *Journal of Neurophysiology* 37: 609–620.

PAVLOV, I. P. 1927. *Conditioned Reflexes*. New York: Dover Publications (reprint).

PERETZ, B., and HOWIESON, D. B. 1973. Central influence on peripherally mediated habituation of an *Aplysia* gill withdrawal response. *Journal of Comparative Physiology* 84: 1–18.

PETERSON, R. P., and ERULKAR, S. D. 1973. Parameters of stimulation of RNA synthesis and characterization by hybridization in a molluscan neuron. *Brain Research* 60: 177–190.

PINSKER, H. M., HENING, W. A., CAREW, T. J., and KANDEL, E. R. 1973. Long-term sensitization of a defensive withdrawal reflex in *Aplysia*. *Science* 182: 1039–1042.

PINSKER, H., KUPFERMANN, I., CASTELLUCCI, V., and KANDEL, E. 1970. Habituation and dishabituation of the gill-withdrawal reflex in *Aplysia*. *Science* 167: 1740–1742.

ROBERTS, A. 1968. Recurrent inhibition in the giant-fibre system of the crayfish and its effect on the excitability of the escape response. *Journal of Experimental Biology* 48: 545–567.

ROBERTS, M. B. V. 1962a. The giant fibre reflex of the earthworm, *Lumbricus terrestris* L. II. Fatigue. *Journal of Experimental Biology* 39: 229–237.

ROBERTS, M. B. V. 1962b. The rapid response of *Myxicola infundibulum* (Grube). *Journal of the Marine Biological Association (United Kingdom)* 42: 527–539.

ROBERTS, M. B. V. 1966. Facilitation in the rapid response of the earthworm, *Lumbricus terrestris* L. *Journal of Experimental Biology* 45: 141–150.

ROEDER, K. D. 1948. Organization of the ascending giant fibre system in the cockroach (*Periplaneta americana* L.) *Journal of Experimental Zoology* 108: 243–261.

ROWELL, C. H. F. 1971a. The orthopteran descending movement detector (DMD) neurones: A characterisation and review. *Zeitschrift für Vergleichende Physiologie* 73: 167–194.

ROWELL, C. H. F. 1971b. Variable responsiveness of a visual interneurone in the free-moving locust, and its relation to behavior and arousal. *Journal of Experimental Biology* 55: 727–747.

ROWELL, C. H. F. 1971c. Antennal cleaning, arousal, and visual interneurone responsiveness in a locust. *Journal of Experimental Biology* 55: 749–761.

RUSHTON, W. A. H. 1946. Reflex conduction in the giant fibers of the earthworm. *Proceedings of the Royal Society (London)* B 133: 109–120.

SCHWARTZ, J. H., CASTELLUCCI, V. F., and KANDEL, E. R. 1971. Functioning of identified neurons and synapses in abdominal ganglion of *Aplysia* in absence of protein synthesis. *Journal of Neurophysiology* 34: 939–954.

SHERMAN, R. G., and ATWOOD, H. L. 1971. Synaptic facilitation: Long-term neuromuscular facilitation in crustaceans. *Science* 171: 1248–1250.

SHERMAN, R. G., and ATWOOD, H. L. 1972. Correlated electrophysiological and ultrastructural studies of a crustacean motor unit. *Journal of General Physiology* 59: 586–615.

SOKOLOVE, P. L., and COOKE, I. M. 1971. Inhibition of impulse activity in a sensory neuron by an electrogenic pump. *Journal of General Physiology* 57: 125–163.

SPENCER, W. A., THOMPSON, R. F., and NEILSON, JR., D. R. 1966. Decrement of ventral root electrotonus and intracellularly recorded PSP's produced by iterated cutaneous afferent volleys. *Journal of Neurophysiology* 29: 253–274.

SPIRA, M. E., and BENNETT, M. V. L. 1971. Synaptic control of electrotonic coupling between neurons. *Brain Research* 37: 294–300.

STENT, G. S. 1973. A physiological mechanism for Hebb's postulate of learning. *Proceedings of the National Academy of Sciences (USA)* 70: 997–1001.

STEPHENS, C. L. 1973a. Relative contribution of synaptic and non-synaptic influences to response decrements in a postsynaptic neurone. *Journal of Experimental Biology* 59: 315–321.

STEPHENS, C. L. 1973b. Progressive decrements in the activity of *Aplysia* neurones following repeated intracellular stimulation: Implications for habituation. *Journal of Experimental Biology* 58: 411–422.

STUART, A. E. 1970. Physiological and morphological properties of motoneurones in the central nervous system of the leech. *Journal of Physiology* 209: 627–646.

TAKEDA, K., and KENNEDY, D. 1964. Soma potentials and modes of activation of crayfish motoneurons. *Journal of Cellular and Comparative Physiology* 64: 165–181.

TAKEUCHI, A. 1958. The long lasting depression in neuromuscular transmission of frog. *Japanese Journal of Physiology* 8: 102–113.

THIES, R. 1965. Neuromuscular depression and the apparent depletion of transmitter in mammalian muscle. *Journal of Neurophysiology* 28: 427–442.

THOMPSON, R. F., and SPENCER, W. A. 1966. Habituation: A model phenomenon for the study of neuronal substrates of behavior. *Psychological Review* 173: 16–43.

VAN ESSEN, D. C. 1973. The contribution of membrane hyperpolarization to adaptation and conduction block in sensory neurones of the leech. *Journal of Physiology* 230: 509–534.

VON FRISCH, K. 1953. *The Dancing Bees*. New York: Harcourt, Brace and Company.

WACHTEL, H., and KANDEL, E. R. 1971. Conversion of synaptic excitation to inhibition at a dual chemical synapse. *Journal of Neurophysiology* 34: 56–68.

WELLS, P. H. 1973. *Honey Bees*. In Corning, Dyal, and Willows (1973), Vol. 2, pp. 173–185.

WICKELGREN, B. 1967a. Habituation of spinal motoneurons. *Journal of Neurophysiology* 30: 1404–1423.

WICKELGREN, B. 1967b. Habituation of spinal interneurons. *Journal of Neurophysiology* 30: 1424–1438.

WIERSMA, C. A. G. 1947. Giant nerve fiber system of the crayfish. A contribution to comparative physiology of synapse. *Journal of Neurophysiology* 10: 23–38.

WILLOWS, A. O. D. 1973. Learning in gastropod mollusks. In Corning, Dyal, and Willows (1973), Vol. 2, pp. 187–273.

WILLOWS, A. O. D., DORSETT, D. A. and HOYLE, G. 1973a. The neuronal basis of behavior in *Tritonia*. I. Functional organization of the central nervous system. *Journal of Neurobiology* 4: 207–237.

WILLOWS, A. O. D., DORSETT, D. A., and HOYLE, G. 1973b. The neuronal basis of behavior in *Tritonia*. III. Neuronal mechanism of a fixed action pattern. *Journal of Neurobiology* 4: 255–285.

WILLOWS, A. O. D., and HOYLE, G. 1969. Neuronal network triggering a fixed action pattern, *Science* 166: 1549–1551.

WINE, J. J. 1971. Escape reflex circuit in crayfish: Interganglionic interneurons activated by the giant command neurons. *Biological Bulletin* 141: 408.

WINE, J. J. 1973. Invertebrate central neurons: Orthograde degeneration and retrograde changes after axonotomy. *Experimental Neurology* 38: 157–169.

WINE, J. J., and KRASNE, F. B. 1969. Independence of inhibition and habituation in the crayfish lateral giant fiber escape reflex. In *Proceedings of the 77th Annual Convention of the American Psychological Association*, pp. 237–238.

WINE, J. J., and KRASNE, F. B. 1972. The organization of escape behavior in the crayfish. *Journal of Experimental Biology* 56: 1–18.

WINE, J. J., KRASNE, F. B., and CHEN, L. 1975. Habituation and inhibition of the crayfish lateral giant fiber escape response. *Journal of Experimental Biology* 62: 771–782.

WOODY, C. D., and BLACK-CLEWORTH, P. 1973. Differences in exitability of cortical neurons as a function of motor projection in conditioned cats. *Journal of Neurophysiology* 36: 1104–1116.

WYERS, E. J., PEEKE, H. V. S., and HERZ, M. J. 1974. Partial reinforcement and resistance to extinction in the earthworm. *Journal of Comparative and Physiological Psychology* 57: 113–116.

YERKES, R. M. 1912. The intelligence of earthworms. *Journal of Animal Behavior* 2: 332–352.

YORK, B., WIERSMA, C. A. G., and YANAGISAWA, K. 1972a. Properties of the optokinetic motor fibers in the rock lobster: Build-up flip back, after discharge, and memory, shown by their firing patterns. *Journal of Experimental Biology* 57: 217.

YORK, B., YANAGISAWA, K., and WIERSMA, C. A. G. 1972b. Input sources and properties of position sensitive oculomotor fibers in the rock lobster, *Panulirus interruptus* (Randall). *Journal of Experimental Biology* 57: 229.

ZELLNER, D. K. 1966. Effects of removal and regeneration of the suprapharyngeal ganglion on learning, retention, extinction and negative movements in the earthworm *Lumbricus terrestris* L. *Physiology and Behavior* 1: 151–159.

ZILBER-GACHELIN, N. F., and CHARTIER, M. P. 1973a. Modification of the motor reflex responses due to repetition of the peripheral stimulus in the cockroach. I. Habituation at the level of an isolated abdominal ganglion. *Journal of Experimental Biology* 59: 359–381.

ZILBER-GACHELIN, N. F., and CHARTIER, M. P. 1973b. Modification of the motor reflex responses due to the repetition of the peripheral stimulus in the cockroach. II. Conditions on activation of the motoneurons. *Journal of Experimental Biology* 59: 383–403.

ZUCKER, R. S. 1973. Crayfish escape behavior and central synapses. I. Neural circuit exciting lateral giant fiber. II. Physiological mechanisms underlying behavioral habituation. III. Electrical junctions and dendritic spikes in fast flexor motoneurons. *Journal of Neurophysiology* 35: 599–651.

ZUCKER, R. S. 1973. Changes in the statistics of transmitter release during facilitation. *Journal of Physiology* 229: 787–810.

ZUCKER, R. S. 1974. Characteristics of crayfish neuromuscular facilitation and their calcium dependence. *Journal of Physiology* 241: 91–110.

ZUCKER, R. S., KENNEDY, D., and SELVERSTON, A. I. 1971. Neuronal circuit mediating escape responses in crayfish. *Science* 173: 645–650.

29

Plasticity in the Invertebrates

WILLIAM J. DAVIS

ABSTRACT Plasticity, the modification of a behavioral or neural output pattern that is produced by experience, is considered from the viewpoint of cellular analysis. Four forms of plasticity are reviewed: habituation, choice and its modification by experience, sensitization, and associative learning.

Habituation is a decrement in behavioral response caused by continuous or repeated stimulation of the same sensory pathway. Studies on both the crayfish tail-flip response and the gill-withdrawal reflex of *Aplysia* have shown that habituation is caused by a decrement in excitatory transmission at central synapses, due in turn, perhaps, to depletion of available transmitter substance.

The second form of plasticity that is reviewed is choice and its modification by experience. In the mollusc *Pleurobranchaea*, choice is dictated by a behavioral hierarchy, defined as the organization of unrelated acts of behavior into a priority sequence. Plasticity is shown by the modification of the behavioral hierarchy by experience, notably food satiation. Behavioral hierarchies may be widespread in the animal kingdom and may be related to psychological phenomena such as attention, selective perception, drive, and motivation. The neurophysiological mechanisms underlying behavioral hierarchies and their modification by experience are not yet known.

The third form of plasticity that is reviewed is sensitization, defined as an increase in the behavioral response to stimulation of one afferent pathway that is caused by activity in a second afferent pathway. The cellular basis of habituation has been analyzed in the gill-withdrawal reflex of *Aplysia* and has been shown to result from a synaptic process known as heterosynaptic facilitation. The same cellular process has been shown to underlie dishabituation. The physiological basis of heterosynaptic facilitation is unknown. Sensitization bears many similarities to, and may represent an evolutionary forerunner of, associative learning.

The fourth form of plasticity that is reviewed is associative learning, defined as a behavioral modification that is caused by reinforced experience; it is clearly distinct from nonassociative learning, which can occur without known reinforcement. Associative learning has been studied by classical and instrumental conditioning in a variety of invertebrates. The most successful demonstrations have involved the use of stimuli that are likely to be associable on ethological grounds in accordance with the "preparedness principle." Neurophysiological correlates of associative learning are not yet known, but promising beginnings have been made in studies of insects and molluscs. Possible cellular mechanisms underlying learning are discussed, and theoretical approaches to learning are summarized.

It is concluded that plasticity is ubiquitous in the animal kingdom, and that invertebrate studies have provided the first cellular explanations of simple forms of behavioral plasticity; that invertebrate studies will most likely provide the first insights into the cellular substrates of more complex forms of plasticity, including associative learning; and that such insights may have general application.

29.1 INTRODUCTION

In the course of evolution animals have been faced with an intriguing dilemma. If a species is to survive, then its members must be reasonably alike in form and function, if only to reproduce successfully. Such homogeneity requires that the genetic blueprint contain a reasonably rigid and stable set of developmental instructions. On the other hand, the survival of a species also requires that its members exhibit considerable behavioral adaptability to cope with the exigencies of day-to-day existence. The dilemma, then, is that a fixed genetic code must give rise to malleable behavioral strategies. The solution is as elegant as it is simple: the genetic code has acquired the capacity to produce an organism that is capable of altering its behavior on the basis of experience acquired during its lifetime. Such behavioral flexibility is termed *plasticity*.

In this article we shall consider plasticity from the viewpoint of cellular analysis. Attention will be focused on four forms of plasticity that can be studied on the cellular level: habituation, choice, sensitization, and associative learning. The conceptual framework for this review is derived largely from studies on vertebrate species, and in some areas, such as mnemochemistry,[1] the invertebrate data are indeed scant. There is now overwhelming evidence that plasticity is universal in the animal kingdom, however, and studies on invertebrate preparations have in fact already provided the first explanations of the cellular basis of simple forms of plasticity. Since the emphasis in this review is on cellular analysis, invertebrate animals, especially molluscs and arthropods, will receive the most complete coverage.

It is no accident that invertebrate preparations have provided the first cellular explanations of plasticity. These animals have a number of important advantages that make them especially suited to cellular analyses of plasticity. First, and prerequisite, invertebrates possess

WILLIAM J. DAVIS, The Thimann Laboratories, University of California, Santa Cruz

---

[1]From the Greek μνήμη (memory). I am indebted to Dr. Jeffrey L. Ram for suggesting this term.

interesting and complex behavioral repertoires that include even the most advanced forms of associative learning. Second, the absolute number of neurons in a typical invertebrate nervous system is small, from about ten thousand in a snail to one hundred thousand in a crayfish, compared to about 10^{10} neurons in the human nervous system. Neurophysiological investigations are correspondingly simplified. Third, unlike vertebrates, invertebrates possess a "distributed" intelligence; that is, their neurons are arranged in numerous discrete ganglia which are often homologous in structure and function (see Frontispiece). These "minibrains" may contain as few as nine neurons, but a more typical number is several hundred to a few thousand. Fourth, invertebrate nerve cells are often large and sometimes brightly pigmented, allowing easy visualization and penetration with stimulating and recording microelectrodes. Fifth, and especially useful, invertebrates possess *identifiable* nerve cells. That is, single neurons occupy the same positions and have the same synaptic connections in all members of a given species, allowing the physiologist multiple access to the "same" neuron. In this article we shall see how these many advantages of invertebrate nervous systems have contributed to cellular analyses of plasticity.

29.2 A DEFINITION OF PLASTICITY

The term plasticity has a long and complex history. It was first employed in the context of neuronal regeneration and development to describe the apparent ability of the nervous system to reorganize its central connections following limb transplantation (Weiss's 1941 hypothesis of myotypic specification; see Gaze, 1970, and Jacobson, 1970, for reviews). Recent experiments, however, suggest that the capacity for myotypic specification of neuronal connection may be limited or absent, at least during the ontogeny of an invertebrate motor system (Davis, 1973; Davis and Davis, 1973). Among invertebrates, the term plasticity was first applied to describe the adaptive modification of a crab's righting behavior that follows limb amputation or incapacitation (Bethe, 1930). In this context plasticity is a term that describes behavior. Subsequent authors, however, used the term to describe modifications of the activity of neuronal networks (e.g., Kristan and Gerstein, 1970; Kristan, 1971) or single nerve cells (e.g., Bureš and Burešová, 1967; see Bliss, Gardner-Medwin, and Lømo, 1973, for a review). In view of these precedents, we are obliged to define plasticity broadly as *a modification of a behavioral or neural output pattern that is acquired because of experience.*

It is important to emphasize that in this definition we are drawing a sharp distinction between *behavioral* plasticity and *neuronal* or *cellular* plasticity. Of course we have faith that the one underlies the other, but the distinction is nonetheless important, because none of the known examples of neuronal plasticity have demonstrated behavioral correlates. Conversely, most forms of behavioral plasticity are not yet understood at the cellular level. To use the same term (e.g., habituation) to describe both behavioral and neuronal events is therefore inappropriate, in that it implies an undemonstrated causal relationship between cellular and behavioral phenomena.

The general definition of plasticity offered above encompasses such an enormous range of complex behavioral and neuronal phenomena that it is bound to be unrestrictive. Applying the definition strictly, for example, qualifies enzyme induction in *E. coli* (Stent, 1967), as well as aging in humans, as forms of plasticity. The definition at least gives us a starting point; it is a necessary but insufficient criterion for plasticity. As will be elaborated in the remainder of this review, the definition can be made more explicit by characterizing the modification that we call plasticity, describing the nature of the experience that causes the modification, and, ultimately, discovering the underlying cellular mechanisms.

29.3 "SIMPLE" FORMS OF PLASTICITY

29.3.1 Habituation

DEFINITION AND CHARACTERISTICS. One of the simplest forms of behavioral plasticity, at least in terms of paradigm, is habituation, defined as a decrement in response that is caused by continuous or repeated stimulation of the same sensory pathway (see Hinde, 1970, for refinements). In terms of the general definition of plasticity offered above, the behavioral modification in habituation is response decrement, while the causal experience is repeated sensory stimulation. A habituated response can frequently be restored to its original amplitude by stimulating a second sensory pathway, a process that is called *dishabituation.*

Habituation has been defined from mammalian studies according to nine operational criteria, all of which involve behavioral rather than cellular measurements (Thompson and Spencer, 1966). Some invertebrate examples that exhibit some, but not all, of these criteria are nevertheless properly classified as habituation. Indeed, some of the nine classical criteria for habituation cannot be applied effectively even to other vertebrate species (e.g., Hinde, 1970; Wyers, Peeke, and Herz, 1973). To become preoccupied with the semantics of definition can obscure conceptual issues and impede the general understanding of mechanism that we seek (see, e.g., Bullock and Quarton, 1966, p. 258). As long as the major criteria for habituation, which certainly include response decrement and the capacity for dishabituation, are met, then an acceptable case for habituation can be made.

Although habituation was first employed as a behavioral term, subsequent investigators have used the term to describe a decrement in synaptic events occurring within central nerve cells (e.g., Bruner and Tauc, 1964, 1965, 1966; Bruner and Kehoe, 1970) or at peripheral neuromuscular junctions (Bruner and Kennedy, 1970). As implied in the preceding section, such dual usage carries the substantial risk of implying an unwarranted or at least undocumented causal connection between behavioral and cellular phenomena. Response decrements in central neurons, for example, could underlie dishabituation rather than habituation if such decrements occur in neurons that inhibit the habituated response. The criteria for demonstrating a causal relation between cellular and behavioral events are necessarily strict and difficult to apply rigorously, as elaborated below.

To term a decrement in response "habituation" requires information on the locus of the decrement. Habituation is generally considered a behavioral phenomenon whose causes lie within the central nervous system; hence, the possibilities of sensory adaptation and muscle fatigue must be eliminated. In the protozoan *Stentor*, for example, which has no central nervous system, "habituation" of a simple response to mechanical stimuli probably results from receptor adaptation (Wood, 1970a,b). In the mollusc *Pleurobranchaea*, habituation of a withdrawal response to light in part reflects sensory adaptation in the eye, although a decline in the responsiveness of central nervous pathways also contributes (Davis and Mpitsos, 1971). In the mollusc *Aplysia*, habituation of the siphon-withdrawal (Lukowiak and Jacklet, 1972) or gill-pinnule-withdrawal (Peretz, 1970) response to mechanical stimulation occurs even when the central nervous system is removed. Such "peripheral habituation" presumably occurs in the peripheral plexus of neurons known to characterize these molluscan motor systems (Peretz and Estes, 1975), but it can be influenced by events in the central nervous system (Peretz and Howieson, 1973). As will be elaborated below, habituation of the gill-withdrawal response of *Aplysia* has been shown to have a strong central component.

Use of the term "habituation" also presupposes a demonstration that the response decrement is selective, i.e., specific to the behavior that is under consideration. Controls for selectivity are especially crucial when the

habituation paradigm entails stimulation beyond that provided by the habituating stimulus. In *Pleurobranchaea*, for example, the feeding response to a jet of liquified squid directed on the oral veil wanes at an interstimulus interval of 1 min, even when sea water is substituted for food stimuli in the habituation paradigm. The "habituation" in this case apparently reflects no more than a nonspecific and unselective decline in responsiveness caused by the excessive mechanical stimulation that is unavoidably associated with making the measurements (Davis, Mpitsos, and Pinneo, 1974a). Generalization of habituation is a potentially interesting and important phenomenon which must be carefully distinguished from selective habituation. The best examples of habituation in invertebrates include controls for selectivity (e.g., Carew, Castellucci, and Kandel, 1971; Carew, Pinsker, and Kandel, 1972).

EXAMPLES OF HABITUATION. Habituation in invertebrates and vertebrates has been reviewed exhaustively in several recent books (Corning, Dyal, and Willows, 1973; Horn and Hinde, 1970; Peeke and Herz, 1973) and review articles (Eisenstein and Peretz, 1973; Kandel, 1974; Kandel and Kupfermann, 1970; Pakula and Sokolov, 1973; Willows, 1973); this substantially lightens my present task. The extensive literature comprises studies of habituation in virtually all of the invertebrate phyla and groups and includes studies on both short-term habituation, lasting seconds to minutes, and long-term habituation, lasting hours to weeks (e.g., Carew, Pinsker, and Kandel, 1971; Carew and Kandel, 1973; Westerman, 1963); studies on behavioral habituation resulting from central mechanisms (e.g., Kupfermann et al., 1970) and from a variety of peripheral causes (e.g., Davis and Mpitsos, 1971; Peretz, 1970); and neurophysiological analyses of habituation (e.g., Davis and Mpitsos, 1971; Horridge, 1959; Roberts, 1962; Zilber-Gachelin and Chartier, 1973a,b). The most complete information on the cellular mechanisms underlying behavioral habituation has resulted from studies on two behaviors: the crayfish tail-flip escape response (Krasne, 1969; Krasne and Bryan, 1973; Krasne and Roberts, 1967; Krasne and Woodsmall, 1969; Wine, 1971; Wine and Krasne, 1969, 1972; Zucker, 1972a-c; Zucker, Kennedy, and Selverston, 1971) and the gill-withdrawal reflex of *Aplysia*. The crayfish example is reviewed in this volume by Krasne, and hence I shall deal mainly with the *Aplysia* example (see Kandel, 1974, for a recent review).

Touching the siphon of *Aplysia* causes a gill-withdrawal response which declines in amplitude with repeated stimuli. The response can be fully restored—dishabituated—by stimulating a different area of the body (Pinsker et al., 1970). The neuronal circuitry that controls the withdrawal response consists of identified sensory neurons, interneurons, and motoneurons located in the abdominal ganglion (Kupfermann et al., 1971; Kupfermann and Kandel, 1969; Peretz, 1969). In a semi-intact preparation, a decrease in the size of the complex excitatory postsynaptic potential (EPSP) recorded from an identified gill-withdrawal motoneuron, L7, invariably accompanied the behavioral habituation of the gill-withdrawal response (Kupfermann et al., 1970; for related studies see Pinsker et al., 1970; Carew, Castellucci, and Kandel, 1971; Carew and Kandel, 1973; Carew, Pinsker, and Kandel, 1972; Kandel et al., 1970; Castellucci et al., 1970). The decrement in EPSP amplitude also occurred in the isolated abdominal ganglion in response to repeated electrical stimulation of the appropriate sensory nerve, presumably corresponding to behavioral habituation; in this case the EPSP could be restored by electrically stimulating another nerve, presumably corresponding to dishabituation (Carew, Castellucci, and Kandel, 1971; Castellucci et al., 1970).

CELLULAR MECHANISMS UNDERLYING HABITUATION. It has long been speculated that the central nervous component of habituation results from a progressive augmentation of inhibitory influences upon the participating neurons (Pavlov, 1927; Holmgren and Frenk, 1961). Some authors apparently regard it as axiomatic that habituation involves an active inhibitory process (e.g., Wyers, Peeke, and Herz, 1973, p. 4). Available data, however, do not support this view. In the *Aplysia* gill-withdrawal preparation the data suggest that habituation results from homosynaptic depression of excitatory synaptic transmission to the participating motoneurons, while dishabituation results from heterosynaptic facilitation of the input to motoneurons (Castellucci et al., 1970). Recent work suggests the possibility of a post-synaptic contribution to habituation in *Aplysia* (Stephens, 1973). Habituation in the gill-withdrawal preparation is not blocked by the application of substances that can inhibit 95 percent of protein synthesis for as long as 30 hr (Schwartz, Castellucci, and Kandel, 1971). Therefore, this simple and relatively short-term form of plasticity, at least, is apparently not directly dependent upon macromolecular synthesis. It remains to be determined whether long-term habituation of the gill-withdrawal response (Carew, Pinsker, and Kandel, 1972) can be influenced by inhibitors of protein synthesis.

Cellular analysis of the crayfish tail-flip escape response also suggests that a decrement in excitatory synaptic transmission, rather than an increment in inhibitory transmission, is the cause of behavioral habituation. Picrotoxin, a substance presumed to block the action of inhibitory transmitter substances, does not eliminate habituation of the tail-flip escape response (Krasne and Roberts, 1967). Moreover, Zucker has directly demonstrated that the habituation of this response can be attributed to a decline in the efficacy of excitatory synaptic transmission (Zucker, 1972a–c). This decline presumably results from a depletion of the transmitter substance involved in carrying messages from the presynaptic terminals of primary afferent inputs to identified interneurons and motoneurons that participate in the behavior (Zucker, 1972a–c; Zucker, Kennedy, and Selverston, 1971). The only demonstrated role for inhibition is to *prevent* habituation by blocking transmitter release at habituation-prone interneuronal synapses during non-escape swimming (Krasne and Bryan, 1973; see also Krasne, this volume).

In both the *Aplysia* and crayfish examples, then, the evidence suggests that behavioral habituation results from a decline in the efficacy of excitatory synaptic transmission in central nervous pathways. This conclusion is necessarily based on correlation between cellular and behavioral data, and it is therefore unavoidably circumstantial, since correlation need not imply causality. In an epistemological sense, however, causality is defined by perfect correlation. In identifying the cellular causes of behavioral plasticity, we can probably do no better than to identify neurons that control the behavior, and then show that these neurons undergo appropriate changes in physiological activity when behavioral plasticity takes place. By these criteria, the hypothesis that the cellular cause of habituation is a response decrement in central nerve cells is adequately documented.

It remains, of course, to discover what causes this decrement in neuronal activity. Recent evidence obtained from the parabolic burster neuron (R15) of *Aplysia* suggests that short-term depression of a unitary EPSP is caused by depletion of a relatively small pool of transmitter substance available for release (Schlapfer et al., 1974). Depletion of transmitter at a rate more rapid than that of replacement is a reasonable but untested candidate hypothesis for behavioral habituation.

There is no generally accepted term for the converse of habituation, i.e., an increment in response caused by repeated stimulation. The term *sensitization* has been used in this sense, but I think this term should be defined more narrowly (see Section 29.3.3). The term *facilitation* has been used to describe the increase in amplitude of a sea anemone's withdrawal response on repeated stimulation (Pantin, 1935), although the same term was applied earlier to neuronal transactions (Lucas, 1917) and is still used to describe an increase in the amplitude of excitatory or inhibitory postsynaptic potentials on repetition. In anemones, a facilitation that is retained over a period of several days has been reported (Wilson, 1959) but has not been found under more carefully controlled conditions (Hoyle, 1960; Ross and Sutton, 1964). Such long-term facilitation has a time course resembling that of learning, but is fundamentally different in paradigm.

Is habituation learning? Habituation originally excited interest not only because it has obvious adaptive value to an organism, but also because it might be considered a simple form of learning. Many authors have subsequently considered habituation in this context (e.g., Applewhite and Gardner, 1971; Eisenstein and Peretz, 1973; Thorpe, 1963; Wyers, Peeke, and Herz, 1973; Willows, 1973; and the most systematic treatment, Petrinovich, 1973).

It is true that habituation always involves a decrease in response, while learning may involve either a decrease or an increase, but this difference need not be troublesome, since the increase in behavioral response that occurs during learning could result from a decrease in the response of inhibitory neurons controlling the behavior. Moreover, there are several more direct parallels between habituation and learning. For example, habituation of the gill-withdrawal response of *Aplysia* can last for several days to weeks (Carew and Kandel, 1973; Carew, Pinsker, and Kandel, 1972), a time course similar to that of learning. Neither short-term learning nor short-term habituation of the gill-withdrawal reflex (Schwartz, Castellucci, and Kandel, 1971) depends upon protein synthesis. Other similarities between habituation and learning are reviewed by Petrinovich (1973).

The above parallels, although undeniable, seem to me unpersuasive in view of the fundamental paradigmatic difference between habituation and learning. The most intriguing and characteristic property of learning is *association*, i.e., the capacity of an organism to form a demonstrable connection between two unrelated and previously unconnected stimuli, one of which is therefore termed reinforcing. The paradigm for habituation excludes the possibility of such association, since only one stimulus is delivered repeatedly. Some investigators argue that the absence of reinforcement in a habituation paradigm in itself constitutes reinforcement (Wyers, Herz, and Peeke, 1973), and it is true that habituation does resemble a form of learning, called temporal conditioning (see p.442), in which absence of reinforcement can be considered a form of reinforcement. Speculation aside, the fact is that we do not yet know the cellular mechanism underlying learning, and until we do, we shall not know the relation between habituation and learning. It is, however, certainly safe to say that most students of plasticity will be disappointed if associative learning involves no more than a depletion of transmitter substance from central synapses.

Even if habituation and learning are unrelated forms of plasticity, cellular studies on habituation in *Aplysia* and in the crayfish have provided two immensely important general lessons for students of plasticity. First, in both cases the dramatic success of the analysis has depended crucially on both carefully controlled behavioral studies and comprehensive neurophysiological information concerning the underlying neuronal circuitry. A combination of these two different but complementary approaches would seem indispensable to cellular analyses of plasticity. Second, studies of habituation in both *Aplysia* and the crayfish have proved that this simple form of plasticity, at least, is entirely tractable to microelectrode analysis at the level of the single nerve cell. This encouraging precedent is of enormous importance to those who seek to understand the cellular basis of more complex forms of plasticity, including learning.

29.3.2 Choice (behavioral hierarchies)

Definition and characteristics. A new form of behavioral plasticity has recently been identified in the carnivorous marine mollusc *Pleurobranchaea*, involving a *behavioral hierarchy* (Davis, Mpitsos, and Pinneo, 1974a,b; Davis et al., 1976a,b). A behavioral hierarchy is defined as the organization of unrelated acts of behavior into a priority sequence that governs behavioral choices. A behavioral hierarchy is demonstrated by a *choice paradigm*, defined as the simultaneous presentation of the releasing stimuli for two different behavioral acts at comparable stimulus strengths. If the animal performs one of the two possible behavioral acts to the partial or complete exclusion of the other, then a behavioral choice has been made in favor of the dominant behavior, and a behavioral hierarchy has been demonstrated.

A behavioral hierarchy is not itself a form of plasticity since it is not associated with an *acquired* modification in behavior. The behavioral hierarchy of *Pleurobranchaea* can be modified by experience, however, and this modification persists for many days after the causal experience. It is in this sense that behavioral hierarchies are relevant to the topic of plasticity.

Examples of choice. The elementary unit of a behavioral hierarchy is a pair of unrelated behavioral acts, one of which takes precedence over the other. For example, *Pleurobranchaea* normally rights itself in 20 sec when turned onto its back, and it normally feeds voraciously when given raw squid or when liquified squid is squirted onto the chemosensory oral veil. If a specimen is inverted and then fed, however, it remains on its back until feeding is completed—in extreme cases, for more than an hour (Davis and Mpitsos, 1971). Righting behavior can also be interrupted by an application of liquified squid, but not sea water, to the oral veil, showing that the chemosensory component of the stimulus mediates the effect (Davis, Mpitsos, and Pinneo, 1974a).

The above results show that feeding behavior is dominant over righting behavior in *Pleurobranchaea*. Feeding also dominates other behavioral acts, including withdrawal of the head and oral veil from tactile stimuli, and mating behavior. For example, quantified tactile stimulation of the oral veil normally causes vigorous withdrawal of the anterior end of the animal. At an interstimulus interval of 1 min, this response does not habituate over several trials, unlike the gill-withdrawal response of *Aplysia*. When the tactile stimulus is accompanied by a presentation of food (raw squid) or an application of liquified squid, however, withdrawal of the head and oral veil is strongly suppressed (Davis et al., 1975a,b). Thus feeding behavior dominates the withdrawal response, presumably guaranteeing that the animals do not pull away from the tactile stimulation associated with food. This effect is highly selective in that the local withdrawal of other parts of the body is not affected by the presence of food stimuli.

Although feeding is normally a dominant behavior in *Pleurobranchaea*, specimens are reluctant to feed when they are laying eggs. Previous work on a closely related gastropod, *Aplysia*, has shown that egg-laying is induced by a hormone contained in "bag cells" within the central nervous system (Kupfermann, 1967, 1970; Strumwasser, Jacklet, and Alvarez, 1969; Toevs and Brackenbury, 1969). Experiments on *Pleurobranchaea* have shown that both egg-laying and the associated suppression of feeding are mediated hormonally, perhaps by the same hormone(s) (Davis, Mpitsos, and Pinneo, 1974b). Therefore, egg-laying occupies a higher position than feeding in the behavioral hierarchy of *Pleurobranchaea*, and it maintains this dominant position hormonally. By this mechanism these voracious carnivores are presumably prevented from eating their own eggs. Only the swimming escape response occupies a higher position than egg-laying in the behavioral hierarchy of *Pleurobranchaea*; indeed, swimming interrupts all other behavioral acts.

The behavioral hierarchy of *Pleurobranchaea* is normally quite stable, but it can be modified by subjecting the animal to various forms of experience. The experience that has been studied most carefully to date is satiation with food. The feeding response threshold of satiated specimens is much higher than that of nonsatiated animals, yet righting behavior is still interrupted or delayed by the application of food stimuli to satiated specimens. In contrast, withdrawal behavior, which is normally suppressed by the application of food stimuli, is unaffected by food stimuli after the animals are satiated (Davis et al., 1975a). Similarly, during egg-laying the dominance of "feeding" over righting is maintained, but the dominance of feeding over withdrawal is abolished (Davis et al., 1975b). Preliminary experiments indicate that the hierarchy can also be modified by conditioning.

The concept of behavioral hierarchy is too new to permit assessment of its generality. There are indications in the literature, however, that such hierarchies may be widespread. Bacteria presented simultaneously with attractant and repellent chemicals "choose" to respond to whichever one is present in more effective concentrations (Adler and Tso, 1974). In the coelenterate *Hydra* the contraction that is normally caused by mechanical stimulation is inhibited in the presence of food (live brine shrimp) or in the presence of glutathione, a substance that induces feeding behavior (Rushforth, Krohn, and Brown 1964; Rushforth, 1973). Thus in *Hydra*, as in *Pleurobranchaea*, feeding appears to dominate withdrawal from tactile stimulation. Similarly, when the escape response of the sea anemone is elicited by aversive stimuli, "all other stimuli become of secondary importance" (Ross, 1965, p. 53). Thus in these coelenterates, as in *Pleurobranchaea*, escape responses apparently take precedence over all other forms of behavior. Wild pigeons also exhibit "choice" in their natural habitats, and this choice can be predictably modified by reinforcement (Baum, 1974).

Differential attentiveness to sensory stimuli, such as may be said to underlie the behavioral hierarchy of *Pleurobranchaea*, has also been examined in flying locusts, where facilitating rather than competing interactions between different motor systems are involved. Changes in wind angle evoke course-correcting reflexes, but only if the insect is actually flying. Nonflying insects do not respond to the identical stimulus. In this case, then, "attentiveness" to sensory stimuli is apparently controlled by a central nervous "switch" or "gate" that is activated by the central flight motor (Camhi, 1970a,b; Camhi and Hinkle, 1972).

The behavioral-hierarchy concept bears some resemblance to Hull's (1943) concept of a habit family, in which different behavioral acts are seen as having different habit strengths. In Hull's formulation, habit strength ($_sH_R$) is a product of interaction between external stimuli from the environment (S_E), including experimental operations such as reinforcement, and internal stimuli, i.e., drives (S_D). Different drives are held to have different "motivational values," much as different behavioral acts in *Pleurobranchaea* occupy different positions in the behavioral hierarchy.

The fundamental difference between Hull's habit family and the behavioral hierarchy is that the former is a theoretical construct, formulated in order to quantify learning theory. As pointed out by Kimble (1967), the theory has little or no factual basis. In contrast, a behavioral hierarchy is an empirical concept, inextricably related to an explicit operational procedure (the choice paradigm). Although a behavioral hierarchy can be *modified* by experience, its existence is presumed to be independent of the organism's learning history.

A behavioral hierarchy implies that an animal "chooses" to perform one behavioral act rather than another when the stimuli for both are present. In an operational sense this kind of choice is indistinguishable from choice in higher animals, including ourselves. Indeed, the phenomenon of behavioral choice bears an obvious paradigmatic relationship to psychological concepts such as attention or selective perception (Hillyard et al., 1973; Horn, 1965; McFarland, 1966) and drive or motivation (Hinde, 1960; Kupfermann, 1974; McFarland and Sibly, 1972). Future research may well reveal that these terms simply represent diverse expressions, both ethological and psychological, of the same basic phenomena. The advantages of the behavioral-hierarchy concept are that it exhibits plasticity, it is operationally explicit, and it is amenable to analysis at the cellular level.

CELLULAR MECHANISMS UNDERLYING CHOICE. The neuronal substrates of behavioral choice are not yet known, but important clues are provided by behavioral observations. When *Pleurobranchaea* is sated, presentation of liquified squid usually fails to elicit the feeding behavior, but the same stimulus nevertheless suppresses righting behavior (Davis et al., 1976a). Therefore, it would appear that this form of choice is, at least in part, programmed at an early stage in central processing. The chemosensory input that elicits the dominant behavior (feeding) may directly inhibit the neurons that cause the subordinate behavior (righting). In contrast, when *Pleurobranchaea* is sated, the dominance of feeding behavior over local withdrawal of the head and oral veil is abolished (Davis et al., 1976a). Since reduced feeding activity accompanies satiation, we may speculate that the execution of the feeding behavior is necessary to the suppression of the withdrawal response to touch. In other words, this aspect of the behavioral hierarchy may be, at least in part, programmed at a later stage in central processing. Perhaps the central interneurons that control the dominant behavior (feeding) directly inhibit neurons that control the subordinate

behavior (withdrawal). The plasticity exhibited by the hierarchy may result simply from the influence of satiation receptors on neurons that mediate withdrawal behavior. Further neurophysiological experimentation is needed to test these hypotheses.

29.3.3 Sensitization

DEFINITION AND CHARACTERISTICS. When a dishabituating stimulus causes an increase in a habituated response to *supra*control levels, sensitization is said to have occurred (Thompson and Spencer, 1966). Sensitization can occur also in the absence of habituation, leading to the more general definition of sensitization as an increase in a response to stimulation of one afferent pathway caused by activity in a second afferent pathway. In terms of the general definition of plasticity offered earlier, the behavioral modification is an increase in response amplitude, while the causal experience is previous, but not necessarily contiguous, activity in a different sensory pathway. Sensitization is thus seen as a kind of "arousal."

Sensitization has frequently been treated as a relatively minor form of behavioral plasticity. Indeed, most examples of sensitization have been discovered simply as a by-product of control experiments for a learning paradigm (e.g., Abraham and Willows, 1972; Wells and Wells, 1971). It is now generally recognized that sensitization is itself an ethologically significant form of plasticity (Wells and Wells, 1971; Dyal and Corning, 1973) and may even bear an important mechanistic relationship to associative learning (see p. 438).

EXAMPLES OF SENSITIZATION. Sensitization has been demonstrated in several invertebrate phyla, including annelids (Evans, 1966a–c), insects (Nelson, 1971), and molluscs (e.g., Pinsker et al., 1973). In the blowfly *Phormia*, for example, stimulation of a single chemoreceptive hair on the mouth parts with sugar solution "arouses" the animal, increasing the likelihood that a normally neutral chemical stimulus delivered to a different sensory hair will cause the feeding response—extension of the proboscis (Dethier, Solomon, and Turner, 1965, 1968). This arousal, interpreted as the production of a "central excitatory state" (CES), is indistinguishable from sensitization.

The most deliberate analysis of sensitization has been performed on the mollusc *Aplysia*. Tactile stimulation of the siphon, which is located on the posterior rim of the mantle shelf, causes the gill to withdraw. Tactile stimulation of the purple gland, on the anterior rim of the mantle shelf, also causes the gill to withdraw. The amplitude of the gill-withdrawal response to either stimulus is larger if the other stimulus has preceded it. In other words, the withdrawal response shows sensitization (Carew, Castellucci, and Kandel, 1971). If either stimulus is delivered repeatedly, the resulting gill-withdrawal response habituates, without, however, altering the response to the other tactile stimulus. A third stimulus that dishabituates the habituated reflex simultaneously sensitizes the unhabituated reflex, providing behavioral evidence that dishabituation and sensitization are manifestations of the same excitatory mechanism (Carew, Castellucci, and Kandel, 1971). According to this interpretation, dishabituation differs from sensitization only in that dishabituation involves a previously habituated response.

Tactile stimulation of the siphon not only causes the gill to withdraw, but also causes the withdrawal of the siphon itself. This siphon-withdrawal response can be sensitized by tactile stimulation of a different mantle region. Removal of the abdominal ganglion promptly and completely abolishes the effects of prior sensitization training, showing that the sensitization is mediated by this ganglion (Pinsker et al., 1973). Sensitization of this siphon withdrawal is retained for longer than three weeks, a time course resembling that of learned behavior (Pinsker et al., 1973).

CELLULAR MECHANISMS UNDERLYING SENSITIZATION. The neural correlates of both dishabituation and short-term sensitization have been studied in *Aplysia* by making intracellular recordings from one of the two major identified motoneurons in the abdominal ganglion that mediate withdrawal of the gill. As might be expected from the behavioral observations described above, this motoneuron receives afferent information from the posterior siphon, via the siphon nerve, and also from the anterior purple gland, via the brachial verve. Stimulation of either the siphon or the brachial nerve causes a complex EPSP in the motoneuron. This EPSP decrements with repeated stimulation, paralleling the behavioral habituation described above. Electrical stimulation of the nerve connective leading from the head ganglia to the abdominal ganglion restores such a decremented EPSP to its original amplitude, and at the same time facilitates a nondecremented EPSP to supracontrol levels (Carew, Castellucci, and Kandel, 1971; Castellucci, Kandel, and Schwartz, 1972; Castellucci et al., 1970). In other words, electrical stimulation of the connective represents a "sensitizing" stimulus which increases the size of the EPSP caused by stimulation of either the siphon nerve or the brachial nerve, by the cellular mechanism of heterosynaptic facilitation.

Heterosynaptic facilitation was first studied by Kandel and Tauc in a giant neuron of unknown behavioral function in *Aplysia* (Kandel and Tauc, 1964, 1965a,b); it has since been analyzed in more detail by several investigators (von Baumgarten and Djahanparwar, 1967; von Baumgarten and Hukuhara, 1969; Epstein and Tauc, 1970; Haigler and von Baumgarten, 1972; Tauc and Epstein, 1967). All of these studies have been performed on molluscs, and all share an important ambiguity. A rigorous demonstration of heterosynaptic facilitation requires proof that activity in one neuronal pathway facilitates the response to activity in a second, *discrete* neuronal pathway. None of the existing analyses of heterosynaptic facilitation clearly eliminates the possibility that the "second" pathway is comprised partly or wholly of neurons from the first pathway. Such redundancy could arise through synaptic interactions between neurons in the two pathways, or through the axonal branching that is known to characterize molluscan nervous systems. If this is the case, then the observed heterosynaptic facilitation may simply represent homosynaptic facilitation, or posttetanic potentiation. The experiments of Tauc and Epstein (1967) and Epstein and Tauc (1970) were addressed to this question, and they showed that the time courses of heterosynaptic facilitation and posttetanic potentiation are different. The experimental design left many unresolved questions, however, and in any case the argument was circumstantial.

Studies on the gill-withdrawal reflex of *Aplysia* are more persuasive, since separate sensory pathways were stimulated to cause the observed heterosynaptic facilitation. In this case, as in the preceding examples, direct depolarization of the neuron exhibiting the facilitated response revealed no parallel change in the conductance of its membrane; hence, heterosynaptic facilitation is not caused by a change in membrane properties of the facilitated neuron, but is instead a presynaptic phenomenon. In the gill-withdrawal reflex it seems likely that heterosynaptic facilitation occurs because the excitatory synapses of presynaptic afferent neurons are, via an unknown mechanism(s), made more efficacious by the sensitizing stimulus (Carew, Castellucci, and Kandel, 1971). Ambiguities remain, however; for example, it has been shown that molluscan tactile sensory neurons can have axonal branches in more than one peripheral nerve (Siegler, Mpitsos, and Davis, 1974), a circumstance that could complicate distinction between heterosynaptic facilitation and posttetanic potentiation. To provide an unambiguous demonstration of heterosynaptic facilitation, and to study the underlying physiological mechanisms, a preparation is needed that consists of three identifiable neurons, all of which can be impaled with stimulating and recording microelectrodes, and two of which show heterosynaptic facilitation of unitary EPSPs on the third. Such an ideal preparation has not yet been dircovered.

Is SENSITIZATION LEARNING? In an operational sense, sensitization resembles associative learning, in that the activity of one afferent pathway facilitates the response to activity in a second pathway. Sensitization differs from most examples of associative learning in that temporal contiguity of the two stimuli is not prerequisite to the behavioral modification. Some behavioral modifications that are accepted as examples of associative learning, however, do not involve temporal contiguity of the two stimuli. In the phenomenon of bait shyness, or Garcia conditioning, for example, learning may take place even when reinforcement is delayed by an hour or more (see Section 29.4.2). Moreover, for many neurons in *Aplysia* the optimum interval of 350 msec between sensitizing and test stimuli produces the strongest and most persistent heterosynaptic facilitation (von Baumgarten and Hukuhara, 1969). The finding of such an optimum interval is reminiscent of the optimum interval of about 0.5 sec in many classical-conditioning paradigms. Finally, it has been shown that sensitization of the gill-withdrawal reflex of *Aplysia* is retained for longer than three weeks (Pinsker et al., 1973), a time course similar to that of learned behavior.

These many similarities between sensitization and learning suggest the possibility that they are mediated by related or even identical cellular mechanisms. Even if sensitization and learning are distinct in terms of mechanisms, sensitization may well represent an evolutionary precursor to true associative learning (Wells, 1968; Razran, 1971), in which case cellular analyses of sensitization should provide insights into the mechanisms underlying learning. As in the case of the relationship between habituation and learning, however, we shall not know the true relationship between sensitization and learning until the cellular basis of learning is understood.

29.4 LEARNING

29.4.1 Associative versus nonassociative learning

Associative learning is an advanced and intriguing form of plasticity in which the temporal contiguity between two events causes an animal to form a demonstrable association between those events. According to the most prevalent theory, the formation of such an association empirically demonstrates that one of the two events has value as a *reinforcer* (Gormezano and Moore, 1969; Hilgard, 1964; Hilgard and Bower, 1966; Kimble, 1961, 1967; Livingston, 1967; Premack, 1959). In an anthropomorphic sense, reinforcement may be considered as the

reward (positive reinforcement) or punishment (negative reinforcement) that necessarily underlies associative learning (see Livingston, 1967, for a cogent discussion of reinforcement). In this context, associative learning may be defined briefly as a behavioral modification caused by reinforced experience. In terms of our general definition of plasticity, the behavioral modification is the acquisition (if the reinforcement is positive) or suppression (if the reinforcement is negative) of a behavioral pattern, while the causal experience is the temporal contiguity of two events, one of which is reinforcing. Different forms of associative learning can then be defined in terms of the characteristics of, and temporal relation between, the two events.

Not all learning requires reinforcement. For example, a rat learns something from running a maze even when electrical shock or food is absent, as shown by the small number of errors made when reinforcement is later introduced (Blodgett, 1929). This phenomenon of "latent learning," or "incidental learning" (Hebb, 1949), is just one example of learning that occurs without reinforcement. An analogous capability is shown by spiders, which can "memorize" a pathway from the web to the retreat without apparent reinforcement (see Lahue, 1973), and bees, which may employ unreinforced learning during foraging behavior (Wells and Wenner, 1973; Wells, 1973). Similarly, certain marine molluscs exhibit homing behavior (Gelperin, 1974), which may have an unreinforced learning component (Willows, 1973). In higher organisms, including humans, efforts to identify reinforcement in language learning, place learning, and the learning of spatial relationships have failed. Clearly, then, there are many forms of plasticity that qualify as learning even though reinforcement is absent. Such learning may be termed *nonassociative learning*.

It is presently impossible to define nonassociative learning rigorously in a way that excludes simpler forms of plasticity, such as habituation, and for this reason many workers prefer to consider habituation as a form of nonassociative learning. All of the examples of nonassociative learning listed above, however, share in common one phenomenon—memory. Assuming that the physiological basis of memory differs from that of habituation, which seems likely, it may eventually prove possible to define nonassociative learning uniquely on this basis. Such a distinction will have to await a better understanding of the physiological mechanisms of memory.

In addition to, or perhaps because of, the difficulty of defining nonassociative learning clearly, the phenomenon seems, for the present, entirely elusive from the viewpoint of cellular analysis. Therefore, even though nonassociative learning may be the most advanced form of learning in a cognitive sense, the following discussion will be confined to associative learning, which is more tractable to neurophysiological analysis. It is probably safe to assume that the cellular mechanisms underlying both types of learning share at least some features in common.

Before discussing the data from specific experiments on associative learning, a review of some basic terminology will be helpful (see also Dyal and Corning, 1973). *Conditioning*, the experimental procedure by which associative learning is usually demonstrated in a laboratory setting, takes two basic forms—classical conditioning (Type I or Pavlovian conditioning) and instrumental conditioning (Type II or operant conditioning).

29.4.2 Classical conditioning

DEFINITION AND CHARACTERISTICS. In a classical-conditioning paradigm, two sensory stimuli (the unconditioned stimulus, or US, and the conditioned stimulus, or CS) are presented together, repeatedly if necessary, until the response formerly caused only by the US (the unconditioned response, or UR) can also be elicited by the CS alone (the conditioned response, or CR).

A variety of temporal relationships between the CS and the US is possible, leading to several different forms of classical conditioning. The CS may precede but not overlap the US (forward trace conditioning), precede and overlap the US (forward delay conditioning, the most widely used paradigm), occur at exactly the same time as the US (simultaneous conditioning), or follow the US (background, or backward, conditioning). The reinforcement (US) may be positive and rewarding (classical reward conditioning), or negative and punishing (classical defense conditioning). Details may be obtained from a variety of sources (Abraham et al., 1972; Bullock and Quarton, 1966; Church, 1963; Dyal and Corning, 1973; Gormezano, 1966; Gormezano and Moore, 1969; Hilgard and Bower, 1966; Hilgard and Marquis, 1940; Kimble, 1961, 1967; Pavlov, 1927; Rescorla, 1967).

The commonest defect in classical-conditioning studies on invertebrates is the lack of sufficient controls for sensitization. It can be claimed that a classical-conditioning paradigm has demonstrated associative learning only if the behavioral modification can be shown to have resulted explicitly from the temporal contiguity between CS and US, i.e., only if the possibility of sensitization is excluded. Suitable control procedures include:

1. presentation of the CS alone;
2. presentation of the US alone (necessarily followed by testing with the CS);
3. unpaired presentation of the CS and the US;

4. randomized presentation of the CS with respect to the US;
5. backward conditioning; and
6. discriminative conditioning.

If the first four of these control procedures do not yield the same behavioral modification that is caused by contiguous CS-US presentation, then the possibility of sensitization is effectively excluded. If the fifth procedure, backward conditioning, yields a negative result (i.e., no behavioral modification), as is often the case in vertebrate preparations, then the positive result obtained by forward conditioning may be assumed to result from the temporal relation between the CS and the US. If backward conditioning yields the same positive result as forward conditioning, however, pseudoconditioning is said to have occurred. The distinction between conditioning and pseudoconditioning may be entirely arbitrary, however, especially if the other sensitization control procedures yield negative results.

The sixth of the above procedures, discriminative conditioning, is the most difficult to apply, but it is also the most conclusive. In this procedure two stimuli comprise the conditioned stimulus, which is therefore termed a compound CS. One of the two stimuli (the CS^+) is made to accompany the US, while the other (the CS^-) is presented at random with respect to the US. In a separate experiment the roles of the two stimuli are reversed; that is, the original CS^+ becomes the CS^-, and conversely. If both experiments yield a conditioned response to the CS^+ but not to the CS^-, then the animal must be capable of discriminating between the CS^+ and the CS^- on the basis of temporal contiguity with the US, and associative learning has thus been unambiguously demonstrated.

EXAMPLES OF CLASSICAL CONDITIONING. Classical conditioning has been demonstrated in most of the major invertebrate phyla, including protozoans, platyhelminths, annelids, arthropods, and molluscs. This literature is reviewed in several recent symposia, books, and review articles (Corning, Dyal, and Willows, 1973; Corning and Lahue, 1972; Eisenstein, 1967; Kandel and Spencer, 1968; McConnell, 1966; Thorpe, 1963; Thorpe and Davenport, 1965; Young, 1965; Wells, 1965, 1966, 1968). The controversial work on classical conditioning in planarians, beginning with Thompson and McConnell (1955), is reviewed in Corning and Ratner (1967), Corning and Riccio (1970), Jacobson (1965), McConnell and Shelby (1970), and especially Corning and Kelly (1973). (The latter authors show that convincing positive reports far outnumber negative reports.) In the present account, therefore, I shall focus on select examples that are either particularly illuminating from a behavioral standpoint or have special potential from the standpoint of cellular analysis.

One of the earliest examples of associative learning in an invertebrate was provided by classical conditioning of a gastropod mollusc more than a half-century ago (Thompson, 1917). Motivated by Pavlov's contemporary experiments on dogs, Thompson applied a classical-conditioning paradigm to the fresh-water snail *Physa*. To train specimens, tactile stimulation of the foot (CS) was paired with the presentation of food (US). Food alone (lettuce) usually caused a characteristic feeding response (the UR: 61 percent of 100 trials on two specimens), and touch did not (3.3 percent feeding responses in 120 trials on six specimens). During paired presentation of the CS and the US, the snails at first showed no feeding response, suggesting that touch inhibits feeding. During the 250 training trials, however, there was a steady increase in the frequency of feeding responses to the CS-US combination. Animals tested with the CS 48 hr after the end of training showed a mean response rate (CR) of 39.6 percent (124 trials on six specimens), compared with 3.3 percent before training. The effects of training persisted for 96 hr.

The study of classical conditioning was in its infancy at the time of Thompson's experiments, and a number of important control procedures were omitted. The interstimulus intervals for paired CS-US presentations and for the repeated presentations of the CS alone were not reported, and the possible effects of habituation or dishabituation to the US or the CS cannot be ascertained from the published data. More serious was the lack of controls for sensitization; in particular, experiments involving unpaired or randomized presentations of the CS with respect to the US were not performed. At the very least, however, Thompson's results did demonstrate long-term sensitization. Moreover, she used a behavior, feeding, which subsequent research has shown to be entirely tractable to detailed neurophysiological analysis at the cellular level (e.g., Berry, 1973; Davis and Mpitsos, 1971; Davis et al., 1974; Davis, Siegler, and Mpitsos, 1973; Kater and Rowell, 1973; Kater, 1974; Kupfermann and Cohen, 1971; Rose, 1971, 1972; Siegler, Mpitsos, and Davis, 1974). Repetition and extension of Thompson's experiments, including appropriate sensitization controls, deserve high priority.

A classical-conditioning paradigm similar to that used on *Physa* has been employed to demonstrate associative learning in the carnivorous marine gastropod *Pleurobranchaea* (Mpitsos and Davis, 1973), and in this case some sensitization controls have been performed. Animals were trained by stroking the anterior oral veil with a glass rod coated with homogenized squid. Thus tactile stimulation (the CS) was paired with food stimuli (the US) in a simultaneous-conditioning paradigm. The combined CS-US caused feeding behavior (UR) in 99 percent of 20,000 trials on 65 experimental animals. In contrast, the CS alone failed to elicit feeding in 95.5 percent of 2,280 trials on 114 naive specimens. In conditioned animals, however, the CS alone elicited feeding behavior (the CR); conventional learning curves and statistical analysis showed that the response was in most cases acquired within five days of the onset of training (20 training trials per day, with an interval between conditioning trials of 1 min or more) and persisted for two weeks (Mpitsos and Davis, 1973).

To control for the effects of habituation and sensitization, control groups were given either the CS alone (touch), the US alone (food, delivered by pouring squid homogenate into the region of the oral veil), or the CS and US unpaired. These procedures caused a weak increase in the frequency of feeding responses to the CS alone, but the increase was invariably less than that caused by paired CS-US presentation. The food sensitization control is open to the criticism that the food was delivered by a different means than that used during conditioning. Regardless of the method of delivery, however, the effect of the food was the same, as evidenced by an equally strong feeding behavior, suggesting that the sensitization control was effective. Consequently, the behavioral modification induced by the classical-conditioning paradigm may be regarded as true associative learning.

In other molluscan studies, classical conditioning of the feeding response in *Aplysia* to a CS of light has been reported in an abstract (Jahan-Parwar, 1971), but the report cannot yet be evaluated because the data have not been published. Attempts to replicate the study using nearly the same procedures have not succeeded (Kupfermann, 1974). The mollusc *Hermissenda* has been exposed to paired light and rotational stimuli, with the result that the subsequent response to light alone was modified (Alkon, 1974). Adequate control procedures for learning were not employed in this experiment, however, and as noted by the author, the result cannot be considered an example of learning because, although the response to light is changed, it does not resemble the normal response to rotation.

Among arthropods, learning studies have focused on the two largest groups, crustaceans and insects. In the Maine lobster, *Homarus americanus*, for example, classical conditioning of heart rate has been accomplished by pairing a tone with electrical shock (Offutt, 1970). Electrical shock normally causes transient cessation of the heartbeat (bradycardia). After a few training trials, the tone alone also caused bradycardia. The number of animals involved in this experiment was small, and adequate control prodecures for sensitization were not performed. This experiment should be pursued vigorously because of the excellent possibilities for cellular analysis. The mechanoreceptors that mediate the response to the CS (the tone) may be readily identifiable, and the UR-CR (bradycardia) is achieved by the action of a single inhibitor neuron supplying the heart (Wiersma and Novitski, 1942). This single, potentially identifiable neuron may be the locus of the physiological changes underlying this possible example of learning.

Classical conditioning has been reported only infrequently in insects (e.g., Frings, 1941; Takeda, 1961), but Nelson (1971) has contributed a convincing study using the blowfly *Phormia*. Nelson performed several different types of classical-conditioning experiments and appropriate control experiments on a total of more than 500 specimens. In her basic paradigm a compound CS was employed, consisting of contact of the feet with water followed by contact of the feet with salt solution. This CS was combined with a US consisting of sugar solution applied to the mouth parts, a stimulus that elicits extension of the feeding proboscis (the UR). In a forward-delay-conditioning paradigm, flies acquired a conditioned proboscis-extension response to the CS alone. The group as a whole showed statistically significant learning, although inspection of individual animals revealed considerable variability. Thirty-nine percent were classified as good learners, 24 percent as fair, and 37 percent as poor. Such findings emphasize the need for large sample sizes and a comparison of mean values in studies on invertebrate learning.

To test for sensitization, Nelson employed a control group that received the CS alone. These animals did not acquire a conditioned proboscis-extension response. Animals exposed to the US alone, however, displayed a heightened responsiveness to water or salt solution, owing to "residual excitation" (i.e., sensitization). To demonstrate associative learning conclusively, Nelson applied a discriminative-conditioning paradigm, using first water and then salt solution as the CS⁺. She found that the flies could be conditioned regardless of which stimulus was used at the CS⁺. Thus the combination of experiments convincingly showed that the behavioral change caused by classical conditioning represented a blend of sensitization and true associative learning. When the sensitizing effect of the US from the preceding conditioning trial was "discharged" by allowing the flies to exercise (walk) in the intertrial interval, the acquisition of the conditioned response was impaired, suggesting that there is a necessary and perhaps causal connection between sensitization and learning in this animal.

BAIT SHYNESS AND GARCIA CONDITIONING. The blowfly

study described above employed a variation of the commonest classical-conditioning paradigm, forward delay conditioning, in which the CS precedes and overlaps the US. In a variety of classical-conditioning studies involving both vertebrate (Gormezano, 1966) and invertebrate (Ratner, 1965) preparations, a CS-US interval (interstimulus interval, ISI) of about 0.5 sec was optimal. Indeed, learning is usually slower and may not occur at all at shorter or longer ISIs. In a historic series of experiments on the white rat, Garcia and his colleagues sparked a minor revolution in psychology by showing that much longer ISIs can be effective in conditioning "bait shyness" (Garcia, Ervin, and Koelling, 1966). Using a classical-conditioning paradigm, these investigators paired a specific taste (salty or saccharin-flavored water; the CS) with exposure to toxic radiation (the US), which causes radiation sickness (the UR). After only one trial, the taste became aversive.[2] Radiation sickness takes an hour to develop, and hence the ISI in this experiment was much longer than the conventional 0.5 sec. Garcia thus rigorously demonstrated what every farmer already knew on the basis of practical experience,[3] namely, that associative learning can occur with delayed reinforcement.

Garcia's experiments demonstrated another property of associative learning that is even more important and relevant to invertebrate studies. When a second CS (an audiovisual stimulus) was employed in the above taste-aversion-conditioning paradigm, it did not become aversive, even though it was also paired with radiation sickness (Garcia and Koelling, 1966). We may conclude that organisms are capable of forming associations between some, but not all, stimuli, and that such selective associability favors contingencies that are likely to have adaptive significance to the organism. In other words, animals may be capable of learning only those tasks for which evolution has "prepared" them. This "preparedness principle" stands in sharp contrast to the "equipotentiality principle" of Pavlov: "It is obvious that the reflex activity of any effector organ can be chosen for the purpose of investigation, since signaling stimuli can get linked up with any of the inborn reflexes" (Pavlov, 1927, p. 7). The preparedness principle has been clearly formulated and documented by Seligman and Hager (1972).

Garcia's experiments furnish two important lessons for students of invertebrate learning. First, we must not be

---

[2]Although training in this experiment takes the form of a classical-defense-conditioning paradigm (Gormezano, 1966), the resulting avoidance conditioning is usually considered a combination of classical and instrumental conditioning.
[3]Many livestock that become ill for nondietary reasons are then reluctant to eat the same, previously acceptable diet.

bound by the conventions developed largely from vertebrate studies. Indeed, Garcia has shown that such conventions are in some cases inapplicable even to vertebrate preparations. Second, and most important, we must select stimuli and responses that are likely to be associable on ethological grounds, in accordance with the preparedness principle. In animals as phylogenetically distant from us as the invertebrates, intuitions based on anthropomorphic extrapolations are likely to be erroneous. A much different insight is required, an insight that can be gained only by patient behavioral observations, combined perhaps with a dash of inspired free association.

I do not know of published accounts of Garcia conditioning in invertebrates, but in an interesting unpublished study, a similar, one-trial learning of taste avoidance has been demonstrated in the terrestrial mollusc *Limax* (A. Gelperin, personal communication). Slugs were fed potatoes (the "safe" food) for eight days and were then presented with mushrooms, accompanied by a five-minute exposure to CO_2 poisoning. The animals normally prefer mushrooms to potatoes when both are freely available, but following the pairing of mushrooms with the aversive stimulus, potatoes became the food of choice. Some specimens avoided mushrooms after a single conditioning trial, and the aversion persisted for two weeks.

At this writing, it has not been determined whether the avoidance of mushrooms represents true associative learning. Perhaps, following aversive stimulation with CO_2, the specimens would have rejected not only the mushrooms but any novel food. In this case the subsequent avoidance could represent a form of sensitization. Alternatively, the result may point the way to an important new form of learning, in which an organism displays a long-term predisposition to reject all novel (potentially unsafe) foods in favor of a familiar (safe) and therefore easily available food. This kind of learning (already known to every parent!) might be related to temporal conditioning, a form of classical conditioning in which repeated presentation of the US alone leads eventually to a UR in anticipation of an undelivered US (Gormezano, 1966). Such learning has a reasonable evolutionary teleology; in some species the development of a preference for an available, safe, and familiar food might be more favorable to survival than indiscriminate sampling of potentially unsafe or only transiently available foods.[4]

---

[4]That "food familiarity" plays a role in the behavior of invertebrates is suggested by the observation of lobster fishermen that crushed mussels are effective bait near mussel beds but not elsewhere (Lindberg, 1955). Similarly, food preferences can apparently be changed and then maintained in captive lobsters (Wilson, 1949).

This possible new form of learning, which may have developmental components (Dethier and Goldrich, 1971), deserves more systematic investigation.

Classical conditioning is sometimes criticized on the ground that it is a laboratory artifact, performed under circumstances that are too contrived and artificial to bear any meaningful relationship to behaviorally significant learning (e.g., John, 1972). This argument has two major flaws. First, ethologically meaningful classical conditioning has been demonstrated: the aversive taste conditioning of slugs to toxic food, described above, is a suggestive example. Second, the fact that a procedure is "artificial" by no means implies that it is incapable of revealing fundamental biological principles. Activation of nerve cells by electronic stimulators is "artificial," yet this procedure has helped to reveal important and general properties of nerve action potentials. Similarly, classical-conditioning studies can presumably reveal general rules governing reinforcement and association, which in turn may be presumed to underlie all forms of associative learning.

29.4.3 Instrumental conditioning

DEFINITION AND CHARACTERISTICS. Instrumental conditioning resembles classical conditioning in that behavioral modification is caused by a temporal association of two events, but it differs in that one of the two events (the reinforcement) is not inevitable, as in classical conditioning, but is instead contingent upon the animal's "voluntary" or "spontaneous" behavior. In instrumental conditioning, as in classical conditioning, the reinforcement may be positive (rewarding) or negative (punishing).

Instrumental conditioning employing a negative reinforcer is often termed avoidance conditioning. Avoidance conditioning takes two different forms: an animal can be taught to suppress a behavior with which punishment is associated (passive avoidance conditioning), or it can be taught to execute a behavior that effectively avoids punishment (active avoidance conditioning). Avoidance conditioning is usually considered to be a combination of classical and instrumental conditioning (e.g., Alloway, 1973; Mowrer, 1947; Solomon and Wynne, 1954). The first stage of avoidance conditioning resembles classical conditioning in that a "neutral" CS reliably precedes or accompanies an aversive US (classical defense conditioning). The second stage resembles instrumental conditioning in that reward (lack of an aversive US) is contingent upon the animal's suppression of a behavioral act (passive avoidance conditioning) or execution of an escape response (active avoidance conditioning). Whatever the etiology of avoidance conditioning, it is considered by most students of conditioning to be an advanced form of learning, inasmuch as the resulting behavioral modification seems "purposeful" and the modification represents an apparent effort to avoid an aversive *future* event.

EXAMPLES OF INSTRUMENTAL-CONDITIONING STUDIES. There are dozens of reports of instrumental conditioning in invertebrates, most of which have been performed in arthropods (for reviews see Alloway, 1973; Best, 1965; Eisenstein, 1972; Lahue, 1973). Among arthropods, crustaceans have been favorite subjects for instrumental conditioning (for a review see Krasne, 1973). For example, Chow and Leiman (1972) used an avoidance-conditioning paradigm to condition crayfish, which are negatively phototrophic, to remain in a lighted area. Animals learned the task equally well using the eyes alone (i.e., with caudal photoreceptor surgically eliminated) or with caudal photoreceptor alone (i.e., with the eyes blindfolded or removed). Animals trained while blindfolded, however, showed no retention of the learned behavior when the blindfold was removed and the caudal photoreceptor was surgically eliminated. These experiments provide the first evidence that the caudal photoreceptor, long used as a model of a simple photoreceptive system (Kennedy, 1963), plays a significant behavioral role. Thus the experiments illustrate the fact that learning paradigms can be profitably employed to explore an animal's sensory capabilities, an approach pioneered by von Frisch (for reviews see von Frisch, 1950, 1967). More important, the experiments of Chow and Leiman demonstrate the principle that two parallel but functionally distinct sensory pathways can mediate the same learning task. The generality of this principle remains to be determined. Krasne (this volume) reviews other examples of learning in crustaceans.

Among insects, recent experiments have shown that the fruit fly *Drosophila*, which has been the subject of creative genetic analyses of behavior (Hotta and Benzer, 1972), is also capable of associative learning (Quinn, Harris, and Benzer, 1974). Populations of flies were presented with two different odors, one of which was accompanied by aversive electrical shock or aversive chemostimulation (quinine sulphate). Flies trained in this differential avoidance-conditioning task learned to avoid selectively the odor associated with aversive stimulation. The task was acquired in one trial and retained for up to one day, although when odors were presented without aversive stimulation, extinction occurred within an hour. Careful control procedures eliminated the possibilities of habituation, sensitization, odor preference, and experimental bias. Similar experiments employing visual cues (colored light) were also

successful. Interestingly, only one-third of the flies learned the task on the first training session, but when the remaining two-thirds were then trained, about one-third again showed learning. This result indicates that each animal has the capacity to learn, and that the learning is apparently probabilistic. There is no evidence for a division of animals into "good learners" and "poor learners." Nelson's (1971) similar data from studies on the blowfly therefore probably do not mean that some flies are smarter than others, but only that the learning paradigms devised to date, while effective, have not yet utilized optimal sensory cues.

Drosophila is not ideal for electrophysiological studies because of its small size. The results of Quinn, Harris, and Benzer (1974) are nevertheless important; this is one of the most carefully controlled studies of learning in an invertebrate, and it also raises the fascinating possibility of using the tools of genetic analysis to gain insight into the physiological mechanisms of learned behavior.

One of the best known and most intensively studied examples of associative learning in the invertebrates is a form of instrumental avoidance conditioning of leg position in insects, studied first by Horridge (1962a,b, 1965; see also Aranda and Luco, 1969; Disterhoft, Haggerty, and Corning, 1971; Disterhoft, Nurnberger, and Corning, 1968; Eisenstein, 1968, 1970a,b; Eisenstein and Cohen, 1965; Eisenstein et al., 1972; Eisenstein and Krasilovsky, 1967; Hoyle, 1965; Pritchatt, 1968; for recent reviews see Eisenstein, 1972; Alloway, 1973). In the basic paradigm an insect (locust or cockroach) is suspended above an electrified saline solution with a wire electrode attached to one of its legs. When the leg extends, the electrode makes contact with the saline, causing the experimental animal to receive an aversive electrical shock. Yoked controls are shocked by the same stimulus, regardless of the position of their own legs. Under such conditions, experimental animals rapidly learn to flex the leg against the pull of gravity in order to avoid the aversive shock. In contrast, control animals show no such learning.

Alloway (1973) argues that this example is not representative of avoidance conditioning, but instead corresponds to a simpler, nonassociative form of learning—"aversive inhibitory conditioning" (Razran, 1971). This view is based on the notion that proprioceptive information on leg position may be unnecessary to leg-position learning, a possibility raised by Hoyle's (1965) finding that in a restrained, headless locust, an electrophysiological analogue of the leg-position learning task could be demonstrated even though the leg was fixed in place and sensory feedback caused by contraction of the single muscle being studied was abolished by severing its tendons. Hoyle's experiment leaves open the possibility of sensory feedback from the contraction of the many remaining muscles in the limb, however, and the implication that avoidance learning in this preparation can occur in the absence of proprioception is unwarranted. As recognized by Hoyle, further experiments, involving more complete deafferentation, need to be performed before the involvement of proprioceptive feedback in this avoidance-conditioning task can be assessed. Even if proprioception is shown to have no role in leg-position learning, other mechanisms by which the nervous system can be informed of motor activity are known, including efference copy (see Kennedy and Davis, 1975). Thus Alloway's argument that leg-position learning is non-associative is unconvincing. The argument is weakened further by Pritchatt's (1968) demonstration that in intact cockroaches, either leg extension *or* leg flexion can be avoidance-conditioned. This result leaves little doubt that the insect is learning to associate a specific leg position with a contingent aversive shock.

Instrumental avoidance conditioning similar to the insect leg-position learning has been attempted in the mollusc *Helix* (Emson, Walker, and Kerkut, 1971). The optic tentacle was electrically shocked whenever it "extruded beyond a certain point," with the result that animals soon "learned" to hold the tentacle in a retracted position, as evidenced by a decline in the number of shocks delivered per unit time. In contrast to experimental animals, "yoked" controls did not acquire the response. This study has several major shortcomings, however. Evaluation of many results are not possible because conclusions are based on comparisons of individual animals, despite the "great variability between animals" reported by the authors (Emson, Walker, and Kerkut, 1971, p. 228). More troublesome, experimental animals were shocked differently from control animals and apparently received a greater number of effective shocks.[5] From the published data it seems entirely possible that the retraction response in experimental animals simply facilitated over time, with the result that the tentacle was

eventually held continuously in a retracted position. That control animals showed no such change is attributable to the fact that they received fewer effective shocks. In view of the biochemical correlates that were identified in this study (see Section 29.4.5), the inadequate behavioral documentation of learning is especially regrettable.

Three reports of instrumental conditioning involving the mollusc *Aplysia* are similarly unconvincing. In the first, Lee (1969) used a battery of photocells to record automatically the positions of specimens within a small lucite chamber. When an experimental animal passed a given position, the behavior was "reinforced" by increasing the water depth in the chamber from 1.0 to 3.5 inches. The major evidence offered for "learning" was that experimental animals spent more time in positions that were reinforced than did control animals that were not exposed to the contingency. Unfortunately, evaluation of many of Lee's results is impossible because for most analyses, data were presented only for select experimental animals. More serious, the temperature in the chambers that contained specimens was neither controlled nor monitored. From Lee's description of methods, it seems likely that when experimental animals were reinforced, they were also substantially cooled. Assuming that locomotor activity declines with decreasing temperature, experimental animals might have remained longer in the "reinforced" position simply because they were cooled while in that position. Such a result would not be expected from control animals, since they were cooled in random positions.[6]

In a related experiment the effects of temperature were examined in *Aplysia* using an operant-conditioning paradigm in which the reinforced behavior consisted of pushing a lever (Downey and Jahan-Parwar, 1972). These authors concluded that reinforcement consisting of "contingent water level change in the absence of a drop in temperature produced response rates near control levels" (p. 511). In other words, and contrary to Lee's conclusion, water level per se is not reinforcing. Downey and Jahan-Parwar found that reinforcing procedures involving decreased temperature caused an

---

[5]The authors write that "the yoke control snail received a shock whenever the experimental animal's tentacle received a shock" (Emson, Walker, and Kerkut, 1971, p. 225). Experimentals, however, were shocked "a few millimetres above the retracted tentacle," while "The yoke control snail's tentacle was loosely looped with a thin silver wire through which it received a shock . . ." (*ibid.*). Experimental animals presumably received an effective aversive shock in every trial (p. 227). In contrast, the yoke control "contracted its tentacle initially when stimulated, but adapted to the stimulation so that low frequency stimulation no longer produced tentacular contraction" (p. 228). It would appear that yoke control animals habituated to the shock, perhaps because they were shocked less intensely than experimentals. The conclusion that experimental animals received a greater number of *effective* shocks than controls seems likely from the published account.

[6]Lee recognized that "When reinforcement occurs, the experimentals may terminate or slow their rate of movement," thus accounting for his data. He argues, however, that the results of a "probe" experiment "nullify this argument" (Lee, 1969, p. 163). In this probe experiment the time required for eight trained experimental animals to return to the reinforced position when replaced into their experimental chambers was measured and compared to corresponding values for eight yoked control animals. The reported means and ranges for experimental and control animals, respectively, were 7.1 sec (1.5 to 35.0 sec) and 17.4 sec (2.2 to 653.3 sec). Statistical comparison of means was not presented, but given the presumably large variance, it is not clear that the differences between experimentals and controls was significant.

apparent difference between experimentals and controls, but the authors concede that "an increase in activity level occurring at the termination of reinforcement could produce higher response rates in experimental animals" (p. 511).[7]

In a third study on *Aplysia* Lickey and Berry (1966) and Lickey (1968) showed that a pair of forceps touched to the lips at first elicits a feeding response, but the number of rejections increases over time. Lickey (1968) concluded that this result could be defended as an example of passive avoidance conditioning, but recognized that "the acquired change could be categorized as the habituation of the ingestion response" (p. 717).[8] We are forced to conclude that instrumental conditioning has not yet been conclusively demonstrated in *Aplysia*.

Avoidance conditioning involving a molluscan feeding behavior has also been investigated in *Pleurobranchaea* (Mpitsos and Davis, 1973). Specimens were first trained to execute feeding behavior in response to tactile stimulation of the oral veil, using the classical-conditioning paradigm described earlier. Specimens were then divided randomly into three groups: experimental, touch control, and shock control. In daily training sessions each member of the experimental group was touched on the oral veil in twenty conditioning trials. In each trial an aversive electrical shock was delivered to the oral veil if the classically conditioned feeding behavior occurred. Animals learned within one day (twenty trials) to suppress the feeding response (passive avoidance conditioning) and execute a withdrawal escape response (active avoidance conditioning). In contrast, touch-control animals, given the same number of tactile stimuli to the oral veil as experimentals but no shocks, continued to exhibit the previously conditioned feeding response for nearly two weeks, despite the absence of reinforcement. Shock-control animals, given the same number of aversive shocks as experimentals but not simultaneous touch, showed no decline in the number of positive feeding responses to touch alone; thus the decline in the response of experimental animals cannot be attributed to shock-induced "amnesia." Moreover,

intense electrical shock to the oral veil of naive specimens does not alter the threshold of the feeding response (Davis Mpitsos, and Pinneo, 1974a), in contrast to the inhibition of feeding caused by shock in *Aplysia* (Kupfermann and Pinsker, 1968). Therefore, the decline in the response of experimental animals cannot be attributed to shock-induced inhibition of feeding behavior. The avoidance-conditioning experiment described above was performed five times on a total of more than fifty animals with the same result.

A form of avoidance conditioning using stimuli deliberately chosen in accord with the preparedness principle has been demonstrated in *Helix* (Stephens and McGaugh, 1972). Specimens learn to climb a vertical glass rod more slowly if trained by placing quinine at the top, and retain both a short-term (24 hr) and long-term (>1 week) memory of the aversive experience. It is notable that this study, like many prior successful demonstrations of learning in molluscs, incorporated a chemical stimulus in the training paradigm, thereby taking good advantage of the well-developed chemical sense of molluscs.

29.4.4 Electrophysiological correlates of learning

We can presumably accept, with Hebb (1949), that learning involves a change in the functional properties of nerve cells and their synapses (but see, for example, John's comment in footnote 11, below). Thus, once learning is demonstrated in a given preparation, identification of neurophysiological correlates is an obvious sequel. Among intact vertebrates, neurophysiological correlates have been found for both classical conditioning (Linseman and Olds, 1973; Olds et al., 1972; Segal, 1973a,b; Segal, Disterhoft, and Olds, 1972; Segal and Olds, 1972, 1973) and instrumental conditioning (Evarts, 1973; Fetz and Baker, 1973; Fetz and Finocchio, 1971; Fuster and Alexander, 1971; John, 1967a; John et al., 1973). However, such changes are distributed widely in hundreds of thousands of neurons in the brain. Cellular analysis of learning in such complex systems is technically infeasible. Plastic changes in vertebrate nervous systems have also been identified in single nerve cells (e.g., Bureš and Burešová, 1967; Keene, 1973; for reviews, see von Baumgarten, 1970, Voronin, 1971, and Weight, 1974), but the relevance of such studies to behaviorally meaningful learning is as yet unclear.

NEUROPHYSIOLOGICAL STUDIES OF CLASSICAL CONDITIONING. The problem of identifying cellular correlates of learning is more tractable with invertebrates. The neuronal circuitry underlying invertebrate behavior can be unraveled with satisfying precision, raising the exciting possibility of studying plastic changes in single,

---

[7]Downey and Jahan-Parwar believe that instrumental conditioning was nevertheless demonstrated, on the basis of a "probe" experiment similar to Lee's. Incomplete data are given for only four experimental animals, however (Downey and Jahan-Parwar, 1972, table 1), and these data in fact suggest that experimental latencies were not significantly different from controls.

[8]When the data in Lickey's Fig. 1 are replotted as the number of positive feeding responses (rather than the number of rejections) vs. cumulative time, the resulting curves bear a striking resemblance to the long-term habituation curves for the gill-withdrawal response of *Aplysia* (Carew, Pinsker, and Kandel, 1972; Carew and Kandel, 1973).

identifiable nerve cells. In *Aplysia*, for example, application of a classical-conditioning paradigm to the isolated nervous system caused plastic changes in single neurons in the pleural or cerebral ganglia (Kandel and Tauc, 1965a; Kristan and Gerstein, 1970; Kristan, 1971). In these cases, however, the behavioral role of the identified neurons was unknown; hence, the relation of the demonstrated plasticity to behavioral learning is uncertain.

In *Pleurobranchaea* a direct electrophysiological correlate to behavioral learning has been identified in the isolated nervous system (Mpitsos and Davis, 1973). Specimens were trained according to the classical-conditioning paradigm described in Section 29.4.2 to exhibit feeding behavior (CR) in response to tactile stimulation of the oral veil (CS). In "double-blind" electrophysiological experiments, nervous systems were removed from 6 classically conditioned specimens, 2 avoidance-conditioned specimens and more than 25 naive (untrained) specimens. These isolated nervous systems were then studied electrophysiologically by stimulating the oral-veil nerves, which normally convey the CS (touch) and the US (food stimuli) to the brain, while extracellularly recording the activity of identified feeding nerves. Such stimulation in nervous systems from naive animals (Davis, Siegler, and Mpitsos, 1973) and from avoidance-conditioned specimens never caused the cyclic motor output that is normally associated with feeding behavior. In contrast, stimulation of the oral-veil nerves in three of the six classically conditioned animals caused strong, rhythmic motor output in feeding nerves; this output could be sustained for many sequential cycles and elicited repeatedly for as long as 24 hr (Mpitsos and Davis, 1973). The probability of this result being caused by chance is less than 0.001 (by t-test comparing the estimated probability of elicited feeding in trained vs. untrained specimens). Presumably the afferent pathways in the stimulated brain become more efficacious in eliciting feeding output when animals are classically conditioned. This finding shows that the changes that occur within the brain of *Pleurobranchaea* during learning are stable enough to survive the removal of the nervous system, thereby encouraging analysis of the physiological correlates of behavioral learning in the isolated brain (Davis et al., 1974).

The *Pleurobranchaea* conditioning preparation may prove especially useful for identifying the neuronal substrates of learning, because the unconditioned response (feeding behavior) is unusually amenable to electrophysiological analysis. It has been shown that the feeding behavior is controlled by four classes of neurons: (1) sensory neurons in the oral veil and stomatogastric nerves (Davis, Siegler, and Mpitsos, 1973); (2) identified motoneurons in the brain and buccal ganglion (Siegler, Mpitsos, and Davis, 1974); (3) identified interneurons in the buccal ganglion that couple the brain and buccal ganglion and perhaps also generate the neuronal oscillation that underlies feeding (Davis et al., 1974); and (4) putative "command" interneurons in the brain (Davis et al., 1974). The last three of these classes of neurons have been identified anatomically by intracellular dye injection and have to some degree been studied electrophysiologically. The putative command neurons are especially likely sites for the neurophysiological changes underlying learning (Davis et al., 1974).

The blowfly classical-conditioning preparation (Nelson, 1971; see Section 29.4.2) represents another potentially favorable preparation for studies on the neurophysiological substrates of classical conditioning. The unconditioned response (extension of feeding proboscis) can be elicited by chemostimulation of single sensory hairs on the mouthparts (Dethier, 1955, 1968), and the neural pathways involved in the unconditioned response are accessible to at least some forms of neurophysiological analysis (e.g., Getting, 1971).

NEUROPHYSIOLOGICAL STUDIES OF INSTRUMENTAL CONDITIONING. Among invertebrates, electrophysiological correlates of instrumental conditioning have been studied only in insects. Luco and Aranda (1964a,b, 1966) showed that when the two forelegs of a cockroach are ablated, the animal "learns" within a week to balance on three of its remaining four legs in order to free one of the middle legs for the task of antennal cleaning. Correlated with this behavioral modification is an increase in responsiveness of the hindlimbs to natural synaptic input caused by electrical stimulation of the nerve cord. As new forelegs are grown, they resume the antennal cleaning role; at the same time, the responsiveness of the hindlimb motoneurons to synaptic activation declines to the original level (Luco and Aranda, 1966). The relevance of these interesting results to learning is unclear, however, since the behavioral change may represent a form of genetically guided developmental or regenerative plasticity that is unrelated to associative learning.

A later study by the same authors employing a similar approach (Aranda and Luco, 1969) is more relevant to instrumental conditioning. Leg-position learning in cockroaches was shown to be accompanied by an increased responsiveness of the participating motoneurons to natural synaptic inputs, as revealed by electrical stimulation of the ventral nerve cord in trained and untrained specimens. Both the behavioral learning and the heightened motoneuron responsiveness declined, however, in 30 min, a much shorter retention than that found in other studies of cockroach leg-position learning (e.g., Oliver, 1973).

Hoyle (1965) has studied the electrophysiology of the leg-position learning preparation in more detail. Using a restrained, headless insect (locust or cockroach), he recorded the activity of single muscles that control leg flexion, usually the metathoracic anterior adductor, which is supplied by a single excitatory motoneuron. Whenever the frequency of impulse discharge in this motoneuron decreased below an arbitrary demand level, punishing shock was delivered to the leg by means of a wire electrode wrapped around its periphery. As a result of this contingency, the motoneuron "learned" to maintain an elevated discharge level. Conversely, when the aversive reinforcement was made contingent upon a high frequency of motoneuron discharge, lower levels of motoneuron activity could be conditioned. This provides a persuasive parallel with Pritchatt's (1968) later behavioral observation that either leg flexion or extension could be avoidance-conditioned. Aversive shocks applied at random with respect to the motoneuron discharge level did not cause changes in the discharge frequency.

Although neither the number of animals nor the reliability of the effects were reported in the above work, the study remains the best example of an electrophysiological correlate to instrumental conditioning. The leg-position learning preparation holds special promise for analysis of the cellular substrates of learning because the underlying neuronal circuitry has been analyzed in detail. The motor patterns that underlie walking and other leg movements in locusts and cockroaches have been described (Delcomyn, 1973; Delcomyn and Usherwood, 1973; Hoyle, 1964, 1970; Iles and Pearson, 1971; Pearson, 1972; Pearson and Iles, 1970, 1973; Wilson, 1966); the leg reflexes are well understood (Delcomyn, 1971; Pearson, 1972; Pearson and Iles, 1973; Pringle, 1940; Runion and Usherwood, 1968; Wilson, 1965); the positions, functional properties, and dendritic architecture of the leg motoneurons have been examined (Burrows, 1973; Burrows and Horridge, 1974; Burrows and Hoyle, 1973; Cohen and Jacklet, 1967; Hoyle and Burrows, 1973a,b); and the central nervous machinery responsible for the generation of locomotor output to the leg has been described for the cockroach (Pearson, Fourtner, and Wong, 1973). Such machinery consists of identified excitatory and inhibitory motoneurons, nonspiking oscillator interneurons that drive the motoneurons, and presumed command interneurons that activate the oscillators. Somewhere in this known neuronal circuitry the electrophysiological and biochemical events that underlie the leg-position learning task should be detectable. The studies of Aranda and Luco (1969) and Hoyle (1965) represent a beginning toward this important and realistic goal.

29.4.5 Cellular mechanisms underlying learning

Given that electrophysiological correlates to learned behavior exist, we must ask how such correlates are related to learning. The information that constitutes the conditioned and unconditioned stimuli is presumed to enter the brain in the form of electrical signals in sensory neurons. It has been considered possible that learned information is also retained as a memory trace in the form of electrical messages (action potentials) that continually reverberate in interneuronal "storage" circuits. We shall refer to this idea as the "reverberation hypothesis." As a second possibility, conditioned and unconditioned stimuli entering the brain as electrical signals might somehow alter the structural/functional properties of central neurons that participate in the learned behavior, rendering such neurons more effective in subsequent trials. We shall refer to this notion as the "circuit-modification hypothesis." Finally, electrical messages entering the central nervous system may trigger biochemical synthesis in central neurons. We shall call this idea the "biochemical hypothesis."

Biochemical changes may be imagined to underlie learning in two subtly distinct ways. First, biochemical changes may mediate structural and functional changes of the kind envisioned in the circuit-modification hypothesis described above. We shall refer to this variation as the "biochemical-antecedent hypothesis." Second, experiential information entering the brain in the form of electrical messages may trigger the synthesis of special macromolecules, the structure of which uniquely codes that information. We shall term this variation the "biochemical-code hypothesis." We shall now examine evidence germane to each of these hypotheses, emphasizing studies on invertebrates.

THE REVERBERATION HYPOTHESIS. If learned information is retained in the nervous system in the form of reverberating action potentials, then any procedure that disrupts or blocks action potentials (e.g., general mechanical stimulation, anesthesia, electroconvulsive shock, cooling) should block learning and memory. Experiments employing this logic have usually been performed on vertebrate preparations, and they have usually shown that although such procedures do interfere with the formation of new memories, they do not disrupt previously established memories (e.g., Andjus et al., 1956; Brooks et al., 1973; Duncan, 1949; Kopp, Bohdanecky, and Jarvik, 1966; Sosenkov and Chirkov, 1970; see McGaugh and Gold, this volume, for a more detailed treatment). Therefore, this hypothesis is not widely accepted.

Related studies on invertebrates have usually dealt with the process of learning rather than with established long-term memories. Both learning and retention of a simple avoidance task in the cockroach were poorer when specimens were cooled to 3–6°C (Hunter, 1932). Similarly, classical conditioning in earthworms was blocked by cooling animals during conditioning, perhaps simply because the CS and US were prevented from reaching the central nervous system (Herz, Peeke, and Wyers, 1964). The rate of leg-position learning in the cockroach increases with increasing temperature (Kerkut et al., 1970b). In contrast, maze learning and retention in the grain beetle were facilitated by cooling the animal to 1.7°C between daily training sessions (Alloway, 1969, 1973; Alloway and Routtenberg, 1967). Mechanical stimulation (enforced treadmill running) immediately after avoidance-conditioning trials in cockroaches impaired retention (Minami and Dallenbach, 1964), while mechanical stimulation (voluntary walking) between classical-conditioning trials in blowflies interfered with acquisition (Nelson, 1971). The latter result, however, has been interpreted to imply that "residual excitation" from the preceding conditioning trial (sensitization) is prerequisite to learning (Nelson, 1971). At the very least, these collective findings suggest that both temperature and activity levels are important variables that should be carefully controlled in studies on invertebrate learning.

THE CIRCUIT-MODIFICATION HYPOTHESIS. A large body of evidence from studies on vertebrate species indicates that the ultrastructure of neurons and their synapses is influenced by experience (for reviews see Greenough, Bennett, this volume; Berry et al., 1973; Horn, Rose, and Bateson, 1973). None of these studies, however, definitely implicates such changes in associative learning, nor have any similar studies been performed on invertebrate species. Until recently the best evidence that learning involves functional changes in neurons consisted of a demonstration of electrophysiological changes concomitant with learning (see section 29.4.4).

A recent study provides additional circumstantial but potentially very important evidence for the circuit-modification hypothesis of learning (Cronly-Dillon, Carden, and Birks, 1974). Goldfish were avoidance-conditioned by shock to discriminate between yellow and blue light. At various times relative to training, colchicine was injected intracranially. Colchicine is a plant alkaloid that disrupts the microtubules of neurons, thereby inter-

fering with axonal growth and elongation and also blocking fast axonal transport. Injecting colchicine 1.25 hr before training did not affect the acquisition of the task, but it blocked long-term retention. Injection immediately after training blocked long-term retention. Injection 1.25 hr after training had little effect on long-term retention. It appears that colchicine prevents the memory of a recently acquired task from entering long-term storage, perhaps by interfering with microtubule formation and thus preventing crucial structural changes at synapses. This important experiment should be replicated and extended to invertebrate learning preparations.

Despite the relative paucity of data directly relevant to the circuit-modification hypothesis, it is difficult to imagine that learning can occur in the absence of changes in the structural and functional properties of neurons. Any such changes, however, will almost certainly result from antecedent biochemical events.

THE BIOCHEMICAL HYPOTHESIS. Numerous recent books and reviews deal with mnemochemistry (e.g., in this volume, the chapters by Dunn, Flood and Jarvik, Quartermain, and Rose, Hambley, and Haywood; Adam, 1971; Ansell and Bradley, 1973; Bogoch, 1968; Bowman and Datta, 1970; Byrne, 1970; Corning and Ratner, 1967; Fjerdingstad, 1971; Glassman, 1969; Gross and Ziegler, 1969; Gurowitz, 1969; Honig and James, 1971; Ingle, 1968; John, 1967b; Lajtha, 1970; Pribram and Broadbent, 1970; Schneider, 1973; Seligman and Hager, 1972; Ungar, 1970). My aim here will be restricted to developing a conceptual framework for discussing this topic and reviewing the few relevant studies on invertebrates.

Three lines of evidence lend support to the biochemical hypothesis. First, and least controversial, de novo biochemical synthesis can be shown to accompany learning. Second, chemical agents that block biochemical synthesis also interfere with learning. Third, and most controversial, there are reports that when macromolecules isolated from trained animals are injected into untrained specimens, the recipient animals behave as if trained. That is, either they learn the specific task for which the donor animals were trained faster than controls, or they exhibit the "learned" behavior with no prior training. In reviewing these three lines of evidence, we shall see that most interpretations of available data favor the biochemical-antecedent hypothesis over the biochemical-code hypothesis, although neither hypothesis is excluded by the available data.

1. DE NOVO MACROMOLECULAR SYNTHESIS DURING LEARNING. Evidence for in vivo, de novo synthesis is the most persuasive that can be marshaled in support of the bio-

chemical hypothesis. The evidence is best developed in vertebrate preparations, where it appears likely that macromolecular synthesis accompanies learning (e.g., Hydén, 1973a,b; Hydén and Lange, 1970a,b; Hydén et al., 1974). The extensive evidence is reviewed in the many recent books and reviews cited earlier. At least some of these studies are careful to distinguish between macromolecular synthesis associated with learning and that associated simply with neuronal activity. An effective control can be provided in principle by analyzing nervous tissue from both experimental and control animals in the learning paradigm, although such efforts have encountered difficulties (see Dunn, and Rose, Hambley, and Haywood, this volume).

Among invertebrates there is good evidence that biochemical synthesis is associated with neuronal *activity* (Berry, 1969; Bocharova et al., 1972; Peterson and Kernell, 1970; Ram, 1972, 1974; see Peterson and Loh, 1973, for a review). Evidence for de novo synthesis accompanying learning is less extensive, but nonetheless interesting. For example, in a potentially important series of studies Kerkut and his colleagues report that changes in protein and RNA synthesis accompany instrumental avoidance conditioning in the cockroach (the leg-position learning task). Incorporation of radioactive amino acid into newly synthesized protein in the metathoracic ganglion of experimental animals was found to be 70 percent greater than in control animals. Similarly, incorporation of labeled uridine into newly synthesized RNA was 44 percent greater in the metathoracic ganglion of experimental animals than in that of control animals, and 69 percent greater in experimental than in resting (unstimulated) animals (Kerkut et al., 1970a,b; Kerkut, Emson, and Beesley, 1972). Autoradiographic techniques showed that uridine incorporation was greatest in that region of the ganglion known to contain the somata of motoneurons supplying the involved limb.

Of greatest potential interest was the finding that synaptic transmitters (GABA, acetylcholine) and related enzymes change activity in association with learning (Oliver et al., 1971; Kerkut et al., 1970a,b; Kerkut, Emson, and Beesley, 1972). For example, it was reported that the activity of acetylcholinesterase, an enzyme that hydrolyzes acetylcholine, declined by more than half in the metathoracic ganglion of experimental animals (Kerkut, Emson, and Beesley, 1972). The time course of the recovery of cholinesterase activity closely paralleled the time course of the disappearance of the learned response (Kerkut et al., 1970a; Oliver, 1973), suggesting the possibility of a causal relationship.

Unfortunately, the reported findings of Kerkut and his colleagues on cholinesterase suffer from a serious inconsistency. It is claimed that K_M, the Michaelis constant, of the enzyme-substrate reaction is changed by training, but V_{max} is not (Kerkut, Emson, and Beesley, 1972).[9] Therefore, determinations of cholinesterase activity made at substrate concentrations much higher than K_M could not possibly reveal differences between experimental and control animals. The reported values of K_M for cholinesterase range from 10^{-4} to 10^{-5} M (Kerkut, Emson, and Beesley, 1972).[10] In their earlier papers, however, substrate concentrations near 10^{-3} M were employed (Kerkut et al., 1970b, 1971). In other words, if the data in the 1972 paper are correct, then the earlier results could not have been obtained.

In two independent studies, the results of Kerkut and his colleagues on changes in cholinesterase activity during learning could not be replicated (Woodson, Schlapfer, and Barondes, 1972; Willner and Mellanby, 1974). Both attempts at replication employed substantially the same behavioral and biochemical procedures as Kerkut, and it is therefore unlikely that the failure to replicate resulted from methodological differences.

If cholinesterase activity is in fact reduced in trained animals, how might this biochemical mechanism mediate learning? It has been suggested that a decrease in cholinesterase activity in the neurons subserving leg movement might increase synaptic efficacies in the corresponding neuronal circuits (Kerkut et al., 1970b; Oliver, 1973; Kerkut, Emson, and Walker, 1973). Possible explanations for the decline in cholinesterase activity were not offered, but Lineweaver-Burk plots for the cholinesterase from experimental and control animals were linear, showed the same V_{max}, but different K_Ms (Kerkut, Emson, and Beesley, 1972, Fig. 9). Such differences are usually ascribed to the action of a competitive enzyme inhibitor (see White, Handler, and Smith, 1968, pp. 236–239). Thus we may speculate that learning in this system involves the synthesis of a competitive inhibitor for cholinesterase, which in turn raises the efficacy of synaptic transmission in the specific neuronal circuits that

[9]A common method of describing the kinetics of an enzyme-catalyzed reaction is to plot the substrate concentration (abscissa) against the velocity of the reaction (ordinate). The resulting curve is typically asymptotic. The maximum velocity occurs at higher substrate concentrations and is the asymptote defined as V_{max}. The substrate concentration that yields a reaction velocity half that of V_{max} is called the K_M, or Michaelis constant (see White, Bandler, and Smith, 1968, for details).

[10]I calculated the Michaelis constants from the Lineweaver-Burk plots in Fig. 9 of Kerkut, Emson, and Beesley (1972) and obtained values of 1.33×10^{-5} and 5.88×10^{-6} for the cholinesterase of experimental and control animals, respectively. In the same figure the authors list values that are one order of magnitude larger. The discrepancy presumably results from a mislabeling of the abscissa; giving the authors the benefit of the doubt for purposes of the argument developed in the text, I have taken the larger value as correct.

mediate the learned task. This hypothetical scheme is conceptually attractive, and it provides an excellent illustration of how associative learning can be approached in invertebrates by using interdisciplinary methods involving mutually supportive and interrelated behavioral, biochemical, and neurophysiological concepts. Unfortunately, the hypothesis must presently be judged improbable owing to the uncertainty surrounding the original data.

Biochemical correlates of instrumental avoidance conditioning have also been studied in the mollusc *Helix* (Emson, Walker, and Kerkut, 1971). In this case, however, a convincing demonstration of associative learning was not made owing to the lack of suitable control procedures (see Section 29.4.3). In particular, experimental and control animals received different numbers of shocks, and controls for the nonspecific effects of shock were not performed. Therefore, the demonstrated differences between RNA and protein synthesis in control and experimental animals may have resulted simply from differences in neural activity, differences in the nonspecific effects of shock, or both.

2. INHIBITION OF MACROMOLECULAR SYNTHESIS. Substantial evidence, including the few invertebrate examples reviewed above, suggests that biochemical synthesis of macromolecules (proteins and RNA) accompanies both neural activity and learning. We must next inquire whether these biochemical changes are necessary for the acquisition and retention of learned tasks. A logical approach is to administer agents known to inhibit macromolecular synthesis and see whether learning is correspondingly inhibited. As with studies of de novo synthesis, the vast majority of experiments employing biochemical inhibitors has involved vertebrate preparations, and these studies are reviewed in the articles and books cited earlier. A major conclusion of such work in vertebrate species is that short-term memory is independent of protein synthesis, but that long-term retention is blocked by inhibitors of protein synthesis (e.g., Squire and Barondes, 1972).

The few invertebrate studies that have been published deal largely with insect leg-position learning. Unfortunately, the majority of these studies contain important ambiguities and therefore are not particularly useful in assessing whether inhibitors of macromolecular synthesis influence learning. For example, Brown and Noble (1967) claim that cycloheximide, an inhibitor of protein synthesis, has an effect on leg-position learning in cockroaches, but in fact their data show no more than an effect of activity levels, as noted by Eisenstein (1968) and Glassman et al. (1970). In studies aimed at determining

the effects of anticholinesterases and other drugs on leg-position learning, Oliver (1973) claims that "the normal control animal [saline injected] learned in 30 minutes whereas the animal injected with physostigmine learned in 10 minutes" (p. 123). However, inspection of the data on which this statement is based (Fig. 7.7, p. 123: one experimental and one control animal) yields a much different conclusion. The control animal in fact learned in 26 minutes, whereas the animal injected with physostigmine learned in 16 minutes. Moreover, differences in the activity levels of the experimental and control animals at the beginning of the experiment completely account for the ten-minute difference in the time to criterion; the *rate* of learning (i.e., the slope of the learning curve) appears identical for experimental and control animals. Oliver's data show simply that animals injected with anticholinesterase are more active than control animals, which is not surprising in view of the function of cholinesterase in hydrolyzing the synaptic transmitter acetylcholine. Oliver's conclusion that "physostigmine therefore facilitated learning" (p. 123) is unsupported, and his conclusions using other drugs are inadmissible on the same grounds.

Kerkut et al. (1970b) present data from three animals that are more convincing (Fig. 8, p. 442), consisting of leg-position avoidance-learning curves in which the slope (i.e., the rate of learning) is decreased by neostigmine (i.e., learning is faster), and increased by cycloheximide (i.e., learning is slower). The remainder of their data (i.e., Figs. 9, 10, pp. 443–445) is presented in the form of either number of shocks or time to criterion, and neither of these parameters effectively distinguishes the effect of the drug on the rate of learning from its effect on initial activity levels. The essential data, i.e., the slopes of the learning curves, are not presented. Therefore, the authors claim that inhibitors and facilitators of macromolecular synthesis influence learning in this preparation cannot be evaluated on the basis of published data.

In the snail *Helix* it is reported that injection of inhibitors of protein and RNA synthesis impairs avoidance learning, and that two "stimulants" (premoline, amphetamine) enhance learning (Emson, Walker, and Kerkut, 1971; Kerkut, Emson, and Walker, 1973). Most of these data are subject to the same ambiguities described above, however. Furthermore, the relevance of these data to learning is questionable, since learning was not convincingly demonstrated in this preparation (see Section 29.4.3).

Invertebrate studies on inhibition of macromolecular synthesis have thus contributed little to date. Such studies, even when performed properly, suffer from a crucial ambiguity; namely, inhibitors that are supposed to be specific in effect may in fact have widespread and in some cases unknown secondary behavioral (e.g., Booth and Pilcher, 1973) or biochemical effects. If learning is in fact blocked by administration of an inhibitor, we can generally not exclude one of these secondary effects as the cause. For example, puromycin, which is widely used to inhibit protein synthesis, is also known to reduce the amplitude of action potentials in the fish spinal cord by 25 percent (Bondeson, Edstrom, and Beriz, 1967), although such side effects are absent in *Aplysia* (Schwartz, Castellucci, and Kandel, 1971). Similarly, inhibitors of RNA synthesis in mice also make the animals sick (Barondes and Cohen, 1967). Even if inhibiting agents are specific, secondary effects of their toxicity may underlie the interference with learning. Thus, although blockage experiments do implicate macromolecular synthesis in learning, the resulting data cannot be considered the strongest source of support for this contention. Moreover, inhibition experiments cannot help to decide between the biochemical-antecedent and the biochemical-code hypothesis.

3. MEMORY TRANSFER. The logic of memory transfer is startling in its simplicity (McConnell and Shelby, 1970): if learning involves the synthesis of new macromolecules, and if these macromolecules are causal to learning or retention, then transferring the macromolecules to a naive animal should make it behave as if trained.

The earliest experiments of this type were performed by McConnell and co-workers using planarians (see Corning and Kelly, 1973, for a review). These experiments claimed to show successful transfer of a classically conditioned light-avoidance response. The transferred substance lost its effect when treated with ribonuclease, implicating RNA as the macromolecular memory "code" (Jacobson, Fried, and Horowitz, 1966). The results of these experiments seemed to require a radical departure from conventional learning theory, for they seemed to imply that neuronal organization per se is quite secondary to memory storage. Perhaps partly for this reason, McConnell's work was disputed, sometimes bitterly, leading to the so-called planarian controversy. The issue is now old enough to be viewed in objective historical perspective, and at least some recent reveiws conclude that the phenomenon of memory transfer of conditioned behavior in planarians is real and reproducible (e.g., Corning and Kelly, 1973). Regardless of one's position on this issue, there can be little disagreement about the originality and impact of McConnell's work. His studies provided impetus for dozens of subsequent investigations on memory transfer. Unfortunately, with the exception of further planarian work, virtually all of these studies have been performed on vertebrate species (e.g., Ungar, 1973; Ungar, Desiderio, and Parr, 1972). Futher experimentation on memory transfer in invertebrates would be welcome.

The ambiguities inherent in experiments involving inhibition of synthesis are to some degree overcome by memory transfer, but an important new ambiguity is introduced. Frank, Stein, and Rosen (1970) have provided an embarrassing demonstration that "memory transfer" of an avoidance task in mice can be accomplished using liver homogenate! They interpret such results in terms of general stress, rather than specific memory transfer, and they caution that controls for specificity of effect are essential in memory-transfer paradigms.

Memory-transfer experiments provide the strongest available support for the biochemical-code hypothesis. In particular, Ungar and his colleagues have isolated and analyzed a polypetide, scotophobin, which is alleged to underlie a dark-avoidance learning task (e.g., Ungar, 1973). Other investigators, however, seem unpersuaded by the interpretation. Thus Glassman and Wilson (1973) write, in the proceedings of a symposium in which Ungar also participated, that "few neurobiologists, if any, believe that experiential information is stored or coded in macromolecules" (p. 81).

If memory transfer exists, this would seem effectively to eliminate the reverberation hypothesis, but the phenomenon does not help us to decide between the biochemical-code hypothesis and the biochemical-antecedent hypothesis. The transferred substance could be a unique "memory molecule," in accordance with the code hypothesis. Alternatively, the substance could influence the organization and functional properties of neuronal circuits, thus mediating the transferred task in the recipient animal in accordance with the antecedent hypothesis. In fact, despite the weighty evidence that macromolecular synthesis *accompanies* learning, available data do not yet prove that macromolecular synthesis *causes* learning. If there is a causal connection between macromolecular synthesis and learning, as we presume, we cannot yet specify its nature. This issue will undoubtedly provide a major focus for learning research in the coming decades.

29.4.6 Theoretical approaches to learning

Learning has attracted considerable attention from theorists, and as a result, learning theories abound. Some theories assume that learning is a "field" or "statistical" phenomenon that is inaccessible to analysis on the cellular level (e.g., John, 1972).[11] Most learning theories,

---

[11]"In view of the absence of any convincing evidence that

however, are based upon Hebb's postulate that learning involves changes in the functional properties of specific neuronal circuits[12] (e.g., Birk, 1970; Briggs and Kitto, 1962; Brindley, 1967, 1968; Burke 1966; Eccles, 1953; Glickman and Schiff, 1967; Griffith, 1966; Grossberg, 1971; Katchalsky and Neumann, 1972; Katchalsky and Oplatka, 1966; Kosower, 1972; Robinson, 1966; Sharpless, 1964; Smith, 1962; Taylor, 1965). Learning theories based on Hebb's postulate have been classified in a review by Kupfermann and Pinsker (1969).

Among the most interesting learning theories are those that involve integration of existing data to develop testable hypotheses on learning mechanisms. For example, Szilard (1964) and Ranck (1964) proposed theories based upon the transport of macromolecules between neurons involved in learning ("transprinting" or "electro-osmosis"). Roitbach (1970) proposes that synapses become "validated" by the addition of myelin to the terminal branches of axons, with the result that current is conserved and conducted more effectively to the terminals. This theory is especially interesting in that it incorporates a role for glial cells (oligodendrocytes) in the learning process. Synaptic "validation" and "invalidation" are also postulated to occur during ontogeny (Jacobson, 1969) and regeneration (Mark, Marotte, and Johnstone, 1970; Marotte and Mark, 1970a,b; Mark and Marotte, 1972; Mark, Marotte, and Mart, 1972), and some learning theories stem directly from such ontogenetic concepts (e.g., Mark, 1970).

One of the more imaginative and synthetic learning theories is that proposed by Stent (1973). The theory was actually developed to explain observations on the plasticity of binocular connections in the cat visual cortex, but it can be extended to include classical conditioning. The theory employs denervation hypersensitivity of neuromuscular junctions as a model (e.g., Lømo and Rosenthal, 1972). It proposes that a neuron (e.g., one mediating the UR in a classical-conditioning paradigm) normally receives contacts from numerous presynaptic neurons (e.g., ones mediating the US and CS), but that most of the corresponding synapses (i.e., those mediating potential CSs) are nonfunctional. Such lability is preserved by action potentials in the postsynaptic neuron, which invade the subsynaptic membrane of labile synapses, cause a reversal in membrane potential, and thereby destroy receptor sites for the synaptic transmitter.[13] Receptor sites associated with active sites (US) are "protected" from the reversal of potential by the subsynaptic permeability change associated with the transmitter action, which tends to "clamp" the membrane potential near zero and thus prevent reversal. During conditioning, the labile synapses (CS) are also afforded such protection because they are activated simultaneously with the postsynaptic neuron (UR) as a direct result of the conditioning procedure. As a consequence of such protection, labile synapses become functional and can eventually cause the postsynaptic cell to discharge (the CR).

The most valuable feature of Stent's theory is that it accounts, in explicit physiological terms and by means of a testable and partially precedented hypothesis, for the effects of contingency. In extending the theory to conditioning, however, as I have done here, a number of problems are encountered. First, it is not clear how the protection of labile synapses can occur during learning, since such protection depends upon the action of active receptor sites that are, according to the theory, absent. Second, the theory predicts that the occurrence of the UR between conditioning trials should interfere with acquisition, and therefore that massed training should be more effective than spaced training. In fact, the converse is true. Third, the theory predicts that learned behavior, once established, is necessarily retained for some time. In fact, conditioned responses can be made to disappear rapidly in the absence of reinforcement (extinction). Fourth, the theory requires that the dendrites of neurons be capable of supporting action potentials. In fact, most dendritic membrane is electrically inexcitable, although exceptions are known (e.g., Zucker, 1972c). Fifth, the theory does not incorporate a role for macromolecular synthesis in learning. Despite these difficulties in extending it to learning, Stent's theory is interesting and provocative. Moreover, it is the kind of theory that may be rigorously testable only by the use of the relatively simple invertebrate preparations discussed in this review.

29.5 OTHER FORMS OF PLASTICITY

In the above treatment I have concentrated on forms of

---

permanent changes in synaptic efficiency actually occur or that new connections are actually established in learning, it seems incongruous that these ideas have come to be so widely accepted"(John, 1972, p. 850).

[12]"When an axon of cell A is near enough to excite cell B and repeatedly and persistently takes part in firing it, some growth or metabolic change takes place in one or both cells such that A's efficiency, as one of the cells firing B, is increased" (Hebb, 1949, p. 62).

---

[13]The hypothesis that reversal in membrane potential destroys receptor sites for synaptic transmitters is based on data such as that of Lømo and Rosenthal (1972) and Drachman and Witzke (1972) showing that the heightened sensitivity to acetylcholine, which spreads over a muscle cell following denervation, is abolished by direct electrical stimulation of the nerve or muscle.

plasticity that are potentially amenable to cellular analysis in invertebrate preparations. As a result of this selective treatment, many forms of plasticity have been omitted. The term plasticity arose in large part in the context of development and regeneration, but these topics are beyond the scope of the present review (see Jacobson, 1969, and Raisman, 1973, for reviews). The important topic of nonassociative learning (i.e., learning without reinforcement) was covered only briefly, owing to the intractability of this form of plasticity to cellular analysis. Many other forms of plasticity in invertebrates that are not covered here are reviewed by Corning, Dyal, and Willows (1973). For example, the phenomenon of "learning sets" has been studied in isopods (Morrow and Smithson, 1969). Many invertebrates exhibit place or "orientation" learning, a form of plasticity that may bear a relation to such an instrumental-conditioning task as maze learning, which has been studied extensively in ants (Weiss and Schneirla, 1967; see Alloway, 1973, for a review).

A form of plasticity often revealed in maze-learning experiments is reactive inhibition. Hull (1943, 1951) used this term as a theoretical component in his theory of behavior, but it has since been employed empirically to describe the tendency of an organism to turn in the opposite direction from a recently made turn (Dingle, 1965; Kupfermann, 1966). McConnell (1966) describes this form of plasticity as a primitive form of learning. More recently, however, Wilson and Hoy (1968) have shown that reactive inhibition in some species probably simply represents a delayed optomotor response. Optokinetic "memory" in crabs (Horridge, 1966a–c) is a related form of plasticity.

A host of additional and related phenomena, seldom studied in the invertebrates, includes attention (McFarland, 1966), selective perception (Horn, 1965; Hillyard et al., 1973), and drive or motivation (Hinde, 1960; McFarland and Sibly, 1972; Kupfermann, 1974). As noted in Section 29.3.2, it is possible that these forms of plasticity represent manifestations of a single, common phenomenon, a behavioral hierarchy. Imprinting (Bateson, 1966; Bateson, Rose, and Horn, 1973; Rose, Bateson, and Horn, 1973), the perhaps related olfactory "memory" (Cooper and Hasler, 1974), and the development or improvement of innate behavior patterns with practice or exposure to appropriate sensory cues (Marler, 1970), are forms of plasticity that have received very little attention in invertebrates. On the cellular level, the circadian rhythm of an endogenously bursting molluscan neuron can be phase-shifted by exposure of the intact animal to a new light/dark cycle (Strumwasser, 1965, and this volume). The same neuron can be entrained to

a non-24-hour period (Lickey, 1969). The bursting rate of the cell can also be influenced by "reinforcement" of certain phases of the cycle with nerve stimulation (Frazier, Waziri, and Kandel, 1965; Pinsker and Kandel, 1967), a cellular analogue of operant conditioning.

29.6 CONCLUSIONS

I would like to end with three general conclusions that seem especially relevant. First, behavioral plasticity, including associative learning, is ubiquitous in the animal kingdom. As reviewed in this article, every major form of behavioral plasticity has now been demonstrated in one or more of the invertebrate phyla. There is a pressing need to replicate successful experiments and to develop additional preparations, especially ones that are amenable to cellular analysis. Toward this end, molluscan and arthropod preparations appear most promising. Given a judicious selection of conditioning and reinforcing stimuli and temporal parameters for learning paradigms, in accordance with the preparedness principle, behavioral experiments on learning in the invertebrates should prove a most fertile area for research in the next decade.

Second, it seems quite likely that the first and most complete cellular explanations of plasticity will come from invertebrate preparations. While it is true that the major conceptual framework has arisen from vertebrate studies, only invertebrates have the relatively limited, accessible nervous systems that permit complete cellular analysis. Workable strategies have already been developed, involving four sequential steps: (1) behavioral analysis of plasticity; (2) description of the neuronal circuits that are involved; (3) identification of the electrophysiological concomitants of plasticity; and (4) investigation of underlying biophysical and biochemical causes. Several invertebrate preparations have already begun to yield answers, including the molluscs *Aplysia* (habituation, sensitization) and *Pleurobranchaea* (choice, associative learning), and the insect leg-position learning preparation (avoidance learning).

Finally, the neuronal substrates of behavioral plasticity are likely to be the same throughout the animal kindom. Some of my colleagues consider this an imprudent suggestion, but I believe that available precedents justify faith in the existence of unifying generalities in the neurosciences. One of the most important general lessons of molecular biology is that evolution has been conservative; protein synthesis, for example, is virtually identical in bacterial and brain cells. For the present, at least, there is every reason to expect that this paradigm (in the sense of Kuhn, 1962) of evolutionary conservatism applies equally well to the operations of the nervous system and, in particular, to the cellular basis of plasticity.

ACKNOWLEDGMENTS

Several colleagues have given generously of their time in reading part or all of this review and offering valuable criticisms, including Samuel Barondes, Bruce Bridgeman, Tom Carew, Donald Kennedy, Frank Krasne, and Jeff Wine. Especially helpful were the comments of Eric Kandel. Jeff Ram provided useful discussions in connection with the section on the biochemistry of learning. I thank my students and postdoctoral colleagues, and especially George Mpitsos, for valuable discussions and for major contributions to the experimental work from this laboratory, which has been supported by NIH Research Grants NS 09050 and MH 23254, NSF Grant GZ 3120, and University of California Faculty Research Grants.

REFERENCES

ABRAHAM, F. D., PALKA, J., PEEKE, H. V. S., and WILLOWS, A. O. D. 1972. Model neural systems and strategies for the neurobiology of learning. *Behavioral Biology* 7: 1–24.

ABRAHAM, F. D., and WILLOWS, A. O. D. 1972. Plasticity of a fixed action pattern in the sea slug *Tritonia diomedia*. *Communications in Behavioral Biology* Part A 6: 271–280.

ADAM, G., ed. 1971. *Biology of Memory*. New York: Plenum Press.

ADLER, J., and TSO, W.-W. 1974. "Decision"-making in bacteria: Chemotactic response of *Escherichia coli* to conflicting stimuli. *Science* 184: 1292–1294.

ALKON, D. L. 1974. Associative training of *Hermissenda*. *Journal of General Physiology* 64: 70–84.

ALLOWAY, T. M. 1969. Effects of low temperature upon acquisition and retention in the grain beetle, *Tenebrio molitor*. *Journal of Comparative and Physiological Psychology* 69: 1–8.

ALLOWAY, T. M. 1973. Learning in insects except *Apoidea*. In Corning, Dyal, and Willows (1973), Vol. 2, pp. 31–185.

ALLOWAY, T. M., and ROUTTENBERG, A. 1967. "Reminiscence" in the cold flour beetle (*Tenebrio molitor*). *Science* 158: 1066–1067.

ANDJUS, R. K., KNOPFELMACHER, F., RUSSELL, R. W., and SMITH, A. U. 1956. Some effects of severe hypothermia on learning and retention. *Quarterly Journal of Experimental Psychology* 8:15–23.

ANSELL, G. B., and BRADLEY, P. B., eds. 1973. *Macromolecules and Behavior*. Baltimore: University Park Press.

APPLEWHITE, P. B., and GARDNER, F. 1971. A theory of protozoan habituation learning. *Nature* 230: 285–287.

ARANDA, L. C., and LUCO, J. V. 1969. Further studies on an electrical correlate to learning: Experiments in an isolated insect ganglion. *Physiology and Behavior* 4: 133–137.

BARONDES, S. H., and COHEN, H. D. 1967. Delayed and sustained effect of acetoxycycloheximide on memory in mice. *Proceedings of the National Academy of Sciences* 58:157–164.

BATESON, P. P. G. 1966. The characteristics and context of imprinting. *Biological Reviews* 41:177–220.

BATESON, P. P. G., ROSE, S. P. R., and HORN, G. 1973. Imprinting: Lasting effects on uracil incorporation into chick brain. *Science* 181: 576–578.

BAUM, W. M. 1974. Choice in free-ranging wild pigeons. *Science* 185: 78–79.

BERRY, M., HOLLINGSWORTH, T., FLINN, R., and ANDERSON, E. M. 1973. Morphological correlates of functional activity in the nervous system. In Ansell and Bradley (1973), pp. 217–240.

BERRY, M. S. 1973. Electrotonic coupling between identified large cells in the buccal ganglia of *Planorbis corneus*. *Journal of Experimental Biology* 57: 173–185.

BERRY, R. W. 1969. Ribonucleic acid metabolism of a single neuron: Correlation with electrical activity. *Science* 166: 1021–1023.

BEST, J. B. 1965. Behavior of Planaria in instrumental learning paradigms. In Thorpe and Davenport (1965), pp. 69–75.

BETHE, A. 1930. Studien über die Plasticität des Nevernsystems. I. Arachoideen und Crustacea. *Pfluegers Archiv für die Gesamte Physiologie des Menschen und der Tiere* 224: 793–820.

BIRK, J. R. 1970. A hypothetical synaptic-neural-behavioral model of operant learning. *Kybernetik* 7: 13–21.

BLISS, T. V. P., GARDNER-MEDWIN, A. R., and LØMO, T. 1973. Synaptic plasticity in the hippocampal formation. In Ansell and Bradley (1973), pp. 193–203.

BLODGETT, H. C. 1929. The effect of the introduction of reward upon the maze performance of rats. *University of California Publications in Psychology* 4: 113–134.

BOCHAROVA, L. S., BOROVYAGIN, V. L., DYAKONOVA, T. L., WARTON, S. S., and VEPRINTSEV, B. N. 1972. Ultrastructure and RNA synthesis in a molluscan giant neuron under electrical stimulation. *Brain Research* 36: 371–384.

BOGOCH, S. 1968. *The Biochemistry of Memory*. Toronto: Oxford University Press.

BONDESON, C., EDSTROM, A., and BERIZ, A. 1967. Effects of different inhibitors of protein synthesis on electrical activity in the spinal cord of fish. *Journal of Neurochemistry* 14: 1032–1034.

BOOTH, D. A., and PILCHER, C. W. T. 1973. Behavioural effects of protein synthesis inhibitors: Consolidation blockage or negative reinforcement? In Ansell and Bradley (1973), pp. 105–112.

BOWMAN, R. E., and DATTA, S. P., eds. 1970. *Biochemistry of Brain and Behavior*. New York: Plenum Press.

BRIGGS, M. H., and KITTO, G. B. 1962. The molecular basis of memory and learning. *Psychological Review* 69: 537–541.

BRINDLEY, G. S. 1967. The classification of modifiable synapses and their use in models for conditioning. *Proceedings of the Royal Society (London)* B 168: 361–376.

BRINDLEY, G. S. 1968. Nerve net models of plausible size that perform many simple learning tasks. *Proceedings of the Royal Society (London)* B 174: 173–191.

BROOKS, V. B., KOZLOVSKAYA, I. B., ATKIN, A., HORVATH, F. E., and UNO, M. 1973. Effect of cooling dentate nucleus on tracking-task performance in monkeys. *Journal of Neurophysiology* 36: 974–995.

BROWN, B. M., and NOBLE, E. P. 1967. Cycloheximide and learning in the isolated cockroach ganglion. *Brain Research* 6: 363–366.

BRUNER, J., and KEHOE, J. 1970. Long-term decrements in the efficacy of synaptic transmission in mollusks and crustaceans. In Horn and Hinde (1970), pp. 323–359.

BRUNER, J., and KENNEDY, D. 1970. Habituation: Occurrence at a neuromuscular junction. *Science* 169: 92–94.

BRUNER, J., and TAUC, L. 1964. Les modifications de l'activité synaptique au cours de l'habituation chez l'Aplysie. *Journal de Physiologie* 56: 306–307.

BRUNER, J., and TAUC, L. 1965. La plasticité synaptique impliquée dans le processus d'habituation chez l'Aplysie. *Journal de Physiologie* 57: 230–231.

BRUNER, J., and TAUC, L. 1966. Long-lasting phenomena in the molluskan nervous system. *Symposia of the Society for Experimental Biology* 20: 457–475.

BULLOCK, T. H., and QUARTON, G. C. 1966. Simple systems for the study of learning mechanisms. *Neurosciences Research Program Bulletin* 4: 203–327.

BUREŠ, J., and BUREŠOVÁ, O. 1967. Plastic changes of unit activity based on reinforcing properties of extracellular stimulation of single neurons. *Journal of Neurophysiology* 30: 98–113.

BURKE, W. 1966. Neuronal models for conditioned reflexes. *Nature* 210: 269–271.

BURROWS, M. 1973. Physiological and morphological properties of the metathoracic common inhibitory neuron of the locust. *Journal of Comparative Physiology* 82: 59–78.

BURROWS, M., and HORRIDGE, G. A. 1974. The organization of inputs to motoneurons of the locust metathoracic leg. *Philosophical Transactions of the Royal Society of London* B 269: 49–94.

BURROWS, M., and HOYLE, G. 1973. Neural mechanisms underlying behavior in the locust *Schistocera gregaria*. III. Topography of limb motoneurons in the metathoracic ganglion. *Journal of Neurobiology* 4: 167–186.

BYRNE, W. L., ed. 1970. *Molecular Approaches to Learning and Memory* New York: Academic Press.

CAMHI, J. M. 1970a. Sensory control of abdomen posture in flying locusts. *Journal of Experimental Biology* 52: 533–537.

CAMHI, J. M. 1970b. Yaw-correcting postural changes in locusts. *Journal of Experimental Biology* 52: 519–531.

CAMHI, J. M., and HINKLE, M. 1972. Attentiveness to sensory stimuli: Central control in locusts. *Science* 175: 550–553.

CAREW, T. J., CASTELLUCCI, V. F., and KANDEL, E. R. 1971. An analysis of dishabituation and sensitization of the gill-withdrawal reflex in *Aplysia*. *International Journal of Neuroscience* 2: 79–98.

CAREW, T. J., and KANDEL, E. R. 1973. Acquisition and retention of long-term habituation in *Aplysia*: Correlation of behavioral and cellular processes. *Science* 182: 1158–1160.

CAREW, T. J., PINSKER, H. M., and KANDEL, E. R. 1972. Long-term habituation of a defensive withdrawal reflex in *Aplysia*. *Science* 175: 451–454.

CASTELLUCCI, V. F., KANDEL, E. R., and SCHWARTZ, J. H. 1972. Macromolecular synthesis and the functioning of neurons and synapses. In G. D. Pappas and D. P. Purpura, eds., *Structure and Function of Synapses*. New York: Raven Press, pp. 193–219.

CASTELLUCCI, V., KUPFERMANN, I., PINSKER, H., and KANDEL, E. R. 1970. Neuronal mechanisms of habituation and dishabituation of the gill withdrawal reflex in *Aplysia*. *Science* 167: 1445–1448.

CHOW, K.-L., and LEIMAN, A. L. 1972. The photo-sensitive organs of crayfish and brightness learning. *Behavioral Biology* 7: 25–35.

CHURCH, R. M. 1963. Effects of punishment on behavior. *Psychological Review* 70: 369–402.

COHEN, M. J., and JACKLET, J. W. 1967. The functional organization of motor neurons in an insect ganglion. *Philosophical Transactions of the Royal Society of London* B 252: 563–571.

COOPER, J. C., and HASLER, A. D. 1974. Electroencephalographic evidence for retention of olfactory cues in homing Coho salmon. *Science* 183: 336–338.

CORNING, W. C., DYAL, J. A., and WILLOWS, A. O. D., eds. 1973. *Invertebrate Learning.* Vol. 1: *Protozoans through Annelids.* Vol. 2: *Arthropods and Gastropod Mollusks.* Vol. 3: *Cephalopods and Echinoderms.* New York: Plenum Press.

CORNING, W. C., and KELLY, S. 1973. Platyhelminthes: The Turbellarians. In Corning, Dyal, and Willows (1973), Vol. 1, pp. 171–224.

CORNING, W. C., and LAHUE, R. 1972. Invertebrate strategies in comparative learning studies. *American Zoologist* 12: 455–469.

CORNING, W. C., and RATNER, S. C., eds. 1967. *Chemistry of Learning: Invertebrate Research.* New York: Plenum Press.

CORNING, W. C., and RICCIO, D. 1970. The planarian controversy. In Byrne (1970), pp. 107–150.

CRONLY-DILLON, J., CARDEN, D., and BIRKS, C. 1974. The possible involvement of brain microtubules in memory fixation. *Journal of Experimental Biology* 61: 443–454.

DAVIS, W. J. 1973. Development of locomotor patterns in absence of peripheral sense organs and muscles. *Proceedings of the National Academy of Sciences* 70: 954–958.

DAVIS, W. J., and DAVIS, K. B. 1973. Ontogeny of a simple locomotor system: Role of the periphery in specifying the development of the central nervous system. *American Zoologist* 13: 409–425.

DAVIS, W. J., and MPITSOS, G. J. 1971. Behavioral choice and habituation in the marine mollusk *Pleurobranchaea californica* MacFarland (Gastropoda, Opisthobranchia). *Zeitschrift fuer Vergleichende Physiologie* 75: 207–232.

DAVIS, W. J., MPITSOS, G. J., and PINNEO, J. M. 1974a. The behavioral hierarchy of the mollusk *Pleurobranchaea*. I. The dominant position of feeding behavior. *Journal of Comparative Physiology* 90: 207–224.

DAVIS, W. J., MPITSOS, G. J., and PINNEO, J. M. 1974b. The behavioral hierarchy of the mollusk *Pleurobranchaea*. II. Hormonal suppression of feeding associated with egg-laying. *Journal of Comparative Physiology* 90: 225–243.

DAVIS, W. J., MPITSOS, G. J., SIEGLER, M. V. S., PINNEO, J. M., and DAVIS, K. B. 1974. Neuronal substrates of behavioral hierarchies and associative learning in *Pleurobranchaea*. *American Zoologist* 14: 1037–1050.

DAVIS, W. J., PINNEO, J. M., MPITSOS, G. J. and RAM, J. L. 1976a. Plasticity in the behavioral hierarchy of *Pleurobranchaea*. I. The effects of food satiation on the dominance of feeding behavior (in preparation).

DAVIS, W. J., PINNEO, J. M., MPITSOS, G. J. and RAM, J. L. 1976b. Plasticity in the behavioral hierarchy of *Pleurobranchaea*. II. The effects of egg-laying hormone on the dominance of feeding behavior (in preparation).

DAVIS, W. J., SIEGLER, M. V. S., and MPITSOS, G. J. 1973. Distributed neuronal oscillators and efference copy in the feeding system of *Pleurobranchaea*. *Journal of Neurophysiology* 36: 258–274.

DELCOMYN, F. 1971. Computer aided analysis of a locomotor leg reflex in the cockroach *Periplaneta americana*. *Zeitschrift fuer Vergleichende Physiologie* 74: 427–445.

DELCOMYN, F. 1973. Motor activity during walking in the

cockroach *Periplaneta americana*. II. Tethered walking. *Journal of Experimental Biology* 59: 643–654.

DELCOMYN, F., and USHERWOOD, P. N. R. 1973. Motor activity during walking in the cockroach *Periplaneta americana*. I. Free walking. *Journal of Experimental Biology* 59: 629–642.

DETHIER, V. G. 1955. The physiology and histology of the contact chemoreceptors of the blowfly. *Quarterly Review of Biology* 30: 348–371.

DETHIER, V. G. 1968. Chemosensory input and taste discrimination in the blowfly. *Science* 161: 389–391.

DETHIER, V. G., and GOLDRICH, N. 1971. Blowflies: Alteration of adult taste response by chemicals present during development. *Science* 173: 242–244.

DETHIER, V. G., SOLOMON, R. L., and TURNER, L. H. 1965. Sensory input and central excitation and inhibition in the blowfly. *Journal of Comparative and Physiological Psychology* 60: 303–313.

DETHIER, V. G., SOLOMON, R. L., and TURNER, L. H. 1968. Central inhibition in the blowfly. *Journal of Comparative and Physiological Psychology* 66: 144–150.

DINGLE, H. 1965. Turn alternation by bugs on causeways as a delayed compensatory response and the effects of varying visual inputs and length of straight paths. *Animal Behaviour* 13: 171–177.

DISTERHOFT, J. F., HAGGERTY, R., and CORNING, W. C. 1971. An analysis of leg position learning in the cockroach yoked control. *Physiology and Behavior* 7: 359–362.

DISTERHOFT, J. F., NURNBERGER, J., and CORNING, W. C. 1968. "P-R" differences in intact cockroaches as a function of testing interval. *Psychonomic Science, Section on Animal and Physiological Psychology* 12: 205–206.

DOWNEY, P., and JAHAN-PARWAR, B. 1972. Cooling as a reinforcing stimulus in *Aplysia*. *American Zoologist* 12: 507–512.

DRACHMAN, D. B., and WITZKE, F. 1972. Trophic regulation of acetylcholine sensitivity of muscle: Effect of electrical stimulation. *Science* 176: 514–516.

DUNCAN, C. P. 1949. The retroactive effect of electroshock on learning. *Journal of Comparative and Physiological Psychology* 42: 32–44.

DYAL, J. A., and CORNING, W. C. 1973. Invertebrate learning and behavior taxonomies. In Corning, Dyal, and Willows (1973), Vol. 1, pp. 1–48.

ECCLES, J. C. 1953. *The Neurophysiological Basis of Mind*. London: Oxford University Press.

EISENSTEIN, E. M. 1967. The use of invertebrate systems for studies on the bases of learning and memory. In G. C. Quarton, T. Melnechuk, and F. O. Schmitt, eds., *The Neurosciences: A Study Program*. New York: Rockefeller University Press, pp. 653–664.

EISENSTEIN, E. M. 1968. Assessing the influence of pharmacological agents on shock avoidance learning in simpler systems. *Brain Research* 11: 471–480.

EISENSTEIN, E. M. 1970a. A comparison of *activity* and *position* response measures of avoidance learning in the cockroach, *P. americana*. *Brain Research* 21: 143–147.

EISENSTEIN, E. M. 1970b. The retention of shock avoidance learning in the cockroach, *P. americana*. *Brain Research* 21: 148–150.

EISENSTEIN, E. M. 1972. Learning and memory in isolated insect ganglia. *Advances in Insect Physiology* 9: 111–181.

EISENSTEIN, E. M., and COHEN, M. J. 1965. Learning in an isolated prothoracic insect ganglion. *Animal Behaviour* 13: 104–108.

EISENSTEIN, E. M., KEMENY, G., SKURNICK, I. D., and HARRIS, J. T. 1972. Transfer of information within the cockroach central nervous system during shock avoidance learning: Is there a nerve impulse code(s) for learned information? *International Journal of Neuroscience* 3: 93–98.

EISENSTEIN, E. M., and KRASILOVSKY, G. H. 1967. Studies of learning in isolated insect ganglia. In C. A. G. Wiersma, ed., *Invertebrate Nervous Systems*. Chicago: The University of Chicago Press, pp. 329–332.

EISENSTEIN, E. M., and PERETZ, B. 1973. Comparative aspects of habituation in invertebrates. In Peeke and Herz (1973), Vol. 2, pp. 1–34.

EMSON, P., WALKER, R. J., and KERKUT, G. A. 1971. Chemical changes in a molluscan ganglion associated with learning. *Comparative Biochemistry and Physiology* 40B: 223–239.

EPSTEIN, R., and TAUC, L. 1970. Heterosynaptic facilitation and posttetanic potentiation in *Aplysia* nervous system. *Journal of Physiology* 209: 1–23.

EVANS, S. M. 1966a. Non-associative avoidance learning in nereid polychaetes. *Animal Behaviour* 14: 102–106.

EVANS, S. M. 1966b. Non-associative behavioral modifications in the polychaete *Nereis diversicolor*. *Animal Behaviour* 14: 107–112.

EVANS, S. M. 1966c. Non-associative behavioral modifications in nereid polychaetes. *Nature* 211: 945–948.

EVARTS, E. V. 1973. Motor cortex reflexes associated with learned movement. *Science* 179: 501–503.

FETZ, E. E., and BAKER, M. A. 1973. Operantly conditioned patterns of precentral unit activity and correlated responses in adjacent cells and contralateral muscles. *Journal of Neurophysiology* 36: 179–204.

FETZ, E. E., and FINOCCHIO, D. V. 1971. Operant conditioning of specific patterns of neural and muscular activity. *Science* 174: 431–435.

FJERDINGSTAD, E. J., ed. 1971. *Chemical Transfer of Learned Information*. Amsterdam: North Holland Publishing Company.

FRANK, B., STEIN, D. G., and ROSEN, J. 1970. Interanimal "memory" transfer: Results from brain and liver homogenates. *Science* 169: 399–402.

FRAZIER, W. T., WAZIRI, R., and KANDEL, E. R. 1965. Alterations in the frequency of spontaneous activity in *Aplysia* neurons with contingent and noncontingent nerve stimulation. *Federation Proceedings* 24: 522.

FRINGS, H. 1941. The loci of olfactory end-organs in the blowfly, *Cynomyia cadaverina* Desvoidy. *Journal of Experimental Zoology* 88: 65–93.

FUSTER, J. M., and ALEXANDER, G. E. 1971. Neuron activity related to short-term memory. *Science* 173: 652–654.

GARCIA, J., ERVIN, F. R., and KOELLING, R. A. 1966. Learning with prolonged delay of reinforcement. *Psychonomic Science, Section on Animal and Physiological Psychology* 5: 121–122.

GARCIA, J., and KOELLING, R. A. 1966. Relation of cue to consequence in avoidance learning. *Psychonomic Science, Section on Animal and Physiological Psychiatry* 4: 123–124.

GAZE, R. M. 1970. *The Formation of Nerve Connections*. New York: Academic Press.

GELPERIN, A. 1974. Olfactory basis of homing behavior in the giant garden slug, *Limax maximus*. *Proceedings of the National Academy of Sciences* 71: 966–970.

GETTING, P. A. 1971. The sensory control of motor output in fly proboscis extension. *Zeitschrift für Vergleichende Physiologie* 74: 103–120.

GLASSMAN, E. 1969. The biochemistry of learning; an evaluation of the role of RNA and protein. *Annual Review of Biochemistry* 37: 605–646.

GLASSMAN, E., HENDERSON, A., CORDLE, H., MOON, H. M., and WILSON, J. E. 1970. Effect of cycloheximide and actinomycin D on the behavior of the headless cockroach. *Nature* 225: 967–968.

GLASSMAN, E., and WILSON, J. E. 1973. RNA and brain function. In Ansell and Bradley (1973), pp. 81–92.

GLICKMAN, S. E., and SCHIFF, B. B. 1967. A biological theory of reinforcement. *Psychological Review* 74: 81–109.

GORMEZANO, I. 1966. Classical conditioning. In J. B. Sidowski, ed., *Experimental Methods and Instrumentation in Psychology*. New York: McGraw-Hill, pp. 385–420.

GORMEZANO, I., and MOORE, J. W. 1969. History and Method. In M. M. Marx, ed., *Learning Processes*. Toronto: Macmillan, pp. 121–203.

GRIFFITH, J. S. 1966. A theory of the nature of memory. *Nature* 211: 1160–1163.

GROSS, C. G., and ZIEGLER, H. P., eds. 1969. *Readings in Physiological Psychology: Learning and Memory*. New York: Harper & Row.

GROSSBERG, S. 1971. On the dynamics of operant conditioning. *Journal of Theoretical Biology* 33: 225–255.

GUROWITZ, E. M. 1969. *The Molecular Basis of Memory*. Englewood Cliffs, N. J.: Prentice-Hall.

HAIGLER, H. J., and VON BAUMGARTEN, R. J. 1972. Facilitation of excitatory post-synaptic potentials in the giant cell in the left pleural ganglion of *Aplysia californica*. *Comparative Biochemistry and Physiology* 41A: 7–16.

HEBB, D. O. 1949. *The Organization of Behavior*. New York: John Wiley & Sons.

HERZ, M. J., PEEKE, H. V. S., and WYERS, E. J. 1964. Temperature and conditioning in the earthworm, *Lumbricus terrestrius*. *Animal Behaviour* 12: 502–507.

HILGARD, E. R. 1964. *Theories of Learning and Instruction*. Chicago: The University of Chicago Press.

HILGARD, E. R., and BOWER, G. H. 1966. *Theories of Learning*. New York: Appleton-Century-Crofts.

HILGARD, E. R., and MARQUIS, D. C. 1940. *Conditioning and Learning*. New York: Appleton-Century.

HILLYARD, S. A., HINK, R. F., SCHWENT, V. L., and PICTON, T. W. 1973. Electrical signs of selective attention in the human brain. *Science* 182: 177–180.

HINDE, R. A. 1960. Energy models of motivation. *Symposia of the Society for Experimental Biology* 14: 199–213.

HINDE, R. A. 1970. Behavioral habituation. In Horn and Hinde (1970), pp. 3–40.

HOLMGREN, B., and FRENK, S. 1961. Inhibitory phenomena and "habituation" at the neuronal level. *Nature* 192: 1294–1295.

HONIG, W. K., and JAMES, P. H. R., eds. 1971. *Animal Memory*. New York: Academic Press.

HORN, G. 1965. Physiological and psychological aspects of selective perception. In D. S. Lehrman, R. A. Hinde, and E. Shaw, eds., *Advances in the Study of Behavior*, Vol. 1. London: Academic Press, pp. 155–215.

HORN, G., and HINDE, R. A., eds. 1970. *Short-Term Changes in Neural Activity and Behaviour*. London: Cambridge University Press.

HORN, G., ROSE, S. P. R., and BATESON, P. P. G. 1973. Experiences and plasticity in the nervous system. *Science* 181: 506–514.

HORRIDGE, G. A. 1959. Analysis of the rapid responses of *Nereis*

and *Harmothoe* (Annelida). *Proceedings of the Royal Society (London)* B 150: 245–262.

HORRIDGE, G. A. 1962a. Learning of leg position by the ventral nerve cord in headless insects. *Proceedings of the Royal Society (London)* B 157: 33–52.

HORRIDGE, G. A. 1962b. Learning of leg position by headless insects. *Nature* 193: 697–698.

HORRIDGE, G. A. 1965. The electrophysiological approach to learning in isolated ganglia. *Animal Behaviour* 12: 163–182.

HORRIDGE, G. A. 1966a. Optokinetic memory in the crab, *Carcinus*. *Journal of Experimental Biology* 44: 233–245.

HORRIDGE, G. A. 1966b. Optokinetic responses of the crab, *Carcinus*, to a single moving light. *Journal of Experimental Biology* 44: 263–274.

HORRIDGE, G. A. 1966c. Direct response of the crab, *Carcinus*, to the movement of the sun. *Journal of Experimental Biology* 44: 275–283.

HOTTA, Y., and BENZER, S. 1972. Mapping of behaviour in *Drosophila* mosaics. *Nature* 240: 527–535.

HOYLE, G. 1960. Neuromuscular activity in the swimming sea anemone, *Stomphia coccinea* (Müller). *Journal of Experimental Biology* 37: 671–688.

HOYLE, G. 1964. Exploration of neuronal mechanisms underlying behavior in insects. In R. F. Reiss, ed., *Neural Theory and Modeling*. Stanford, Calif.: Stanford University Press, pp. 346–376.

HOYLE, G. 1965. Neurophysiological studies of "learning" in headless insects. In J. E. Treherne and J. W. L. Beament, ed., *The Physiology of the Insect Central Nervous System*. New York: Academic Press, pp. 203–232.

HOYLE, G. 1970. Cellular mechanisms underlying behavior-neuroethology. *Advances in Insect Physiology* 7: 349–444.

HOYLE, G., and BURROWS, M. 1973a. Neural mechanisms underlying behavior in the locust *Shistocerca gregaria*. I. Physiology of identified motoneurons in the metathoracic ganglion. *Journal of Neurobiology*. 4: 3–41.

HOYLE, G., and BURROWS, M. 1973b. Neural mechanisms underlying behavior in the locust *Shistocerca gregaria*. II. Integrative activity in metathoracic neurons. *Journal of Neurobiology* 4: 43–67.

HULL, C. L. 1943. *Principles of Behavior*. New York: Appleton-Century-Crofts.

HULL, C. L. 1951. *Essentials of Behavior*. New Haven: Yale University Press.

HUNTER, W. S. 1932. The effect of inactivity produced by cold upon learning and retention in the cockroach, *Blatella germanica*. *Journal of Genetic Psychology* 41: 253–266.

HYDÉN, H. 1973a. Changes in brain protein during learning. In Ansell and Bradley (1973), pp. 3–26.

HYDÉN, H. 1973b. RNA changes in brain cells during changes in behavior and function. In Ansell and Bradley (1973), pp. 51–75.

HYDÉN, H., and LANGE, P. W. 1970a. S100 brain protein: Correlation with behavior. *Proceedings of the National Academy of Sciences* 67: 1959–1966.

HYDÉN, H., and LANGE, P. W. 1970b. Brain cell protein synthesis specifically related to learning. *Proceedings of the National Academy of Sciences* 65: 898–904.

HYDÉN, H., LANGE, P. W., MIHAILOVIĆ, L. J., and PETROVIĆ-MINIĆ, B. 1974. Changes of RNA base composition in nerve cells of monkeys subjected to visual discrimination and delayed alternation performance. *Brain Research* 65: 215–230.

ILES, J. F., and PEARSON, K. G. 1971. Coxal depressor muscles of the cockroach and the role of peripheral inhibition. *Journal of Experimental Biology* 55: 151–164.

INGLE, D., ed. 1968. *The Central Nervous System and Fish Behavior.* Chicago: University of Chicago Press.

JACOBSON, A. L. 1965. Learning in planarians: Current status. In Thorpe and Davenport (1965), pp. 76–81.

JACOBSON, A. L., FRIED, C., and HOROWITZ, S. D. 1966. Planarians and memory. I. Transfer of learning by injection of RNA. *Nature* 209: 599–601.

JACOBSON, M. 1969. Development of specific neuronal connections. *Science* 163: 543–547.

JACOBSON, M. 1970. *Developmental Neurobiology.* New York: Holt, Rinehart and Winston.

JAHAN-PARWAR, B. 1971. Conditioned responses in *Aplysia californica. American Zoologist* 10: 287.

JOHN, E. R. 1967a. Electrophysiological studies of conditioning. In G. C. Quarton, T. Melnechuk and F. O. Schmitt, eds., *The Neurosciences: A Study Program.* New York: Rockefeller University Press, pp. 690–704.

JOHN, E. R. 1967b. *Mechanisms of Memory.* New York: Academic Press.

JOHN, E. R. 1972. Switchboard versus statistical theories of learning and memory. *Science* 177: 850–864.

JOHN, E. R., BARTLETT, F., SHIMOKOCHI, M., and KLEINMAN, D. 1973. Neural readout from memory. *Journal of Neurophysiology* 36: 893–924.

KANDEL, E. R. 1967. Cellular studies of learning. In G. C. Quarton, T. Melnechuk, and F. O. Schmitt, eds., *The Neurosciences: A Study Program.* New York: Rockefeller University Press, pp. 666–689.

KANDEL, E. R. 1974. An invertebrate system for the cellular analysis of simple behaviors and their modifications. In F. O. Schmitt and F. G. Worden, eds., *The Neurosciences: Third Study Program.* Cambridge, Mass.: MIT Press, pp. 347–370.

KANDEL, E. R., CASTELLUCCI, V., PINSKER, H., and KUPFERMANN, I. 1970. The role of synaptic plasticity in the short-term modification of behavior. In Horn and Hinde (1970), pp. 281–322.

KANDEL, E. R., and KUPFERMANN, I. 1970. The functional organization of invertebrate ganglia. *Annual Review of Physiology* 32: 193–258.

KANDEL, E. R., and SPENCER, W. A. 1968. Cellular and neurophysiological approaches in the study of learning. *Physiological Review* 48: 65–134.

KANDEL, E. R., and TAUC, L. 1964. Mechanisms of prolonged heterosynaptic facilitation. *Nature* 202: 145–147.

KANDEL, E. R., and TAUC, L. 1965a. Heterosynaptic facilitation in neurons of the abdominal ganglion of *Aplysia depilans. Journal of Physiology* 181: 1–27.

KANDEL, E. R., and TUAC, L. 1965b. Mechanisms of heterosynaptic facilitation in the giant cell of the abdominal ganglion of *Aplysia depilans. Journal of Physiology* 181: 28–47.

KATCHALSKY, A., and NEUMANN, E. 1972. Hysteresis and molecular memory record. *International Journal of Neuroscience* 3: 175–182.

KATCHALSKY, A., and OPLATKA, A. 1966. Hysteresis and macromolecular memory. *Neurosciences Research Program Bulletin* 4: 71–93.

KATER, S. B. 1974. Feeding in *Helisoma trivolvis*: The morphological and physiological basis of a fixed action pattern. *American Zoologist* 14: 1017–1036.

KATER, S. B., and ROWELL, C. H. F. 1973. Integration of sensory and centrally programmed components in the gener-ation of cyclical feeding activity of *Helisoma trivolvis. Journal of Neurophysiology* 36: 142–155.

KEENE, J. J. 1973. Reward-associated inhibition and pain-associated excitation lasting seconds in single intralaminar thalamic units. *Brain Research* 64: 211–224.

KENNEDY, D. 1963. Physiology of photoreceptor neurons in the abdominal nerve cord of the crayfish. *Journal of General Physiology* 46: 551–572.

KENNEDY, D., and DAVIS, W. J. 1975. The organization of invertebrate motor systems. In E. R. Kandel, ed., *Handbook of Physiology: Neurophysiology.* Bethesda: American Physiological Society (in press).

KERKUT, G. A., BEESLEY, P., EMSON, P., OLIVER, G., and WALKER, R. J. 1971. Reduction in ChE during avoidance learning in the cockroach CNS. *Comparative Biochemistry and Physiology* 39B: 423–424.

KERKUT, G. A., EMSON, P. C., and BEESLEY, P. W. 1972. Effect of leg-raising learning on protein synthesis and ChE activity in the cockroach CNS. *Comparative Biochemistry and Physiology* 41B: 635–645.

KERKUT, G. A., EMSON, P., and WALKER, R. J. 1973. Learning in the lower animals. In Ansell and Bradley (1973), pp. 241–257.

KERKUT, G. A., OLIVER, G. W. O., RICK, J. T., and WALKER, R. J. 1970a. Biochemical changes during learning in an insect ganglion. *Nature* 227: 722–723.

KERKUT, G. A., OLIVER, G. W. O., RICK, J. T., and WALKER, R. J. 1970b. The effects of drugs on learning in a simple preparation. *Comparative and General Pharmacology* 1: 437–483.

KIMBLE, G. A. 1961. *Hilgard and Marquis' Conditioning and Learning.* New York: Appleton-Century-Crofts.

KIMBLE, G. A. 1967. *Foundations of Conditioning and Learning.* New York: Appleton-Century-Crofts.

KOPP, R. Z., BOHDANECKY, Z., and JARVIK, M. E. 1966. Long temporal gradient of retrograde amnesia for a well-discriminated stimulus. *Science* 153: 1547–1549.

KOSOWER, E. M. 1972. A molecular basis for learning and memory. *Proceedings of the National Academy of Sciences* 69: 3292–3296.

KRASNE, F. B. 1969. Excitation and habituation of the crayfish escape reflex: The depolarizing response in lateral giant fibers of the isolated abdomen. *Journal of Experimental Biology* 50: 29–46.

KRASNE, F. B. 1973. Learning in crustacea. In Corning, Dyal, and Willows (1973), Vol. 2, pp. 49–130.

KRASNE, F. B., and BRYAN, J. S. 1973. Habituation: Regulation through presynaptic inhibition. *Science* 182: 590–592.

KRASNE, F. B., and ROBERTS, A. 1967. Habituation of crayfish escape response during release from inhibition induced by picrotoxin. *Nature* 215: 769–770.

KRASNE, F. B., and WOODSMALL, K. S. 1969. Waning of the crayfish escape response as a result of repeated stimulation. *Animal Behaviour* 17: 416–424.

KRISTAN, W. B. 1971. Plasticity of firing patterns in neurons of *Aplysia* pleural ganglion. *Journal of Neurophysiology* 34: 321–336.

KRISTAN, W. B., and GERSTEIN, G. 1970. Plasticity of synchronous activity in a small neural net. *Science* 169: 1336–1339.

KUHN, T. S. 1962. *The Structure of Scientific Revolutions.* Chicago: The University of Chicago Press.

KUPFERMANN, I. 1966. Turn alternation in the pill bug (*Armadillidium vulgare*). *Animal Behaviour* 14: 68–72.

KUPFERMANN, I. 1967. Stimulation of egg laying: Possible

neuroendocrine function of bag cells of abdominal ganglion of *Aplysia californica. Nature* 216: 814–815.

KUPFERMANN, I. 1970. Stimulation of egg laying by extract of neuroendocrine cells (bag cells) of abdominal ganglion of *Aplysia. Journal of Neurophysiology* 33: 877–881.

KUPFERMANN, I. 1974. Feeding behavior in *Aplysia*. A simple system for the study of motivation. *Behavioral Biology* 10: 1–26.

KUPFERMANN, I., CASTELLUCCI, V., PINSKER, H., and KANDEL, E.1970. Neuronal correlates of habituation and dishabituation of the gill-withdrawal reflex in *Aplysia. Science* 167: 1743–1745.

KUPFERMANN, I., and COHEN, J. 1971. The control of feeding by identified neurons in the buccal ganglion of *Aplysia. American Zoologist* 11: 667.

KUPFERMANN, I., and KANDEL, E. R. 1969. Neural controls of a behavioral response mediated by the abdominal ganglion of *Aplysia. Science* 164: 847–850.

KUPFERMANN, I., and PINSKER, H. 1968. A behavioral modification of the feeding reflex in *Aplysia californica. Communications in Behavioral Biology* 2A: 13–17.

KUPFERMANN, I., and PINSKER, H. 1969. Plasticity in *Aplysia* neurons and some simple neuronal models of learning. In J. T. Tapp, ed., *Reinforcement and Behavior*. New York: Academic Press, pp. 356–386.

KUPFERMANN, I., PINSKER, H., CASTELLUCCI, V., and KANDEL, E. R. 1971. Central and peripheral control of gill movements in *Aplysia. Science* 174: 1252–1256.

LAHUE, R. 1973. The chelicerates. In Corning, Dyal, and Willows (1973), Vol. 2, pp. 1–48.

LAJTHA, A., ed. 1970. *Protein Metabolism of the Nervous System*. New York: Plenum Press.

LEE, R. M. 1969. *Aplysia* behavior: Effects of contingent water level variation. *Communications in Behavioral Biology* 4A: 157–164.

LICKEY, M. E. 1968. Learned behavior in *Aplysia vaccaria. Journal of Comparative and Physiological Psychology* 66: 712–718.

LICKEY, M. E. 1969. Seasonal modulation and non-24-hour entrainment of a circadian rhythm in a single neuron. *Journal of Comparative and Physiological Psychology* 68: 9–17.

LICKEY, M. E., and BERRY, R. N. 1966. Learned behavioral discrimination of food objects by *Aplysia californica. Physiologist* 9: 230.

LINDBERG, R. G. 1955. Growth, population, dynamics and field behavior in the spiny lobster *Panulirus interruptus* (Randell). *University of California Publications in Zoology* 59: 157–247.

LINSEMAN, M. A., and OLDS, J. 1973. Activity changes in rat hypothalamus, preoptic area, and striatum associated with Pavlovian conditioning. *Journal of Neurophysiology* 36: 1038–1050.

LIVINGSTON, R. B. 1967. Reinforcement. In G. C. Quarton, T. Melnechuk, and F. O. Schmitt, eds., *The Neurosciences: A Study Program*. New York: Rockefeller Press, pp. 568–577.

LØMO, T., and ROSENTHAL, J. 1972. Control of ACh sensitivity by muscle activity in the rat. *Journal of Physiology* 221: 493–513.

LUCAS, K. 1917. *The Conduction of the Nervous Impulse*. London: Longmans and Green.

LUCO, J. V., and ARANDA, L. C. 1964a. An electrical correlate to the process of learning. *Acta Physiologica Latino Americana* 14: 274–288.

LUCO, J. V., and ARANDA, L. C. 1964b. An electrical correlate

to the process of learning. Experiments in *Blatta orientalis. Nature* 201: 1330–1331.

LUCO, J. V., and ARANDA, J. C. 1966. Reversibility of an electrical correlate to the process of learning. *Nature* 209: 205–206.

LUKOWIAK, K., and JACKLET, J. W. 1972. Habituation and dishabituation: Interactions between peripheral and central nervous systems in *Aplysia. Science* 178: 1306–1308.

MARK R. F. 1970. Chemospecific synaptic repression as a possible memory store. *Nature* 225: 5228.

MARK, R. F., and MAROTTE, L. R. 1972. The mechanism of selective reinnervation of fish eye muscles. III. Functional, electrophysiological and anatomical analysis of recovery from section of the IIIrd and IVth nerves. *Brain Research* 46: 131–148.

MARK, R. F., MAROTTE, L. R. and JOHNSTONE, J. R. 1970. Reinnervated eye muscles do not respond to impulses in foreign nerves. *Science* 170: 193–194.

MARK, R. F., MAROTTE, L. R., and MART, P. E. 1972. The mechanism of selective reinnervation of fish eye muscles. IV. Identification of repressed synapses. *Brain Research* 46: 149–157.

MAROTTE, L. R., and MARK, R. F., 1970a. The mechanism of selective reinnervation of fish eye muscles. I. Evidence from muscle function during recovery. *Brain Research* 19: 41–51.

MAROTTE, L. R., and MARK, R. F. 1970b. The mechanism of selective reinnervation of fish eye muscles. II. Evidence from electron microscopy of nerve endings. *Brain Research* 19: 53–69.

McCONNELL, J. V. 1966. Comparative physiology of learning in invertebrates. *Annual Review of Physiology* 28: 107–136.

McCONNELL, J. V., and SHELBY, J. 1970. Memory transfer in invertebrates. In Ungar (1970), pp. 71–101.

McFARLAND, D. 1966. The role of attention in the disinhibition of displacement activity. *Quarterly Journal of Experimental Psychology* 18: 19–30.

McFARLAND, D., and SIBLY, R. 1972. "Unitary drives" revisited. *Animal Behaviour* 20: 548–563.

MARLER, P. 1970. A comparative approach to vocal learning: Song development in white-crowned sparrows. *Journal of Comparative and Physiological Psychology* 71: 1–25.

MINAMI, H., and DALLENBACH, K. M. 1946. The effect of activity upon learning and retention in the cockroach, *Periplaneta americana. American Journal of Psychology* 59: 1–58.

MORROW, J. E., and SMITHSON, B. L. 1969. Learning sets in an invertebrate. *Science* 164: 850–851.

MOWRER, O. H. 1947. On the dual nature of learning—A reinterpretation of "conditioning" and "problem-solving." *Harvard Educational Reviews* 17: 102–148.

MPITSOS, G. J., and DAVIS, W. J. 1973. Learning: Classical and avoidance conditioning in the mollusk *Pleurobranchaea. Science* 180: 317–321.

NELSON, M. C. 1971. Classical conditioning in the blowfly (*Phormia regina*): Associative and excitatory factors. *Journal of Comparative and Physiological Psychology* 77: 353–368.

OFFUTT, G. C. 1970. Acoustic stimulus perception by the American lobster *Homarus americanus* (Decapoda). *Experientia* 26: 1276–1278.

OLDS, J., DISTERHOFT, J. F., SEGAL, M., KORNBLITH, C. L., and HIRSH, R. 1972. Learning centers of rat brain mapped by measuring latencies of conditional unit responses. *Journal of Neurophysiology* 35: 202–219.

OLIVER, G. W. O. 1973. Neurochemical aspects of shock-avoidance learning in cockroaches. In Ansell and Bradley (1973), pp. 113–131.

OLIVER, G. W. O., TABERNER, P. B., RICK, J. T., and KERKUT, G. A. 1971. Changes in GABA level, GAD and ChE activity in CNS of an insect during learning. *Comparative Biochemistry and Physiology* 38B: 529–535.

PAKULA, A., and SOKOLOV, E. N. 1973. Habituation in Gastropoda: Behavioral, interneuronal and endoneuronal aspects. In Peeke and Herz (1973), Vol. 2, pp. 35–107.

PANTIN, C. F. A. 1935. The nerve net of the Actinozoa. I. Facilitation. *Journal of Experimental Biology* 12: 119–138.

PAVLOV, I. P. 1927. *Conditioned Reflexes*. New York: Dover Publications (reprint).

PEARSON, K. G. 1972. Central programming and reflex control of walking in the cockroach. *Journal of Experimental Biology* 56: 173–193.

PEARSON, K. G., FOURTNER, C. R., and WONG, R. K. 1973. Nervous control of walking in the cockroach. In R. B. Stein, K. G. Pearson, R. S. Smith, and J. B. Redford, eds., *Control of Posture and Locomotion*. New York: Plenum Press, pp. 495–514.

PEARSON, K. G., and ILES, J. F. 1970. Discharge patterns of coxal levator and depressor motoneurons of the cockroach,, *Periplaneta americana*. *Journal of Experimental Biology* 52: 139–165.

PEARSON, K. G., and ILES, J. F. 1973. Nervous mechanisms underlying intersegmental coordination of leg movements during walking in the cockroach. *Journal of Experimental Biology* 58: 725–744.

PEEKE, H. V. S., and HERZ, M. J., eds. 1973. *Habituation*. Vol. 1: *Behavioral Studies*. Vol. 2: *Physiological Substrates*. New York: Academic Press.

PERETZ, B. 1969. Central neuron initiation of periodic gill movements. *Science* 166: 1167–1172.

PERETZ, B. 1970. Habituation and dishabituation in the absence of a central nervous system. *Science* 169: 379–381.

PERETZ, B., and ESTES, J. 1975. Histology and histochemistry of the peripheral neural plexus in the *Aplysia* gill. *Journal of Neurobiology* 5: 3–19.

PERETZ, B., and HOWIESON, D. B. 1973. Central influence on peripherally mediated habituation of an *Aplysia* gill withdrawal response. *Journal of Comparative Physiology* 84: 1–18.

PETERSON, R. P., and KERNELL, D. 1970. Effects of nerve stimulation on the metabolism of ribonucleic acid in a molluscan giant neurone. *Journal of Neurochemistry* 17: 1075–1085.

PETERSON, R. P., and LOH, Y. P. 1973. The role of macromolecules in neuronal function in *Aplysia*. In G. A. Kerkut and J. W. Phillis, eds., *Progress in Neurobiology*, Vol. 2, Part 2. New York: Pergamon Press, pp. 179–203.

PETRINOVICH, L. 1973. A species-meaningful analysis of habituation. In Peeke and Herz (1973), Vol. 1, pp. 141–162.

PINSKER, H. M., HENIG, W. A., CAREW, T. J., and KANDEL, E. R. 1973. Long-term sensitization of a defensive withdrawal reflex in *Aplysia*. *Science* 182: 1039–1042.

PINSKER, H., and KANDEL, E. R. 1967. Contingent modification of an endogenous bursting rhythm by monosynaptic inhibition. *Physiologist* 10: 279.

PINSKER, H., KUPFERMANN, I., CASTELLUCCI, V., and KANDEL, E. 1970. Habituation and dishabituation of the gill-withdrawal reflex in *Aplysia*. *Science* 167: 1740–1742.

PREMACK, D. 1959. Toward empirical behavior laws. I. Positive reinforcement. *Psychological Review* 66: 219–233.

PRIBRAM, K. H., and BROADBENT, D. E., eds. 1970. *Biology of Memory*. New York: Academic Press.

PRINGLE, J. W. S. 1940. The reflex mechanism of the insect leg. *Journal of Experimental Biology* 17: 8–17.

PRITCHATT, D. 1968. Avoidance of electric shock by the cockroach *Periplaneta americana*. *Animal Behaviour* 16: 178–185.

QUINN, W. G., HARRIS, W. A., and BENZER, S. 1974. Conditioned behavior in *Drosophila melanogaster*. *Proceedings of the National Academy of Sciences* 71: 708–712.

RAISMAN, G. 1973. Anatomical evidence for plasticity in the central nervous system in the adult rat. In Ansell and Bradley (1973), pp. 183–191.

RAM, J. L. 1972. Effects of high potassium media on radioactive leucine incorporation into *Aplysia* nervous tissue. *Physiologist* 15: 242.

RAM, J. L. 1974. High [K+] effects on the molecular weight distribution of proteins synthesized in *Aplysia* nervous tissue. *Brain Research* 76: 281–296.

RANCK, J. B. 1964. Synaptic "learning" due to electroosmosis: A theory. *Science* 144: 187–189.

RATNER, S. C. 1965. Research and theory on conditioning of annelids. In Thorpe and Davenport (1965), pp. 101–108.

RAZRAN, G. 1971. *Mind in Evolution: An East-West Synthesis of Learned Behavior and Cognition*. Boston: Houghton-Mifflin.

RESCORLA, R. A. 1967. Pavlovian conditioning and its proper control procedures. *Psychological Review* 74: 71–80.

ROBERTS, M. B. V. 1962. The giant fibre reflex of the earthworm, *Lumbricus terrestris* L. II. Fatigue. *Journal of Experimental Biology* 39: 229–237.

ROBINSON, C. E. 1966. A chemical model of long-term memory and recall. In O. Walaas, ed., *Molecular Basis of Some Aspects of Mental Activity*. New York: Academic Press, pp. 29–35.

ROITBACH, A. I. 1970. A new hypothesis concerning the mechanism of function of the conditioned reflex. *Acta Neurobiologiae Experimentalis (Warsaw)* 30: 81–94.

ROSE, R. M. 1971. Patterned activity of the buccal ganglion in the nudibranch mollusc *Archidoris pseudoargus*. *Journal of Experimental Biology* 55: 185–204.

ROSE, R. M. 1972. Burst activity of the buccal ganglion of *Aplysia depilans*. *Journal of Experimental Biology* 56: 735–754.

ROSE, S. P. R., BATESON, P. P. G., and HORN, G. 1973. Biochemistry and behavior in the chick. In Ansell and Bradley (1973), pp. 93–104.

ROSS, D. M. 1965. The behavior of sessile coelenterates in relation to some conditioning experiments. In Thorpe and Davenport (1965), pp. 43–55.

ROSS, D. M., and SUTTON, L. 1964. The swimming response of the sea anemone, *Stomphia coccinea* to electrical stimulation. *Journal of Experimental Biology* 41: 735–749.

RUNION, H. I., and USHERWOOD, P. N. R. 1968. Tarsal receptors and leg reflexes in the locust and grasshopper. *Journal of Experimental Biology* 49: 421–436.

RUSHFORTH, N. B. 1973. Behavioral modifications in coelenterates. In Corning, Dyal, and Willows (1973), Vol. 1, pp. 123–169.

RUSHFORTH, N. B., KROHN, I. T., and BROWN, L. K. 1964. Behavior in *Hydra*: Inhibition of the contraction response of *Hydra pirardi*. *Science* 145: 602–604.

SCHLAPFER, W. T., WOODSON, P. B. J., TREMBLAY, J. P., and BARONDES, S. H. 1974. Depression and frequency facilitation at a synapse in *Aplysia californica*: Evidence for regulation by availability of transmitter. *Brain Research* 76: 267–280.

SCHNEIDER, D. J., ed. 1973. *Protein of the Nervous System.* New York: Raven Press.

SCHWARTZ, J. H., CASTELLUCCI, V. F., and KANDEL, E. R. 1971. Functioning of identified neurons and synapses in abdominal ganglion of *Aplysia* in absence of protein synthesis. *Journal of Neurophysiology* 34: 939–954.

SEGAL, M. 1973a. Flow of conditioned responses in limbic telencephalic system of the rat. *Journal of Neurophysiology* 36: 840–854.

SEGAL, M. 1973b. Dissecting a short-term memory circuit in the rat brain. I. Changes in entorhinal unit activity and responsiveness of hippocampal units in the process of classical conditioning. *Brain Research* 64: 281–292.

SEGAL, M., DISTERHOFT, J. F., and OLDS, J. 1972. Hippocampal unit activity during classical aversive and appetitive conditioning. *Science* 175: 792–794.

SEGAL, M., and OLDS, J. 1972. The behavior of units in the hippocampal circuit of the rat during learning. *Journal of Neurophysiology* 35: 680–690.

SEGAL, M., and OLDS, J. 1973. The activity of units in the hippocampal circuit of the rat during differential classical conditioning. *Journal of Comparative and Physiological Psychology* 82: 195–204.

SELIGMAN, M. E. P., and HAGER, J. L., eds. 1972. *Biological Boundaries of Learning.* New York: Appleton-Century-Crofts.

SHARPLESS, S. K. 1964. Reorganization of function in the nervous system—use and disuse. *Annual Review of Physiology* 26: 357–388.

SIEGLER, M. V. S., MPITSOS, G. J., and DAVIS, W. J. 1974. Motor organization and generation of rhythmic feeding output in the buccal ganglion of *Pleurobranchaea*. *Journal of Neurophysiology* 37: 1173–1196.

SMITH, C. E. 1962. Is memory a matter of enzyme induction? *Science* 38: 889–890.

SOLOMON, R. L., and WYNNE, L. C. 1954. Traumatic avoidance learning: The principles of anxiety conservation and partial irreversibility. *Psychological Review* 61: 353–385.

SOSENKOV, V. A., and CHIRKOV, V. D. 1970. Electrical activity of neurons on the cat cortex during cooling. *Neurophysiology* 2: 46–49.

SQUIRE, L. R., and BARONDES, S. H. 1972. Variable decay of memory and its recovery in cycloheximide-treated mice. *Proceedings of The National Academy of Sciences* 69: 1416–1420.

STENT, G. 1967. Induction and repression of enzyme synthesis. In G. C. Quarton, T. Melnechuk, and F. O. Schmitt, eds., *The Neurosciences: A Study Program.* New York: Rockefeller University Press, pp. 152–161.

STENT, G. S. 1973. A physiological mechanism for Hebb's postulate of learning. *Proceedings of the National Academy of Sciences* 70: 997–1001.

STEPHENS, C. L. 1973. Relative contribution of synaptic and nonsynaptic influences to response decrements in a post-synaptic neurone. *Journal of Experimental Biology* 59: 315–321.

STEPHENS, G. L., and McGAUGH, J. L. 1972. Biological factors related to learning in the land snail (*Helix aspersa* Müller). *Animal Behaviour* 20: 309–315.

STRUMWASSER, F. 1965. The demonstration and manipulation of a circadian rhythm in a single neuron. In J. A. Schoff, ed., *Circadian Clocks.* Amsterdam: North Holland Publishing Company, pp. 442–462.

STRUMWASSER, F., JACKLET, J. W., and ALVAREZ, R. B. 1969. A seasonal rhythm in the neural extract induction of behavioral egg-laying in *Aplysia*. *Comparative Biochemistry and Physiology* 29: 197–206.

SZILARD, L. 1964. On memory and recall. *Proceedings of the National Academy of Science* 51: 1092–1099.

TAKEDA, K. 1961. Classical conditioned response in the honey bee. *Journal of Insect Physiology* 6: 168–179.

TAUC, L., and EPSTEIN, R. 1967. Heterosynaptic facilitation as a distinct mechanism in *Aplysia*. *Nature* 214: 724–725.

TAYLOR, W. K. 1965. A model of learning mechanisms in the brain. *Progress in Brain Research* 17: 369–397.

THOMPSON, E. L. 1917. An analysis of the learning process in the snail, *Physa gyrina* Say. *Behavior Monographs* 3: 1–89.

THOMPSON, R., and McCONNELL, J. V. 1955. Classical conditioning in the planarian, *Dugesia dorotocephala*. *Journal of Comparative and Physiological Psychology* 48: 65–68.

THOMPSON, R. F., and SPENCER, W. A. 1966. Habituation: A model phenomenon for the study of neuronal substrates of behavior. *Psychological Review* 73: 16–43.

THORPE, W. H. 1963. *Learning and Instinct in Animals.* Cambridge, Mass.: Harvard University Press.

THORPE, W. H., and DAVENPORT, D., eds. 1965. Learning and associated phenomena in invertebrates. *Animal Behaviour* suppl. 1: 1–190.

TOEVS, L. A., and BRACKENBURY, R. W. 1969. Bag cell-specific proteins and the humoral control of egg laying in *Aplysia californica*. *Comparative Biochemistry and Physiology* 29: 207–216.

UNGAR, G., ed. 1970. *Molecular Mechanisms in Memory and Learning.* New York: Plenum Press.

UNGAR, G. 1973. Molecular mechanisms in central nervous system coding. In Ansell and Bradley (1973), pp. 151–162.

UNGAR, G., DESIDERIO, D. M., and PARR, W. 1972. Isolation, identification and synthesis of a specific-behavior-inducing brain peptide. *Nature* 238: 198–202.

VON BAUMGARTEN, R. 1970. Plasticity in the nervous system at the unitary level. In F. O. Schmitt, ed., *The Neurosciences: Second Study Program.* New York: Rockefeller University Press, pp. 260–271.

VON BAUMGARTEN, R., and DJAHANPARWAR, B. 1967. Time course of repetitive heterosynaptic facilitation in *Aplysia californica*. *Brain Research* 4: 295–297.

VON BAUMGARTEN, R., and HUKUHARA, T. 1969. The role of interstimulus interval in heterosynaptic facilitation in *Aplysia californica*. *Brain Research* 16: 369–381.

VON FRISCH, K. 1950. *Bees: Their Vision, Chemical Senses and Language.* Ithaca, N. Y.: Cornell University Press.

VON FRISCH, K. 1967. *The Dance Language and Orientation of Bees.* Cambridge, Mass.: Harvard University Press.

VORONIN, L. L. 1971. Microelectrode investigations of cellular analogs of learning. *Soviet Neurological Psychiatry* 4 (2): 99–125.

WEIGHT, F. F. 1974. Physiological mechanisms of synaptic modulation. In F. O. Schmitt and F. G. Worden, eds., *The Neurosciences: Third Study Program.* Cambridge, Mass.: MIT Press, pp. 929–941.

WEISS, P. 1941. Self-differentiation of the basic patterns of coordination. *Comparative Psychology Monographs* 17: 1–46.

WEISS, P. A., and SCHNEIRLA, T. C. 1967. Inter-situational transfer in the ant *Formica schaufussi* as tested in a two-phase single choice point maze. *Behavior* 28: 269–279.

WELLS, M. J. 1965. Learning by marine invertebrates. *Advances in Marine Biology* 3: 1–62.

WELLS, M. J. 1966. Learning in the octopus. *Symposia of the Society for Experimental Biology* 20: 477–508.

WELLS, M. J. 1968. Sensitization and the evolution of associative learning. In J. Salánki, ed., *Symposium on Neurobiology of Invertebrates*. New York: Plenum Press, pp. 391–411.

WELLS, M. J., and WELLS, J. 1971. Conditioning and sensitization in snails. *Animal Behaviour* 19: 305–312.

WELLS, P. H. 1973. Honey bees. In Corning, Dyal, and Willows (1973), Vol. 2, pp. 173–185.

WELLS, P. H., and WENNER, A. M. 1973. Do honey bees have a language? *Nature* 141: 171–175.

WESTERMAN, R. A. 1963. Somatic inheritance of habituation of responses to light in planarians. *Science* 140: 676–677.

WHITE, A., HANDLER, P., and SMITH, E. L. 1968. *Principles of Biochemistry*. New York: McGraw-Hill.

WIERSMA, C. A. G., and NOVITSKI, E. 1942. The mechanism of the nervous regulation of the crayfish heart. *Journal of Experimental Biology* 19: 255–265. .

WILLNER, P., and MELLANBY, J. 1974. Cholinesterase activity in the cockroach CNS does not change with training. *Brain Research* 66: 481–490.

WILLOWS, A. O. D. 1973. Learning in gastropod mollusks. In Corning, Dyal, and Willows (1973), Vol. 2, pp. 187–273.

WILSON, D. M. 1959. Long-term facilitation in a swimming sea anemone. *Journal of Experimental Bilology* 36:526–532.

WILSON, D. M. 1965. Proprioceptive leg reflexes in cockroaches. *Journal of Experimental Biology* 43:397–409.

WILSON, D. M. 1966. Insect walking. *Annual Review of Entomology* 11: 103–123.

WILSON, D. M., and HOY, R. R. 1968. Optomotor reaction, locomotory bias and reactive inhibition in the milkweed bug *Oncopeltus* and the beetle *Zophobas*. *Zeitschrift für Vergleichende Physiologie* 58: 136–152.

WILSON, D. P. 1949. Notes from the Plymouth Aquarium. *Journal of the Marine Biological Association (United Kingdom)* 29: 345–351.

WINE, J. J. 1971. Escape reflex circuit in crayfish: Interganglionic interneurons activated by the giant command neurons. *Biological Bulletin* 141: 408.

WINE, J. J., and KRASNE, F. B. 1969. Independence of inhibition and habituation in the crayfish lateral giant fiber escape reflex. In *Proceedings of the 77th Annual Convention of the American Psychological Association*, pp. 237–238.

WINE, J. J., and KRASNE, F. B. 1972. The organization of escape behavior in the crayfish. *Journal of Experimental Biology* 56: 1–18.

WOOD, D. C. 1970a. Electrophysiological studies of the protozoan, *Stentor coeruleus*. *Journal of Neurobiology* 1: 363–377.

WOOD, D. C. 1970b. Electrophysiological correlates of the response decrement produced by mechanical stimuli in the protozoan *Stentor coeruleus*. *Journal of Neurobiology* 2: 1–11.

WOODSON, P. B. J., SCHLAPFER, W. T., and BARONDES, S. H. 1972. Postural avoidance learning in the headless cockroach without detectable changes in ganglionic cholinesterase. *Brain Research* 37: 348–352.

WYERS, E. J., PEEKE, H. V. S., and HERZ, M. J. 1973. Behavioral habituation in invertebrates. In Peeke and Herz (1973), Vol. 1, pp. 1–57.

YOUNG, J. Z. 1965. The organization of a memory system. *Proceedings of the Royal Society (London)* B163: 285–320.

ZILBER-GACHELIN, N. F., and CHARTIER, M. P. 1973a. Modification of the motor reflex responses due to repetition of the peripheral stimulus in the cockroach. I. Habituation at the level of an isolated abdominal ganglion. *Journal of Experimental Biology* 59: 359–381.

ZILBER-GACHELIN, N. F., and CHARTIER, M. P. 1973b. Modification of the motor reflex responses due to the repetition of the peripheral stimulus in the cockroach. II. Conditions of activation of the motoneurons. *Journal of Experimental Biology* 59: 383–403.

ZUCKER, R. S. 1972a. Crayfish escape behavior and central synapses. I. Neural circuit exciting lateral giant fiber. *Journal of Neurophysiology* 35: 599–620.

ZUCKER, R. S. 1972b. Crayfish escape behavior and central synapses. II. Physiological mechanisms underlying behavioral habituation. *Journal of Neurophysiology* 35: 621–637.

ZUCKER, R. S. 1972c. Crayfish escape behavior and central synapses. III. Electrical junctions and dendrite spikes in fast flexor motoneurons. *Journal of Neurophysiology* 35: 638–651.

ZUCKER, R. S., KENNEDY, D., and SELVERSTON, A. I. 1971. Neuronal circuit mediating escape responses in crayfish. *Science* 173: 645–650.

30

Small-System Neurophysiology and the Study of Plasticity

HUGH FRASER ROWELL

ABSTRACT Only two classes of preparation allow a factual resolution of cellular mechanisms of plasticity: these are (1) arrays of cells with extensive lateral replication (e.g., the vertebrate visual system) and (2) neural circuits consisting of repeatedly identifiable individual neurons, as in some invertebrates. Little progress has so far been made; this reflects both the small number of circuit analyses attempted and our basic ignorance of fundamental neurophysiological processes. Until these factors are corrected, most understanding of plastic processes will arise by serendipity during the analysis of technically accessible neural circuits which are not selected primarily for their plastic properties.

At a behavioral level, a labile relationship between stimulus and response is a biological necessity, and it is virtually universal. This lability subsumes much of the so-called plasticity of behavior. Analysis of the neural circuitry of a conspicuously labile behavior pattern (the escape jump of a locust in response to a visual input) shows that the bases of lability are in this case widely distributed throughout the circuit. They are found in at least five different synapses, and include the processes of summation, inhibition, and gating, and the habituation and dishabituation of synaptic transmission. Interaction with other sensory inputs takes place on at least three different levels.

I want first to take this opportunity to place in perspective, relative to other approaches to the problems of neural plasticity, studies in cellular neurophysiology. The first point I would like to make is that the cellular mechanisms of plastic processes, while possibly fundamental in an academic sense, are not necessarily the most important things we might wish to know about these processes. For some purposes, indeed, they may not be even very useful. An earlier speaker drew the analogy between small invertebrate nervous systems and the pocket electronic calculator; shouldn't we be looking instead at the big computer installation, he asked? Instead of answering that question directly, I intend to pursue his analogy a little further, to see if the question is still relevant.

If presented with a new and complex electronic instrument in the laboratory, the questions most people would ask are, "What does it do?", "How do you operate it?", and "What are its limitations?" Such questions, which are functionally the most important ones, form the proper field of inquiry of psychology when asked of

HUGH FRASER ROWELL, Department of Zoology, University of California, Berkeley

the mammalian brain. For some purposes, and especially as an aid to understanding the answers to this first category of questions, a block circuit diagram of the instrument is also very useful. Obtaining this block diagram for the brain is approximately the level of endeavor of the physiological psychologist. One does not strictly have to know what components are connected to what, or how a semiconductor device operates, unless it becomes necessary to repair the instrument, modify its function, or build a new one, though if one has this knowledge, one's understanding of the instrument's normal mode of operation is undeniably deeper. This level, analogous to that of cellular neurophysiology, is not essential for understanding the commonest and most functional questions.

This being said, the fact remains that if one wishes to understand cellular mechanisms of plasticity, very few approaches will yield facts, as opposed to theories. The basic constraint is that it is very difficult to understand the function of any cell from a single recording, and impossible to ascertain its connectivity and the mechanisms of its functioning. For this, it is absolutely necessary to be able to record from effectively the same site on a number of different occasions; in our work on arthropod interneurons, we find between 10 and 100 penetrations of the same cell necessary.

At the present technical level, there are only two broad classes of preparations that can fulfill this requirement. One consists of those areas of higher nervous systems that exhibit arrays of cells with extensive lateral replication, the individuals of which differ only in their spatial address. Here one can justifiably make the assumption that the results of previous experiments are applicable to the cell currently being recorded. In this way one can obtain almost the rigor of a preparation of identified cells. The validity of this approach has been most strikingly demonstrated in the vertebrate retina (and it is currently being used by workers on other elaborate retinas too). It is hoped that it also applies to the basal and cortical projections of the visual system, to the cerebellum, and to parts of the spinal cord, but the assumptions made are clearly larger in these instances. The second category of viable preparations for the study of cellular mechanisms consists of identifiable cells, in the sense that a given cell can be routinely identified as an individual on both physiological and anatomical grounds (see Davis, this volume). Aside from a very few vertebrate instances, such as Mauthner cells and supramedullary cells of fishes and amphibians, these systems are found only in the invertebrates. Even within the invertebrates, as Krasne (this volume) has pointed out, the fact that an animal shows plastic behavior does not necessarily imply that it is a good preparation for cellular analysis. Most such animals will either fail to meet the numerous peripheral requirements of a good preparation (such as hardiness, availability, attractiveness to funding, resistance to experimental trauma, and the existence of general biological knowledge about it) or lack the accessible nerve cells and readily describable behavior that are directly required for cellular neurophysiology. It is perhaps worth stressing that any use of vertebrate nerve cells for cellular research purposes, outside of the arrays mentioned above, has usually only our natural species-chauvinism as its justification. The proof of this can be seen by considering the cephalopods, a group in which the central nervous system is as complex and as technically difficult as that of mammals—but as we are not cephalopods, no cellular neurophysiologist works on them. The cephalopod mantle giant system, of course, is the exact parallel of the Mauthner fibers, and equally unrepresentative of the group.

I have little but amen to say to the greater part of the excellent reviews of Krasne and Davis. They give lucid accounts of the progress in understanding cellular mechanisms of plasticity that has resulted from the recent intensive use of a few invertebrate preparations. I want to play devil's advocate and note that despite this progress, despite the skillful public-relations activity of some of the invertebrate neurophysiologists, despite the almost religious conviction of righteousness with which all workers with identifiable cells, not least myself, regard their sphere of endeavor, this conference is clear demonstration that invertebrate neurophysiology has not yet solved any of the major problems of neural plasticity.

There are perhaps three categories of explanation for this state of affairs. First, as I have already noted, interesting questions do not necessarily demand cellular answers. Second, and self-evidently, the work is hard, difficult, and slow, and there are still not so many experienced workers engaged in it. Third, and this is perhaps worthy of more consideration, our basic knowledge of neural processes is astonishingly incomplete, both at the level of cellular processes and at that of neural circuitry. Here, for example, is a selection of findings, either recently accepted or apparently about to be so, that provide new "circuit components," any of which

can transform our understanding of a neural configuration:

—spontaneously oscillating DC potentials in nonspiking neurons;

—chemical synapses whose output is controlled by graded, nonspiking potentials;

—propagation of graded signals down long thin processes formerly thought to require action potentials;

—persistent electrical and enzymatic function in enucleate, or transected, neurons;

—electrical synapses of restricted bandpass and determined polarity;

—modulation of transmission across electrical synapses through a shunting of current, brought about by changes in pre- or postsynaptic membrane conductance caused by accessory synaptic activity;

—the emerging variety of transmitter substances and the variety of ionic fluxes that each can mediate via different receptors.

Further, many of the fundamental cellular processes commonly invoked in discussions of the mechanisms of plasticity are not causally understood. Many of the cellular neurophysiological terms are merely reifications of descriptions, and as causal explanations they are no more sophisticated than, say, Lorenzian hydraulic models of motivation, though they may have been similarly useful. Examples of such terms are these:

—sodium (or potassium, etc.) inactivation

—accumulating refractoriness

—postinhibitory rebound

—presynaptic inhibition

—accommodation.

There are partial theories of causation for these and similar phenomena, but none that are complete and substantiated.

To all this must be added our ignorance of control of development of individual neurons or of connectivity patterns between neurons, and of what may subsequently modify these patterns, or even of whether or not they *are* subsequently modified. In the face of this overwhelming inadequacy, it seems likely that advances in the study of the mechanisms of learning must await advances in basic neurophysiology and circuit analysis—or serendipity. Serendipity has in fact been responsible for most of our progress to date. The interesting findings have emerged from the process of solving neural circuits which have been chosen for purely technical reasons, not for their specifically plastic behavior. Fortunately, plasticity is so common and fundamental a property of nervous systems, at least in its simpler manifestations, that even the relatively unpromising circuits so far investigated have been richly informative. Krasne has pointed out that the commonest circuits to attract the physiologist are the escape circuits, which are characterized by high conduction velocity and large cells; yet even these have yielded valuable information in the crayfish, the sea hare, the locust, and other preparations. This is a very encouraging sign, and presumably when the circuitry of more plastic behavior patterns, such as grooming, is investigated, much more profound effects will be found. Such systems, however, by virtue of their smaller neurons, will be more difficult to investigate, and I personally think that the most fruitful approach for some time to come is likely to remain what it is now: analyze an accessible circuit, then look for plasticity once the components are known. The circumstances in which animals show plastic modification of behavior are usually apparent only after ethological analysis (see Manning, this volume), and this is likely to be even more than usually true of the invertebrate animals, where learning ability is probably confined within each species to a few situations of biological importance, rather than being a general property. The experimental neurophysiologist in search of the bases of plastic change in the nervous system must be prepared to respect, learn, and utilize ethological techniques to find plasticity, and psychological ones to control for behavioral artifacts generated by his experimental technique.

If the physiologist working in this area has much to learn from these disciplines, it is also true that psychologists sometimes forget that plastic change in the nervous system can be subsumed under different descriptive headings, and "learning" is only one of these. To a zoologist, perhaps the most impressive feature of animal behavior is its adaptiveness, and to the physiologist, its lability. The relation between stimulus and response is unendingly variable, the "Harvard Law of Animal Behavior"—that under precisely controlled experimental conditions the animal does what it damn well pleases— being one realization of this fact. This lability is a necessary consequence of the need to couple a restricted range of motor outputs to a barrage of sensory input of almost unbelievable size, complexity, and transience. If the relation between stimulus and response were indeed a fixed one, behavior could not be adaptive: absolutely identical sensory situations never recur, and, further, no action once initiated would ever be completed, because of the change in stimulus situation brought about by the response itself.

Now behavioral lability, in this sense, arises from all the different forms of plasticity mentioned at this conference, and also from several different, additional forms of neural mechanism. To illustrate this, and some additional points that arise from other papers of this conference, I shall describe briefly the results of work by myself and my colleagues on the system that controls

visually elicited escape jumps in the locust (Burrows and Rowell, 1973; O'Shea and Rowell, 1975a,b; O'Shea, Rowell and Williams, 1974; O'Shea and Williams, 1974; Rowell, 1971a,b). This system is a typical example of a labile behavior pattern, and also of the way in which invertebrate preparations are selected. No one who has ever attempted to catch alert grasshoppers in their natural environment has any doubt that they respond to sudden novel movements in the visual field by jumping, nor can one doubt the adaptive nature of the response. The relationship between the stimulus and the response is a very imprecise one, however, if one uses only behavioral measures: under laboratory conditions an experimentally produced visual input elicits a jump only rarely.

When we started to work on this system (the descending movement-detector, or DMD, system) we did not even know its function. It was originally selected for analysis because of the size of its participating neurons, and only with some six years' work have we elucidated much of its circuitry and behavioral singificance, and quantified its response to a variety of stimulus situations. During this work it has been found to show some classical plastic properties, including habituation, dishabituation, and "facultative nonresponsiveness." These properties seem to be behaviorally relevant. Because of the accumulated knowledge of the circuit and its identified cells, it seems likely that we shall be able to explain these three phenomena at the cellular level in this system. It is clearly not going to tell us "how animals learn," but the known complexity of the system, which is steadily increasing, does show how much of the lability of animal behavior can be due to the interplay of basically very simple elements.

A block diagram of the DMD system is shown in Figure 30.1; only half of the bilaterally symmetrical system is shown. At least three different outputs of the optic lobe are utilized by the DMD system, and they all synapse onto the interneuron we call the lobular giant movement detector (LGMD). One input, sensitive to the dimming or brightening of even single ommatidia, consists of a retinotopic array of thousands of afferents projecting onto the major dendritic fan of the LGMD, which is the site of convergence of that system. Each of these synapses produces EPSPs that wane if evoked faster than once every few minutes. These inputs are prevented from functioning when the changes in illumination cover large areas of the retina by the presence of a lateral inhibition network between the afferents. Lateral inhibition networks of this sort cannot block responses to *transient* large-field stimuli, however, and such stimuli do indeed produce EPSPs in the LGMD. The LGMD, however, is prevented from responding

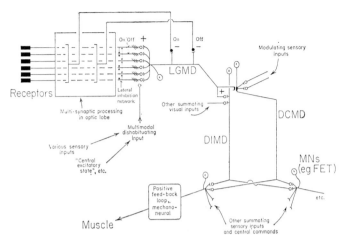

FIGURE 30.1 A diagrammatic presentation of one-half of the bilaterally symmetrical descending movement-detector system in locusts. Several additional factors affecting the system are omitted for the sake of clarity (e.g., the mutual inhibition between ipsi- and contralateral systems referred to in the text). DCMD: descending contralateral movement detector. DIMD: descending ipsilateral movement detector. LGMD: lobula giant movement detector. MNs: motoneurons. FET: fast extensor of the tibia.

appreciably to these EPSPs by the action of two other, inhibitory, inputs. These derive by summation over medium-sized areas of the retinotopic array from an earlier stage in the optic lobe, and provide compound IPSPs in the LGMD in response to transient changes in illumination of the retina; the larger the area affected, the larger the IPSP. There are two sets of such inhibitory inputs, one driven by dimming and one by brightening of the retina, and in contrast to the excitatory inputs to the LGMD, they show little or no habituation. The summed effect of these three classes of inputs is to produce a system specifically sensitive to the novel movement of small contrasting objects anywhere in the visual field, and relatively insensitive to all other forms of visual input.

Habituation of the DMD system to repeated stimuli appears to be due solely to response decrement at the excitatory chemical synapses onto the LGMD, and the process appears to be a presynaptic one. This localization has some inherent interest. In the few other cases of habituation that both have a behavioral significance and have been analyzed neurophysiologically, the decremental process was localized at the primary afferent synapses (see Krasne, this volume). There has been a tendency to generalize, conceivably too far, from these observations. The probability of the decremental process being located at primary afferent synapses must in any specific case be modified by at least two factors:

1. the amount of sensory processing required to abstract significant information from the receptor array;

2. the number of independent behavioral systems to which the receptors contribute.

Both of these qualities are likely to be at their lowest in the crayfish tail-flip circuit or the sea hare gill-withdrawal circuit, which are initiated by discontinuously active tactile sense organs of little other function. At perhaps the other extreme are circuits that derive their input from sophisticated eyes. In these circuits the raw retinal-cell output is processed and extensive lateral interaction occurs. There are often gain-control circuits to compress the dynamic range of the stimulus within that of the neural network, a process clearly incompatible with decremental responses. The final output is differentiated for many purposes; form, movement, direction, color, distance information, plane of polarization, and other parameters are all abstracted. Further, in some of these abstractions retinotopic information is preserved, while in others it is not. When habituation is detected in one such output, the primary afferent synapses would seem an unlikely choice of site for this process, and they are clearly not the site in the DMD system. The two most proximal ganglionic layers in the insect optic lobe, the medulla and the lobula, contain many other fan-shaped "tangential" cells of the same general type as the LGMD, and these are presumably the output of other forms of visual information derived from the retinotopic projection. Not all of these can be expected to show habituation (for example, those that are sensitive to directional movement and drive the optomotor system are known not to do so), but where they do, it can be expected that the site will be found either subsequent to the point of convergence onto the interneuron if stimulus generalization is required, or at that point if it is not.

The rate of decrement of the small-field dimming response can be shown to be dependent on the level of tonic sensory input to the animal as a whole. Similarly, the system can be dishabituated by a variety of strong novel stimuli, including those arising from the animal's own activity, restoring the original transmission properties. These are thought to represent tonic and phasic aspects of the same functional input to the DMD system. If recordings are made from the LGMD dendrite fan during dishabituation, one sees a total restoration of the EPSP amplitude that was lost during habituation. This supports previous, less direct, evidence suggesting that in this preparation dishabituation corresponds to a resetting of the habituated synapse, not to a compensatory enhancement of transmission elsewhere in the system (see Krasne, this volume, for some comment on this hypothesis). We currently lean to the hypothesis that this modulation is effected by an efferent multimodal tangential cell (probably of linear, as opposed to fan-shaped, morphological type) that synapses on the presynaptic terminals. We postulate that hyperpolarization of the terminals by this input causes increased entry of calcium during subsequent depolarization, by analogy with suggested explanations of postinhibitory rebound, and that transmitter release is thereby restored. To be fully explanatory, this theory would thus imply that diminishing release of transmitter substance during habituation is a function of a decrease in available intracellular calcium within the terminal, which I believe to be a new proposition. So far, however, we lack the morphological identification of the efferent neuron that is required to test these hypotheses.

The afferent synapse onto the LGMD is, however, by no means the only place where the DMD system can be modulated, even though it so far appears to be the only one responsible for response-generated effects. The LGMD is connected to at least two further interneurons that transmit its signals to the motor cells of the thorax. The synapse to one of these, the descending contralateral movement detector (DCMD), is a spike-transmitting electrical junction, normally transmitting 1:1. There is, however, evidence that this transmission can be gated by accessory chemical inputs that modulate the membrane conductance of the postsynaptic cell but do not cause it to spike. The LGMD also drives an ipsilateral cerebrothoracic neuron, the DIMD, this time via a labile chemical synapse; this cell also receives other visual input, as yet uncharacterized, with which the LGMD input summates. Both the DIMD and the DCMD synapse on at least six different sets of motor cells involved in the escape jump in the metathorax, and they probably make similar connections in the remaining thoracic ganglia. The EPSPs within the most important motoneuron (the fast extensor of the tibia) show marked spatial summation, but little or no temporal summation, with respect to these two movement-detector inputs. The efficacy at the motoneuron of a given output from the LGMD is thus dependent on simultaneous transmission at two different cerebral synapses, where transmission may be either gated or enhanced by other sensory inputs. At the motor cells there is extensive convergence from many other sensory sources, and summation with these is required to bring the fast extensor of the tibia to fire: the DMD input alone is not adequate, but in life a variety of other sensory inputs will always be present. Finally, we have been able to show mutually inhibitory relations between the DMD systems of the two eyes. This inhibition affects both the DCMD and the LGMD; its function is presumably to eliminate responses to stimulus situations that affect both eyes simultaneously.

Reviewing what we know about the circuit so far, it comes as no surprise that the relationship between visual stimulus and escape jump is so elusive when one is confined to behavioral measures. The "plastic" properties of the circuit are not the only ones responsible for lability; their role has to be seen against the functioning of the system as a whole before a proper appreciation of their function can be obtained. They are merely some of the many ways in which the stimulus-response linkage is modified, all contributing to the overall lability of the behavior pattern.

REFERENCES

BURROWS, M., and ROWELL, C. H. F. 1973. Connections between descending visual interneurones and metathoracic motoneurones in the locust. *Journal of Comparative Physiology* 85:221–234.

O'SHEA, M., and ROWELL, C. H. F. 1975a. A spike-transmitting electrical synapse between visual interneurones in the locust movement detector system. *Journal of Comparative Physiology* 97: 143–158.

O'SHEA, M., and ROWELL, C. H. F. 1975b. Protection from habituation by lateral inhibition. *Nature* 254: 53–55.

O'SHEA, M., ROWELL, C. H. F., and WILLIAMS, J. L. D. 1974. The anatomy of a locust visual interneuron: The descending contralateral movement detector. *Journal of Experimental Biology* 60: 1–12.

O'SHEA, M., and WILLIAMS, J. L. D. 1974. Anatomy and output connections of the lobular giant movement detector neuron (LGMD) of the locust. *Journal of Comparative Physiology* 91: 257–266.

ROWELL, C. H. F. 1971a. The orthopteran descending movement detector (DMD) neurones: A characterization and review. *Zeitschrift für vergleichende Physiologie* 73: 167–194.

ROWELL, C. H. F. 1971b. Variable responsiveness of the DCMD neurone in freely moving locusts, and its relation to behaviour and arousal. *Journal of Experimental Biology* 55: 749–762.

31

Properties of Neurons and Their Relationship to Concepts of Plasticity

FELIX STRUMWASSER

ABSTRACT The possible mechanisms of habituation and of associative forms of learning at the level of synapses and single neurons are analyzed. Presynaptic and postsynaptic regulatory controls are examined. It is suggested that the regulation of density and topography of transmitter release sites, transmitter and hormonal receptors, ion channels and ion pumps could all play important roles in the plasticity of the nervous system. The field is at a stage where we are still ignorant of how such components are selectively synthesized, inserted into, and removed from membranes, nor do we know the nature of their regulatory signals. It is pointed out that the existence of endogenous 24-hour clocks in certain specialized neurons offers the possibility of examining how intracellular mechanisms couple to excitable membranes to allow read-out and resetting of these rhythms which constitute a form of highly patterned information.

It is the purpose of this article to comment on those properties of neurons that hold some promise for yielding insight into the mechanisms of learning and memory. Davis and Krasne, in their chapters, have described the invertebrate preparations in which substantial progress has been made in demonstrating habituation, sensitization, and associative forms of learning and in defining their parameters. In some cases of habituation—gill withdrawal in *Aplysia*, tail flip in crayfish—a fair amount of detailed knowledge has been uncovered about the identifiable neurons and the pathways involved. While electrical measurements indicate that postsynaptic potentials decrease in the "motor" neurons driving these two different systems during habituation to a periodic stimulus, the mechanism of these decreases is not understood. Carew and Kandel (1974) state, "If one can determine that the change is presynaptic, it will be necessary to distinguish further between a change in the availability of transmitter, in the probability of release, or in the number of release sites."

31.1 PRESYNAPTIC CONTROLS

It is generally (but not universally) accepted that at chemical synapses, transmitter release is dependent on

the sequence: action potential (or electrotonic depolarization) $\rightarrow$ Ca^{++} influx in presynaptic membrane $\rightarrow$ increase in release sites on inner membrane surface $\rightarrow$ release of transmitter into synaptic cleft from vesicles bound to release sites. A decrement in transmitter release with repetition of a stimulus could occur by any of the following six processes:

1. The presynaptic terminal is invaded by a smaller-amplitude action potential with each stimulus.

2. Less Ca^{++} influx occurs with each impulse.

3. Ca^{++} influx is normal, but release sites are refractory and require a long time to recover normal function.

4. The pool of transmitter-charged vesicles in the terminal is small.

5. Recycling (Heuser and Reese, 1973) and recharging of spent vesicles is slow and rate-limiting.

6. Reuptake of relased transmitter (or its precursor) from the synaptic cleft by the presynaptic terminal is reduced.

It is somewhat ironic that the most studied synapses—vertebrate neuromuscular synapses and the squid giant synapse—do not show habituation; they also have a large quantum content per impulse. In the former synapse quantal synaptic events can be directly observed by recording from the postsynaptic (muscle) structure, but the presynaptic terminal cannot be impaled and directly voltage-controlled. In the latter synapse the presynaptic terminal is large enough to be impaled (and hence, to be directly manipulated), but quantal events cannot be observed, presumably because the postsynaptic membrane input resistance is too low. The prospects for gaining insight into synaptic habituation will depend upon the discovery of preparations in which either a quantal analysis can be performed or, at least, the presynaptic terminal can be impaled. Processes 4 and 5, above, could be studied if a quantal analysis were possible (ideally by observing the amplitude and frequency of miniature synaptic potentials), while processes 1 to 3 could be evaluated if the presynaptic terminal could be impaled. Aequorin, a protein from the bioluminescent jellyfish *Aequorea*, is a sensitive luminescent indicator of free Ca^{++} and has already been used to detect intracel-

FELIX STRUMWASSER, Division of Biology, California Institute of Technology, Pasadena, CA

lular Ca^{++} changes in a variety of systems (Ashley and Ridgway, 1970; Llinás, Blinks, and Nicholson, 1972; Stinnakre and Tauc, 1973; Chang, Gelperin, and Johnson, 1974).

There are at least two other presynaptic controls that could account for synaptic habituation:

7. Free Ca^{++} is sequestered in mitochondria.

8. An intracellular inactivator or degrader of transmitter is released.

There is certainly evidence that each of these factors can influence synaptic function.

Ruthenium Red, an inhibitor of mitochondrial Ca^{++} pumping, will increase the frequency of miniature endplate potentials at the frog neuromuscular junction. This finding is interpreted by Rahamimoff and Alnaes (1973) as indicating that the mitochondria play an important role in regulating [Ca^{++}] in the nerve terminal. For habituation to be accounted for by a mitochondrial mechanism, it would be required that the mitochondria in habituating synapses be located very close to the presynaptic membrane, and perhaps in addition receive a regulating signal for controlling the rate of Ca^{++} pumping. Ca^{++}, in itself, could be a very important regulator in the nerve terminal since, when injected into cell bodies, it increases K$^+$ conductance and clamps the membrane at a hyperpolarized level (Meech and Strumwasser, 1970; Meech, 1972). It has recently been found (Parnas and Strumwasser, 1974) that a long-lasting synaptically induced inhibition in the R15 neuron of *Aplysia* is blocked by EGTA (a calcium chelator) intracellularly applied. Any mechanism that clamps the presynaptic terminal membrane (due to a conductance increase) will shunt and hence reduce the terminal action potential, which in turn will reduce transmitter release (e.g., presynaptic inhibition).

The release of an intracellular inactivator or degrader of transmitter could operate in the manner recently demonstrated by Tauc et al. (1974), who injected acetylcholinesterase into known cholinergic neuron cell bodies in *Aplysia* and found abolition of evoked (mono)synaptic transmission within 2–4 hours. (Tauc and his colleagues use this finding to argue against the vesicular-release theory, but that is not of concern to us here.) Dishabituation should not be immediately demonstrable if such a mechanism is to account for some forms of habituation. The natural production and release of the inactivator or degrader of transmitter could be within the terminal itself, which would circumvent delays due to transport from a cell-body site of production and release. (Monoamine oxidase, a mitochondrial enzyme, is involved in catecholamine catabolism and is known to exist in synaptic terminals.) Such a drastic mechanism would have

the advantage that a synaptic connection could be incapacitated for hours or even days, depending on the relative rates of synthesis and degradation of the inactivator and transmitter.

31.2 POSTSYNAPTIC CONTROLS

Hebb (1949) proposed that in associative learning the conditioned stimulus, initially a weak convergent stimulus onto a neuron (or neuron pool), comes to have stronger properties by its repeated temporal overlap with the action potential caused by the unconditioned stimulus, in the postsynaptic cells. Marr (1969) has used this proposition in asserting that the cerebellum learns to perform motor skills. At the single-neuron level he visualizes that "if a parallel fibre is active at about the same time as the climbing fibre to a Purkinje cell with which that parallel fibre makes synaptic contact, then the efficacy of that synapse is increased towards some fixed maximum value." There are now two explicit physiological models that have been put forth to account for Hebb's postulate.

Stent (1973) theorizes that each time a postsynaptic neuron fires an action potential, transmitter receptors (TRs) are lost from the membrane, with the exception of those in the zone that caused the action potential. I believe a more useful way of describing the postulated physiological process would be to say that postsynaptic action potentials tend to displace TRs when these are not bound to transmitters of any class, since a single neuron may have more than one class of TR. One consequence would then be that any single input that fires frequently will diminish the present and future effectiveness of all other nonfiring inputs. If two of the inputs that converge onto the postsynaptic cell overlap in time, even if only one produces action potentials, then these two inputs will become dominant because all TRs for other inputs will be slowly reduced or eliminated, while those for the two active inputs will be strengthened.

Mark (1974), on the basis of neuromuscular-regeneration experiments in fish and salamanders, has postulated the repression by the postsynaptic cell of transmission from nonactive inputs via a recognition process. That is, more "marker" molecules are synthesized in the active presynaptic unit and inserted into its synaptic membrane. The postsynaptic cell then recognizes the elevated level of marker molecules and represses all other synapses not bearing these presumably elevated levels. This is a more complex mechanism than that proposed by Stent. Recently, however, Frank et al. (1974) have found in the rat that a foreign nerve (the superficial fibular nerve) will innervate a denervated muscle (soleus) and remain functional even after the proper nerve (tibial) has reinnervated the muscle. Hence, the generality of the findings of Mark and his colleagues is in question at the moment.

Stent's hypothesis, that the overshoot of the action potential of a postsynaptic cell regulates the topography of its TRs by displacing those that are not bound to transmitters, is an imaginative idea for which there is no evidence at present. It is known that the kinetics of the closing of the ion channel for acetylcholine (ACh) activation in the frog muscle membrane is sensitive to membrane voltage (faster with depolarization, slower with hyperpolarization; see Kordaš, 1969; Magleby and Stevens, 1972), but there is no evidence that ACh sensitivity decreases with membrane depolarization at either extrasynaptic or end-plate sites. Stent's theory is really based on the observation of Lømo and Rosenthal (1972) that directly stimulated denervated leg muscles in rats will not develop extrasynaptic ACh receptors, and that if such stimulation is performed after these receptors develop, they disappear. Stent suggested that the overshooting action potentials in these muscles eliminate ACh receptors, but he was careful to point out that he was assuming lack of "a mechanical or chemical effect of the muscle contractions initiated by these action potentials." However, there is already in the literature a claim that voltage pulses just *below* mechanical threshold prevent development of ACh supersensitivity in the same rat muscles (Gruener, Baumbach, and Coffee, 1974). This finding certainly implies that it is not action potentials (nor muscle contractions) that prevent receptor development—at least in the latter experiments. Frankly this finding also causes concern as to what the applied currents themselves might be doing.

If muscle action potentials were really directly displacing TRs, one would expect that prolonging the action potential would produce an even larger effect, as happens with transmitter release (Kusano, Livengood, and Werman, 1967; Katz and Miledi, 1967). If denervated rat diaphragm strips are stimulated under organ-culture conditions at 36°C, after 6–7 days of stimulation, muscle fibers, responding to both polarities of the stimulation paradigm, show a 95 percent decrease in ACh (iontophoretic) sensitivity in comparison with nonstimulated control strips (Purves and Sakmann, 1974). In separate experiments, $[^{125}I]\alpha$-bungarotoxin (α-BuTX) was used to assay ACh receptors, and it was found that stimulated diaphragm strips bound 30–35 percent less α-BuTX than control strips (Strumwasser and Dreifuss, unpublished data). However, if similar experiments are performed at 25°C, where the action potential should be 2–3 times longer in duration, stimulated diaphragm strips bind about 25 percent *more* α-BuTX than control

strips. This finding, for the moment, suggests that Stent's hypothesis is inadequate—at least in its present form—in that it cannot account for how action potentials might directly cause an increase in TRs.

31.3 REGULATION OF THE SURFACE PROPERTIES OF CELLS

Very little is known, in neurons or muscle cells, about how TRs, their associated ion channels, the electrically excitable Na and K channels, and the various ion pumps are synthesized and inserted into the membrane; there is essentially no information on their lifetime or stability. Nothing is known about the regulation of the topography of these membrane elements or the nature of the controlling signals. It seems unlikely that much progress concerning plasticity in the nervous system will be made until such fundamental knowledge is available.

There is evidence that a presynaptic neuron, perhaps through trophic factors, regulates the topography of some of these elements. In frog, some components of the iliofibularis and pyriformis muscles, "slow" extrafusal muscle fibers, normally do not produce action potentials, but after their nerve supply is cut, the muscle membrane is, within two weeks, capable of producing action potentials (Miledi, Stefani, and Steinbach, 1971). Actinomycin D (in vivo), an inhibitor of DNA-dependent RNA synthesis, blocks the development of this membrane reaction to denervation (Schmidt and Tong, 1973). Another example in which it seems likely that trophic control by presynaptic neurons exists is demonstrable in tissue culture. Neurons derived from a neuroblastoma can be selected in culture for very low (or absent) ACh and choline acetylase levels. When such neurons make contact with mouse muscle cells, although they cannot release ACh, they induce in the muscle cell a region of high sensitivity to ACh at the contact zone (Harris, 1974). Botulinus toxin applied before the contact is made will block the induction, but it has no effect on the high-sensitivity zone after the contact is made. It seems likely that Botulinus toxin binds to some (non-TR) membrane sites blocking release (presynaptic) and/or reception (postsynaptic) of a trophic factor.

The nature of the controlling forces that account for the orderly topographical arrangement of the functional elements (TRs, ion channels, pumps, trophic factor and hormone receptors) in neuronal and muscle membranes may be gleaned from recent research dealing with "single" cellular systems. Singer and Nicolson (1972) propose that (membrane) proteins (structural and functional) are free to diffuse in the lipid of the membrane—their "fluid-mosaic" model of cell surfaces. The behavior of the photoreceptor protein rhodopsin in isolated retinal rods suggests that it is free to diffuse; this is indicated by measurements of circular dichroism (Cone, 1972) and by the fact that a very small bleaching by light in one part of a single rod will be transmitted (with the right speed for free diffusion of a 15–30 Å globule) along the axis of orientation of the retinal discs (Poo and Cone, 1974). Synaptosomes prepared from rat neocortex have membranes, at least in regions immediately outside the synaptic cleft, that appear to satisfy the fluid-mosaic model. Concanavalin A-ferritin will bind the membranes of fixed synaptosomes homogeneously, suggesting a random topographical distribution of glycoprotein sites on the membrane. These sites are free to move in unfixed synaptosomes because concanavalin A-ferritin binding followed by incubation with (rabbit) antiferritin antibody causes discrete patches of concanavalin A-ferritin to form, due to cross-linking (Matus, de Petris, and Raff, 1973). If the nerve (and muscle) membrane is for the most part a fluid mosaic, with the probable exception of synaptic zones, then signal molecules collected on the membrane surface (bound to protein) can travel by free diffusion within the membrane until they run into the appropriate membrane device for triggering intracellular mechanisms such as synthesis, degradation, and the unmasking of membrane components. While the nature of such molecular signals or membrane devices is presently obscure, the collision frequencies are sufficiently high for membrane particles (10^5–10^6 per second estimated for rhodopsin) to make the mechanism feasible.

Colchicine, an agent known to bind microtubule protein, blocks the internalization of concanavalin A-membrane binding sites that normally arises from induced phagocytosis in polymorphonuclear leukocytes (Oliver, Ukena, and Berlin, 1974). In the same system phagocytosis, while removing external membrane, does not alter the transport of nonelectrolytes, implying that the transport carriers are (selectively) not internalized; after colchicine treatment, however, phagocytosis leads to a marked reduction in nonelectrolyte transport, implying that the colchicine has interfered with the selection procedure (Ukena and Berlin, 1972). It is quite interesting that in the rat colchicine appears to prevent the dramatic reduction of ACh sensitivity in stimulated denervated muscles in vivo (Lømo, 1974). It is conceivable that colchicine may, in muscle, interfere with the membrane devices that control the internalization of certain membrane components and not others, as in the case of polymorphonuclear leukocytes. It may thus be expected that further investigations of the action of such compounds as colchicine will yield clues to the connection, in muscle, between the membrane action potential or its sequelae and the topography of ACh receptors.

31.4 NEURAL IMPULSES THAT READ OUT TEMPORAL INFORMATION

Some neurons are specialized to provide recurring activity cycles with a period of about one day (the circadian rhythm, CR). The fact that the phase of these cycles can be set by an external light-dark cycle, a phenomenon called entrainment, would suggest that such systems might provide clues as to how environmental information can be stored (and read out) in other neuronal systems.

The mollusc *Aplysia californica* is a day-active species, as determined by measurements of locomotor activity in the laboratory (Strumwasser, 1967; Kupfermann, 1967; Jacklet, 1972). At 350 lux about 60 percent of the animals require their paired eyes to entrain to a light-dark cycle (see Figs. 2,3,4, in Strumwasser, 1973). In our laboratory three circadian systems have been discovered in the nervous system of *Aplysia*. One circadian system exists in the paired eyes and can be expressed in vitro under conditions of total darkness and isolation from the rest of the organism (Jacklet, 1969; Eskin, 1971). Under these conditions the impulse frequency of compound action potentials in the optic nerve cycles with a period slightly less than 24 hours if the medium is sea water, and greater than 24 hours if the medium is enriched with amino acids, vitamins, glucose, and *Aplysia* serum. Under organ-culture conditions the CR of the eye may be maintained for up to two weeks (Eskin, 1971). The first cycle (in vitro) reads out the position of the dawn (dark-to-light transition) that the intact organism had been entrained to; it is thus clearly a kind of memory. An isolated eye shows little or no optic-nerve activity during the projected dark period, but becomes active before projected dawn and peaks at 1.4 ($\pm$1.1) hours after projected dawn (standard deviation: n=13; see Fig. 7 in Strumwasser, 1973). Entrainment of the CR is possible in vitro by applying light-dark cycles, an 11-hour phase advance requiring 3–5 days to be completed (Eskin, 1971).

Two other circadian systems can be directly measured, at the level of single neurons, in the isolated parieto-visceral (abdominal) ganglion (PVG) of *Aplysia*. Intracellular recordings from a neurosecretory neuron, R15, over a two-day period show that this neuron can produce at least two cycles of spike output in a sea-water medium with periods ranging from 21.4 to 28.6 hours (Strumwasser, 1965). If dissection and impalement are performed during the early part of the dark phase of the entraining light-dark cycle, then the spike output of R15 is at a maximum around projected dawn. Audesirk (1974) has recently found that the position of the R15 peak is a function of both the past light-dark cycle and the time of dissection. He has also found that the eyes are necessary for the entrainment of R15 in the intact animal, that is, the peaks of R15 (studied in vitro)only shift with a shifted light schedule when the eyes are present (see Table 31.1).

Under conditions of organ culture (Strumwasser and Bahr, 1966; Strumwasser, 1971) and of extracellular recording from output axons in either the pericardial or genital nerves of the isolated PVG, CRs are found in four or five neuronal units whose cell bodies are unidentified at the moment. The CRs in these units can be observed during at least the second and third weeks in organ culture, either by multiunit recording (Strumwasser, 1967) or by automatic reliable sorting of single units from such recordings (Strumwasser, 1973). With the latter technique it is possible to state confidently that the CRs so far observed in simultaneously recorded units have different periods and are not found to be in phase with one another.

In summary, we can conclude that long-term (cyclic) programs of impulse activity (with memory of the timing of a past environmental event) are possible in neurons in ganglia or eyes removed from the organism without any known sensory or hormonal inputs. Furthermore, in vitro entrainment (by light) can occur in the eyes, and the eyes appear to be necessary in the intact organism to entrain the CR in the R15 neuron.

Three major questions emerge concerning these systems: (1) What is the nature of entrainment? (2) Is the CR a network property? (3) If the CR is a property within a single cell, how is it generated? Only the crudest

answers can be given to these questions at the present time.

The nature of entrainment has been studied in the CR of the isolated eye. Eskin (1972) has shown that depolarization of all the cells in the eye by a four-hour pulse of 100 mM K^+ (a tenfold increase from normal medium) produces systematic phase advances or delays depending on the time in the cycle at which the pulse is delivered. Spiking is quickly inactivated during the high-K^+ treatment and since a high Mg^{++} and low Ca^{++} treatment in the presence of high K^+ does not prevent the phase shift, it seems likely that membrane depolarization per se—rather than either impulses or transmitter release—mediates the high-K^+ effect. Thus one clue to entrainment of a neuronal circadian oscillator is the fact that the membrane potential (depolarization) can reset the phase of the oscillator. The nature of the signal that couples the membrane potential to the phase of the oscillator is not known, but it may be a temperature-sensitive step since modest heat pulses (10°C rise for 2–4 hours) applied to the isolated PVG during the early projected night will phase-advance the CR in R15 (Strumwasser, 1965).

It appears unlikely that the CR is a neuronal-network property. Under conditions where impulses and synaptic transmission are blocked in the isolated PVG, with tetrodotoxin and zero calcium in the artificial sea water, intracellular recordings from R15 show that at least one cycle of CR is expressed (Strumwasser, 1971, 1973). In the absence of impulse production, the driving pacemaker waves in R15 (which would have produced impulses) are uncovered. Such recordings reveal that in the first 24-hour period, R15 shows about 10–12 hours of inactivity followed by a similar period of activity (pacemaker waves) if the PVG comes from previously entrained *Aplysia*.

It is also doubtful that the CR in the eye of *Aplysia* is a network property. There is certainly no definitive experiment that proves this point for the eye; however, eyes that are surgically reduced to less than 20 percent of normal size (to the region where the optic nerve emerges) still produce a normal CR (see Fig. 7, Strumwasser, 1973). Clarification of the CR in the eye must await a more detailed study of the cellular organization of the eye than presently exists (Jacklet, Alvarez, and Bernstein, 1972; Strumwasser and Alvarez have undertaken such a study).

An eventual understanding of entrainment will depend upon an unraveling of the mechanism of the CR in single neurons, since all the present evidence indicates that the CR can in fact be a property of a single neuron. The CR represents, in the course of evolution, a mechanism by which (environmentally entrainable) information stored within a cell can be read out cyclically. How is the

TABLE 13.1

Effects of blinding and sham operations on the timing of the maximum spike output to a six-hour phase advance in the light-dark schedule (R15 in isolated PVG)

	Control[a]	Normal shift[b]	Blind shift[b]	Sham shift[b]
Time of peak[c]	+0030	−1530	−2030	−1430
(PDT)	+0230	−1800	−2130	−1530
	−2230	−1530	−2400	−1800
	−2130	−1600	−2000	−2100
	−2000	−1900	−2330	−1300
Mean ±S.D.	−2300	−1648	−2154	−1624
	±0233	±0136	±0147	±0309
Predicted peak[d]		−1700	−1700	−1700

a. Control light schedule: 12 hr light: 12 hr dark; lights on at 0800 hr, off at 2000 hr.
b. Shifted light schedule: 12 hr light: 12 hr dark; lights on at 0200 hr, off at 1400 hr.
c. Positive times occurred on the day after dissection; negative times occurred on the day of dissection.
d. Predicted peak times are based on a six-hour advance over the control peak average.
Source: Audesirk (1974).

472   FELIX STRUMWASSER

CR generated? There are at least three different explanatory models in the literature. Ehret and Trucco (1967) suggest that the 24-hour cycle is generated by a controlled rate of gene transcription in DNA, which in turn, through translation of messenger RNA into protein, causes a fixed sequence of biochemical events, a full cycle being circadian. Pavlidis (1969) conceives of a number of biochemical oscillators within the cell, each of which, although fully independent and with periods considerably less than 24 hours, interact (i.e., they are strongly coupled) to produce the circadian period. Njus, Sulzman, and Hastings (1974) have recently proposed a highly qualitative model in which the CR resides entirely within the membrane (presumably the external membrane) of the cell and in which "time-dependent cooperative phenomena may account for accurate timekeeping." A comparison of these various models and their relationship to reality is beyond the scope of this particular paper, but the reader will note that the three models can be respectively classified as nuclear (Ehret and Trucco), cytoplasmic (Pavlidis), and membranal (Njus, Sulzman, and Hastings) in orientation and emphasis. None of these models is easily testable, so all three may stand for some time until substantially new data are brought into the field.

My own view is that within a neuron with a CR, readout (of a temporal pattern of impulses) is probably mediated by the intracellular production of depolarizing or hyperpolarizing substances that activate or inactivate the surface-membrane ion channels and pumps by acting on the inner surface of the cell (Strumwasser, 1965, 1967). A quantitative model constructed with Dr. M. Kim (quoted in Strumwasser, 1971) shows how self-sustained oscillations of electrical potential, with periods of minutes, can be generated without the use of electrically excitable ion channels. This model can account for many of the properties of the pacemaker waves in R15—however, it can not account for a CR. The dramatic abolition of the CR of the *Aplysia* eye with Actinomycin D or Aflatoxin Bl (Rothman and Strumwasser, 1973), both inhibitors of DNA-dependent RNA synthesis, suggests that new RNA and protein synthesis is part of the CR mechanism, contrary to the model of Njus, Sulzman, and Hastings mentioned above. More recent studies indicate dose-dependent phase shifts of the CR of this eye with puromycin and cycloheximide, two inhibitors of protein synthesis in this system (Rothman and Strumwasser, in preparation).

In pacemaker neurons in *Aplysia* most of the newly synthesized protein has a molecular weight of about 12,000 and 6,000–9,000 (Wilson, 1971; Strumwasser, 1973), whereas in nonpacemaker neurons there is little synthesis of these components. This finding suggests that these SDS-soluble (presumably membrane) proteins may be involved in the control and function of the pacemaker mechanism. The readout of the entrained CR in R15, as a modulation of the pacemaker mechanism, could involve the *selective* production (and degradation) of controlling and functional polypeptides within the cell whose targets would be the cell membrane. These ideas appear, at least, to be testable.

ACKNOWLEDGMENTS

This paper was written while the author was in residence in the Department of Biophysics, University College, London. While there, he was supported by a fellowship from the Muscular Dystrophy Associations of America. Travel to England was supported by a NATO senior fellowship. Original research (on *Aplysia*) reported in this paper has been supported by grants from the NIH (NS07071) and the Alfred P. Sloan Foundation. The author wishes to thank Professor B. Katz and Dr. G. Audesirk ior their comments on this paper.

REFERENCES

ASHLEY, C. C., and RIDGWAY, E. B. 1970. On the relationships between membrane potential, calcium transient, and tension in single barnacle muscle fibers. *Journal of Physiology* 209: 105–130.

AUDESIRK, G. 1974. Studies on the interrelationship between two neuronal circadian oscillators in *Aplysia californica*. Unpublished Ph.D. dissertation, California Institute of Technology.

CAREW, T. J., and KANDEL, E. R. 1974. Synaptic analysis of the interrelationships between behavioral modifications in *Aplysia*. In M. V. L. Bennett, ed., *Synaptic Transmission and Neuronal Interaction*. New York: Raven Press, pp. 339–383.

CHANG, J. J., GELPERIN, A., and JOHNSON, F. H. 1974. Intracellularly injected aequorin detects transmembrane calcium flux during action potentials in an identified neuron from the terrestrial slug, *Limax maximus*. *Brain Research* 77: 431–442.

CONE, R. A. 1972. Rotational diffusion of rhodopsin in the visual receptor membrane. *Nature; New Biology* 236: 39–43.

EHRET, C. F., and TRUCCO, E. 1967. Molecular models for the circadian clock. I. The Chronon concept. *Journal of Theoretical Biology* 15: 240–262.

ESKIN, A. 1971. Properties of the *Aplysia* visual system: *In vitro* entrainment of the circadian rhythm and centrifugal regulation of the eye. *Zeitschrift für Vergleichende Physiologie* 74: 353–371.

ESKIN, A. 1972. Phase shifting a circadian rhythm in the eye of the *Aplysia* by high potassium pulses. *Journal of Comparative Physiology* 80: 353–376.

FRANK, E., JANSEN, J. K. S., LØMO, T., and WESTGAARD, R. 1974. Maintained function of foreign synapses on hyperinnervated skeletal muscle fibres of the rat. *Nature* 247:375.

GRUENER, R., BAUMBACH, N., and COFFEE, D. 1974. Reduction of denervation supersensitivity of muscle by submechanical threshold stimulation. *Nature* 248: 68–69.

HARRIS, A. J. 1974. Inductive functions of the nervous system. *Annual Review of Physiology* 36: 251–305.

HEBB, D. O. 1949. *The Organization of Behavior*. New York: John Wiley & Sons.

HEUSER, J. E., and REESE, T. S. 1973. Evidence for recycling of synaptic vesicle membrane during transmitter release at the frog neuromuscular junction. *Journal of Cell Biology* 57: 315–344.

JACKLET, J. W. 1969. A circadian rhythm of optic nerve impulses recorded in darkness from the isolated eye of *Aplysia*. *Science* 164: 562–564.

JACKLET, J. W. 1972. Circadian locomotor acrtivity in *Aplysia*. *Journal of Comparative Physiology* 79: 325–341.

JACKLET, J. W., ALVAREZ, R., and BERNSTEIN, B. 1972. Ultrastructure of the eye of *Aplysia*. *Journal of Ultrastructure Research* 38: 246–261.

KATZ, B., and MILEDI, R. 1967. A study of synaptic transmission in the absence of nerve impulses. *Journal of Physiology* 192: 407–436.

KORDAŠ, M. 1969. The effect of membrane polarization on the time course of the end-plate current in frog sartorius muscle. *Journal of Physiology* 204: 493–502.

KUPFERMANN, I. 1967. A circadian locomotor rhythm in *Aplysia californica*. *Physiology and Behavior* 3: 179–182.

KUSANO, K., LIVENGOOD, D. R., and WERMAN, R. 1967. Correlation of transmitter release with membrane properties of the presynaptic fiber of the squid giant synapse. *Journal of General Physiology* 50: 2579–2601.

LLINÁS, R., BLINKS, J. R., and NICHOLSON, C. 1972. Calcium transient in presynaptic terminal of squid giant synapse determined with aequorin. *Science* 176: 1127–1129.

LØMO, T. 1974. Neurotrophic control of colchicine effects on muscle? *Nature* 249: 473–474.

LØMO, T., and ROSENTHAL, J. 1972. Control of ACh sensitivity by muscle activity in the rat. *Journal of Physiology* 221: 493–513.

MAGLEBY, K. L., and STEVENS, C. F. 1972. The effect of voltage on the time course of end-plate currents. *Journal of Physiology* 223: 151–171.

MARK, R. 1974. *Memory and Nerve Cell Connections*. Oxford: Clarendon Press.

MARR, D. 1969. A theory of cerebellar cortex. *Journal of Physiology* 202: 437–470.

MATUS, A., DE PETRIS, S., and RAFF, M. C. 1973. Mobility of concanavalin A receptors in myelin and synaptic membranes. *Nature; New Biology* 244: 278–280.

MEECH, R. W. 1972. Intracellular calcium injection causes increased potassium conductance in *Aplysia* nerve cells. *Comparative Biochemistry and Physiology* 42: 493–499.

MEECH, R. W., and STRUMWASSER, F. 1970. Intracellular calcium injection activates potassium conductance in *Aplysia* nerve cells. *Federation Proceedings* 29: 834.

MILEDI, R., STEFANI, E., and STEINBACH, A. B. 1971. Induction of the action potential mechanisms in slow muscle fibres of the frog. *Journal of Physiology* 217: 737–754.

NJUS, D., SULZMAN, F. M., and HASTINGS, J. W. 1974. Membrane model for the circadian clock. *Nature* 248: 116–120.

OLIVER, J. M., UKENA, T. E., and BERLIN, R. D. 1974. Effects of phagocytosis and colchicine on the distribution of lectin-binding sites on cell surfaces. *Proceedings of the National Academy of Sciences (USA)* 71: 394–398.

PARNAS, I., and STRUMWASSER, F. 1974. Mechanisms of long

lasting inhibition of a bursting pacemaker neuron. *Journal of Neurophysiology* 37: 609–620.

PAVLIDIS, T. 1969. Populations of interacting oscillators and circadian rhythms. *Journal of Theoretical Biology* 22: 418–436.

POO, M., and CONE, R. A. 1974. Lateral diffusion of rhodopsin in the photoreceptor membrane. *Nature* 247: 438–441.

PURVES, D., and SAKMANN, B. 1974. The effect of contractile activity on fibrillation and extrajunctional acetylcholine-sensitivity in rat muscle maintained in organ culture. *Journal of Physiology* 237: 157–182.

RAHAMIMOFF, R., and ALNAES, E. 1973. Inhibitory action of Ruthenium Red on neuromuscular transmission. *Proceedings of the National Academy of Sciences (USA)* 70: 3613–3616.

ROTHMAN, B., and STRUMWASSER, F. 1973. Aflatoxin Bl blocks the circadian rhythm in the isolated eye of *Aplysia*. *Federation Proceedings* 32: 365.

SCHMIDT, H., and TONG, E. Y. 1973. Inhibition by actinomycin D of the denervation-induced action potential in frog slow muscle fibres. *Proceedings of the Royal Society (London)* B184: 91–95.

SINGER, S. J., and NICOLSON, G. L. 1972. The fluid mosaic model of the structure of cell membranes. *Science* 175: 720–731.

STENT, G. S. 1973. A physiological mechanism for Hebb's postulate of learning. *Proceedings of the National Academy of Sciences (USA)* 70: 997–1001.

STINNAKRE, J., and TAUC, L. 1973. Calcium influx in active *Aplysia* neurones detected by injected aequorin. *Nature; New Biology* 242: 113–115.

STRUMWASSER, F. 1965. The demonstration and manipulation of a circadian rhythm in a single neuron. In J. Aschoff, ed., *Circadian Clocks*. Amsterdam: North Holland Publishing Company, pp. 442–462.

STRUMWASSER, F. 1967. Neurophysiological aspects of rhythms. In G. C. Quarton, T. Melnechuk, and F. O. Schmitt, eds., *The Neurosciences: A Study Program*. New York: Rockefeller University Press, pp. 516–528.

STRUMWASSER, F. 1971. The cellular basis of behavior in *Aplysia*. *Journal of Psychiatric Research* 8: 237–257.

STRUMWASSER, F. 1973. Neural and humoral factors in the temporal organization of behavior (The 17th Bowditch lecture). *The Physiologist* 16: 9–42.

STRUMWASSER, F., and BAHR, R. 1966. Prolonged *in vitro* culture and autoradiographic studies of neurons in *Aplysia*. *Federation Proceedings* 25: 512.

TAUC, L., HOFFMANN, A., TSUJI, S., HINZEN, D. H., and FAILLE, L. 1974. Transmission abolished on a cholinergic synapse after injection of acetylcholinesterase into the presynaptic neurone. *Nature* 250: 496–498.

UKENA, T. E., and BERLIN, R. D. 1972. Effect of colchicine and vinblastine on the topographical separation of membrane functions. *Journal of Experimental Medicine* 136: 1–7.

WILSON, D. L. 1971. Molecular weight distribution of proteins synthesized in single identified neurons of *Aplysia*. *Journal of General Physiology* 57: 26–40.

32

Learning and Memory: Habituation as Negative Learning

EUGENE N. SOKOLOV

ABSTRACT The selective diminution of behavioral and neuronal responses due to repeated presentation of a stimulus is called habituation and is regarded as learning for "not responding" (negative learning). The results of behavioral, extracellular, and intracellular studies of habituation of the response to novelty (orienting response) can be interpreted in the following way: during repeated stimulus presentation a "neuronal model of the stimulus" is elaborated which selectively blocks the responses to stimuli coinciding with the elaborated model. At the level of single hippocampal neurons the neuronal model is represented as a set of modified synapses reflecting the feature detectors involved in the perception of a given stimulus. At the intracellular level the neuronal model can be represented as a set of modified membrane loci.

Each of the preceding papers has focused mainly on problems at a single level. Some have been restricted to the behavioral level, some to the level of single units, and some to the level of intracellular mechanisms. At each of these levels of analysis we can distinguish different types of learning, such as habituation, classical conditioning, and operant conditioning. I now propose to make a vertical analysis of the phenomenon of habituation, summarizing relevant data from the behavioral level, the level of single-unit studies, and the level of intracellular recordings.

Habituation is an effect that can be observed in many different situations, including the vestibular, ocular, and motor responses, but if we are to understand its role in conditioning exactly, I believe we must start by returning to the conditioned-reflex procedure of Pavlov (1927). Within this procedure we can differentiate two relatively independent aspects. The first aspect is extension of the receptive fields of the unconditioned response. In other words, due to the conditioning procedure certain receptive surfaces, which at first were not involved in the triggering of a given unconditioned response, are now combined with this response and can trigger it. The second aspect is continuous limitation of the receptive surfaces, that is, the possibility of mapping receptive surfaces and, by using the procedure of nonreinforcement, rendering only selected, limited subsets of the surfaces capable of triggering the unconditioned response.

Having differentiated these two aspects of the condi-

EUGENE N. SOKOLOV, Department of Psychology, Moscow State University, Moscow, U.S.S.R.

tioned-reflex procedure, we can now ask the following two questions: First, can we find an unconditioned response that initially has a very extensive receptor surface? Second, if we can find such an unconditioned response, can we develop a procedure for limiting the receptive surface that will allow us to study the second aspect of the conditioned response?

A response with an initially extended receptive surface is available—this is the so-called orienting response that is made to novel stimuli and that consists of eye movements, galvanic skin responses, and EEG depression (Sokolov, 1963). This response can be elicited by all stimuli for which receptive surfaces are available. Using it, we can therefore concentrate our attention on the second aspect of the conditioned response, studying only limitations of the receptive surface of the unconditioned orienting response. Habituation is in this case an example of conditioned inhibition produced by nonreinforcement of the conditioned response; that is, it refers to a limitation of the initially very widely distributed receptive surface of the orienting response. From this point of view we can study the selectivity of the habituation as the most important feature of negative learning.

If a specific stimulus is given several times and then test stimuli are presented, we may find that the response to the given stimulus is selectively depressed and that the other new signals can still evoke responses. We express this by saying that the nervous system can elaborate self-adjustable filters which are particularly tuned to the repeated stimulus under certain conditions. Now, each stimulus has a variety of parameters—duration, intensity, color, frequency (of sounds), and so forth. In the nervous system there will thus be elaborated, in parallel, a series of filters, each selectively adjusted to a specific parameter of the repeated stimulus. The end result is a multidimensional filter that blocks only the neural signals arising from the particular stimulus. Thus a stimulus that can be defined by a particular duration, intensity, and color combination, for example, will produce a certain region in a three-dimensional "characteristic space" such that all neural signals coming from this region are blocked. This blockage can be studied using EEG or galvanic skin responses.

Our problem is whether such filters are elaborated in

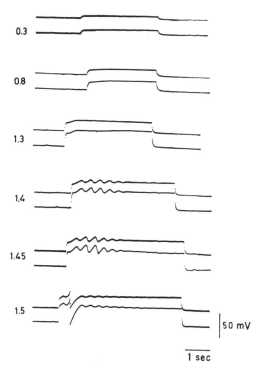

FIGURE 32.1 The dependence of the pacemaker potential on applied depolarizing current. With the increase of intensity the amplitudes of pacemaker oscillation rise, and there is an increase of frequency. The response of the neuron is prolonged mainly during initial part of the stimulation.

Two microelectrodes were placed in latent pacemaker cell of *Helix pomatia*, and recordings were made from the stimulating electrode through the bridge circuit. Numbers on the left show the intensity of the depolarizing current in nanoamperes (na).

most neurons. Our studies have shown that no habituation is present in the afferent neurons. Only in hippocampal neurons have we found some characteristics that can be observed at the behavioral level in the orienting response. Single hippocampal neurons show a convergence of signals from all modalities of all the body's receptive surfaces, including vision and hearing. Another relevant feature of the hippocampal neuron is a selective habituation similar to the habituation of the orienting response. The main model that can be suggested is that different feature detectors send their axons directly or by means of interneurons to hippocampal neurons, and each hippocampal neuron then forms a representation on a portion of its membrane of the parts of the receptive surfaces due to each feature detector. Thus formation of the selective filter in the hippocampal neuron is due to some modifications either in the feature detector itself, or between the feature detector and the hippocampal neuron, or in the hippocampal neuron itself.

Observations have shown that cortical neurons are very stable; even during six hours of continuous stimulation practically no habituation is found. Thus the filters

must be located in either the interneurons or the hippocampal neurons (Sokolov, 1969).

The next question is, what is the mechanism of this selective habituation or selective depression of particular inputs? Our attempts to record intracellularly from hippocampal neurons over a long period of time have not been successful. This is why we have moved to a study of giant neurons of molluscs, where, as was shown by Humphrey (1933), selective habituation at the behavioral level is very prominent. There are two different types of habituation shown by molluscan neurons. The first—presynaptic depression of the release of transmitter—is known mainly from the studies of Bruner and Tauc (1966) and Kandel and Spencer (1968). The other type of habituation, which is not so well known, is related to a specific potential recorded in giant cells of molluscan neurons—the pacemaker potential (Pakula and Sokolov, 1973).

The pacemaker potential can be recorded in neurons that are completely isolated mechanically. This intrinsic mechanism is not modulated through a change in the resistance of the membrane. It is mainly dependent upon the electrogenic effects of active ionic transport and is due to the neuron's use of its internal energy. If this oscillation reaches the threshold, the spike is triggered. The most interesting feature of the pacemaker potential in our context is a very high sensitivity to applied current (Figure 32.1). The change produced by such a current is principally nonlinear; that is, the current changes the frequency rather than the amplitude of the pacemaker potential. If, however, internal current is applied several times to the cell body, we can observe a decrease in the amplitude of the pacemaker-potential response (Figure

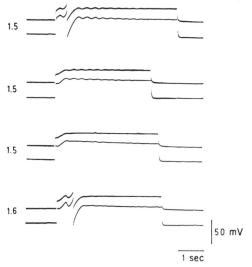

FIGURE 32.2 Modification of the pacemaker response due to repeated intracellular presentation of depolarizing current (in nanoamperes) and reestablishment of the response due to the increase of intensity. (Cf. Figure 32.1.)

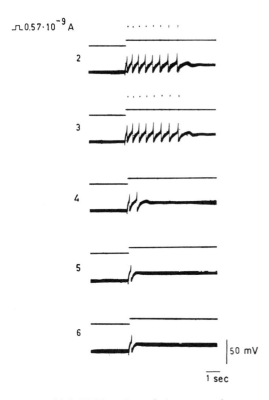

$\text{JL } 0.57 \cdot 10^{-9} \text{ A}$

50 mV

1 sec

FIGURE 32.3 Habituation of the pacemaker response of the latent pacemaker neuron of *Helix pomatia* under repeated (6) presentations of the stimulus. The level of depolarization is not changed under repeated stimulus presentation; however, the influence on the pacemaker potential is reduced. Current intensity, 0.33 na. Stimulus duration, 7 sec. Intervals, 10 sec. Recordings were made from the stimulating electrode through the bridge circuit.

32.2). This habituation is not dependent upon the level of depolarization induced by direct application of the current, which is stable (Figures 32.3–32.5). The resting membrane potential and the resistance of the membrane are also stable. The process of habituation is directly related to the locus of the pacemaker potential, manifesting itself in a reduction in the number of spikes (Figure 32.6).

At first glance, the pacemaker potential does not seem directly related to behavioral effects. We have found, however, that the depolarization produced by synaptic input to a neuron can trigger the pacemaker potential in much the same way as can the application of current through an intracellular microelectrode. Thus synaptic events can modulate the pacemaker potential. The neuron is in this case a regulated generator, and habituation takes place only in the link between the stable post-synaptic potential and the plastic pacemaker mechanism. Moreover, local application of acetylcholine (ACh) on the membrane of the giant neuron has shown us that even when no desensitization of the membrane is present and

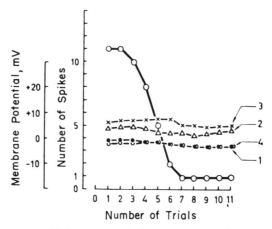

FIGURE 32.4 Number of spikes per stimulus (larger circles) and membrane potentials (numbered curves) as a function of successive injections of depolarizing current. Measures of membrane potential were taken (1) just before each stimulus, (2) early during the stimulus, (3) late during the stimulus, and (4) just after the stimulus.

the shape of the membrane potential produced by ACh is stable, we can still observe a diminution in the number of spikes generated by the neuron. This habituation, which differs from desensitization, is dependent upon the decrease in pacemaker-potential response to the current induced by the change in membrane resistance that follows application of ACh (Figures 32.7–32.10).

$\text{JL } 0.33 \cdot 10^{-9} \text{ A}$

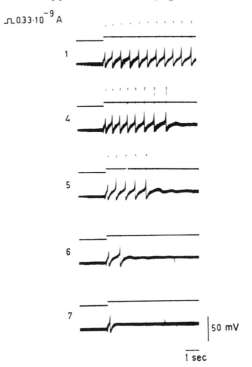

50 mV

1 sec

FIGURE 32.5 Habituation of the pacemaker response under repeated presentation of the stimulus (Series II). The interval between series I and II was 10 min. Current intensity, 0.57 na. (Cf. Figure 32.3.)

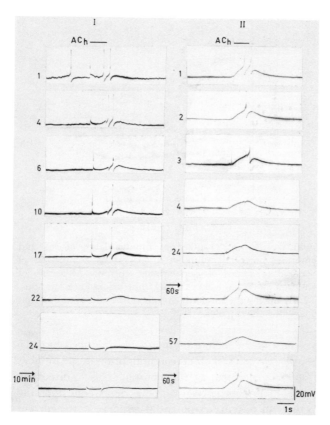

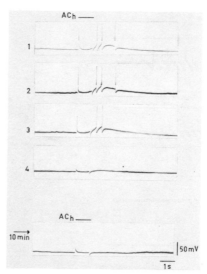

FIGURE 32.7 Initial habituation and subsequent desensitization of the membrane to ACh application. Each of the first three presentations of ACh results in diminution of the number of pacemaker spikes without a marked change in the depolarizing wave. Desensitization occurs on presentations 4–10. The response is not recovered even after 10 min of rest.

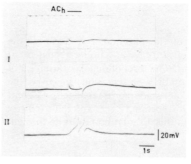

FIGURE 32.8 Selective membrane modification. After desensitization in one locus (I), the increase of the ACh application from 110 to 270 na in the same locus results in no marked effect, as shown in the top and middle records. The locus 50 μ away (II) responds to 110-na ACh application with depolarizing wave and pacemaker spikes. (Cf. Figure 32.6.)

FIGURE 32.6 Desensitization (I) and habituation (II) of the pacemaker potential evoked in two different loci at the membrane of the neuron in the *Helix pomatia*. Stimulus duration, 1 sec. Intervals, 10 sec. Current of ACh application, 100 na. In the case of desensitization, the amplitude of the depolarizing wave is reduced, and response is not recovered even after 10-min rest. In the case of habituation, the depolarizing wave is stable; however, the pacemaker oscillations are habituated. The response is recovered after 60 sec. On the left in each row is the number of the stimulus presentation.

This habituation was found to be selective in respect to the locus of ACh application on the membrane. A further experiment was designed to study the extent to which the pacemaker potential can participate in the behavioral act. We have studied muscle responses from the animal and the number of synaptic and pacemaker spikes that are generated by the neurons directly involved in the reflex arc. It turns out that the pacemaker potential acts as a powerful amplifier, prolonging the response and intensifying the muscle activities. The habituation of the motor response corresponds to the decrease of pacemaker action potentials contributing to the behavioral response.

The selective habituation of the pacemaker in respect to the locus of ACh application on the membrane seems to depend upon selective modification of membrane loci. A similar effect is suggested when different feature detec-

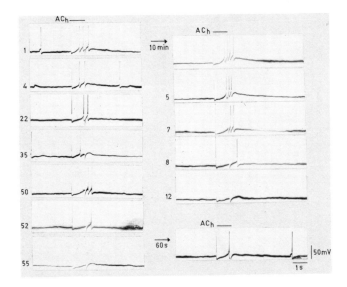

FIGURE 32.9 Habituation of the pacemaker response to ACh without depolarizing-wave modification. *Left* (1–55): Series I of applications. *Right* (1–12): Series II of applications. The reduction of pacemaker spikes is due to the habituation in the pacemaker mechanism. Complete recovery after 10 min. Partial recovery after 60 sec. (Cf. Figure 32.6.)

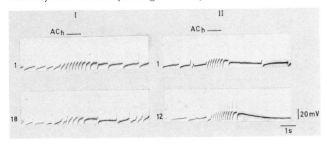

FIGURE 32.10 Habituation (I) and facilitation (II) of the pacemaker potentials under repeated presentations of ACh in two different loci of the same cell. (Cf. Figure 32.6.)

tors converge on single hippocampal neurons characterized by selective habituation.

Habituation thus occurs through the elaboration of a set of neural filters, a process that establishes a neural model of the stimulus. This model consists of a set of modified membrane loci selectively blocking signals coming from repeatedly stimulated feature detectors.

REFERENCES

BRUNER, J., and TAUC, L. 1966. Habituation at the synaptic level in *Aplysia. Nature* 210: 37–39.

HUMPHREY, G. 1933. *The Nature of Learning in Its Relation to Living Systems.* New York: Harcourt, Brace and Company.

KANDEL, E. R., and SPENCER, W. A. 1968. Cellular neurophysiological approaches in the study of learning. *Physiological Review* 48: 65–134.

PAKULA, A., and SOKOLOV, E. 1973. Habituation in gastropoda: Behavioral, interneuronal, and endoneuronal aspects. In H. V. Peeke and M. J. Herz, eds., *Habituation.* Vol. 2: *Electrophysiological Substrates.* New York: Academic Press.

PAVLOV, I. P. 1927. *Conditioned Reflexes.* Oxford: Clarendon Press.

SOKOLOV, YE. N. 1963. *Perception and the Conditioned Reflexes.* New York: Macmillan.

SOKOLOV, YE. N. 1969. *Mekhanismy pamjati.* Moscow: Isdatelstvo Moskouskogo Universiteta.

CNS Manipulation in the
Study of Memory: Drugs

33

Drug Influences on Learning and Memory

JAMES F. FLOOD AND MURRAY E. JARVIK

ABSTRACT Recent psychopharmacological research on memory formation is reviewed. Research on short-term memory indicates that drugs or treatments that modify membrane conductance cause a more rapid onset of amnesia, with a shorter temporal gradient, than do drugs that inhibit protein synthesis. This is interpreted to mean that short-term memory depends on membrane conductance and electrical changes that last for only a short time after training, whereas protein synthesis is important for the formation of long-term memories. A reversible inhibitor of RNA synthesis has been reported to block memory formation in goldfish, and administration of uridine monophosphate directly into the brain has been shown to slow extinction of a learned response. Parameters of training and of the inhibition of protein synthesis have been found to influence the amnesic effect obtained in passive- and active-avoidance situations. Catecholamines have been found to influence both memory formation and retrieval. High catecholamine levels after training or prior to a retention test can relieve amnesia. Low norepinephrine levels have been found to block recall of passive avoidance and appetitive training. ACTH peptide fragments not having hormonal effects have been found to relieve the amnesia caused by CO_2 and electroconvulsive shock. The target areas for these peptide fragments are closely related to the reticular formation and its projections. This raises the question of whether the peptide is a stimulant that improves recall of poorly remembered training. d-Amphetamine has been found to restore memory to amnesic subjects if at least some evidence of a weak memory is present. The drug had the same effect on subjects made amnesic with drugs as on saline controls that had simply forgotten. Problems of analysis and interpretation involved in determining the inhibition level of RNA synthesis, the permanence of amnesia, and drug and hormonal modifications of memory-retrieval, as distinct from memory-formation, processes, are discussed.

33.1 INTRODUCTION

Even though it has been observed that learning and memory are psychological functions that are relatively resistant to drug effects (Jarvik, 1972), there are circumstances in which it can be demonstrated that drugs can influence the registration, retention, or retrieval of memory traces. There are several reasons why the use of drugs should be considered as a means of clarifying the role of neural mechanisms in learning and memory:

1. Today neuroanatomists and neurophysiologists recognize that the brain is a complex chemical factory and that even the chemical bricks constituting its structure are in a continual state of flux. Drugs can be considered chemical tools for evaluating the nature of this flux. They provide a convenient and necessary supplement to the techniques of the histologist and the electrophysiologist because they can be used in the intact, performing animal and they usually do not require surgical invasion or sacrifice of the animal.

2. Drugs are frequently reversible in their actions. This permits repeated use of the same subject; and the use of human subjects becomes feasible if confidence in the reversibility can be established.

3. Drugs are usually inexpensive, and it ordinarily does not take special skill to administer them by the usual oral or parenteral routes.

4. Finally, there is intense interest in the practical application of drugs for therapeutic purposes and even for recreational use. Thus it is important to assay the possibility that drugs might be employed to facilitate learning and memory and, conversely, to become cognizant of the ways in which drugs might impair learning and memory.

The present review will concentrate on a few classes of drugs that have been the subject of the greatest interest in psychopharmacological studies of learning and memory in recent years. There has been a growing literature on macromolecules and memory, with interest, naturally enough, centering upon proteins and nucleic acids. Implicit in many of these studies is the idea that the structure of the nervous system changes as a result of experience and that the change is manifested in the synthesis of these macromolecules.

The other group of endogenous substances that has concerned researchers in the field of memory psychobiology consists of those chemicals whose function is to transmit information from one part of the body to another. Thus the hormones, which carry messages over long distances in the body via the bloodstream, have been shown to be involved in learning. Similarly, neurotransmitters, which carry messages over short distances without using the blood stream, also seem to have something to do with learning and memory. We are not going to be able to consider other classes of drugs except in passing, but these have been covered in other reviews

JAMES F. FLOOD and MURRAY E. JARVIK, Department of Psychiatry, University of California, Los Angeles

(Thompson, Patterson, and Teyler, 1972; Deutsch, 1969; McGaugh, 1973).

33.1 The physiological basis of short-term memory

That a short-term memory exists has been inferred from experiments showing that memory may be present for a few hours after a subject has received an amnestic treatment (e.g., electroconvulsive shock, amygdaloid stimulation, RNA-synthesis inhibition, protein-synthesis inhibition, CO_2, or anesthesia). Whether the nature of this short-term memory is electrophysiological or biochemical is the question that the studies included in this section are trying to answer.

Watts and Mark (1971) compared the effects of ouabain and cycloheximide on forgetting starting immediately after a single-trial, passive-avoidance task for chickens (Cherkin and Lee-Teng, 1965), In this task a shiny object is presented to the chicken. The object is coated with methylanthranilate "which is particularly distasteful to chickens . . . as they characteristically shook their heads vigorously" (Watts and Mark, 1971). The retention test consisted of presenting the shiny object again and seeing if the chicken would peck at it. Saline, ouabain, or cycloheximide was administered 5 min prior to training; retention tests were given 10, 30, 60, or 90 min after training. The saline-injected chickens showed little sign of forgetting. The cycloheximide-injected chicks showed a slow rate of forgetting, and at the end of 90 min only 50 percent pecked at the object. But chickens given ouabain showed a rapid loss of retention that was essentially complete within 60 min of training with the highest dose used (0.55 mg/chicken) (Figure 33.1).

The effective doses of ouabain, a digitalislike drug that has been used clinically to treat heart failure, did not cause drowsiness, EEG changes, or convulsions. According to Watts and Mark, ouabain at the doses used inhibited the Na^+/K^+ adenosine triphosphatase in the nerve membranes, on which the sodium pump is dependent. It is known to abolish the afterpotential sequence generated by the Na^+ pump activity in some neurons after repeated discharge, and it also blocks posttetanic potentiation. At higher doses than those used in this report, ouabain depolarizes and eventually blocks action potentials.

Watts and Mark suggest that the faster and more complete forgetting caused by ouabain indicates that short-term memory is dependent on electrophysiological events such as posttetanic potentiation. The persistence of memory during the inhibition of protein synthesis caused by cycloheximide is interpreted by these authors as meaning that the early phases of memory formation

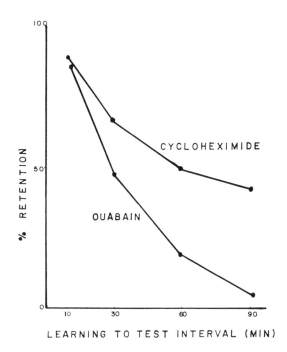

FIGURE 33.1 The effect of a pretraining injection of ouabain or cycloheximide on short-term retention for passive-avoidance training. Ouabain caused a more rapid loss of short-term retention than did cycloheximide. Based on material in Watts and Mark (1971).

are not dependent on protein synthesis. Thus "ouabain and cycloheximide . . . interfere with memory in different ways. We suggest that they do so at successive stages and that memory begins with a membrane store of limited time-span involving ionic metabolism and this is soon supplemented by a process dependent on synthesis of proteins which perhaps alter synaptic properties" (Watts and Mark, 1971).

In a previous study (Watts and Mark, 1970) it was reported that ouabain and lithium given shortly before passive-avoidance training produced retention deficits 24 or 72 hr later, but a 10-min posttraining injection was not effective. Cycloheximide produced a retention deficit when administered prior to or 10 min after training, but not when given 30 min after training. It was concluded—and the two reports support the idea—that membrane mechanisms are required for the initiation of long-term memory but not for the consolidation process that occurs later.

Another investigation comparing the electrophysiological and biochemical time course of memory formation employed electroconvulsive shock (ECS) and cycloheximide (Andry and Luttges, 1972). Mice trained on a one-trial, step-through, passive-avoidance task were given cycloheximide or saline 30 min prior to training and ECS or sham ECS 0, 30, 60, or 180 min after

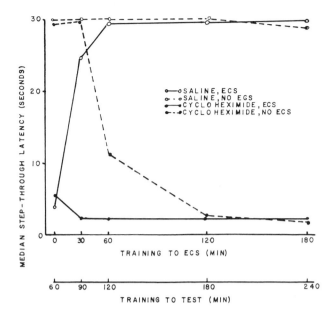

FIGURE 33.2 Effect of ECS and cycloheximide on retention for passive-avoidance training. The combination of ECS given immediately after training and cycloheximide given shortly prior to training caused the most immediate loss of retention when compared to the effect of cycloheximide or ECS given alone. From Andry and Luttges (1972). Copyright 1972 by the American Association for the Advancement of Science.

training. The retention test was given 60 min after ECS or sham-ECS treatment. The results were as follows (Figure 33.2): (1) saline + ECS caused amnesia only if ECS was given immediately after training. (2) Cycloheximide + no ECS resulted in amnesia when subjects were tested 60 min or more after training. (3) The cycloheximide + ECS group was found to be amnesic at all times tested. An interaction between cycloheximide and ECS is apparent when ECS is given 30 or 60 min after training; that is, the amnesia was greater than when either ECS or cycloheximide were given alone. (4) The saline + no ECS group had uniformly good retention.

To control for possible effects of ECS and cycloheximide on the retrieval rather than the formation of memories, mice were subjected to the four treatments 24 hours after training, with the retention test again following 60 min after ECS or sham ECS. None of the groups treated 24 hr after training showed memory disruption. Thus the memory deficits observed were not due to effects of ECS or cycloheximide on retrieval.

Andry and Luttges interpreted their findings as supporting the dual-trace hypothesis of memory formation, in that (1) the cycloheximide + ECS group was found to be amnesic immediately after training because ECS blocked the cycloheximide-resistant short-term memory,

and (2) since protein-synthesis-dependent long-term memory was impaired by cycloheximide, ECS effects could be demonstrated to occur with treatments given at longer times after training than would otherwise be expected.

33.2 NEW WORK ON THE ROLE OF RNA AND PROTEIN SYNTHESIS IN MEMORY FORMATION

33.2.1 Inhibition of RNA synthesis

In the past it has not been possible to test the role of RNA synthesis in memory formation critically using inhibitors of RNA synthesis because of their toxic side effects. Actinomycin-D has been tested behaviorally and found to make mice very ill about 4 to 6 hr after it is injected intracerebrally; the dose used caused a high percentage inhibition of precursor uptake (thought to reflect an inhibition of RNA synthesis), but it also proved to be lethal. Barondes and Jarvik (1964) reported that actinomycin-D did not affect retention for a passive-avoidance task measured 4 hr after training. A failure to find amnesia at this time could mean that short-term memory is not dependent on RNA synthesis. It does not rule out the possibility that long-term memory is dependent on RNA synthesis. Agranoff, Davis, and Brink (1966) administered actinomycin-D intracerebrally to goldfish

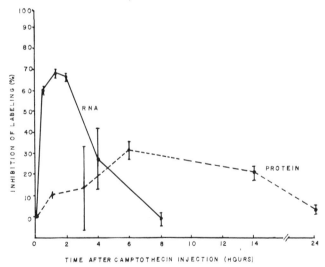

FIGURE 33.3 Effect of camptothecin on RNA and protein synthesis. A 50 μg dose of camptothecin given to goldfish inhibited the uptake of labeled uridine into RNA shortly after injection. Inhibition reached a peak of 75%, followed by recovery within 4 hr of administration. A significant inhibition of protein synthesis followed the inhibition of RNA synthesis; however, from previous work, this level of inhibition seems too low to be the main cause of the reported amnesia. From Neale, Klinger, and Agranoff (1973). Copyright 1973 by the American Association for the Advancement of Science.

immediately or 3 hr after shuttlebox training. Retention tested 4 days later was disrupted by the immediate posttraining injection of actinomycin-D but not by the injection given 3 hr after training. However, the drug proved to be lethal by the eleventh day.

Neale, Klinger, and Agranoff (1973) used camptothecin, a plant alkaloid, to block RNA synthesis in goldfish. This inhibitor, injected intracerebrally, caused reversible inhibition of RNA synthesis (Figure 33.3), and unlike actinomycin-D, it could be used at doses that were not lethal. RNA synthesis, measured by the incorporation of labeled uridine, was rapidly inhibited, and the effect lasted about 2 hr at between 65 and 70 percent inhibition. An inhibition of protein synthesis followed about 4 hr after the peak of inhibition of RNA synthesis but only reached 30 percent. Recovery of RNA synthesis occurred between 2 and 4 hr after the administration of camptothecin and seemed to be complete within 8 hr.

In a behavioral test of effects of camptothecin, fish were trained in a shuttlebox to avoid shock. Either 0, 1.5, 5, or 24 hr after the training session, camptothecin was administered at different doses intracerebrally. Retention was tested on the eighth day. The results showed that if camptothecin was administered immediately after training, about a 50 percent loss of expected retention occurred. This effect was nearly dose-independent within the range of 10 to 50 μg (Figure 33.4). The authors reported that administering the inhibitor 1.5 hr after training had an effect; however, it is clear that this group differed only slightly from the controls. Camptothecin had no effect on retention when given 5 or 24 hr after training. Thus it did not produce brain damage or any other long-lasting effect sufficient to account for the retention deficit observed in those fish receiving the drug immediately after training.

Kobiler and Allweis (1974) reported that 2, 6-diaminopurine (DAP) inhibited the uptake of labeled uridine into RNA by 75 percent. The speed and duration of inhibition of uridine incorporation were influenced by the dose of DAP (60 or 120 μg/rat). The peak of inhibition was not influenced. Rats were given intracisternal injections of DAP dissolved in sodium bicarbonate or just sodium-bicarbonate solution (control group) 90 min prior to training. DAP had no detectable effect on the acquisition of a training task consisting of one-way active avoidance of footshock. It was found that retention was poor for long-term memory (tested 5 hr to 4 days after training) but did not affect short-term memory (tested 1–4 hr after training). The degree of training influenced amnesia: the amnestic treatment was less effective with a high training criterion (10/10 correct responses) than with a low criterion (5/5).

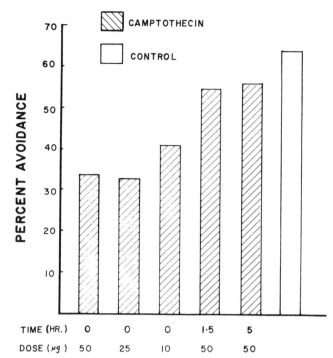

FIGURE 33.4 Effect of camptothecin on retention for shuttlebox training in goldfish. The time listings are times after training at which camptothecin was administered. The major effect on retention is seen when camptothecin is injected immediately after training. Based on data from Neale, Klinger, and Agranoff (1973).

The duration of inhibition also influenced amnesia: a longer duration of inhibition (9 hr) had a greater amnesic effect than a shorter duration (4 hr). In the last experiment in the series adenosine was administered intracisternally 30 min to 3 hr after training to rats that had been given DAP prior to training. Under these conditions the adenosine, which rapidly reverses the inhibition of RNA synthesis by DAP, prevented amnesia. Amnesia was not prevented when adenosine was given more than 3 hr after training. These results show a time-dependent process at work and show that DAP did not interfere with acquisition sufficiently to account for the amnesia.

Reiniš (1971) has also reported that intracerebral injections of DAP impaired retention for step-through, passive-avoidance training in mice. Injections given 48 hr prior to training and 2 or 24 hr after training were not effective in disrupting retention. When DAP was administered 24 hr prior to or 1 hr after training, it did interfere with retention; however, the deficit in retention was not present at 24 hr after training, but reached significance only 3 days or 1 week after training and drug treatment. This delayed onset of amnesia was also reported to be characteristic of other mutagenic antimetabolites tested: 5-iodouracil, 6-mercaptopurine, 6-

thioguanine, and 5-bromouracil. Reiniš suggested that the effectiveness of the injection of DAP 24 hr prior to training may be accounted for by the fact that DAP is rather insoluble at the body's pH, and therefore the DAP may have remained around for some time. This suggestion does not agree with the inhibition data of Kobiler and Allweis (1974), who reported recovery from DAP-induced RNA-synthesis inhibition in about 9–10 hr. Between the reports a major question seems in need of answering: Does DAP interfere with retention by inhibition of RNA synthesis or by its mutagenic action, or both?

33.2.2 Effect of RNA precursors on memory formation

Interest in the relationship between RNA precursors and memory was probably stimulated by early reports indicating that RNA rations fed to aged human volunteers improved mental functioning, increased alertness, reduced psychogenic confusion, and improved memory (Cameron and Solyom, 1961). In the animal literature, Cook et al. (1963) reported that injections of yeast RNA facilitated performance by rats on a conditioned avoidance task.

Additional new evidence for the role of RNA synthesis in the formation of memory has been furnished by Ott and Matthies (1973a,b), who administered uridine monophosphate (UMP) to rats. The rats were implanted with cannulas aimed at the dorsal hippocampus. They were then trained on a Y-shaped shuttlebox to escape footshock by making a light-dark discrimination until they made ten successive correct responses; this took from 30 to 45 min. In this task the rat starts in one of the three alleys and must move to the one alley of the remaining two that is dark. On succeeding trials the previously correct alley becomes the new starting point, and the rat must again discriminate between the other two alleys. The rats received a 1.0-μl injection containing 40μg of UMP 30 min prior to training or 1 or 60 min after training. Three control groups were included: one was sham-operated, one vehicle-injected, and one received UMP into the frontal cortex. (This last group was included in order to see if any effect was specific to the dorsal hippocampus.) The results were determined on the basis of five daily extinction sessions of 31 trials each, beginning 24 hr after the end of training. The assumption behind this use of the extinction test is that rats with better "memory formation" will be more resistant to extinction. The results showed that when UMP was injected 30 min prior to training or 1 min after training, extinction was delayed (Figure 33.5 A, B). Amazingly, rats receiving injections of UMP 30 min before training showed no significant tendency to ex-

tinguish over the five extinction days (Figure 33.5A). When UMP was administered 60 min after training, the effect on extinction was significant only over the first and second extinction sessions (Figure 33.5C). Injecting UMP into the frontal cortex did not alter extinction relative to the sham-operated or vehicle-injected rats.

Since extinction can be viewed as a form of learning, it might be argued that the UMP damages the hippocampus in such a way that learning not to respond is difficult. If this were true, however, the injection given 60 min after training should also have delayed extinction: it did not. This work has at least one important advantage over previous RNA-precursor studies: since the drug was injected directly into the brain, rather than intraperitoneally (IP), and autoradiographs were taken, we can at least be sure that the RNA precursor reached the desired area of the brain. Previously those who have tried to test RNA-extract and RNA-precursor effects on learning and memory have used the IP route of administration, which left considerable doubt as to whether the material injected actually crossed the blood-brain barrier sufficiently intact to carry information about memory storage. In Ott and Matthies's study no biochemical measures of RNA or protein synthesis were obtained; thus we cannot be sure that the UMP entered the nerve cells and, if it did enter, that it actually stimulated RNA synthesis, and thereby protein synthesis, as suggested by the authors. It will be important for the interpretation of this work to determine whether the administration of RNA precursors can increase the rate of RNA synthesis.

In a follow-up of this study Ott and Matthies (1973b) showed that rats trained in a one-way, active-avoidance task and given 100 μg of UMP (probably after training) required fewer footshocks to reach a performance criterion when retrained 24 hr later. However, when UMP and cycloheximide were administered together, the retention scores (number of shocks to regain criterion) did not significantly differ from those of controls (Figure 33.6): cycloheximide blocked the beneficial effect of UMP on retention performance. The authors concluded that "it is reasonable to suppose that pharmacologically induced improvement in long-term storage is accompanied by increased protein synthesis in the CNS." They suggested that the increased UMP supply facilitated the protein synthesis via an accelerated RNA synthesis.

33.2.3 Effects of protein-synthesis inhibition on memory formation

A considerable literature has been reviewed on the effect of protein-synthesis inhibition on memory formation (Rahwan, 1971; Spear, 1973; Roberts and Flexner, 1969; Squire and Barondes, 1972). If one assumes that

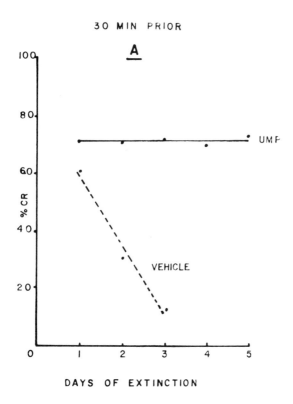

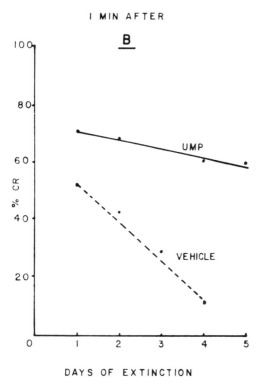

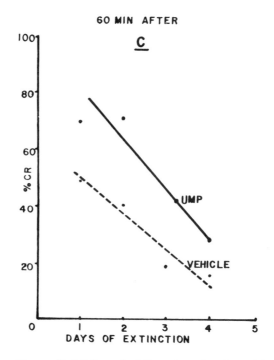

FIGURE 33.5 Effect of uridine monophosphate (UMP) on the rate of extinction following active-avoidance training on footshock. UMP significantly delayed extinction when given 30 min prior to training (A) or 1 min after training (B), but not when administered 60 min after training (C). From Ott and Matthies (1973a). Reproduced with the permission of Springer-Verlag.

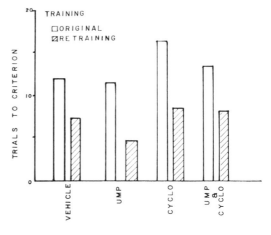

FIGURE 33.6 The effect of UMP and cycloheximide on retention for one-way active-avoidance training. UMP-injected rats reached criterion in fewer trials when retrained than rats given either saline or cycloheximide and UMP at the same time. Presumably UMP enhances retention by causing greater protein synthesis, but when cycloheximide and UMP are given at the same time, cycloheximide blocks the synthesis of protein, so that UMP has no effect. Based on data from Ott and Matthies (1973b).

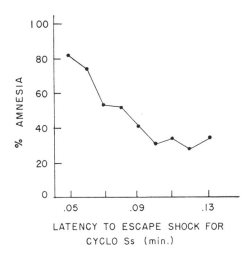

FIGURE 33.7 Effect of variation in escape latency on retention of training in cycloheximide-injected mice. As the escape latency increased, the probability of amnesia decreased significantly ($\chi^2 = 8.89$, $p < 0.005$ for 0.06 min vs. 0.13 min). However, even at 0.13 min cycloheximide-injected mice differ significantly from controls ($p = 0.01$). From Flood et al. (1972). Reproduced with the permission of Pergamon Press.

inhibition of protein synthesis is the cause of amnesia, rather than a side effect of the drugs, then one can conclude that protein-synthesis inhibition can disrupt memory formation in mice, rats, birds, and goldfish. In most cases the inhibitor is administered prior to training, but in a few cases impaired retention has been reported with posttraining injections (Geller et al., 1969; Agranoff, 1972; Barondes and Cohen, 1968). A common observation is that too much training will block the amnesic effect of protein-synthesis inhibition (Barondes, 1970).

We shall consider here only some of the most recent findings on the role of protein synthesis and memory

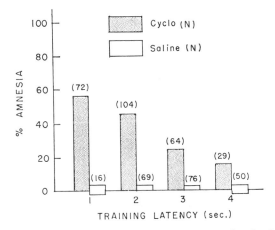

FIGURE 33.8 Effect of the latency to enter the shock compartment on the training day for saline- and cycloheximide-injected mice. As the latency to enter increased from 1 to 4 sec, the probability of amnesia decreased for cycloheximide-injected mice. From Flood et al. (1972). Reproduced with the permission of Pergamon Press.

formation. In an effort to determine if overtraining totally blocks the amnesic effect of protein-synthesis inhibition by cycloheximide, as reported by Barondes (1970), Flood et al. (1972) undertook an investigation into the parameters of passive-avoidance training and testing that influence cycloheximide-induced amnesia. Mice were trained on a one-trial, step-through, passive-avoidance task 15 min after receiving a single injection of cycloheximide or saline. The latencies to enter and escape from the shock compartment were recorded.

By classifying the mice according to the combination of latencies obtained during training, it was possible to show that the degree of amnesia was directly related to the degree of training. Training strength was varied by altering the shock intensity or by considering different combinations of latencies to enter and escape from the shock compartment. Amnesia was defined as any latency under 20 sec to reenter the shock compartment on the test day (this was the range of naive subjects' latencies to enter the shock compartment).

The percentage of amnesic mice decreased as the shock intensity increased. Shock duration also had a significant effect on amnesia: the longer the escape latency on the

TABLE 33.1
Distribution of retention test latencies

Test latency	Cyclo		Saline	
(sec)	N	%	N	%
0–20	104	47.3	4	1.8
21–40	10	4.5	3	1.4
41–60	6	2.7	1	0.5
61–80	7	3.2	0	
81–100	5	2.3	2	0.9
101–120	5	2.3	3	1.4
121–140	3	1.4	2	0.9
141–160	5	2.3	2	0.9
161–180	7	4.2	2	0.9
181–200	1	0.5	5	2.3
201–220	0		1	0.5
221–240	1	0.5	2	0.9
241–260	2	0.9	0	
261–280	0		3	1.4
281–300 +	64	29.1	189	85.9
	220		219	

Test latencies of 0–20 sec are the range of scores representing amnesia. Cyclo caused significantly more cases of amnesia than did saline ($\chi^2 = 122.2$, df = 1, $p < 0.001$). If latencies of 21–200 sec are taken to show impaired memory, 22% of the Cyclo subjects compared to 9% of the control subjects showed impaired memory ($\chi^2 = 14.3$, df = 1, $p < 0.001$).
Source: Flood et al. (1972). Reprinted with the permission of Pergamon Press.

training day, the lower the percentage of amnesic mice (Figure 33.7). The latency to enter on the training day also affected the percentage of amnesics: the longer the latency to enter, the lower the percentage of amnesics (Figure 33.8).

A distribution of all test latencies (Table 33.1) showed that cycloheximide-injected mice tended either to forget (47 percent) or to obtain close to the maximum score of 300 sec (29 percent). In all, few saline-injected mice showed amnesia—only 4 out of 219 had retention latencies of 20 sec or less. In this experiment the subjects were overtrained; thus it was not possible to see whether the distribution was peculiar to the drug-treated mice or whether less well trained controls would have shown a similar distribution. In a later study Flood et al. (1974) showed that under lower training strength, saline-injected mice show a distribution of retention scores similar to that of cycloheximide-injected mice.

The retention interval was also manipulated: mice were tested 24 hr or 1, 2, or 3 weeks after training. The test scores showed that the percentage of amnesic mice tended to increase over the three-week retention period (Figure 33.9).

Several important observations were made by the authors:

1. Highly consistent amnesic effects can be obtained with pretraining injections of cycloheximide if the parameters affecting acquisition are measured and controlled.

2. The measurement of these parameters is important, since cycloheximide-injected mice tend to enter the shock compartment faster than saline controls and also tend to have longer escape latencies. Since the latencies to enter and to escape from the shock compartment affect learning of the passive-avoidance task (Flood et al., 1972, 1974), in the absence of controls misleading conclusions might be drawn concerning the magnitude of the cycloheximide-induced amnesia.

3. "Overtraining" can be rigorously defined here as that level of training for which control subjects' retention is on the asymptote to the acquisition-retention curve.

Acetoxycycloheximide is generally not available today, but recently Ungerer (1973) trained mice on a lever-press task for food reward. Acetoxycycloheximide was administered 3, 30, 60, or 180 min after a single training session. Training consisted of learning that a lever press would deliver food reward only within a 5-sec signaled period. The measures of retention were the number of reinforcements and the total amount of time before receiving the first reinforcement. Retention was tested 6 days after training. When acetoxycycloheximide was administered within 3 min after training, it caused a deficit in responding at the retention test: these mice received fewer total reinforcements, pressed more times before receiving their first reinforcement, and took longer to make their first successful conditioned response. The other injections given at 30, 60, or 180 min after training produced slight or no effect (Figure 33.10).

In appetitive tasks one must be wary of "bait shyness" (Garcia et al., 1972). Since many protein-inhibiting drugs cause some illness, the apparent amnesia may in fact be conditioned aversion due to the negative reinforcement of illness. However, since Ungerer's group that

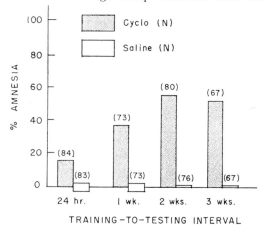

FIGURE 33.9 The influence of the duration of the retention period on the percent amnesia. As the retention period increased, the cycloheximide-injected subjects showed an increased percent amnesia up to 2 weeks; saline-injected mice showed no significant loss in retention over the same time period. From Flood et al. (1972). Reproduced with the permission of Pergamon Press.

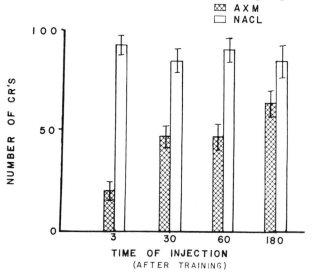

FIGURE 33.10 Effect of acetoxycycloheximide (AXM) on retention for a food-rewarded lever-pressing task in mice. AXM significantly impaired retention when administered 3 min after training but not when administered 30, 60, or 180 min after training. From Ungerer (1973). Reproduced with the permission of Pergamon Press.

received an injection 30 min after training did not show impaired performance on the retention test, it seems unlikely that bait shyness can explain these results.

Gervai and Csányi (1973) reported that cycloheximide did not prevent imprinting in chickens, but did prevent approach conditioning. With respect to imprinting, the maximal interval at which retention was tested was only 3 hr. It has been previously reported that cycloheximide-induced amnesia does not begin to occur until 3–6 hr after training (Barondes and Cohen, 1968; Cohen and Barondes, 1968; Agranoff, 1972; Davis and Klinger, 1969). Flood et al. (1972) showed that, depending on the degree of training, the full extent of anmesia may not appear for 2 or 3 weeks after training and treatment. Thus the results of Gervai and Csányi may show only that short-term memory is not dependent on protein synthesis. Longer retention intervals will have to be employed before one can evaluate the importance of protein synthesis for memory in imprinting.

Squire and Barondes (1973) and Squire, Smith, and Barondes (1973) reported that cycloheximide caused an impairment in learning within 3 to 4 min after the beginning of training (trials 15–21). This impairment was interpreted by the authors to mean that part of short-term memory is protein-synthesis-dependent. Mice were trained to escape shock on an automated task involving the discrimination between a small rod and a large rod. The intertrial interval was about 15 sec. In the first report it was shown that cycloheximide-injected mice learned as rapidly as saline-injected subjects through trials 15–21. Thereafter the cycloheximide-injected mice made about 25 percent fewer correct choices. However, the acquisition curves were parallel, indicating that cycloheximide-injected mice were still learning. The results could thus be explained by assuming that, with time, the cycloheximide was making the subjects ill and less attentive to the learning task. An isocycloheximide group was used to control for possible behavioral depression caused by cycloheximide, and the authors reported that saline- and isocycloheximide-injected mice showed no decrease in the rate of acquisition. However, isocycloheximide does not inhibit protein synthesis and therefore is not likely to make the subjects ill.

To address the question of illness versus inhibition of protein synthesis more directly, Squire, Smith, and Barondes (1973) adminstered cycloheximide subcutaneously either 10, 30, or 210 min prior to training on the small-rod-versus-large-rod discrimination task. Inhibition of protein synthesis reached 80 percent or more within 2–5 min of injection. If illness due to the duration of high levels of inhibition of protein synthesis were responsible for the observed decrement in acquisition,

then impairment should be noticed immediately in the 210-min group and should appear after fewer training trials in the 30-min group than in the 10-min group. The results showed that in mice receiving cycloheximide either 10 or 30 min prior to training, impairment of acquisition appeared after training trials 15–25 (Figure 33.11). The group receiving cycloheximide 210 min prior to training did not show significant impairment of acquisition. Thus it appears that the impairment is related to profound inhibition of protein synthesis and is not due to illness or changes in motor activity.

The authors concluded that the "expression of normal memory may depend on cerebral protein synthesis within minutes after the beginning of training" (Squire and Barondes, 1973), and "that a memory storage process dependent on protein synthesis may be required for improvement within minutes after the onset of training" (Squire, Smith, and Barondes, 1973).

Andry and Luttges (1973) also reported that pre-training injections of cycloheximide impaired acquisition for long-term training (50 training trials in a single session) on a wheel-turning task to avoid footshock. However, it was noted that cycloheximide and saline controls performed equally well on the retention test. If we believe that the cycloheximide-injected mice actually learn less on original training, then we must conclude also that cycloheximide improves retention, since the percent difference in percent avoidances was greater for the cycloheximide-injected mice than for the saline-injected mice. Clearly, a dissociation has occurred between learning and performance.

This report by Andry and Luttges suggests that the effect reported by Squire, Smith, and Barondes (1973) might be interpreted in terms of an impaired ability to manifest learning behaviorally during high levels of protein-synthesis inhibition. The nature of the deficit might be related to a protein-synthesis-dependent short-term memory or to motor, arousal, or motivational systems that are not functioning optimally during high levels of protein-synthesis inhibition.

Randt, Korein, and Levidow (1973) reported abnormal brain electrophysiological activity from the parietal cortex, midbrain reticular formation, and dorsal hippocampus of cycloheximide-injected mice. The onset of this abnormal electrical behavior is such that training tasks involving only a few trials would be completed before the abnormal activity begins to occur. The intervals used to determine the onset of the abnormal activity were not spaced closely enough to permit any clear evaluation of whether cycloheximide impairment performance coincides with the onset of the altered brain electrical activity.

Anisomycin (Ani) is an inhibitor of brain protein

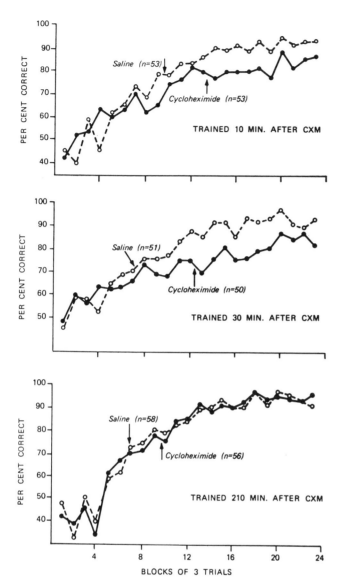

FIGURE 33.11 Effect of cycloheximide or saline on acquisition of an object-discrimination task to escape footshock in mice. Cycloheximide given either 10 min (A) or 30 min (B) prior to training slowed down the rate of acquisition. Cycloheximide given 210 min (C) prior to training did not affect the rate of acquisition. High levels of inhibition of protein synthesis are still present at training in groups injected 10 and 30 min prior to training, but a substantial degree of recovery from inhibition is present at training in the group injected 210 min prior to training. From Squire et al. (1973). Reproduced with the permission of Macmillan Journals Ltd.

synthesis that has recently been introduced in the study of memory formation (Flood et al., 1973). Ani given at a dose of 0.5 mg/mouse rapidly inhibits protein synthesis after subcutaneous administration; the inhibition remains at a level of 80 percent or more for 2 hr. Doses greater than 0.5 mg/mouse did not significantly influence the peak or duration of inhibition; also, no significant strain differences in inhibition occurred (Flood et al., 1973). The duration and time course of this inhibition was similar to that of cycloheximide (Cyclo). The principal advantages that Ani offers over Cyclo are that (1) it is used at a level that is at least twenty times below the 50 percent lethal dose, while Cyclo must be used at very near the lethal dose, and (2) Ani causes significantly less illness and no death. By using successive injections of Ani, the authors were able to prolong the duration of inhibition of protein synthesis. When Ani was administered subcutaneously at 2-hr intervals, inhibition was maintained at 80 percent or more for two additional hours with each injection. It was reported that no deaths or prolonged illnesses occurred as a result of the long periods of inhibition of brain protein synthesis (up to 14 hr of inhibition were used).

Flood et al. studied the effect of Ani on one-trial, step-through, passive-avoidance training in the mouse. A single injection of Ani was given 15 min prior to training, and additional injections were given at 2-hr intervals thereafter. On the basis of the test latency to reenter the shock compartment, subjects were classified as amnesic or not-amnesic. A latency of 20 sec or less was defined as amnesia.

The most important finding was that, training remaining constant (i.e., same shock intensity and range of latencies to enter and escape the shock compartment), the longer the duration of inhibition, the greater the amnesia (Figure 33.12). Since longer periods of inhibition were caused by injections of Ani given several hours after training (e.g., $1\frac{3}{4}$ or $3\frac{3}{4}$ hr after training), the additional injections could not have interfered with acquisition and are not likely to have had proactive effects at the time of the retention test given one or two weeks after training. In some of the experiments a single pretraining injection caused no significant amnesia, while three successive injections caused 95–100 percent amnesia.

The amnesic effect of Ani was also replicated across six genetically distinct strains of mice (Flood et al., 1974). An interesting feature of this study was that each strain was trained on one-trial passive avoidance under those conditions of shock duration and intensity that produced 90–100 percent avoidance in undrugged subjects of that strain. Once the minimal training conditions needed to achieve this level of retention in the

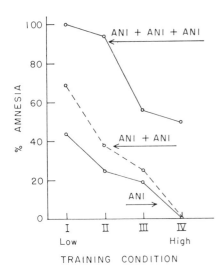

FIGURE 33.12 Effect of the interaction of training strength and duration of inhibition on the percent amnesia in anisomycin-injected mice. At a given training level (e.g., I), as the duration of inhibition increased from 2 to 6 hr (Ani to Ani + Ani + Ani), amnesia increased. For a given duration of inhibition, as the training strength increased, the probability that a subject would be amnesic decreased. From Flood et al. (1973). Reprinted with the permission of Pergamon Press.

control mice were determined, the effect of one or two injections of Ani was tested in each strain. The amnesic effect of Ani was similar in each strain in spite of the fact that actual training values for shock duration and intensity differed considerably (Tables 33.2 and 33.3).

Evidence was also presented that Cyclo may impair acquisition relative to Ani. In an experiment in which two successive injections were given (i.e., Ani + Ani, Ani + Cyclo), no significant difference in the level of amnesia occurred. However, a single cycloheximide injection given prior to training caused a greater percent amnesia than a single pretraining injection of Ani (80 versus 36 percent amnesia). The authors concluded that since the parameters of the inhibition of protein synthesis did not differ significantly between the two drugs, the discrepancy between the effects of pre- and posttraining injections could probably be accounted for by assuming that Cyclo has some subtle effect on acquisition.

Control experiments demonstrated that the multiple-injection procedure itself did not have an effect on retention and that when Ani was injected for the first time $1\frac{3}{4}$ hrs after training as a second injection (saline + Ani), it had no amnesic effect.

After completion of these experiments on passive avoidance, protein-synthesis inhibition by Ani was shown to disrupt memory formation for escape conditioning and for active avoidance (Flood et al., 1975a). The apparatus consisted of a T maze with a brass grid

TABLE 33.2

Amnesic effect of anisomycin across strains of mice

Strain	T.C.	Shock intensity (ma)	% Amnesia Saline	% Amnesia Ani
CB	I	0.18	10	70
C57B1/Jf	I	0.18	0	45 (Ani + Ani 85)
C57B1/6J	I	0.18	10	90
Swiss (CD-1)	I	0.38	10	80
C57Br/cdJ	II	0.23	10	80
BALB/cJ	II	0.28	15	85

Clear amnesic effects were obtained in all strains with a single pretraining injection of Ani. Given similar degrees of learning (as demonstrated by the scores of saline control groups), the amnesic effects are about the same for five strains in spite of large differences in training strengths. The exception is C57B1/Jf strain, in which two injections were required to produce a high level of amnesia. T. C. is the training condition: I is weak training obtained with shock durations of 1–4.4 sec; II is stronger training with shock durations of 4.5–8 sec. Amnesia is defined by a test latency $\leq$ 20 sec. N = 20/strain/injection group. The smallest percentage differences are in the C57B1/Jf strain, and even these are significant: Ani vs. saline, p < 0.001 by Fisher Exact Probability Test.

Source: Flood et al. (1974). Reprinted with the permission of Academic Press, Inc.

TABLE 33.3

Effects of doubling the duration of protein-synthesis inhibition on percentage amnesia

Strain	T.C.	Shock intensity (ma)	% Amnesia saline + saline	Ani+Ani	Ani
CB	I	0.23	0	95	20
C57B1/Jf	I	0.23	0	70	15
C57B1/6J	I	0.23	0	70	30
Swiss (CD-1)	I	0.42	0	80	20
C57Br/cdJ	II	0.28	0	95	30
BALB/cJ	II	0.33	0	95	65

Two injections of Ani clearly had a greater amnesic effect than a single injection. By comparing Table 33.2 with this table, it can be seen that increasing the shock intensity decreased the effectiveness of Ani as an amnestic agent, but giving two successive injections of Ani restored the high level of amnesia.

Source: Flood et al. (1974). Reprinted with the permission of Academic Press, Inc.

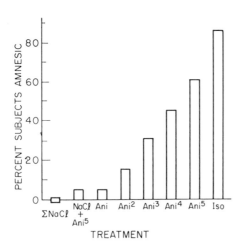

FIGURE 33.13 Effect of the duration of inhibition of protein synthesis on retention for active-avoidance training in mice. The superscripts indicate the number of successive injections given at 2-hr intervals. Thus Ani⁵ received 5 successive injections of Ani. Each injection of Ani extends inhibition 2 hr; thus Ani caused 2 hr of inhibition and Ani⁵ 10 hr of inhibition. NaCl + Ani⁵ received a pretraining injection of saline followed 2 hr later by a series of 5 Ani injections. The $\sum$NaCl group represents the average for 3 saline groups given 1, 3, or 5 successive saline injections; the combined groups showed 0% amnesia. The graph shows that as the duration of inhibition increased, the percent amnesia increased. The NaCl + Ani⁵ group showed that a long series of injections is not sufficient to cause amnesia and that long inhibition does not cause brain damage or illness that can interfere with retention. The Iso group is a group that was isolated and trained for the first time when the other groups were being retrained; this group serves as the naive baseline. From Flood et al. (1975a). Reproduced with the permission of Pergamon Press.

floor through which a shock could be administered. The mice were trained against their first-trial preference in a left-right shock-avoidance situation with a 1-min intertrial interval; all mice received five trials. Injections of Ani or saline were given 15 min prior to training, and additional injections were given at 2-hr intervals. The results presented in Figure 33.13 show that there is a linear trend for longer inhibition to cause greater memory loss of active avoidance. None of the saline-injected mice was classed as amnesic (amnesia was defined as a savings score of less than 30 percent). The Ani injections also had a significant effect upon retention for which side to escape to. In the Ani⁴ and Ani⁵ groups (4 and 5 successive injections of Ani, respectively), a significant number of subjects made an error by escaping to the wrong side of the T maze. (Those mice making an avoidance on the first retention trial were not included in the analysis.) Few subjects injected with Ani, saline + Ani⁵, or saline made discrimination errors (Table 33.4).

TABLE 33.4
Effects of Ani on retention for the left-or-right escape response

$\sum$NaCl	NaCl+Ani⁵	Ani	Ani²	Ani³	Ani⁴	Ani⁵
11.7%	15%	15%	20%	20%	35%	55%

Naive subjects showed no left or right preference (54% went to the right side of a T maze on the first training trial); thus 50% errors could be considered complete amnesia. One assumption being made is that if one could repeatedly test a single subject to see what its first choice would be, it would show no preference. However, it cannot be determined if an individual mouse has a side preference. In the groups receiving 4 or 5 Ani injections, significant numbers of the subjects forgot which side was correct. The Ani⁵ group may be completely amnesic for the escape-response portion of this training task. All the groups have N = 20 except $\sum$NaCl, which contains 20 each for saline subjects given 1, 3, or 5 successive saline injections.

Source: Flood et al. (1975a). Reprinted with the permission of Pergamon Press.

In a second experiment on active avoidance, mice were given a fixed number of training trials (6, 8, or 10), and these groups were further subdivided on the basis of the trial on which the first conditioned response was made. Across these groups the effect of 0, 2, 8, 10, 12, or 14 hr of inhibition of protein synthesis was studied. To achieve these long periods of inhibition a combination of Ani and acetoxycycloheximide (AXM) injections was used. Ani (0.5 mg/mouse) was always the first injection and occurred 15 min prior to training. Retention was found to be a function of the rate of acquisition, the number of training trials, and the duration of inhibition. Amnesia was high when the rate of acquisition was low (Table 33.5), the number of trials few (Table 33.6), and the duration of protein-synthesis inhibition long (Table 33.7). In Table 33.7 one can also see that there was an interaction between the number of training trials and the duration of inhibition, such that amnesia was highest for subjects that had been given the fewest number of trials and that had had the longest duration of inhibition. To

TABLE 33.5
The effect of the rate of acquisition on the percent amnesia

Made 1st CR on trial no.	Percent mice amnesic
7	73% (N = 37)
6	63% (N = 43)
5	54% (N = 41)
4	10% (N = 21)

In the T-maze footshock-avoidance task it took an average of 5 trials for the mice to make their first avoidance response. In this table one can see that for mice learning more slowly, the inhibition of protein synthesis had a greater amnesic effect, while those learning faster than the average were not affected by the amnestic treatment. Amnesia was defined as a savings score of 30% or less. (Unpublished data)

TABLE 33.6
The effect of the number of training trials on the percent amnesia

Number of training trials	Percent mice amnesic
6	77% (N = 44)
8	60% (N = 35)
10	50% (N = 42)

The number of training trials in the T maze had some effect on the ability of Ani to block memory formation. The fewer the number of training trials, the greater the amnesic effect. (Unpublished data)

control for possible permanent brain damage to the mice, a control group was employed in which a saline injection was given prior to training and 14 hr of inhibition of protein synthesis followed $1\frac{3}{4}$ after training; this group was not found to differ significantly from the saline controls. Thus the amnesia observed in the experimental groups could not be accounted for as being the result of physiological damage, prolonged illness, interference with acquisition, or proactive effects that might impair the subject's performance at retraining.

Squire and Davis (in preparation) have reported that high doses of Ani (30 mg/kg or 210 mg/kg) impaired memory for an object-discrimination task to escape footshock. However, they did not find that multiple 30-mg/kg injections had any greater amnesic effect than a single dose of 30 mg/kg. Their lower-dose injections caused significantly less amnesia than the larger dose of 210 mg/kg. Flood et al. (1975a) also found that a pre-training dose of Ani (2.5 mg, or 83 mg/kg/mouse) caused greater amnesia than five successive low-dose injections (0.5 mg, or 17 mg/kg/mouse/injection). But the five successive injections caused greater amnesia than a

TABLE 33.7
The effect of the duration of inhibition and the number of training trials

TT	Duration of inhibition (hours)					
	0	2	8	10	12	14
6	0%	10%	77%	73%	70%	90%
	(N=13)	(N=10)	(N=13)	(N=11)	(N=10)	(N=10)
8	0%	10%	44%	50%	71%	77%
	(N=10)	(N=10)	(N= 9)	(N=10)	(N= 7)	(N= 9)
10	0%	0%	36%	38%	60%	62%
	(N=16)	(N=10)	(N=11)	(N=8)	(N=10)	(N=13)

TT: Number of training trials.
The table shows that an interaction exists such that the more trials a subject is given and the shorter the duration of inhibition, the lower the probability that a subject will be amnesic at retraining.
Source: Flood et al. (1975a). Reprinted with the permission of Pergamon Press.

single 0.5-mg dose. An interesting finding was that if the small dose was given prior to training and the high dose was given as a second injection 2 hr after the first injection, the amnesia was no greater than if two low-dose injections had been given. But when the injections were reversed, with the high dose being given prior to training and the low dose after training, the degree of amnesia was unexpectedly high (80 percent). While it is clear that the large dose is more effective, it is not clear how this is accomplished, since the parameters of inhibition do not differ greatly for high or low dose.

The object-discrimination task employed by Squire and Davis differs considerably from the tasks employed by Flood et al. (passive avoidance and active avoidance in a T maze). The object-discrimination task involves twenty trials, on most of which subjects receive foot-shock. The T maze employs a maximum of ten trials, of which only about five involve shock. A position habit in a T maze to escape shock is learned in two trials or less, and active avoidance is learned in another three trials on the average. By comparison, the object discrimination is learned very slowly over twenty trials, and even at the end of training the percent correct avoidances has only changed from 30 percent correct (object bias) to 62 percent correct.

In our laboratory we have recently found that the jump-pole task employed by Greven and de Wied (1973) is sensitive to the effects of multiple injections of Ani. The task is learned in two trials if the mice are not handled. Mice were subjected to 0, 2, 5, or 7 hr of inhibition by injections of Ani and Ani + Cyclo. The percentage of amnesics increased almost linearly as the duration of inhibition increased.

Possibly the difficulty of the task used by Squire and Davis necessitates more profound inhibition at the time of training to obtain a high percentage of amnesic mice. Also, the large number of training trials necessitated by the slow rate of acquisition might interfere with the amnesic effect of long periods of inhibition of protein synthesis.

The effects of controlled periods of posttrial protein synthesis were studied (Flood et al., 1975b). The design employed two or more successive injections of Ani, one injection given prior to training and one or more given after training. A delay beyond the usual 2-hr interinjection interval was used to create a pulse of protein synthesis, due to a partial recovery from inhibition, against a background of inhibition. The task in this case was step-through passive avoidance with mice. In Figure 33.14 the results of this experiment are shown. The longer the pulse of protein synthesis (40 to 90 min), the lower the percentage of amnesic mice (60 to 15

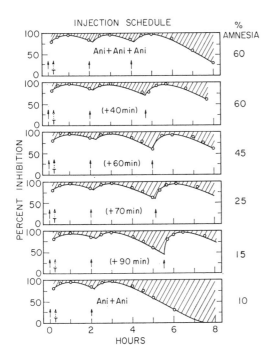

FIGURE 33.14 The effect of pulses of protein synthesis on the percent amnesia for passive-avoidance training in mice. A third injection of Ani caused significantly greater amnesia than just two successive Ani injections. This indicates that protein synthesis relevant to memory formation was occurring over 4 to 6 hr after training. Delays in the injection of Ani caused pulses of protein synthesis (40, 60, 70, or 90 min duration) during the period of 4 to 6 hr after training. Protein synthesis occurring at this time reduced amnesia such that the longer the pulse of protein synthesis, the lower the percentage of amnesic mice. From Flood et al. (1975b). Reprinted with the permission of Pergamon Press.

percent). Evidence was also found that a delay period is less likely to reduce amnesia, the further in time from training that it occurs. For example, a delay period of 40 min between injections 1 and 2, 2 and 3, or 3 and 4 resulted in 35, 40, or 65 percent amnesia, respectively, in a treatment involving four successive injections of Ani.

These studies suggest that the better a subject is trained, the longer memory-related protein synthesis occurs after training. An interesting paradox in this work is that very long periods of protein-synthesis inhibition may be required to cause amnesia, while brief periods of controlled protein synthesis may permit memory to be established. Thus more protein may normally be synthesized than is needed to guarantee memory one week after training. A possible reason for this "extra" protein being synthesized is suggested by some pilot data showing that for a given delay period (i.e., a given pulse of protein synthesis), retention was unaffected over the first week, but over the remaining six weeks retention decreased to zero. The saline controls

over the same period of time showed 0 and 10 percent amnesia for tests given at 24 hr and 6 weeks, respectively. Thus a possible reason for the "extra" protein is to establish a memory that will last essentially for the life of the mouse.

Recently the effects of Ani on retention reported by Flood et al. have been to some extent replicated and extended by Squire and Barondes (1974). In their experiment mice were trained to discriminate between a large and small rod to escape footshock. Ani was injected 30 min prior to training at a dose of 150mg/kg (approximately nine times greater than that used by Flood et al.). The retention tests given 1, 7, or 14 days after training revealed significant impairment of retention. There was a trend for greater impairment of retention as the retention interval increased. In the same study Cyclo was injected in a similar manner, and effects on retention approximately equal to those of Ani were obtained. Flood et al. (1973) reported that with passive avoidance Cyclo caused greater amnesia than Ani when given prior to training, but not when given after training as a second injection.

Squire and Barondes also used a low dose of Ani approximately equal to that used by Flood et al., but found that it did not affect retention. The finding that a low dose of Ani does not produce amnesia is not inconsistent with the report of Flood et al. (1975a) in which it was found that up to four successive injections of Ani were required to cause significant amnesia in a multiple-trial training task (i.e., footshock-avoidance training).

The effect of Ani on habituation to mouse "shrieks" was tested in a drink task (Squire and Becker, 1974). Consumption of water was suppressed by the presentation of "recorded mouse shrieks" during the drinking session. Control mice, when tested three days later, showed no suppression of drinking when the mouse shrieks were presented, which indicated that they had habituated to the shrieks. Mice given Ani immediately following the drink task failed to habituate to the mouse shrieks, as indicated by continued drink suppression, but those injected 8 hr later did habituate.

In another study Squire et al. (1975) studied the possibility that bait shyness could account for the amnesia induced by Ani. Ani and lithium chloride were used to induce illness and to cause bait shyness of a saccharin solution. Illness was judged to be equivalent for Ani and lithium chloride injections when both caused an equal aversion to the saccharin solution. A dose of 30 mg/kg of Ani was found to induce as much avoidance of saccharin solution as lithium chloride. However, in a second part of that study Ani and lithium chloride were given to mice trained on an automated object-discrimination task. Doses of 30 mg/kg or 150 mg/kg of Ani induced amnesia, but the lithium chloride treatment did not. Thus the amnesia due to an Ani injection is not the result of an illness or an aversion, since otherwise the mice injected with lithium chloride would have been amnesic.

33.3 INTERPRETATION OF THE ROLE OF RNA AND PROTEIN SYNTHESIS IN MEMORY FORMATION

33.3.1 The role of RNA synthesis in memory formation

While a large body of research employing the uptake of RNA precursors has suggested that increases in RNA synthesis may be involved in memory processing, a better understanding of what is being measured by the uptake of labeled RNA precursors will be important to evaluating the evidence suggesting that RNA synthesis is necessary for memory formation. Dunn (this volume) has discussed the problem of determining changes in RNA synthesis by using uptake of RNA precursor as the assay method, and he has indicated that much of the assay indicates only changes in pool size.

Until recently it was not possible to evaluate the role of RNA synthesis critically using inhibitors of RNA synthesis because of their toxicity. Camptothecin is an inhibitor of RNA synthesis whose effects seem to be reversible, but the interpretation that camptothecin actually inhibits mRNA relies upon the validity of the assay technique of measuring the uptake of labeled RNA precursor. From our earlier discussion of Neale, Klinger, and Agranoff (1973), it is clear that camptothecin administered to goldfish shortly after training can interfere with long-term memory processing; whether this is accomplished by the inhibition of RNA synthesis will have to await an evaluation by biochemists as to what method of assay is appropriate.

The effects of intracerebral administration of uridine monophosphate (UMP) on extinction also suggest that new RNA synthesis needs to occur shortly after training if long-term memories are to be formed. The reports by Ott and Matthies (1973a,b) require a biochemical confirmation that UMP administration can stimulate RNA and protein synthesis before a complete interpretation is possible. As with the Neale study, modification of RNA metabolism had to occur within 1 min of training to yield a sizeable effect. Supposedly, the UMP caused a stronger memory trace to be formed and this made the rats more resistant to extinction, in much the same way that overtraining produces high resistance to extinction.

The report that Cyclo blocks UMP resistance to extinction suggests that UMP is ultimately influencing the mechanisms of memory-related protein synthesis (Ott and Matthies, 1973b). It is possible, of course, that UMP

has a nonspecific action unrelated to its role in RNA synthesis. For example, it may resemble caffeine or other purines in enhancing the activity of cyclic AMP, or there might be other, general, CNS-stimulating actions. The cycloheximide effect might thus simply have antagonized the UMP effect through unrelated mechanisms.

Two reports suggest that new mRNA synthesis may not be necessary for long-term memory formation on the basis of the speed with which memory-related protein is formed. Squire and Barondes (1972, 1973) showed that Cyclo can impair acquisition when prolonged training is involved. This was interpreted to mean that phases of memory (short-term memory) may be dependent on protein synthesis. The observed decrement in acquisition begins to occur within 4–6 min of training. Flood, Bennett, Rosenzweig, and Orme have found that if protein synthesis is permitted to occur only for a period of 1 min after training, retention for passive-avoidance training can be shown to exist on a test given one week after training. One minute is probably too short a time for new mRNA synthesis followed by protein synthesis to have occurred in mammals. It was suggested that, due to the almost constant activity of neurons, pools of mRNA may exist that can serve as a template for the protein needed to modify synaptic relationships. Thus only activation and not synthesis of mRNA would be required for memory-related protein synthesis to occur.

At present, the exact role of RNA and its relationship to the electrophysiological events of learning and to memory-related protein synthesis remain somewhat obscure.

33.3.2 Permanence of amnesia

The most serious challenge to the interpretation that protein-synthesis inhibitors affect memory formation has come from reports that inhibition of protein synthesis does not lead to permanent amnesia. We would now like to examine the conditions under which temporary amnesia has been reported.

Serota, Roberts, and Flexner (1972) claim transient amnesic effects from inhibition of protein synthesis. However, an examination of their retention data does not suggest that memory recovered to an appreciable extent. Rats were trained on a shock-avoidance, brightness-discrimination task in a Y maze. AXM or saline was administered prior to training. Controls showed 87 percent mean savings on retraining to a criterion of 9 out of 10 avoidances. The AXM group, tested 24 hr after training, showed 6.6 percent mean savings, which increased to 20.3 percent by day 6. The difference between the AXM groups (24 hr versus 6 days) was statistically significant (p < 0.001), so some recovery of memory or learning ability occurred between 24 hr and 6 days after the drug treatment. Yet a clear amnesic effect still remained in the AXM 6-day subjects when compared to the saline group (20 versus 87 percent). Thus the amnesia was not completely transient, as implied by Serota, Roberts, and Flexner.

Squire and Barondes (1972) also reported a transient amnesic effect using Cyclo and mice trained to escape shock by making a large-versus-small-rod discrimination. The Cyclo-injected mice showed significantly poorer retention 24 to 48 hr after training (p < 0.05). By the third day retention did not differ significantly between Cyclo- and saline-injected mice. A control for illness was included. The control mice received Cyclo 30 min after training; their retention scores did not differ significantly from those of the saline controls.

Squire and Barondes (1972) are the only investigators who have controlled for illness as a possible explanation for the transient amnesia. Their control may not have been adequate, however, as it was assumed that Cyclo is as likely to cause illness when given after training as when given prior to training.

The extent to which illness is likely to affect relearning or other test procedures is not easily determined. It may be harder yet to reach agreement about the degree of illness present shortly after training and drug treatment. By way of a demonstration, we would like to present some data indicating that Cyclo is more toxic when given prior to training and is more toxic in multiple-trial than in single-trial learning situations. The measure of toxicity is the percentage of mice that die. C57Bl/Jf female mice weighing between 18 and 21 grams were given 0.27 mg of Cyclo either 15 min prior to training or 15 min after training in either a passive-avoidance or a T-maze, active-avoidance paradigm. The results indicated that Cyclo was more toxic when given prior to training in either task and was more toxic in active than in passive avoidance. In passive avoidance, pretraining injections caused death in 50 percent of the mice, while none of the mice given a posttraining injection of Cyclo died. In active avoidance 85 percent of the mice given pretraining injections but only 13 percent of those given posttraining injections died. With active-avoidance training an interaction occurred between toxicity, rate of learning, and the time of the injection. Cyclo was more toxic to slow learners (those taking more than 5 trials to make an avoidance response—all mice received 15 training trials) than to fast learners (67 versus 25 percent dead). Among the slow learners Cyclo was more toxic when given prior to training (100 percent dead) than when given after training (22 percent dead). While most of the mice died within 24 hr of the drug treatment, some did not die until 3 days posttreatment. Thus illness in Cyclo-injected mice can exist for a considerable time after treatment is given, depending on the type of train-

ing and how rapidly the mice learn. Thus the control of Squire and Barondes (1972) is not valid against illness as a cause of transient amnesia.

In addition, it might be mentioned that permanent amnesia has been reported more frequently than transient amnesia: e.g., by Squire and Barondes (1973), Squire, Smith, and Barondes (1973), Squire and Davis (in preparation), Flood et al. (1972, 1973, 1974, 1975a, b), Agranoff (1971), and Geller et al. (1969), to cite just a few using either Cyclo or Ani.

On the other hand, Quartermain and McEwen (1970) reported a dramatic recovery of retention in mice trained on step-through passive avoidance and treated with Cyclo. Two shock intensities were used—1.6 ma and 0.16 ma. No recovery of retention was observed in the Cyclo-injected mice tested 24 to 48 hr after training with the 0.16-ma footshock. But the Cyclo-injected mice in the high-shock-intensity group showed very poor retention at 24 hr and no amnesia at 48 hr after training (Figure 33.15).

It seems strange that "transient amnesia" is reported to occur only 1–2 days after training and drug treatment,

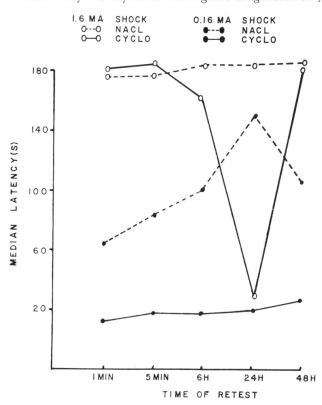

FIGURE 33.15 The effect of training shock level and cyclo-heximide on retention. Training with 1.6-ma shock caused a trainsient amnesia 6 and 24 hr after training in cycloheximide-injected mice. But training at 0.16 ma caused a persistent amnesia in cycloheximide-injected mice. From Quartermain and McEwen (1970). Reproduced with the permission of Macmillan Journals Ltd.

a time at which it is reasonable to expect that subjects have not fully recovered from the effects of the inhibitors. Indeed, Quartermain and his associates have recently been investigating the pharmacological basis of transient amnesia. Botwinick and Quartermain (1974) reported that amnesia for one-trial passive avoidance induced by Cyclo treatment was reversed by administering either pheniprazine (catron) or pargyline 1 to 2 hr prior to the retention test. Pheniprazine and pargyline were used to block the oxidative deamination of norepinephrine and dopamine, thus causing an increase in brain levels of catecholamine transmitters. Randt et al. (1971) reported that diethyldithiocarbamate (DDC), a dopamine-β-hydroxylase inhibitor that decreases norepinephrine biosynthesis, blocked retention for passive-avoidance training. When DDC was administered either 30 min prior to or 1 min after one-trial, passive-avoidance training, mice were found to have poor retention. However, posttrial injections of DDC have elsewhere been shown to cause a memory deficit for passive avoidance but to enhance retention for active avoidance (Haycock and McGaugh, personal communication). Quartermain has suggested that other amnestic treatments such as inhibition of protein synthesis might achieve their effects by altering brain catecholamine levels as does DDC.

At this point we should stop and examine the paradigm used by Quartermain's group and the hypotheses that follow therefrom. In their experiment the subject is trained under the low-catecholamine drug state and tested under one of two conditions: (1) low catecholamine levels, or (2) normal or elevated catecholamine levels. Retention tests are given at various times from 24 to 48 or more hours after the training and drug treatment.

There are two possible explanations for the amnesia found in this paradigm: (1) The amnesia resulted from impaired learning or memory storage during or shortly after acquisition, due to low levels of catecholamine transmitters. (2) Amnesia resulted from impaired retrieval due to low catecholamine levels at testing. Since the critical factor in the first hypothesis is the drug state during or shortly after acquisition, the amnesia should be permanent regardless of the interval between drug treatment and testing. This hypothesis could thus account for permanent amnesia and suggests that long-term memory requires protein synthesis, but only if hypothesis 2 is incorrect. Hypothesis 2 suggests that the amnesia should be transient, with poor retention shortly after training but good retention after recovery of normal catecholamine levels (48 or more hours after the drug treatment). This hypothesis also implies that low levels of brain catecholamines do not necessarily interfere with

memory formation, since retention should then be permanently disrupted. Hypothesis 2 cannot account for reports of persistent amnesia (i.e., amnesia lasting one or more weeks after training and drug treatment).

The evidence supporting the general hypothesis that transient amnesia is due to low catecholamine levels is discussed below and summarized in Table 33.8.

Randt et al. (1971) injected DDC prior to training and reported amnesia in mice tested 24 hr later. This result supports hypothesis 2. Quartermain and McEwen (1970) administered Cyclo prior to training and tested retention 24 and 48 hr after training. The mice were given no injections prior to the retention test. Retention was found to be very poor 24 hr after training and drug treatment, but normal at 48 hr when catecholamine levels would presumably be nearly normal. This supports hypothesis 2. Botwinick and Quartermain (1974) gave Cyclo prior to training and 24 hr later tested retention. Before the retention test the Cyclo-injected mice were given saline, catron, or pargyline. Catron and pargyline reversed the amnesia, and similar results were shown for DDC. This again supports hypothesis 2.

Table 33.8

A summary of studies dealing with catecholamines and memory

Study	Injection	Time of test (hr)	Test treatment	Retention
Randt et al. (1971)	DDC	24	none	poor
Quartermain and McEwen (1970)	Cyclo	24	none	poor
		48	none	good
Botwinick and Quartermain (1974)	Cyclo	24	saline	poor
			catron	good
			pargyline	good
Quartermain and Botwinick (1975):				
Exp. 2	Cyclo	24	none	poor
		36	none	fair
		48	none	good
Exp. 3	Cyclo	24	catron	good
			pargyline	good
Exp. 6b	AMPT	24	saline	poor
			pargyline	good

Studies relating memory-retrieval deficits in transient amnesia to the low level of catecholamines that may exist during the 24–36 hr following the use of Cyclo or DDC. Injections were given prior to training; test treaments involving injections were given prior to testing. The task used differs: the first three used passive avoidance, and the last used an appetitive-training task.

Quartermain and Botwinick (1975) in an experiment with several parts presented some relevant data. In their Experiment 2 Cyclo was administered to mice prior to training in an appetitive task, and retention was tested 24, 36, or 48 hr later. No injections were given prior to the retention test. The mice showed a marked amnesia at 24 hr after training, nearly normal retention at 36 hr, and normal memory at 48 hr. In Experiment 3 mice trained on the same task were given Cyclo prior to training, and retention was tested 24 hr later. Prior to the retention test mice were injected with pheniprazine, pargyline, or saline. Pheniprazine and pargyline reversed the amnesia, but the saline-injected mice still showed a strong memory impairment. It is interesting that pheniprazine given to saline controls prior to the retention test has a disrupting effect on retention. In Experiment 6b α-methyl-p-tyrosine (AMPT), which also inhibits tyrosine hydroxylase activity and depletes norepinephrine (NE), was injected prior to appetitive training, and the subjects were tested 24 hr later. Prior to the retention test pargyline or saline was injected. The AMPT-injected mice given saline prior to the retention test showed poor retention, while those given pargyline prior to the 24-hr retention test showed good retention.

Thus the data presented by Quartermain and his associates strongly suggest that low catecholamine levels impair memory retrieval, resulting in a transient amnesia. No evidence presented among these papers can be interpreted to mean that amnesia that persists for days or weeks after drug treatment is due to catecholamine depletion. In fact, the evidence is to the contrary since retention tests given 48 hr after training all showed that subjects had good retention. Clearly, the bases of transient amnesia and permanent amnesia differ in that the former seems to depend on low levels of brain NE or catecholamines in general, while the latter persists even though normal levels of NE are present. Presumably, unless long-term depletion can be demonstrated due to some side effect of protein-synthesis inhibition, it is still a good working hypothesis that protein synthesis is necessary for long-term memory formation.

Another type of study by Rigter, van Riezen, and de Wied (1974) and Greven and de Wied (1973) raises a similar question as to whether amnesia is due to poor memory formation or poor retrieval. However, in these studies a reversal of amnesia is being reported for a long-term memory deficit. Rigter, van Riezen, and de Wied (1974) trained rats on a one-trial, step-through, passive-avoidance task. Amnesia was induced by either CO_2 or ECS given shortly after training. $ACTH_{4-10}$, a fragment of the ACTH molecule which does not have ACTH-like hormonal properties, administered 1 hr

prior to retest, blocked the amnesia caused by CO_2 or ECS. A similar finding occurred in a thirst-motivated task, where CO_2 caused amnesia and $ACTH_{4-10}$ alleviated the amnesia. The results suggested to the authors that $ACTH_{4-10}$ reverses the disturbance of retrieval induced by amnesia treatment.

In the experiments reported by Rigter, van Riezen, and de Wied (1974) and by Botwinick and Quartermain (1974), the effect of the drugs was not tested on *poorly* trained control subjects. If it is the case that controls with poor retention due to weak training also have better retention after ACTH, pheniprazine, or pargyline treatment, then one could interpret the findings as indicating that these drugs have the ability to improve the recall of poorly remembered tasks. Greven and de Wied (1973) provide evidence that nondrugged, weakly trained rats had better recall if they were given ACTH or some of its peptide fragments prior to testing. Using the rate of extinction from shuttlebox training as a measure of ACTH effect on retention, Greven and de Wied showed that rats treated with ACTH, α-melanocyte-stimulating hormone (MSH), $ACTH_{1-10}$, β-MSH, or $ACTH_{4-10}$ made at least 50 percent more responses during shuttlebox extinction than placebo-treated rats. Placebo-treated rats showed very poor retention on passive avoidance, while ACTH-treated subjects had test scores at least ten times greater in most cases. Thus it appears that reversal of amnesia is not uniquely associated with any of the amnestic treatments used, but, rather, that amnestic treatments permit only a weak memory trace to be formed, and only with special treatment can retention be detected. It is interesting that each of the drugs used to reverse amnesia eventually has a stimulating effect on CNS electrical activity.

Our laboratory has recently found that d-amphetamine, injected IP (2 mg/kg) into mice 15 min prior to a retention test for passive-avoidance training, will reverse Ani's amnesic effect. Mice were given two successive injection of Ani, the first 15 min prior to training, the second $1\frac{3}{4}$ hr after training. One week later the subjects were tested for passive avoidance; those with test latencies of 0.1–9.0 sec or 9.1–20.0 sec were given a second retention test 3–4 days later. d-Amphetamine or saline was injected IP 15 min prior to the second retention test. The d-amphetamine- and saline-injected subjects with short retest latencies (0.1–9.0 sec) did not differ significantly (70 versus 80 percent amnesia). However, d-amphetamine-injected mice with long test latencies (9.1–20.0 sec) showed a substantial reduction of amnesia, compared to the saline control group with long latencies (10 versus 80 percent amnesia). One might conclude that treatments such as those described here can improve recall of poorly stored information, but that below a certain threshold even this type of treatment is not effective in improving retention.

33.4 THE ROLE OF HORMONES IN RETENTION AND PERFORMANCE

Since the early 1960s a great deal of research has been done on the role of the pituitary-adrenocortical axis in learning motivated primarily by footshock (for a review, see de Wied, 1969). More recently attention has turned to the effects of adrenocorticotropic hormone (ACTH) and related compounds on extinction. The appearance of extinction is in many cases difficult to class exclusively as learning, since changes in motivation or arousal may well influence the rate of extinction. We shall describe some of the effects of ACTH and related compounds on retention and examine recent claims that ACTH reverses amnesia caused by CO_2, ECS, and puromycin.

Rigter, van Riezen, and de Wied (1974) trained rats on a one-trial, step-through, passive-avoidance task and then induced amnesia by administering either CO_2 or ECS immediately after training. In both cases amnesia could be alleviated by $ACTH_{4-10}$ administered 1 hr prior to the retrieval test. When this peptide was given 1 hr prior to the acquisition trial, it did not affect the amnesia. It was also reported that CO_2 could induce amnesia for a thirst-motivated learning task and that when $ACTH_{4-10}$ was administered 1 hr prior to the retention test, it reversed the amnesia. However, it is possible that $ACTH_{4-10}$ simply improves recall and that this phenomenon has nothing to do with the particular method by which poor memory traces are obtained (e.g., inhibition of RNA or protein synthesis, CO_2, ECS, or just poor training). Lande, Flexner, and Flexner (1972) trained mice in a Y maze to avoid footshock. A puromycin injection given 24 hr after training caused amnesia. But ACTH or desglycinamide[9]-lysine vasopressin (DGVP) administered prior to training or 12, but not 24, hr after training blocked puromycin's amnesic effect.

33.4.1 Effects on extinction

Van Wimersma Greidanus and de Wied (1971) reported that young adult rats trained to avoid footshock by jumping onto a pole showed slower rates of extinction if $ACTH_{1-10}$ was given subcutaneously prior to the extinction session. Under the same conditions $ACTH_{1-10}$ D-Phe[7] (the isomer with D-Phe as the seventh amino acid —the L isomer being the normal form of Phe in ACTH) facilitated extinction. These compounds were also administered intracerebrally in the crystalline form to several areas of the brain, primarily along the midline in the diencephalon and rhinencephalon. Of particular interest to these authors was the observation that application of these drugs into the thalamic midline nuclei (thalamic diffuse projection system) reproduced the subcutaneous effects of the drugs. The suggestion was made that the midline area of the thalamus might be the target for the ACTH peptides. Other suggested target areas were in the caudal regions of the reticular formation. For the most part, the specific sensory nuclei of the thalamus and motor nuclei of the brainstem were not effective sites for altering the rates of extinction. The authors interpreted their findings in terms of memory formation; it would seem, though, that since the rats were tested in the drug state, this work could best be interpreted in terms of retrieval processes and pathways. Also, it should be pointed out that the diffuse thalamic projection is intimately related to the reticular formation of the brainstem, and ACTH effects in these areas may be altering arousal.

Bohus and de Wied (1966) reported that for shuttlebox training, $ACTH_{1-10}$ slowed down the rate of extinction and $ACTH_{1-10}$ D-Phe[7] increased the rate of extinction. Greven and de Wied (1973) studied different peptide fragments of ACTH to determine the shortest possible fragment that would still have effects on extinction but would hopefully not have hormonal effects. $ACTH_{4-10}$ was reported to be as effective as ACTH in delaying extinction of shuttlebox performance, jump-pole response, and passive avoidance. $ACTH_{4-10}$ D-Phe[7] facilitated shuttlebox and jump-pole extinction but delayed extinction for passive avoidance. The $ACTH_{4-10}$ peptide possesses almost none of the adrenocorticotropic effects of the parent molecule ACTH (de Wied, 1969). Greven and de Wied (1973) suggested that the ACTH peptide acts on membranes of specific target cells and, by inducing conformational changes, stimulates cyclic AMP production. This in turn stimulates protein synthesis and leads to the establishment of new synaptic junctions.

33.4.2 Effects of adrenocorticosteroids

Cortisol administration to intact rats suppresses pituitary secretion of ACTH. Thus one would expect opposite behavioral effects from ACTH and cortisol: ACTH retards extinction and cortisol enhances extinction. Bohus (1968) trained rats on a shelf-escape task to a footshock-avoidance criterion. After training, the rats were implanted with cannulas aimed at the median eminence (ME) or the rostral midbrain reticular formation (MRF). Crystalline cortisol was administered via the cannulas, and cholesterol was used as a vehicle control. The rats were then retrained and then given extinction tests. The cortisol, cholesterol and unoperated groups showed no significant differences in the mean number of conditioned responses on retraining. Cortisol but not cholesterol in the MRF greatly increased the rate of extinction. The control performance decreased to 70 percent responding, while cortisol in the MRF decreased responding to about 20 percent. Cortisol in the ME had a moderate effect, with the response rate decreasing to about 45 percent.

Cortisol was found to reduce ACTH release by about 50 percent of control levels in the ME and 32 percent in the MRF. A correlation between total number of responses and ACTH level showed that the stronger the suppression of ACTH, the faster the extinction (correlation coefficient 0.79, p < 0.001) for rats with cortisol in the ME. Strangely, no correlation was observed for rats with MRF implants.

Weiss et al. (1970) suggested that ACTH and corticosterone may affect the central nervous system in a generalized manner by altering arousal or emotionality. Evidence exists that cortisol depresses the activity of the ascending pathways of the reticular formation (Ruf and Steiner, 1967) and depresses cortisol-evoked potentials (Slusher, Hyde, and Laufer, 1966). This might suggest that cortisol and ACTH have their effects via arousal mechanisms, with cortisol decreasing arousal and facilitating extinction and ACTH increasing arousal and delaying extinction. In part, the target areas suggested for ACTH action should raise some concern as to whether it is motivational or memory-retrieval effects that are being studied.

In line with the arousal explanation, it should be pointed out that there are many studies in the literature indicating that extinction of a conditioned response can be increased by administering depressant drugs such as barbiturate or phenothiazine and decreased by administering stimulant drugs such as amphetamine. However, it would be useful to obtain some independent measure of arousal caused by either ACTH peptides or steroids.

33.5 THE ROLE OF NEUROTRANSMITTERS IN MEMORY FORMATION

Since the time of Cajal the idea that synapses in the central nervous system might have something to do with the formation of new memories has been an attractive one. Since many synapses operate by means of chemical transmitter agents, it is reasonable to assume that neurotransmitters have something to do with the strengthening and weaking of these connections and therefore of traces (Sharpless, 1964; Ungerstedt, 1974). The anatomical evidence that synaptic changes occur with experience is discussed in several chapters in this volume and seems convincing. We shall now review the pharmacological

evidence for transmitter involvement in learning and memory.

33.5.1 Acetylcholine
The most firmly established neurotransmitter in the central nervous system is acetylcholine. Unfortunately, it is difficult to measure this substance directly due to its rapid enzymatic destruction in brain tissue. However, drugs may be employed to alter acetylcholine levels in the brain. Posttrial injections of physostigmine, an anticholinesterase, can facilitate memory (Greenough, Yuwiler, and Dollinger, 1973; McGaugh, 1973), while posttrial injections of scopolamine impair memory (Glick and Zimmerberg, 1972). Other side effects of these drugs on motor activity, arousal, and brain electrophysiology may in some experimental designs be the primary cause of the effect. Posttrial administration of nicotine can facilitate memory, but it is not certain whether the cholinergic or adrenergic effects of this drug are responsible for its actions (McGaugh, 1973).

33.5.2 Catecholamines
Possibly the most widely investigated putative transmitters are the catecholamines—dopamine, norepinephrine, and epinephrine. Many studies indicate that some or all of these are involved in learning in important ways. However, it is not as clear that memory can be significantly influenced since few studies have employed posttraining injections and thus ruled out an influence of these drugs on acquisition.

Randt et al. (1971) used diethyldithiocarbamic acid (DDC), a dopamine-β-hydroxylase inhibitor, to suppress norepinephrine formation either 30 min before or immediately after training; they found that the performance on a one-trial, passive-avoidance test was severely depressed 24 hr later. This and other work from Quartermain's laboratory, already discussed, strongly supports the role of catecholamines in the retrieval of stored memory.

Rake's laboratory has reported, in a series of experiments (Dismukes and Rake, 1972; Rake 1973; Allen, Allen, and Rake, 1974), a pharmacological distinction between memory formation for passive and active avoidance. Table 33.9 summarizes the results of these experiments. It was found that posttrial reduction in the brain levels of catecholamines and indoleamines (serotonin) by reserpine causes retention deficits for passive avoidance and one-way and two-way active avoidance. If 5-HTP or dopa was administered, brain levels of serotonin or catecholamines were selectively increased. When posttraining catecholamine levels were low and indoleamine levels normal, retention for passive avoidance 8 days after training was found to be normal, but retention for both

TABLE 33.9

Summary of studies by A. V. Rake and associates distinguishing between memory formation for passive and active avoidance

Posttraining injection (immediate)	Effect on catechol- amines	Effect on indole- amines	Task	Effect on retention
Reserpine	low	low	PA	deficient
	low	low	one-way AAR	deficient
	low	low	two-way AAR	deficient
Reserpine +5-HTP	low	normal	PA	normal
	low	normal	one-way AAR	deficient
	low	normal	two-way AAR	deficient
Reserpine +dopa	normal	low	PA	deficient
	normal	low	one-way AAR	normal
	normal	low	two-way AAR	normal
PCPA (pretraining)	normal	low	two-way AAR	normal

Results of studies by Dismukes and Rake (1972), Rake (1973), and Allen, Allen, and Rake (1974). "Low" means brain levels were reduced; "normal" means levels were raised and presumed to be near normal. PA = passive avoidance; AAR = active-avoidance responding (two-way AAR is also known as shuttlebox conditioning).

one- and two-way active avoidance was deficient. When catecholamine levels were normal and indoleamine levels low (immediately after training), subsequent retention tests found passive avoidance deficient and one- and two-way active avoidance normal. The authors concluded that "the simplest explanation of these results . . . is that indoleamines are necessary for the formation of memory in a passive event and that catecholamines are necessary for memory formation in an active training event" (Allen, Allen, and Rake, 1974).

This work greatly strengthens the results of Quartermain and his associates, discussed in Section 33.3.2, suggesting an important role for biogenic amine pathways in memory formation and retrieval. However, we have little information about the effect of altering the brain levels of other putative transmitters. Thus we have yet to determine the degree of pharmacological specificity associated with different training tasks or any particular transmitter's role in memory formation or retrieval. It is possible that inhibitors of protein synthesis are causing amnesia by disrupting the metabolism of biogenic amines. It will be important for the interpretation of both lines of research to determine the extent to which inhibitors of protein synthesis are capable of producing decreases in catecholamines and indoleamines or impairing their ability to function.

Another explanation is that protein synthesis is required in some of the adrenergic, dopaminergic, and serotonergic pathways for memory formation. If activation of these pathways results in the release of neurotransmitters, which in turn stimulate memory-related protein synthesis, then retention would be disrupted by either depleting biogenic amines or by blocking the protein synthesis resulting from activation of these neurons.

Quartermain's results might be explained by such a model. When training activates neurons in the biogenic pathways, some of the neurons are normally modified—thus storing memory. But because of the inhibition of protein synthesis, the neuronal activity does not lead to a sufficient change for memory to be expressed. Since inhibition of protein synthesis is never complete and may not have lasted long enough, a small change in the CNS may have taken place; but the degree of change is normally below the threshold for memory to express itself in the retention test. If the brain levels of biogenic amines are increased, neuronal excitability might increase to the point that retrieval of this weak trace is possible. It is interesting and possibly significant that the neuron cell bodies synthesizing most of the catecholamines and indoleamines are located in important pathways that are found to influence arousal in the brainstem and diencephalon.

Employing another approach, Anlezark, Crow, and Greenway (1973) showed that lesions in the locus ceruleus that destroy neurons synthesizing norepinephrine, also diminish the rate of increase of running for food reward in a simple L-shaped runway (Figure 33.16). Running speed can be taken as a measure of motivation or learning, in that (1) the level of hunger will influence running speed, and (2) as the subject remembers where the food is located, the running speed should increase. The authors claimed that there was no impairment in motivation and that weight gain was normal in these animals; they simply seemed incapable of learning where the food was located. This, as well as much of the work already cited, is in line with Kety's suggestion (1972, and this volume) that norepinephrine plays an important role in learning.

Coyle, Wender, and Lipsky (1973) compared genetic differences in learning ability with catecholamine metabolism in different strains of rats. They found that poor learners in a two-way avoidance situation had low adrenal levels of tyrosine hydroxylase, dopamine-β-hydroxylase, and phenylethanolamine methyltransferase. In the assay of brain tissue, poor learners were found to have higher levels of dopamine-β-hydroxylase activity. Such a finding is not what one would expect given the results of Rake's and Quartermain's studies, in which the brain levels of tyrosine hydroxylase activity were not

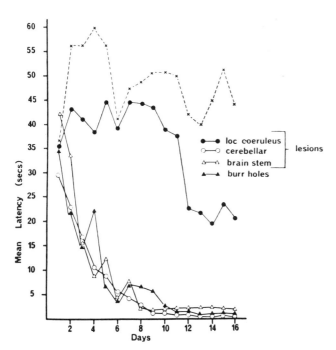

FIGURE 33.16 The mean latencies (time taken to run 120 cm) in the initial arm of an L-shaped runway for four groups of rats. The dotted line shows mean latencies for the three rats with the most bilateral ablation of the nucleus locus ceruleus. From Anlezark, Crow, and Greenway (1973). Copyright 1973 by the American Association for the Advancement of Sicence.

different in normal and poor learners. This may indicate a learning deficit due to poor conversion of dopamine to norepinephrine in the brain. It was found by Moore and Rech (1967) and Fuxe and Hanson (1967) that inhibition of the synthesis of central catecholamines impaired avoidance conditioning. Hanson (1967) found that amphetamine could reverse a response decrement caused by inhibitors of catecholamine synthesis. Pretrial injections of amphetamine have been known for some time to improve avoidance conditioning in animals that show poor performance.

Cooper, Grant, and Breese (1973) found that 6-hydroxydopamine alone did not cause a deficit in a continuously reinforced bar-pressing task in rats; however, when AMPT or reserpine was superimposed upon these 6-hydroxydopamine-treated animals, they did show a behavioral deficit. These investigators have demonstrated that it is possible to deplete dopamine preferentially by pretreating the animals with desipramine and then following with intracisternal injections of 200 μg of 6-hydroxydopamine. This treatment reduced brain dopamine by approximately 74 percent and norepinephrine by only 16 percent. Intracisternally administered 6-hydroxydopamine alone reduced brain norepinephrine by 51 percent and dopamine by 12 percent. On the other

hand, injection of 200 μg of 6-hydroxydopamine after 50 mg/kg of pargyline caused a depletion of norepinephrine by 72 percent and of dopamine by 84 percent. Behavioral responding in rats preferentially depleted of norepinephrine was slightly reduced, but not to the extent observed in animals depleted of dopamine. This experiment points up the importance of dopamine in maintaining a motor habit, but it does not reveal whether retention of the conditioned reponse requires dopamine at all times.

Brown, Davis, and Carlsson (1973) reported that dopa under certain circumstances could reverse the hypoxia-induced disruption of a conditioned-avoidance response in rats. It was, however, necessary to use the peripheral decarboxylase inhibitor RO-4-4602 plus dopa to bring the shuttlebox behavior of hypoxia animals back toward normal. It appears that this effect is related to the level of arousal or of motor ability, both of which are mediated by dopaminergic or possibly noradrenergic neurons.

Deficiency of brain catecholamine levels impairs discrimination performance, while an excess seems to facilitate performance. Kitsikis, Roberge, and Frenette (1972) found that L-dopa improved the performance of cats in a delayed-response, visual-discrimination situation. Since catecholamines mediate arousal and also reward, facilitation of learning may follow potentiation of these functions. Cooper, Black, and Paolino (1971) found that AMPT, which decreases brain catecholamine levels by blocking synthesis of dopa and norepinephrine, decreased the responding of rats to rewarding brain electrical stimulation in the septal forebrain and the lateral hypothalamic areas. p-Chlorophenylalanine (PCPA), which reduces brain levels of serotonin, did not produce any change in performance in this task. This supports the view of Stein (1971) that reward is a noradrenergically mediated process.

There is a surprising report by Saper and Sweeney (1973) showing that AMPT facilitates learning of an appetitive discrimination task but does not affect memory of that task. Since AMPT increased the response time, it may be that the slowness of responding is enough to give the animal more time to "think" and thus make the proper decision.

It is interesting that behavior may also influence norepinephrine levels. For example, rats working at performing a lever-press response for water reward showed an increase in brain norepinephrine metabolism with respect to controls (Lewy and Seiden, 1972). In humans a similar result was reported by Post and Goodwin (1973), who found that volunteers simulating hypomanic behavior showed an increased excretion of catecholamines.

33.5.3 Serotonin

While catecholamines have been generally found to exert a positive effect on acquisition and performance, the effect of serotonin on acquisition and performance is not so clear. Riege (1971) found that decreasing serotonin with PCPA protected rats from the amnesic effect of ECS in a one-trial avoidance task (Table 33.10). It has been shown by others that PCPA facilitates active avoidance (Schlesinger, Schreiber, and Pryor, 1968; Tenen, 1967). Brody (1970) found that a reduction of brain indoleamines improved learning in both active- and passive-avoidance situations. But Rake and his co-workers reported low serotonin levels due to administration of PCPA or reserpine + dopa caused a deficiency in retest performance of two-way active avoidance.

There is a long list of candidate transmitters for the central nervous system. However, only a few of these have been studied for their role in behavior. Probably because the analytical methods for their determination have been so successfully worked out, the biogenic amines (dopamine, norepinephrine, epinephrine, and 5-hydroxytryptamine) have been investigated extensively, and these have been discussed here. Acetylcholine has been the subject of a smaller but still respectable number of psychopharmacological investigations. The inhibitory substances, γ-aminobutyric acid (GABA) and glycine, have been relatively ignored by psychologists, and there is practically no behavioral literature on the putative transmitters glutamate, aspartate, and taurine. As more is learned about these and other possible transmitters, it can be expected that they will be studied along with their precursors and metabolites.

TABLE 33.10.

Median step-through latencies in a one-trial avoidance task (sec)

Group	N	Before footshock	After footshock 1 hr	1 day	4 days
CPA + ECS	9	6.8	34.8	27.2	24.4
CPA	9	7.2	24.0	32.8	28.6
Saline + ECS	9	11.4	18.6*	12.6*	14.2*
Saline	9	12.2	50.2	41.4	33.6

The protective effect of p-chlorophenylalanine (PCPA or CPA) for amnesia caused by electroconvulsive shock (ECS). ECS caused amnesia at 1 hr, 1 day, and 4 days after passive-avoidance training (saline + ECS), but CPA blocked the amnesia at each of the retention tests.

*These values differ significantly from the saline controls (Mann-Whitney U Test).

Source: Riege (1971). Reprinted with the permission of Gordon and Breach Science Publishers, Inc.

REFERENCES

AGRANOFF, B. W. 1972. Effects of antibiotics in long-term memory formation in the goldfish. In W. K. Honig and P. H. James, eds., *Animal Memory*. New York: Academic Press, pp. 243–258.

AGRANOFF, B. W., DAVIS, R. E., and BRINK, J. J. 1966. Effects of puromycin, acetoxycycloheximide and actinomycin D on protein synthesis in goldfish brain. *Journal of Neurochemistry* 13: 899.

ALLEN, C., ALLEN, B. S., and RAKE, A. V. 1974. Pharmacological distinctions between "active" and "passive" avoidance memory formation as shown by manipulation of biogenic amine active compounds. *Psychopharmacologia (Berlin)* 34: 1–10.

ANDRY, D. K., and LUTTGES, M. W. 1972. Memory traces: Experimental separation by cycloheximide and electroconvulsive shock. *Science* 178: 518–520.

ANDRY, D. K., and LUTTGES, M. W. 1973. Time variables affecting the permanence of amnesia produced by combined cycloheximide and electroconvulsive shock treatments. *Pharmacology and Biochemistry of Behavior* 1: 301–306.

ANLEZARK, G. M., CROW, T. J., and GREENWAY, A. P. 1973. Impaired learning and decreased cortical norepinephrine after bilateral locus coeruleus lesions. *Science* 181: 682–684.

BARONDES, S. H. 1970. Some critical variables in studies of the effect of inhibitors of protein synthesis on memory. In W. L. Byrne, ed., *Molecular Approaches to Learning and Memory*. New York: Academic Press, pp. 27–34.

BARONDES, S. H., and COHEN, H. D. 1968. Memory impairment after subcutaneous injection of acetoxycycloheximide. *Science* 160: 556–557.

BARONDES, S. H., and JARVIK, M. E. 1964. The influence of actinomycin D on brain RNA synthesis and on memory. *Journal of Neurochemistry* 11: 187–195.

BOHUS, B. 1968. Pituitary ACTH release and avoidance behaviour of rats with cortisol implants in mesencephalic reticular formation and median eminence. *Neuroendocrinology* 3: 355–365.

BOHUS, B. 1973. Pituitary-adrenal influences on avoidance and approach behavior of the rat. In E. Zimmerman, W. H. Gispen, B. E. Marks, and D. de Wied, eds., *Progress in Brain Research*. Vol. 39: *Drug Effects on Neuroendocrine Regulation*. Amsterdam: Elsevier Scientific Publishing Company, pp. 407–420.

BOHUS, B., and DE WIED, D. 1966. Inhibitory and facilitatory effects of two related peptides on extinction of avoidance behavior. *Science* 153: 318–320.

BOTWINICK, C. Y., and QUARTERMAIN, D. 1974. Recovery from amnesia induced by pre-test injections of monoamine oxidase inhibitors. *Pharmacology, Biochemistry and Behavior* 2: 375–379.

BRODY, J. F. 1970. Behavioral effects of serotonin depletion and of p-chlorophenylalanine (serotonin depletion) in rats. *Psychopharmacologia (Berlin)* 17: 14–33.

BROWN, R., DAVIS, J. N., and CARLSSON, A. 1973. Dopa reversal of hypoxia-induced disruption of the conditioned avoidance response. *Journal of Pharmacy and Pharmacology (London)* 25: 412–414.

CAMERON, D. E., and SOLYOM, L. 1961. Effects of ribonucleic acid on memory. *Geriatrics* 16: 74–81.

CHERKIN, A., and LEE-TENG, E. 1965. Interruption by halothane of memory consolidation in chicks. *Federation Proceedings* 24: 328.

COHEN, H. D., and BARONDES, S. H. 1968. Effects of acetoxy-cycloheximide on learning and memory of a light-dark discrimination. *Nature* 218: 271–273.

COOK, L., DAVIDSON, A. B., DAVIS, D. J., GREEN, H., and FELLOWS, E. J. 1963. Ribonucleic acid: Effect on conditioned behavior in rats. *Science* 41: 268–269.

COOPER, B. R., BLACK, W. C., and PAOLINO, R. M. 1971. Decreased septal forebrain and lateral hypothalamic reward after alpha methyl-p-tyrosine. *Physiology and Behavior* 6: 425–429.

COOPER, B. R., GRANT, L. D., and BREESE, G. R. 1973. Comparison of the behavioral depressant effects of biogenic amine depleting and neuroleptic agents following various 6-hydroxydopamine treatments. *Psychopharmacologia (Berlin)* 31: 95–109.

COYLE, J. T., WENDER, P., and LIPSKY, A. 1973. Avoidance conditioning in different strains of rats: Neurochemical correlates. *Psychopharmacologia (Berlin)* 31: 25–34.

DAVIS, R. E., and KLINGER, P. D. 1969. Environmental control of amnestic effects of various agents in goldfish. *Physiology and Behavior* 4: 269–271.

DEUTSCH, J. A. 1969. The physiological basis of memory. *Annual Review of Psychology* 20: 85–104.

DE WIED, D. 1969. Effects of peptide hormones on behavior. In W. F. Ganong and L. Martin, eds., *Frontiers in Neuroendocrinology*. New York: Oxford University Press, pp. 97–140.

DE WIED, D. 1971. Long term effect of vasopressin on the maintenance of a conditioned avoidance response in rats. *Nature* 232: 58–60.

DE WIED, D. and BOHUS, B. 1966. Long term and short term effects on retention of a conditioned avoidance response in rats by treatment with long acting pitressin and α-MSH. *Nature* 212: 1484–1486.

DISMUKES, R. K., and RAKE, A. V. 1972. Involvement of biogenic amines in memory formation. *Psychopharmacologia (Berlin)* 23: 17–25.

FLOOD, J. F., BENNETT, E. L., ORME, A.E., and ROSENZWEIG, M. R. 1975a. Effects of protein synthesis inhibition on memory for active avoidance training. *Physiology and Behavior* 14: 177–184.

FLOOD, J. F., BENNETT, E. L., ORME, A. E., and ROSENZWEIG, M. R. 1975b. The relation of memory formation to controlled amounts of brain protein synthesis. *Physiology and Behavior* 15: 97–102.

FLOOD, J. F., BENNETT, E. L., ROSENZWEIG, M. R., and ORME, A. D. 1972. Influence of training strength on amnesia induced by pretraining injections of cycloheximide. *Physiology and Behavior* 9: 589–600.

FLOOD, J. F., BENNETT, E. L., ROSENZWEIG, M. R., and ORME, A. E. 1973. The influence of duration of protein synthesis inhibition on memory. *Physiology and Behavior* 10: 555–562.

FLOOD, J. F., BENNETT, E. L., ROSENZWEIG, M. R., and ORME, A. E. 1974. Comparison of the effects of anisomycin on memory across six strains of mice. *Behavioral Biology* 10: 147–160.

FUXE, K., and HANSON, L. C. F. 1967. Central catecholamine neurons and conditioned avoidance behavior. *Psychopharmacologia (Berlin)* 11: 439.

GARCIA, J., HANKINS, W., ROBINSON, J., and VOGT, J. 1972. Baitshyness: Tests of CS-US mediation. *Physiology and Behavior* 3: 807–810.

GELLER, A., ROBUSTELLI, F., BARONDES, S. H., COHEN, H. D., and JARVIK, M. E. 1969. Impaired performance by post-trial injections of cycloheximide in a passive avoidance task. *Psychopharmacologia (Berlin)* 14: 371–376.

GERVAI, J., and CSÁNYI, V. 1973. The effects of protein synthesis inhibitors in imprinting. *Brain Research* 53: 151–160.

GLICK, S. D., and ZIMMERBERG, B. 1972. Amnestic effects of scopolamine. *Behavioral Biology* 7 (2): 245–254.

GREENOUGH, W. T., YUWILER, A., and DOLLINGER, M. 1973. Effects of post-trial eserine administration on learning in "enriched"- and "impoverished"-reared rats. *Behavioral Biology* 8: 261–272.

GREVEN, H. M., and DE WIED, D. 1973. The influence of peptides derived from corticotrophin (ACTH) on performance, structure activity studies. In E. Zimmerman, W. H. Gispen, B. H. Marks, and D. de Wied, eds., *Progress in Brain Research*. Vol 39: *Drug Effects on Neuroendocrine Regulation*. Amsterdam: Elsevier Scientific Publishing Company, pp. 429–442.

HANSON, L. C. F. 1967. Evidence that the central action of (+)-amphetamine is mediated via catecholamines. *Psychopharmacologia (Berlin)* 10: 289.

JARVIK, M. E. 1972. Effects of chemical and physical treatments on learning and memory. *Annual Review of Psychology* 23: 457–486.

KETY, S. 1972. Brain catecholamines, affective states and memory. In J. McGaugh, ed., *The Chemistry of Mood, Motivation and Memory*. New York: Plenum Press, pp. 65–80.

KITSIKIS, A., ROBERGE, A. G., and FRENETTE, G. 1972. Effect of L-dopa on delayed response and visual discrimination in cats and its relation to brain chemistry. *Experimental Brain Research* 15: 305–317.

KOBILER, D., and ALLWEIS, C. 1974. The prevention of long-term memory formation by 2,6 diaminopurine. *Pharmacology, Biochemistry and Behavior* 2: 9–17.

LANDE, S., FLEXNER, J. B., and FLEXNER, L. B. 1972. Effect of corticotrophin and desglycinamide-lysine vasopressin on suppression on memory by puromycin. *Proceedings of the National Academy of Sciences (USA)* 69: 558–560.

LEWY, A. J., and SEIDEN, L. S. 1972. Operant behavior changes norepinephrine metabolism in rat brain. *Science* 175: 454–456.

McGAUGH, J. 1973. Drug facilitation of learning and memory. *Annual Review of Physiology* 13: 229–242.

MOORE, K. E., and RECH, R. 1967. Antagonism by monoamine oxidase inhibitors of alphamethyltyrosin induced catecholamine depletion and behavioral depression. *Journal of Pharmacology and Experimental Therapeutics* 156: 70–75.

NEALE, J. H., KLINGER, P. D., and AGRANOFF, B. W. 1973. Camptothecin blocks memory of conditioned avoidance in the goldfish. *Science* 179: 1243–1246.

OTT, T., and MATTHIES, H. 1973a. Some effects of RNA precursors on development and maintenance of long-term memory: Hippocampal and cortical pre- and post-training application of RNA precursors. *Psychopharmacologia (Berlin)* 28: 195–204.

OTT, T., and MATTHIES, H. 1973b. Suppression of uridine monophosphate-induced improvement in long-term storage by cycloheximide. *Psychopharmacologia (Berlin)* 28: 103–106.

POST, R. M., and GOODWIN, F. K. 1973. Simulated behavior states: An approach to specificity in psychobiological research. *Biological Psychiatry* 7: 237–254.

QUARTERMAIN, D., and BOTWINICK, C. Y. 1975. The role of

biogenic amines in the reversal of cycloheximide-induced amnesia. *Journal of Comparative and Physiological Psychology* 88: 386–401.

QUARTERMAIN, D., and McEWEN, B. S. 1970. Temporal characteristics of amnesia induced by protein synthesis inhibitor: Determination by shock level. *Nature* 228: 677–678.

QUARTERMAIN, D., McEWEN, B. S., and AZMITIA, JR., E. C. 1970. Amnesia produced by electroconvulsive shock or cycloheximide: Conditions for recovery. *Science* 169: 683–686.

RAHWAN, R. G. 1971. Chemical and pharmacological basis of learning and memory. *Agents and Actions: Swiss Journal of Pharmacology* 27: 87–102.

RAKE, A. V. 1973. Involvement of biogenic amines in memory formation: The central nervous system indole amine involvement. *Psychopharmacologia (Berlin)* 29: 91–100.

RANDT, C. T., KOREIN, J., and LEVIDOW, L. 1973. Localization of action of two amnesia producing drugs in freely moving mice. *Experimental Neurology* 41: 628–634.

RANDT, C. T., QUARTERMAIN, D., GOLDSTEIN, M., and ANAGNOSTE, B. 1971. Norepinephrine biosynthesis inhibition: Effects on memory in mice. *Science* 172: 498–499.

REINIŠ, S. 1971. Effects of 5-iodouracil and 2,6-diaminopurine on passive avoidance task. *Psychopharmacologia (Berlin)* 19: 34–39.

RIEGE, W. H. 1971. One-trial learning and brain serotonin depletion by parachlorophenylalanine. *International Journal of Neuroscience* 2: 237–240.

RIGTER, H., VAN RIEZEN, H., and DE WIED, D. 1974. The effects of ACTH—and vasopressin—analogues on CO$_2$-induced retrograde amnesia in rats. *Physiology and Behavior* 13: 381–388.

ROBERTS, R. B., and FLEXNER, L. B. 1969. The biochemical basis of long-term memory. *Quarterly Review of Biophysics* 2: 135–173.

RUF, K., and STEINER, F. A. 1967. Steroid-sensitive single neurons in rat hypothalamus and midbrain: Identification by microelectrophoresis. *Science* 156: 667–669.

SAPER, C. B., and SWEENEY, D. C. 1973. Enhanced appetitive discrimination learning in rats treated with alphamethyltyrosine. *Psychopharmacologia (Berlin)* 30: 37–44.

SCHLESINGER, K., SCHREIBER, R. A., and PRYOR, G. T. 1968. Effects of p-chlorophenylalanine on conditioned avoidance learning. *Psychonomic Science* 11: 225–226.

SEROTA, G. R., ROBERTS, R. B., and FLEXNER, L. B. 1972. Acetoxycycloheximide-induced transient amnesia: Protective effects of adrenergic stimulants. *Proceedings of the National Academy of Sciences (USA)* 2: 340–342.

SHARPLESS, S. K. 1964. Reorganization of function in the nervous system use and disuse. *Annual Review of Physiology* 26: 357–388.

SLUSHER, M. A., HYDE, J. E., and LAUFER, M. 1966. Effect of intracerebral hydrocortisone on unit activity of diencephalon and midbrain in cats. *Journal of Neurophysiology* 29: 157–169.

SPEAR, N. E. 1973. Retrieval of memory in animals. *Psychological Review* 80: 163–194.

SQUIRE, L. R., and BARONDES, S. H. 1972. Variable decay of memory and its recovery in cycloheximide-treated mice. *Proceedings of the National Academy of Sciences (USA)* 69: 1416–1420.

SQUIRE, L. R., and BARONDES, S. H. 1973. Memory impairment during prolonged training in mice given inhibitors of cerebral protein synthesis. *Brain Research* 56: 215–225.

SQUIRE, L. R., and BARONDES, S. H. 1974. Anisomycin, like other inhibitors of cerebral protein synthesis, impairs "long-term" memory of a discrimination task. *Brain Research* 66: 301–308.

SQUIRE, L. R., and BECKER, C. 1974. Protein synthesis inhibition impairs long-term habituation. *Society for Neurosciences, Fourth Annual Meeting* (St. Louis, 1974), Abstract 650, p. 433.

SQUIRE, L. R., EMANUEL, C. A., DAVIS, H. P., and DEUTSCH, J. A. 1975. Inhibition of cerebral protein synthesis: Dissociation of aversive and amnesic effects. *Behavioral Biology* (in press).

SQUIRE, L. R., SMITH, G. A., and BARONDES, S. H. 1973. Cycloheximide affects memory within minutes after the onset of training. *Nature* 242: 201–202.

STEIN, L. 1971. Neurochemistry of reward and punishment: Some implications for the etiology of schizophrenia. *Journal of Psychiatric Research* 8: 345–361.

TENEN, S. S. 1967. The effects of p-chlorophenylalanine, a serotonin depletor, on avoidance acquisition, pain sensitivity, and related behavior in the rat. *Psychopharmacologia (Berlin)* 10: 204–219.

THOMPSON, R. F., PATTERSON, M. M., and TEYLER, T. J. 1972. The neurophysiology of learning. *Annual Review of Psychology* 23: 73–104.

UNGERER, A. 1973. Nature et ampleur des effets de l'acétoxycycloheximide sur la retention d'un apprentissage instrumental chez la souris. *Physiology and Behavior* 11: 323–327.

UNGERSTEDT, U. 1974. Brain dopamine neurons and behavior. in F. O. Schmitt and F. G. Worden, eds., *The Neurosciences: Third Study Program.* Cambridge, Mass.: MIT Press, pp. 979–988.

VAN WIMERSMA GREIDANUS, TJ. B., and DE WIED, D. 1971. Effects of systemic and intracerebral administration of two opposite acting ACTH-related peptides on extinction of conditioned avoidance behavior. *Neuroendocrinology* 7: 291–301.

WATTS, M. E., and MARK, R. F. 1970. The initiation of memory. *Proceedings of the Australian Physiological and Pharmacological Society* 1: 26.

WATTS, M. E., and MARK, R. F. 1971. Separate actions of ouabain and cycloheximide on memory. *Brain Research* 25: 420–423.

WEISS, J. M., McEWEN, B. S., WILVA, M. T., and KALKUT, M. 1970. Pituitary-adrenal alterations and fear responding. *American Journal of Physiology* 218: 864–868.

34

The Influence of Drugs on Learning and Memory

DAVID QUARTERMAIN

ABSTRACT Two general issues relevant to the interpretation of drug effects on memory and learning are briefly discussed. The first concerns the frequently encountered difficulty of evaluating the nonspecific effects of drugs, such as activity changes or illness and debilitation. An experimental procedure that includes a built-in control for such side effects is described. The second general point concerns the need for systematic variation of training and testing parameters in order to characterize the full range of effects that a particular drug may have on learning and memory.

The effect of protein-synthesis inhibition on memory is then discussed in detail. Experiments are reviewed which show that the amnesic effects of cycloheximide are blocked by increases in training strength. It is concluded that retention is impaired only when habits are learned to a low level of mastery. The issue of the permanence of amnesia following protein-synthesis inhibition is reviewed. Evidence indicates that in many cases memory may recover spontaneously or recovery may be induced by pharmacological manipulations. It is suggested that since amnesias are often temporary and since posttraining cycloheximide treatments can induce anmesia, the memory deficit can be most readily accounted for in terms of an impairment of retrieval mechanisms. However, in view of the limited training conditions under which retrieval deficits can be produced, protein synthesis may play a less important role in memory than has been commonly believed.

Finally, the role of the biogenic amines in memory is briefly discussed. Compounds that deplete brain catecholamines induce temporary amnesias only for poorly learned habits. In this respect, they closely resemble cycloheximide-induced amnesias.

34.1 INTRODUCTION

Before discussing some specific issues raised by Flood and Jarvik's review, I would like to make two general points relevant to the interpretation of studies in which drugs are used either to impair or to enhance learning and memory. The first concerns the evaluation of side effects. The fact that drugs have a number of effects besides the ones usually studied is well recognized but is frequently ignored in practice. Two examples will highlight some of the problems that nonspecific drug effects present for the analysis of memory.

Inhibitors of protein synthesis have complex effects on locomotor activity, and it is frequently difficult to be sure whether a drug is directly affecting learning or retention or merely changing activity levels. It has been shown, for instance, that pretraining injections of cycloheximide (Cyclo) induce amnesia when retention is tested as early as one minute after one-trial, passive-avoidance training (Quartermain and McEwen, 1970). Such findings suggest that Cyclo may be influencing short-term memory, but the short step-out latencies could be an artifact resulting from Cyclo's general enhancement of activity (Squire, Geller, and Jarvik, 1970). Inclusion of control groups to evaluate the influence of activity changes is necessary in order to characterize adequately the effect of Cyclo on short-term memory. A number of recent studies have included such controls and have concluded that Cyclo's effects on locomotor activity are separate from its effects on short-term memory (Segal, Squire, and Barondes, 1971; Gutwein, Quartermain, and McEwen, 1974). Activity changes are a potential source of confusion in all drug-behavior studies, and appropriate controls need to be included for their evaluation.

The fact that all drugs are potentially capable of inducing illness or general debilitation introduces similar problems. Many of the protein-synthesis inhibitors, for example, are highly toxic and are administered in relatively high doses, so that animals may be sick in varying degrees during learning or at the time of testing. Flood and Jarvik (this volume) have suggested that illness might account for the transient amnesia following Cyclo administration found by some investigators (Quartermain and McEwen, 1970; Serota, Roberts, and Flexner, 1972; Squire and Barondes, 1972). It is clear that adequate controls must be included to evaluate the role of drug-induced illness in amnesia and recovery from amnesia. This is an especially important consideration in experiments where memory blockade typically results in diminished responding.

An experimental procedure has recently been developed in our laboratory which is designed to study the effects of protein-synthesis inhibition on memory and which includes a built-in control for the effects of illness or general debilitation (Quartermain and Botwinick, 1975a). This procedure has been applied to both position- and brightness-discrimination tasks motivated by food reward and by shock avoidance. Briefly, the procedure

DAVID QUARTERMAIN, Departments of Neurology and Physiology, New York University School of Medicine, New York, NY

is as follows. Thirty minutes after drug treatment, animals are trained to go to either the right or the left (or to the bright or the dark side of a maze) to obtain food or avoid shock. Retention is tested 24 hr later. If animals are retrained to the same side that was reinforced the previous day, saline control animals show good retention and Cyclo-treated animals show amnesia, that is, no savings. If, however, the retention test consists of a reversal to the side opposite that rewarded on training, the Cyclo-treated mice now perform significantly better than the saline controls, presumably because the amnesia has eliminated the source of proactive interference. Typical data from both approach and avoidance experiments are shown in Table 34.1. These data indicate that Cyclo produces a true amnesia and thus clearly eliminate the possibility that sickness, general debilitation, or inability to relearn the task are responsible for the typical performance decrement.

The use of this reversal procedure is also a good control for general enhancement of learning ability or motivation, which becomes a relevant consideration in experiments that purport to demonstrate a recovery from amnesia induced by pharmacological manipulations. For example, Serota, Roberts, and Flexner (1972) have shown that drugs that increase the activity of the catecholaminergic neuron, such as imipramine, d-amphetamine, and tranylcyproamine, restore memory loss due to puromycin and acetoxycycloheximide (AXM)

TABLE 34.1

Mean trials to criterion for initial discrimination and reversal in mice treated with cycloheximide or saline

		Mean trials to criterion		
	N	Initial discrimination	Retest, same side	Retest, reversal
Shock avoidance, Y maze, brightness discrimination				
Cyclo	12	8.8	9.9	7.6
Saline	12	9.5	8.0	10.7
Appetitive incentive, T maze, spatial discrimination				
Cyclo	10	28.7	29.1	26.2
Saline	11	28.3	27.2	30.2

Mice were trained to a criterion of 4 correct avoidances or escapes, or 17 correct appetitive discriminations. Cyclo or saline was injected 30 min before the initial discrimination, and animals were reversed 24 hr after initial training. Typical scores for mice retested to the side reinforced during the initial discrimination are given for comparison.

administration. These authors, however, fail to demonstrate conclusively that the enhanced performance represents a recovery of memory rather than a general improvement in relearning. We have recently used the reversal procedure to test for recovery of memory. Cyclo-treated animals who show improved performance following pretest injections of monoamine oxidase inhibitors (MAOIs) and amphetamine when the retention test consists of relearning the original discrimination, show impaired performance when the retention test is a reversal to the opposite side. This shows that the drugs are recovering some part of the memory of the original discrimination, rather than generally enhancing learning or motivation.

The second point I would like to discuss concerns the dependence of drug effects on the particular training and testing parameters employed. One major determinant of the effects of drugs on memory is the strength of the habit at the time of drug treatment. For example, it has been demonstrated that treatment with imipramine results in retention decrements only in cases where the habit is well learned (Leftoff, 1973). On the other hand, there is evidence (to be discussed in Sections 34.2 and 34.3) that amnesias induced by protein-synthesis inhibition or depletion of biogenic amines can be blocked by increases in training strength. Although these amnesias are often fragile, in that they can be antagonized by relatively minor changes in training variables, highly reliable amnesic effects can be obtained through the selection of appropriate training parameters (Quartermain and Botwinick, 1975a; Flood et al., 1972).

Since habit strength generally varies with time following learning, the age of the habit at the time of drug treatment is an important consideration. Drugs that fail to disrupt memory when injected before or immediately after training, may produce amnesia if they are administered at a later time when the habit has been weakened by normal forgetting. For example, it has been recently shown that in a particular experimental paradigm, Cyclo is not effective when injected immediately or 3 days after training, but produces amnesia when injected 6 days after training (Quartermain and Botwinick, 1975b). Furthermore, the same drug may either block or facilitate memory, depending on the age of the habit. Deutsch (1971) has shown that the anticholinesterase drug di-isopropyl fluorophosphate (DFP) produces amnesia for a 14-day-old memory, but facilitates the recall of a 28-day-old memory. There is also recent evidence that the MAOI pheniprazine can induce amnesia in a 1-day-old memory, but facilitates a 7-day-old memory (Quartermain and Botwinick, 1975a, b). These data indicate that the influence of a particular drug on memory depends on a number of training and testing parameters. This points up the need for systematic variation of both training parameters and treatment-to-training intervals in order to discover the full range of effects that a particular drug may have on memory and learning.

34.2 PROTEIN-SYNTHESIS INHIBITION AND MEMORY

34.2.1 The role of habit strength

One of the most striking behavioral characteristics of protein-synthesis inhibitors is that they do not produce amnesia in well-trained or even moderately well trained animals. Although there are some data (mostly from experiments employing intracerebral puromycin) showing that amnesia can occur when animals are trained in a discrimination task to a criterion of 9 out of 10 correct choices (e.g., Flexner, Flexner, and Roberts, 1967; Flexner and Flexner, 1967, 1968, 1969), the majority of studies employing Cyclo or AXM as protein-synthesis inhibitors have found that much lower criteria are necessary to obtain amnesia (e.g., 3 out of 4 in Cohen and Barondes, 1968; 4 out of 5 in Daniels, 1971; 5 out of 6 in Barondes and Cohen, 1968b).

We have recently studied the effect of changes in training strength on the magnitude of Cyclo-induced amnesia for a shock-avoidance brightness-discrimination response in a Y maze (Gutwein and Quartermain, in preparation). Table 34.2 shows that no amnesia occurs when animals are trained to a criterion of 7 out of 10 or

9 out of 10. With a criterion of 6 out of 7 there is a significant difference between the percent savings in Cyclo- and saline-injected animals, but the percent savings in the Cyclo group is relatively high. Substantial amnesia begins to occur with a criterion of 3 out of 4 correct. The greatest magnitude of amnesia, in terms of the lowest percent savings, occurs in the group trained to a criterion of any 4 correct. The number of trials to reach this criterion also shows less variability than the number to reach the other criteria tested.

Similar data have been reported by Quartermain and Botwinick (1975a) for an appetitively motivated position-discrimination task. The basic procedure consisted of training on the inital right-left discrimination on day 1. Cyclo and saline treatment was given on day 2, 30 minutes before a reversal to the side opposite that rewarded on day 1. Relearning to criterion was carried out on day 3. Initial exploratory data indicated that the magnitude of amnesia was greatest if animals were given 20 trials on day 1 followed by a reversal on day 2 until they had attained a total of 17 correct choices. Table 34.3 shows the effects of some of the possible variations in day-1 training on the magnitude of amnesia observed on day 3. Groups 1 and 2 confirm the exploratory data and indicate that this combination of training and reversal conditions produces a marked amnesia which is highly reliable and characteristically low in variability. Of the several hundred mice we have trained using these parameters, less than 5 percent have failed to show total amnesia. Table 34.3 indicates that increasing or decreasing amount of day-1 training influences the magnitude of amnesia. Eliminating the 20 trials on day 1 reduces the amnesic effect, while increasing amount of training (Group 7) obliterates the amnesia entirely. Apparently, the 20 trials on day 1 proactively interfere with day-2 reversal learning to a sufficient degree to make it optimally susceptible to disruption by Cyclo. We have recently shown that a substantial amnesia can be obtained when the 20 trials on day 1 are eliminated if the day-2 reversal-training criterion is reduced to 10 correct choices rather than 17. Although the reversal is not a necessary condition for the production of amnesia in this task, its use results in a greater magnitude of amnesia and less variability than can be produced by any other training procedure we have yet tried.

Variations in amount of training on the day Cyclo is administered (day 2) also influence the magnitude of amnesia. If no day-2 training is given, no amnesia results. Figure 34.1 shows the effects of allowing mice to make 9, 17, or 35 correct responses on day 2, day-1 training being held constant at 20 trials. It can be seen from 34.1 that Cyclo-treated animals have significantly poorer savings scores than saline controls at all criterion

TABLE 34.2

Mean trials to criterion for different training criteria in a shock-avoidance brightness-discrimination task.

Training criterion	Treatment	Mean trials to criterion Training	Test	Mean % savings*
Any 4	Cyclo	8.5	9.9	−10
	saline	9.8	8.0	29
3 out of 4	Cyclo	17.4	17.4	0
	saline	15.4	12.1	26
5 out of 6	Cyclo	18.1	13.3	37
	saline	20.2	10.3	67
6 out of 7	Cyclo	17.4	12.6	40
	saline	18.4	7.9	81
7 out of 10	Cyclo	25.8	11.3	77
	saline	24.4	9.4	86
9 out of 10	Cyclo	41.8	13.8	84
	saline	42.2	13.7	86

*Percent savings is calculated by the formula $100 \times (R - T)/(R - C)$, where R is number of trials to reach criterion on the reversal day, T is number of trials to criterion on the test day, and C is criterion.

TABLE 34.3
Effect on the magnitude of amnesia of variations in the amount of training on the initial position discrimination in a T-maze reversal task

| Group | N | Treatment | Day 1 | Day 2* | Day 3** | Mean trials to criterion | | Percent savings† |
						Reversal day	Test day	
1	10	Cyclo	20 trials	reverse to 17 correct trials	test reversal	28.2	28.8	−5
2	10	saline	20 trials	reverse to 17 correct trials	test reversal	26.1	22.5	40
3	17	Cyclo	no training	17 correct trials	test	29.9	28.9	6
4	17	saline	no training	17 correct trials	test	29.2	27.6	13
5	11	Cyclo	20 trials	no training	reverse to 17 correct trials	28.9	24.2	28
6	10	saline	20 trials	no training	reverse to 17 correct trials	28.9	24.5	37
7	9	Cyclo	17 correct trials	reverse to 17 correct trials	test reversal	28.6	26.6	16
8	9	saline	17 correct trials	reverse to 17 correct trials	test reversal	28.2	26.1	18

*Cyclo was administered 30 min before training on day 2.
**Groups 5 and 6 were tested for retention of the reversal on day 4 instead of day 3.
†See note to Table 34.2.

levels, but the magnitude of the amnesia is greatest by far with the 17-correct criterion.

The training variable that most decisively eliminates the amnesic effect of Cyclo in this task is an increase in the intertrial interval (ITI) (Quartermain and Botwinick, 1975a). Using the optimal number of trials (20 on day 1, 17 correct discriminations on day 2), good amnesia occurs if animals are reversed with a 30-sec ITI, but no amnesia at all occurs if the ITI during reversal is 80 sec. Apparently, ITI during training is the critical variable, since mice trained with a 30-sec ITI and tested with an 80-sec ITI show amnesia. The basis of this effect is probably an increase in training strength that results from distributed practice.

I have described the effects of varying training parameters at some length because they clearly indicate the fragile nature of Cyclo-induced amnesia. The demonstration that all but the weakest habits can be stored and retrieved despite greater than 90 percent inhibition of protein synthesis during training indicates that Cyclo is effective in blocking only a narrow class of memories. Evidence to be presented in Section 34.2.2 demonstrates that in most cases where Cyclo does produce amnesia, the memory can be recovered. The temporary nature of

the amnesia, coupled with the narrow range of training conditions under which it can be produced, seems to suggest a somewhat diminished role for protein synthesis as a general mechanism involved in the storage and retrieval of memory.

It is, however, possible that a greater duration of protein-synthesis inhibition than commonly results from a single pretraining injection is necessary to produce more robust and durable effects of Cyclo on memory

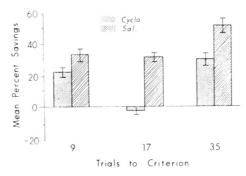

FIGURE 34.1 Mean percent savings for mice reversed to a criterion of 9, 17, or 35 correct discriminations 30 min following Cyclo or saline injection. All animals were given 20 trials on day 1. N = 15 in each group.

processes. We have recently completed an experiment designed to test the effects of long durations of protein-synthesis inhibition on memory in a multiple-trial task in the T maze. The experiment was designed to determine whether increasing the duration of protein-synthesis inhibition prior to learning could overcome the effect of increasing the ITI to 80 sec. Extending the duration of protein-synthesis inhibition prior to learning should result in a greater net depletion of functional proteins, some of which might be involved in the registration stage of memory storage.

Animals were initially injected with 2.5 mg of anisomycin (Ani), and every 2 hr for the next 8 hr they were given a further 0.5-mg injection of Ani. Control animals were injected with saline. Based on data by Flood et al. (1973b), this schedule of injections results in approximately 85 percent inhibition of protein synthesis for an 8-hr period. All animals were trained 15 min after the final injection. An ITI of 80 sec was employed, and animals were run until they had achieved a criterion of 17 correct discriminations. Mean trials to criterion on training were not significantly different for the two groups. When animals were retrained 24 hr later, there was no evidence of amnesia in the Ani-treated group. Mean trials to criterion on the test day was 23.0 for the Ani mice and 22.5 for the saline controls. These data indicate that increasing the duration of protein-synthesis inhibition prior to training does not counteract the effects of increased habit strength. On the other hand, Flood et al. (1973) have shown that multiple post-training injections of Ani can counter the effects of increases in training strength in a one-trial, passive-avoidance task, and it is possible that sustained posttraining inhibition of protein synthesis might be similarly effective in overcoming the effects of the increased ITIs in the present discrimination task.

34.2.2 Permanence of amnesia

Considerable controversy surrounds the issue of whether amnesias induced by protein-synthesis inhibitors are permanent. Several studies have failed to demonstrate recovery of memory following Cyclo treatment (Flood et al., 1972; Barondes and Cohen, 1967), but there are a sufficient number of studies in which recovery occurs spontaneously or can be induced by reminder shock or pharmacological manipulation to indicate that at least some of the amnesias induced by protein-synthesis inhibition are temporary (Squire and Barondes, 1972; Quartermain and Botwinick, 1975a; Serota, 1971; Botwinick and Quartermain, 1974; Quartermain, McEwen, and Azmitia, 1972). In this section I propose to describe some experiments in which recovery of memory can unequivocally be shown to occur and to outline some

of the conditions under which this recovery appears to take place.

Spontaneous recovery from Cyclo-induced amnesia has been demonstrated for both food-motivated and shock-avoidance multiple-trial tasks. Squire and Barondes (1972) have shown a spontaneous recovery of memory, for a multiple-trial, shock-avoidance task, that is practically complete by 3 days after training. Serota (1971) has also demonstrated that intracerebral AXM reliably produces amnesia in rats 24 hr after training, but that memory spontaneously recovers within 6 days. In neither of these studies does drug-induced illness appear to account for the amnesia.

Figure 34.2 shows recovery from amnesia in a food-rewarded position-discrimination task in a T maze (Quartermain and Botwinick, 1975a). Animals were trained using the optimum conditions for the production of amnesia in this task, described in Section 34.2.1. Cyclo was injected 30 min before reversal training on day 2. Different groups of mice were tested 24, 36, and 48 hr after training. Figure 34.2 shows that substantial recovery had occurred at 36 hr and that by 48 hr there was a total recovery from the amnesia. Sickness cannot account for these data since it has been shown that Cyclo-treated animals tested at 24 hr perform significantly better than saline controls if the retention test is a second reversal.

The variables that determine spontaneous recovery from amnesia remain largely unspecified. In the multiple-trial studies reviewed above, no environmental triggering was necessary to induce recovery. There is, however, some evidence that in a one-trial, passive-avoidance task, recovery may not occur until animals are reexposed to the training situation (Quartermain, McEwen, and Azmitia, 1972; Herz and Peeke, 1967). Also, there is some suggestion that spontaneous recovery is more common in multiple-trial, than in single-trial, passive-avoidance tasks, but this remains to be carefully

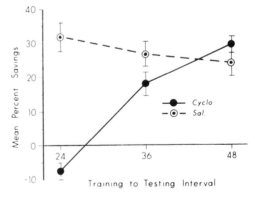

FIGURE 34.2 Mean percent savings scores for groups tested 24 ($N_C = 10$; $N_S = 10$), 36 ($N_C = 20$; $N_S = 19$), and 48 hrs ($N_C = 20$; $N_S = 19$) following training.

investigated. One variable that may determine recovery is the completeness of the induced amnesia. It has been argued (Cherkin, 1972; Gold et al., 1973) that a noncontingent reminder shock is effective in inducing recovery only if the amnesia is incomplete. Evidence against this proposition as an explanation for spontaneous recovery comes from the results shown in Figure 34.2. Cyclo-treated mice trained under optimal conditions and tested at 24 hr routinely show complete amnesia (i.e., zero or negative savings). Despite this, recovery always occurs in this task.

It is possible that the occasional failure of Cyclo to produce permanent amnesia may be the result of an insufficient duration of protein-synthesis inhibition. We have some preliminary data on the effects of sustaining protein-synthesis inhibition for an 8-hr period prior to training by repeated injections of Ani. Animals were trained using the optimal conditions for the production of amnesia in this task described above. On day 2 injections of Ani and saline were scheduled as described in the last section. Half of the animals were tested at 24 hr and the remaining half at 48 hr after training. The repeated injections of Ani produced amnesia 24 hr after training (7 percent savings, as opposed to 21.6 percent for saline controls), but considerable recovery had occurred by 48 hr (Ani, 16 percent; saline, 25 percent). These data do not encourage the view that extending the duration of inhibition prior to training can prevent spontaneous recovery of memory. We are currently investigating the effect of increasing the duration of protein-synthesis inhibition following training on spontaneous recovery.

Recent evidence indicates that recovery of memory following protein-synthesis inhibition can be induced pharmacologically. Roberts, Flexner, and Flexner (1970) and Serota, Roberts, and Flexner (1972) have shown that adrenergic stimulants can induce memory recovery following puromycin and AXM treatment in a multiple-trial, shock-avoidance task. Botwinick and Quartermain (1974) have shown that Cyclo-induced amnesia for a one-trial, passive-avoidance response can be reversed by pretest injections of two MAOIs, pheniprazine and pargyline.

The interpretation of these findings, however, is not clear. In cases where stimulants are administered shortly before retention testing, it is necessary to show that the enhanced performance is not a reflection of either enhanced ability to learn the task or increased motivation. Not all of the studies have included adequate controls for this possibility. Botwinick and Quartermain (1974) did include a control group that was given Cyclo and a noncontingent footshock. These mice failed to show increased latencies following pretest treatment with MAOIs, and this indicates that the recovery was specific

to animals trained in the passive-avoidance apparatus. However, none of the studies has controlled for the possibility that the pharmacological agents that induce recovery might nonspecifically enhance performance on any poorly learned response. As Flood and Jarvik point out in their review, this possibility must be controlled for by the inclusion of poorly trained saline-treated animals.

Two recent studies have included control groups to evaluate the role of drug-induced enhancement of learning and motivation and the possibility of nonspecific drug enhancement of a weak habit. Quartermain and Botwinick (1975a) have shown that the amnesia that occurs under optimal training conditions in the T maze can be reversed by injecting pheniprazine or pargyline 1–2 hr before the retention test on day 3 (see Figure 34.3). In order to control for enhanced learning ability, an additional group of mice was injected with pheniprazine but given a second reversal. We noted previously that with this testing procedure, Cyclo-injected animals perform significantly better than saline controls. Thus, if the MAOIs are recovering memory, Cyclo mice treated with pheniprazine should perform more poorly on the second reversal than Cyclo mice treated with saline. Results confirmed this prediction. The mean trials to criterion on the retention test was 26.25 for the Cyclo-saline group and 27.60 for the Cyclo-pheniprazine group ($p < 0.02$). This result would seem to rule out the possibility that MAOI treatments are merely acting as general enhancers of performance.

In a second study (Quartermain and Botwinick, 1975b) saline-treated mice were trained to a criterion of either 5 or 9 correct choices on the reversal day (the standard criterion is 17 correct discriminations) and injected with pheniprazine 1 hr before the retention test, which was either the regular test to the same side as training or a second reversal to the opposite side. These

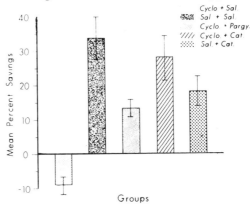

FIGURE 34.3 Mean percent savings scores for Cyclo and saline groups treated with the MAOIs catron (pheniprazine·HCl) and pargyline. Ns are, from left to right, 28, 18, 14, 13, and 17.

groups were designed to evaluate the possibility that pheniprazine would nonspecifically enhance the performance of poorly trained control animals. Table 34.4 shows the results of this experiment. It is clear that there is no tendency for pheniprazine to enhance performance on either training criterion. These data suggest that pheniprazine acts to improve the retrieval of memories temporarily blocked by protein-synthesis inhibition.

These experiments with MAOIs, along with the studies of Flexner and his associates, suggest the involvement of the biogenic amines in Cyclo-induced amnesia. The exact role that they play is, however, not clear. Serota, Roberts, and Flexner (1972) believe that protein-synthesis inhibitors may be producing their amnesic effects by reducing the amount of available norepinephrine (NE). They propose that NE released during training facilitates networks of synapses that are associated with training and that, during testing, released NE reactivates this previously facilitated network. Treatment with protein-synthesis inhibitors such as Cyclo or AXM may reduce the rate of NE release so that, 24 hr after learning, insufficient quantities are available to facilitate retrieval. By day 6 the NE system has recovered and the memory can be retrieved.

Direct evidence in support of this hypothesis is meager. There are some data indicating that both Cyclo and AXM inhibit the activity of tyrosine hydroxylase (Flexner, Serota, and Goodman, 1973). However, the inhibitory effects were relatively small, and considerable recovery had begun to occur 4 hr after treatment. It would appear unlikely from these data that the NE system would be inhibited 24 hr after Cyclo treatment. It should, however, be pointed out that these biochem-

TABLE 34.4
Mean trials to criterion on training and testing for two undertrained saline groups treated with catron before testing

Group	N	Treatment	Training criterion	Mean trials to criterion— day 1	Mean trials to criterion— day 2
1*	7	saline	5	9.3	7.1
2*	7	catron	5	9.3	7.0
3*	7	saline	9	16.6	12.3
4*	7	catron	9	16.4	12.3
5**	7	saline	5	9.3	7.6
6**	7	catron	5	9.0	7.1
7**	7	saline	9	16.6	13.7
8**	7	catron	9	16.7	13.3

*Animals is groups 1–4 were retrained to the same side that had been rewarded in the initial training.
**Animals in groups 5–8 were reveresd to the side opposite that rewarded initially.

ical data were obtained from large samples of cerebral hemisphere, and it is possible that specific regions critical for memory retrieval may have been more profoundly depleted. More recent preliminary data (Flexner and Goodman, personal communication) indicate that amnestic doses of AXM, Cyclo, Ani, and puromycin significantly inhibit rates of synthesis of both NE and dopamine in the first 3 hr following treatment.

It is possible, of course, that adrenergic compounds induce memory recovery by virtue of their role as general CNS stimulants rather than through restoration of functional levels of amine stores, as seems to be suggested by the Flexners' hypothesis. For example, Barondes and Cohen (1968a) have shown that Cyclo-induced amnesia can be prevented by brief footshock, amphetamine, and corticosteroids if these treatments are administered 3 hr after training. They interpret these findings to mean that stimuli that produce generalized arousal can establish long-term memory. This recovery from amnesia fails to occur if the treatments are given 6 hr after training, by which time, Barondes and Cohen suggest, short-term memory has terminated and long-term memory has begun. The reminder-shock experiments also suggest a role for CNS arousal in the recovery of memory. These studies (Quartermain, McEwen, and Azmitia, 1970, 1972) indicate that a brief footshock administered outside the training apparatus can reverse Cyclo-induced amnesia.

It is also possible that treatments that increase arousal induce recovery by increasing functional levels of brain catecholamines or by increasing the rate of release or utilization of catecholamines. Further biochemical studies on both enzyme activity and rate of turnover of catecholamines will be necessary if the role played by depletion of biogenic amines in the induction of Cyclo-induced amnesia is to be adequately characterized.

34.2.3 Storage versus retrieval deficit

Previous studies have attempted to account for the impairment of memory after Cyclo treatment in terms of interference with the formation of long-term memory (Barondes and Cohen, 1967) However, recent experiments that have shown clear evidence of spontaneous or induced memory recovery following amnesia have directed attention to the possibility that an impairment of retrieval rather than storage mechanisms may underlie the memory deficit following protein-synthesis inhibition. The major difficulty with a strict retrieval interpretation of amnesia is that protein-synthesis inhibitors are usually ineffective when administered after learning. If the memory deficit is just the result of an impairment of retrieval, Cyclo administered 30 min before and 30 min after training should be equally effective in producing amnesia. Evidence clearly indicates that this is not the case. Squire and Barondes (1972) argue that the ineffectiveness of posttraining Cyclo treatments compels the conclusion that temporary amnesia is due to a specific impairment in memory-storage processes. In order to account for memory recovery following Cyclo-induced amnesia, they postulate a discrete memory process that develops gradually in the days following training.

It may not, however, be necessary to postulate the existence of such a mechanism in order to account for recovery of memory following Cyclo-induced amnesia. It is possible that the dependence of amnesia on pretraining Cyclo treatment (which is the basis for the belief that a specific storage impairment is involved) is an artifact resulting from Cyclo's peculiar sensitivity to increases in training strength. Material reviewed in Section 34.2.1 has indicated that relatively small increases in the strength of a habit can antagonize the amnesic effects of Cyclo. Since in multiple-trial tasks habit strength is increasing during training and may increase for some hours thereafter (Jaffard et al., 1974), the posttraining habit may have increased in strength beyond the point where it can be significantly influenced by Cyclo treatment. Thus posttraining Cyclo may be ineffective because of the inability of the drug to overcome increased habit strength, rather than because the memory trace has passed into a storage state where it is no longer vulnerable to disruption. This proposition differs from conventional consolidation interpretations in that it regards the resistance of the posttraining habit to amnesia as temporary; any reduction in the strength of the posttraining habit brought about either by extinction or by allowing forgetting to occur should permit Cyclo to disrupt the memory.

We have recently attempted to test this hypothesis by using normal forgetting as a means of weakening the posttraining habit. Mice were trained in a T maze for a food reward using the procedure and training parameters previously described. Groups of mice were injected with Cyclo or saline 30 min before training ($N_C = 10$, $N_S = 10$), or immediately ($N_C = 16$, $N_S = 15$), 3 days ($N_C = 15$, $N_S = 14$), 6 days ($N_C = 23$, $N_S = 19$), or 9 days ($N_C = 9$, $N_S = 11$) after training. All animals were tested 24 hr after drug treatment. The results are shown in Figure 34.4. It can be seen that no amnesia occurred in groups injected immediately or 3 days after training. However, the group injected with Cyclo 6 days following training and tested on day 7 show a marked amnesia. This finding has been replicated on several occasions and appears to be a robust phenomenon. The amnesia can also be reversed by treatment with the MAOI pheniprazine administered 1 hr before the retention test on day 7 (Figure 34.4). These data suggest that amnesias

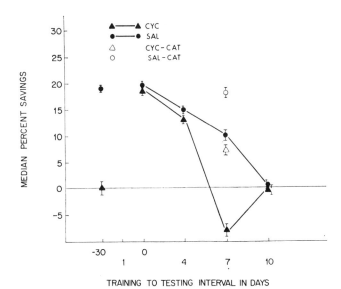

FIGURE 34.4 Median percent savings for the groups injected with Cyclo or saline at various times before and after training. Animals were tested at times indicated on the abscissa. Cyclo and saline were injected 24 hr before testing. Two groups were tested 1 day following training: one group was injected 30 min before training and the other immediately after. The effect of injection of the MAOI catron on saline- and Cyclo-treated mice is also shown. Cyclo and saline were injected on day 6 and catron 1 hr before retention test on day 7.

may be routinely produced with posttraining Cyclo administration if habit strength is reduced before drug treatment. Such a conclusion would in turn suggest that a pure retrieval deficit may underlie all Cyclo-induced amnesias.

It thus appears that although memory storage is independent of cerebral protein synthesis, the normal operation of retrieval mechanisms is not. Transient impairment of retrieval processes may be the result of metabolic disturbances, which lead to a deficiency in the synthesis of enzymes required for neurotransmitter functions. The recovery from such metabolic disturbances may underlie the recovery of memory following amnesia. It should be remembered, however, that these retrieval deficits occur for a very narrow range of memories: those that are weakly represented in the nervous system or that have been poorly learned. Retrieval of the great majority of well-learned responses is unaffected by profound inhibition of cerebral protein synthesis.

34.3 THE ROLE OF THE BIOGENIC AMINES IN MEMORY

Much recent theory and research has centered around the possible role of the biogenic amines in learning and memory. The experimental literature, which is rapidly increasing in this area, has been well reviewed in Flood and Jarvik's chapter. I would like to comment on several aspects of this research.

It is of interest that catecholamine-depleting compounds have behavioral effects similar to those shown by protein-synthesis inhibitors such as Cyclo. For example, both α-methyl-p-tyrosine (AMPT), which inhibits tyrosine hydroxylase activity, and diethyldithiocarbamate (DDC) which inhibits dopamine-β-hydroxylase activity produce amnesia only when the habit is poorly learned (Quartermain and Botwinick, 1975a,b). Neither of these drugs influences retention of well-learned or even moderately well learned habits. Figure 34.5 shows an example of this. It has been previously demonstrated that increasing the number of correct discriminations in the T maze on the reversal day from 17 to 35 greatly attenuates the amnesic effect of Cyclo. Figure 34.5 shows that this is also true for AMPT and DDC. We also have data indicating that increasing the training intertrial interval to 80 sec eliminates the amnesic effects of DDC and AMPT in the same way as it does with Cyclo (Quartermain and Botwinick, unpublished data).

Amnesias resulting from inhibition of NE biosynthesis show spontaneous recovery in the appetitive T-maze task. Figure 34.6 indicates that amnesia induced by pretraining injections of two inhibitors of dopamine-β-hydroxylase, DDC and bis-(4-methyl-1-homopiperazinylthiocarbonyl)-disulfide (FLA-63), shows spontaneous recovery 48 hr after learning. It can be shown by the use of appropriate control groups that drug-induced illness cannot account for the spontaneous recovery.

The effects of longer durations of NE inhibition have also recently been studied (Quartermain, Botwinick, Freedman, and Hallock, in preparation). In order to produce a sustained inhibition of dopamine-β-hydroxylase activity, mice were given two injections of DDC (250 mg/kg) 12 hr apart. We had previously shown (Randt et al., 1970) that a single injection of DDC produces a marked inhibition of dopamine-β-hydroxylase (as measured by conversion of [14C]dopamine to [14C]norepinephrine), which is still apparent $8\frac{1}{2}$ hr after injection. A second injection 12 hr after the first would be expected to potentiate the inhibitory effects by extending the duration of inhibition for a further 8–12 hr. Animals were trained 3 hr after the second injection. Control animals received either a single injection of DDC 3 hr after training, or two saline injections 12 hr apart. Mice were tested 24, 48, or 72 hr after training.

Results are shown in Figure 34.7. Percent savings of saline controls show the expected regular decline over the 3-day period. The group receiving the single DDC injection essentially replicates previous findings from this laboratory. Mice show total amnesia 24 hr after treatment and a full recovery by 48 hr. The group that re-

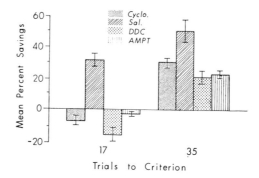

FIGURE 34.5 Effect of increasing training strength on amnesia induced by AMPT and DDC. Cyclo data are included for comparison. N = 15 in each group.

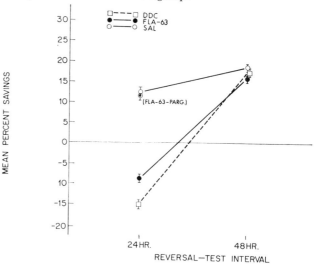

FIGURE 34.6 Spontaneous recovery of memory following amnesia induced by FLA-63 and DDC. The MAOI pargyline (75 mg/kg), injected 2 hr prior to the 24-hr retention test, also produced memory recovery. N = 12 in all groups.

ceived two injections of DDC shows amnesia at 24 hr and at 48 hr, but recovery at 72 hr. The difference between the groups that received one and two DDC injections at 24 hr results from the effect of the two injections on reversal learning. Reversal learning is significantly enhanced by two DDC injections. Mean trials to criterion for this group is 24.5, as opposed to 27.0 for the single-injection group (t = 3.88, p < 0.001). Mean trials for saline control animals is 27.5. Since both of the DDC groups require approximately 29 trials to learn on the test day (this is the score made by naive mice learning the reversal for the first time), there is a greater apparent decrement in the group receiving two injections when percent savings is calculated by the standard formula. This enhanced performance following prolonged NE depletion should be investigated further. The recovery data indicate that increasing the duration of NE inhibition prolongs the period during which the

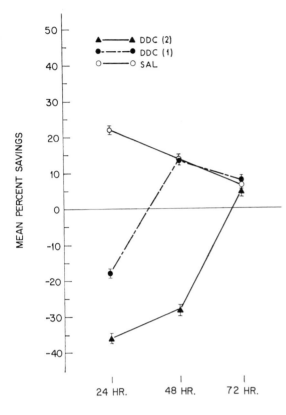

FIGURE 34.7 Mean percent savings for groups which received one or two DDC injections prior to reversal training. Different groups were tested 24, 48, and 72 hr after training. N = 10 in each group.

memory is inaccessible; that recovery eventually occurs indicates that the memory-storage mechanisms have not been impaired. (Two DDC injections *following* reversal training do not impair retrieval.)

There is also evidence that these amnesias can be reversed by the same pharmacological manipulations that restore memory following Cyclo treatment. Quartermain and Botwinick (1975a) have shown that the amnesias induced by AMPT in the T maze can be reversed by pretest injections of the MAOI pargyline. Amnesia resulting from inhibition of NE by FLA-63 can also be reversed by treatment with pargyline (see Figure 34.6). Botwinick and Quartermain (1974) have shown that amnesia in a one-trial, passive-avoidance task induced by DDC can be reversed by both pheniprazine and pargyline. These data suggest that amnesias resulting from inhibition of the synthesis of biogenic amines are both fragile and temporary. In both of these respects they closely resemble memory deficits resulting from protein-synthesis inhibitors such as Cyclo.

Compounds that increase tissue concentrations of catecholamines produce amnesias with different char-

acteristics. For example, it has been shown that increasing the levels of biogenic amines with imipramine produces amnesias only at times when the habit is well remembered (Leftoff, 1973). Similarly, we have shown that treatment with the MAOI pheniprazine produces amnesia for a 1-day-old habit but markedly facilitates a 7-day-old habit that is poorly remembered (Quartermain and Botwinick, 1975a,b). These effects of pheniprazine are similar in a number of respects to the effects of DFP reported by Deutsch (1971) in the cholinergic system.

In sum, then, compounds that influence biogenic amines have complex effects on memory which depend upon both the characteristics of the habit and the mechanism of action of the drug. In order to understand the role that the biogenic amines play in memory retrieval, experiments must be designed to study the effects of both enhancement and depletion of these putative transmitters on habits of different strengths and different ages.

ACKNOWLEDGMENT

The research described in this chapter was supported by The Grant Foundation Inc.

REFERENCES

BARONDES, S. H., and COHEN, H. D. 1967. Delayed and substained effects of acetoxycycloheximide on memory in mice. *Proceedings of National Academy of Sciences (USA)* 58: 157–162.

BARONDES, S. H., and COHEN, H. D. 1968a. Arousal and the conversion of "short-term" to "long-term" memory. *Proceedings of National Academy of Sciences (USA)* 61: 923–929.

BARONDES, S. H., and COHEN, H. D. 1968b. Memory impairment after subcutaneous injection of acetoxycycloheximide. *Science* 160: 556–557.

BOTWINICK, C. Y., and QUARTERMAIN, D. 1974. Recovery from amnesia induced by pre-test injections of monoamine oxidase inhibitors. *Pharmacology, Biochemistry and Behavior* 2: 375–379.

CHERKIN, A. 1972. Retrograde amnesia in the chick: Resistance to the reminder effect. *Physiology and Behavior* 8: 949–955.

COHEN, H. D., and BARONDES, S. H. 1968. Cycloheximide impairs memory of an appetitive task. *Behavioral Biology* 1: 337–340.

DANIELS, D. 1971. Acquisition, storage, and recall of memory for brightness discrimination by rats following intracerebral infusion of acetoxycycloheximide. *Journal of Comparative and Physiological Psychology* 76: 110–118.

DEUTSCH, J. A. 1971. The cholinergic synapse and the site of memory. *Science* 174: 788–794.

FLEXNER, J. B., and FLEXNER, L. B. 1967. Restoration of expression of memory lost after treatment with puromycin. *Proceedings of National Academy of Sciences (USA)* 57: 1651–1654.

FLEXNER, J. B., and FLEXNER, L. B. 1969. Studies on memory: Evidence for a widespread memory trace in the neocortex after the suppression of recent memory by puromycin.

Proceedings of National Academy of Sciences (USA) 62: 729–732.

FLEXNER, L. B., and FLEXNER, J. B. 1968. Intracerebral saline: Effect on memory of trained mice treated with puromycin. *Science* 159: 330–331.

FLEXNER, L. B., FLEXNER, J. B., and ROBERTS, R. B. 1967. Memory in mice analyzed with antibiotics. *Science* 155: 1377–1383.

FLEXNER, L. B., SEROTA, F. G., and GOODMAN, R. H. 1973. Cycloheximide and acetoxycycloheximide: Inhibition of tyrosine hydroxylase activity and amnestic effects. *Proceedings of National Academy of Sciences (USA)* 70: 354–356.

FLOOD, J. F., BENNETT, E. L., ROSENZWEIG, M. R., and ORME A. E. 1972. Influence of training strength on amnesia induced by pretraining injections of cycloheximide. *Physiology and Behavior* 9: 589–600.

FLOOD, J. F., BENNETT, E. L., ROSENZWEIG, M. R., and ORME, A. E. 1973. The influence of duration of protein synthesis inhibition on memory. *Physiology and Behavior* 10: 555–562.

GOLD, P. E., HAYCOCK, J. W., MARCI, J., and McGAUGH, J. 1973. Retrograde amnesia and the "reminder effect": An alternative interpretation. *Science* 180: 1199–1201.

GUTWEIN, B. M., QUARTERMAIN, D., and McEWEN, B. S. 1974. Dissociation of cycloheximide's effects on activity from its effects on memory. *Pharmacology, Biochemistry and Behavior* (in press).

HERZ, M. J., and PEEKE, H. V. S. 1967. Permanence of retrograde amnesia produced by electroconvulsive shock. *Science* 156: 1396–1397.

JAFFARD, R., DESTRADE, C., SOUMILHEU-MOURAT, B. S., and CARDO, B. 1974. Time dependent improvement of performance on appetitive tasks in mice. *Behavioral Biology* 11: 89–100.

LEFTOFF, S. 1973. Time-dependent memory retrieval effects following peripheral and hippocampal treatments to increase synaptic biogenic amines. Unpublished Ph.D. dissertation, New York University.

QUARTERMAIN, D., and BOTWINICK, C. Y. 1975a. The role of biogenic amines in the reversal of cycloheximide-induced amnesia. *Journal of Comparative and Physiological Psychology* 88: 386–401.

QUARTERMAIN, D., and BOTWINICK, C. Y. 1975b. Effect of age of habit on susceptibility to cycloheximide-induced amnesia. *Journal of Comparative and Physiological Psychology* 89: 803–809.

QUARTERMAIN, D., and McEWEN, B. S. 1970. Temporal characteristics of amnesia induced by protein synthesis inhibitor: Determination by shock level. *Nature* 228: 677–678.

QUARTERMAIN, D., McEWEN, B. S., and AZMITIA, E. C. 1970. Amnesia produced by electroconvulsive shock or cycloheximide: Conditions for recovery. *Science* 169: 683–686.

QUARTERMAIN, D. McEWEN, B. S., and AZMITIA, E. C. 1972. Recovery of memory following amnesia in the rat and mouse. *Journal of Comparative and Physiological Psychology* 79: 360–370.

RANDT, C. T., QUARTERMAIN, D., GOLDSTEIN, M., and ANAGNOSTE, B. 1971. Norepinephrine biosynthesis inhibition: Effects on memory in mice. *Science* 172: 498–499.

ROBERTS, R. B., FLEXNER, J. B., and FLEXNER, L. B. 1970. Some evidence for the involvement of adrenergic sites in the memory trace. *Proceedings of National Academy of Sciences (USA)* 66: 310–313.

SEGAL, D. S., SQUIRE, L. R., and BARONDES, S. H. 1971. Cycloheximide: Its effects on activity are dissociable from its effects on memory. *Science* 172: 82–84.

SEROTA, R. G. 1971. Acetoxycycloheximide and transient amnesia in the rat. *Proceedings of National Academy of Sciences (USA)* 68: 1249–1250.

SEROTA, R. G., ROBERTS, R. B., and FLEXNER, L. B. 1972. Acetoxycycloheximide-induced transient amnesia: Protective effects of adrenergic stimulants. *Proceedings of National Academy of Sciences (USA)* 69: 340–342.

SQUIRE, L. R., and BARONDES, S. H. 1972. Variable decay of memory and its recovery in cycloheximide treated mice. *Proceedings of National Academy of Sciences (USA)* 69: 1416–1420.

SQUIRE, L. R., GELLER, A., and JARVIK, M. E. 1970. Habituation and activity as affected by cycloheximide. *Communications in Behavioral Biology* 4: 249–254.

CNS Manipulation in the
Study of Memory: Lesions

35

Experimental Brain Lesions and Memory

ROBERT L. ISAACSON

ABSTRACT Although experimental brain damage is followed by behavioral changes, it is difficult to establish that a disruption of memory is the correct interpretation of any of these changes. This review places emphasis on alternative explanations—changes in motivation, incentives, sensory effectiveness, and other nonmnemonic qualities and factors that can influence performance. Reports of experimental studies dealing with the effects of localized brain damage on retention of different types of tasks are examined critically. From this review it is concluded that there is little evidence that any restricted form of brain damage produces deficits in information storage. Damage to certain systems of the brain seems capable of altering retrieval of information, often by altering the animal's perception of the environment, but it also produces many other types of performance change. Disturbances of information storage seem to result from rather general disturbances of brain function and are most likely to do so in the period immediately after learning.

35.1 INTRODUCTORY COMMENTS

Pierre Flourens (1794–1867) is considered to be the first scientist to use systematically produced brain damage to study brain function, and I have been asked to review here the results stemming from the application of his method—surgical ablations of brain tissue—as they may be related to a particular "faculty" of behavior —memory. In its present usage, "memory" is a concept which would please phrenologists like Gall and Spurzheim who tried to localize in the brain various types of psychological faculties, such as physical love, combativeness, self-esteem, wit, etc. Phrenologists tried to isolate universal attributes of behavior and correlate them with special prominences of the skull. These bulges of the skull were thought to be related to an exaggerated development of certain regions of the underlying brain.

Flourens is credited with discrediting the phrenologists (see Krech, 1962) and with supplanting their doctrine with newer views that had a far-reaching impact on psychology and related fields. One of these is that the intellectual abilities exist in the cerebrum "coextensively," inseparable from each other. According to Flourens, the functions of the cortex depend upon activities in many or all regions, even though there may be redundancy of functions within the brain. Flourens

ROBERT L. ISAACSON, Department of Psychology, University of Florida, Gainesville, FL

assumed a "nonlocalization-of-function" approach, but it was not absolute.

In the century and more since Flourens's work, the balance of scientific thought has wavered back and forth between positions of localization and nonlocalization of faculties, processes, and abilities. Fritsch and Hitzig, Ferrier, Sherrington, and others were influential in producing movement of the collective scientific mind, but it was the work of S. I. Franz and Karl Lashley that shaped the thinking of neurobehavioral scientists in the first half of this century. Franz reported that newly acquired habits were lost after destruction of the neocortex, whereas instinctive acts and "long-standing" habits were unaffected. Furthermore, he found that habits acquired after the initial damage could be disrupted by a second invasion of the cortex. In general, Franz believed that while there were differences among the activities of various systems of the brain, this did not imply that mental processes were discretely localized. This view was supported by Lashley, who felt that the (then) known facts of localization might be only accidents of growth and development of the nervous system and that attempts to localize mental activities should be abandoned (Lashley, 1937). Lashley also believed that the more complex and difficult the task given an animal, the more diffusely would the neural representations of that activity be scattered through the brain.

It is fair to say that "localization of function" tends to be more heavily emphasized by investigators working with nonhuman primates than those working with rodents. Nevertheless, it should be noted that even H. F. Harlow (1952), the distinguished investigator of the contributions of the primate brain to behavior, reached a conclusion quite in keeping with the views of Lashley and Franz, namely, that it has yet to be shown that the destruction of any given association area brings about the destruction of a particular intellectual function.

These historical comments are relevant to this review since it, as any review, must be read and interpreted in light of the writer's biases, attitudes, and beliefs. No one is entirely objective despite the best of intentions. Overall, when beginning this review my sentiments were with the ablationists. I anticipated that the effects of past learning would be found to be distributed widely over many, if not all, regions of the brain and perhaps over other areas of the central nervous system. Indeed, it would be odd if any biological system could not be modified by experience.

What about memory? Should it be considered as *a* faculty or as a set of faculties? Is it a functional entity which can be assigned to particular regions or systems of the brain? Frankly, I do not find myself sympathetic to references to memory as a "thing" or to "memory circuits," "storage locations," or the like. These were my biases at the start of this review, and the reader should consider himself or herself forewarned.

35.2 THOUGHTS ABOUT EXPERIMENTAL PROCEDURES

Basically, the experimental paradigm for attempting to determine the effects of brain damage on memory involves training an animal in a task, imposing some form of brain damage, allowing the animal to recover, and retesting the animal on the original task. Control procedures or subjects must be used to ensure that the brain damage has in fact produced an effect upon memory exceeding any effect that might follow from the mere passage of time, from the trauma of surgery, or from sensory or perceptual alterations, motor debilities, or more general behavioral changes produced by the brain damage.

Controls for the effects of the trauma and stress of surgery often involve the study of the behavior of sham-operated animals or animals with other forms of brain damage relative to the behavior of animals not subjected to any surgical manipulation. Determination of the effects due to the simple passage of time is usually made by comparisons among normal, sham-operated, and other groups of lesioned animals who have been away from the testing situation for equal amounts of time.

Sometimes a technique is used whereby an animal is intended to serve as its own control: After the original training, a delay is introduced that is as long as the recovery period to be allowed after surgery, and the animal is retested. If an animal shows good retention over the first delay period, it is then assumed able to remember the problem for such a period of time. However, this assumption that memory will be maintained over the second of two time gaps in the same way it was over the first is itself in need of testing. Furthermore, brain-damaged animals that experience training periods with imposed vacations from training may be differently affected by the vacations than are intact animals.

The method of testing used in evaluating retention also deserves consideration. After the recovery period,

animals can be tested under conditions in which they are exposed to the training paradigm and allowed to respond without being rewarded for any response (extinction conditions), or they can be retrained in the task with rewards provided for correct responses. There are problems inherent in both techniques. If the animal is tested without rewards, it may in normal circumstances eventually stop responding entirely. If a brain lesion were to alter an animal's ability to continue responding without reward, this could be misinterpreted as an alteration in memory. On the other hand, if the animal is retrained on the original task with rewards, changes in learning ability, attention, motivation, and the value of incentives could affect performance. Some forms of brain damage produce animals that can learn certain problems very rapidly. Other forms of brain damage make the acquisition of tasks difficult.

35.2.1 Motivation and incentives

Lesions of several parts of the brain have been shown to influence food and water consumption, and other lesions affect reactions to electrical shocks. Yet other lesions could also alter the incentive value of rewards related to these motives. The finicky eating habits of animals after hypothalamic lesions would be one such example. Even if the brain damage does not directly involve areas known to affect biological motives or reactions to incentives, unanticipated changes in them could be mistaken for changes in memory.

Procedures should thus include a demonstration that the lesioned animals work as hard and as diligently after surgery for the rewards provided, under an appropriate deprivation regime, as do control animals.

It is important to recognize that appropriate controls for alterations in motives and incentives may not be easy to achieve. The effects produced by brain damage in the animals may be subtle. For example, consider the progressive changes in deprivation that occur over a prolonged food-deprivation program. Rats are often kept at 80–90 percent of their *initial* body weights during a training program despite the natural tendency of animals to gain weight throughout life. This means that the animals are being subjected to increasing food deprivation throughout the entire experiment. Animals with brain damage may have different metabolic requirements than intact animals, and this could alter the value of incentives used in the experiment or change the general energy levels of the animals. One possibility would be for the experimenter to demonstrate that the task being studied is relatively insensitive to changes in the motivation or incentive value.

Some subtle aspects of motivational and incentive changes induced by brain damage on performance were shown by studies of Freeman, Mikulka, and D'Auteuil (1974). These authors have shown that the effect of hippocampal destruction on the suppression of appetitive behaviors by punishment depends upon incentive value. Van Hartesveldt (1973) has found differential responsiveness to changes in reward magnitude by animals with hippocampal destruction.

35.2.2 Performance

Although distinctions among learning, memory, and performance have been emphasized by many authors over the years, they are still too often forgotten.

The traditional distinctions among these factors are based upon changes in motivation, incentives, and other experimental variables which are thought to energize learned associations between stimuli and responses. In the past, learning and memory were thought to be made up of S-R associations that lie dormant until activated by motives, incentives, and the like. On the other hand, it is clear that we have information about the world, often referred to as "knowledge," that is hard to characterize in terms of S-R bonds. Animals can, and probably often do, learn about the consequences of actions rather than about specific responses to be used in obtaining them. Rats can roll or swim through a maze to get to the goal. It is getting to the goal that is important, not the responses made to get there.

Gestalt psychologists distinguished between the learning of habits and the reorganization of experiences that results in the rapid changes in behavior called "insight." The acquisition of habits was thought to be based upon the slow accumulation of S-R associations. In the 1930s and 1940s monotonic relationships were assumed between habits and rewards, trials, and the amount of incentives provided. For Gestalt psychologists, insight did not stand in a monotonic relationship with these variables. Past experiences were important, of course, since they determined the "world" of the animal, but changes in this world could cause the relationships of the world to be altered quickly, and performance would change just as rapidly.

Maier (1932) was one of the first to argue for this type of distinction at the animal level He had the audacity to suggest that rats could "reason" as well as "learn." Reasoning, for Maier, was much the same as "insight" for the Gestalt psychologists who studied human perceptual phenomena. Moreover, he found that even small amounts of neocortical destruction caused a switch from performance in accordance with "reasoning" to performance based upon the number of prior responses and rewards.

From the point of view of memory, the distinction between habits and insight suggests that damage to different parts of the brain might produce quite different effects on performances depending on which of these two bases of behavioral changes is affected.

35.2.3 Changes in sensory and peripheral processes

Brain damage can alter, distort, or destroy the perception of the environment, and such changes can be mistaken for changes in memory. In the simplest example, lesions that blind an animal would rather adversely affect retention scores on a test of visual discrimination. However, more subtle changes could also be produced by brain damage. Indeed, as will be discussed below, Bauer and Cooper (1964) have shown that certain effects thought to be a consequence of cerebral damage in the rat can be attributed to a loss of resolution in the animal's visual system. Brain damage might also alter the somatic and autonomic peripheral nervous systems or induce changes in the ways in which tastes and smells are perceived. If such changes do occur as a consequence of brain damage, it would be like testing the animal under new conditions, and a performance decrement would be anticipated. Therefore, in experiments attempting to demonstrate changes in memory, it is necessary to show that the changes cannot be explained on the basis of sensory or perceptual alterations.

It is, of course, impossible to test animals under every possible kind of environmental change. Some kind of selectivity must be instituted on the basis of the changes that can be expected from the lesions. The estimation of such changes must be based upon our overall knowledge of the contributions of the damaged brain region.

35.2.4 "States"

State-dependent phenomena are now a commonplace in the study of the effects of drugs upon behavior (see Overton, 1971). In essence, state-dependency refers to the fact that any demonstration of memory is contingent upon possible differences between the state of the subject during acquisition and that during testing. Learning of many problems may occur in either a drugged or an undrugged state, but later expression of the learning depends on a reinstatement of the conditions existing during acquisition. State-dependent phenomena are different from changes in sensory or perceptual processes in that they cannot be explained on the basis of peripheral changes induced by the drugs. Presumably they depend upon alterations of central neural mechanisms.

As far as I know, Girden (1940) was the first to propose a specific neural model for state-dependent phenomena. He proposed that both cortical and subcortical systems of the dog could subserve the acquisition of a behavioral task. In the normal dog the neocortex was presumed to be predominant, and its actions were thought to inhibit subcortical systems. However, if the cortex was rendered inactive by a drug (erythroidine), the subcortical systems could be used to acquire the task. When the cortex was released from the drug's effects, it inhibited the subcortical mechanisms again, and the animal behaved as if it had not been trained. Girden found that decortication eliminated the dissociation effect, but more recent research has shown that neocortical destruction in the rat does not eliminate state-dependent behaviors induced by phenobarbital (reported in Overton, 1971).

It seems likely that any damage to the central nervous system can produce a chronically different state of the individual which could be similar to the temporarily different states produced by some drugs. This new state might interfere with the expression of previously acquired responses.

An appropriate control for lesion-induced state-dependent effects is difficult to devise. Perhaps the best approach would be to keep the possibility of such effects in mind when interpreting the data from all experiments and, when appropriate, to control for changes in "arousal levels" in the experimental design. Many of the drugs that are most effective in inducing state-dependent effects are hypnotics, and this suggests that changes in arousal level could form at least one part of the basis of the dissociation effect.

35.2.5 Reactions to the environment
A peculiar type of state-dependent effect that is related to species-typical behavioral tendencies can be observed. For example, damage to the posterior neocortex of the rat has the effect of eliminating aversions to light or to bright stimuli in visual-discrimination tasks. Intact rats learn to approach the black stimulus more readily than the white stimulus in such problems. After posterior neocortical damage, this differential ease of learning is lost, and it is just as easy to learn to go to the white stimulus as to the black stimulus. P. M. Meyer (1973) has suggested that this change in behavior often hides the fact that relearning a brightness discrimination after neocortical damage is more difficult than before surgery, since animals are usually trained to approach the white stimulus.

This species-typical tendency to approach dark places or stimuli *could* be the basis on which some discriminations are acquired. Animals may learn to do what they don't want to do, i.e., they may learn to do what "feels bad." If lesions eliminate the basis of some species-typical behaviors, then postoperatively there may be no basis for performance on some problems.

Another way in which brain lesions could affect behavior would be by altering an animal's orientation to its surroundings. Lesions of several brain regions, especially the amygdala and the hippocampus, alter methods used to search the environment and perhaps spatial orientation as well. Depending on the nature of the task requirements, these changes could impair or facilitate performance.

35.2.6 The willingness to respond
Destruction of certain regions of the brain can influence animals in such a way that they are reluctant to undertake either single responses or sequences of responses. It is unlikely that these changes can be explained on the basis of a reduction in motivation or a decrease in the value of incentives, since once responses are initiated, new behaviors are quickly acquired and are maintained at normal levels. In general, the behavior of the lesioned animals is "sluggish." The animals do not show much inclination to change their response styles in the face of alterations of the environment. A few examples may be helpful. Animals with damage to the amygdala have difficulty acquiring a two-way active-avoidance response because in the early stages of training, no avoidance responses are made. Once avoidance responding is begun, however, conditioning progresses as rapidly as in intact animals (Kling et al., 1960). In another context, the unwillingness of monkeys with amygdala lesions to undertake new responses has been described as an essential part of the syndrome (Pribram, Douglas, and Pribram, 1969).

Another example of a reluctance to undertake new responses stems from the work of Krieckhaus and his associates on animals with damage to the mammillothalamic tracts (Krieckhaus et al., 1968; Krieckhaus and Randall, 1968). A reluctance to undertake new responses explains many of the deficits found after these and other brain lesions, and there is some evidence that amphetamine can counteract this lesion-produced behavioral change.

This is a most important result since the original deficit reported to follow lesions of the mammillothalamic tracts was an impairment in retention of an active-avoidance problem. It turned out that this retention deficit could be eliminated by amphetamine, which indicated that an inability of the lesioned animals to begin new responses had been misconstrued as a memory deficit. Once the drug made the animals capable of initiating responding, the memory for the task could be expressed. This suggests yet another control procedure for studies of retention after brain damage, namely, testing the subjects, or subgroups of them, under stimulants that can help energize behaviors sufficiently to allow the expression of what has been acquired and retained.

Animals with amygdala lesions are not only loathe to undertake new responses, they are also quick to give them up. They quickly stop responding in active-avoidance tasks (rapid extinction) and sometimes stop making any choice responses at all during reversal training in discrimination tasks. These behavioral changes could affect performance during retention tests, especially under conditions in which extinction or reversal procedures are used.

While some brain lesions make animals reluctant to undertake responses, other lesions can seem to make them overly eager to do so. This alteration in behavior is frequently described in terms of a release from inhibitory influences of one kind or another, and it often appears as a result of damage to prefrontal, hippocampal, or septal areas. In studying the postoperative retention of an auditory-discrimination problem, Brutkowski and Dabrowska (1966), for example, have found that after prefrontal damage in dogs, many more responses are made to a stimulus signaling a period in which no rewards will be forthcoming (S^Δ), but there is no change in the number of responses following a signal indicating that responses will be followed by rewards (S^D). Prefrontal damage can increase both positive responses to food and aversive reactions to punishment (see Brutkowski, 1964).

There is some evidence that the effects of some lesions can be interpreted as a potentiation of prepotent responses to a situation, whether they are active or passive in nature. Galef (1970) has found that septal lesions potentiate either approach or withdrawal responses, depending on which are predominant in the situation. This suggests that explanations of lesion-produced behavioral changes should go beyond a simple "release from inhibition." Damage to the brain produces a host of behavioral changes, many of which are complicated and subtle. All can produce changes in performance that can readily be confused with alterations in memory. Because so many types of changes can follow brain damage, a demonstration of a memory loss is especially difficult to establish. Convincing evidence of a disturbance of memory or retention must be based upon studies in which appropriate controls for other types of changes have been made.

35.3 STUDIES ATTEMPTING TO RELATE BRAIN LESIONS TO MEMORY

For over a hundred years the primary basis for the assumption that memories are reducible to physiological changes in the brain has been the belief that brain lesions can disturb or destroy the retention of past experiences. If this is true, then it suggests that an individual will not "remember" if his brain is not in an adequate condition. It shows that an appropriate functional state of the brain or some of its systems is necessary for retention of the past, but it does not allow the conclusion that a certain state of the brain is *sufficient* to produce a particular memory of the past. To do so would require a demonstration of differences in brain structure and function that correspond to differences in past experiences. Such direct evidence is lacking. Therefore, analysis must be made of changes in performance after brain damage with consideration given to the control measures that have been discussed above.

A review of the studies that have been done relating brain lesions to memory can begin with any number of topics, but perhaps the most appropriate place is with studies of the effects of damage to the neocortex. It was with studies of rats with such damage that Franz and Lashley began the modern era of research on the effects of brain damage on retention, and most of the research to date has concentrated on the neocortical mantle.

35.3.1 Neocortical lesions and memory

BRIGHTNESS-DISCRIMINATION TASKS. The appropriate point to begin a review of work on the retention of brightness-discrimination problems after neocortical destruction in the rat is with the work of Karl Lashley. Because of his pervasive influence, some comments about his methods may be in order. In Lashley's experiments the destruction of the cortical surface of the rat was usually accomplished by a thermocautery. A wire was sometimes applied while red hot, but at other times it was inserted cold and then heated. This last technique was said to be preferable in that fewer postoperative complications seemed to result from it. A postoperative recovery period of ten days was frequently provided but longer times were allowed if an animal did not seem healthy. Histological evaluation of the neocortical damage was provided by sketches of the extent of the surface lesion made on drawings of the dorsal and lateral surfaces of the brain. These sketches were based upon histologically prepared cross sections of the brains. Subcortical landmarks were used as guides for the reconstruction of cortical damage. The drawings of brain damage prepared by this technique cannot be compared directly with photographs of either the dorsal or lateral surfaces of the brain taken before processing for histological study.

In testing for brightness-discrimination abilities (as reported in Lashley, 1929), a Yerkes box was used in which the animals left a small start box and stepped into a wide area. They were confronted by two short alleys separated by a partition. Each alley had a grid floor which could be electrified individually. At the far end of each alley was a round window through which light could come from a "light box" behind. Light always came from the window of one alley and not the other, and the rats were trained to approach the illuminated alley. If the animal approached the illuminated alley, it could make a turn and push open a celluloid door leading to a side alley that gave access to a compartment where food was provided. The grid floor in front of the unlit alley was electrified, and the door leading to the side alley was locked. Therefore, behavior on the problem was motivated both by food as reward and by footshock as punishment.

In one study Lashley (1929) trained animals on a series of problems after extensive damage to the posterior third of the neocortex. These included maze and brightness-discrimination problems, and some of the problems were repeated in the series. The brightness-discrimination problem was the fourth test in the series. It was relearned as the eighth test of the postoperative testing series. Maze and other tests intervened. The lesioned animals were not impaired in learning the brightness problem or in its retention. Indeed, if anything, they were slightly superior to the intact control animals. This demonstrated that the animals with posterior neocortical damage were able to learn the brightness problem and to retain it despite training on other behavioral problems between acquisition and retraining.

In 1935 Lashley reported data, which have since been widely accepted as conclusive, showing that retention of a brightness discrimination was lost if destruction of the posterior third of the neocortex intervened between acquisition and relearning. Relearning of the discrimination task after surgery took about as many trials as was required by the same animals during original learning.

Subsequently, Horel et al. (1966) have studied the retention of a brightness discrimination in a Thompson-Bryant apparatus. This apparatus is one in which behavior is motivated solely by electrical footshock. A choice is made between two doors that can be made to vary in brightness or in the patterns on them. Electrical shocks are used to urge the animal to leave the start box and to approach one or the other of the doors, and to punish the animal for incorrect responses. The apparatus is similar to the Yerkes box used by Lashley except that there are more opportunities for punishment and no food reward is provided. The results obtained by Horel et al. were in close agreement with those of Lashley. Animals with posterior neocortical destruction seemed to lose the brightness-discrimination habit but could relearn it. There was a slight improvement over original learning, but this was probably due to a loss of aversion for the brighter stimulus. The retention of a pattern discrimination was also impaired postoperatively, and it could not be relearned. The relearning of the brightness

problem did not depend on the integrity of frontal neocortical areas since relearning in animals without the frontal regions progressed as well as in animals with these areas intact. This stressed the possibility that relearning after posterior neocortical destruction occurs subcortically. If the relearning after posterior neocortical damage is subcortical, what structures are involved? This question will be considered in greater detail below.

Destruction of the anterior neocortex of the rat can impair retention of several, primarily visual, tasks (Horel et al., 1966; Saavedra and Pinto-Hamuy, 1963). The study of Thompson (1960) failed to reveal a deficit as a consequence of anterior neocortical lesions, but strain differences may account for this discrepancy (e.g., Meyer Yutzey, and Meyer, 1966). Deficits have also been reported to follow damage to the middorsal rat neocortex which spares both the extreme frontal and extreme posterior regions (Petrinovich and Bliss, 1966).

There are many procedural and methodological variables which may contribute to the deficit seen in visually guided problems after destruction of the posterior neocortex of the rat and other animals. It is not simply a case of the surgical intervention producing a categorical loss of memory for visual problems of a particular kind.

The amount of preoperative training and the amount of time allowed for postoperative recovery have been found to influence the degree of retention for a visually signaled active-avoidance task (Worthington and Isaac, 1967). In this study the longer the postoperative recovery (20 versus 5 days) and the higher the preoperative criterion of learning, the greater the postoperative retention. Previously, Lashley (1929) had not found that increasing postoperative recovery times had helped animals in the Yerkes discrimination apparatus, but he had not studied this in a systematic fashion.

The type of behavioral problem offered to the subjects seems to be of special importance. When retention is measured in avoidance tasks signaled by visual cues, the results are different from those obtained when retention is measured in two-choice problems such as the Yerkes or Thompson-Bryant boxes.

The behavioral effects of serial (multistage) destruction of the posterior neocortex are task- and procedure-dependent, and consideration of the tasks used by different investigators helps to explain some of the discrepancies in the results that have been reported.

When a region of the brain is removed serially, the experiences of the animal between the operations may be critical to the effects measured after the second operation. Thompson (1960) argued that animals have to receive training on the specific task being measured in the interoperation period for any benefit of serial destruction to be observed. On the other hand, Meyer, Isaac, and

Maher (1958) and Isaac (1964) found that general sensory stimulation not related to the specific behavioral problem can benefit the animals when imposed between operations. Cole, Sullins, and Isaac (1967) reported that the administration of a stimulant between the two surgical procedures suffices to enhance retention: sensory stimulation per se is not even required. Kirchner et al. (1970) found that serial destruction of the posterior neocortex failed to improve performance on a brightness discrimination in a Thompson-Bryant box even with the administration of stimulants between operations. No specific training was given between the two operations, and the authors concluded that retention scores are improved in two-choice discrimination problems after multiple-stage lesions only if such training is provided. Nonspecific stimulation between operations seems to be sufficient to aid animals in avoidance tasks.

Petrinovich and Bliss (1966) reported a savings in the retention of a brightness discrimination measured in a Thompson-Bryant box after serial destruction of posterior neocortex in the rat. However, their lesions were quite small and did not approach complete destruction of the visual area. They found disturbances of retention only if the animals in the two-stage group were kept in darkness between the operations. Petrinovich and Carew (1969) suggest that serial destruction of the neocortex provides a benefit in retention only if the lesions are small. Probably, both the nature of the tasks given the animals and the size of the lesions play important roles in determining the losses found after neocortical destruction.

If the effects of neocortical damage, whether it be of frontal, middle, or posterior areas, are best explained in terms of a disruption of memory, then this should be reflected in all types of tests for the preoperatively learned task. Breen and Thompson (1966) trained rats to make a shuttlebox response to a visual cue to obtain water when thirsty. They found a most surprising result: posterior neocortical lesions did not disturb this habit, while anterior neocortical lesions did. In addition, lesions involving the hippocampus, superior colliculi, pretectal area, septal area, or medial thalamus also failed to affect retention. The only lesions that did impair retention were those of the frontal necortex and the lateral geniculate nucleus. While it may be that the frontal lesions produced behavioral effects by disturbing sensorimotor abilities, as Breen and Thompson suggest, the failure to find deficits after posterior neocortical lesions is most important.

LeVere and Morlock (1973) have questioned the interpretation of the effects of neocortical damage as a retention deficit. In their experiment the animals were retrained on the *reversal* of a preoperatively established brightness discrimination. A Y maze was used, and the animals were trained to avoid footshock. The authors argued that if memory for the preoperatively, trained brightness discrimination is abolished by the lesion, then reversal learning should proceed as if it were being learned for the first time. They found the lesioned animals to be severely impaired on the reversal task. These results suggest that the memory of the preoperatively learned task is not lost after neocortical insult, but, for unknown reasons, it fails to express itself fully during the usual conditions of postoperative training.

The work of Braun, Meyer, and Meyer (1966) is also relevant to this point. They found that amphetamine could facilitate the postoperative expression of a previously learned brightness-discrimination task, although the same drug level did not improve the original acquisition of the same task. Some degree of arousal, probably mediated by posterior hypothalamic regions or the reticular formation, is necessary for the performance of conditioned responses (Doty, Beck, and Kooi, 1959), since conditioned responses can usually be demonstrated only when fast electrical activity occurs in neocortical areas after these lesions. The results of Braun, Meyer, and Meyer support the view of LeVere and Morlock that preoperatively established memories remain but do not gain expression in behavior unless special pharmacological or behavioral procedures are used. Following this line of reasoning, D. R Meyer (1972) has synthesized the results of many studies, a substantial number of which have come from his own laboratory, and reached the conclusion that the problem resulting from neocortical damage is one of retrieval rather than memory storage.

There is yet another serious difficulty for those who would believe that destruction of the rat posterior neocortex disrupts retention of visual memories, namely, the possibility that damage to visual neocortical regions produces a loss of "resolution" in the visual abilities of the animals (e.g., Pinto-Hamuy, Santibañez-H, and Rojas, 1963). Following this hypothesis, Bauer and Cooper (1964) reported a series of studies in which the behavioral effects of destruction of about the posterior half of the rat neocortex were investigated. All of their results are more easily explained on the basis of a loss of sensory capacities than on the basis of an alteration in memory. For example, they found small losses in postoperative performance on a brightness discrimination if the positive stimulus was emitted light coming through the correct door, but a great disruption if the discrimination was based upon light reflected off stimulus cards placed on the doors. Lesioned animals previously tested on a discrimination problem using reflected light acquired the flux-discrimination problem more quickly than did intact control animals. Bauer and Cooper also showed the importance of ambient illumination in another experiment. Animals with posterior neocortical destruction were made worse than nonlesioned controls in the flux discrimination simply by increasing the overall illumination of the room in which testing took place.

In an experiment in which translucent cups were sewn around their eyes, animals were somewhat impaired in learning the flux problem. Their performance was about that of animals in the reflected-light problem. However, when trained with the translucent eye cups, there was no loss in performance of the task after destruction of the posterior neocortex. In fact, the lesioned animals seemed to retain the flux problem somewhat better than intact control animals who had had a two-week vacation from training.

In some ways these results are quite similar to those found 22 years earlier by Klüver (1942) in the monkey. Most important, for present purposes, is the fact that these observations cast serious doubt upon assertions that a memory loss is involved in deficits observed on visual tasks following posterior neocortical destruction in the rat. If there is a retrieval deficit, the basis for the deficit could easily arise from the distorted and imperfect sensory world of the brain-damaged animals.

MULTIPLE VISUAL-MEMORY SYSTEMS. Many researchers investigating the role of central-nervous-system structures in visually guided behaviors have felt it necessary to assume the existence of several systems. Horel et al. (1966), for example, felt this to be the case because the extirpation of the visual areas destroyed the tendency of intact rats to learn "approach-the-white-stimulus" more slowly than it did their tendency to learn "approach-the-black-stimulus." As a result, brain-damaged rats learned the black-white discrimination more readily than did intact animals. The differences in acquisition rate suggested to these investigators that two (or more) different learning mechanisms might be used by rats with and without posterior neocortex. The same conclusion can be justified by the differences found in how animals with or without posterior neocortex reach successively more difficult performance criteria in a brightness-discrimination task (Horel et al., 1966; Spear and Braun, 1969).

Thompson, Baumeister, and Rich (1962) argued that two brain systems must be involved in the retention and postoperative relearning of a visual-discrimination problem. The first was a "posterior system" responsible for maintaining a simultaneous discrimination. This system included the visual cortex, the posterior thalamus, the lateral hypothalamic areas, the habenulo-interpeduncular tract, and the interpeduncular nucleus. For a successive discrimination task, the posterior system was thought to require supplementation by an anterior system that included the anterior neocortex, the globus pallidus, and the anterior thalamus. This second, anterior, system was thought to be necessary for responses based on the spatial location of visual stimuli.

In an elaboration of their earlier models, Thompson, Rich, and Langer (1964) suggested that visually guided behaviors motivated by shock avoidance depended upon a convergence of two systems, one conveying information about the specific sensory signals and the other indicating the motivational circumstances. The convergence was presumed to occur in the lateral hypothalamic–ventral tegmental region, including the area of the central gray and red nucleus (see also McNew, 1968). The substrates of specific visual signals were thought to involve the posterior system, described above, and the frontal neocortical, limbic, and diffusely projecting thalamic systems. These conclusions were based in part upon the observation that conditioned-avoidance reactions can be affected by damage to frontal cortex (Saavedra and Pinto-Hamuy, 1963; Thompson, 1963) as well as to subcortical sites.

In 1969 Thompson proposed that the performance of visual habits depends upon descending pathways from striate cortex to the ventral lateral geniculate bodies, from there to the posterior nucleus of the thalamus, and from there to the region of the red nucleus. Data supporting the importance of this system come from work in his laboratory and others in which discrete knife cuts have been made in the brainstem (Horel, 1968a,b; Thompson, Truax, and Thorne, 1969). In a more recent publication, Petit and Thompson (1974) propose that a descending corticoreticular projection system is also involved in visual-discrimination performance.

The work of Thompson and his collaborators has provided a tentative basis for considering different systems and different memory-stage models for the rat, but their approach is not the only one. For visual phenomena, two systems have been postulated to deal with a possible distinction between how the nervous system decides "What is it?" and "Where is it?" (e.g., Schneider, 1969). Disturbances in either mechanism could lead to difficulties in performance that might be interpreted as memory failures. P. M. Meyer (1973) has suggested that animals with extensive destruction of the visual neocortex may be able to make discriminations among contours of different lengths even if they are a deficient in pattern discrimination. In addition, she suggests that it is possible that animals with damage to the geniculostriate system can distinguish a visual field filled with some objects from one not so filled, but they may not be able to differentiate the forms of particular objects (see also Dalby, Meyer, and Meyer, 1970). These suggestions are based on the assumption of separate systems mediating the perception of specific patterns, and a more general ability related to the presence or absence of poorly defined "figures."

The locations of the subcortical regions that are essentially related to performance on visual tasks after necortical damage is not completely known; probably, they are related to specific motivational and procedural factors found in a particular experiment. The lateral pretectal area and accessory optic nucleus have been implicated by Pasik and Pasik (1973), and the posterior thalamic nucleus by Horel (1968). Although the superior colliculi have not been found to be involved in visual discriminations in rats, they have been in cats (Norton and Clark, 1963).

However, lesions of the superior colliculi or the areas ahead of it which interrupt the tectothalamic tract can produce an altered responsiveness to stimuli presented on the side opposite the lesions and an enhancement of approach responses to stimuli presented on the same side (Sprague and Meikle, 1965). These changes may not indicate a sensory defect, but rather, may reflect alterations in progressive motor responsiveness (Cooper et al., 1970).

As mentioned, Thompson and his colleagues have argued for a memory system related to visually guided problems in the rat and other species. This system is said to include the posterior neocortex, the posterior thalamus, the area around the interpeduncular nucleus, the red nucleus, the substantia nigra, and the brainstem reticular formation. It is defined on the basis of losses in performance measured after lesions in these areas. Often, the postoperative relearning of a problem requires many more trials than were needed for original learning, and this suggests a loss in capacity as well as a possible retention deficit.

As mentioned above, there are many reasons to question whether destruction of the posterior neocortex actually produces any retention loss in brightness-discrimination problems, and there must therefore be reservations about any memory system in which the posterior neocortex serves as a vital link. Lesions of the subcortical sites of the system may or may not impair sensory capacities, but they probably alter the behavioral reactions (or reactiveness) of the individual.

Other "memory systems" have been proposed by Thompson and his co-workers for different types of behavioral tasks, e.g., a conditioned-avoidance memory system, a kinesthetic memory system, and a "manipulative-response" memory system. In my opinion, the criticisms directed against the idea of multiple visual-memory systems can also be directed against these other memory systems. Consider, for example, the manipulative memory system as reported by Spiliotis and Thompson (1973) In this study a retention loss in three manipulative latchbox problems was found after destruction of the anterior neocortex. All of the three animals with anterior neocortical damage failed to learn one problem and were markedly impaired on the others. This suggests a loss in skill or capacity, rather than an impairment of memory, as the primary cause of the performance deficits.

In an unpublished study Nick Masi and I studied the postoperative retention of the forepaw-manipulation problem developed by Castro (1972). In conformity with Castro's results, we found substantial deficits after damage to the frontal neocortex in many (but not all) of the rats studied. Some animals recovered their ability to respond, while others did not. "Recovery" could not be related to the size or location of the damage in the frontal regions. Manual dexterity was substantially reduced in all animals, but some continued trying to obtain the pellets and ultimtely achieved some degree of success. Other rats just seemed to give up, and stopped trying after a few attempts. We decided not to publish this study because we realized that we had not adequately controlled for this giving-up effect. We should repeat the experiment, providing frustrative nonreward on an intermittent basis and controlling the use of each paw before surgery. Without such controls, conclusions about the nature of the degree of manual impairment or retention of the task cannot be made. The reduction in motor skill was obvious, however, and I would expect that a similar reduction of skill could account for the results obtained by Spiliotis and Thompson.

Thompson and Myers (1971) studied the effects of lesions in many areas of the brains of Rhesus monkeys on the retention of three visual-discrimination problems. The animals were trained in a Wisconsin General Test Apparatus, with pieces of banana used as rewards. None of the lesions produced a serious deficit in a color discrimination—the easiest problem. Lesions of the posterior nucleus produced a substantial postoperative deficit in a triangle-disc form discrimination, and lesions of the pretectal area produced deficits so large that the animals required about twice as many trials to relearn the problem postoperatively as they did during original learning. A number of lesions produced deficits in the most difficult discrimination: a horizontal versus a vertical line painted on blocks of wood. These areas were the pulvinar, the posterior nucleus, the pretectal region, the magnocellular portion of the red nucleus, and the reticular formation. It is somewhat surprising that the posterior-nucleus lesion and the pretectal lesion caused a greater deficit in the moderately difficult task than in the hardest task. This could be due to a practice effect, since testing on the triangle-disc form discrimination came before testing on the horizontal-vertical stripe discrimination.

Let us consider the performance of individual animals: Animals with damage to the posterior nucleus and the pretectal areas were impaired on at least the two more difficult problems, and animals in both groups showed an oculomotor defect—a reluctance to move head or eyes downward. This defect continued throughout the postoperative testing period. In only one other animal of the series were these symptoms found in a mild form. This animal had a tegmental lesion but did not show a retention deficit.

Four of seven animals with damage to the area below the red nucleus were impaired on the most difficult discrimination. These animals also maintained their heads in a peculiar tilted position postoperatively. Animals in this group that did not have the head tilt were not impaired. Animals with behavioral deficits following red-nucleus lesions also had a disturbance of head orientation.

Three out of four monkeys with pulvinar damage showed a deficit on the hardest discrimination problem (horizontal versus vertical stripes). One monkey showed almost perfect retention. The animal with the greatest deficit on this problem had some incidental damage to the visual radiations and was also impaired on the triangle-disc problem. These results are in contrast to an earlier report of Chow (1954), who failed to find an effect of pulvinar lesions on retention of a visual task. It is also possible that the use of a more sensitive measure of retention by Thompson and Myers might have accounted for this discrepancy.

What do the observations of Thompson and Myers tell us about the memory systems related to vision? First, animals with posterior-nucleus or pretectal lesions seemed to suffer from deficiencies in visual capacities, as indicated by the much greater number of trials required for relearning than for original learning. This could also be related to motor disturbances affecting vision. Furthermore, these areas have been considered to be involved in the regulation of forebrain arousal in a diffuse fashion. Therefore, animals with these lesions reveal nothing about memory per se. Second, animals in all other lesion groups were impaired only on the most difficult discrimination task. The performances of all subcortical-lesion groups on color and form problems were intact. Therefore, the lesion-induced behavioral deficits cannot be considered to pertain to visual memories in general. Third, lesions of the pulvinar do not always produce deficits (e.g., Chow, 1954), and it may well be that the changes in temperament can be related

to changes in performance during testing for retention. Moreover, the lesions in the pulvinar might disturb fibers passing to pretectal areas from inferotemporal cortex, since Reitz and Pribram (1969) have found that fibers from inferotemporal cortex pass through the pulvinar. Inferotemporal lesions disrupt performance on visual tasks, and impairments were found in two monkeys tested by Thompson and Myers with such cortical lesions. Therefore, it would appear that the effects ascribed to pulvinar damage may in fact be attributable to inferotemporal damage and not to the pulvinar damage itself. Fourth, the impairments found after damage to the red nucleus were generally slight, were found only in a minority of animals, and were probably correlated with changes in the tilting of the head found postoperatively. This suggests that damage to the red nucleus, and to the regions around it, produces changes in performance that are related not to memory but to mechanisms associated with the orientation of the body and head. Fifth, the only other animals with retention deficits were the three (of five) animals with lesions of the reticular formation. However, there were varying degrees of damage to the red nucleus and to the posterior nucleus of the thalamus in these subjects. The animal with the greatest debilitation had the greatest damage to the posterior nucleus.

Given these considerations, there seems to be no basis on which to conclude that damage to any of the subcortical regions discussed above affects the memory for visual experiences. All of the behavioral deficits could result from changes in the animals' analysis of the visual environment.

It should also be noted that lesions of many other regions failed to produce any deficit in retention of the visual problems. These include the centromedial and dorsomedial nuclei of the thalamus, the subthalamic area, the lateral hypothalamus, the substantia nigra, the central tegmental area, the superior colliculus, and the subcollicular area.

The work of Thompson and his colleagues (e.g., Mc-New and Thompson, 1966; Thompson et al., 1967; Thompson and Rich, 1961) in nonprimates has revealed structures important for the maintenance of normal performance on visually guided tasks, but it appears that these studies are not directly relevant to the analysis of memory.

PATTERN DISCRIMINATIONS. Typically, removal of the "visual areas" of the brain leads to deficits in pattern discriminations that are similar to those found in brightness problems, except that relearning of the tasks is seldom possible. For this reason, the testing of visual-pattern abilities is of less interest for the study of memory. If the capacity to solve a problem has been lost, then impaired performance cannot be used as an indicator of storage or retrieval losses.

However, in recent years there have been reports that rats (e.g., Lewellyn, Lowes, and Isaacson, 1969), cats (e.g., Wetzel, 1969), and monkeys (e.g., Weiskrantz, 1963) with extirpation of the visual neocortex can show some forms of pattern discrimination. Dalby, Meyer, and Meyer (1970) have shown that cats with visual-neocortex destruction can respond on the basis of the lengths of lines and contours and they can even solve some tasks in which the different patterns have equal contours.

Amphetamine can influence the "retrieval" of responses that have apparently been lost for a prolonged period of time. Meyer, Horel, and Meyer (1963) found that the administration of amphetamine to cats reinstated visually guided placing responses that had not been exhibited for months after damage to the striate areas. On the other hand, Jonason et al.(1970) were not able to find improvement in the retention of an equal-flux, equal-contour, pattern-discrimination problem after amphetamine. They concluded that the facilitation of retrieval produced by the drug may be beneficial only to certain specific types of visual performance. However, in the study by Jonason et al. only one dosage of amphetamine was used, and it is possible that improvements could have been found with other dosages. From these considerations it seems that animals with extensive or nearly complete damage to the neocortical visual system are deficient in pattern-discrimination capabilities, but that amphetamine can enhance performance, probably by supporting access or retrieval mechanisms.

The complicated roles played by the neocortex in various types of visual problems are really little understood. Maier (1941) found that lesions of the neocortex produced substantial increases in the number of visual stimuli seen as "equivalent" to stimuli used in training.

A high correlation was found between the number of equivalent stimuli and the amount of neocortical damage, suggesting that after cerebral damage details of the stimuli become less important to the animals.

MAZES. After performing surgery aimed primarily at the neocortical surface, Lashley (1929) administered a series of ten tests to his animals, the first of which involved his Maze III (a maze with 8 culs-de-sac). He retested them on maze III 40 days later to determine retention. Two other maze tests and the brightness-discrimination problem were interposed between learning and retention testing. The animals with neocortical damage showed impaired retention, and Lashley concluded that this loss in retention could not be explained only on the basis of the impaired learning capacities demonstrated during original training. He believed that the neocortical lesions produced a loss of the ability to retain the information.

This conclusion was based upon an analysis of the data presented in his Tables I and II (Lashley, 1929, pp. 36–39). However, if the amount of damage to subcortical structures is taken into consideration, the interpretation of the data from this study becomes entirely different. I have reorganized his data pertaining to the learning and relearning of Maze III in Table 35.1 using information from his Table VIII (p. 64). Animals with neocortical damage but without limbic-system damage are considered separately from those with "slight" damage to the hippocampus. Another group is made up of animals with "moderate" or "severe" damage to the hippocampus and animals with septal-area involvement, with or without damage to the hippocampus.

The effect of the neocortical destruction on the original learning of the maze problem can be seen from Table 35.1. It took rats with neocortical damage (NC) over three times as many trials to learn the problem as the intact animals. Retention, however, was quite good, although not quite as good as that demonstrated by the

TABLE 35.1
Median numbers of errors and trials in the learning and relearning of Maze III by normal and impaired animals

Group*	Median percent of cortex destroyed	Original learning		Relearning		Percent not learning†	Percent failing to relearn (if learned)†	Percent relearning
		Errors	Trials†	Errors	Trials†			
N	0	43	20 (22)	4	2 (15)	0	0	100
NC	11.2	147	51 (10)	9.5	6 (8)	9 (1)	20 (2)	73
NCh	27.9	297	77 (6)	7	9 (1)	14.3 (1)	83 (5)	14.3
NCH	34.8	436	75 (4)	115	18 (2)	55 (5)	50 (2)	22

*Abbreviations: N, normal; NC, neocortical damage but no limbic-system damage; NCh, neocortical and "slight" hippocampal damage; NCH, "moderate" and "severe" hippocampal and/or septal damage.
†Number of subjects is given in parentheses.
Data from Lashley (1929).

intact animals. Eight of the ten animals with neocortical damage that learned the problem relearned it. Overall, 73 percent of the animals in the neocortical-lesion group were capable of relearning it. The difference between Groups NC and N in the number of errors and trials required for relearning is probably related to differences in the learning capacities of the animals that showed up during original training. The effect of even "slight" limbic-system damage (NCh) was a much greater incapacity for learning and retention. Only about one-fifth of the animals with any type of limbic damage mastered the problem on the retention tests. If there was moderate to severe damage to the limbic system (NCH), more than half of the animals failed to learn the maze during original training.

The amount of neocortical destruction is confounded with limbic-system damage in this study. The greater the neocortical damage, the more likely it is that hippocampal or septal damage will also be found. This confounding cannot be untangled by Lashley's own data, but there are animals with limbic-system damage the extent of whose neocortical destruction lies in the same range as that of animals with only neocortical destruction. The behavior of these animals is similar to that of animals with moderate to severe hippocampal destruction.

All animals in the "limbic-system groups," i.e., NCh and NCH, make more "errors" than would be expected on the basis of the number of trials required for learning. It is quite possible that errors were accumulated by the perseverative retracing of incorrect maze pathways, which generated many errors on a single trial. This sort of result was found by Kimble (1963) in testing animals with large hippocampal lesions but with much less neocortical damage than in most of Lashley's subjects. Lashley commented that the animals with the largest lesions had a tendency to exhibit stereotyped reactions that impaired their proficiency. It would appear likely that it was the incidental involvement of the septo-hippocampal systems in animals with large lesions of the neocortex that led to the retention deficits in Lashley's animals. Therefore, it is likely that this behavioral deficit stems from alterations in performance-related variables rather than memory, since Kimble found that the length of the culs-de-sac of the maze affected the tendency of animals to make repetitive errors.

In another experiment reported by Lashley (1929), animals were trained in Maze III before surgery. They were given one retention test before surgery after a 10-day vacation from training. Ten days was also the length of the postoperative recovery interval. Preoperatively, the animals required about 25 trials and made about 54 errors prior to learning. When tested for retention pre-

operatively, they required about 3.5 trials and 4 errors to regain criterion. On this basis it would be reasonable to consider postoperative retention to be nearly perfect if 5 or fewer trials are required for relearning. Impaired retention might be inferred if relearning requires more than 5 trials.

A question arises when animals do make more than 5 errors: What number of errors or trials should be used as criterion for the demonstration of a change in their ability to perform the problem rather than merely a loss of memory? The most severe criterion would be a failure to relearn the maze after the maximum of 125 trials allowed; but what about animals that ultimately learn the problem yet require many more trials than during original learning? With this problem in mind, I reexamined Lashley's data (Table XIV, pp. 92–93) on the basis of amount of neocortex destroyed, the degree of limbic system damage, and whether retention was perfect (requiring 5 trials or less to relearn), impaired (requiring more than 5 trials but only about the number of trials required for original learning), or greatly impaired (requiring many more trials than in original learning). The results are presented in Table 35.2.

Only 7 of the 59 animals showed deficits in the range that might be considered related to retention. These animals took more than 5 trials during relearning but

TABLE 35.2

Types of performance changes found after surgery, based upon the amount of neocortex destroyed and incidental damage to subcortical structures

Amount of neocortex destroyed	Type of performance change*	Additional damage**				
		None	H(uni)	F or H(bi)	Septal area	Striatum
<12%	P	12				1
	I	1		1		
	C		1			
12–18%	P	6				1
	I	4				
	C	2		2	1	
18–30%	P	5	1			
	I			1		
	C	7	1	3	1	2
>30%	P			1		
	I					
	C			4	1	
Total		37	3	12	3	4

*Abbreviations: P, perfect retention; I, impaired rentention; C, change in capacity to perform the Maze-III task.
**H, hippocampus; F, fornix; uni, unilateral; bi, bilateral.
Data from Lashley (1929).

required only about the same number of trials as had been needed for original learning. Five of these animals had damage restricted to the neocortex, and 2 had neocortical and hippocampal damage. Twenty-four animals made many more errors and took many more trials during relearning than had been needed for original learning; I interpret this as a loss in the ability to perform the maze problem. Two of the 37 animals with only neocortical damage failed to learn the problem in the 150 trials allotted, as did 3 of the 12 animals with bilateral hippocampal damage, 2 of the 4 animals with striatal involvement, and 2 of the 3 animals with damage to the septal area.

While this analysis makes it likely that Lashley confused changes in performance abilities with memory for the maze problem, there are 7 animals with behavioral alterations that could be related to a memory deficit. All of these animals had damage to the posterolateral neocortex. None had damage to the frontal regions. The lesions of animals with impaired capacities tended to be scattered, but about half of them had damage to midline cortex. Whether these are true deficits in memory for the maze is not certain. It may be that the deficits reflected disturbances of the visual capacities of animals that had previously relied heavily on visual cues in solving the problem. If this is the case, then similar sensory disturbances in animals that did not rely heavily on visual cues would have produced much less debilitation.

The learning by rats of complex mazes like Lashley's Maze III seems to require only limited use of visual cues by only a small proportion of the animals (Lansdell, 1953; Thompson, 1959a). Pursuing this question further, Thompson (1959b) studied the retention of a Maze-III problem in peripherally blinded rats that were subjected to either anterior or posterior cortical damage. The maze was adapted so that the animals had to escape from water. There was no difference in the retention scores of animals with anterior or posterior lesions. The animals required about half as many trials to relearn the task after brain damage as they did to learn the problem originally. Unfortunately, there were no control groups made up of blind animals that received sham operations or merely a ten-day vacation from training. Therefore, it is not possible to determine whether the anterior or posterior lesions produced any memory impairment in these blind animals.

In the same study other groups of animals were blinded after learning the maze. When tested three days later, these animals showed considerable retention of the maze. They were then subjected to anterior or posterior neocortical lesions. Those receiving anterior neocortical lesions were more impaired than those receiving posterior lesions. Indeed, they required more trials to relearn the problem than they did in their initial learning and made almost five times as many errors in relearning than in learning.

Thompson indicated that these results could be explained on the basis of the cues used in performing the maze problem. He believes that the water-filled maze induced the animals to use visual cues more than did the normal Lashley Maze III. Therefore, posterior neocortical lesions produced great difficulty for the animals with vision. However, if animals were forced to rely on nonvisual cues, there was no selective debilitation by the posterior lesions. If it can be assumed that animals without vision use proprioceptive information, then anterior lesions might produce difficulty by hampering the ability to use response-produced information. However, this difficulty cannot be considered to be solely a loss of retention. The great number of errors, which far exceeded the number made in original learning, indicates that the animals had not forgotten the maze but, rather, had difficulty using the available cues to aid their performance.

These studies underscore the point that inquiries into retention after any surgical intervention must take into consideration the possibility that the changes made have affected the ability of the animals to use cues in their environment. If the animal cannot use a set of environmental cues, it cannot use information from the past related to them.

35.3.2 Association areas
Over the years a number of different investigators have pursued the behavioral contributions made by those areas of the neocortex to which primary sensory or motor functions cannot be ascribed. Most of this work has used the monkey as a subject, although some work has involved cats, dogs, and other animals in which there is agreement about the anatomical locations of the association areas. In the monkey some association areas have been more or less closely tied to information arriving over a particular sensory modality: e.g., parts of the inferotemporal cortex have been related to vision, and the parietal association cortex has been tied to somatosensory information. The goal of many researchers has been to describe just how the association areas influence behavior mediated by information from particular sensory modalities. To determine the perceptual capacities remaining after brain damage, investigators must rule out changes in memory as a cause of the performance changes. If an animal is trained on a somesthetic discrimination task every day for a month and doesn't show

improvement over the course of training, this could be due to a poor memory over days, or within a day, for somesthetic information, as well as to reduced sensory capacities. In order to show that the relevant change is in sensory capacities, memory effects need to be controlled. The problem is the opposite of that faced by investigators who are interested in ascribing performance changes to losses in memory; they must demonstrate that the behavioral changes are not due to alterations in sensory capabilities. Therefore, procedures are often incorporated into studies of the functions of association areas to eliminate the possibility that a memory deficit has produced the results.

Frequently, such memory control procedures occur in the context of the paradigm of "double dissociation of function" (Teuber, 1955). In this paradigm two types of brain lesions and two tasks are used. One type of lesion produces its effects only on one of the tasks, while the second type of lesion produces effects only on the second task. The idea is to show specific lesion effects, as opposed to more general effects that may follow brain damage to many regions and may be found in many behavioral problems.

A representative experimental paradigm is that used by M. Wilson (1957). The effects of lesions in the parietal and inferotemporal association areas were studied on visual and tactual problems. The animals were trained on all tasks preoperatively. After they achieved criterion performance levels, a preoperative retention test was given after a two-week pause in the testing regime. After these retention tests animals underwent surgery and a two-week recovery period before being tested for postoperative retention by the relearning of the problems. As would be expected, animals with inferotemporal lesions were impaired on the visual problem, and animals with parietal lesions were impaired on the tactual discrimination. The question for the present chapter is whether or not these results reveal anything about memory.

The use of the double-dissociation paradigm can provide information about memory under certain conditions. Over and above the conditions that have been described earlier as the necessary control procedures for establishing a memory disturbance, "order-of-testing" effects must be carefully controlled and evaluated.

The results obtained by Wilson on testing retention of the most difficult visual and tactual problems could be explained on the basis of a loss of sensory capacities by animals with inferotemporal or parietal lesions, respectively. However, on less difficult problems one animal in each lesion group had some difficulty in retention despite a demonstrated capacity to perform the problem. It can be asked whether this represents a memory deficit for the

particular task which occurs in some, but not all, animals after the brain damage.

It is increasingly apparent that the effects of brain damage are often probabilistic in nature; that is, they increase the likelihood of a particular form of behavioral change but do not guarantee that it will occur in all subjects (see Isaacson, 1975). One explanation of the probabilistic results found in brain-lesion studies is that they are due to alterations in the tolerance for failures on a problem. Increased failures could result from diminished capabilities. In the study under examination it is not possible to determine if the two animals with retention difficulties did have a memory disturbance related to particular sensory modalities or whether another explanation of the results would be more suitable.

Research on the localization of functional systems within the prefrontal areas has revealed a dissociation of retention deficits. Goldman and Rosvold (1970) found that a lesion of the depths and banks of the arcuate sulcus produced a severe retention deficit in the performance of a "conditioned positional response" (learning to respond to one location in a Wisconsin General Test Apparatus if a tone comes from above and to other location if the tone comes from below). Lesions of the depths and banks of the principal sulcus did not produce this retention deficit. large lesions of the prefrontal areas (excepting the area of the principal sulcus) and the premotor areas did produce some deficit, but these deficits were not as great as those resulting from destruction of the arcuate-sulcus region. The observations of Goldman and Rosvold also reveal a dissociation phenomenon in that the principal-sulcus lesions produced a delayed response deficit, whereas the arcuate lesion produced only a mildly deleterious effect on this task. This supports the observation that damage to the region of the principal sulcus in the prefrontal lobe results in deficits in delayed-response and delayed-alternation problems (Mishkin, 1957; Gross and Weiskrantz, 1962).

While other hypotheses can be considered, Goldman and Rosvold examined the possibility that deficiencies in memory could explain their results. As they point out, this would only be possible if memory is not considered in a global way. The main argument against a memory deficit as the primary explanation of frontal-lobe deficits was the experiment of Mishkin et al. (1969). These authors found that animals with lateral prefrontal lesions performed well on a test requiring memory, namely, delayed object alternation. Previously, Gross (1963a) had failed to find a postoperative retention deficit on an object-discrimination task after frontal-lobe injury. A failure to find a deficit in some types of problems requiring retention of previous experiences need not mean that other forms of memory cannot be impaired however, if the notion of a general memory is rejected in favor of multiple specific memory systems. Goldman and Rosvold suggest that either a specific memory for spatial discriminations or a specific memory for response-produced information would have to have been affected by principal-sulcus lesions. The lesion of the arcuate sulcus may produce deficits when performances are based upon auditory signals or when "directional responses" must be made. In general, Goldman and Rosvold did not feel that the effects of this lesion reflected an impairment of memory systems.

Other authors have thought that specific memory losses could be the basis of the behavioral deficits found in monkeys after prefrontal-lobe damage. For example, Pinto-Hamuy and Linck (1965) suggested that such animals could not remember their progress through a sequence of behaviors if external cues were not present to guide them. They believed that the animals could not develop a plan for a series of acts that could be used to guide and direct the series. Without such a plan, information could be retained but behavior would be chaotic: Responses would be repeated, and the sequence would be begun again and again. As a result, an external observer could infer a deficiency in memory. This suggestion follows from prior work and analysis by Pribram (1961) in which it was shown that monkeys with prefrontal damage did not have special trouble with the localization of signals in space, proprioception, or visual performances. They did show behavioral disturbances when the cues guiding behavior became unreliable, and they had trouble organizing behavior toward relevant goals.

The delayed-response performance of animals with prefrontal-lobe damage can be improved by increasing their food deprivation (Pribram, 1950). Gross (1963b) extended this finding by showing that increased deprivation produced its beneficial effect by enhancing the value of the incentives used in baiting food wells.

Buddington, King, and Roberts (1969) also found that the performance of monkeys with prefrontal damage could be improved by changing the method by which the correct response was signaled. In their paradigm food was not shown the animals in the baiting period; instead, plastic cubes were illuminated in different ways to signal the correct response. Certain ways of signaling benefited the brain-damaged animals. In his dissertation, Buddington (1971) suggested that the method of cuing, the introduction of a delay before the response, and the method of restraining the subjects may all be influential in determining the degree of impairment.

Sensory impairments of a complex nature have been found after frontal lobe damage. The behavior of the lesioned animals often resembles what would be expected on the basis of a hemianopia, in which objects are disregarded rather than not seen (Kennard and Ectors, 1938). This effect has been found to be associated with damage to the superior limb of the arcuate sulcus by Welch and Stuteville (1958). This type of deficit, sometimes called "sensory neglect," has been found in man after parietal-lobe and frontal-lobe damage (Heilman and Valenstein, 1972). The perceptual deficit found after prefrontal-lobe damage may not be restricted to visual events since a loss in cutaneous sensitivity has been reported by Kennard (1939). These observations of a perceptual deficit after prefrontal damage may be an important factor, if not the determining factor, of the impairment on the delayed-response problem.

The importance of the method of indicating the correct response for animals with prefrontal-lobe damage on the delayed-response task is further emphasized by the work of Mishkin and Pribram (1956). If the cue indicating which of two responses wil be rewarded after the delay is presented at a single spatial location, no deficit is found. This would suggest that if a memory model is to explain the effects of the prefrontal-lobe damage on delayed-response problems, it must be restricted to memories based on cues from two positions (rather than one) and to specific signals and methods of restraint, and it must relate the strength of memories to the saliency of the incentives or signals presented. This would be a most specific sort of memory, indeed, and while such a restricted memory system cannot be ruled out, it would seem that other forms of explanation based upon goal-related "plans" or attentional factors are of greater value.

Iversen (1973) has reviewed many studies of brain lesions as they may be related to presumed memory functions, devoting considerable attention to the generation of memory models and to the reconciliation of memory-deficiency studies in man with studies at the animal level. Early in her report she traces the history of theorizing about the structural correlates of memory, including Lashley's inability to find the engram (see Lashley, 1950) and the resurgence of attempts to find such correlates as more and more localization of functions has been reported for the primate neocortex. Localization of other functions has led to the presumption of a localization of "memory." She also points out the wide variety of behavioral deficits found after brain damage whose effects could mimic deficits produced by a disturbance of memory. These include deficits in organizing material in sequential orders, changes in object or stimulus preferences, changes in response abilities (e.g., impairments found after orbitofrontal damage on "go/no-go" tasks but not on left-right spatial tasks, as reported in Lawicka, Mishkin, and Rosvold, 1966), aberrant visual searching, disruptions of spatial orientations, alterations in learning abilities, and alterations in "perceptual processing." Yet, despite this analysis of the difficulties in establishing memory losses because of possible confounding with other changes in performance, Iversen concludes by assuming that changes in memory do occur after prefrontal- and temporal-lobe damage.

Butler (1969) found that retention for object discriminations is adequate over 15-min and 24-hr retention periods, but there is evidence that interference produced by training on similar tasks between learning and retention training does produce a retention deficit. This has been reported even when the training occurs a long time after surgery, when no acquisition deficit can be detected (Iversen, 1970). No greater impairment was found after lesions of the temporal lobe and hippocampus than after lesions of the inferotemporal cortex alone.

Studying baboons, which are not "sophisticated" subjects, Iversen and Weiskrantz (1970) found that temporal-lobe lesions produced an impairment in learning an object discrimination. The animals had trouble retaining the problem over an interval of 24 hr. This result is likely due to the inadequate sampling of the visual world by inferotemporal operates, who tend to have abnormally strong responses to certain salient cues (Butter, 1968: Butter, Mishkin, and Rosvold, 1965). The results of Iversen and Weiskrantz suggest that impaired performances during retention testing will be found when the discriminations allow for the perseveration of responses to salient cues and when opportunities for interference by similar problems is maximized.

35.3.3 Overtraining

From the time of William James, and probably before, it has been thought that well-practiced responses are retained in a somewhat different fashion from those on which only limited training has been given. Little attention needs to be directed toward the execution of well-practiced habits. Just after the turn of the last century, the general impression was formed that well-trained responses are somehow transferred from neocortical to subcortical systems and thus become automatic. Lashley and Franz (1917) studied this problem in rats with extensive destruction of the frontal pole. They found, however, that postoperative performance on the maze problem they used was not greatly affected by the lesions, regardless of the amount of pretraining. Because of his success in disrupting visual habits with posterior neocortical destruction in the rat, Lashley turned to studies using this sort of lesion to evaluate whether extensive preoperative training would produce a decrease in "neocortical localization" (Lashley, 1921). Overtraining should produce greater retention of a brightness discrimination in animals after destruction of posterior neo-

cortical areas than is found in less well trained subjects.

In his study four animals were given at least 1,200 trials after learning a light-alley/dark-alley discrimination. Food was given for correct responses, and an undefined punishment was given after mistakes. The animals were always trained to approach the lighted alley. They were then subjected to destruction of the posterior neocortex produced by the heating of a wire coil placed into the brain. Testing began 24 hr after the lesion for three of the rats and on the sixth postoperative day for the fourth (a female rat which remained stuporous for five days after surgery). The results were not conclusive, due perhaps to differences in the location of the neocortical lesions, the involvement of subcortical structures, or the occurrence of postoperative shock. Overall, the subjects did not perform well in the discrimination task, and Lashley concluded that the overtraining had not protected the animals from the disturbance caused by posterior neocortical destruction. He concluded that the extended training did not transfer the visual habit presumably established in the neocortex to subcortical sites.

A related approach was undertaken by Orbach and Fantz (1958). They wanted to determine if discrepancies among reports pertaining to the effects of lesions of the inferotemporal cortex of monkeys could be resolved on the basis of "overtraining" given the subjects by some investigators but not others. Perhaps the overtraining protected the animals against the lesion-produced effects. Six rhesus monkeys were trained to criterion on three visual problems (brightness, color, and pattern) and then were given 245 additional trials on one of these problems. That is, two monkeys were overtrained on the brightness discrimination, two on the color discrimination, and two on pattern. Lesions were then made in the inferotemporal cortex, and after a two-week recovery period, the animals were retested on all three problems. The monkeys' performance was best on the problem on which they had been overtrained, and the authors concluded that the highly trained habits were "resistant" to the lesions.

However, this conclusion cannot be accepted with certainty because the problem on which an ainmal was overtrained was also the most recent one on which training had been given before the lesion. During the period of the 245 overtraining trials (about 30 trials per training session), no other training was given. It is, therefore, impossible to conclude anything about the effects of simple overtraining, uncontaminated by "recency" effects. It should be pointed out that Orbach and Fantz were interested in the effects of inferotemporal lesions on the visual capabilities of their subjects and not in memory. Their experimental design was created to evaluate *differential* memory capacities related to vision and not to demonstrate a generalized loss in memory. No control groups were run with sham operations, destruction of other brain regions, or varying periods of postoperative recovery. Therefore, conclusions about overtraining and even memory itself cannot be made from these data.

35.3.4 The limbic system

Recently, I have suggested that all of the various structures of the limbic system operate to regulate more fundamental mechanisms of the protoreptilian brain (to use the metaphor of MacLean and Elliot Smith) and that the functional distinctions among the structures primarily concern the conditions under which this regulation is exerted (Isaacson, 1974). This suggestion arose, in part, from an examination of the many and varied effects produced by damage to the limbic system—effects which are difficult to categorize under conventional behavioral classification systems. In general, the effects of damage to the limbic system seem to be related to changes in performance but not to learning and memory per se.

AMYGDALA. In considering the behavioral changes that follow destruction of the amygdala, Goddard (1964) has written as follows: "The amygdala is primarily involved in the active suppression of motivated approach behavior. Once an amygdalectomized animal has overcome the initial postoperative depression and lethargy, it overeats, responds sexually to all stimuli even remotely resembling a receptive female, approaches all stimuli whether dangerous or not with curiosity, and is unresponsive to variations in deprivation and food reward. In other words, it does not know when to stop" (p. 102). Accepting this general description of the effects of amygdala damage means that postoperative testing of such animals will be done within a greatly changed behavioral context. If testing is begun shortly after surgery, the animals are lethargic and have a lowered body temperature. They are reluctant to do much of anything, including grooming and eating. Frequently, the animals must be maintained through forced feeding. If tested later, they are hyperactive, impulsive, and unable to inhibit responses based upon the basic biological motives. However, these descriptions should be recognized as oversimplifications. The amygdala is a heterogeneous structure, and different portions of it act to affect behavior in different, and sometimes antagonistic, ways. Furthermore, the effects usually produced by damage to one part of the amygdala can be changed or reversed by lesions in another part (Fonberg 1973). This suggests that whether animals are hyper- or hyporeactive, and whether they exhibit other, correlated behavioral changes, depends upon the relative damage to the several subregions of the amygdala.

Destruction of the amygdala has been reported not to affect retention of an active-avoidance response (Brady et al., 1954) despite its well-known effect on the acquisition of this sort of response. Even here, however, exceptions can be found, since Horvath (1963) has reported a deficit in the retention of a preoperatively learned active-avoidance task after amygdala damage. No retention loss of an active-avoidance response to a light cue was found after interruption of fibers connecting the amygdala with the hypothalamus over the ansa lenticularis. Animals with these lesions who were given original training in the task postoperatively did show acquisition deficits (Caruthers, 1968). Fonberg, Brutkowski, and Mempel (1962) found that overtraining protected the animals from the loss of defensive leg-flexion response, otherwise disrupted by damage to the amygdala. Since the deficit in acquiring an active-avoidance response produced by amygdala destruction can be offset by the administration of ACTH an hour before training (Bush, Lovely, and Pagano, 1973), it would be of interest to determine whether the mobilization of the corticosteroids influences postoperative retention of the leg-flexion response.

Lesions of the amygdala in the monkey fail to influence the retention of a discrimination based upon the sizes of two stimulus sequences, although postoperatively there is a reduction in the number of stimuli seen as equivalent to the training stimuli (Bagshaw and Pribram, 1965).

Destruction of the tissue between the amygdala and the hippocampus in the cat results in a deficit in two-way active avoidance that is much greater for a visual cue (flicker) than for an auditory one (tone). However, this deficit probably reflects an impairment in the abilities required to perform the response, since retraining often required many more trials than did original learning (Caruthers, 1969). Damage in the same general area (ventral temporal lobe) has previously been reported not to affect the retention of an avoidance response utilizing an auditory cue (Brady et al., 1954).

Schwartzbaum, Thompson, and Kellicutt (1964) reported a deficit in the retention of an auditory discrimination after damage to the amygdaloid region in the rat. However, such deficits can be found in animals trained entirely postoperatively in the task (Freeman and Kramarcy, 1974), and the deficit therefore seems to result from an inability to perform the discrimination task rather than from an inability to retain it in memory.

SEPTAL AREA. Carey (1967) found that septal lesions *reduced* the number of responses made during postoperative extinction testing by animals that had been trained preoperatively in an operant task. But animals that first underwent surgery and were then trained on the task and placed on an extinction schedule were *more* resistant to extinction than controls. The decreased resistance to extinction found when the lesioned animals were trained before surgery and placed on extinction afterwards may reflect a deficit in retention, but it could also reflect changes in the perception of the environment related to differential drive-associated stimuli or to alterations in emotionality. While not a definitive study in regard to memory, this work does point out that a perseveration of acquired responses is not the inevitable consequence of septal-area destruction.

Carey (1968) reports a deficit in retention of a multiple-choice maze demanding alternating left and right turns. After surgery the animals performed poorly, but it is not clear what effect the surgery might have had on the ability to use spatial or response-produced information. The importance of the septal area in the use of spatial information was suggested by Donovick and Schwartzbaum (1966) and by Kasper (1965), and this proposal was supported by Schwartzbaum and Donovick (1968). The last authors found three types of performance changes after septal lesions: (1) a spatial disorientation; (2) a perseveration of responses; and (3) a tendency to respond quickly. One or more of these types of behavioral changes could probably account for the "retention deficits" found in Carey's maze study.

Holdstock and Edelson (1969) failed to find a deficit in the retention of a discriminated operant task based upon the degree to which an operant chamber was tilted, although the animals with septal lesions did not make as fine discriminations in the degree of tilt as did control animals. Other failures to find retention deficits after septal lesions include studies involving visual-discrimination tasks (Breen and Thompson, 1966; Kleiner, Meyer, and Meyer, 1967) and a straight-alley runway (Raphelson, Isaacson, and Douglas, 1966).

Moore (1964) reported deficits in the retention of a two-way active-avoidance task by cats after septal-area damage, and a more accentuated deficit after combined septal-hippocampal damage. These results are difficult to explain, given the rapid acquisition of this sort of task after such destruction found in other studies; they may be related to a loss of the ability to make the necessary instrumental responses, a loss which was clearly seen in some of Moore's subjects.

The fact that the tendencies or sets established before surgery carry over to affect postoperative performance in passive-avoidance tasks indicates that septal (or hippocampal) damage does not obliterate aversive memories (e.g., Wishart and Mogenson, 1970; Kimble, Kirk-

by and Stein, 1966; Kimura, 1958). Therefore, as with damage to the amygdala, most studies related to the retention of learned behaviors after septal-area damage fail to support the view that memory has been disrupted by the lesions.

HIPPOCAMPUS. Buerger (1970) failed to find any postoperative retention deficit in the relearning of a visual-discrimination problem after hippocampal destruction. Cats newly trained on this problem postoperatively were found to have impaired acquisition. Winocur and Salzen (1968) failed to find evidence for retention deficits in a task in which circles of two sizes had to be discriminated, although an impaired transfer of the conditioned response to similar sets of stimuli was found in other animals after dorsal hippocampal damage. Hippocampal damage in monkeys does not affect retention of delayed-response (Correll and Scoville, 1960) or delayed matching-to-sample problems (Correll and Scoville, 1965b).

In a study of monkeys with medial-temporal-lobe damage Correll and Scoville (1965a) found deficits suggesting difficulty in the retention of "serial tasks." This difficulty may have been related to excessive interference among test problems for the lesioned subjects. This increased sensitivity to interfering events could help account for the discrepancies among other studies (e.g., Orbach, Milner, and Rasmussen, 1960), although it probably is but one of several consequences of medial-temporal-lobe damage and may not be uniquely associated with hippocampal destruction.

The ordering of behaviors after hippocampal or medial-temporal-lobe damage can be difficult, as further evidenced by the impairments found after such damage on delayed-alternation problems (e.g., Mahut and Cordeau, 1963; Pribram, Wilson, and Connors, 1962; Rosvold and Szwarcbart, 1964; Racine and Kimble, 1965). As is found after damage to the prefrontal lobes, a disruption of the proper ordering of events can easily be mistaken for an impairment in memory.

35.4 CONCLUSIONS

From my review of the literature pertaining to the effects of experimental brain damage as it might affect memory, I conclude that no type of localized brain damage yet studied has produced deficits in information-storage mechanisms. Experiments that have produced results seemingly consistent with information-storage deficiencies have had to assume memory systems of such a specialized and restricted nature (e.g., in a specific behavioral task, with a certain type of signal used for the correct response, with a single type of response demanded, under specified conditions of deprivation, and with a particular incentive provided) that explanations based upon other sorts of changes seem to be much more parsimonious and to encompass more of the data.

However, even though brain damage does not seem to influence the storage of information, it does seem capable of influencing the expression of previously acquired information in two ways: (1) by making the retrieval of information difficult, and (2) by altering the ability of animals to stop responding on the basis of previous established habits. The first of these ways can be seen in studies in which damage is inflicted upon some part of a sensory system. The world is perceived differently, and probably less clearly, after such lesions. As a consequence, cues that indicate the correct pathways, responses, or goals are less effective in guiding behavior. Retrieval is hampered by a reduction in the resolution of the signals that direct behavior. It is as if the signal-to-noise ratio of the cues needed for performing the learned response had been reduced, although most likely the brain damage produces distortions in the animal's perception of the environment as well as a reduction in efficiency. These distortions undoubtedly also lead to confusion and impaired retrieval. The effects of damage to components of sensory systems could be likened to testing animals with less articulated and intense signals in weirdly distorted circumstances. Changes in the expression of previously acquired responses would not be unexpected under such circumstances, and if some basic sensory capacity is affected by the damage, relearning requiring that capacity would obviously be forever lost.

It is more difficult to describe changes in behavior that reflect a perseveration of previously acquired ways of responding. In many ways, damage to the limbic system, or to neocortical systems more or less closely associated with the limbic system, makes it difficult for animals to change their old ways of responding. This amounts to a deficiency in inhibitory regulation of previously acquired responses, and it produces a greatly exaggerated proactive interference. This proactive interference may also account for at least some of the retrieval deficits found in human amnesic disorders (Warrington and Weiskrantz, 1973). The memory defect is one in which access to past memories or retrieval of stored information is affected by changes in the behavioral dispositions of the animals. Thus the effect on memory is secondary to these other changes.

If they occur at all, disturbances of information storage seem to be a consequence of general disruptions of brain function rather than damage to isolated areas. The disruptions produced by electroconvulsive shock, inhibitors of protein synthesis, and spreading depression are well known, even if there are still questions as to whether storage or retrieval mechanisms are the most

affected. Probably the most convincing demonstration of changes in memory brought about by manipulations of the general state of the nervous system is the production of time-dependent effects by the administration of stimulants after a learning experience (McGaugh, 1968). In this paradigm the traces of the experience seem to be enhanced, since the drug could not have affected the animals during the acquisition period. Furthermore, the beneficial effects are only found if the drug is given shortly after training. Similar time-dependent effects have seldom been studied with brain lesions. However, a deficit in the retention of a step-through passive-avoidance task measured 24 hr after training has been reported to follow stab wounds to the neocortex, provided the damage is inflicted immediately after training. If the hippocampus is also penetrated by the stab, the retention deficit can be observed if the procedure is administered up to 1 hr after training (Dorfman et al., 1969). Some localization may be involved, since wounds to the cerebellum fail to induce the amnesic effects. Uretsky and McCleary (1969) found that "isolation" of the hippocampus by section of the fornix and damage to the entorhinal area produced a deficit in retention of an avoidance task, as measured by relearning, if the lesions were made three hours after acquisition of the task. Lesions made several days after acquisition did not affect retention. (Lesions of the fornix or the entorhinal area, by themselves, did not affect retention at either postacquisition interval.)

Fried and Goddard (1967) found that the emotional state of an animal at the time of surgery helps determine postoperative behavior, especially in regard to aversive tasks. They initiated surgery after various amounts of experience with an approach-avoidance problem and found that the consequences of the surgery depended upon the emotional "set" of the animals at the time of the operation. Although the experiment did not investigate time-dependent effects per se, it does suggest that time-dependent effects can be related to the "fixation" of sets in the animals at the time of surgery.

The representations of past experiences tend to survive many, if not all, forms of damage to the brain except, perhaps, insults that occur shortly after learning. Even in these cases, the damage may influence retrieval rather than storage, and relatively little has been done in investigating time-dependent effects of brain damage. This review suggests that the storage of information may be a ubiquitous quality of nervous-system tissue, if not of all living matter. After all, learning and memory have been demonstrated in animals made up of but a few cells and with no known nervous system. Brain damage seems to be effective only in altering access to the stored information, through disturbances in sensory and perceptual systems and changes in the animal's ability to modify its previously established response tendencies.

REFERENCES

BAGSHAW, J. H., and PRIBRAM, K. H. 1965. Effect of amygdalectomy on transfer of training in monkeys. *Journal of Comparative and Physiological Psychology* 59: 118–121.

BAUER, J. H., and COOPER, R. M. 1964. Effects of posterior cortical lesions on performance of a brightness-discrimination task. *Journal of Comparative and Physiological Psychology* 58: 84–92.

BRADY, J. V., SCHREINER, L., GELLER, J., and KLING, A. 1954. Subcortical mechanisms in emotional behavior: The effect of rhinencephalic injury upon the acquisition of a conditioned avoidance response in cats. *Journal of Comparative and Physiological Psychology* 47: 179–196.

BRAUN, J. J., MEYER, P. M., and MEYER, D. R. 1966. Sparing of a brightness habit in rats following visual decortication. *Journal of Comparative and Physiological Psychology* 61: 70–82.

BREEN, T., and THOMPSON, R. 1966. Cortical and subcortical structures mediating a visual conditioned response motivated by thirst. *Journal of Comparative and Physiological Psychology* 61: 146–150.

BRUTKOWSKI, S. 1964. Prefrontal cortex and drive inhibition. In J. M. Warren and K. Akert, eds., *The Frontal Granular Cortex and Behavior*. New York: McGraw-Hill, p. 242.

BRUTKOWSKI, S., and DABROWSKA, J. 1966. Prefrontal cortex control of differentiation behavior in dogs. *Acta Biologiae Experimentalis (Warsaw)* 26: 425–439.

BUDDINGTON, R. W. 1971. Intratrial cue observations and delayed response performance in normal and prefrontal monkeys. Unpublished Ph.D. dissertation, University of Florida.

BUDDINGTON, R. W., KING, F. A., and ROBERTS, L. 1969. Analysis of changes in indirect delayed response performance in monkeys with prefrontal lesions. *Journal of Comparative and Physiological Psychology* 68: 147–154.

BUERGER, A. A. 1970. Effects of preoperative training on relearning a successive discrimination by cats with hippocampal lesions. *Journal of Comparative and Physiological Psychology* 72: 462–466.

BUSH, D. F., LOVELY, R. H., and PAGANO, R. R. 1973. Injection of ACTH induces recovery from shuttle-box avoidance deficits in rats with amygdaloid lesions. *Journal of Comparative and Physiological Psychology* 83: 168–172.

BUTLER, C. R. 1969. Is there a memory impairment in monkeys after inferior temporal lesions? *Brain Research* 13: 383–393.

BUTTER, C. M. 1968. The effect of discrimination training on pattern equivalence in monkeys with inferotemporal and lateral striate lesions. *Neuropsychologia* 6: 27–40.

BUTTER, C. M., MISHKIN, M., and ROSVOLD, H. E. 1965. Stimulus generalization in monkeys with inferotemporal and lateral occipital lesions. In D.J. Mostofsky, ed., *Stimulus Generalization*. Stanford, Calif.: Stanford University Press, pp. 119–133.

CAREY, R. J. 1967. A retention loss following septal ablations in the rat. *Psychonomic Science* 7: 307–308.

CAREY, R. J. 1968. Impairment of maze retention resulting from septal injury. *Physiology and Behavior* 3: 495–497.

CARUTHERS, R. P. 1968. Ansa lenticularis area tractotomy and shuttle avoidance learning. *Journal of Comparative and Physiological Psychology* 65: 295–302.

CARUTHERS, R. P. 1969. Deficits in shock-avoidance performance after amygdala-hippocampus separation. *Journal of Comparative and Physiological Psychology* 67: 547–554.

CASTRO, A. J. 1972. The effects of cortical ablations on digital usage in the rat. *Brain Research* 37: 173–186.

CHOW, K. L. 1954. Lack of behavioral effects following destruction of some thalamic association nuclei in monkeys. *Archives of Neurology and Psychiatry* 71: 762–771.

COLE, D., SULLINS, W. R., and ISAAC, W. 1967. Pharmacological modification of the effects of spaced occipital ablations. *Psychopharmacologia (Berlin)* 11: 311–316.

COOPER, R. M., BLAND, B. H., GILLESPIE, L. A., and WHITAKER, R. H. 1970. Unilateral posterior cortical and unilateral collicular lesions and visually guided behavior in the rat. *Journal of Comparative and Physiological Psychology* 72: 286–295.

CORRELL, R. E., and SCOVILLE, W. B. 1960. Effects of medial temporal lesions on delayed reactions. Paper read at the meeting of the American Psychological Association, Chicago, September 1960.

CORRELL, R. E., and SCOVILLE, W. B. 1965a. Effects of medial temporal lesions on visual discrimination performance. *Journal of Comparative and Physiological Psychology* 60: 175–181.

CORRELL, R. E., and SCOVILLE, W. B. 1965b. Performance on delayed match following lesions of medial temporal lobe structures. *Journal of Comparative and Physiological Psychology* 60: 360–367.

DALBY, D. A., MEYER, D. R., and MEYER, P. M. 1970. Effects of occipital neocortical lesions upon visual discriminations in the cat. *Physiology and Behavior* 5: 727–734.

DONOVICK, P. J., and SCHWARTZBAUM, J. S. 1966. Effects of low-level stimulation of the septal area on two types of discrimination reversal in the rat. *Physchonomic Science* 6: 3–4.

DORFMAN, L. J., BOHDANECKA, M., BOHDANECKY, Z., and JARVIK, M. E. 1969. Retrograde amnesia produced by small cortical stab wounds in the mouse. *Journal of Comparative and Physiological Psychology* 69: 324–328.

DOTY, R. W., BECK, E. C., and KOOI, K. A. 1959. Effect of brainstem lesions on conditioned responses of cats. *Experimental Neurology* 1: 360–385.

FONBERG, E. 1973. The normalizing effect of lateral amygdalar lesions upon the dorsomedial amygdalar syndrome in dogs. *Acta Biologiae Experimentalis (Warsaw)* 33: 449–466.

FONBERG, E., BRUTKOWSKI, S., and MEMPEL, E. 1962. Defensive conditioned reflexes and neurotic motor reactions following amygdalectomy in dogs. *Acta Biologiae Experimentalis (Warsaw)* 22: 51–57.

FREEMAN, F. G., and KRAMARCY, N. R. 1974. Stimulus control of behavior and limbic lesions in rats. *Behavioral Biology* 13: 609–615.

FREEMAN, F. G., MIKULKA, P. J., and D'AUTEUIL, P. D. 1974. Conditioned suppression of a licking response in rats with hippocampal damage. *Behavioral Biology* 12: 257–263.

FRIED, P. A., and GODDARD, G. V. 1967. The effects of hippocampal lesions at different stages of conflict in the rat. *Physiology and Behavior* 2: 325–330.

GALEF, B. G. 1970. Aggression and timidity: Responses to novelty in feral Norway rats. *Journal of Comparative and Physiological Psychology* 70: 370–381.

GIRDEN, E. 1940. Cerebral mechanisms in conditioning under curare. *American Journal of Psychology* 53: 397–406.

GODDARD, G. V. 1964. Functions of the amygdala. *Psychological Bulletin* 62: 89–109.

GOLDMAN, P. S., and ROSVOLD, H. E. 1970. Localization of function within the dorsolateral prefrontal cortex of the rhesus monkey. *Experimental Neurology* 27: 291–304.

GROSS, C. G. 1963a. A comparison of the effects of partial and total lateral frontal lesions on test performance by monkeys. *Journal of Comparative and Physiological Psychology* 56: 41–47.

GROSS, C. G. 1963b. Effect of deprivation on delayed response and delayed alternation performance by normal and brain operated monkeys. *Journal of Comparative and Physiological Psychology* 56: 48–51.

GROSS, C. G., and WEISKRANTZ, L. 1962. Evidence for dissociation of impairment on auditory discrimination and delayed response following lateral frontal lesions in monkeys. *Experimental Neurology* 4: 453–47.

HARLOW, H. F. 1952. Functional organization of the brain in relation to mentation and behavior. In *The Biology of Mental Health and Disease*. New York: Paul B. Hoeber.

HEILMAN, K. M., and VALENSTEIN, E. 1972. Frontal lobe neglect in man. *Neurology* 22: 660–664.

HOLDSTOCK, T. L., and EDELSON, A. 1969. Retention of a geotaxic discrimination task following septal lesions in rats. *Psychonomic Science* 15: 169–170.

HOREL, J. A. 1968a. A visual function for the ventral nucleus of the lateral geniculate body. *Anatomical Record* 160: 367.

HOREL, J. A. 1968b. Effects of subcortical lesions on brightness discrimination acquired by rats without visual cortex. *Journal of Comparative and Physiological Psychology* 65: 103–109.

HOREL, J. A., BETTINGER, L. A., ROYCE, G. J., and MEYER, D. R. 1966. Role of neocortex in the learning and relearning of two visual habits by the rat. *Journal of Comparative and Physiological Psychology* 61: 66–78.

HORVATH, F. E. 1963. Effects of basolateral amygdalectomy on three types of avoidance behavior in cats. *Journal of Comparative and Physiological Psychology* 56: 380–389.

ISAAC, W. 1964. Role of stimulation and time in the effects of spaced occipital ablations. *Psychology Reports* 14: 151–154.

ISAACSON, R. L. 1974. *The Limbic System*. New York: Plenum Publishing Corporation.

ISAACSON, R. L. 1975. The myth of recovery from early brain damage. In N. R. Ellis, ed., *Aberrant Development in Infancy. Human and Animal Studies*. Potomac, Md.: Lawrence Erlbaum Associates.

IVERSEN, S. D. 1970. Interference and inferotemporal memory deficits. *Brain Research* 19: 277–289.

IVERSEN, S. D. 1973. Brain lesions and memory in animals. In J. A. Deutsch, ed., *The Physiological Basis of Memory*. New York: Academic Press, pp. 305–364.

IVERSEN, S. D., and WEISKRANTZ, L. 1970. An investigation of a possible memory defect produced by inferotemporal lesions in the baboon. *Neuropsychologia* 8: 21–36.

JONASON, K. R., LAUBER, S., ROBBINS, M. J., MEYER, P. M., and MEYER, D. R. 1970. The effects of dl-amphetamine upon discrimination behaviors in rats with cortical lesions. *Journal of Comparative and Physiological Psychology* 73: 47–55.

KASPER, P. 1965. Disruption of position habit reversal by septal stimulation. *Psychonomic Science* 3: 111–112.

KENNARD, M. A. 1939. Alterations in response to visual stimuli following lesions of frontal lobes in monkeys. *Archives of Neurology and Psychiatry* 41: 1153.

KENNARD, M. A., and ECTORS, L. 1938. Forced circling movements in monkeys following lesions of the frontal lobes. *Journal of Neurophysiology* 1: 45.

KIMBLE, D. P. 1963. The effect of bilateral hippocampal lesions in rats. *Journal of Comparative and Physiological Psychology* 56: 273–283.

KIMBLE, D. P., KIRKBY, R. J., and STEIN, D. G. 1966. Response perseveration interpretation of passive avoidance deficits in hippocampectomized rats. *Journal of Comparative and Physiological Psychology* 61: 141–143.

KIMURA, D. 1958. Effects of selective hippocampal damage on avoidance behavior in the rat. *Canadian Journal of Psychology* 12: 213–218.

KIRCHNER, K. A., BRAUN, J. J., MEYER, D. R., and MEYER, P. M. 1970. Equivalence of simultaneous and successive neocortical ablations in production of impairments of retention. *Journal of Comparative and Physiological Psychology* 73: 47–55.

KLEINER, F. B., MEYER, P. M., and MEYER, D. R. 1967. Effects of simultaneous septal and amygdaloid lesions upon emotionality and retention of a black-white discrimination. *Brain Research* 5: 459–468.

KLING, A. J., ORBACH, J., SCHWARZ, N., and TOWNE, J. 1960. Injury to the limbic system and associated structures in cats. *Archives of General Psychiatry* 3: 391–340.

KLÜVER, H. 1942. Functional significance of the geniculostriate system. In H. Klüver, ed., *Visual Mechanisms*. Lancaster, Pa.: Jacques Cattell Press, pp. 253–299.

KRECH, D. 1962. Cortical localization of function. In L. Postman, ed., *Psychology in the Making*. New York: Alfred A. Knopf.

KRIECKHAUS, E. E. 1964. Decrements in avoidance behavior following mammillothalamic tractotomy in cats. *Journal of Neurophysiology* 27: 753–767.

KRIECKHAUS, E. E., COONS, E. E., GREENSPON, T., WEISS, J., and LORENZ, R. L. 1968. Retention of choice behavior in rats following mammillothalamic tractotomy. *Physiology and Behavior* 3: 125–131.

KRIECKHAUS, E. E., and RANDALL, D. 1968. Lesions of mammillothalamic tract in rat produce no decrements in recent memory. *Brain* 91: 369–378.

LANSDELL, H. D. 1953. Effect of brain damage on intelligence in rats. *Journal of Comparative and Physiological Psychology* 46: 461–464.

LASHLEY, K. S. 1921. Studies of cerebral function in learning. II. The effects of long continued practice upon cerebral localization. *Journal of Comparative Psychology* 1: 453–468.

LASHLEY, K. S. 1929. *Brain Mechanisms and Intelligence*. Chicago: The University of Chicago Press.

LASHLEY, K. S. 1935. The mechanism of vision. XII. Nervous structures concerned in habits based on reactions to light. *Comparative Psychology Monographs* 11: (Whole No. 52).

LASHLEY, K. S. 1937. Functional determinants of cerebral localization. *Archives of Neurology and Psychiatry* 38: 371–387.

LASHLEY, K. S. 1950. In search of the engram. *Symposia of the Society for Experimental Biology* 4: 454–482.

LASHLEY, K. S., and FRANZ, S. I. 1917. The effects of cerebral destruction upon habit formation and retention in the albino rat. *Psychobiology* 1: 71–139.

LAWICKA, W., MISHKIN, M., and ROSVOLD, H. E. 1966. Dissociation of impairment on auditory tasks following orbital and dorsolateral frontal lesions in monkeys. *Congress Polish Physiological Society Lectures* (Symposium abstracts). Lublin: Polish Physiological Society, p. 178.

LeVere, T. E., and Morlock, G. W. 1973. Nature of visual recovery following posterior neodecortication in the hooded rat. *Journal of Comparative and Physiological Psychology* 83: 62–67.

Lewellyn, D., Lowes, G., and Isaacson, R. L. 1969. Visually mediated behaviors following neocortical destruction in the rat. *Journal of Comparative and Physiological Psychology* 69: 25–32.

McGaugh, J. L. 1968. Drug facilitation of memory and learning. In D. H. Efron et al., eds., *Psychopharmacology: A Review of Progress, 1957–1967*. Washington, D.C.: U. S. Public Health Service Publication No. 1836, pp. 891–904.

McNew, J. J. 1963. Role of the red nucleus in visually guided behavior in the rat. *Journal of Comparative and Physiological Psychology* 56: 60–65.

McNew, R. B., and Thompson, R. 1966. Effect of posterior thalamic lesions on retention of a brightness discrimination motivated by thirst. *Journal of Comparative and Physiological Psychology* 62: 125–128.

Mahut, H., and Cordeau, J. P. 1963. Spatial reversal deficit in monkeys with amygdalohippocampal ablations. *Experimental Neurology* 7: 426–434.

Maier, N. R. F. 1932. The effect of cerebral destruction on reasoning and learning in rats. *Journal of Comparative Neurology* 54: 45–75.

Maier, N. R. F. 1941. The effect of cortical injury on equivalence reactions in rats. *The Journal of Comparative Psychology* 32: 165–188.

Meyer, D. R. 1972. Access to engrams. *American Psychologist* 27: 124–133.

Meyer, D. R., Isaac, W., and Maher, B. 1958. The role of stimulation in spontaneous reorganization of visual habits. *Journal of Comparative and Physiological Psychology* 51: 546–548.

Meyer, D. R., Yutzey, D. A., and Meyer, P. M. 1966. Effects of neocortical ablations on relearning of a black-white discrimination habit by two strains of rats. *Journal of Comparative and Physiological Psychology* 61: 83–86.

Meyer, P. M. 1973. Recovery from neocortical damage. In G. M. French, ed., *Cortical Functioning in Behavior*. Glenview, Ill.: Scott, Foresman.

Meyer, P. M., Horel, J. A., and Meyer, D. R. 1963. Effects of dl-amphetamine upon placing responses in neodecorticate cats. *Journal of Comparative and Physiological Psychology* 56: 402–404.

Meyer, P. M., Johnson, D., and Vaughn, D. 1970. The consequences of septal and neocortical ablations upon learning a two-way conditioned avoidance response. *Brain Research* 22: 113–120.

Mishkin, M. 1957. Effects of small frontal lesions on delayed alternation in monkeys. *Journal of Neurophysiology* 20: 615–622.

Mishkin, M., and Pribram, K. H. 1956. Analysis of the effects of frontal lesions in monkey. II. Variations of delayed response. *Journal of Comparative and Physiological Psychology* 49: 36–40.

Mishkin, M., Vest, B., Waxler, M., and Rosvold, H. E. 1969. A reexamination of the effects of frontal lesions on object alternation. *Neuropsychologia* 7: 357–364.

Moore, R. Y. 1964. Effects of some rhinencephalic lesions on retention of conditioned avoidance behavior in cats. *Journal of Comparative and Physiological Psychology* 57: 65–71.

Norton, A. C., and Clark, G. 1963. Effects of cortical and collicular lesions on brightness and flicker discrimination in the cat. *Vision Research* 3: 29–44.

Orbach, J., and Fantz, R. L. 1958. Differential effects of temporal neocortical resections on overtrained and nonovertrained visual habits in monkeys. *Journal of Comparative and Physiological Psychology* 51: 126–129.

Orbach, J., Milner, B., and Rasmussen, T. 1960. Learning and retention in monkeys after amygdal-hippocampus resection. *Archives of Neurology* 3: 220–251.

Overton, D. A. 1971. Commentary. In J. A. Harvey, ed., *Behavioral Analysis of Drug Action*. Glenview, Ill.: Scott, Foresman.

Pasik, T., and Pasik, P. 1973. Extrageniculostriate vision in the monkey. IV. Critical structures for light vs. no-light discrimination. *Brain Research* 56: 165–182.

Petit, T. L., and Thompson, R. 1974. Nucleus cunieformis lesions: Amnestic effects on visual pattern discrimination in the rat. *Physiological Psychology* 2: 126–132.

Petrinovich, L., and Bliss, D. 1966. Retention of a learned brightness discrimination following ablations of the occipital cortex in the rat. *Journal of Comparative and Physiological Psychology* 61:136–138.

Petrinovich, L., and Carew, T. J. 1969. Interaction of neocortical lesion size and interoperative experience in retention of a learned brightness discrimination. *Journal of Comparative and Physiological Psychology* 68: 451–454.

Pinto-Hamuy, T., Santibañez-H, G., and Rojas, A. 1963. Learning and retention of a visual conditioned response in neodecorticate rats. *Journal of Comparative and Physiological Psychology* 56: 19–24.

Pinto-Hamuy, T., and Linck, P. 1965. Effect of frontal lesions on performance of sequential tasks by monkeys. *Experimental Neurology* 12: 96–107.

Pribram, K. H. 1950. Some physical and pharmacological factors affecting delayed response performance of baboons following frontal lobotomy. *Journal of Neurophysiology* 13: 373–382.

Pribram, K. H. 1961. A further experimental analysis of the behavioral deficit that follows injury to the primate frontal cortex. *Experimental Neurology* 3: 432–466.

Pribram, K. H., Douglas, R. J., and Pribram, B. J. 1969. The nature of nonlimbic learning. *Journal of Comparative and Physiological Psychology* 69: 765–772.

Pribram, K. H., Wilson, W. A., and Connors, J. 1962. Effects of lesions of the medial forebrain on alternation behavior of rhesus monkeys. *Experimental Neurology* 6: 36–47.

Racine, R. J., and Kimble, D. P. 1965. Hippocampal lesions and delayed alternation in the rat. *Psychonomic Science* 3: 295–286.

Raphelson, A. C., Isaacson, R. L., and Douglas, R. J. 1966. The effect of limbic damage on the retention and performance of a runway response. *Neuropsychologia* 4: 253–264.

Reitz, S. L., and Pribram, K. H. 1969. Some subcortical connections of the inferotemporal gyrus of the monkey. *Experimental Neurology* 25: 632–645.

Rosvold, H. E., and Szwarcbart, M. 1964. Neural structures involved in delayed-response performance. In J. M. Warren and K. Akert, eds., *The Frontal Granular Cortex and Behavior*. New York: McGraw-Hill, pp. 1–15.

Saavedra, M. A., and Pinto-Hamuy, T. 1963. Effects of removal of the anterior or posterior portions of the neocortex on learning and retention of a visual habit. *Journal of Comparative and Physiological Psychology* 56: 25–30.

SCHNEIDER, G. E. 1969. Two visual systems. *Science* 163: 895–902.

SCHWARTZBAUM, J. S., and DONOVICK, P. J. 1968. Discrimination reversal and spatial alternation associated with septal and caudate dysfunction in rats. *Journal of Comparative and Physiological Psychology* 65: 83–92.

SCHWARTZBAUM, J. S., THOMPSON, J. B., and KELLICUTT. M. H. 1964. Auditory frequency discrimination and generalization following lesions of the amygdaloid area. *Journal of Comparative and Physiological Psychology* 57: 257–266.

SPEAR, P. D., and BRAUN, J. J. 1969. Nonequivalence on normal and posteriorly neodecorticated rats on two brightness discrimination problems. *Journal of Comparative and Physiological Psychology* 67: 235–239.

SPILIOTIS, P. H., and THOMPSON, R. 1973. The "manipulative response memory system" in the white rat. *Physiological Psychology* 1: 101–114.

SPRAGUE, J. M., and MEIKLE, JR., T. H. 1965. The role of the superior colliculus in visually guided behavior. *Experimental Neurology* 11: 115–146.

TEUBER, H.-L. 1955. Physiological psychology. *Annual Reviews of Psychology* 6: 267–296.

THOMPSON, R. 1959a. Learning and retentiveness in brain-damaged rats. *Journal of Comparative and Physiological Psychology* 52: 501–505.

THOMPSON, R. 1959b. The comparative effects of anterior and posterior cortical lesions on maze retention. *Journal of Comparative and Physiological Psychology* 52: 506–508.

THOMPSON, R. 1960. Retention of a brightness discrimination following neocortical damage in the rat. *Journal of Comparative and Physiological Psychology* 53: 212–215.

THOMPSON, R. 1963. Differential effects of posterior thalamic lesions on retention of various visual habits. *Journal of Comparative and Physiological Psychology* 56: 60–65.

THOMPSON, R. 1969. Localization of the "visual memory system" in the white rat. *Journal of Comparative and Physiological Psychology*, Monograph 69: 1–29.

THOMPSON, R., BAUMEISTER, A. A., and RICH, I. 1962. Subcortical mechanisms in a successive brightness discrimination habit in the rat. *Journal of Comparative and Physiological Psychology* 55: 478–481.

THOMPSON, R. LUKASZEWSKA, I., SCHWEIGERDT, A., and McNEW, J. J. 1967. Retention of visual and kinesthetic discriminations in rats following pretectodiencephalic and ventral mesencephalic damage. *Journal of Comparative and Physiological Psychology* 63: 458–468.

THOMPSON, R. and MYERS, R. E. 1971. Brainstem mechanisms underlying visually guided responses in the Rhesus monkey. *Journal of Comparative and Physiological Psychology* 74: 479–512.

THOMPSON, R. and RICH, I. 1961. A discrete diencephalic pretectal area critical for the retention of visual habits in the rat. *Experimental Neurology* 4: 436–443.

THOMPSON, R., RICH, I., and LANGER, S. K. 1964. Lesion studies on the functional significance of the posterior thalamo-mesencephalic tract. *Journal of Comparative Neurology* 123: 29–44.

THOMPSON, R., TRUAX, T., and THORNE, M. 1969. Retention of visual learning following ventromedial midbrain transections in rats. Paper presented at the Conference on the Subcortical Visual Systems, Cambridge, June 1969.

URETSKY, E., and McCLEARY, R. A. 1969. Effect of hippocampal isolation on retention. *Journal of Comparative and Physiological Psychology* 68: 1–8.

VAN HARTESVELDT, C. 1973. Size of reinforcement and operant responding in hippocampectomized rats. *Behavioral Biology* 8: 347–356.

WARRINGTON, E. K., and WEISKRANTZ, L. 1973. An analysis of short-term and long-term memory defects in man. In J. A. Deutsch, ed., *The Physiological Basis of Memory*. New York: Academic Press, pp. 356–396.

WEISKRANTZ, L. 1963. Contour discrimination in a young monkey with striate cortex ablation. *Neuropsychologia* 1: 145–164.

WELCH, K., and STUTEVILLE, P. 1958. Experimental production of neglect in monkeys. *Brain* 81: 341.

WETZEL, A. B. 1969. Visual cortical lesions in the cat: A study of depth and pattern discrimination. *Journal of Comparative and Physiological Psychology* 68: 580–588.

WILSON, M. 1957. Effects of circumscribed cortical lesions upon somesthetic and visual discrimination in the monkey. *Journal of Comparative and Physiological Psychology* 50: 630–635.

WINOCUR, G., and SALZEN, E. A. 1968. Hippocampal lesions and transfer behavior in the rat. *Journal of Comparative and Physiological Psychology* 65: 303–310.

WISHART, T., and MOGENSON, G. 1970. Effects of lesions of the hippocampus and septum before and after passive avoidance training. *Physiology and Behavior* 5: 31–34.

WORTHINGTON, C. S., and ISAAC, W. 1967. Occipital ablation and retention of a visual conditioned avoidance response in the rat. *Psychonomic Science* 8: 289–290.

36

Some Difficulties Associated with the Use of Lesion Techniques in the Study of Memory

GARY LYNCH

ABSTRACT The pronounced biochemical and morphological changes which occur in the various cellular elements of areas connected to damaged brain regions are reviewed briefly, and the difficulties these create for the interpretation of the locus of action of lesions are considered. The argument is made that these difficulties, combined with the apparently dispersed localization of memory storage sites in the brain, must cause us to question the logic of using lesion techniques to search for these sites.

Recent work has shown that certain cellular components of the brain possess remarkable plasticity and will show striking alterations in the face of changing circumstances. For example, it appears that axons can sprout new terminals (Moore, this volume) and that the morphology of dendrites reflects to some degree events occurring in their afferents (e.g., Globus and Scheibel, 1966; Parnavalas et al., 1974). I think it is fair to say that much of our interest in topics of this sort derives from a hope that some of these neuronal capabilities are the ones used by the brain to store memories, and indeed this seems plausible.

However, before attacking the problem of whether our favorite type of neuronal plasticity is actually a substrate of learning or memory, it seems apparent that we must first have some idea of where in the brain these elusive psychological processess take place. It is for this reason that I find Isaacson's review of brain lesions and memory (this volume) most timely, for as he points out, the central question in that hoary literature is precisely that of where experiences are stored in the brain.

In my discussion of Isaacson's paper I shall first add to his list of the difficulties that attend any interpretation of the behavioral effects of brain lesions, and then, with these problems in mind, I shall add some comments on what lesions have told us about the localization of memory.

Isaacson has done an impressive job in detailing the controls that must be employed if any psychological study using lesions is to be at all useful. I should like to argue now that in any lesion study, not only will there be great difficulty in establishing which behavioral process

is responsible for induced disturbances, but it will be equally difficult to deduce which brain systems are involved. More specifically, I would like to suggest that any change in behavior seen after brain damage can be attributed to a loss of tissue or to irreversible disturbances in regions not directly affected by the lesion.

A brain lesion, no matter how discrete, initiates biochemical and morphological reactions in the regions connected to the damaged area; and in some cases these reactions develop quite rapidly and persist indefinitely. They will be found in regions that send fibers to the target area as well as in areas that receive afferents from it. Unless an incredible amount of secondary compensation takes place, the net result of all this will be to produce brain systems that function in a radically abnormal fashion.

Changes in cells that project to a damaged area have been the subject of anatomical studies for nearly a century. These cells undergo a syndrome called retrograde degeneration, which includes displacement of the nucleus, aberrations in the Nissl substance, and a variety of enzymatic changes.

Furthermore, recent ultrastructural work has demonstrated that in some cases intact synaptic terminals are displaced from the soma of these cells by glial processes (Blinzinger and Kreutzberg, 1968; Kerns and Hinsman, 1973). Glial reactions in the vicinity of reactive neurons are quite pronounced and include reactions in astrocytes and a massive invasion by a mysterious type of cell usually called "microglia" (e.g., Kerns and Hinsman, 1973).

In some cases these effects result in a massive cell loss. More commonly, however, the process stops before this stage is reached, and a disturbed but still viable brain region results. If some cells in this region project to areas other than the site of the lesion, a situation is created in which grossly abnormal cells are influencing still operative brain circuitry. This would presumably cause behavioral effects which might be falsely attributed to the removal of tissue by the lesion.

The problem of retrograde morphological changes resulting from the severing of axons and the possible functional significance of this for intact circuitry was

GARY LYNCH, Department of Psychobiology, University of California, Irvine considered by Ramón y Cajal (1959). He found that if a lesion was made in month-old cats just beyond the initial collaterals of the axon, cells in the cerebellum and cortex would not only survive but would hyperdevelop their remaining collateral branches. It was his thought that the loss of the primary axon, combined with the hypertrophy of the initial collaterals, transformed the cell into a type of interneuron. Through their newly hyperdeveloped collaterals, these new interneurons could exert powerful influences over wide areas containing cells not initially affected by the lesion (See Fig. 245 in Ramón y Cajal, 1959).

Retrograde changes are not restricted to the regions whose cells project to the area involved in the lesion; they are spread more widely through the brain. Recent experiments show that transmitter enzymes in the collaterals of axons that have lost branches because of lesions are greatly affected by the damage (Reis and Ross, 1973). Thus brainstem projections to the cerebellum are altered by lesions that interrupt their collaterals to the forebrain. This raises the startling possibility that a hypothalamic lesion might have behavioral effects that are actually caused by imbalances in the cerebellum.

In immature animals it is known that the retrograde consequences of lesions can cross synapses and affect brain regions many steps removed from the damaged area. Whether qualitatively similar effects are to be found in adults is not known, but certainly the possibility exists (see the review by Cowan, 1970).

Dramatic anatomical changes also take place in brain areas that receive afferents from the damaged region, and these are found in at least three different cellular elements: in the dendrites of the cells that have lost afferents; in the remaining intact afferents to those cells; and in the neuroglia. These effects have been found throughout the brain, but for purposes of brevity I shall restrict my remarks to the area in which my collaborator Carl Cotman and I have focused our efforts, namely, the dentate gyrus of the rat hippocampus. Following removal of the major input to that structure (the fibers of the entorhinal cortex), there appears to be a marked reduction in the number of dendritic spines in the deafferented dendritic zones. Over several postoperative weeks these lost spines are to some degree apparently replaced (Parnavalas et al., 1974). An alternative interpretation is that spines are losing their staining properties and then regaining them. Whichever explanation is correct, some alteration is taking place in the postsynaptic cell. With regard to remaining afferent systems to the hippocampus, four different fiber systems including associational, commissural, and extrinsic afferents—show reactive anatomical changes; in some cases the changes include growth or "sprouting" into the dendritic zones that have been denervated by the lesions (Cotman et al., 1973; Lynch et al., 1972; Lynch, Deadwyler, and Cotman, 1973; Lynch, Stanfield, and Cotman, 1973; Lynch, 1974; Steward, Cotman, and Lynch, 1974). In two cases we have been able to establish that these new connections are functional (Lynch, Deadwyler, and Cotman, 1973; Steward, Cotman, and Lynch, 1974). It should be emphasized that these effects are obtained after lesions in both adult and immature rats, although developmental differences in the extent of growth have been found (Lynch, Stanfield, and Cotman, 1973; Zimmer, 1973). With regard to glial changes we have only preliminary data, but these suggest that the rapid astroglial reaction and subsequent "microglial" invasion reported by others also occurs in the dentate gyrus.

This spectrum of changes convinces me that the dentate gyrus is transformed into a very unusual but still operative structure within a few days after the entorhinal lesion. To emphasize this, consider the fact that normally the rostral end of this structure receives little input from the contralateral cortex, but after removal of the ipsilateral entorhinal cortex, crossed fibers appear to be the dominant extrinsic afferent.

In view of the fact that the dentate gyrus is the first relay in the series of connections that make up the hippocampal circuitry, it seems apparent that these anatomical changes must produce profound behavioral alterations. This, then, is the problem facing anyone attempting to correlate psychological function with brain locus on the basis of results with lesions: Are the observed effects due to the loss of neural tissue, or are they a consequence of rewiring in areas distant to the lesion?

Having considered some of the difficulties associated with interpreting the behavioral consequences of brain damage, I would now like to make some comments on Isaacson's review of the effects of lesions on memory. Isaacson points out that lesions have been used primarily to identify the anatomical locus of memory and that very early in this enterprise disagreements arose between those who felt that there existed specialized sites for the storage of memories of many types and those who believed that memories were scattered throughout the brain. Gradually, the weight of evidence has forced us to accept the latter position. Isaacson finds no evidence in his analysis that a single localized lesion ever knocks out memories of many different types, and while this is not emphasized, reviews of brain damage in humans indicate that long-term memory (as opposed to memories) is rarely eliminated by any but the most drastic of lesions (Rozin, this volume).

These observations can only direct us to the conclusion that brain evolution has not produced specialized structures that serve as general storage bins for memories. Isaacson does not find this particularly surprising and neither do I; I would suggest, however, that the search for such depositories of experiences had to be made if the investigations into the molecular bases of memory were to have direction. The unhappy realization that the components of memory are likely to be found dispersed among the countless subdivisions of the brain indicates a strategy for future investigations that will be very different from the course we might have followed had we believed in general storage sites.

Unfortunately, the criticisms of the use of lesions in memory research become most pertinent if we accept the idea of the scattered memory system. For if memories represent a lasting change in a system that has primary, nonmemorial functions, then a lesion must necessarily eliminate these functions along with the memory. Note that this would not be the case if memories were stored in some conveniently specialized, isolated locus.

While the history of lesion studies has forced us to accept this dispersal of memory and thereby question the logic of using lesions to look for memory, the above conclusions do not necessarily support Isaacson's radical position that pieces of memory are to be found in every neuron in the brain. Within each system we may yet find components, possibly segregated from their neighbors, that are specialized for change. These components might be scattered throughout the system, or, more hopefully, they might be localized to particular nuclei or regions. Neurophysiological research seems to be heading toward a test of this idea, and I suggest that in doing so, it is making use of the legacy of the many neuropsychologists who have used lesions to search for engrams.

REFERENCES

Blinzinger, K. H., and Kreutzberg, G. W. 1968. Displacement of synaptic terminals from regenerating motoneurones by microglial cell. *Zeitschrift für Zellforschung und Mikroskopische Anatomie* 85: 147–157.

Cotman, C. W., Matthews, D. A., Taylor, D., and Lynch, G. 1973. Synaptic rearrangement in the dentate gyrus: Histochemical evidence of adjustments after lesions in immature and adult rats. *Proceedings of the National Academy of Sciences (USA)* 70: 3473–3477.

Cowan, W. M. 1970. Anterograde and retrograde transneuronal degeneration in the central and peripheral nervous system. In W. J. H. Nauta and S. O. E. Ebbesson, eds., *Contemporary Research Methods in Neuroanatomy*. New York: Springer-Verlag, pp. 217-252.

Globus, A., and Scheibel, A. 1966. Loss of dendritic spines as an index of presynaptic terminal patterns: An experimental application of the Golgi method. *Nature* 212:463–465.

Kerns, J. M., and Hinsman, E. J. 1973. Neuroglial response to sciatic neurectomy. II. Electron microscopy. *Journal of Comparative Neurology* 151: 255–280.

Lynch, G. 1974. The formation of new synaptic connections after brain damage and their possible role in recovery of function. *Neurosciences Research Program Bulletin* 12: 228–233.

Lynch, G., Deadwyler, S., and Cotman, C. 1973. Post-lesion axonal growth produces permanent functional connections. *Science* 180: 1364–1366.

Lynch, G., Matthews, D. A., Mosko, S., Parks, T., and Cotman, C. 1972. Induced acetylcholinesterase-rich layer in rat dentate gyrus following entorhinal lesion. *Brain Research* 42: 311–318.

Lynch, G., Stanfield, B., and Cotman, C. 1973. Developmental differences in post-lesion axonal growth in hippocampus. *Brain Research* 59: 155–168.

Parnavalas, J. G., Lynch, G., Brecha, N., Cotman, C. W., and Globus, A. 1974. Spine loss and regrowth in hippocampus following deafferentation. *Nature* 248: 71–73.

Ramón y Cajal, S. 1959. *Degeneration and Regeneration in the Nervous System*, Vol. 2. Translated by R. May. New York: Hafner Publishing.

Reis, D. J., and Ross, R. A. 1973. Dynamic changes in brain dopamine-β-hydroxylase activity during anterograde and retrograde reactions to injury of central noradrenergic axons. *Brain research* 57: 307–326.

Steward, O., Cotman, C. W., and Lynch, G. 1974. Growth of a new fiber projection in the brain of adult rats: Reinnervation of the dentate gyrus by the contralateral entorhinal cortex follwing ipsilateral entorhinal lesions. *Experimental Brain Research* 20: 42–66.

Zimmer, J. 1973. Extended commissural and ipsilateral projections in postnatally de-entorhinated hippocampus and fascia dentate demonstrated in rats by silver impregnation. *Brain Research* 64: 293–311.

CNS Manipulation in
the Study of Memory:
Electrical Stimulation

37

Modulation of Memory by Electrical Stimulation of the Brain

JAMES L. McGAUGH AND PAUL E. GOLD

ABSTRACT This paper reviews recent studies of the effects of electrical stimulation of the brain on memory-storage processes. Emphasis is placed on studies in which the stimulation is administered to animals shortly after training. Two general findings emerge. First, the effectiveness of the electrical stimulation in altering retention performance varies inversely with the time between training and treatment. Second, for each treatment the length of the gradient of retrograde amnesia or memory enhancement varies directly with the intensity of the treatment.

The primary goal of most of these studies is to understand the nature of alterations in brain function that influence memory-storage processes. It is not yet clear just what neurobiological alterations are critical in this regard. The findings of several studies indicate, for example, that brain seizures are correlated with amnesia only under limited conditions. Furthermore, it is possible to alter memory storage by administering subseizure direct brain stimulation to many brain regions, including the amygdala, hippocampus, caudate nucleus, substantia nigra, and midbrain reticular formation. One interpretation of such findings is that the effective stimulation sites may be brain regions in which memory processing occurs after training. According to this view, electrical stimulation disrupts the localized information processing. However, it is also possible that the effects of even well-localized brain stimulation are actually due to more general influences on brain activity. For example, localized brain stimulation may alter memory processes via trophic influences, which can affect widespread neural systems, including systems that do not have direct anatomical connections with the stimulated site. Possible mechanisms might include alterations in neurotransmitters, or hormones. The understanding of such modulating influences should provide some insight into the neurobiological bases of memory storage.

Electrical stimulation of the brain is used extensively as a technique for investigating the neurobiological bases of behavior. While most of the research using brain stimulation has focused on brain systems involved in motivation and emotion, the procedure has also been used in studies of learning and memory. For example, brain stimulation has been used as a conditioned or unconditioned stimulus, or as a means of modifying the acquisition and performance of learned responses (Doty, 1969; Kesner and Wilburn, 1974). Further, there is extensive evidence that brain stimulation can modulate—that is, either enhance or disrupt—memory-storage processes (McGaugh and Herz, 1972).

JAMES L. McGAUGH and PAUL E. GOLD, Department of Psychobiology, University of California, Irvine

We shall review here some findings from recent studies of the effects of electrical stimulation of the brain on memory-storage processes. Three types of brain stimulation are considered: electroconvulsive shock (ECS) administered through corneal or pinneal electrodes, direct stimulation of the brain through cortical electrodes, and direct stimulation of subcortical brain regions. Studies using ECS were the first to demonstrate that learning and memory can be influenced by passing a current through the brain (Duncan, 1949; Gerard, 1949). Some of the issues raised by ECS studies are relevant to the effects of more specific brain stimulation, and we shall therefore look closely at some of the evidence provided by ECS studies. The studies using direct cortical and subcortical stimulation have investigated neural correlates of the modified retention. In addition, they have attempted to determine whether effects on memory can be produced by stimulation of specific brain regions. Research in this area has been reviewed in a number of recent papers (Gold, Zornetzer, and McGaugh, 1974; Bloch, 1970; Kesner, 1973; Kesner and Wilburn, 1974). Consequently, this chapter will focus on some of the central issues raised by the search and will emphasize recent findings.

37.1 TIME-DEPENDENT EFFECTS: GRADIENTS OF RETROGRADE AMNESIA

Evidence from studies using a variety of experimental procedures indicates that the retention of learned responses is influenced by treatments administered after the learning experience (Glickman, 1961; McGaugh, 1968, 1973; Jarvik, 1972; McGaugh and Herz, 1972; Gibbs and Mark, 1973). Treatments that are effective include antibiotic drugs, convulsant drugs, cortical spreading depression, and, as we shall consider in detail in this chapter, electrical stimulation of the brain (McGaugh, 1974; Zornetzer, 1974).

A general finding of the research is that the treatments are most effective if they are administered shortly after a training experience. The degree of modification of retention decreases as the interval between the training and treatment is increased. Most of the research in this area is concerned with retention impairment produced by posttraining treatments, that is, with retrograde amnesia; in these studies the time-dependent nature of the effect is referred to as a retrograde-amnesia (RA) gradient. Posttraining treatments that enhance retention also decrease in effectiveness as the interval between the training and treatment is increased (McGaugh, 1973; McGaugh and Dawson, 1971). RA gradients merely indicate the effectiveness of a given treatment, administered at a particular time, on retention performance measured at a subsequent time. RA gradients do not provide a direct measure of the time required for the consolidation of long-term memory. It seems reasonable to assume that the longest time after training at which a treatment can significantly modulate subsequent retention should vary with the treatment, as well as with the degree to which the treatment affects the neural systems involved in the hypothesized consolidation processes. In addition, there is no a priori reason to expect that comparable "consolidation times" are initiated under different training conditions. According to this view, experimental studies of retrograde disruption and enhancement of retention should not be expected to yield any time constant for consolidation.

The results of RA studies are consistent with the general view. Under some conditions, for example, treatments such as ECS and convulsant drugs affect retention only if they are administered within a few seconds or minutes after training (Chorover and Schiller, 1965). Under other conditions effects are obtained with treatments administered as long as two or three days after training (McGaugh and Herz, 1972; Mah and Albert, 1973; Jamieson, 1972). Such findings are, of course, perplexing only if it is assumed that RA directly reflects the time needed for the completion of consolidation processes. However, there is extensive evidence that the gradients depend upon the specific experimental conditions used. Cherkin (1969) has shown, for example, that the RA gradients produced by treating neonatal chicks with the convulsant gas flurothyl varies directly with the concentration of the flurothyl and the duration of the treatment. Similarly, several studies (Alpern and McGaugh, 1968; Haycock and McGaugh, 1973; Buckholtz and Bowman, 1972) have shown that the lengths of the RA gradients vary directly with the intensity and duration of ECS.

Gold, Macri, and McGaugh (1973a) have obtained comparable results with direct electrical stimulation of the cortex in rats. Current intensities ranging from 1 to 8 mA (0.5 sec, 60 Hz) were administered directly to either frontal or posterior cortex in rats at various times after training on a one-trial inhibitory (passive) avoidance task. The results, shown in Figure 37.1, indicate

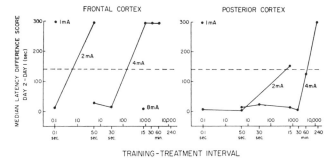

FIGURE 37.1 Median retention scores for crossing into a shock compartment after training on a one-trial inhibitory (passive) avoidance task and then receiving either frontal- or posterior-cortex stimulation at various intensities and training-treatment intervals. The retention scores are based on the difference between the latencies to cross on the training and test trials. All median latencies below 140 seconds (dashed line) are significantly lower (p < 0.05) than those of the nonstimulated foot-shock control group (median = 300 sec). Note that the lengths of the RA gradients vary directly with the intensity of the stimulation. From Gold, Macri, and McGaugh (1973a). Copyright 1973 by the American Association for the Advancement of Science.

that the retention performance, tested 24 hr later, varied with the site of stimulation, the intensity of the stimulation, and the training-treatment interval. The important point here is that with stimulation of either frontal or posterior cortex, the RA gradient varied directly with the stimulation intensity. For example, 2-mA frontal-cortex stimulation produced RA when administered immediately after training but not if delayed by 5 sec. However, 4-mA frontal-cortex stimulation produced amnesia when delayed by 5 sec or even 30 sec after training. When 4 mA was administered 15 min after training, the treatment did not affect retention, but 8-mA stimulation of frontal cortex delayed by 15 min did produce amnesia.

These findings indicate that RA gradients may reflect time-dependent changes in the disruptive threshold for producing amnesia. At a theoretical level, such results imply that memory-storage processes may remain susceptible to modulating influence over long posttraining intervals if appropriate treatments are used (e.g., Mah and Albert, 1973; Alpern and Crabbe, 1972). On the other hand, increasing the intensity of a particular treatment does not necessarily extend the RA gradient. For example, under some conditions very intense cortical stimulation (10–100 mA) produces only short amnesia gradients (< 30 sec) (Paolino and Hine, 1973; Gold, McDonald, and McGaugh, 1974). These results need not imply that there is a maximal amnesia gradient, but may simply indicate that the disruptive effectiveness of a given treatment is limited under the particular experimental conditions used.

Whatever the interpretation of these results, it is clear on both empirical and logical grounds that RA gradients do not directly or precisely reflect the time course of the underlying memory processes that are modulated by amnestic treatments. Memory-disruption studies provide direct information only about the susceptibility of memory to disruption; they do not provide direct information about the underlying memory processes (Weiskrantz, 1966; McGaugh and Dawson, 1971; Gold and McGaugh, 1975).

Thus the major principle derived from these studies is that the treatment effects are time-dependent: the effectiveness of a particular amnestic treatment varies inversely with the training treatment interval and directly with the severity of the treatment used.

37.1.1 Alternative interpretations of the retention deficits produced by posttrial treatments

The findings of studies of the effects on retention of posttrial treatments, such as direct electrical stimulation of the brain, are generally quite consistent with the interpretation that the treatments modulate time-dependent processes underlying memory. However, several alternative interpretations of the basic findings of these studies have been proposed. Since some of these interpretations are considered in other recent papers (McGaugh and Herz, 1972; McGaugh and Dawson, 1971; Mah and Albert, 1973; Lewis, 1969; Miller and Springer, 1973; Gold and King, 1974), we shall not review them in detail here.

A common assumption of several alternative interpretations is that the treatments produce amnesia by affecting retrieval processes rather than by disrupting memory storage. In view of the facts of time dependency, however, it cannot be assumed that the treatments have a general effect on memory retrieval. It must be assumed that the treatments affect the retrievability of recently stored information without affecting the storage processes. Without additional evidence, such an interpretation would be very difficult to assess, since it is not clear how one could distinguish time-dependent storage effects from time-dependent retrieval effects. However, the retrieval hypothesis need not assume that the information is permanently irretrievable. It might be that the information can be retrieved if special experimental procedures are used.

For example, several studies (Lewis, Misanin, and Miller, 1968; Quartermain, McEwen, and Azmitia, 1970; cf. Miller and Springer, 1973) have suggested that rats rendered amnesic by a posttrial treatment can subsequently display retention of the response if they are given some kind of treatment that "reminds" them of the original training. However, in assessing this "reminder"

effect it is important to examine in detail the specific experimental procedures being used. Typically, the animals are trained on a one-trial inhibitory avoidance task. They are punished with a footshock for stepping from one compartment to another. Retention is indexed by high response latencies on the retention test trial. The reminder treatment is usually a footshock administered in a different apparatus. Evidence from several recent studies (Cherkin, 1972; Gold et al., 1973; Haycock, Gold, Macri, and McGaugh, 1973) indicates that the reminder treatment can have punishing effects that influence response latencies on the retention test. Further, reminder treatments are effective only if the animals have some residual memory of the original training. The reminder effect can be readily explained as resulting from the combination, through generalization, of the punishing effects of the reminder stimulus with a weak memory of the original inhibitory avoidance training. It is not necessary to assume that the reminder treatment acts on retrieval processes.

Of course, such evidence is not proof that reminders do not act as proposed by a retrieval hypothesis. The evidence does indicate that it is at least equally reasonable to assume that reminders affect behavior simply because they are mildly punishing. If this is the case, then reminder effects do not shed any light on the question as to whether the effects of posttrial treatment are due to influences on storage or on retrieval of memory.

Another interpretation of the effects of posttrial treatment on retention is that the memory has been stored under the brain state produced by the treatment and, consequently, is irretrievable under normal conditions. Evidence supporting this "state-dependency" hypothesis has been obtained by several investigators (Nielson, 1968; Thompson and Neely, 1970). In our laboratory, however, we have not obtained support for the state-dependent interpretation of posttrial effects (Zornetzer and McGaugh, 1969; McGaugh and Landfield, 1970). In one study, for example, mice were first given a single training trial on an inhibitory avoidance task. Some of the mice were then given a transcorneal ECS treatment 20 sec after the training trial. A retention test was given six days later. One hour before the test half the animals in each group received an ECS. Thus the ECS-treated animals were tested under a brain state comparable to that elicited by the posttrial ECS treatment. The results of this study were contrary to the prediction of the state-dependency hypothesis. The ECS treatment given before the retention test did not attenuate the amnesia produced by the posttrial treatment and did not cause amnesia in animals that had received no ECS following the original training. Of course, our findings do not rule out the possibility that there might be conditions under which posttrial treatments can produce "state-dependent" learning. They do, however, indicate that such an interpretation does not provide a general explanation of retrograde amnesia produced by posttrial treatments.

In summary, the basic finding of studies of the effects of posttrial treatments on memory is that the effects are time-dependent. While there have been many alternative interpretations of the time-dependent effects, experimental tests of these interpretations have not produced critical evidence against the view that the treatments affect retention by modulating memory-storage processes.

37.2 NEUROBIOLOGICAL ASPECTS OF MEMORY MODULATION BY POSTTRIAL ELECTRICAL STIMULATION OF THE BRAIN

While the question of the nature of the retention deficits produced by brain stimulation has generated controversy, it is clear that brain stimulation does affect retention. Much recent research has attempted to determine the neurobiological bases of the effects. The research has focused on two questions. First, what physiological changes are necessary and sufficient conditions for producing memory modulation by brain stimulation? Second, are there specific brain regions in which electrical stimulation is particularly effective in altering retention?

37.2.1 Correlates of retrograde amnesia
In a series of studies using ECS and direct brain stimulation in rats and mice, we have investigated the relationship between brain seizures and amnesia. The basic strategy was to vary the stimulation intensity and to examine concurrently the brain-seizure and RA thresholds. In mice we found that the threshold for producing retrograde amnesia was generally very close to the brain-seizure threshold. Furthermore, if the brain-seizure threshold was elevated with diethyl ether, the RA threshold was also elevated to the same extent (McGaugh and Zornetzer, 1970; Zornetzer and McGaugh, 1971a). Gehres et al. (1973) have obtained similar results in an experiment using hypothermia as the amnestic treatment. The amnesic effect was blocked by drugs that prevented the brain seizures normally produced by hypothermia. However, under some conditions electrical stimulation administered at intensities somewhat below that necessary for brain seizure is sufficient to produce amnesia (Zornetzer and McGaugh, 1971b). Conversely, in certain strains of mice light ether elevates the amnesia threshold far above the brain-seizure threshold (Van Buskirk and McGaugh, 1974).

Similar results have been obtained in studies with rats. Under a variety of conditions RA is produced by direct stimulation of the cortex if the stimulation elicits brain seizures. That is, the thresholds for seizures and RA are similar (Zornetzer, 1974). Under other conditions, however, direct stimulation of the brain does not result in RA even if the current intensity is well above the brain-seizure threshold (Zornetzer, 1972; Gold and McGaugh, 1973; Gold, Macri, and McGaugh, 1973a; Gold, McDonald, and McGaugh, 1974). These results clearly indicate that the brain-seizure threshold and the amnesia threshold can be dissociated.

An important variable that influences the relationship between brain seizures and RA is the training-treatment interval. The brain-seizure threshold for both frontal and posterior cortex is between 1 and 2 mA. However, as was shown in Figure 37.1, the current intensity necessary for producing RA varies directly with the time at which the treatment is administered after training. Thus, although the brain seizure and amnesia thresholds are coupled at the shortest training-treatment intervals, they are dissociated at longer intervals.

A further major variable (or set of variables) which must be considered is the precise nature of the behavioral task. As shown in Figure 37.2, the thresholds for producing amnesia (with a 5-sec training-treatment interval) with frontal- or posterior-cortex stimulation varies in two different inhibitory avoidance tasks. It is important to remember that the brain-seizure threshold is 2 mA for

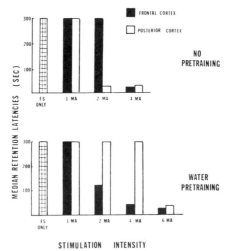

FIGURE 37.2 Retention latencies of rats trained in an inhibitory avoidance task under different behavioral conditions before receiving posttrial stimulation in the frontal or posterior cortex (5-sec training-treatment interval). RA thresholds for frontal and posterior cortex vary with the behavioral conditions. Under conditions of no water deprivation or pretraining exposure to the apparatus (upper graph), the frontal-cortex RA threshold is lower than that of posterior cortex. However, when rats are water-deprived and pretrained to drink prior to inhibitory avoidance training, the frontal-cortex RA threshold is higher than that of posterior cortex. Data from Gold, Bueno, and McGaugh (1973).

both stimulation sites and is stable under these behavioral conditions. However, the threshold for producing RA varies with the particular motivational and training procedures used in the two tasks (Gold, Bueno, and McGaugh, 1973).

In summary, our studies indicate that while in many cases amnesia and seizure thresholds are closely coupled, seizures are neither necessary nor sufficient for producing amnesia. There are, of course, other neurobiological effects of ECS and cortical stimulation that may be related to retrograde amnesia. For example, ECS at an intensity that produces both brain seizures and amnesia also produces a modest degree of inhibition of protein synthesis (approximately 30 percent; see Cotman et al., 1971; Dunn, 1971). Also, cortical stimulation that produces both seizures and amnesia decreases the amount of cortically recorded theta activity (4–7 Hz) for several minutes after stimulation (Landfield, McGaugh, and Tusa, 1972). Rebert, Pryor, and Schaeffer (1974) report that cortical stimulation produces a slow, positive cortical potential which lasts for several minutes after the stimulation. Thus, although there are several potential candidates for neural correlates of amnesia, causal relationships have not been determined. Furthermore, some of the data obtained suggest that it may not be possible to find a causal relationship with these methods (see Gold, Zornetzer, and McGaugh, 1974). Because there are many physiological events that accompany brain seizures, the findings described above suggest that subseizure stimulation of specific brain sites may be a more useful technique for investigating the neurobiology of retrograde amnesia.

37.2.2 Disruption of memory-storage processes by subseizure stimulation

There is considerable evidence that memory is influenced by posttrial electrical stimulation of several brain regions. At one level, the approach may provide little information not already available. For example, if gross electrical brain stimulation (i.e., ECS) can produce amnesia, surely, it might be argued, sufficiently intense stimulation of any brain structure should have the same effect. Indeed, we expect this to be the case, and there is considerable evidence that direct electrical stimulation does produce retrograde amnesia when administered to any of several brain structures. Many studies have used stimulation intensities that produce brain seizures. Because of the possible loss of anatomical and physiological specificity, these studies are not included here (for reviews that do include such studies, see McGaugh and Herz, 1972; Kesner and Wilburn, 1974; and Gold, Zornetzer, and McGaugh, 1974). However, many recent studies of the effects of posttrial electrical

stimulation of the brain on memory have used stimulation below the brain-seizure threshold. A major advantage of such studies is that, in addition to providing further information about time-dependent memory processes, they can determine the brain structures in which electrical stimulation is most effective in modulating memory. In this way, the approach may potentially provide useful information about the neural systems that modulate memory.

A review of these studies indicates that posttrial subseizure electrical stimulation is an effective amnestic treatment if administered to the hippocampus (Wyers et al., 1968; Haycock, Deadwyler, Sideroff, and McGaugh, 1973; McDonough and Kesner, 1971; Kesner and Conner, 1972, 1974; Zornetzer and Chronister, 1973; Zornetzer, Chronister, and Ross, 1973), caudate nucleus (Thompson, 1958; Wyers et al., 1968; Wyers and Deadwyler, 1971; Peeke and Herz, 1971; Haycock, Deadwyler, Sideroff, and McGaugh, 1973; Wilburn and Kesner, 1972), substantia nigra (Routtenberg and Holzman, 1973), thalamus (Mahut, 1962, 1964; Wilburn and Kesner, 1972), midbrain reticular formation (Glickman, 1958), and amygdala (McDonough and Kesner, 1971; Ilyutchenok and Vinnitsky, 1971; Bresnahan and Routtenberg, 1972; Gold, Macri, and McGaugh, 1973b; Kesner and Conner, 1974; Handwerker, Gold, and McGaugh, 1974; Gold, Edwards, and McGaugh, 1975; Gold, Rose, Spanis, and McGaugh, in preparation).

Although there is some disagreement, for example, as to whether subseizure stimulation of the caudate (Gold and King, 1972), midbrain reticular formation (Zornetzer, 1972), or amygdala (Lidsky et al., 1970) produces retrograde amnesia in all cases, there is for the most part considerable general consistency in these findings. First, at least in many cases, localized brain stimulation can produce amnesia in the absence of brain seizures. Second, the amnestic effectiveness of these treatments, as of other treatments, varies inversely with the time after training. Third, there appears to be generality of these findings across behavioral tasks. For example, caudate stimulation disrupts retention of inhibitory avoidance (Wyers et al., 1968; Haycock, Deadwyler, Sideroff, and McGaugh, 1973; McDonough and Kesner, 1971; Kesner and Conner, 1972, 1974; Zornetzer and Chronister, 1973), discriminated avoidance (Thompson, 1958), maze learning (Peeke and Herz, 1971), one-trial appetitive learning (Zornetzer and Chronister, 1973), habituation (Deadwyler and Wyers, 1972), and extinction (Herz and Peeke, 1971). Similarly, amygdala stimulation disrupts retention of a variety of avoidance tasks. Task generality has not been examined to the same extent for stimulation of other structures.

This degree of success in producing amnesia with low-level electrical brain stimulation suggests that such studies may be valuable for determining specific neural systems in which electrical stimulation is effective in modulating memory-storage processing. For example, we recently examined the effects on retention of posttrial subseizure electrical stimulation of several brain regions. Of various structures stimulated, including the dorsal hippocampus, septum, preoptic area, and dorsal thalamus, only amygdala stimulation produced retrograde amnesia in our situation. This finding was of interest in view of other findings indicating that the amygdala is a particularly effective region for producing RA by direct brain stimulation with current intensities that are above as well as below the seizure threshold (Kesner and Wilburn, 1974). Subsequently, we have conducted a series of studies of the effects of stimulation of the amygdala. In one study (Figure 37.3) bilateral amygdala stimulation (25 μA, 0.1 msec, 100 Hz, 10-sec train) produced retrograde amnesia if the stimulation was administered within 1 hr after training on a one-trial passive avoidance task. However, the stimulation had no effect on retention when delayed by 6 hr after training (Gold, Macri, and McGaugh, 1973b). We have found that posttrial unilateral amygdala stimulation can also produce amnesia in this same training situation (Gold, Edwards, and Mc Gaugh, 1975). With unilateral stimulation, it is possible to examine with more precision the relationship between the site of stimulation and the effect on memory. The results of this study, which are shown in Figure 37.4 indicate that stimulation in or near the basomedial nucleus produces the greatest degree of amnesia. Thus the basomedial nucleus of the amygdala is a very effective brain site for producing amnesia with low-level stimulation.

Results of two other recent studies in our laboratory

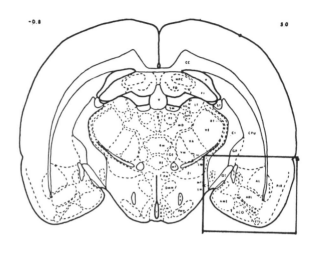

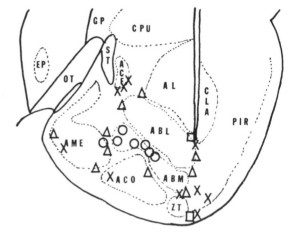

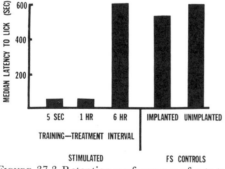

FIGURE 37.3 Retention performance of rats trained on a one-trial inhibitory (passive) avoidance task. After training, animals received bilateral amygdala stimulation (25 μA, 0.1 msec, 100 Hz, 10-sec train) at times indicated. Retention was measured 24 hr later. Groups receiving posttrial stimulation 5 sec or 1 hr after training had latencies that were significantly lower than those of either the control group or the group stimulated 6 hr after training. From Gold, Macri, and McGaugh (1973b).

LEGEND FOR LATENCIES	MEAN DISTANCE FROM BASOMEDIAL NUCLEUS (ABM)
O = 0 – 30 SEC	0.0 MM
△ = 30 – 150	0.3
□ = 150 – 300	0.4
X = 300 – 600	0.6

FIGURE 37.4 The effects of posttrial unilateral stimulation of the amygdala (50 μA, 0.1 msec, 100 Hz, 10–30-sec train) on retention of one-trial inhibitory (passive) avoidance training. Electrode placements are illustrated by figures which indicate the retention performances of individual animals. The lowest retention latencies (i.e., greatest amnesia) were obtained with stimulation in or near the basomedial nucleus. From McGaugh and Gold (1974).

support the anatomical localization just described. In an attempt to examine the behavioral generality of the amnesia produced by amygdala stimulation, rats were trained on either a one-way active-avoidance task (Handwerker, Gold, and McGaugh, 1974) or a discriminated-avoidance task (Gold, Rose, Spanis, and McGaugh, in preparation). Significant retrograde amnesia was produced by the stimulation in both cases. For example, in the one-way active-avoidance task, animals received nine training trials. Stimulation was administered either immediately or 3 hr later. Retention was measured the next day by examining the improvement in avoidance scores on another nine trials (Day 2 − Day 1 avoidances). As shown in Figure 37.5, animals that received the stimulation immediately after training had a significant retention deficit compared to either the implanted or unimplanted controls. Stimulation delayed 3 hr after training had no significant effect on retention. In this study nearly all electrodes were within the amygdala. In order to examine the relationship between the electrode placements and the retention deficit, we compared the difference score, for each animal, with the average distance of the two electrodes from the basomedial nucleus. The correlation was highly significant; that is, the greatest improvement in retention was found in animals with electrodes outside the region of the basomedial nucleus. Results comparable to these were also obtained in the discriminated-avoidance task. In this task amnesia was produced by stimulation administered as long as 4 hr, but not 10 hr, after training. Consistent with previous findings, the greatest degree of amnesia produced with immediate posttrial stimulation was observed in those animals in which the electrodes were near the basomedial nucleus. However, the amnesia produced by stimulation delayed by 4 hr after training, though approximately equivalent to that produced by immediate posttrial stimulation, was not related to the distance between the stimulating electrodes and the basomedial nucleus. With a 4-hr posttraining interval, the most effective stimulation site appears to be the basolateral nucleus. While these latter results are only preliminary, they suggest the intriguing possibility that the brain regions in which electrical stimulation is most effective as an amnestic treatment may vary with the training-treatment interval.

The results described thus far in this section indicate that subseizure electrical stimulation of several subcortical areas can modulate memory-storage processes. There is some localization of the areas in which electrical stimulation is most effective; furthermore, the effects of the brain stimulation on memory are time-dependent. We turn now to the important consideration of why some areas are more effective stimulation sites than others. This basic problem—that of determining critical structures—is more easily stated than solved. There are important assumptions here that are often ignored. When comparing two brain structures in terms of the amnestic effectiveness of the stimulation, it is not possible to choose stimulation parameters that are equally effective in each structure, unless effectiveness is defined in terms of the dependent variable (retention performance), in which case comparisons become meaningless. The usual resolution of the problem is to compare the stimulation intensities, train durations, frequencies, or number of pulses needed to produce amnesia. However, it should be clear that the distinctions made at the operational level need not apply at the neurobiological level.

However, aside from this issue, there is the even more basic problem of defining what it is that comprises a "critical" neural structure. There are at least two major types of interpretation that may be offered for these data. First, an effective stimulation site may be part of a neural system involved in the memory-storage process. The major assumption underlying this interpretation is that the important neurobiological effects of the electrical stimulation are localized to the neural system that is directly stimulated. Thus the interpretation requires the view that direct brain stimulation produces localized, transient neural alterations that interfere with memory processing. This localizationist position is described in detail by Kesner and Wilburn (1974), and the conclusions that can be derived from it are illustrated by the studies of Kesner and Conner (1972, 1974). In these

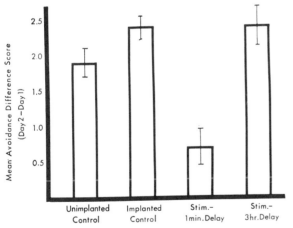

FIGURE 37.5 Retrograde amnesia for one-way active-avoidance training produced by posttrial electrical stimulation of the amygdala. Rats received 8 trials on each of 2 consecutive days. The figure illustrates the mean difference scores (Day 2 − Day 1) for all groups tested. Bilateral amygdala stimulation (50 μA, 0.1-msec pulses, 100 Hz, 10-sec train) produced amnesia when administered 1 min, but not 3 hr, after training. From Handwerker, Gold, and McGaugh (1974). Reproduced with the permission of ASP Biological and Medical Press (Elsevier division).

studies rats were trained on a one-trial inhibitory avoidance task. After training, the animals received either hippocampal or midbrain-reticular-formation (MRF) stimulation. Animals that received hippocampal stimulation showed good retention 1 min later and poor retention a day later. In contrast, animals that received MRF stimulation showed poor retention 1 min later and good retention the next day. On the basis of these findings, Kesner and Conner proposed that the MRF is part of a neural system mediating short-term memory and the hippocampus is part of a system mediating long-term memory.

Although the interpretation offered by Kesner and Conner is consistent with their findings, the results of this study as well as others are open to other interpretations (Gold, Zornetzer, and McGaugh, 1974). It seems equally likely that electrical stimulation of a well-localized site may affect memory storage through mechanisms that involve alterations of neural function in diffuse brain regions. For example, the stimulation may cause relatively nonspecific neural alterations by influencing arousal or hormonal systems. In fact, we have recently found that posttrial hormonal treatments can facilitate or impair later retention. It seems likely that different brain regions have different roles in the processing and utilization of memory. However, the function of a given region is not easily determined by studying the behavioral effects of treatments applied to the region. It may well be that stimulation of some regions directly affects the processes involved in memory storage in the region stimulated, while stimulation of other regions produces indirect or general influences that modulate memory-storage processes throughout the brain.

As we discussed in the section on RA gradients, it has become apparent in recent years that studies of the disruption and facilitation of memory provide direct information only about the modulating influences of the treatments on memory, not about the underlying memory processes (Weiskrantz, 1966; McGaugh and Dawson, 1971; Gold and McGaugh, 1975). This conclusion does not alter the potential value of the study of the effects of brain stimulation on memory. However, it does significantly alter the focus of these studies, which may better be described as attempts to learn about neural systems that may modulate memory processing. Further systematic study of the critical changes necessary for producing memory modulation by stimulation of specific brain regions should provide useful leads to understanding the neurobiological bases of memory.

37.2.3 Facilitation of memory-storage processes by posttrial subseizure stimulation

According to the view that localization studies examine areas in which electrical stimulation *modulates* memory-storage processes, rather than directly tapping the neural systems involved in storage, it becomes less surprising that electrical stimulation may in some cases facilitate retention (Doty, 1969). The majority of the studies that have used electrical brain stimulation to facilitate memory processes have been conducted by Bloch and his colleagues (Bloch, 1970). In these studies posttrial electrical stimulation of the MRF was found to facilitate later retention of a variety of tasks, including one-trial discrimination learning (Bloch, Deweer, and Hennevin, 1970), multitrial appetitive learning (Bloch and Deweer, 1968), avoidance training with weak punishment (Bloch and Denti, 1966), and extinction (Deweer, 1970). In our laboratory we also found that posttrial MRF stimulation improved retention above the level of implanted controls (Denti et al., 1970). Parenthetically, this series of experiments emphasized the need for implanted control animals. Under some conditions electrodes implanted in the MRF produce deficits in the active-avoidance tasks and facilitation must be measured against these poorly performing controls (Bloch, Denti, and Schmaltz, 1966; Denti et al., 1970). However, in other cases (Deweer, 1970; Bloch, 1970) retention is facilitated even when the electrode-implanted control animals do not show a retention deficit. Thus the facilitation cannot be attributed entirely to a compensation for a lesion-produced deficit.

In all cases the effectiveness of the stimulation in facilitating retention varies inversely with the time after training. Such results indicate that the treatments modulate time-dependent memory processing. It is also possible to use posttrial hippocampal stimulation to facilitate retention for maze learning (Stein and Chorover, 1968), and active- and discriminated-avoidance learning (Erickson and Patel, 1969; Landfield, Tusa, and McGaugh, 1973; Destrade, Soumireu-Mourat, and Cardo, 1973).

Bloch (1970) has pointed out that it is necessary to use tasks which are not themselves arousal-producing in order to obtain memory facilitation with MRF stimulation. In most studies of the effect of brain stimulation on memory, avoidance training with intense footshock has been used, and this must produce considerable arousal. In a practical sense, high footshock levels are used so that amnesia, if produced, is obvious when compared to the good performance of the control groups. We have recently obtained preliminary evidence that the effect on memory of brain stimulation, whether facilitation or interference, may vary with the motivational level. For example, in a passive avoidance task, posttrial amygdala stimulation appears to facilitate retention of a weak footshock (Gold et al., 1975), although, as we

556   J. L. McGAUGH AND P. E. GOLD

described earlier, it is a potent amnestic treatment for high footshock. These findings are consistent with a study by Lidsky et al. (1970), in which subseizure amygdala stimulation failed to produce retrograde amnesia. This experiment, which used a conditioned-emotional-response task involving training with a footshock lower than that used in other studies, is the only previous study, to our knowledge, in which amygdala stimulation failed to produce amnesia. Comparable results have also been obtained using posttrial injections of pentylenetetrazol (Krivanek, 1971) and ACTH or epinephrine (Van Buskirk and Gold, in preparation). These results indicate that there may be important interactions between the physiological state of the animal after training and the effect of the posttrial treatments on memory (Gold and McGaugh, 1975). This possible interaction between the motivational level and the nature of the effect on memory has generally been ignored. However, the few results available indicate that the interaction may be a very important variable. At the very least, these findings emphasize the necessity of considering the organism's response to the treatments rather than merely the parameters of the treatments.

37.3 CONCLUDING COMMENTS

Twenty-five years have passed since Duncan (1949) and Gerard (1949) first reported evidence suggesting that ECS interferes with the storage of recent experience. There is little doubt that ECS and less intense electrical stimulation of the brain can modify retention. And on the basis of most of the recent research, it seems likely that the stimulation administered after training influences retention because it alters time-dependent memory-storage processes. While there have been many alternative interpretations of the effects of brain stimulation on memory, the research findings remain generally consistent with the view that the treatments alter storage processes. These findings are also consistent with those of studies using other types of treatments that alter retention. However, even if this general interpretation proves to be incorrect and if some alternative interpretation of the basis of the retention effects turns out to be correct, the fundamental problem will still be to find the neurobiological basis (or bases) of the effects. Why does brain stimulation produce retrograde amnesia and retrograde facilitation of retention? We have discussed two possibilities. The stimulation may directly alter storage processes in cells stimulated by the current. Or the stimulation may cause effects in other brain regions either through neuronal pathways or by affecting hormonal systems. Obviously, the effects of the stimulation will depend upon the brain region stimulated. But

since no brain region exists in isolation, discovering the specific effects responsible for producing altered retention by stimulation of any specific brain region will no doubt be a difficult task.

Brain seizures appear to be neither necessary nor sufficient conditions for producing memory effects. There is evidence that ECS alters brain activity for some time (minutes) following the treatment. It may be that milder forms of stimulation also produce such changes. The arousing effects of MRF stimulation are well known. It is also known that stimulation of the amygdala results in a release of pituitary hormones. Bloch and his colleagues (Leconte and Bloch, 1971; Leconte, Hennevin, and Bloch, 1973; Leconte and Hennevin, 1973; Bloch, this volume) have reported that in rats, the degree of retention of a response varies closely with the amount of REM sleep that occurs following training. Further, Fishbein, McGaugh, and Swarz (1971) have reported that in mice, REM-sleep deprivation extends the RA gradient produced by posttraining ECS. Thus it might be that treatments affect retention because they alter the degree of REM sleep that occurs between the training and the retention test.

In a previous paper (Gold and McGaugh, 1975) we suggested that the strength of memory for an experience may depend upon the motivational or arousing consequences of the experience. Conceptually, this view is similar to the hypothesis proposed by Kety (1972 and this volume), according to which normal variations in retention are assisted by variations in the physiological processes (e.g., arousal, release of pituitary and adrenal hormones) elicited by the experience. Treatments that alter such processes, either by attenuating them or potentiating them, would be expected to modulate the storage of experiences preceding those treatments. Stimulation of some regions of the brain might be affective in influencing retention because of such "nonspecific" effects, while stimulation of other brain regions might directly modify the activity of cells participating in the storage processes. Understanding the bases of the effects of electrical stimulation of the brain on memory will require careful study of the specific physiological consequences of stimulation of each brain region and a determination of which of the effects are necessary and sufficient for producing the effects on retention.

Another approach to the problem is to search for other treatments that produce alterations suspected of contributing to the modulating influences of brain stimulation. For example, recent studies have shown that retention is influenced by posttraining administration of pituitary hormones, adrenal hormones, and drugs that affect catecholamines (Gold and Van Buskirk, 1975; Randt et al., 1971; Van Buskirk and Gold, in preparation).

Understanding the neurobiological bases of the modulating influences of brain stimulation on retention should contribute significantly to an eventual understanding of the neurobiological bases of memory.

ACKNOWLEDGMENT

Original research reported in this chapter has been supported by Research Grants MH12526, HD07981-01, and MH25384-01 from the National Institute of Mental Health, USPHS, and Grant GB-42746 from the National Science Foundation.

REFERENCES

ALPERN, H. P., and CRABBE, L. 1972. Facilitation of the long-term store of memory with strychnine. *Science* 177: 722–724.

ALPERN, H. P., and MCGAUGH, J. L. 1968. Retrograde amnesia as a function of duration of electroshock stimulation. *Journal of Comparative and Physiological Psychology* 65: 265–269.

BLOCH, V. 1970. Facts and hypotheses concerning memory consolidation. *Brain Research* 24: 561–575.

BLOCH, V., and DENTI, A. 1966. Facilitation de la fixation amnésique par stimulation réticulaire. *Proceedings of the 18th International Congress (Moscow)* 4: 187.

BLOCH, V., DENTI, A., and SCHMALTZ, G. 1966. Effets de la stimulation réticulaire sur la phase de consolidation de la trace amnésique. *Journal de Physiologie* 58: 469–470.

BLOCH, V., and DEWEER, B. 1968. Rôle accelerateur de la stimulation réticulaire sur la phase de consolidation d'un apprentissage en un seul essai. *Comptes Rendus de l'Académie des Sciences (Paris)* 266D: 384–387.

BLOCH, V., DEWEER, B., and HENNEVIN, E. 1970. Suppression de l'amnésie rétrograde et consolidation d'un apprentissage à essai unique par stimulation réticulaire. *Physiology and Behavior* 5: 1235–1241.

BRESNAHAN, E., and ROUTTENBERG, A. 1972. Memory disruption by unilateral low levels, sub-seizure stimulation of the medial amygdaloid nucleus. *Physiology and Behavior* 9: 513–525.

BUCKHOLTZ, N. S., and BOWMAN, R. E. 1972. Incubation and retrograde amnesia studies with various ECS intensities and durations. *Physiology and Behavior* 8: 113–117.

CHERKIN, A. 1969. Kinetics of memory consolidation: Role of amnesic treatment parameters. *Proceedings of the National Academy of Sciences (USA)* 63: 1094–1101.

CHERKIN, A. 1972. Retrograde amnesia in the chick: Resistance to the reminder effects. *Physiology and Behavior* 8: 949–955.

CHOROVER, S. L., and SCHILLER, P. H. 1965. Short-term retrograde amnesia in rats. *Journal of Comparative and Physiological Psychology* 59: 73–78.

COTMAN, C., BANKER, G., ZORNETZER, S., and MCGAUGH, J. L. 1971. Electroshock effects on brain protein synthesis: Relation to brain seizures and retrograde amnesia. *Science* 173: 454–456.

DAWSON, R. G., and MCGAUGH, J. L. 1973. Drug facilitation of learning and memory. In J. A. Deutsch, ed., *The Physiological Basis of Memory*. New York: Academic Press.

DEADWYLER, S. A., and WYERS, E. J. 1972. Disruption of habituation by caudate nuclear stimulation in the rat. *Behavioral Biology* 7: 55–64.

DENTI, A., MCGAUGH, J. L., LANDFIELD, P. W., and SHINKMAN, P. 1970. Effects of posttrial electrical stimulation of the mesencephalic reticular formation on avoidance learning in rats. *Physiology and Behavior* 5: 659–662.

DESTRADE, C., SOUMIREU-MOURAT, B., and CARDO, B. 1973. Effects of posttrial hippocampal stimulation on acquisition. *Behavioral Biology* 8: 713–724.

DEWEER, B. 1970. Accélération de l'extinction d'un conditionnement par stimulation réticulaire chez le rat. *Journal de Physiologie* 62: 270–271.

DOTY, R. W. 1969. Electrical stimulation of the brain in behavioral context. *Annual Review of Psychology* 20: 289–320.

DUNCAN, C. P. 1949. The retroactive effect of electroshock on learning. *Journal of Comparative and Physiological Psychology* 42: 32–44.

DUNN, A. 1971. Brain protein synthesis after electroshock. *Brain Research* 35: 254–259.

ERICKSON, C. K., and PATEL, J. B. 1969. Facilitation of avoidance learning by posttrial hippocampal stimulation. *Journal of Comparative and Physiological Psychology* 68: 400–406.

FISHBEIN, W., MCGAUGH, J. L., and SWARZ, J. R. 1971. Retrograde amnesia: Electroconvulsive shock effects after termination of rapid eye movement sleep deprivation. *Science* 172: 80–82.

GEHRES, L. D., RANDALL, C. L., RICCIO, D. C., and VARDARIS, R. M. 1973. Attenuation of hypothermic retrograde amnesia produced by pharmacologic blockage of brain seizures. *Physiology and Behavior* 10: 1011–1017.

GERARD, R. W. 1949. Physiology and psychiatry. *American Journal of Psychiatry* 106: 161–173.

GIBBS, M. E., and MARK, R. F. 1973. *Inhibition of Memory Formation*. New York: Plenum Press.

GLICKMAN, S. 1958. Deficits in avoidance learning produced by stimulation of the ascending reticular formation. *Canadian Journal of Psychology* 12: 97–102.

GLICKMAN, S. E. 1961. Preservative neural processes and consolidation of the memory trace. *Psychological Bulletin* 58: 218–233.

GOLD, P. E., BUENO, O. F., and MCGAUGH, J. L. 1973. Training and task-related differences in retrograde amnesia thresholds determined by direct electrical stimulation of the cortex in rats. *Physiology and Behavior* 11: 57–63.

GOLD, P. E., EDWARDS, R., and MCGAUGH, J. L. 1975. Retrograde amnesia produced by unilateral stimulation of the amygdala. *Behavioral Biology* 15: 95–105.

GOLD, P. E., HANKINS, L., EDWARDS, R., CHESTER, J., and MCGAUGH, J. L. 1975. Memory interference and facilitation with posttrial amygdala stimulation: Effect on memory varies with footshock level. *Brain Research* 86: 509–513.

GOLD, P. E., HAYCOCK, J. W., MACRI, J. and MCGAUGH, J. L. 1973. Retrograde amnesia and the "reminder effect": An alternative interpretation. *Science* 180: 1199–1201.

GOLD, P. E., and KING, R. A., 1972. Caudate stimulation and retrograde amnesia: Amnesia threshold and gradient. *Behavioral Biology* 7: 709–715.

GOLD, P. E., and KING, R. A. 1974. Retrograde amnesia: Storage failure vs. retrieval failure. *Psychological Review* 81: 465–469.

GOLD, P. E., MCDONALD, R., and MCGAUGH, J. L. 1975. Direct cortical stimulation: A further study of treatment intensity effects on retrograde amnesia gradients. *Behavioral Biology* 10: 485–490.

GOLD, P. E., and MCGAUGH, J. L. 1973. Relationship between

amnesia and brain seizure thresholds in rats. *Physiology and Behavior* 10: 41–46.

GOLD, P. E., and McGAUGH, J. L. 1975. A single-trace, two-process view of memory storage processes. In D. Deutsch and A. J. Deutsch, eds., *Short Term Memory*. New York: Academic Press.

GOLD, P. E., MACRI, J., and McGAUGH, J. L. 1973a. Retrograde amnesia gradients: Effects of direct cortical stimulation. *Science* 179: 1343–1345.

GOLD, P. E., MACRI, J., and McGAUGH, J. L. 1973b. Retrograde amnesia produced by subseizure amygdala stimulation. *Behavioral Biology* 9: 671–680.

GOLD, P. E., and VAN BUSKIRK, R. B. 1975. Facilitation of time-dependent memory processes with posttrial epinephrine injections. *Behavioral Biology* 13: 145–153.

GOLD, P. E., ZORNETZER, S. F., and McGAUGH, J. L. 1974. Electrical stimulation of the brain: Effects on memory storage. In G. Newton and A. Riesen, eds., *Advances in Psychobiology*, Vol. 2. New York: Wiley Interscience.

HANDWERKER, M., GOLD, P. E., and McGAUGH, J. L. 1974. Effects of posttrial electrical stimulation of the amygdala on retention of an active avoidance response. *Brain Research* 75: 324–327.

HAYCOCK, J. W., DEADWYLER, S. A., SIDEROFF, S. I., and McGAUGH, J. L. 1973. Retrograde amnesia and cholinergic systems in the caudate-putamen complex and dorsal hippocampus of the rat. *Experimental Neurology* 41: 201–213.

HAYCOCK, J. W., GOLD, P. E., MACRI, J., and McGAUGH, J. L. 1973. Noncontingent footshock "attenuation" of retrograde amnesia: A generalization effect. *Physiology and Behavior* 11: 99–102.

HAYCOCK, J. W., and McGAUGH, J. L. 1973. Retrograde amnesia gradients as a function of ECS-intensity. *Behavioral Biology* 9: 123–127.

HERZ, M. J., and PEEKE, H. V. S. 1971. Impairment of extinction with caudate nucleus stimulation. *Brain Research* 33: 519–522.

ILYUTCHENOK, R. Y., and VINNITSKY, I. M. 1971. Influence of high frequency stimulation of the amygdaloid complex on memory in rats. *Zhurnal Vysshei Nervnoi Deyatel'nosti* 21: 1220–1222.

JAMIESON, J. L. 1972. Temporal patterning of electroshock and retrograde amnesia. Unpublished Ph.D. dissertation, University of British Columbia.

JARVIK, M. E. 1972. Effects of chemical and physical treatments on learning and memory. *Annual Review of Psychology* 23: 457–486.

KESNER, R. 1973. A neural system analysis of memory storage and retrieval. *Psychological Bulletin* 80: 177–203.

KESNER, R. P., and CONNER, H. S. 1972. Independence of short- and long-term memory: A neural systems approach. *Science* 176: 432–434.

KESNER, R. P., and CONNER, H. S. 1974. Effects of electrical stimulation of rat limbic system and midbrain reticular formation upon short- and long-term memory. *Physiology and Behavior* 12: 5–12.

KESNER, R. P., and WILBURN, M. W. 1974. A review of electrical stimulation of the brain in the context of learning and retention. *Behavioral Biology* 10: 259–293.

KETY, S. S. 1972. Brain catecholamine, affective states and memory. In J. L. McGaugh, ed., *The Chemistry of Mood, Motivation and Memory*. New York: Plenum Press.

KRIVANEK, J. 1971. Facilitation of avoidance learning by

pentylenetetrazol as a function of task difficulty, deprivation and shock level. *Psychopharmacologia (Berlin)* 20: 213–229.

LANDFIELD, P. W., McGAUGH, J. L., and TUSA, R. J. 1972. Theta rhythm: A temporal correlate of memory storage processes in the rat. *Science* 175: 87–89.

LANDFIELD, P. W., TUSA, R., and McGAUGH, J. L. 1973. Effects of posttrial hippocampal stimulation on memory storage and EEG activity. *Behavioral Biology* 8: 485–505.

LECONTE, P., and BLOCH, V. 1971. Déficit de la rétention d'un conditionnement après privation de sommeil paradoxal chez le rat. *Comptes Rendus de l'Académie des Sciences (Paris)* 271 D: 226–229.

LECONTE, P., and HENNEVIN, E. 1973. Charactéristiques temporelles de l'augmentation de sommeil paradoxal consécutif à l'apprentissage chez le rat. *Physiology and Behavior* 11: 677–686.

LECONTE, P., HENNEVIN, E., and BLOCH, V. 1973. Analyse des effets d'un apprentissage et de son niveau d'acquisition sur le sommeil paradoxal consécutif. *Brain Research* 49: 367–379.

LEWIS, D. J. 1969. Sources of experimental amnesia. *Psychological Review* 76: 461–472.

LEWIS, D. L., MISANIN, J. R., and MILLER, R. R. 1968. Recovery of memory following amnesia. *Nature* 220: 704–705.

LIDSKY, T. I., LEVINE, M. S., KREINICK, C. J., and SCHWARTZBAUM, J. 1970. Retrograde effects of amygdaloid stimulation on conditioned suppression (CER) in rats. *Journal of Comparative and Physiological Psychology* 73: 135–149.

MAH, C. J., and ALBERT, D. J. 1973. Electroconvulsive shock-induced retrograde amnesia: An analysis of the variation in the length of the amnesia gradient. *Behavioral Biology* 9: 517–540.

MAHUT, H. 1962. Effects of subcortical electrical stimulation on learning in the rat. *Journal of Comparative and Physiological Psychology* 55: 472–477.

MAHUT, H. 1964. Effects of subcortical electrical stimulation on discrimination learning in cats. *Journal of Comparative and Physiological Psychology* 58: 390–395.

McDONOUGH, J. H., and KESNER, R. P. 1971. Amnesia produced by brief electrical stimulation of the amygdala or dorsal hippocampus in cats. *Journal of Comparative and Physiological Psychology* 77: 171–178.

McGAUGH, J. L. 1968. Drug facilitation of memory and learning. In D. H. Efron et al., eds., *Psychopharmacology: A Review of Progress, 1957–1967*. Washington, D.C.: U.S. Public Health Service Publication No. 1836, pp. 891–904.

McGAUGH, J. L. 1973. Drug facilitation of learning and memory. *Annual Review of Pharmacology* 13: 229–241.

McGAUGH, J. L. 1974. Electroconvulsive shock: Effects on learning and memory in animals. In M. FINK, S. S. KETY, J. L. McGAUGH, and T. A. WILLIAMS, eds., *The Psychobiology of Convulsive Therapy*. Washington, D.C.: V. H. Winston & Sons.

McGAUGH, J. L., and DAWSON, R. G. 1971. Modification of memory storage processes. *Behavioral Science* 16: 45–63.

McGAUGH, J. L., and GOLD, P. E. 1974. The effects of drugs and electrical stimulation of the brain on memory storage processes. In R. D. Myers and R. R. Drucker-Colin, eds., *Neurohumoral Coding of Brain Function*. New York: Plenum Press, pp. 189–206.

McGAUGH, J. L., and HERZ, M. J. 1972. *Memory Consolidation*. San Francisco: Albion Publishing Company.

McGAUGH, J. L., and LANDFIELD, P. W. 1970. Delayed development of amnesia following electroconvulsive shock. *Physiology and Behavior* 5: 1109–1113.

McGaugh, J. L., and Zornetzer, S. 1970. Amnesia and brain seizure activity in mice: Effects of diethyl ether anesthesia prior to electroshock stimulation. *Communications in Behavioral Biology* Part A, 5: 243–248.

Miller, R. R., and Springer, A. D. 1973. Amnesia, consolidation and retrieval. *Psychological Review* 80: 69–79.

Nielson, H. C. 1968. Evidence that electroconvulsive shock alters memory retrieval rather than memory consolidation. *Experimental Neurology* 20: 3–20.

Paolino, R. M., and Hine, B. 1973. EEG seizure anomalies following supramaximal intensities of cortical stimulation: Relationships with passive-avoidance retention in rats. *Journal of Comparative and Physiological Psychology* 83: 285–293.

Peeke, H. V. S., and Herz, M. J. 1971. Caudate nucleus stimulation retroactivity impairs complex maze learning in the rat. *Science* 173: 80–82.

Quartermain, D., McEwen, B. S., and Azmitia, Jr., E. C. 1970. Amnesia produced by electroconvulsive shock or cycloheximide: Conditions for recovery. *Science* 169: 683–686.

Randt, C. T., Quartermain, D., Goldstein, M., and Anagnosti, B. 1971. Norepinephrine biosynthesis inhibition: Effects on memory in mice. *Science* 172: 498–499.

Rebert, C. S., Pryor, G. T., and Schaeffer, J. 1974. Slow cortical potential consequences of electroconvulsive shock in rats. *Physiology and Behavior* 12: 131–134.

Routtenberg, A., and Holzman, N. 1973. Memory disruption by electrical stimulation of substantia nigra, pars compacta. *Science* 181: 83–86.

Stein, D. G., and Chorover, S. L. 1968. Effects of posttrial electrical stimulation of hippocampus and caudate nucleus on maze learning in the rat. *Physiology and Behavior* 3: 781–791.

Thompson, C. I., and Neely, J. E. 1970. Dissociated learning in rats produced by electroconvulsive shock. *Physiology and Behavior* 5: 783–786.

Thompson, R. 1958. The effects of intracranial stimulation on memory in cats. *Journal of Comparative and Physiological Psychology* 51: 421–426.

Van Buskirk, R., and McGaugh, J. L. 1974. Pentylenetetrazol-induced retrograde amnesia and brain seizures in mice. *Psychopharmacologia (Berlin)* 40: 77–90.

Weiskrantz, L. 1966. Experimental studies of amnesia. In C. W. M. Whitty and A. L. Zangwill, eds., *Amnesia*. London: Butterworth & Company.

Wilburn, M. W., and Kesner, R. P. 1972. Differential amnesia effects produced by electrical stimulation of the caudate nucleus and nonspecific thalamic systems. *Experimental Neurology* 34: 45–50.

Wyers, E. J., and Deadwyler, S. A. 1971. Duration and nature of retrograde amnesia produced by stimulation of caudate nucleus. *Physiology and Behavior* 6: 97–103.

Wyers, E. J., Peeke, H. V. S., Welliston, J. S., and Herz, M. J. 1968. Retroactive impairment of passive avoidance learning by stimulation of the caudate nucleus. *Experimental Neurology* 22: 350–366.

Zornetzer, S. F. 1972. Brain stem and RA in rats. A neuroanatomical approach. *Physiology and Behavior* 8: 239–244.

Zornetzer, S. F. 1974. Retrograde amnesia and brain seizures in rodents: Electrophysiological and neuroanatomical analyses. In M. Fink, S. S. Kety, J. L. McGaugh, and T. A. Williams, eds., *The Pyschobiology of Convulsive Therapy*. Washington, D.C.: V. H. Winston & Sons.

Zornetzer, S. F., and Chronister, R. B. 1973. Neuroanatomical localization of memory disruption: Relationships between brain structure and learning task. *Physiology and Behavior* 10: 747–750.

Zornetzer, S. F., Chronister, R. B., and Ross, B. 1973. The hippocampus and retrograde amnesia: Localization of some positive and negative memory disruptive sites. *Behavioral Biology* 8: 507–518.

Zornetzer, S. F., and McGaugh, J. L. 1969. Effects of electroconvulsive shock upon inhibitory avoidance: The persistence and stability of amnesia. *Communications in Behavioral Biology* Part A 3: 173–180.

Zornetzer, S. F., and McGaugh, J. L. 1971a. Retrograde amnesia and brain seizures in mice. *Physiology and Behavior* 7: 401–408.

Zornetzer, S. F., and McGaugh, J. L. 1971b. Retrograde amnesia and brain seizures in mice: A further analysis. *Physiology and Behavior* 7: 841–845.

38

An Experimental Critique of the "Consolidation Studies" and an Alternative "Model-Systems" Approach to the Biophysiology of Memory

STEPHAN CHOROVER

ABSTRACT In behavioral experiments performed mainly with rats, gross electroconvulsive shock (ECS) and electrical stimulation of discrete brain regions (ESB) have been used to study the time course of retrograde amnesia (RA) and to evaluate other effects upon retention-test performance in various one-trial training paradigms. Such experiments have established some reliable and critical empirical findings and have demonstrated that it is possible to dissociate several classes of treatment effects. However, the outcomes of such purely behavioral experiments have several inherent limitations. For example, they have at best only an indirect bearing on the so-called consolidation hypothesis, and they do not permit any inferences regarding the time course of memory-trace initiation. Furthermore, they shed no light on the crucial psychobiological problem of specifying the physiological mechanisms responsible for either the RA phenomenon or the process of normal memory fixation.

A recognition of these limitations led us to perform experiments in which electrophysiological recordings were made in human subjects and laboratory animals. The results of these studies have some important implications for the analysis of naturally occurring memory interference, and they may help to produce a conceptual unification of sensory and mnemonic processes which are generally viewed as being quite dissimilar.

Taken together, the results reported here have led us away from the traditional "frontal" attack upon the problem of memory-trace initiation and have prompted us to search for a more fruitful "model-systems" approach.

38.1 INTRODUCTION

When Plato likened the fixation of memory to the process of imparting an impression to a block of wax, he was speaking without the benefit of any detailed knowledge of the central nervous system. It is therefore all the more remarkable that he was able to grasp one of the most important ideas underlying the search for biological foundations of learning and remembering: that every aspect of behavior derives from certain anatomical and physiological conditions, or that all the activities of

STEPHAN CHOROVER, Department of Psychology, Massachusetts Institute of Technology, Cambridge, MA

organisms have a structural basis. A somewhat more specific counterpart of Plato's metaphor is the concept of the "engram": the fundamental neuropsychological postulate which holds that some more or less enduring change in the structure of the nervous system must underlie the phenomenon of experiential memory.

How does experience (e.g., learning) give rise to memory? What is the nature of the engram? Where, when, and how are engrams formed? To what degree do those phenomena that we generally designate as "neural information processing" involve the gross electrical activity of the nervous system? What processes are involved in the initiation of memory "traces" or engrams? What events intervene between memory-trace initiation (during learning) and memory "retrieval" (during retention, recall, or recognition trials)? Questions such as these lie behind most attempts to understand the biological basis of experiential plasticity. They have guided the work of our laboratory for the past ten years.

It may be useful to emphasize at the outset of this review that our overall perspective on the problem of memory-trace initiation has changed quite substantially during the past decade. At the outset, our principal point of departure was the familiar "consolidation hypothesis" (Müller and Pilzecker, 1900; Hebb, 1949), according to which memory fixation (or engram formation) is a more or less protracted affair involving at least two concurrent or sequential stages (see McGaugh, 1966). During the first stage (often assumed to coincide with short-term memory) some transitory (reverberatory?) aftereffects of stimulus presentation are postulated in the form of a dynamic, labile, "memory trace" which is highly susceptible to interference or modification by various treatments. During the second stage a relatively permanent (or long-term) memory is presumably established, through a process still unspecified, with the result that retention of previous experience becomes relatively stable and impervious to various disruptive treatments.

Guided by this general notion, our initial experimental interest was focused upon the time-dependent behavioral effects of such treatments. Accordingly, we performed a series of experiments in which electroconvulsive shock (ECS) or direct electrical stimulation of specific brain areas (ESB) was administered to animals at various times after single training trials in order to study the temporal characteristics and nature of the resulting retention-test deficit. Although reliable and interesting results were obtained in these experiments, we came eventually to realize that our findings about the time course of certain treatments were actually irrelevant to the more important problem of discovering the underlying physiological events. The following section describes the findings that led us to conclude that purely behavioral studies of "consolidation" need to be drastically modified (or perhaps even abandoned) by those who seek to understand what goes on in the nervous system during learning.

38.2 "CONSOLIDATION STUDIES" IN RETROSPECT

During the past several years a number of laboratories—including ours—have been involved in research concerned with various aspects of the consolidation problem. A principal objective of such research has been to shed light upon the processes involved in memory-trace initiation by providing reliable measures of their temporal characteristics. The most notable feature of this period has been the production of a large body of data concerning the time-dependent effects of various posttrial treatments upon retention-test performance in animals (see McGaugh and Gold, this volume).

Like most of the experiments in this field, ours were undertaken with three objectives in mind: (1) to evaluate the consolidation hypothesis, (2) to estimate the temporal characteristics of neural processes involved in memory-trace formation, and (3) to identify behavioral effects specifically due to interference with memory processes and to dissociate these from other treatment effects. In retrospect, it seems apparent that we achieved only the latter objective and were rather naive to imagine that the former ones could be attained through such experiments.

38.2.1 Temporal characteristic of ECS-induced RA

The phenomenon of retrograde amnesia (RA) is the principal source of experimental support for the consolidation hypotheses (see, e.g., Glickman, 1961; McGaugh, 1966). In operational terms, RA may be described as a time-dependent performance deficit which can be produced by administering certain treatments to individuals at varying time intervals following an ex-

perience (e.g., a single training trial on a learning task). The usual finding in such cases is an inverse relationship between the *severity* of retention-test impairment and the *duration* of the time interval between training and treatment. Examples of RA derived from many species, tasks, and treatments have been adduced in support of the consolidation hypothesis for many years.

After reviewing the evidence available to us at the outset, we were forced to acknowledge, with Coons and Miller (1960), that many alleged examples of RA (particularly those produced by ECS) could be accounted for more simply on grounds other than memory interference.

In order to determine whether ECS does indeed produce RA, we devised and conducted a series of experiments intended to avoid the pitfalls that had been pointed out by Coons and Miller. Briefly, we administered single ECS treatments to rats at varying times after completion of single training trials in a number of one-trial learning paradigms. The results of several experiments (Chorover, 1965; Chorover and Schiller, 1965a,b, c, 1966; Schiller and Chorover, 1967) convinced us that posttrial treatments with ECS produced a reliable and significant impairment, characterized—in most cases—by a temporal gradient of severity. In other words, we confirmed the general finding of an inverse relationship between the *duration* of the training-ECS interval on the one hand and the *degree* of retention-test impairment on the other hand. We also succeeded in showing that certain disruptive effects of posttrial ECS were due to factors other than memory interference, but that the actual RA phenomenon was real and could not be adequately accounted for by alternative interpretations involving "conflict" (Coons and Miller, 1960), "competing response" (Adams and Lewis, 1962a,b) or "conditioned inhibition" (Lewis and Maher, 1965).

In our initial experiments we consistently failed to find evidence for ECS-induced RA in animals that had received the convulsive treatments more than 10–15 seconds after completion of a single learning trial. Our finding of a "short-term ECS-induced RA" was reproduced several times in our own laboratory and was repeatedly confirmed by others (e.g., Quartermain, Paolino, and Miller, 1965; M.E. Jarvik, personal communication; W. Sherman and E. Stellar, personal communication; Suboski et al., 1969; Schneider and Sherman, 1968; Carew, 1970).

We were naturally aware of the fact that our finding of a shortterm RA was at odds with the results of others who had found the duration of ECS-induced RA to vary from a few minutes (e.g., Madsen and McGaugh, 1961; Heriot and Coleman, 1962; McGaugh and Alpern, 1966) to several hours (e.g. Bureš and Burešová, 1963; Kopp,

Bohdanecky, and Jarvik, 1966). We at first attached a great deal of theoretical importance to the remarkable diversity of time constants reflected in the various "consolidation curves" obtained in different experiments (see Figure 38.1). Based on the belief that the temporal characteristics of the RA gradient reflected the time course of processes involved in memory-trace consolidation, the enormous range of results led some observers to interpret each curve as a different "estimate of consolidation time" (see, e.g., Lewis and Maher, 1965, and almost every current textbook of physiological psychology).

We, too, felt that certain contradictions were implied by the diversity of results. Accordingly, we undertook to repeat several experiments, including those of McGaugh and Alpern (1966), Heriot and Coleman (1962), and Bureš and Burešová (1963). In each case we were able to replicate the reported results in most essential respects. Moreover, in several instances (see esp. Chorover and Schiller, 1966; Schiller and Chorover, 1967) we were able to suggest a way of resolving the disparities (either by showing that the effects of ECS might be due to factors other than RA, or by demonstrating that seemingly trivial procedural variations can exert profound effects on the outcome of experiments in this area). In agreement with others (e.g., McGaugh, 1966), we found that numerous experimental variables can modify the duration of the critical interval during which a posttrial treatment is effective in producing deficient retention-test performance. For example, we observed differences in the duration of ECS-induced RA that were attributable to the following factors: the strain, sexual status, and previous experience of the subject; the nature and com-

plexity of the learning task, the kind and amount of deprivation and reinforcement used; and of course, the physical parameters of the ECS stimulus (e.g., waveform, intensity, frequency, duration) as well as its route and mode of administration (e.g., transpinnate, transcorneal, or transcortical in animals that were restrained or freely moving, awake or asleep, etc.).

From our experience with the behavioral effects of ECS, and from a reexamination of previously published reports, we finally concluded that factors such as those listed above—rather than statistical disparities or some mysterious differences in "consolidation times"—were responsible for the differences illustrated in Figure 38.1. From our success in rationalizing the apparent disparities, we were led to reexamine the fundamental assumption that the temporal characteristics of ECS-induced RA are relevant to questions about consolidation and/or the time course of the processes involved in memory formation. These are our principal conclusions:

1. In a fundamental sense, the idea of consolidation is inescapable—and must necessarily be correct in outline. If one accepts the premise that memory must ultimately depend upon some kind of change in the nervous system, one must by the same token acknowledge that changes in such a system cannot occur except in real time.

2. In a certain sense, therefore, the question is not whether consolidation occurs, but, rather, what it is, where it happens, and how long it takes. "Consolidation experiments" are obviously addressed to the last of these three important questions. But can they answer it? We think not, for at least four reasons:

a. Consider the results illustrated in Figure 38.1 and the fact that seemingly minor procedural variations account for many of the apparent disparities. If the illustrated differences are real (we say they are), then it follows either that "consolidation time" is not a constant, but varies from case to case, or that "consolidation time" is constant, but may be irrelevant to the experimental results.

b. In any event, it should be clear that one simply cannot draw any general inferences about the temporal characteristics of memory-trace initiation per se on the basis of results obtained with a given treatment in a given situation. At best, even the most reliable behavioral data, obtained under ideal conditions, can do no more than provide an accurate estimate of the temporal characteristics of RA produced by *that* treatment under those conditions.

c. Nor is the situation substantially improved by studying the behavioral effects of the same treatment in several different contexts. Under such conditions, one readily confirms that the treatment effects are strongly context-

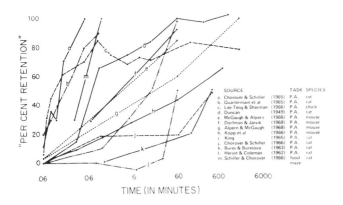

FIGURE 38.1 "Consolidation curves" from various experiments, illustrating the wide range of results obtained using ECS with a variety of tasks, techniques, and species. Data were obtained from sources listed on the figure and recalculated to conform with this semilogarithmic plot. PA: passive avoidance. (Note that Duncan, 1949, should be active avoidance rather than PA.)

dependent, but one cannot resolve the dilemma alluded to in 2a.

d. Finally, it must be acknowledged that attempts to study consolidation take many forms. The ECS-RA experiments predominate, but they represent only one aspect of a broad enterprise and deal with only one amnestic agent. When one goes on to consider other relevant time-dependent effects of head trauma, brain disease, concussion, discrete brain stimulation, convulsions, ablation, anesthesia, hypothermia, stimulant drug treatments, etc., in human patients and in animal subjects, one is obviously faced with an overwhelming set of complex variables and a baffling range of putative "RA values." In sum, we simply lack the means of resolving the inevitable confusion that has arisen from the use of different species, training, and treatment variables.

3. The confusion just alluded to is not superficial, but final. It cannot be resolved by doing more of the same or even by doing the same thing better. Our behavioral RA experiments have unequivocally demonstrated the very great importance of context-dependent and treatment-dependent factors. In so doing, they have taught us at last that we cannot hope to shed light upon the time course (let alone the physiological details) of critical neural events in memory consolidation by behavioral studies of RA, any more than we can hope to learn the details of what is going on inside a house by observing who goes in the door and what comes out the chimney.

4. We have failed in our initial attempts to specify precisely the time course of neural events in memory fixation (indeed, we have concluded that our behavioral experiments are irrelevant to this problem). If the question itself has any validity (and we believe it does), it seems inescapable that we must carry our search directly into the nervous system and try to focus our attention upon critical events going on there during—and shortly after—learning trials.

To the extent that it is possible to be a bit more specific about the kinds of neural events likely to be involved in memory-trace initiation, it appears possible now to revise and update our initial working hypothesis. Rather than supporting a two-stage process, the weight of evidence argues strongly against this simple, dichotomous classification. More specifically, we now prefer the concept of memory as an "addressable" interneuronal process, tending to exhibit self-regulatory (i.e., homeostatic) properties and subject to continuous or periodic "reprogramming," mediated by transient alterations in neuroelectrical activity correlated with the information content of "messages" (familiar and novel stimuli, etc.) (see Arbib, Kilmer, and Spinelli, this volume).

More specifically, we take "long-term memory" to be a variable, rather than an asymptotic state, presumably based upon some relatively enduring (or readily reproduced) biochemical and/or morphological change. No assumptions can be made at this point as to whether this state is achieved through "stimulogenous proliferation" (Eccles, 1963; Hebb, 1949) of some intracellular or transsynaptic trace, or through the equally plausible (but rarely considered) alternative of "stimulogenous depletion" (e.g., Young, 1966; Dawkins, 1971). In any case, we assume that the condition of the resulting "homeostat" is subject to continuous alteration on the basis of the events involved in memory-trace initiation. These events we may arbitrarily divide into two categories, according to their apparent temporal characteristics: The first consists of brief, transient events relevant to the "on-line" processing of neural information. The "correlates" of these events include evoked potentials related to the stimulus or response, changes in frequency and/or patterns of unit activity, etc. The second category (which may overlap the first to some extent, but which generally outlasts it by some time) includes events correlated with more prolonged neuroelectrical changes, including steady-potential shifts, polarization phenomena, protracted EEG activation, changes in neural excitability cycles, etc. A substantial amount of effort has been devoted to the problem of devising appropriate techniques and experimental paradigms with which to study and redefine these categories.

38.2.2 Effects of discrete electrical brain stimulation upon learning and performance in rats

ECS is a crude, gross, and traumatic instrument, poorly suited to the fine-grained analysis of neural information processing. Like McGaugh and his colleagues, we have sought more refined approaches and have tried to determine whether, and to what extent, localized electrical stimulation of specific brain structures would occasion the kind of retrograde amnesia that is produced by more generalized ECS.

In one such experiment (Stein and Chorover, 1968) we employed an appetitive learning task (a modified Hebb-Williams maze) and a variant of a one-trial training procedure that we had previously shown to be susceptible to disruption by ECS. Using rats, we studied the effects upon performance of posttrial electrical stimulation applied bilaterally to the caudate nucleus and dorsal hippocampus. These structures were chosen because of our prior findings implicating them in this type of behavior (Chorover and Gross, 1963; Gross, Chorover, and Cohen, 1965; Gross, Black, and Chorover, 1968). The results of this experiment indicated that localized posttrial electrical stimulation of brain areas presumably involved in memory fixation may facilitate or disrupt subsequent performance. More specifically, the performance of animals that received massed-trial training was disrupted by hippocampal stimulation and slightly facilitated by caudate stimulation, whereas the performance of animals that received spaced-trial training was facilitated by hippocampal stimulation and unaffected by caudate stimulation. These effects were complementary to those produced by ECS in the sense of being due primarily to alterations in the activity of brain mechanisms involved in the processing of experiential information.

A second line of research on the effect of brain stimulation was undertaken using anodal and cathodal currents applied to the posterior (visual) cortex in rats. This work was conducted on rats that had been trained in a Hebb-Williams maze (an apparatus in which performance is particularly susceptible to disruption following posterior cortical lesions). The DC stimulation was intended to produce relatively prolonged alterations in cortical excitability and thereby focus upon the second (i.e., tonic) phase of the hypothetical consolidation process. During this time we were also engaged in a series of experiments concerning the effects of cortical spreading depression (SD) upon memory. We therefore began the stimulation experiments by using DC currents, which might be expected to produce polarizing effects comparable to those resulting from the application of KCl solutions to the dural surface.

Animals were fitted with special stainless-steel disk electrodes (3–5 mm diameter), and an indifferent electrode (a wound clip) was attached to the neck muscle. We found that after 1 min of cathodal stimulation applied to cortex, SD could be demonstrated by the electrocorticogram (ECoG). The current necessary to induce SD in this way was 3.0mA (5 volts). This rather high level of stimulation, although only slightly higher than that previously found adequate by Marshall (1959), invariably produced gross and permanent damage to the cortex.

Since SD could be produced only at the expense of marked cortical damage, and since the threshold for such damage was found to be 0.06mA (one-fiftieth that necessary to evoke SD), we decided to shift to biphasic square-wave stimulation in order to avoid the frankly injurious effects of DC stimulation.

We first determined that there was no injurious effect of biphasic square-wave stimulation (300 Hz), up to and including levels sufficient to produce an overt motor response. There was never any ECoG evidence that such stimulation produced SD. All stimulation during behavioral testing was carried out below the level that produced motor effects (0.4 mA).

During tests of the effect of stimulation upon lever-pressing for food, there was a significant drop in performance during 2-min periods of cortical stimulation as compared with equal intervals when no stimulus was given ($p < 0.02$). Tests for possible reinforcing effects of the stimulation were negative.

Animals trained in accordance with our one-trial maze-learning paradigm reliably showed savings on the second trial on a novel maze problem. Such animals were stimulated for 5 sec during initial exposure to a novel maze problem, immediately upon reaching the goal box on trial 1, or immediately after being allowed to feed in the goals box for 5 sec on trial 1; control animals were not stimulated. Animals stimulated immediately upon reaching the goal box made significantly fewer errors on trial 2 (6 hr later) than animals that received no stimulation or were stimulated at other times during or after trial 1 ($p < 0.02$). Other groups showed no effects of the stimulation, as compared with unstimulated controls. These results are generally consistent with those reported by McGaugh and Gold (this volume).

38.3 "PERCEPTUAL AMNESIA"

An insight into the conceptual difficulties surrounding the consolidation hypothesis is afforded by a reinterpretation of a well-known "perceptual" phenomenon.

When two equally intense visual stimuli with adjacent contours are presented in rapid succession, the brightness of the first stimulus appears greatly reduced. This type of brightness suppression, generally referred to as "metacontrast" (Stigler, 1910), is one of several visual phenomena showing that brightness can be modified by a temporal interaction between stimuli.

Metacontrast has been extensively studied by psychophysical methods (Raab 1963). It is readily observed under the following conditions: a disk is presented very briefly and is followed, after a variable interval, by a surrounding ring of equal area, intensity, and duration. When the interval between disk and ring is short (0 to 10 msec), both are clearly seen. As the interval is increased, the brightness of the disk diminishes. At interstimulus intervals between 40 and 100 msec, metacontrast suppression becomes maximal and the disk virtually disappears. With further increases in the interstimulus interval, the disk becomes progressively brighter again. When the two stimuli are separated by 200 to 250 msec, the disk appears to have regained its original brightness. Throughout a sequence of such presentations, the appearance of the ring remains relatively unchanged.

Several different theories have been proposed to explain metacontrast suppression in terms of retinal (Alpern, 1953), subcortical (Fry, 1934; Piéron, 1935), and cortical (Werner, 1935; Baumgardt and Segal, 1942) interactions between neural responses to the two stimuli. In order to evaluate such interpretations, one should be able to specify the neural correlates of brightness perception. This is not yet possible, but recent work with evoked potentials recorded from the scalp in man has shown that the amplitude of evoked potentials increases, and their latency decreases, as stimulus intensity (and therefore brightness) is increased (Tepas and Armington, 1962; Vaughan, Hull, and Hull, 1965). Are these covariations due to the altered stimulus intensity, or to the change in brightness, or both?

In attempting to answer this question, Peter Schiller and I wished to know whether the brightness reduction observed under metacontrast conditions (where the subject reports that he has seen a relatively dim flash, although the intensity has remained constant) is accompanied by evoked-potential changes comparable to those that normally occur when stimulus intensity is varied. If metacontrast suppression (like intensity reduction) were accompanied by a decrease in amplitude and an increase in latency of the evoked potential to the initial stimulus, this would suggest that these aspects of the cortical evoked response correlate with the psychological variable of brightness perception, rather than with physical variations in stimulus intensity per se. However, if evoked potentials were to change only when brightness and intensity covary, and not when brightness alone is reduced (as in metacontrast), this would suggest that while the amplitude and latency of the evoked response may correlate with physical aspects of the stimulus, they do not necessarily correlate with the perceptual response of the subject.

The subject was seated with his head on a chin rest, facing the stimulus display unit 150 cm away. He was instructed to fixate binocularly on a faint red light 12 cm to the right of the center of the stimulus display. The experiment was carried out in a darkened room. Each subject was dark-adapted for at least 10 min before the beginning of a session.

We recorded evoked potentials to flashes of varying intensity (from 1.35 to 135 ft-lam) and confirmed earlier reports of a characteristic reduction in amplitude and increase in latency of initial components as the intensity is decreased. Initial observations had shown that during optimal metacontrast suppression, a disk at 135 ft-lam actually appears less bright than a disk presented alone at 1.35 ft-lam. This striking observation is consistent with psychophysical data obtained at lower luminance levels (Schiller and Smith, 1966).

Therefore, if the brightness reduction during metacontrast suppression is accompanied by evoked-potential changes like those occurring when stimulus intensity is reduced, the amplitude and latency of the average evoked response to the 135-ft-lam disk under metacon-

trast conditions should be similar to the amplitude and latency of the evoked response to the 1.35-ft-lam disk presented alone.

Data obtained during paired presentations of the disk-ring sequence and the disk and ring separately reveal no change in the initial components of the evoked response with interstimulus interval when metacontrast suppression is maximal. For example, at interstimulus intervals of 60 and 100 msec, the subject reports that the disk is "virtually invisible," yet the amplitude and latency of relevant components of the visual evoked response to the disk do not diminish as they do when disk intensity is reduced (Schiller and Chorover, 1966).

The finding that the evoked response to the first stimulus is relatively unchanged at interstimulus intervals producing maximal metacontrast suppression helps to explain two observations that have previously been made in metacontrast experiments: (1) reaction time to the first stimulus is not affected by metacontrast suppression (although reaction time normally increases as stimulus intensity is decreased); and (2) in a forced-choice paradigm, the first stimulus is equally detectable at all interstimulus intervals (Schiller and Smith, 1966).

Although metacontrast suppression is generally referred to as a "perceptual" phenomenon, the results of this experiment can be interpreted in terms of a curious, modality-specific, and very brief retrograde amnesia. In effect, the results show that the disk is "perceived" (in terms of *both* the evoked potential and the reaction time), but that the subject *does not remember it* (!). This interpretation has two interesting implications: (1) It suggests that very short term effects of normal sensory stimuli may imitate longer-term effects of traumatic stimuli, and that perception and memory may be intimately related in this sense. (2) It adds further weight to our argument that it is meaningless to search for a specific "consolidation time" per se. In the present instance, for example, one might say that the memory trace for the disk becomes impervious to interference by the ring in about 150 msec. Should one conclude, therefore, that "visual-information processing" is "consolidated" in that brief period? We think not.

38.4 ELECTROCORTICOGRAPHIC SIGNS OF LEARNING AND ECS

A first aspect of our consolidation research extends the ECS experiments described at the outset of this review. In discussing the RA experiments, we emphasized the occurrence of disparities in the *absolute* value of observed RAs, but we noted that under otherwise constant conditions, the relative degree of RA is generally found to vary inversely with the duration of the training-ECS interval. It is, accordingly, undeniable that RA is due to an *interaction* between some aspect of the convulsive treatment and some neural aftereffect of the training experience. What aspects of the convulsive treatment are critical in this regard? Which are the relevant aftereffects? Although there are various speculations inherent in theoretical conceptualizations of the consolidation process (see, e.g., Hebb, 1949; Glickman, 1961; McGaugh, 1966), it must be acknowledged that we actually know very little about the crucial neural events inolved in learning and still less about how their sequelae may interact with ECS. In fact, until we performed such an experiment (Chorover and DeLuca, 1969), there had apparently been no conjoint experimental investigations of this problem using electrophysiological techniques. Some have been done since (e.g., Zornetzer and McGaugh, 1970; McGaugh and Gold, this volume).

What we did was simply to observe the overt behavior and the gross electrical activity of the cerebral cortex in rats under conditions comparable to those commonly employed to study ECS-induced RA. At the outset of the experiment we assumed—as all who conduct ECS-RA experiments must—that the direct and immediate physiological effect of ECS upon the brain is a variable whose specific value in any given case may be taken as a *constant* (i.e., whose value is selected and controlled solely by the appropriate physical stimulus parameters, such as waveform, intensity, duration, route of administration, circuit resistance, etc.). Let us restate this point for emphasis: if one wishes to study the behavioral (amnesic) effects of ECS, that is, if one wishes to attribute variations in the experimental results either to specific time-dependent effects of ECS upon the neural aftereffects of training (McGaugh and Alpern, 1966) or to the formation of an association bond (a conditioned response) between antecedent sensory stimuli and the convulsive consequences of ECS stimulation (Lewis and Maher, 1966), one must assume that the *only* relevant independent variable in the experiment is the training-ECS interval. Accordingly, one must either hold constant or assume the invariance of all relevant conditions except the aforementioned interval. One such condition that is presumed to remain constant is the direct physiological response to passage of the ECS current.

This presumption, which is routinely taken for granted in ECS-RA experiments, is at least indirectly supported by a common observation: a specific ECS stimulus of adequate intensity, duration, etc., tends to produce a constant and highly stereotyped overt convulsion in most cases. In any event, the view has been generally accepted that a given ECS stimulus exerts a constant, stereotyped, and uniform effect upon the brain, irrespective of the prevailing background neural activity. In the experiment

under consideration here, however, we obtained direct and unequivocal electrocorticographic evidence that the *direct response* to a constant ECS stimulus varies significantly as a function of the occurrence or timing of neural events during the training-treatment interval.

Administration of a brief, painful footshock (FS) stimulus was found to produce an immediate and transient behavioral arousal, and a corresponding desynchronization (activation) of the ECoG. A surprising finding was that the ECoG reaction to a subsequent ECS varied in nature and duration as a function of the occurrence and/or timing of the antecedent FS (Figure 38.2). This shows that factors other than the physical parameters of the ECS affect the neural response to convulsive treatment. It was found that the nature (and, hence, the duration) of the arousal reaction to FS was a more important determinant of this effect than was the duration between FS and ECS per se.

The finding that the neural aftereffects of FS influence the epileptogenic efficacy of a constant ECS stimulus suggests that a decrease in seizure susceptibility accompanies electrocortical activation. This general conclusion has been reported previously, but it has never been recognized that the effect is sufficiently pronounced to influence the reaction to as apparently prepotent an epileptogenic agent as ECS.

Three aspects of this experiment merit particular consideration: (1) the finding of a dissociation between the electrocortical and behavioral reactions to ECS; (2) the nature of the interaction between the convulsive treatment and the aftereffects of antecedent stimuli; and (3) the possible implications of these findings for the interpretation of ECS-induced RA.

1. A dissociation between the neural mechanisms responsible for convulsive movements and those presumably involved in the mediation of ECS-induced RA is implied by several earlier findings. It has been shown, for example, that the brain itself is unnecessary for the production of such movements and that the spinal cord suffices (Esplin and Freston, 1960). Also, RA is not prevented when the overt convulsive reaction to ECS is blocked by drugs (Ottoson, 1960; Weissman, 1965; McGaugh and Alpern, 1966). However, what was not previously known, and what the present results indicate, is that such a dissociation may also occur in intact, unanesthetized, unrestrained rats and that it may develop as a natural consequence of prior stimulus events. A similar dissociation between overt and electrographic patterns of convulsive activity has been observed in epileptic patients (Gastaut and Fischer-Williams, 1959). Taken together, the available evidence appears to argue against the direct relevance of the overt, convulsive response for an understanding of the behavioral effects of

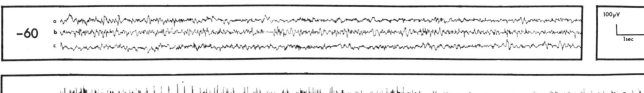

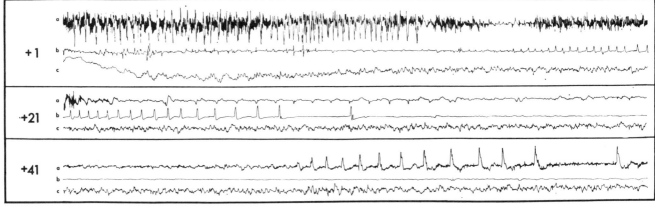

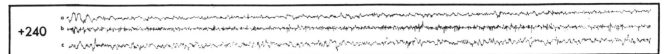

FIGURE 38.2 Three basic types of ECoG reaction to ECS. (a) No footshock (FS); response to ECS is a synchronous and symmetrical convulsive pattern. (b) FS 5 sec prior to ECS; asynchronous and asymmetrical seizure activity and marked postic-tal depression. (c) FS 30 sec prior to ECS; absence of ECoG seizure signs during normal overt convulsion. Numerals at left indicate time (in sec) of sweep onset relative to time of ECS administration.

ECS. Accordingly, the remainder of this discussion will focus primarily on other factors.

2. A finding of particular interest is that the ECoG reaction to ECS is altered as a consequence of prior FS. In general, the frequency of occurrence of such alterations tended to decline as the FS-ECS interval increased. However, a comparison of the behavioral reactions to FS and the ECoG response to ECS in individual animals suggests that the occurrence and nature of the abnormal ECoG reaction to ECS depends more upon the momentary state of the animal at the time of ECS administration (i.e., upon the severity and, hence, the duration of the behavioral reaction to FS) than it does upon the time interval, per se, between FS and ECS. Thus the most pronounced alterations in seizure pattern (random spiking, long postictal phase, etc.) were observed when ECS was given very soon after FS. During this time the animals were very likely to be highly aroused and actively moving as an immediate consequence of the noxious stimulus. The onset of such movements was usually immediate, and their duration was relatively short. The most pronounced inhibitory effects (no significant ECoG change due to ECS) were obtained, irrespective of the actual time interval, in animals that were showing strong signs of emotionality or fear at the moment of ECS administration. Such signs may develop slowly and may persist for relatively long periods under the conditions used in the present experiment. For example, all but one of the animals that had received FS 300 sec prior to ECS, appeared to have recovered from the noxious effects of the stimulus and were either standing quietly or moving slowly about the enclosure at the time ECS was given. All of these animals showed normal ECoG seizure. The lone exception was a severely frightened animal that remained frozen and trembling in the same position throughout the FS-ECS interval. The ECoG of this animal showed a complete inhibition of cortical seizure activity throughout an otherwise typical convulsive episode. Many similar instances of this type were observed in the course of the experiment. The overall results suggest, therefore, that arousal and/or fear are prominent among the neural aftereffects of FS and that they may, therefore, play a role in the alteration of inhibition of the normal ECoG reaction to ECS.

The implication of arousal mechanisms in these effects is consistent with the observation that the FS employed did actually have a desynchronizing effect on the ECoG. There is, furthermore, considerable clinical evidence that the cortical desynchronization which accompanies normal behavioral arousal, attention, or sensory stimulation may inhibit the development of hypersynchronous seizure activity in epileptic patients (Penfield and Jasper,

1954). Alertness or arousal in experimental animals will usually abolish or attenuate recruiting responses and wave/spike discharges produced by thalamic stimulation (Moruzzi and Magoun, 1949). Similar anticonvulsant effects can be produced in experimental animals by electrical stimulation of the mesencephalic reticular formation (Fernandez-Guardiala, Alcaraz, and Guzman, 1961).

3. On the basis of this evidence, the following interpretation is offered to account for the findings of the present experiment and for the apparent time-dependent effects commonly obtained in studies of ECS-induced RA.

A painful FS, or equivalent discriminative stimulus, initiates an arousal reaction as its immediate and natural consequence. The magnitude and duration of this reaction vary from task to task and from animal to animal in response to several factors, such as stimulus intensity and novelty. The numerous physiological manifestations of the arousal reaction may include a varying degree of autonomic activation, but they will also invariably entail a transient increase in cortical desynchronization, mediated primarily via the reticular activating system and varying in degree and duration according to the factors already mentioned. One aspect of this increased cortical desynchronization is a corresponding decrease in susceptibility to cortical seizure, which ultimately results in a transient decrease in the epileptogenic efficacy of a constant ECS stimulus. Given the assumption that the magnitude of a given arousal reaction will at first increase (as "fear" increases) and then eventually decline monotonically with time, it follows that the epileptogenic efficacy of a given convulsive stimulus will vary correspondingly. Thus, in the case of a typical ECS-RA experiment, where the time of ECS administration is varied with respect to an antecedent FS, the normal statistical distribution of arousal-response durations tends to produce results consistent with a possible interference by time-dependent processes involved in memory consolidation. However, closer observation of each individual case would probably reveal that variations in the behavioral effects of ECS are closely related to response-dependent effects of prior stimuli upon the epileptogenic efficacy of the constant ECS stimulus.

In conclusion, neither the finding of interactions between FS and ECS, nor the interpretation offered to account for it, assumes or denies the possibility that time-dependent neural processes are involved in memory fixation. (Whether such processes are or are not reflected in the transient arousal reaction to significant stimuli in a learning situation remains an interesting question for future research). The demonstration of this interaction does, however, challenge the views that ECS-induced RA is due to the electric current per se (McGaugh and Alpern, 1966), to the overt convulsive reaction per se (Lewis and Maher, 1966), or even to the electrocortical seizure activity per se. Furthermore, the arousal interpretation offered to account for this interaction rests upon neural mechanisms which are known to exist and whose details are open to further investigation by available physiological and anatomical methods. Finally, although future research will surely dictate its revision or abandonment, this interpretation seems to require few, if any, additional assumptions or hypothetical constructs in order to encompass a large body of current experimental data on ECS-induced RA.

A further series of experiments on the ECoG signs of seizure activity in relation to arousal level confirmed and extended the development of arousal-produced inhibition of convulsive reactions in rats with focal and non-focal experimental epilepsy (Pinel and Chorover, 1972). Nonfocal epilepsy was produced by daily systemic injections (12 mg/kg) of the nitrogen-mustard derivative chlorambucil; focal epilepsy was induced by subdural applications of ethyl chloride in chlorambucil-treated animals. The cortical EcoG was monitored conventionally over a period of 11 days following treatment. Both focal and nonfocal epileptiform activity was reliably suppressed during periods marked by ECoG activation and behavioral arousal. Thus, in addition to blocking the *onset* of ECS seizures, stimuli that produce arousal are capable of *interrupting* (i.e., terminating) ongoing epileptiform activity. Moreover, the inhibition of this activity was found to persist for several minutes or more following stimulus termination.

A further series of experiments was conducted to determine the duration and severity of proactive ECS effects (DeLuca and Chorover, unpublished). Of particular interest in this respect were cortical steady potentials and sleep-wakefulness patterns. Rats were implanted with chronic nonpolarizable electrodes and were studied for extended periods of time before and after ECS administration. Administration of a single ECS treatment was found to produce several electrophysiological and behavioral aftereffects. For example, transiently large DC potential shifts of 4 to 10 mV (posterior cortical surface negative) were observed immediately after ECS. A similar finding has recently been reported by Rebert, Pryor, and Schaeffer (1974). In our animals the effect recurred periodically for up to 48 hr and was accompanied by a disruption, lasting 2–4 days, in the normal circadian sleep-wakefulness and activity cycle. Furthermore, we found an appreciable reduction in REM sleep times (see also Bloch, this volume), followed by a marked rebound.

These findings are in accord with those of Bloch (this

volume) in suggesting that some ECS-produced changes in learning and memory might be indirect (i.e., might reflect effects of convulsive treatment upon various mechanisms involved in maintaining electrocortical homeostasis).

38.5 SUMMARY CONCERNING CONSOLIDATION

In the consolidation experiments described thus far, we followed what might be called a "frontal assault" on the problem of memory formation. Our experiments were predicated largely upon traditional behavioristic concepts of learning and memory and relied exclusively upon conventional neuropsychological research methods. We have gradually come to the view that our frontal assault failed to attain its intended objective because we knew neither *how* our treatments actually affect the nervous system nor *what* neural mechanisms are actually involved in memory-trace initiation. Furthermore, we have learned enough about the problem to realize that all similar efforts, aimed at identifying specific morphological or functional changes in the mammalian brain in relation to "experience," are likewise bound to remain unsuccessful to the extent that they continue to be based solely upon the narrow conceptual foundations of operational neobehaviorism.

Although this conclusion may appear rather harsh, it hardly seems unwarranted. In any event, it has led us to seek ways of replacing our prior emphasis upon "99.44 percent pure learning" (Miller, 1965) with a broader concern with more general types of "neurobehavioral plasticity," including such ubiquitous and important phenomena as sensitization and habituation. Furthermore, we have sought a fundamental simplification of the problem by employing a suitably reduced experimental preparation.

38.6 AN ALTERNATE "MODEL-SYSTEMS" APPROACH

During the past decade a promising line of attack upon the problems of learning and memory has been opened by researchers who have adopted much less restrictive definitions of these phenomena and have then been able to devise fruitful "model systems" with which to study them. Perhaps the most familiar examples of these systems are the ones based upon the use of invertebrates—or of reduced or isolated preparations thereof. Several reports in this volume attest to the power and elegance of this approach. But, however attractive such invertebrate "simple systems" may be, it seems inescapable that the key to understanding the biological basis of

mammalian learning and memory must ultimately be sought within the mammalian brain itself. That being so, we have chosen a model system based upon (1) a reduced and relatively simple mammalian brain preparation and (2) the fundamental phenomena of sensitization and habituation.

There is nothing particularly novel in the idea that a simple-systems approach is needed in order to permit effective analysis of neurobehavioral plasticity in the mammalian central nervous system. On the contrary, there are numerous precedents, including studies of the sensitization and habituation of isolated spinal-cord reflexes, experimental focal epileptogenesis (and the elaboration of "mirror foci") in the cerebral cortex, effects of synaptic use and disuse in the spinal cord, and post-tetanic potentiation. We think that there is something new, however, in the particular simple-systems approach that we are pursuing.

We aim to be able, eventually, to localize, identify, and characterize specific changes in the brain due to experience. Toward that end, we are focusing upon the rodent olfactory bulb—a critically important brain structure that has been shown to exhibit several unique and particularly attractive morphological and functional features. The neural organization of the rodent olfactory bulb—already revealed in great detail by light- and electron-microscopic studies in normal animals—offers some unusual possibilities for correlating the results of electrophysiological and behavioral experiments with morphological findings. Correlative studies of this general type have been attempted previously in the cerebellar cortex (Eccles, Ito, and Szentágothai, 1967; Fox et al., 1967), in the lateral geniculate nucleus (Colonnier and Guillery, 1964; Szentágothai, Hamari, and Tömhäl, 1966; Peters and Palay, 1966), in the retina (Dowling and Boycott, 1966), and in the olfactory bulb (Willey, 1969; Price and Powell, 1970a–d; Shepherd, 1970; Rall, 1970; Freeman, 1972). However, most of those experiments were primarily intended to characterize the normative ultrastructure and functional activity of these regions. Scant attention has thus far been paid to the possibility of correlating changes in functional activity with changes in morphology. That is our eventual aim. Few structures seem as well suited for this purpose as the olfactory bulb of macrosmatic mammals.

38.6.1 Olfaction and mammalian adaptation
The olfactory bulb of macrosmatic mammals is an appealing structure, first of all, from the point of view of mammalian adaptation. It is a phylogenetically old brain region whose general features of neuronal organization are clearly recognizable throughout the vertebrate series. From the perspective of neurobehavior-

al plasticity, the olfactory system—and the olfactory bulb in particular—plays a critical role in many of the complex adaptive behavior patterns upon which individual and species survival depend.

In macrosmatic mammals from mouse (Whitten, 1966) to monkey (Michael, 1971), there are many examples of olfactory functions related to species-specific behavior patterns. Among the macrosmatic rodents, pheromonelike odors (as yet undefined chemically) serve important purposes in many spheres of social and reproductive behavior:

1. Female rats and hamsters produce an odorous vaginal secretion that varies in copiousness and chemical composition with daily fluctuations in the estrous cycle. Male conspecific rats prefer the odor of estrous over anestrous females (LeMagnen, 1952; Carr, Loeb, and Dissinger, 1966; Pfaff and Pfaffman, 1969b; Macrides and Chorover, 1972), but hamsters seem to find the odors of estrous and anestrous females equally attractive (Darby, Devor, and Chorover, 1975).

2. Male hamsters possess a specialized flank gland, and some species of rabbits possess a specialized chin gland. In both cases the secretions are dependent upon systemic androgen levels and are generally repellent to male conspecifics. The secretions are used extensively by these animals to mark environmental objects within their territories. Similarly specialized exocrine organs are found among various other species of rodentia, including the nonmurid deer mouse and the Mongolian gerbil.

3. Certain odorous secretions of rodents have profound effects upon the neuroendocrine status of other conspecifics. Three instances are of particular significance in the present context because they epitomize the importance of olfactory habituation and sensitization in species survival: First, the absence of male odors from a colony of aggregated female mice tends to cause a significant increase in the incidence of spontaneous pseudopregnancies and induces other abnormalities in the estrous rhythm (the Lee-Boot effect). Second, the introduction of odors from a sexually mature male conspecific into such a colony of aggregated females tends to accelerate and synchronize their estrous cycles (the Whitten effect). Third, the odor of an unfamiliar male is sufficient, under certain circumstances, to inhibit uterine implantation of fertilized ova in recently inseminated female mice (the Bruce effect). The latter effect, which has been observed in other species of rodentia (including the field vole, which, like the rabbit, is an induced ovulator), is of especial interest as an instance of the kind of naturally occurring learning to which too little attention has previously been paid. (Obviously, the differential reaction of a female to odors from a strange male implies more than a mere sensitivity to olfactory stimuli of natural origin. It shows, furthermore, the existence of a highly specific, experientially acquired discrimination between individual conspecifics on the basis of their smell. Moreover, the fact that two or three days may intervene between exposure to the stud male and the strange male implies the presence of a memory mechanism capable of storing the relevant information during the interval.)

It has also been shown that destruction of the olfactory bulbs exerts dire effects on the adaptive behavior of several species of macrosmatic mammals (see, e.g., Pribram and Kruger, 1954; Signoret, 1962; Heimer and Larsson, 1967; Murphy and Schneider, 1970; Gandelman et al., 1971).

Although the stimulus-coding problem has been notoriously refractory to solution in the olfactory system, some progress has recently been made in electrophysiological studies aimed at characterizing the effects of animal secretions upon neuronal unit activity in the olfactory bulb (Macrides, 1970; Macrides and Chorover, 1972) and in other parts of the olfactory system (Pfaff and Pfaffman, 1969a,b).

A further indication of the importance of the olfactory bulb in rodents may be seen in the fact that the primary distribution field of olfactory-bulb fibers encompasses most of the basal aspect of the brain and is closely related to the amygdala, the mediodorsal thalamus, the hypothalamus, and the hippocampal formation. These limbic structures are implicated in a wide range of innate and acquired behavior patterns and are among the critical brain sites where electrical and chemical stimulation has been shown to exert potent effects upon response acquisition, retention, and emotional reactivity (see, e.g., Papez, 1937; Pribram and Kruger, 1954; Ramón y Cajal, 1911, 1955; Brady and Nauta, 1953; Adey, 1959; Powell, Cowan, and Raisman, 1963; McCleary and Moore, 1965; Heimer, 1968; Stein and Chorover, 1968). As Freeman (1972) has pointed out, there are only two synaptic surfaces interposed between the olfactory receptors in the nasal cavity and the various limbic brain sites in which stimulation with current or chemicals produces "teleologically significant patterns of behavior." One obvious implication of this functional proximity is that many "fundamental neurosensory transformations must therefore take place in the bulb and prepyriform cortex" (Freeman, 1972, p. 1).

38.6.2 Morphological and functional aspects of the rodent olfactory system

Beyond the idea of its adaptive importance and beyond the fact of its intimate association with other brain areas that are critically involved with various aspects of neurobehavioral plasticity, the olfactory bulb of macrosmatic mammals is an attractive object for our purposes because it exhibits a unique combination of unusual morphological and functional features.

INTRINSIC MORPHOLOGY. The structure of the rodent olfactory bulb has been extensively studied at the macroscopic, light-microscopic, and electron-microscopic levels. In rats and rabbits (Figure 38.3) the bulb is a large, well-defined, and readily accessible structure. It is notable, first of all, because its pattern of intrinsic elements and extrinsic interconnection exhibits the distinctive features of cortical organization commonly seen in many regions of the mammalian brain. Like all cortical structures, it possesses several distinct types of neurons whose cell bodies and processes are arranged in a regular and nonrepeating laminar order, and it includes some relatively large and specialized output neurons whose processes span most layers and whose axons extend to other parts of the nervous system while sending off collaterals that may form a basis for local recurrent activity within the structure itself.

While it is tempting to suggest that cortical organization per se may constitute a prototypical morphological response of neural tissue to the adaptive pressures arising in nature for brain mechanisms capable of mediating learning and memory, we need not make this explicit claim here. What we do want to stress, however, is that common principles of functional organization are likely to apply to different neuronal systems possessing comparable features of cortical organization. Thus, in viewing the rodent olfactory bulb as a model cortical system, we invoke the same kind of reasoning that has recently been used by others in analyzing other brain regions as information-processing systems (e.g., Eccles, Ito, and Szentágothai, 1967). This is an important point for, as we shall try to show in a moment, the rodent olfactory bulb is an exceptionally simple structure in comparison with other cortical regions of the mammalian central nervous system. This point is stressed also by Shepherd (1970), who spiritedly proclaims the rodent olfactory bulb to be "an *E. coli* for cortical physiology" (p. 539).

The pattern of anatomical interconnections and functional interactions within the rodent olfactory bulb may be summarized with respect to Figure 38.4 as follows:

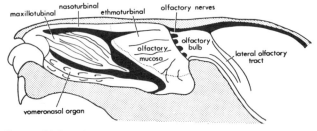

FIGURE 38.3 Peripheral olfactory structures in rabbit (parasagittal view). From Shepherd (1970).

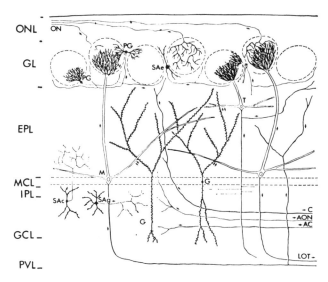

FIGURE 38.4 Principal neuronal arrangement of mammalian olfactory bulb. Based upon Golgi-stained material. Modified slightly from Shepherd (1970). For abbreviations, see text.

Olfactory sensory input, arising from the receptor surface within the nasal cavity, reaches the bulb from below via the primary olfactory neurons (ON), of which there are approximately 10^8 in the rabbit (Allison and Warwick, 1949; LeGros Clark, 1956). The olfactory nerve layer (ONL) is the most superficial layer of the bulb; from it, the nerves penetrate in bundles before ramifying in a single uniform layer of glomeruli (GL), where they synapse upon the terminal branches of the primary dendrites of the mitral (M) and tufted (T) cells. Many small cells, termed external granule or periglomerular cells (PG) surround the glomeruli. Immediately deep to the glomerular layer lies the external plexiform layer (EPL), which contains secondary dendrites of the mitral and tufted cells, together with peripheral processes of granule cells. Deep to the external plexiform layer lie the perikarya of the mitral cells, which form a compact lamina (MCL) only one or two cells thick. The mitral cells, as previously noted, send their primary dendrites to the glomerular level, where they synapse with the primary olfactory neurons. The secondary dendrites of the mitral cells extend obliquely into the external plexiform layer, where they branch and appear to form a second—and completely independent—dendritic field with the peripheral processes of more deeply situated granule cells. From their deep poles the mitral cells and tufted cells project long axons, which pass deeply into the periventricular layer (PVL) and eventually extend to more caudal parts of the brain via the lateral olfactory tract (LOT). The axons of mitral and tufted cells give off at least two classes of collaterals: one to the internal plexiform layer (IPL), which lies immediately deep to the mitral-cell layer, and the other to the external plexiform layer. Within the glomerular and internal plexiform layers are situated various short-axon cells (SAc, SAe, and SAg). Deep to the internal plexiform layer lies the granule-cell layer (GCL). The granule cells (C) are relatively small and are by far the most numerous neuron cell type in the olfactory bulb.

Their peripheral processes, which extend to the external plexiform layer, are dendritic in form (Rall et al., 1966; Price and Powell, 1970a) and have been termed "gemmules." They are believed to form reciprocal (dendrodendritic) synapses with the secondary dendrites of mitral and tufted cells. Note that the external plexiform layer exhibits morphological features capable of supporting at least two kinds of recurrent circuitry: (1) axodendritic synapses between mitral-cell axon collaterals and mitral secondary dendrites—the type of circuitry that Ramón y Cajal (1911) suggested as a possible basis for "avalanche conduction"—and (2) dendrodendritic synapses between granule-cell gemmules and mitral secondary dendrites; Shepherd (1970) and Rall (1970) have recently suggested that these may be inhibitory synapses comprising an intrabulbar system for recurrent inhibition similar to that found in other sensory systems. From their deeper aspects the granule cells send smaller dendrites toward the center of the bulb. The deepest layer of the bulb, the periventricular layer, surrounds the rostral remnant of the lateral ventricle and contains only ependymal and glial cells, in addition to the axons of mitral and tufted cells and the deep dendrites of the deepest granule cells. Terminations of centrifugal fibers, including those from the anterior commissure (AC) and anterior olfactory nucleus (AON), are located at various points throughout the intermediate levels of the bulb.

AFFERENT AND EFFERENT PATHWAYS. In addition to the primary olfactory neurons, which project from the nasal mucosa to the glomerular layer of the olfactory bulb, there are at least three different fiber pathways to the bulb from more caudal parts of the cerebral hemisphere:

1. Fibers arising in the contralateral anterior olfactory nucleus cross in the anterior limb of the anterior commissure (Lohman, 1963) and appear to terminate sparsely within the granule-cell layer of the bulb (Price and Powell, 1970c).

2. Fibers arising in the ipsilateral anterior olfactory nucleus enter the bulb along with the commissural fibers from the contralateral side (Valverde, 1965) and have been found to terminate upon the spines and gemmules of granule cells (i.e., in the internal and external plexiform layers) (Price and Powell, 1970c).

3. Fibers arising in the ipsilateral nucleus of the horizontal limb of the diagonal band (area inominata) pass forward in close association with the main efferent tract from the bulb (the lateral olfactory tract) (Heimer, 1968; Price, 1969) and appear to terminate mainly in the vicinity of gemmules in the external plexiform layer (Price and Powell, 1970c).

The sole centripetal pathway from the olfactory bulb to more caudal regions of the brain is via the lateral olfactory tract. According to both White (1965) and Heimer (1968), almost the entire basal aspect of the brain represents primary olfactory cortex in the rat. Following lesions of the olfactory bulb or transections of the lateral olfactory tract, reduced silver methods reveal dense terminal degeneration in the plexiform layer of the olfactory peduncle, the olfactory tubercle, the prepyriform and periamygdaloid cortices, the cortical amygdaloid nucleus, and the ventrolateral entorhinal area. Moderate terminal degeneration is also found in the multiform layer of the prepyriform cortex (Heimer, 1968).

FUNCTIONAL INTERRELATIONS. There is a substantial body of electrophysiological evidence for mutual influences among the brain regions that receive inputs from—and send fibers to—the rodent olfactory bulb. For example, stimulation of the anterior limb of the anterior commissure has been shown to inhibit evoked potentials in the bulb and prepyriform cortex (Kerr and Hagbarth, 1955; Yamamoto, 1961; Mancia, von Baumgarten, and Green, 1962; von Baumgarten, Green, and Mancia, 1962; Yamamoto, Yamamoto, and Iwama, 1963; Boisacq-Scheppens and Cathens, 1963). Unilateral stimulation of the bulb or nasal mucosa inhibits evoked activity in the contralateral bulb and prepyriform cortex; this effect is mediated by the anterior limb of the anterior commissure (Kerr and Hagbarth, 1955; Kerr, 1960; Mancia, von Baumgarten, and Green, 1962; Fujita et al., 1964), but it is not due to any direct interbulbar connections, since no such connections have been found (Lohman, 1963; Lohman and Lammers, 1963). Stimulation of the amygdala and stimulation of the mesencephalic reticular formation also exert centrifugal inhibitory effects upon evoked activity in the rabbit olfactory bulb, but these two effects are exerted via different routes (Fujita et al., 1964).

It is pertinent to stress several additional anatomical features of experimental interest. By virtue of its location—in front of the forebrain and just beneath an overlying layer of bone—the rodent olfactory bulb is easily reached for study. Furthermore, the spatial separation of its input and output pathways endows the bulb with some of the same experimental advantages found in the spinal cord (a structure that is considerably more difficult to reach). As noted previously, the main sensory input to the bulb is via the olfactory nerve fibers from the nasal cavity, and the only way in which olfactory nerve activity (whether induced by odor stimuli or by electrical shocks) can set up impulses in the axons of the lateral olfactory tract is by way of the mitral primary dendrites. At the same time, the bulb may be activated by stimulating the lateral olfactory tract to produce a combined orthodromic and antidromic input to the bulb. Thus the bulb can be activated over at least two completely independent pathways, both of which lie fully exposed on the brain surface. Even the presence of centrifugal fibers in the lateral olfactory tract does not significantly compromise the effective segregation of olfactory-bulb inputs, since it is possible to activate the two main populations of fibers independently (e.g., the centrifugal fibers orthodromically by stimulating the area inominata and the axons of the lateral olfactory tract antidromically by stimulating at various points along the basal aspect of the brain). Several fairly simple and reliable experimental techniques have been developed for studying functional interactions in the bulb by stimulating separate input and output pathways and recording the extracellular currents generated around the activated cells within the bulb (e.g., Phillips, Powell, and Shepherd, 1963; Shepherd, 1963; Freeman, 1972).

From some initial studies of single-unit activity in the rodent olfactory bulb in response to animal secretions, we obtained preliminary evidence for the existence of enduring changes in the excitability of olfactory-bulb units as a result of experience. For example, we found that mitral cells in the mouse and hamster show both transient (phasic) and prolonged (tonic) changes in the rate and patterning of firing in response to both pure chemical odors and chemically unspecified odors of animal origin. By and large, the latter produce more clear-cut and longer-lasting effects and are influenced more by the prior experiential history of the test animal. In several cases we have recorded prolonged changes in olfactory-bulb unit activity under conditions closely resembling those where sensitization and habituation have been observed in reflexes of isolated spinal cord (see below). Our findings of prolonged changes in olfactory-bulb activity following alterations in sensory input are complemented by the recent data of Willey (1969), who observed some remarkably protracted changes in neuronal activity in the cat olfactory bulb as a result of long-term stimulation of the lateral olfactory tract with a 40-Hz electrical current. Although obtained in a different species, and under very different conditions from those we have employed, Willey's results lend further support to the idea that enduring changes in neural activity should be demonstrable in the olfactory bulb following the application of appropriate forms of stimulation.

The work described in the following paragraphs has a single unifying theme: the attempt to exploit the rodent olfactory system in studies of neurobehavioral plasticity. Our approach is predicated upon the biological significance of putative mammalian pheromones and seeks to understand the roles of prior experience, exposure history, and endocrine status in sensitization or habituation to olfactory and other stimuli.

38.6.3 Sensitization and habituation experiments

In order to maximize the inherent advantages of the rodent olfactory-bulb preparation, we are exploiting it in relation to phenomena which are themselves as simple and straightforward as possible. We are studying sensitization and habituation, which we take to refer, respectively, to the increased and decreased responsiveness to repeated stimulation that is manifested by an organism, system, tissue, etc. Both of these phenomena have been extensively studied in behaving organisms from paramecium (Jennings, 1906; Jensen, 1965) to man (Sokolov, 1963). The literature has been reviewed recently in considerable detail by Thompson and Spencer (1966), Horn (1967), and Groves and Thompson (1970). A good deal of relevant electrophysiological research on sensitization and habituation has been done with invertebrates (see, e.g., chapters by Davis and Krasne, this volume), but we shall restrict the present discussion to pertinent data obtained from work with mammals.

The terms habituation and sensitization encompass several other descriptors of response decrement (extinction, stimulus satiation, reactive inhibition, fatigue, etc.) and increment (dishabituation, pseudoconditioning, priming, "kindling," etc.). Interest in these phenomena during the past decade has been largely stimulated by the important contributions of Sharpless and Jasper (1956) and Sokolov (1963). There are now several general models of neuronal systems that deal with habituation (e.g., Sokolov, 1963; Konorski, 1967; Carlton, 1968; Groves and Thompson, 1970) and a number of contrasting theories couched in terms of synaptic physiology. The latter are hardly less speculative than the former, since there are still no available methods for analyzing mammalian synaptic activity in sufficient detail to establish their validity. In any event, the candidates that have been proposed to date include postsynaptic desensitization (Sharpless, 1964), monosynaptic low-frequency depression, presumably due to presynaptic or postsynaptic changes in transmitter action comparable to those that have been found in *Aplysia* neurons (Thompson and Spencer, 1966; Horn, 1967; Kandel and Spencer 1968), and postsynaptic inhibition (Wickelgren, 1967a,b).

Groves and Thompson (1970) argue that habituation and sensitization may be mediated by different populations of interneurons. They rely heavily upon studies of changes in spinal-cord interneuron activity in the acute spinal cat and describe three kinds of interneurons that they have observed with equal frequency, but in different loci, within the lumbosacral cord. Two of the three types of interneurons are termed "plastic" and are said to subserve habituation and sensitization, respectively. Groves and Thompson suggest that there may be at least three "fundamentally different types of excitatory synaptic actions in the central nervous system," and they argue, by extension, "that similar classes of interneurons may exist in the brain to mediate habituation and sensitization in the intact organism" (p. 431).

Transient excitability changes in reduced preparations of the mammalian central nervous system have been widely reported over the years. The commonly recognized examples include posttetanic potentiation (Lloyd, 1949) and low-frequency depression (Jefferson and Schlapp, 1953; Curtis and Eccles, 1960) in the spinal cord. In addition, Wall (1967) has reported finding "novelty detectors" in the lumbosacral cord of decerebrate cats. These are units that respond initially to cutaneous stimuli, but eventually cease responding if the stimulus is repeated. The habituation patterns of such units have been carefully studied by Wickelgren (1967a, b). By contrast, progressive *increases* in evoked spinal-cord activity with repetitive stimulation were observed by Mendell and Wall (1965) and Mendell (1966). They report what they call "windup" (i.e., sensitization) of units (putatively C fibers) in the spinocervical tract. Similar changes were described earlier by Frank and Fuortes (1956) for interneurons of the lumbosacral cord. Horn (1965) describes units that exhibit both sensitization and habituation in the tectotegmental region in the rabbit. Surprisingly, few similar findings have been obtained from more rostral structures, although units showing habituation and sensitization have been recorded from the rabbit visual cortex (Sokolov, Polyanskii, and Bagdonas, 1968) and from the hamster olfactory bulb (Macrides, 1970; Macrides and Chorover, 1972).

Various neurobehavioral effects have been observed following direct electrical stimulation at sites within the mammalian brain. For example, an increased disposition to develop seizures and epileptiform discharges has been demonstrated following repeated low-level stimulation of limbic-system structures. Goddard, McIntyre, and Leech (1969) term this effect "kindling." The basic finding is that brief trains of electrical current, delivered daily at levels below the threshold for overt behavioral reactions, may eventually come to elicit bilateral grand-mal epileptiform convulsions. This effect, which they produced with unilateral stimulation of the amygdala, undoubtedly involves a progressive change in the brain's response to periodically applied focal stimuli and presumably entails a correspondingly enduring change in the morphology and/or chemical organization of the affected neurons. The effect is long-lasting, robust, reliable, and stimulus-dependent. Goddard believes that the effect is transsynaptic and due to nondegenerative morphological changes at or near the stimulated site,

but evidence on these points is still rather unconvincing, in our view.

Similar electrophysiological effects have been reported to follow low-level electrical stimulation of other brain structures, including the hippocampus in cat (Delgado and Sevillano, 1961) and rat (Racine, 1972a,b; Racine, Okujava, and Chipashvili, 1972), the thalamus and septal forebrain in rat (Tress and Herberg, 1972) and the amygdala in rat (Racine, Okujava, and Chipashvili, 1972; McIntyre and Goddard, 1973; Bobington and Wedeking, 1973).

Goddard and his colleagues stress the apparent similarity between "kindling" and "learning." They note that "each is a relatively permanent change resulting from repeated experience, the limbic system is implicated in both. . . both involve transfer from one stimulus to another, and in both cases, the acquisition of a new response results in retroactive interference with old responses" (p. 328). Questions about the relevance of this effect to "99.44 percent pure" learning obviously cannot be answered in factual terms at this time. But there is reason to believe that studies of such models are likely to lead to a constructive reformation of the learning and memory problem.

The sensitization of neural activity by means of electrical stimulation bears an obvious resemblance to another model system that has been employed in the mammalian brain to study neurobehavioral plasticity, namely, the development of primary and secondary (mirror) epileptic foci (e.g., Morrell, 1969). The "kindling" effect is said to lead to the development of comparable secondary foci (i.e., to other electrophysiologically defined areas of paroxysmal discharge at least one synapse removed from the primary epileptogenic zone and presumably connected to that zone by a relatively massive fiber pathway). Furthermore, the use of electrical stimuli appears to offer some practical advantages over more conventional methods of producing experimental epileptogenic lesions. Unlike alumina cream, cobalt, penicillin, ethyl chloride, etc., electrical stimuli are easy to apply, control, and quantify because the electrical current itself can be measured and administered in well-localized and periodic doses.

In the sensitization experiments thus far mentioned, electrical stimuli were applied to brain sites possessing extremely complex intrinsic organization and extrinsic interconnections. It has been difficult, therefore, to determine whether the elaboration of epileptiform activity reflects events at the locus of stimulation (Racine, Okujava, and Chipashvili, 1972) or entails the development of new synaptic connections elsewhere (Goddard, McIntyre, and Leech, 1969).

PLASTICITY IN OLFACTORY-BULB UNIT ACTIVITY. In their experiments Goddard, McIntyre, and Leech (1969) obtained the clearest "kindling" effect with electrodes in the amygdala, which, as we have previously noted, receives a substantial input from the olfactory bulb, is an important center of the limbic system, and, when stimulated, exerts effects upon memory (McGaugh and Gold, this volume) and upon the neuroelectric activity of the olfactory bulb.

In several respects, therefore, the induction of epileptiform activity by means of electrical stimulation of the olfactory bulb appeared to us to provide a particularly appealing method for investigating mammalian brain mechanisms involved in neurobehavioral plasticity.

In experiments presently underway, we are using electrical stimuli to trigger epileptiform activity in the intact or isolated rodent olfactory bulb in situ. At the outset we attempted to record both slow-wave and unit potentials in acute and chronically implanted animals with fine-wire electrodes, ranging in diameter from 68 to 85 μm, according to the general methods of Strumwasser (1958) and Hirano, Best, and Olds (1970). Although single units were detectable and could occasionally be isolated sufficiently for short periods, the same unit(s) could rarely be held for periods exceeding a few hours. (Those who have reported better success with this technique have generally been recording from deeper brain regions populated by somewhat larger cells than those of the mitral-cell layer of the olfactory bulb; see, e.g., Olds et al., 1972; O'Keefe and Bouma, 1969.) After considerable trial and error, we discovered that it was possible to employ individually insulated platinum-iridium (Pt-Ir) wires of approximately one-third the diameter previously used (the finest we have been able to obtain has a diameter of 25 μm). We have incorporated these wires in an electrode assembly that seems to solve the difficult problem of long-term mechanical stability in vivo.

A detailed description of our multiple fine-wire semimicroelectrode has been published elsewhere (Chorover and DeLuca, 1972). Briefly, the device consists of a set of individually insulated Pt-Ir wires that are simultaneously implanted in a preselected brain area, using conventional stereotaxic methods. Among the virtues of design, construction, and performance that distinguish our electrode from previous fine-wire designs are the following: (1) It is entirely prefabricated prior to surgical implantation. No delicate and time-consuming assembly or soldering steps are required during surgery. (2) Seven (or more) of the 25-μm wires may be inserted through the lumen of a single 26-gauge stainless-steel hypodermic tube. Although the individual monofila-ments would normally be too fine and flexible to penetrate even the softest tissue, they are rendered reversibly rigid by being fused into a shaft coated with melted dextrose. (3) The sugar coating is hard and smooth, and it provides adequate mechanical stiffness to permit brain penetration. The sugar is chemically innocuous and dissolves rapidly, thereby freeing each of the wires to assume a position of minimum mechanical stress. (4) Within a few days after implantation, most electrodes come to exhibit a high degree of neutral bouyancy and imperviousness to mechanical displacement with respect to the immediately surrounding brain tissue. As a result, long-term electrical stability is achieved, and it is possible to record activity from the same unit(s) over prolonged periods of time. At present, a standard seven-wire assembly is in routine use in our laboratory. Through an improvement in our sugar-coating technique, we are now able to produce multiple electrodes with an overall tip diameter considerably smaller than the one illustrated in the published description.

So far, semimicroelectrode assemblies have been implanted in the olfactory bulbs and other brain areas of more than 24 rats and rabbits. In eighteen cases electrode performance was studied in vivo for periods ranging up to ten months. In all but two animals (both of them rabbits), we succeeded in obtaining stable single- or multiple-unit recordings from one or more pairs of electrodes. We obtain on-line oscillographic display of unit activity and several other signals. Our principal dependent variables are: unit potentials falling within some preset operating range of a window discriminator; the cortical electroencephalogram (ECoG); and slow-wave potentials recorded from the semimicroelectrode. These data are preserved on a strip chart, together with integrated signals analyzed during a given sampling epoch (usually 10 sec). The strip-chart records in Fig. 38.5 illustrate typical data displays. Note that

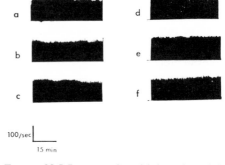

FIGURE 38.5 Integrated multiple-unit activity recorded from a pair of chronically implanted semimicroelectrodes in the mitral-cell layer of rabbit olfactory bulb. Each block represents recordings made under identical baseline conditions on 6 consecutive days.

under baseline conditions, the data exhibit a high degree of day-to-day stability. All variables are recorded on magnetic tape to permit subsequent reexamination and analysis of results.

Using brief trains of biphasic square wave pulses (100 Hz for 5 sec, once daily) at current levels well below the initial threshold for detectable overt or electrographic aftereffects (usually in the range of 1–5 μA), we succeeded in producing the basic sensitization effect within a few days by stimulating the olfactory bulb. Fig 38.6 illustrates some results obtained from a placement in the olfactory bulb of a male Dutch-Belted rabbit. Stimulation was applied via the recording electrode pair at the points indicated. Note the long-lasting effects upon subsequently recorded unit activity. Preliminary examinations of the brains of implanted and stimulated animals have revealed no evidence of adverse tissue reactions due to either the sugar or the low current levels involved (see Fig. 38.7). Equally compelling evidence that our implantation and stimulation procedures are relatively nontraumatic comes from the fact that we are generally able to obtain excellent recordings from many placements over extremely long periods of time.

In cases like the one illustrated in Figure 38.6, five or six stimulations of the intact olfactory bulb are required to produce a detectable change in the unit activity derived from the stimulating/recording electrodes. The degree and direction of the effect is somewhat variable, but it clearly suggests that periodic stimulation is capable of effecting a prolonged alteration in the firing pattern of olfactory-bulb units.

PLASTICITY IN THE ISOLATED OLFACTORY BULB. As noted previously, rodent olfactory-bulb fibers project extensively to many regions of the basal forebrain, and the bulb receives various centrifugal inputs from more caudal brain regions. The possibility therefore remains that the effects of stimulation upon unit activity in the intact olfactory bulb are not due to changes in the functional activity of intrinsic bulb units, but reflect a transsynaptic effect occurring elsewhere. In order to determine whether comparable changes can be observed when extrinsic synaptic pathways are eliminated, slow-wave and unit potentials were recorded from the isolated olfactory bulbs of two animals. In two others the bulb contralateral to the stimulated one was isolated, and two additional animals served as unoperated controls.

Recordings made without stimulation for 2–10 weeks after olfactory-bulb isolation and electrode implantation showed that slow-wave activity is generally depressed in the isolated bulb but there continue to be units with stable firing patterns.

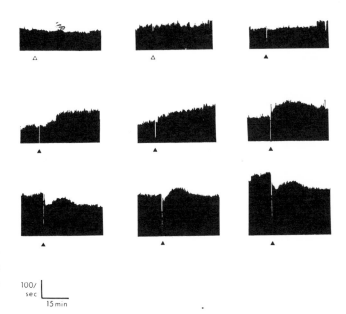

FIGURE 38.6 Continued recording from the same electrodes as in Figure 38.5, showing a response to low-level electrical stimulation applied to the bulb on 7 successive days. Open triangles indicate sham stimulation; closed triangles indicate the point at which a 5-sec current was applied.

Unit and slow-wave responses to stimulation of the isolated bulb showed an exaggeration of the pattern seen in recordings from intact animals. At the stimulus levels employed, several successive stimulations were required to provoke a change in unit activity in the intact animals. By contrast, a single exposure to the stimulating current was sufficient to produce such a change in animals with isolated olfactory bulbs. This was the case whether the electrodes were implanted in the bulb ipsi- or contralateral to the transection.

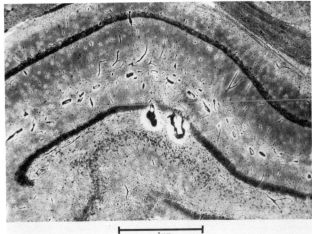

FIGURE 38.7 Tip localization of a stimulating/recording electrode pair in rabbit hippocampus.

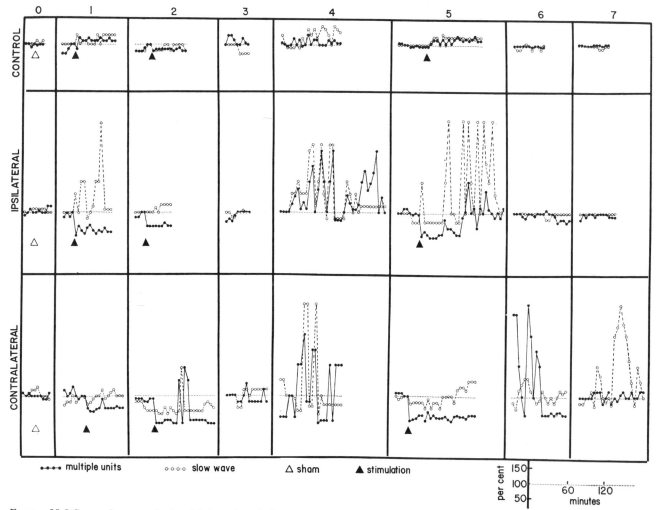

FIGURE 38.8 Seven-day record of multiple-unit and slow-wave activity in rabbit olfactory bulb. Control: both bulbs intact. Ipsilateral: electrode in isolated olfactory bulb. Contralateral: electrode in intact bulb; contralateral bulb isolated. Open triangles: sham stimulation. Closed triangles: stimulation. Responses are expressed as a percentage of baseline (prestimulus) level.

Fig. 38.8 shows the levels of unit and slow-wave activity before and after the first stimulation in three animals with electrodes in their left olfactory bulbs. In the first case both bulbs were intact, in the second the left olfactory bulb was isolated, and in the third the right bulb was isolated. In all three cases stable baseline recordings had been obtained as already described for at least three weeks prior to the session in which stimulation was applied.

The stimulation was without detectable effect in the intact animal, but all four of the subjects with isolated bulbs showed an immediate and marked change in both unit and slow-wave activity following stimulation. Following a few interpolated sham stimulation sessions, during which the recorded activity returned to baseline levels, the stimulation treatment was repeated with essentially the same results. After two stimulations,

however, the records obtained from the isolated animals showed persistent alterations. In all cases spike and wave seizure activity and marked fluctuations in unit discharge patterns were observed in the absence of stimulation for from one to three days following each stimulation session. In two cases (both with the left bulb isolated) the seizure activity observed after the second stimulation was found to persist for five days without further treatment. From these results we conclude that the isolated olfactory bulb retains an ability to exhibit long-term changes in unit and slow-wave activity following a brief period of low-level electrical stimulation. Although the effects of stimulation are somewhat more variable than in the intact preparation, the influence of more caudal brain regions is excluded by the transection, and it seems inescapable that the electrophysiological changes observed in the isolated bulb are due solely to events occurring within the isolated tissue itself. Since the isolated bulb retains both its normal input from primary receptor cells and its extensive pattern of reciprocal interconnections between the secondary receptor (mitral) cells from which we have been recording and other cell types within the bulb itself, the more likely mechanisms responsible for the development of long-term sensitization or habituation following stimulation are: (1) mitral-cell axon collaterals, which have been shown to form reciprocal axodendritic synapses among large numbers of mitral cells (Price and Powell, 1970a), and (2) reciprocal dendrodendritic synapses between granule-cell gemmules (Rall et al., 1966) and mitral-cell secondary dendrites. It has been suggested that the latter may comprise intrabulbar systems capable of generating recurrent inhibition (Shepherd, 1970; Rall, 1970) and may play a role in those cases in which olfactory-bulb stimulation leads to a reduction (rather than to an increase) in unit activity.

Additional work will be required to characterize further and identify the basis of transient excitability changes produced by electrical stimulation of the isolated rodent olfactory bulb in situ. The results obtained thus far, however, show that the olfactory bulb, which exhibits intrinsic morphological features generally associated with "cortical" tissues (Shepherd, 1970), also possesses an inherent ability to mediate the kind of functional plasticity most commonly associated with the phenomena of learning and memory within the mammalian brain. Taken together, the adaptive importance of olfaction in rodent behavior, the relative accessibility of the olfactory bulb, its intimate involvement with the limbic system and associated basal forebrain mechanisms critical for normal learning and memory, and the ease with which the bulb may be isolated in situ, comprise a persuasive case for using this region of the brain in further studies aimed at identifying a morphological basis for experimental learning and memory.

REFERENCES

ADAMS, H. E., and LEWIS, D. J. 1962a. Electroconvulsive shock, retrograde amnesia and competing responses. *Journal of Comparative and Physiological Psychology* 55: 299–301.

ADAMS, H. E., and LEWIS, D. J. 1962b. Retrograde amnesia and competing responses. *Journal of Comparative and Psyiological Psychology* 55: 302–305.

ADEY, W. R. 1959. The sense of smell. In J. Field, H. W. Magoun, and V. E. Hall, eds., *Handbook of Physiology*. Section 1: *Neurophysiology*, Vol. 1. Washington D.C.: American Physiological Society, pp. 535–548.

ALLISON, A. C. 1953. The structure of the olfactory bulb and its relationship to the olfactory pathways in the rabbit and the rat. *Journal of Comparative Neurology* 98: 309–353.

ALLISON, A. C., and WARWICK, R. T. T. 1949. Quantitative observations on the olfactory system of the rabbit. *Brain* 72: 186–197.

ALPERN, H. P., and McGAUGH, J. L. 1968. Retrograde amnesia as a function of duration of electroshock stimulation. *Journal of Comparative and Psyiological Psychology* 65: 265–269.

ALPERN, M. 1953. Metacontrast. *Journal of the Optical Society of America* 43: 648–657.

BAUMGARDT, E., and SEGAL, J. 1942. Facilitation et inhibition parametres de la fonction visuelle. *Année Psychologique* 43: 54–102.

BOBINGTON, R. G., and WEDEKING, P. W. 1973. The pharmacology of seizures induced by sensitization with low intensity brain stimulation. *Pharmacology, Biochemistry and Behavior* 1: 461–467.

BOISACQ-SCHEPPENS, N., and CATHENS, M. 1963. Caractéristiques électrophysiologiques des connexions entre les bulbes olfactifs. *Archives Internationales de Physiologie* 71: 618–620.

BRADY, J. V., and NAUTA, W. J. H. 1953. Subcortical mechanisms in emotional behavior: Affective changes following septal forebrain lesions in the albino rat. *Journal of Comparative and Physiological Psychology* 46: 339–346.

BUREŠ, J., and BUREŠOVÁ, O. 1963. Cortical spreading depression as a memory distrubing factor. *Journal of Comparative and Physiological Psychology* 56: 268–272.

CAREW, T. J. 1970. Do passive avoidance tasks permit assessment of retrograde amnesia in rats? *Journal of Comparative and Physiological Psychology* 72: 267–271.

CARLTON, P. L. 1968. Brain acetylcholine and habituation. In P. B. Bradley and M. Fink, eds., *Progress in Brain Research*. Vol. 28: *Anticholinergic Drugs and Brain Functions in Animals and Man*. Amsterdam: Elsevier Publishing Company.

CARR, W. J., LOEB, L. S., and DISSINGER, M. L. 1965. Responses of rats to sex odors. *Journal of Comparative and Physiological Psychology* 59: 370–377.

CHOROVER, S. L. 1965. Electroshock and memory. In D. P. Kimble, ed., *The Anatomy of Memory*, Vol. 1. Palo Alto, Calif.: Science and Behavior Books.

CHOROVER, S. L., and DeLUCA, A. M. 1969. Transient change in electrocorticographic reaction to ECS in the rat following footshock. *Journal of Comparative and Physiological Psychology* 69: 141–149.

CHOROVER, S. L., and DeLUCA, A. M. 1972. A sweet new multiple electrode for chronic single unit recording in moving animals. *Psychology and Behavior* 9: 671–674.

CHOROVER, S. L., and GROSS, C. G. 1963. Caudate nucleus lesions: Behavioral effects in the rat. *Science* 141: 826–827.

CHOROVER, S. L., and SCHILLER, P. H. 1965a. Neural information processing and memory. *Technical Engineering* 1: 43–55.

CHOROVER, S. L., and SCHILLER, P. H. 1965b. Short-term retrograde amnesia in rats. *Journal of Comparative and Physiological Psychology* 59: 73–78.

CHOROVER, S. L., and SCHILLER, P. H. 1965c. Retrograde amnesia. *Science* 149: 1521.

CHOROVER, S. L., and SCHILLER, P. H. 1966. Reexamination of prolonged retrograde amnesia in one-trial learning. *Journal of Comparative and Physiological Psychology* 61: 34–41.

COLONNIER, M., and GUILLERY, R. W. 1964. Synaptic organization in the lateral geniculate nucleus of the monkey. *Zeitschrift für Zellforschung und Mikroskopische Anatomie* 62: 333–335.

COONS, E. E., and MILLER, N. E. 1960. Conflict versus consolidation of memory traces to explain "retrograde amnesia" produced by electroconvulsive shock. *Journal of Comparative and Physiological Psychology* 53: 524–531.

CURTIS, D. R., and ECCLES, J. C. 1960. Synaptic action during and after repetitive stimulation. *Journal of Physiology* 150: 374–398.

DARBY, M., DEVOR, M., and CHOROVER, S. L. 1975. A presumptive sex phenome in the hamster: Some behavioral effects. *Journal of Comparative and Physiological Psychology* 88: 496–502.

DARFNON, L. J., and JARVIK, M. E. 1968. A parametric study of electroshock-induced retrograde anmesia in mice. *Neuropsychologia* 6: 373–380.

DAWKINS, R. 1971. Selective neurondeath as a possible memory mechanism. *Nature* 229: 118–119.

DELGADO, J. M. R., and SEVILLANO, M. 1961. Evolution of repeated hippocampal seizures in the cat. *Electroencephalography and Clinical Neurophysiology* 13: 722–733.

DOWLING, J. E., and BOYCOTT, B. B. 1966. Organization of the primate retina: Electron microscopy. *Proceedings of the Royal Society (London)* B 166: 80–111.

DUNCAN, C. P. 1949. The retroactive effect of electroshock on learning. *Journal of Comparative and Physiological Psychology* 42: 32–44.

ECCLES, J. C. 1965. In D. P. Kimble, ed., *Anatomy of Memory*. Palo Alto, Calif.: Science and Behavior Books.

ECCLES, J. C., ITO, M., and SZENTÁGOTHAI, J. 1967. *The Cerebellum as a Neuronal Machine*. New York: Springer-Verlag.

ESPLIN, D. W., and FRESTON, J. W. 1960. Physiological and pharmacological analysis of spinal cord convulsions. *Journal of Pharmacology and Experimental Therapeutics* 130: 68–80.

FERNANDEZ-GUARDIALA, A., ALCARAZ, V., and GUZMAN, F. 1961. Inhibition of convulsive activity by the reticular formation. *Acta Neurologica Latino Americana* 7: 30–36.

FOX, C. A., HILLMAN, D. E., SIEGESMUND, K. A., and DUTTA, C. R. 1967. The primate cerebellar cortex: A Golgi and electron microscope study. *Progress in Brain Research* 25: 174–225.

FRANK, K., and FUORTES, M. G. F. 1965. Unitary activity of spinal interneurons of cats. *Journal of Physiology* 131: 424–436.

FREEMAN, W. J. 1972. Spatial and temporal dispersion in primary olfactory nerve of cat. *Journal of Neurophysiology* 35: 733–744.

FRY, G. A. 1934. Modulation of the optic nerve current as a base for color-vision. *American Journal of Physiology* 108: 701–707.

FUJITA, H., OIKAWA, I., IHARA, H., and TAKAGI, S. F. 1964. Centrifugal regulation of olfactory bulb activity as studied by stimulation of the amygdala and the anterior limb of the anterior commissure. *Japanese Journal of Physiology* 14: 615–629.

GANDELMAN, K., ZARROW, M. X., DENENBERG, V. H., and MYERS, M. 1971. Olfactory bulb removal eliminates maternal behavior in the mouse. *Science* 171: 210–211.

GASTAUT, H., and FISCHER-WILLIAMS, M. 1959. In J. Field, H. W. Magoun, and V. E. Hall, eds., *Handbook of Physiology*. Section 1: *Neurophysiology*, Vol. 1. Washington D.C.: American Physiological Society.

GLICKMAN, S. E. 1961. Perseverative neural processes and consolidation of the neural trace. *Psychology Bulletin* 58: 218–233.

GODDARD, G. V., McINTYRE, D. C., and LEECH, C. K. 1969. A permanent change in brain function resulting from daily electrical stimulation. *Experimental Neurology* 25: 295–330.

GROSS, C. G., BLACK, P., and CHOROVER, S. L. 1968. Hippocam-

pal lesions: Effects on memory in rats. *Psychonomic Science* 12: 165–166.

GROSS, C. G., CHOROVER, S. L., and COHEN, S. M. 1965. Caudate, cortical, hippocampal and dorsal thalamic lesions in rats: Alternation and Hebb-Williams maze performance. *Neuropsychologia* 3: 53–68.

GROVES, P. M., and THOMPSON, R. F. 1970. Habituation: A dual-process theory. *Psychological Review* 77: 419–450.

HEBB, D. O. 1949. *The Organization of Behavior*. New York: J. Wiley & Sons.

HEIMER, L. 1968. Synaptic distribution of centripetal and centrifugal nerve fibers in the olfactory system of the rat. An experimental anatomical study. *Journal of Anatomy* 103: 413–432.

HEIMER, L., and LARSSON, K. 1967. Mating behavior of male rats after olfactory bulb lesions. *Psychology and Behavior* 2: 207–209.

HERIOT, J. T., and COLEMAN, P. D. 1962. The effect of electroconvulsive shock on retention of a modified "one-trial" conditioned avoidance. *Journal of Comparative and Physiological Psychology* 55: 1082–1084.

HIRANO, T., BEST, P. and OLDS, J. 1970. Units during habituation, discrimination learning and extinction. *Electroencephalography and Clinical Neurophysiology* 28: 127–135.

HORN, G. 1965. Physiological and psychological aspects of selective perception. In D. S. Lehrman, R. A. Hinde, and E. Shaw, eds., *Advances in the Study of Behavior*, Vol. 1. New York: Academic Press.

HORN, G. 1967. Neuronal mechanisms of habituation. *Nature* 215: 707–711.

JEFFERSON, A. A., and SCHLAPP, W. 1953. Some effects of repetitive stimulation of afferents on reflex conduction. In J. L. Malcolm and A. B. Gray, eds., *Ciba Foundation Symposium. The Spinal Cord*. London: J. & A. Churchill.

JENNINGS, H. S. 1906. *Behavior of the Lower Organisms*. Bloomington, Ind.: Indiana University Press (New edition, 1962).

JENSEN, D. D. 1965. Paramecia, planaria, and pseudo-learning. In *Learning and Associated Phenomena in Invertebrates* (*Animal Behaviour* Suppl.), pp. 9–20.

KANDEL, E. R., and SPENCER, W. A. 1968. Cellular neurophysiological approaches in the study of learning. *Psychological Reviews* 48: 65–134.

KERR, D. I. B. 1960. Properties of the olfactory efferent system. *Australian Journal of Experimental Biology* 38: 29–36.

KERR, D. I. B., and HAGBARTH, K. E. 1955. An investigation of the olfactory centrifugal fiber system. *Journal of Neurophysiology* 18: 362–374.

KING, R. A. 1965. Consolidation of the neural trace in memory: Investigation with one-trial avoidance conditioning and electroconvulsive shock. *Journal of Comparative and Physiological Psychology* 59: 283–284.

KONORSKI, J. 1967. *Integrative Activity of the Brain: An Interdisciplinary Approach*. Chicago: The University of Chicago Press.

KOPP, R,. BOHDANECKY, Z., and JARVIK, M. E. 1966. Long temporal gradient of retrograde amnesia for a well discriminated stimulus. *Science* 153: 1547–1549.

LEE-TENG, E., and SHERMAN, S. M. 1966. Memory consolidation of one-trial learning in chicks. *Proceedings of the National Academy of Sciences* (*USA*) 56: 926–931.

LEGROS CLARK, W. E. 1956. Observation on the structure and organization of olfactory receptors in the rabbit. *Yale Journal of Biology and Medicine* 29: 83–95.

LeMagnen, J. 1952. Les pheromones olfacto-sexuels chez le rat blanc. *Archives des Sciences Physiologiques* 6: 295–332.

Lewis, D. J., and Maher, B. A. 1965. Neural consolidation and electroconvulsive shock. *Psychological Review* 72: 225–239.

Lewis, D. J., and Maher, B. A. 1966. Electroconvulsive shock and inhibition: Some problems considered. *Psychological Review* 73: 388–392.

Lloyd, D. P. C. 1949. Post-tetanic potentiation of response in monosynaptic reflex pathways of the spinal cord. *Journal of General Physiology* 33: 147–170.

Lohman, A. H. M. 1963. The anterior olfactory lobe of the guinea pig. A descriptive and experimental anatomical study. *Acta Anatomica* 49: 53.

Lohman, A. H. M., and Lammers, H. J. 1963. On the connections of the olfactory bulb and the anterior olfactory nucleus in some mammals. An experimental study. *Progress in Brain Research* 3: 149–162.

Macrides, F. 1970. Single unit activity in the hamster olfactory bulb: Response to animal and pure chemical odors. Unpublished Ph.D. dissertation, Massachusetts Institute of Technology.

Macrides, F., and Chorover, S. L. 1972. Olfactory bulb units: Activity correlated with inhalation cycles and odor quality. *Science* 175: 84–87.

Madsen, M. C., and McGaugh, J. L. 1961. The effect of electroconvulsive shock on one trial avoidance learning. *Journal of Comparative and Physiological Psychology* 54: 522–523.

Mancia, M., von Baumgarten, R., and Green, J. D. 1962. Response patterns of olfactory bulb neurons. *Archives Italiennes de Biologie* 100: 449–462.

Marshall, W. H. 1959. Spreading cortical depression of Leao. *Physiological Reviews* 39: 239–279.

McCleary, R. A., and Moore, R. Y. 1965. *Subcortical Mechanisms of Behavior*. New York: Basic Books.

McGaugh, J. L. 1966. Time-dependent processes in memory storage. *Science* 153: 1351–1358.

McGaugh, J. L., and Alpern, H. P. 1966. Effects of electroshock on memory: Amnesia without convulsion. *Science* 152: 665–666.

McIntyre, D. C., and Goddard, G. V. 1973. Transfer, interference and spontaneous recovery of convulsions kindled from the rat amygdala. *Electroencephalography and Clinical Neurophysiology* 35: 533–543.

Mendell, L. M. 1966. Physiological properties of unmyelinated fiber projections to the spinal cord. *Experimental Neurology* 16: 316–332.

Mendell, L. M., and Wall, P. D. 1965. Responses of single dorsal horn cells to peripheral cutaneous unmyelinated fibers. *Nature* 206: 97–99.

Michael, R. P. 1971. Neuroendocrine factors regulating primate behavior. In L. Martini and W. F. Ganong, eds., *Frontiers in Neuroendocrinology*. New York: Oxford University Press.

Miller, N. E. 1965. Discussion. In D. P. Kimble, ed., *The Anatomy of Memory*, Vol. 1. Palo Alto, Calif.: Science and Behavior Books.

Morrell, F. 1969. Physiology and histochemistry of the mirror focus. In H. H. Jasper et al., eds. *Basic Mechanisms of the Epilepsies*. Boston: Little, Brown, pp. 357–374.

Moruzzi, G., and Magoun, H. W. 1949. Brain stem reticular formation and activation of the EEG. *Electroencephalography and Clinical Neurophysiology* 1: 445–473.

Müller, G. E., and Pilzecker, A. 1900. Experimentale Beiträge zur Lehre vom Gedächtnis. *Zeitschrift für Psychologie* Suppl.: 1–288.

Murphy, M. R., and Schneider, G. E. 1970. Olfactory bulb removal eliminates mating behavior in the male golden hamster. *Science* 167: 302–304.

O'Keefe, J., and Bouma, H. 1969. Complex sensory properties of certain amygdala units in the freely moving cat. *Experimental Neurology* 23: 384–398.

Olds, J., Disterhoft, J. F., Segal, M., Kornblith, C. L., and Hirsh, R. 1972. Learning centers of rat brain mapped by measuring latencies of conditioned unit responses. *Journal of Neurophysiology* 35: 202–219.

Ottoson, J. O. 1960. Experimental studies of memory impairment after electroconvulsive therapy: The role of the electrical stimulation and of the seizure by variation of cerebral responses in man. *Acta Psychiatrica Scandinavica* 35: 7–32.

Papez, J. W. 1937. A proposed mechanism of emotion. *Archives of Neurology and Psychiatry* 38: 725–744.

Penfield, W., and Jasper, H. H. 1954. *Epilepsy and the Functional Anatomy of the Human Brain*. Boston: Little, Brown.

Peters, A., and Palay, S. L. 1966. The morphology of lamine A & AI of the dorsal lateral geniculate body of the cat. *Journal of Anatomy* 100: 451–486.

Pfaff, D. W., and Pfaffman, D. 1969a. Olfactory and hormonal influences on the basal forebrain of the male rat. *Brain Research* 15: 137–156.

Pfaff, D. W., and Pfaffmann, D. 1969b. Behavioral and electrophysiological responses of male rats to female rat urine odors. In C. Pfaffmann, ed., *Olfaction and Taste*. New York: Rockefeller University Press.

Phillips, C. G., Powell, T. P. S., and Shepherd, G. M., 1963. Responses of mitral cells to stimulation of the lateral olfactory tract in the rabbit. *Journal of Physiology* 168: 65–88.

Piéron, H. 1935. Le processus de metacontraste. *Journal de Psychologie, Normale et Pathologique* 32: 5–24.

Pinel, J. P. J., and Chorover, S. L. 1972. Inhibition by arousal of epilepsy induced by chloroambucil in rats. *Nature* 236: 232–234.

Powell, T. P. S., Cowan, W. M., and Raisman, G. 1963. Olfactory relationships of the diencephalon. *Nature* 199: 710–712.

Pribram, K. H., and Kruger, L. 1954. Functions of the "olfactory brain." *Annals of the New York Academy of Sciences* 58: 109–138.

Price, J. L. 1969. The origin of the centrifugal fibres to the olfactory bulb. *Brain Research* 14: 542–545.

Price, J. L., and Powell, T. P. S. 1970a. An experimental study of the origin and the course of the centrifugal fibres to the olfactory bulb in the rat. *Journal of Anatomy* 107: 215–237.

Price, J. L., and Powell, T. P. S. 1970b. The morphology of the granule cells of the olfactory bulb. *Journal of Cell Science* 7: 91–123.

Price, J. L., and Powell, T. P. S. 1970c. The synaptology of the granule cells of the olfactory bulb. *Journal of Cell Science* 7: 125–155.

Price, J. L., and Powell, T. P. S. 1970d. An electron-microscopic study of the termination of the afferent fibres to the olfactory bulb from the cerebral hemisphere. *Journal of Cell Science*: 7: 157–187.

Quartermain, D., Paolino, R. M., and Miller, N. E. 1965.

A brief temporal gradient of retrograde amnesia independent of situational change. *Science* 149: 1116–1118.

Raab, D. H. 1963. Backward masking. *Psychology Bulletin* 60: 118–129.

Racine, R. J. 1972a. Modification of seizure activity by electrical stimulation: I. After discharge threshold. *Electroencephalography and Clinical Neurophysiology* 32: 269–279.

Racine, R. J. 1972b. Modification of seizure activity by electrical stimulation: II. Motor seizure. *Electroencephalography and Clinical Neurophysiology* 32: 281–294.

Racine, R. J., Okujava, V., and Chipashvili, S. 1972. Modification of seizure activity by electrical stimulation. III. Mechanisms. *Electroencephalography and Clinical Neurophysiology* 32: 295–299.

Rall, W. 1970. Dendritic neuron theory and dendrodendritic synapses in a simple cortical system. In F. O. Schmitt, ed., *The Neurosciences: Second Study Program*. New York: Rockefeller University Press, pp. 552–565.

Rall, W., Shepherd, G. M., Reese, T. S., and Brightman, M. W. 1966. Dendrodendritic synaptic pathway for inhibition in the olfactory bulb. *Experimental Neurology* 14: 44–56.

Ramón y Cajal, S. 1911. *Histologie du Système Nerveux de l'Homme et des Vertébrés*. Paris: Maloine.

Ramón y Cajal, S. 1955. *Studies on the Cerebral Cortex*. Translated by L. M. Kraft. Chicago: Yearbook Publishers.

Rebert, C. S., Pryor, G. T., and Schaeffer, J. A. 1974. Slow cortical potential consequences of electro-convulsive shock in rats. *Physiology and Behavior* 12: 131–134.

Schiller, P. H., and Chorover, S. L. 1966. Metacontrast: Its relation to evoked potentials. *Science* 153: 1398–1400.

Schiller, P. H., and Chorover, S. L. 1967. Short-term amnestic effects of electroconvulsive shock in a one-trial maze learning paradigm. *Neuropsychologia* 5: 155–163.

Schiller, P. H., and Smith, M. 1966. Detection in metacontrast. *Journal of Experimental Psychology* 71: 32.

Schneider, A., and Sherman, W. 1968. Amnesia: A function of the temporal relation of footshock to electroconvulsive shock. *Science* 159: 219–221.

Sharpless, S. K. 1964. Reorganization of function in the nervous system—use and disuse. *Annual Review of Physiology* 26: 357–388.

Sharpless, S. K., and Jasper, H. 1956. Habituation of the arousal reaction. *Brain* 79: 655–680.

Shepherd, G. M. 1963. Responses of mitral cells to olfactory nerve volleys in the rabbit. *Journal of Physiology* 168: 89–100.

Shepherd, G. M. 1970. The olfactory bulb as a simple cortical system: Experimental analysis and functional implications. In F. O. Schmitt, ed., *The Neurosciences: Second Study Program*. New York: Rockefeller University Press, pp. 539–552.

Signoret, J. P. 1962. Action de l'ablation des bulbes olfactifs sur les mecanismes de la reproduction chez la truie. *Annales de Biologie Animale, Biochimie, Biophysique* 2: 67–174.

Sokolov, E. N. 1963. *Perception and the Conditioned Reflex*. Translated by S. W. Waydenfeld. Oxford: Pergamon Press.

Sokolov, E. N., Polyanskii, V. B., and Bagdonas, A. 1968. Stabilization of single unit responses of the visual cortex in unanesthetized rabbits to repeated photic stimulation. *Zhurnal Vyssher Nervnoi Deyatel'nosti imeni I.P. Pavlova* 18: 701–707.

Stein, D. G., and Chorover, S. L. 1968. Effects of posttrial electrical stimulation of hippocampus and caudate nucleus on maze learning in the rat. *Physiology and Behavior* 3: 787–791.

Stigler, R. 1910. Chronophetische Studien über den Umgeb-

ungskontrast. *Pflügers Archiv für die Gesamte Physiologie des Menschen und der Tiere* 134: 365–435.

Strumwasser, F. 1958. Long-term recording from single neurons in brain of unrestrained mammals. *Science* 127: 469–470.

Suboski, M. D., Black, M., Litner, J., Greener, R. T., and Spevack, A. A. 1969. Long and short term effects of electroconvulsive shock following one-trial discriminated avoidance conditioning. *Neuropsychologia* 7: 349–356.

Szentágothai, J., Hamari, J., and Tömhál, T. 1966. Degeneration and electron microscope analysis of the synaptic glomeruli in the lateral geniculate body. *Experimental Brain Research* 2: 283–301.

Tepas, D. I., and Armington, J. C. 1962. Properties of evoked visual potentials. *Vision Research* 2: 449–461.

Thompson, R. F., and Spencer, W. A. 1966. Habituation: A model phenomenon for the study of neuronal substrates of behavior. *Psychological Review* 73: 16–43.

Tress, K. H., and Herberg, L. J. 1972. Permanent reduction in seizure threshold resulting from repeated electrical stimulation. *Experimental Neurology* 37: 347–359.

Valverde, F. 1965. *Studies on the Piriform Lobe*. Cambridge, Mass.: Harvard University Press.

Vaughan, Jr., H., Hull, H. G., and Hull, R. C. 1965. Functional relation between stimulus intensity and photically evoked stimulus intensity and modification by lidocaine of seizure discharge. *Nature* 206: 720–722.

von Baugarten, R., Green, J. D., and Mancia, M. 1962. Recurrent inhibition of the olfactory bulb. II. Effects of antidromic stimulation of commissural fibers. *Journal of Neurophysiology* 25: 489–500.

Wall, P. D. 1967. The laminar organization of dorsal horn and effects of descending impulses. *Journal of Physiology* 188: 403–423.

Weissman, A. 1965. Effects of anticonvulsive drugs on electroconvulsive shock-induced retrograde amnesia. *Archives Internationales de Pharmacodynamie et de Therapie* 154: 122–130.

Werner, H. 1935. Studies on contour I qualitative analysis. *American Journal of Psychology* 47: 40–64.

White, Jr., L. E. 1965. Olfactory bulb projections of the rat. *Anatomical Record* 152: 465–480.

Whitten, W. K. 1966. Pheromones and mammalian reproduction. *Advances in Reproductive Physiology* 1: 155–177.

Wickelgren, B. G. 1967a. Habituation of spinal motoneurons. *Journal of Neurophysiology* 30: 1404–1423.

Wickelgren, B. G. 1967b. Habituation of spinal interneurons. *Journal of Neurophysiology* 30: 1424–1438.

Willey, T. J. 1969. Effects of long-term electrical stimulation of the lateral olfactory tract on olfactory bulb and cortex. Unpublished Ph.D. dissertation, University of California, Berkeley.

Yamamoto, C. 1961. Olfactory bulb potentials to electrical stimulation of the olfactory mucosa. *Japanese Journal of Physiology* 11: 545–554.

Yamamoto, C., Yamamoto, T., and Iwama, K. 1963. The inhibitory systems in the olfactory bulb studied by intracellular recording. *Journal of Neurophysiology* 26: 403–415.

Young, J. Z. 1966. *Memory Systems of the Brain*. Berkeley: University of California Press.

Zornetzer, S. F., and McGaugh, J. L. 1970. Effects of frontal brain electroshock stimulation on EEG activity and memory in rats: Relationship to ECS-produced retrograde amnesia. *Journal of Neurobiology* 1: 379–394.

39

Brain Activation and Memory Consolidation

VINCENT BLOCH

ABSTRACT The sensory encoding of information is followed by a perseveration of brain activity which is indispensable for the storage of this information. While we do not know the exact nature of the processing mechanism, we can demonstrate in the rat that the condition for efficient processing is an intensification of cerebral function. Immediately after the encoding, in the few minutes known as the consolidation time, artificial brain activation provoked by electrical stimulation of the reticular formation facilitates the retention of information. On the other hand, learning sessions with no electrical reticular stimulation are always followed in the subsequent spontaneous sleep by an increase in the amount of time spent in paradoxical sleep, the main characteristic of which is brain activation. This increase is correlated with the degree of learning achieved, being maximal while learning is progressing and diminishing when the memory trace is stabilized. This increase of paradoxical sleep disappears when reticular stimulation is given during the consolidation time, suggesting that the brain activation provided by reticular stimulation fulfills the need for processing. In both cases we suspect that a massive neuronal output from the reticular activating system facilitates the formation of the spatiotemporal configurations of neuronal activity.

Contemporary research has focused on the chronology of the events that lie between the sensory encoding (registration) and the retrieval of information. It appears that the memory trace is not built up instantaneously. On the contrary, storage requires information processing, which can demand a rather long time.

At the beginning of the century, Müller and Pilzecker (1900) suggested that the nervous activity triggered by a perception did not stop immediately, and that this perseveration of the activity was indispensable for the consolidation of new information. As a consequence, any other activity that occurred during this phase, and that disturbed the continuing brain activity, would prevent retention. This hypothesis was supported by a large body of experimental work, starting with Duncan (1949), which provided much evidence that any agent that disrupts brain functioning prevents memory fixation when it is delivered shortly after the learning session. However, even though we know that something important goes on in the brain starting immediately after the registration of information, we still have little idea of the

VINCENT BLOCH, Université de Paris-Sud, and Laboratoire de Physiologie Nerveuse, Département de Psychophysiologie, CNRS, Gif-sur-Yvette, France

nature of this process (see Bloch, 1970). Nevertheless, we do know that in the rat this process normally takes place during more than one relatively short period and that these periods can occur either during wakefulness or during sleep; we know also that a major condition for the efficiency of the processing is brain arousal.

The first period of processing is known as the phase of memory consolidation, but it would be better named the phase of information processing because the word "consolidation" implies some sort of a priming mechanism acting on an already established trace (Bloch, 1970). Many data demonstrate that processing is not completed at the end of the "consolidation" phase, and we shall see later that there exists a subsequent period of processing, occurring in paradoxical sleep, which also seems necessary for the efficient storage of long-term memory. I hope to demonstrate that the important factor seems to be that these two phases are dependent upon some sort of brain activation, either artificially enchanced by reticular stimulation during wakefulness or naturally present in paradoxical sleep.

39.1 THE EFFECT OF RETICULAR STIMULATION ON CONSOLIDATION

On the basis of a large body of data, we know that storage of new information requires a high level of arousal. The possibility of acquisition of information during sleep has never been supported by scientific evidence. In the few cases where positive results have been obtained, it has been shown later, when the level of vigilance has been monitored, that the stimuli were delivered during a short period of arousal, or that they provoked arousal themselves. During wakefulness, Lehmann and Koukkou (1974) have found in man that significantly higher and longer EEG activation is provoked by the presentation of sentences when learning is successful than when it is not. This indicates a systematic relationship between the level of EEG activation after presentation of the material and the degree of subsequent retention. Along the same lines, it is well known that emotional arousal increases the probability of memory fixation. Finally, we know from animal work on consolidation time that drugs such as barbiturates inhibit consolidation, while excitatory drugs facilitate it. For example, Rabe and Gerard (1959) showed that in rats which have received an injection of barbiturates, electroshock still interferes with retention when given over an hour after learning, but it has no effect after the same delay in uninjected animals. On the other hand, drugs which have excitatory properties, such as strychnine, picrotoxin, nicotine, amphetamine, etc., seem to shorten the consolidation period, as has been shown principally in McGaugh's laboratory (see McGaugh, 1973).

If memory consolidation depends upon the intensification of a cerebral process, we may assume that this process is partly subject to the activity of the mesencephalic reticular system. If this holds true, it seems most likely that drugs which lengthen or shorten the consolidation period do so by acting on the reticular system. However, we cannot determine the exact moment at which such drugs start to take effect, and we cannot rule out the possibility of long-lasting effects. For these reasons, we have tried in our laboratory, since 1965, to influence the level of cerebral excitability more directly by means of electrical stimulation of the reticular formation delivered exclusively during the consolidation period, i.e., immediately after information registration and until the time when the effects of agents that perturb cerebral functioning are known to decrease. In our experiments, which use a fast-acting anesthetic, fluothane, as the interrupting agent for consolidation, this time is about one or two minutes. This value was found in rats for various learning tasks involving positive or negative reinforcement and multitrial or one-trial procedures. For this reason, we use a 90-sec reticular stimulation delivered immediately after the trial. Since we want to bring about very small changes in observable activity, we have had to use extremely weak electrical stimulation. We have also had to choose learning tasks in which the reinforcing agent itself does not lead to an abrupt increase in the arousal level.

We have met the first condition by using a sine-wave stimulus, 300 Hz, for 90 sec, interrupted for 3 sec every 6 sec. This is done in order to avoid cortical habituation to long-lasting arousing stimuli, which involves a bulbar negative feedback demonstrated previously in cats (Bonvallet and Bloch, 1961). The value of the stimulus is determined individually for each animal by preliminary cortical and behavioral measurement of arousal thresholds, based on psychophysical methods. We take the average of these two values and use in the experiment a value 10 percent below this average. Under these conditions the stimulus is extremely weak, with a mean value of 5 μA, and has no overt effect.

To meet the second condition we have always used either learning tasks based on negative reinforcements of low emotional value (Denti, 1965; Bloch, Denti, and Schmaltz, 1966) or, more often, on positive reinforcement (Bloch and Deweer, 1968).

Under these conditions we have demonstrated that posttrial reticular stimulation considerably enhances retention in several different situations:

1. one-trial discrimination learning (Figure 39.1), in which one posttrial stimulation facilitates retention as measured by tests one or five days later (Bloch, Deweer, and Hennevin, 1970; Leconte, Deweer, and Bloch, 1969);

2. multitrial avoidance learning (Bloch, Denti, and Schmaltz, 1966);

3. positively reinforced learning of a T maze or multichoice maze (unpublished);

4. extinction of a Skinnerian conditioning, which, like learning, requires a consolidation period.

In the last case posttrial reticular stimulation accelerated extinction, while fluothane anesthesia given 90 sec after the trial slowed extinction (Deweer, 1970).

In addition, stimulation that precedes fluothane annuls the effect of the anesthetic (Bloch, Deweer, and Hennevin, 1970). This is not due to an increase in the resistance of the brain to the anesthetic, since if a delay is introduced between the end of the stimulation and the anesthetization, the stimulation is still able to annul the subsequent effect of the fluothane. Thus reticular

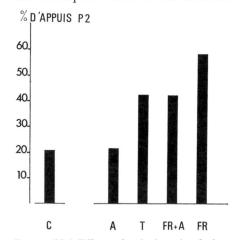

FIGURE 39.1 Effects of reticular stimulation on consolidation of a one-trial learning task (positive reinforcement). Performance on a retention test after 24 hr, as shown by % presses ("appuis") on P2, the reinforced pedal. C: no training. T: control group, one-trial learning. A: fluothane anesthesia 90 sec after the trial (no evidence of memory; compare with C). FR + A: reticular stimulation for 90 sec, then anesthesia (the stimulation annuls the effect of fluothane; compare with T). FR: reticular stimulation alone for 90 sec (consolidation is enhanced). From Bloch, Deweer, and Hennevin (1970).

stimulation abolishes the retrograde amnesia by annulling the effect of an agent that normally prevents consolidation.

Thus a very weak reticular stimulation, even when it is applied only once, enhances the amount of information memorized and shortens the duration of consolidation.

This facilitation of memory fixation is not greater when the stimulation is prolonged beyond 90 sec, and the effect of the stimulation is lowered when it is delayed and begins 90 sec after the trial. Thus reticular arousal exerts its effect on a mechanism which is relatively well delimited in time and which under our experimental conditions is active during the period of maximum lability of the memory trace. In contrast, reticular stimulation (with the same parameters as are used in consolidation experiments) has no effect on performance when it is applied during retrieval (Granger and Bloch, unpublished data).

Several hypotheses, not mutually exclusive, can be made to explain the nature of the consolidation phase and the facilitation of its mechanisms by reticular stimulation. We could assume a consolidation process in the sense of a priming mechanism and propose that reticular arousal, by increasing brain metabolism, stabilizes an already established trace at the level of synaptic organization or at the molecular level. Such a view would be close to principles of the reinforcement theory, and Hebb (1972) has pointed out the similarities between the notions of consolidation and reinforcement.

But it is unlikely that reticular stimulation has a rewarding effect, since we were unable to obtain self-stimulation at the same electrode site in the mesencephalic tegmentum (Bloch, Denti, and Schmaltz, 1966). Moreover, we compared the self-stimulation rates in these animals with the rates in animals with electrodes implanted in the medial forebrain bundle, which is known to give a high rate of self-stimulation. The rate for the hypothalamic rats was 3,700 bar presses per hour, while that for the reticular rats was only 5.3. In addition, if one increases the current strength of the reticular stimulation, it becomes definitely aversive. Finally, we have recently seen that the effect of reticular stimulation on consolidation is equally efficient, if it is applied at the end of the trial, whether or not the animal is rewarded during the stimulation. Thus the beneficial effect of induced brain arousal upon retention seems to be relatively independent of motivational factors.

The question now has to be raised whether the reticular stimulation exerts its effect through a nonspecific arousal involving the whole brain or through a specific activation of some localized circuit involved in information processing.

In this context we naturally think first of the hippocampus. Posttrial hippocampal stimulation has been reported to facilitate retention (Stein and Chorover, 1968; Erickson and Patel, 1969; Landfield, Tusa, and McGaugh, 1973; Destrade and Cardo, 1974). It should be noted that Destrade and Cardo have obtained maximum facilitative effects upon retention with durations of stimulation very similar to ours.

In the hippocampal model proposed by Vinogrodova (1970), "when a stimulus which is not registered in the memory system appears, the inhibitory control (exerted on reticular formation) occurs and the process of registration starts. . . . Thus the hippocampus plays a double role, comparing the signals, and blocking or unblocking the reticular activating mechanisms which are necessary for registration of information on the basis of such comparison" (i.e., of novel versus familiar signals). Thus we could say that reticular stimulation overrides the tonic inhibitory influence exerted by the hippocampus and especially by the "identity-detector" neurons, and that direct hippocampal stimulation either facilitates the function of "novelty detectors" or, on the contrary, disrupts the organization of the inhibitory circuit.

Future research will say more about the relationship between hippocampus and reticular formation in memory consolidation, but it is also possible to make another assumption: any stimulation that arouses the brain can increase the temporal coherence of activity patterns in cooperative neuronal ensembles which, according to John (1972), involve the linking together of such groupings in different brain areas.

All the evidence discussed above shows that there is a relatively well defined period of "consolidation" and that this process depends upon brain activation. But the evidence does not show that information processing is completed during this period. On the contrary, the so-called consolidation cannot be considered as some definitive fixation of an already established trace. Rusinov (1962) and Albert (1966) have shown that cathodal polarization of the cortical surface can be used to interrupt the consolidation phase, and Albert has claimed to be able to reactivate the trace using anodal polarization. Moreover, after the interruption of the consolidation phase, McGaugh (1967) was able to reactivate the trace by injection of strychnine. Thus we must consider the first phase of consolidation as the critical period of information processing, but we must realize that the processing probably remains active for a long period of time. We shall see in the next section that a second critical phase of this processing seems to occur during sleep—more exactly, during paradoxical sleep—in which another type of brain arousal occurs.

39.2 MEMORY CONSOLIDATION AND PARADOXICAL SLEEP

The beneficial effect of sleep upon the retention of information acquired during wakefulness was shown long ago, in man, by experimental psychologists (Jenkins and Dallenbach, 1924; Van Ormer, 1932). Two hypotheses have been proposed: The "passive" hypothesis is that sleep prevents activities that interfere with memory. The "active" hypothesis is that during sleep there is some sort of consolidation mechanism at work or some kind of information processing. When paradoxical sleep (PS) was discovered, the "active" hypothesis was reinforced because of the considerable brain activity recorded during this phase, the increase in cerebral blood flow, and the intense activity of cortical and reticular cells, all of which point to the existence of an active functional process. In addition, the sensory isolation during this sleep—isolation revealed by very high thresholds—would suggest that any processing during this phase must involve information that has been previously registered during wakefulness. Also, the fact that the amount of PS is greater during early life, which is a critical time for basic learning, reinforces the hypothesis of a relationship between memory and information processing during PS.

Several attempts have been made to see whether selective deprivation of PS would impair retention. Leconte and Bloch (1970) have shown that 48 hr of selective deprivation of paradoxical sleep in the rat produces a retention deficit without affecting subsequent relearning. Pearlman and Greenberg (1973) have presented evidence that only 2 hr of paradoxical-sleep deprivation is sufficient to produce a retention deficit. By combining procedures of interruption of consolidation and sleep deprivation, Fishbein, McGaugh, and Swarz (1971) found that in animals deprived of paradoxical sleep during 2 days after learning, subsequent electroshock was still able to produce disruption in consolidation, showing that in this case the length of the consolidation period is extended from several minutes to several days. Wolfowitz and Holdstock (1971), who obtained similar results, suggested that the memory trace is maintained in a labile form during sleep deprivation and is only consolidated when the effects of deprivation are over.

If PS has a functional role in the process of fixation of the memory trace, it seems likely that there should be an increase of PS after learning. In fact, we have accumulated, in our laboratory, considerable evidence showing that different types of learning produce an increase in the amount of PS during the period of sleep following the training period. Lucero (1970) was the first investigator to publish data about an augmentation of PS following learning. He trained rats in a maze and demonstrated a

significant increase in PS, with respect to controls, during the 3 hr immediately after learning. At the same time, in our laboratory, we performed several studies investigating the PS-augmentation phenomenon in rats (Leconte and Hennevin, 1971, 1973; Bloch, 1973; Hennevin, Leconte, and Bloch, 1974; Leconte, Hennevin, and Bloch, 1973, 1974). These studies were primarily centered on the relationship between the level of acquisition in several different tasks and the subsequent time spent in PS. We showed that in the course of distributed learning, each learning session is followed by an immediate and short-term augmentation of PS (Figure 39.2). What is most interesting is that the increase of PS is related to the degree of learning achieved, but when performance reaches the asymptote of the learning curve, the time spent in PS returns to the reference level. On the other hand, slow-wave sleep is unaffected throughout the experiment. We also found that if the animals face a new situation, such as a stimulus differentiation, this new task is followed by a new increase of PS (Fig. 39.3). Finally, when no learning occurs, as in a group of "poor learners," there is no PS augmentation.

Furthermore, the augmentation appears to be a function of the increase in the number of PS phases, whereas the average duration of each PS phase remains invariable. This finding suggested to us that a PS trigger mechanism (or mechanisms) had been primed by the learning, and that the trigger is much more likely to be tripped

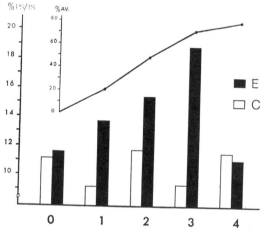

FIGURE 39.2 Paradoxical-sleep augmentation after learning. Ratio of paradoxical sleep to total sleep (% PS/TS) during a 3-hr recording period after each daily block of trials in avoidance conditioning (conditioning, black columns, group E; pseudoconditioning, white columns, group C). Column marked 0 shows the PS/TS ratio before treatment. The learning curve for group E is shown above the histogram. Note the gradual increase in PS ratio in relation to the level of learning and the return to the prelearning level when the learning "plateau" is reached. From Leconte, Hennevin, and Bloch (1973). Reproduced with the permission of ASP Biological and Medical Press (Elsevier division).

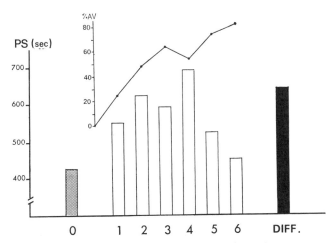

FIGURE 39.3 Paradoxical-sleep augmentation after a complication of the learning task. PS duration during a 3-hr recording period after each daily learning session. 0: PS duration before treatment. The learning curve is shown above the histogram. DIFF.: differentiation experiment with the presentation of two tones, one being the CS. Note the immediate increase of PS, which had returned to the reference level.

during sleep. We were able to see this augmentation phenomenon for a wide variety of learning tasks, such as avoidance learning with massed or distributed practice, bar pressing for water, maze learning, and even extinction.

Some of these findings have been replicated by Smith et al. (1974) in their study with mice trained in a multiple-trial discrimination task. They have also found that the PS-augmentation phenomenon dissipates as the learning curve approaches its asymptote.

It is also interesting that the PS augmentation appears to be instantaneous, counting either from sleep onset or from the first phase of PS. This characteristic is a relative phenomenon, since we have found that we can artificially delay sleep onset by 90 min without altering the augmentation effect or producing a learning deficit, but if we delay sleep onset for 3 hr, the acquisition of the learned response is impaired, and PS augmentation is not observed (Leconte and Hennevin, 1973).

Regarding the useful duration of PS augmentation, 90 min of free sleep following each learning session appears to be sufficient for good retention to occur, but 30 min of free sleep during which PS increase is not observed does not allow the learned material to be established in long-term memory. Sixty minutes of free sleep, with PS increase, only slightly disturbs the learning curve (Leconte, Hennevin, and Bloch, 1974). Therefore, the period consecutive to learning during which time the integrity of sleep seems necessary is, in rats, between 60 and 90 min. It would thus appear that one of the essential elements of memory fixation is the presence of PS, in sufficient quantity, occurring quickly after learning.

So it seems that PS does play a role in information processing, particularly while learning is in progress and diminishing when the memory trace is stabilized. Furthermore, the amplitude of PS augmentation seems to reflect variations in the degree of difficulty of the different steps of memorization. Thus this phenomenon does not reflect some sort of a consolidation of an already established trace, but seems to be linked with the elaboration of this trace. This is very similar to the conclusion we made when we discussed the nature of the consolidation phase in wakefulness.

In addition, we have emphasized that this is not the only consolidation phase, though it might be a critical period of a process that can be periodically reactivated. Similarly, the PS-augmentation process may not be limited only to the short period of time immediately following learning, but may continue for a prolonged period of time. In support of this idea, Smith et al. (1974) and Fishbein, Kastaniotis, and Chattman (1974) have observed that learning in mice induces, in addition to the immediate PS augmentation, a small but protracted augmentation of PS time lasting 24 hr.

From our point of view, it is possible that the information processing necessary for memory storage encompasses a period starting in wakefulness, during the so-called consolidation phase, and continuing during the first episodes of PS as well as subsequent episodes. The important factor appears to be that these phases are dependent upon some sort of brain activation, either enhanced by reticular stimulation during wakefulness or naturally present in PS.

We shall give direct evidence for the relationship between these two phenomena in the next section.

39.3 THE RELATIONSHIP BETWEEN MEMORY CONSOLIDATION IN WAKEFULNESS AND IN PARADOXICAL SLEEP

The phase of memory consolidation occurring immediately after learning and the phenomenon of PS augmentation in the subsequent period of sleep are both very susceptible to experimental perturbation; the suppression of one or the other either prevents or perturbs the fixation of information. Both are dependent upon brain arousal, since the first can be facilitated by reticular stimulation and the second occurs in a state that is characterized by reticular and cortical activation.

In order to investigate this similarity, and to see if there is an interaction between these two events, we have recently performed the following experiment (Bloch, Hennevin, and Leconte, 1975): In a maze-learning experiment with one trial a day, two groups of rats were compared. The first group received the usual postrial 5-μA reticular stimulation (see Section 39.1), and the other received no stimulation. The animals of both groups were returned to their home cages after each trial, and the sleep phases were monitored for 3 hr. The records were compared with reference values for the duration of slow-wave sleep, paradoxical sleep, and total sleep obtained previously under the same conditions. The nonstimulated group showed the PS augmentation after each trial, with the maximum amplitude just before the asymptote of the learning curve (Fig 39.4). But in the stimulated group, in which performance was slightly enhanced by reticular stimulation, there was no PS augmentation (with the exception of a small increase just after the trial preceding the asymptote).

Thereafter, both groups were trained in a new task involving another configuration of gates in the maze, with no reticular stimulation after the trials. Under these conditions PS augmentation was present with the same amplitude in both groups after the trial. Thus it must in fact have been the reticular stimulation which in the first experiment prevented the PS-augmentation phenomenon. An important point is that reticular stimulation alone produced no modification of PS in the subsequent sleep episode. Therefore, it seems that some part of the need for arousal in the processing of new information is fulfilled by reticular stimulation immediately after registration, so that a supplementary PS period is no longer necessary in the subsequent sleep. The latter data also reinforce the idea that information processing is triggered after registration and continues during sleep in the periods when the necessary brain activation normally occurs.

While we think that the information-processing hypothesis accounts for our observations, it is also possible that paradoxical sleep is not directly implicated in the process of memorization, and that its increase is a consequence of the memory process rather than its cause. Moruzzi (1966) has suggested that one function of sleep could possibly be to restore the activity of the neurons implicated in learning. When we consider the special case of paradoxical sleep, we might assume that the high metabolic rate characteristic of this state is correlated with a high level of chemical synthesis. Therefore, as we have discussed elsewhere (Bloch, 1973), it could be assumed that the amount of paradoxical sleep increases as a function of the neuronal material utilized, during wakefulness, in the memorizing process.

Stern and Morgane (1974) have hypothesized that the function of PS is to maintain catecholamine availability in the central nervous system. Normal periodic PS would allow recovery from the "synaptic fatigue" produced by waking activity, and PS augmentation would be triggered by a supplementary decreased availability

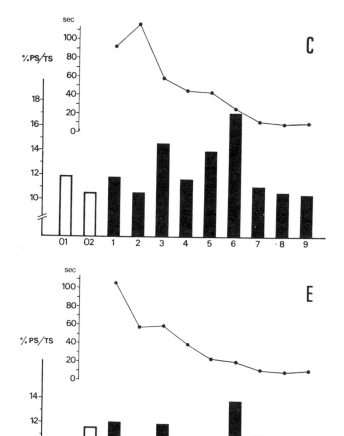

FIGURE 39.4 Suppression of PS augmentation after learning by posttrial reticular stimulation. The PS ratio is shown for a 3-hr recording period after each daily trial in a maze-learning task. 01, 02: PS ratios before treatment. The learning curves (time) are shown above the histograms. C: control group, with no reticular stimulation. E: experimental group, which receives posttrial reticular stimulation. Note the almost total suppression of PS augmentation in E.

of free catecholamine induced by learning activity. However, in order to account for the effect of PS deprivation—which acts, as we have shown, not on the acquisition but on the consolidation of memory—we are obliged to assume that PS does not serve only a repair function. Moreover, in the present state of our knowledge, it would be difficult to understand why reticular stimulation, which probably activates noradrenergic ascending pathways, would suppress a restorative function of catecholamines. On the contrary, if we assume that reticular stimulation facilitates some neurophysiological events that are normally replayed during PS, we could understand that this stimulation suppresses the PS augmentation.

It has been argued, notably by John (1972), that the

essential event taking place during learning is the elaboration and occurrence of spatiotemporal configurations of neuronal activity characterizing large populations of neurons ("memory readout"). The time span for the occurrence of such patterns is compatible with the time span of a few minutes that characterizes the early phase of consolidation. These dynamic patterns could possibly be reactivated by the neuronal bombardment originating from the reticular formation during PS, with a consequent increase in their coherence. Following a similar argument, Feinberg and Evarts (1969) have emphasized the fact that the high level of temporal organization of reticular activation during PS suggests a functional role for this type of activity.

Thus it appears that the occurrence of a memory trace for a particular event implies a long and continuous process with some critical periods. Immediately after the period of acquisition, the information is processed during a relatively short period that has become known as the phase of consolidation. This processing continues during the first episode of PS and may also be present in subsequent ones. These events might be related in a hierarchical manner such that the PS augmentation is dependent upon the rate of consolidation of the memory trace during wakefulness. We know that experimental enhancement of memory consolidation during wakefulness suppresses the PS augmentation during subsequent sleep. But this does not imply that the mechanisms of PS constitute a part of the memory mechanism. Rather, it means that PS plays an important role in the *conditions* that serve to enhance and help maintain the soundness of a memory trace. These conditions seem to depend upon brain activation.

REFERENCES

ALBERT, D. J. 1966. The effects of polarizing currents on the consolidation of learning. *Neuropsychologia* 4: 65–77.

BLOCH, V. 1970. Facts and hypotheses concerning memory consolidation processes. *Brain Research* 24: 561–575.

BLOCH, V. 1973. L'activation cérébrale et al fixation mnésique. *Archives Italiennes de Biologie* 111: 577–590.

BLOCH, V., DENTI, A., and SCHMALTZ, G. 1966. Effets de la stimulation réticulaire sur la phase de consolidation de la trace mnésique. *Journal de Physiologie* 58: 469–470.

BLOCH, V., and DEWEER, B. 1968. Role accélérateur de la stimulation réticulaire sur la phase de consolidation d'un apprentissage en un seul essai. *Comptes Rendus de l'Académie des Sciences (Paris)* 266D: 384–387.

BLOCH, V., DEWEER, B., and HENNEVIN, E. 1970. Suppression de l'amnésie rétrograde et consolidation d'un apprentissage à essai unique par stimulation réticulaire. *Physiology and Behavior* 5: 1235–1241.

BLOCH, V., HENNEVIN, E., and LECONTE, P. 1975. Post-trial reticular stimulation effect on paradoxical sleep augmentation following learning in the rat. Paper read at the Second International Congress of Sleep Research, Edinburgh.

BONVALLET, M., and BLOCH, V. 1961. Bulbar control of cortical arousal. *Science* 133: 1133–1134.

DENTI, A. 1965. Facilitation d'un conditionnement par stimulation réticulaire lors de la phase de fixation mnésique. Thèse d'Université, Paris.

DESTRADE, C., and CARDO, B. 1974. Effects of post-trial hippocampal stimulation on time-dependent improvement of performance in mice. *Brain Research* 78: 447–454.

DEWEER, B. 1970. Accélération de l'extinction d'un conditionnement par stimulation réticulaire chez le rat. *Journal de Physiologie* 62: 270–271.

DUNCAN, C. P. 1949. The retroactive effect of electroschock on learning. *Journal of Comparative and Physiological Psychology* 42: 32–44.

ERICKSON, C., and PATEL, J. B. 1969. Facilitation of avoidance learning by post-trial hippocampal electrical stimulation. *Journal of Comparative and Physiological Psychology* 68: 400–406.

FEINBERG, I., and EVARTS, E. 1969. Changing concepts of the function of sleep: Discovery of intense brain activity during sleep calls for revision of hypothesis as to its function. *Biological Psychiatry* 1: 331–348.

FISHBEIN, W., KASTANIOTIS, C., and CHATTMAN, D. 1974. Paradoxical sleep: Prolonged augmentation following learning. *Brain Research* 76: 61–75

FISHBEIN, W., McGAUGH, J. L. and SWARZ, J. R. 1971. Retrograde amnesia: Electroconvulsive shock effects after termination of rapid eye movement sleep deprivation. *Science* 172: 80–82.

HEBB, D. O. 1972. *Textbook of Psychology*. Philadelphia, Pa.: W. B. Saunders.

HENNEVIN, E., LECONTE, P., and BLOCH, V. 1974. Augmentation du sommeil paradoxal provoquée par l'acquisition, l'extinction et la réacquisition d'un apprentissage à renforcement positif. *Brain Research* 70: 43–54.

JENKINS, J., and DALLENBACH, K. 1924. Obliviscence during sleep and waking. *American Journal of Psychology* 35: 605–612.

JOHN, E. R. 1972. Switchboard versus statistical theories of learning and memory. *Science* 177: 850–864.

LANDFIELD, P. W., TUSA, R., and McGAUGH, J. L. 1973. Effects of post-trial hippocampal stimulation on memory storage and EEG activity. *Behavioral Biology* 8: 485–505.

LECONTE, P., and BLOCH, V. 1970. Déficit de la rétention d'un conditionnement après privation de sommeil paradoxal chez le rat. *Comptes Rendus de l'Académie des Sciences (Paris)* 271D: 226–229.

LECONTE, P., DEWEER, B., and BLOCH, V. 1969. Consolidation et conservation de la trace mnésique: Effets respectifs de la stimulation réticulaire. *Journal de Physiologie* 61: 334–335.

LECONTE, P., and HENNEVIN, E. 1971. Augmentation de la durée du sommeil paradoxal consécutive à un apprentissage chez le rat. *Comptes Rendus de l'Académie des Sciences (Paris)* 273D: 86–88.

LECONTE, P., and HENNEVIN, E. 1973. Caractéristiques temporelles de l'augmentation de sommeil paradoxal consécutif à l'apprentissage chez le rat. *Physiology and Behavior* 11: 677–686.

LECONTE, P., HENNEVIN, E., and BLOCH, V. 1973. Analyse des effets d'un apprentissage et de son niveau d'acquisition sur le sommeil paradoxal consécutif. *Brain Research* 49: 367–379.

LECONTE, P., HENNEVIN, E., and BLOCH, V. 1974. Duration of paradoxical sleep necessary for the acquisition of conditioned avoidance in the rat. *Physiology and Behavior* 13: 675–681.

LEHMANN, D., and KOUKKOU, M. 1974. Computer analysis of

EEG wakefulness-sleep patterns during learning of novel and familiar sentences. *Electroencephalography and Clinical Neurophysiology* 37: 73–84.

LUCERO, M. 1970. Lengthening of REM sleep duration consecutive to learning in the rat. *Brain Research* 20: 319–322.

MCGAUGH, J. L. 1967. A multi-trace view of memory storage processes. Communication, International Symposium of Recent Advances in Learning and Retention, Rome.

MCGAUGH, J. L. 1973. Drug facilitation of learning and memory. *Annual Review of Pharmacology* 13: 229–241.

MORUZZI, G. 1966. The functional significance of sleep with particular regard to the brain mechanisms underlying consciousness. In J. C. Eccles, ed., *Brain and Conscious Experience*. New York: Springer-Verlag, pp. 345–388.

MÜLLER, G. E., and PILZECKER, A. 1900. Experimentelle Beiträge zur Lehre von Gedächtnis. *Zeitschrift für Psychologie und Physiologie der Sinnesorgane* 1: 1–300.

PEARLMAN, J. R., and GREENBERG, R. 1973. Post-trial REM sleep: A critical period for consolidation of shuttlebox avoidance. *Animal Learning and Behavior* 1: 49–51.

RABE, A., and GERARD, W. 1959. The influence of drugs on memory fixation time. *American Psychologist* 14: 423.

RUSINOV, V. S. 1962. Electrophysiological studies during the formation of a temporary connection. *Proceedings of the 22nd International Congress, Union of Physiological Sciences* 1: 882–887.

SMITH, C., KITAHAMA, K., VALATX, J. L., and JOUVET, M. 1974. Increased paradoxical sleep in mice during acquisition of a shock avoidance task. *Brain Research* 77: 221–230.

STEIN, D. G., and CHOROVER, S. L. 1968. Effects of post-trial electrical stimulation of hippocampus and caudate nucleus on maze learning in the rat. *Physiology and Behavior* 3: 781–791.

STERN, W. C., and MORGANE, P. J. 1974. Theoretical view of REM sleep function: Maintenance of catecholamine systems in the central nervous system. *Behavioral Biology* 11: 1–32.

VAN ORMER, G. B. 1932. Retention after intervals of sleep and waking. *Archives of Psychology* 21, No. 137.

VINOGRADOVA, O. S. 1970. Registration of information and the limbic system. In G. Horn and R. A. Hinde, eds., *Short-Term Changes in Neuronal Activity and Behaviour*. London: Cambridge University Press, pp. 95–140.

WOLFOWITZ, B. E., and HOLDSTOCK, T. L. 1971. Paradoxical sleep deprivation and memory in rats. *Communications in Behavioral Biology* 6: 281–284.

Conference Summary

40
Conference Summary

MARK R. ROSENZWEIG

Can we use some of the varied advice we have received during the conference to help us remember the material of the conference itself? If we consider the findings on paradoxical sleep presented by the last participant, Vincent Bloch, perhaps a good sleep would be advisable at this time. On the other hand, some of the psychologists of learning tell us that repetition is the best way to guarantee memory. Perhaps what we should do now is read rapidly through the abstracts at the head of each chapter. But considering that procedure reminds me of something that happened recently to a student on our campus. Having worked hard—perhaps a little too hard—right down to the end of the quarter the student was asked by his professor on the last day of class to describe the difference between ignorance and apathy. He drawled back, "I don't know and I don't care."

Other investigators assure us that memory is favored when material is processed, when it is grouped into easily recognized chunks. It might be useful, therefore, to identify some of the main themes—some explicit and some implicit—that have occurred in several of the papers. Some of these were stated in similar or complementary form by several participants; others proved to be topics of divergence or even dissension. Let us review, then, several of these themes of the conference, noting some of the progress, some of the problems, and some of the prospects in this area.

40.1 PERSISTENCE AND CHANGE IN PROBLEMS AND APPROACHES

40.1.1 Early research: The golden decade

Paul Rozin started the conference by pointing out some enduring themes that arose during what he called the Golden Decade of memory research, beginning in 1882. The first contribution he mentioned was Ribot's book on the *Diseases of Memory*; then came Hughling Jackson's concept of levels of function of the nervous system and behavioral hierarchies in 1884; then Ebbinghaus's important work, the first experimental measurements of memory in 1885; then Korsakoff's paper in 1889; and the decade ended with William James's great book, the

Mark R. Rosenzweig, Department of Psychology, University of California, Berkeley

Principles of Psychology (1890), with its important chapters on memory.

That was a Golden Decade, but it seems to me that the next decade was almost equally fruitful. In the 1890s and the first years of the present century, investigators started to bear down upon problems of learning and memory, to find how to work on some of the principles that had been enunciated and how to attack them experimentally. Right at the beginning of that next decade, in 1891, there was the enunciation of the neuron doctrine, which had been proved by Ramón y Cajal's work. Just two years later, Tanzi, an Italian neurologist, pointed out that the plastic changes involved in learning would very likely be found at the junctions between neurons. These junctions didn't even have a name yet, but a little later in that same decade, Sherrington, in his chapter in Foster's *Neurophysiology* (1887), gave them the name "synapse." Sherrington also stated that the synapse was likely to be strategic for learning. He put it in this picturesque way:

Shut off from all opportunity of reproducing itself and adding to its number by mitosis or otherwise, the nerve cell directs its pent-up energy towards amplifying its connections with its fellows, in response to the events which stir it up. Hence, it is capable of an education unknown to other tissues. (p. 1117)

Concerning the experimental attack on learning, 1898 was the date of Thorndike's important work on animal learning, to be followed shortly, but quite independently, by Pavlov's work on conditioning. In 1900 Müller and Pilzecker published an important book on studies on verbal memory, following up Ebbinghaus's work. In the course of that book they put forward what they called the "perseveration-consolidation hypothesis," which has engendered so much work since then. That is, they suggested that once activity was started up in the nervous system, it boiled around for awhile, perseverated, and this led to the consolidation of a stable memory trace. In reviewing that book the next year, William McDougall pointed out that this hypothesis might very well account for retrograde amnesia following a blow to the head; the blow would prevent the information from circulating and so prevent consolidation from taking place. McDougall commented on how important this book was from the point of view of human verbal learning and also for possible insights about what happens in the nervous system during learning. In fact, McDougall felt it was unfortunate that Müller and Pilzecker didn't spend more of their time on the neural events; their ideas were so good that they should have pushed ahead further and wrapped up the question of neural events during learning. With hindsight, we can see that McDougall, like Tanzi, was expecting things to happen too rapidly.

At the end of the Silver Decade of memory research, in 1902, Shepard I. Franz put out an important article in which he brought together two techniques: the new technique, learned from Thorndike, of training animals, and the technique of making experimental brain lesions. His procedure allowed him to study the effects on learning and memory of interfering with brain processes. That, of course, set the stage for all of the interesting studies presented at this conference on the effects of manipulation of the central nervous system on learning and memory—not only the varied effects of brain lesions that Robert Isaacson reviewed and that Gary Lynch discussed, but also the striking effects of drugs presented by James Flood and Murray Jarvik and by David Quartermain, and the noteworthy effects of electrical stimulation of the brain on memory that James McGaugh and Paul Gold reviewed and that were discussed by Stephan Chorover and Vincent Bloch.

When Paul Rozin reviewed his Golden Decade, he asked what has been accomplished since then, and we can now ask the same question about the twenty-year period that ended in 1902. Rozin found a great increase in detailed knowledge over the succeeding years, but without a corresponding increase in theoretical approaches. But this conference indicates that things have been improving recently. Let us review a few areas in which there has been a great deal of activity, quite a bit of progress, and some new problems. It seems to me that both psychology and neurology, the disciplines that were originally concerned with learning and memory, have really made extensive progress, as reflected in the chapters of our volume. Detailed and powerful methods of experimental psychology and information processing have provided not only descriptions but also penetrating analyses of the processes of learning and memory. Methods have been devised for the study of animal behavior that have also turned out to be helpful in studying human behavior. Consider, for example, the progress made by applying such methods to split-brain patients and to preverbal children. Having developed means to communicate with animals that cannot talk, we can use them to communicate with very young children and find out about their cognitive processes. And, of course, some methods that were elaborated to study human behavior have proved to be extremely effective with animals, as Donald Riley pointed out in his chapter. Also, as Robert Rescorla and Peter Holland have shown, the concepts of learning have been generalized and freed from the restricted definitions that used to hem them in. Nevertheless, it is clear that there are plenty of basic problems that remain at the level of the behavioral analysis of memory.

One of the controversies that was taken up here concerns whether there really are multiple memory stores, as Herbert Simon holds, or whether, as Riley maintains, the duration of memory depends upon the level of processing, there being really only one kind of store. Rozin presented and discussed findings bearing on this issue, pointing out that patients such as H. M. may not be restricted to short-term memory, provided certain cuing techniques are employed. Clearly, this is a critical area for further research.

40.1.2 The entry of new disciplines

New disciplines have joined those that originally shared this area, and this has been a big part of the history of research on learning and memory in the last thirty years or so. Electrophysiology is a prominent example. In the 1940s it looked as though electrophysiological research might provide the key to unlock the secrets of memory. That didn't prove to be correct then, but now we are finding refined techniques of intercellular recording becoming a major tool, as the reports of Davis, of Krasne, of Eisenstein, and of Sokolov have testified. But of course, as some of the contributors have pointed out, on the electrophysiological level, too, there are still basic problems. What is the nature of accommodation? What is really meant by rebound? What is the link between the axon potential and the release of the synaptic transmitter?

Anatomists have also contributed immensely valuable techniques and talents. For one thing, neuroanatomy has become quantitative. Recall the 1959 book of Siegfried Bok, the Dutch neuroanatomist. In the foreword Bok pointed out that just as civilization progressed historically from astrology to astronomy, so he hoped that we would now be advancing from histology to histonomy, and he entitled his book *Histonomy*. Bok didn't receive much attention at that time, but anatomy has been growing more quantitative ever since. I might note, too, that we have had the Psychonomic Society since 1959.

Through the techniques of quantitative neuroanatomy as well as of neurochemistry, it has become clear that training and enriched experience bring about many significant changes in the brain. This was demonstrated in the reviews of William Greenough and Les Rutledge and in Edward Bennett's discussion. Bennett and Greenough showed that simply placing rats for a few days or weeks in differential environments (enriched or impoverished) leads to significant changes in their brains. Among these changes are differences in activities of brain enzymes, amounts of nucleic acids, weights of parts of the brain, and aspects of neural circuitry including branching of dendrites, numbers of dendritic spines, and sizes of synaptic contacts. Other work, too, is showing that the brain is much more plastic anatomically than would have been supposed a dozen years ago. Striking evidence for this plasticity is found in the chapters by Moore, Raisman, and Lynch. They report the sprouting of new neuronal contacts when tracts of brain fibers are cut or when tissue is implanted in the brain. Reports of measurable changes in the brain as a consequence of experience—reports that seemed startling and controversial when we first announced them in the early 1960s—have now been generally accepted. Subsequent reports of neural sprouting and of the formation of new contacts in the brains of even adult animals, while not obtained in learning situations, nevertheless demonstrate capacities for plasticity that may well underlie learning. Moreover, work cited here and research in progress indicate that functional changes in neural connections may occur rapidly enough to encode long-term memories.

Electron microscopy is now finally permitting the sort of work on the synapse that Tanzi called for in 1893. But in this and other attempts to do quantitative neuroanatomy, the detailed work remains prohibitive, and breakthroughs are needed. There have been important recent advances in staining techniques and intracellular dyes, but much staining still remains a "cookbook" affair. (A rather special contribution of electron microscopy has been evidence for the homunculus!—see Rozin's postscript.)

Biochemists have also entered the fray, becoming interested in recent years in learning and memory. They can analyze now for specific materials in very small samples of tissue, in some cases even in single cells. But the chapters of Rose, Hambley, and Haywood, and of Dunn have revealed unsolved problems in the identification and interpretation of the biochemical changes that occur with experience. Some of these problems are caused by the multiplicity of cellular components, and some occur because the grain of the analyses still remains too coarse to identify the specific proteins involved. Edward Bennett suggested in conversation at the conference the attractive analogy that consolidation of long-term memory is something like the development of the new Polaroid color film: a process gets under way and goes through a number of steps, and the picture becomes clearer and clearer, changing colors until eventually it reaches the final state and is fixed for all time. There are several aspects of this analogy that make it attractive: There is, for example, the succession of cordinated chemical steps that is involved, and also the fact that one can trigger these processes immediately after the picture is taken, which is usually the case, or one can prevent this from occurring and have the development take place later on. Flood and Jarvik gave evidence here indicating that there can be a delay in some of the consolidation processes. For example, if certain inhibitors of protein synthesis are given, the consolidation process, or at least certain biochemical processes necessary for long-term memory, can be delayed for up to several hours and nevertheless occur successfully later on. What initiates these processes may well be a chemical trigger, as Adrian Dunn and David Quartermain discussed. Similar concepts, although phrased in terms of arousal or affective state, were offered by James McGaugh and Paul Gold, and by Seymour Kety. But then again, as Rose pointed out, it may be oversimple to think in terms of a linear sequence of biochemical stages that would account for all of the aspects of memory consolidation.

In the reports of Manning, Garcia and Levine, and Rowell, we learned about work of ethologists and zoologists who are determining the place of learning in the life of diverse species of animals. If, as it is sometimes said, there is one best species to study any research problem, then there are millions of species whose behavior needs careful scrutiny. Are there some ethological principles that could help us here? What kinds of ethological niches favor the development of an ability for rapid and powerful learning? On the other hand, are there ethological niches that make learning a dispensable luxury and plasticity unnecessary?

While new disciplines and techniques are brought to bear, older techniques have come under question. Thus Robert Isaacson in his review raised doubts about the value of experimental brain lesions for the study of memory, and Gary Lynch added further criticism of this technique in his discussion. Isaacson concluded "that no type of brain damage yet studied has produced deficits in information-storage mechanisms." This is not to deny that brain lesions cause impairment on tests of memory, but rather to point out that the deficits are likely to reflect processes other than storage of information. Thus some lesions alter perception and thereby interfere with retrieval, while others affect the ability of animals to stop responding to stimuli as they could do preoperatively. Lynch showed that even localized lesions cause widespread biochemical and morphological reactions in the brain, so that changes in behavior may involve quite different regions from those lesioned. In spite of these cautions, such participants as Rozin, Signoret and Lhermitte, and Gazzaniga drew far-reaching conclusions about mechanisms of memory storage from the study of brains damaged by disease or by surgical intervention. Have the results and implications of detailed experimental studies based on animal subjects failed to reach the clinical investigators? Are those who deal with brain-injured human beings less critical than the experimenters with animal subjects? This seems doubtful, especially since researchers such as Gazzaniga and Rozin conduct experimental studies with animals as well as with human subjects. Was the conclusion of Isaacson unduly pessimistic? Unfortunately, the reports on effects of brain damage in human subjects were scheduled for the initial session of the conference, while those on studies of brain lesions in animals came four days later, and a direct confrontation of views was not demanded. The papers of Rozin and Gazzaniga did draw upon animal as well as human data, and Isaacson cited results of some research on human subjects, but although we have cogent reviews and discussions of research in this area, we do not have a full critical evaluation of the two approaches in terms of each other.

With the entry of many disciplines into this field of research, the diversity of preparations being studied has also expanded. Consider the variety of subjects or preparations discussed in the papers of this conference. These range from normal adult human beings (Simon) to cultures of nerve cells (Mandel; Nelson and Christian). Other subjects include human beings with various forms of brain damage or disease (Rozin; Signoret and Lhermitte) and persons in whom the corpus callosum has been severed, creating a split brain (Gazzaniga). Normal mammals are studied under field conditions (Manning; Garcia) and under laboratory conditions (Rescorla; McGaugh and Gold; Flood and Jarvik; Riley; Greenough; Bennett). Mammals with a variety of brain lesions are investigated (Isaacson) and are compared with certain types of brain-lesioned human beings. Invertebrates of many species are being studied for the relative simplicity of their nervous systems (Krasne), and in many cases still further simplification is obtained by working with only portions of the nervous system (Davis; Eisenstein; Sokolov; Strumwasser). Portions of the nervous system are grown in culture and studied in terms of their anatomical development and electrical activity (Seil and Leiman). Extending this scale, or perhaps off in another dimension, are the artificial brains of the neural modelers (Arbib, Kilmer, and Spinelli; Cowan). This is a challenging new approach, even if its applica-

tion to learning is premature, as Arbib and his colleagues suggested; but on the other hand, the reports of Arbib and his colleagues, and of Cowan indicate that this is probably an overmodest evaluation.

40.2 UNITY OR DIVERSITY?

This impressive variety of subjects and neural preparations may reflect in part the determination to sample widely the phenomena of learning and memory throughout the animal kingdom. But beyond the desire for representative sampling, the variety of subjects studied reflects two opposed theoretical approaches. On the one hand, there is the assumption of a basic unity of processes underlying learning and memory. From this point of view, whatever is learned from the study of one kind of preparation will apply to all others, so that the clearest, most readily analyzed example should be the one studied. On the other hand, there is the belief that different basic processes will be found to be responsible for learning and memory in different kinds of animals and that a number of processes probably occur in more complex animals. Several participants in this conference came down strongly on the side of unity and parsimony (Davis; Eisenstein; Gazzaniga; Krasne). Thus Krasne stated, "Indeed, it is entirely possible that the nervous system is highly parsimonious in its use of plastic processes and that but a single kind of persistent and input-inducible functional change in nerve cells underlies all types of learning" (p. 408). The moral for Krasne is to study these processes in invertebrates. Certainly, some discoveries made with invertebrates have later been shown to be true for vertebrates as well. For example, synapses where transmission is electrical rather than chemical were first demonstrated in invertebrates but are now an active subject of research in vertebrates. On a behavioral level, the concept of central programming of motor functions, first worked out with reference to invertebrates, was later found useful for the understanding of mammalian behavior. Perhaps the same route will be followed in the study of learning and memory. But Gazzaniga, although also a proponent of unity, took the opposite point of view: "It is my guess that real insight into the biology of memory can be best obtained at this time by considering clinical and human experimental data" (p. 57). Other participants took issue with the assumption of the unitary nature of learning. For example, recall this statement of Seymour Kety:

I have always been impressed with the prolific diversity of nature, and the unity of memory processes, like the unity of biochemistry, seems to be something of an oversimplification. . . .

So profound and powerful an adaptation as learning

or memory is not apt to rest upon a single modality. Rather, I suspect that advantage is taken of every opportunity provided by evolution. There were forms of memory before organisms developed nervous systems, and after that remarkable leap forward it is likely that every new pathway and neural complexity, every new neurotransmitter, hormone, or metabolic process that played upon the nervous system and subserved a learning process was preserved and incorporated.

Invertebrate learning has much to teach us, especially since it can be studied more rigorously than the processes occurring in the mammalian brain. We must be aware, however, that it gives us only one part of a remarkable concert of memory processes that are possible and that have come into play in nervous systems of greater complexity and with more varied behavioral options. (pp. 321–322)

So important and basic a theme as unity versus diversity of basic processes involved in learning and memory was not, of course, resolved at this conference. But you will find cogent statements on both sides in these papers, and you will also find much data with which to evaluate the claims made on both sides.

40.2.1 Age as a variable

Age is another variable considered here. Byron Campbell and Xenia Coulter reviewed the intriguing problem of "infantile amnesia"—why children can't recall events from their first few years even though they are clearly learning at the time. Rats are also poor at recall during their early weeks, even though they learn simple material as rapidly as do adults. Guinea pigs, which unlike the rat are born relatively mature, do not show deficits of early memory. Thus it appears that capacities for learning and for memory show different rates of development, and this may provide useful clues to determining the neural mechanisms involved in learning and memory. The Scheibels pointed to early anatomical changes in neural circuits that could provide a basis for memory storage. Joseph Altman and Fatma Bulut considered the types of impairment that can be inflicted upon the developing nervous system; they also explored behavioral tests that can be employed to measure the capacities of very young rodents.

40.3 SHARED ASSUMPTIONS—AND LIMITATIONS

Certain widely shared assumptions may limit or restrict research at any given time. Such prevailing views undoubtedly exist even at a conference like this one, where many disciplines and points of view are represented. It is not easy to identify such assumptions, since they often go unstated and form an accepted common ground, but let me try to indicate one. (The reader may perceive others, and more will undoubtedly be seen later by hindsight.) I refer to the implicit assumption in many papers that THE problem of the neural basis of learning and memory is how information can be stored in neural terms. In other words, what is the form of the engram? An equally important problem is how stored information can be retrieved, in terms of neural processes. This may well be a more difficult problem than that of storage, especially since few investigators have addressed the question or seem to have a handle on it. A few of the participants did consider or allude to the problem of retrieval (Rozin; Arbib, Kilmer, and Spinelli; Quartermain). What happens in neural terms when information cannot be retrieved on one occasion, although it can on a subsequent occasion? If we knew, perhaps we could uncover rich stores of hidden memories.

40.4 MULTIDISCIPLINARY RESEARCH— PROBLEMS AND POTENTIALITIES

The contribution of many disciplines to this research has meant a powerful and multipronged attack. But such an attack is not without its own problems. Many of us do benefit in our research from techniques developed in sister disciplines, but there is usually a time lag in such borrowings, and sometimes one field will be using techniques that have been superseded in another. The group that gathered for this conference was obviously a select group of researchers in its willingness to cohabit for a week to try to teach each other, and perhaps even to learn. But even here there were some traces of nervousness and unease, and some cases of clear misunderstandings. The friendly interaction and informal exchanges were, I think, helpful in clearing the air. Some of these problems between disciplines can be alleviated by the understanding that many of us are really working at different levels of analysis, as Herbert Simon expressed so clearly in his paper. To quote just one sentence, "In this world there is need for chemistry as well as physics, biology as well as chemistry, and information-processing psychology as well as physiological psychology." Solving problems at one level does not necessarily solve them at another, although it should provide help and encouragement.

One of the bywords of the conference—John Garcia was the person to introduce it—was that most researchers early learn their own song, like the Oregon junco, and are then incapable of learning any other song, and maybe even any other dialect. Hopefully, part of the result of conferences such as this one will be to encourage further interdisciplinary collaboration. Several members of our group already do move easily among different levels and disciplines. It seems to me that in reading some of the chapters of the conference, it is rather hard to tell whether the author is a psychologist, a zoologist, or a physiologist. If many of these types of learning can interact within one skull, this is obviously advantageous. We might think, too, about training students who will be capable of fruitful interdisciplinary exchange as well as having a firm basis in their own discipline. That is, how can we help to prepare investigators who will join the chorus as well as singing their own song? This may be a tall order, but it is vital; as Hallowell Davis put it at another meeting, "We're down on what we're not up on."

40.5 LEVELS OF ANALYSIS

Several of the disciplines represented here work at different levels of analysis. This suggests that a useful alternative way to summarize or at least to outline the themes of this conference is in terms of the levels of the phenomena being considered and the scope or precision of the questions being asked. As Herbert Simon pointed out in his paper, "There are numerous examples in modern science of the need for multiple explanations of complex phenomena at different levels of fineness of detail." Arnold Leiman and I have prepared Table 40.1, which attempts to indicate some of the levels of analysis employed at this conference, from purely behavioral descriptions of learning and memory to the study of synaptic plasticity in cultures of nerve cells. Along with each level are shown typical questions being asked and the names of some participants who took up questions at the various levels. Like most classificatory schemes, this one relies on individual judgments, and different but equally useful alternatives could undoubtedly be prepared. This is probably not exactly the table that Simon would have drawn up, nor may all those named agree with their location in the table; but the scheme may be helpful to the reader, and it can be used to bring out certain features that have not yet been commented upon and to reinforce some other points that have been mentioned.

It appears that the fullest available treatments are at the top level, that of behavioral description. Most individuals restrict their work to a single level or to adjacent levels of analysis. Simultaneous work is going on relatively independently at the different levels, often with little mutual knowledge or interaction. The long-run goal is to discover the rules or transformations that permit translation from one level of analysis to another. Accomplishing this is as formidable as it is desirable. A major purpose of our conference and of its publication is to foster and facilitate work in this direction.

40.6 APPLICATIONS OF RESEARCH ON NEURAL BASES OF LEARNING AND MEMORY

Application of this research is the final topic we should consider in this summary. The reports at this conference have hewed quite closely to the level of research and conceptualization, with little explicit attention to applications. Most of us are convinced that our work will eventually lead to human betterment, but we rarely take time to develop this theme. It therefore seems appropriate for me to put a few of our social concerns on the record briefly at this point. Among the major contributions to be expected from advances in this kind of research are methods of preventing the decline of learning and memory in older people and the retardation of learning in young people, and techniques to help cases of decline or retardation when they do occur. Studies in this area should lead to means of aiding recovery of function after damage to the brain caused by accident or disease. They should also contribute to education by providing better understanding of the basic processes involved. One can foresee, for example, a clear mandate for promoting early experiences that will make children most capable of efficient later learning. Understanding the neural bases of learning should eventually improve the diagnosis and overcoming of difficulties in learning. It should prevent establishment of permanent sensory defects by eliminating deficient or distorted early experience, as, for example, in cases of astigmatism or hearing impairments. As well as these specific applications that we can foresee, I think that we promote others by fostering sensitivity to this area of learning and memory among our own students. We can keep such human problems before our students, as well as preparing them in their own specialized fields.

The question of communicating with the public cannot be separated from the question of applications of research. We have obligations there, certainly—obligations to the educated public to respond to their general curiosity, obligations to the public who in the long run foot the bill for the interesting research to which we are devoted, obligations to prepare our fellow citizens to make informed policy choices about education and about forms of clinical treatment. It is certainly our ongoing responsibility to communicate our research, and to try to do this in such a way as to prevent misuse of our findings, to prevent misunderstanding, and to prevent attempts to use biological shortcuts to solve long-term social problems. We are fortunate that at this conference we did not have to bear the whole brunt of communication with the public ourselves, many of us not having as much skill or experience in that area as would be desirable. Luckily we were able to recruit Irving Bengelsdorf to prepare a public account of our conference. The notebooks that he filled all during the week were the basis for an informative press release and brochure distributed by the National Institute of Education. We have also communicated at other levels through this conference. To our professional colleagues we present this volume as a statement of the art as it exists at this time. To the members of the National Institute of Education and of other institutes and foundations who spent the week with us at Asilomar, we have also presented a picture of current research and of future prospects. NIE has sponsored this conference because it is defining its own policy of research support in this area and needs the informed background of communication with researchers.

To conclude, it seems to me that a feeling of progress and optimism has pervaded our discussions, even as we acknowledge the problems that we still have to face. This is in strong contrast to the situation in 1950 when Lashley wrote his scathing paper "In Search of the Engram." Lashley, having apparently demolished all existing theories of biology of memory, including his own, was almost ready to conclude that learning was in fact impossible. Agranoff has stated that Lashley subjected the area to such an overkill that for years others were discouraged from entering the field. It is the same Lashley, of course, who was unable by techniques available to him to find any important deficits in split-brain animal preparations and who concluded wryly that apparently the corpus callosum was there just to hold the two hemispheres together mechanically. There has been progress since that time. Michael Gazzaniga has shown us how far psychologists have gone beyond Lashley's despair. I believe that some current researchers will be successful in finding engrams, if not The Engram. Meanwhile, others will have found ways of investigating how the engram is retrieved, and new problems will have been perceived. An end to the process of discovery cannot be foreseen, but many applied questions will undoubtedly be solved along the way, leading to enhancement of human capacities to learn and remember and to understand.

TABLE 40.1

Levels of analysis of learning and memory and the neural processes involved: Some investigators and some typical questions

A. Behavioral Descriptions of Learning and Memory (Rescorla and Holland; Manning; Garcia; Riley)

How do learning and memory occur? That is, what are adequate formal descriptions of stimulus conditions or manipulations under which learning occurs? What are the typologies of behaviors that allow us to infer learning and memory?

What rules relate changes of behavior to stimuli and to the events intervening between presentations of stimuli?

How do adaptive specializations that have occurred during evolution constrain or limit learning and memory? Can an ethological analysis of the behavior of a particular species in its environmental niche lead us to predict features of its learning and memory, including novel or unusual forms of adaptiveness?

B. Formal Systems Approaches to Learning and Memory (Block Diagrams) (Simon; Riley; Arbib, Kilmer, and Spinelli; Cowan)

What hypothetical processes could account for the observed features of learning and memory? The range of efforts extends from rather general descriptions to formal mathematical or network specifications to hardware devices.

C. Molar or General Neural Processes (Rose, Hambley, and Haywood; Flood and Jarvik; Dunn; Quartermain; Kety; McGaugh and Gold; Chorover; Bloch)

Are there generalized chemical processes occurring in all or many cells and underlying learning and memory? Are there systemic or regional chemical modifications that mediate learning and memory?

What are the time dependencies of such processes? (This question also goes under the name of "consolidation of memory.")

Similar questions are asked about molar anatomical and electrophysiological events that may encode memories.

D. Regional Localization of Neural Processes Involved in Learning and Memory (Rozin; Signoret and Lhermitte; Gazzaniga; Isaacson; Lynch; McGaugh and Gold)

Are certain regions of the brain differentially involved in learning and memory? What can be learned about regional brain functions in learning and memory from study of brain injury or brain disease in human beings? Are some processes revealed more clearly when the brain is "simplified" or "reduced" by injury? Can tests of learning and memory aid in differential diagnoses of brain injury and in establishing programs of reeducation?

Utilizing the advantages of animal experimentation (e.g., precise location of lesions, opportunities for repetitive testing and for control of environment, accurate comparisons with control animals), what can be learned about regional functions of the brain in learning and memory? Can the bases of compensation and recovery after brain lesions be determined?

E. Changes in Synapses and in Neural Circuits as Bases of Learning and Memory (Rutledge; Raisman; Moore; the Scheibels; Greenough; Bennett; Pettigrew)

Can evidence be found for development or changes in complex neural circuits that could underlie memory in adult as well as in young individuals? How can observed neural changes be tested for relations to learning and memory?

F. Use of Simpler Systems for Detailed Study of Neural Processes in Learning and Memory (Krasne; Davis; Rowell; Eisenstein; Sokolov; Strumwasser; Nelson and Christian; Mandel; Seil and Leiman)

Can synaptic changes be identified that account for examples of learning and memory in simpler systems? Can simpler organisms, parts of organisms, or tissue preparations be found in which the synaptic processes underlying learning and memory can be identified exhaustively? Using these simpler systems, can one develop a molecular biology of learning?

G. Study of Learning, Memory, and Neural Changes in Developing Subjects (Campbell and Coulter; Altman and Bulut; Greenough; Bennett; the Scheibels; Seil and Leiman; Pettigrew; Spinelli)

This is not a separate level of analysis but represents a different approach which can be studied at a number of levels including behavioral, regional, network, and cellular.

Can a developmental perspective help to solve questions about neural processes involved in learning and memory, either because of the relative simplicity of younger organisms or because asynchronies of growth help to separate out factors that seem to be inextricably entwined in the adult?

List of Authors

Professor Joseph Altman
Department of Biological Sciences
Purdue University
West Lafayette, IN 47907

Professor Michael Arbib
Department of Computer and Information Science
Center for Systems Neuroscience
University of Massachusetts
Amherst, MA 01002

Dr. Edward L. Bennett
Laboratory of Chemical Biodynamics
Lawrence Berkeley Laboratory
University of California, Berkeley
Berkeley, CA 94720

Professeur Vincent Bloch
Laboratoire de Physiologie Nerveuse
Département de Psychophysiologie
Centre National de la Recherche Scientifique
91190 Gif-sur-Yvette, France

Dr. Fatma G. Bulut
Department of Biological Sciences
Purdue University
West Lafayette, IN 47907

Professor Byron A. Campbell
Department of Psychology
Princeton University
Princeton, NJ 08540

Professor Stephan Chorover
Department of Psychology
Massachusetts Institute of Technology
Cambridge, MA 02139

Dr. Clifford N. Christian
Behavioral Biology Branch
National Institute of Child Health and Human
    Development
Bethesda, MD 20014

Professor Xenia Coulter
Department of Psychology
Princeton University
Princeton, NJ 08540

Professor Jack D. Cowan
Department of Biophysics and Theoretical Biology
University of Chicago
Chicago, IL 60637

Professor William J. Davis
The Thimann Laboratories
University of California, Santa Cruz
Santa Cruz, CA 95064

Professor Adrian J. Dunn
Department of Neuroscience
University of Florida
College of Medicine
Gainesville, FL 32601

Professor E. M. Eisenstein
Department of Biophysics
Michigan State University
East Lansing, MI 48823

Dr. James F. Flood
Department of Psychiatry
University of California, Los Angeles
Los Angeles, CA 90024

Professor John Garcia
Department of Psychology
University of California, Los Angeles
Los Angeles, CA 90024

Professor Michael S. Gazzaniga
Department of Psychology
State University of New York at Stony Brook
Stony Brook, NY 11790

Dr. Paul Gold
Department of Psychobiology
University of California, Irvine
Irvine, CA 92650

Professor William T. Greenough
Department of Psychology
University of Illinois
Champaign, IL 61820

Mr. John Hambley
Department of Behavioral Biology
Research School of Biological Sciences
Australian National University
Canberra, Australia

Mr. Jeff Haywood
Department of Biochemistry
University of Leeds
Leeds, United Kingdom

Dr. Peter Holland
Department of Psychology
Yale University
New Haven, CT 06510

Professor Robert L. Isaacson
Department of Psychology
University of Florida
Gainesville, FL 32601

Professor Murray E. Jarvik
Department of Psychiatry
University of California, Los Angeles
Los Angeles, CA 90024

Professor Seymour S. Kety
Department of Psychiatry
Harvard Medical School and
Massachusetts General Hospital
Boston, MA 02114

Dr. William L. Kilmer
Department of Computer and Information Science
Center for Systems Neuroscience
University of Massachusetts
Amherst, MA 01002

Professor Franklin B. Krasne
Department of Psychology
University of California, Los Angeles
Los Angeles, CA 90024

Professor Arnold L. Leiman
Department of Psychology
University of California, Berkeley
Berkeley, CA 94720

Dr. Michael S. Levine
Department of Psychiatry
University of California, Los Angeles
Los Angeles, CA 90024

Professeur F. Lhermitte
Neurologie et Neuropsychologie
I.N.S.E.R.M. U 84
Hôpital de la Salpêtrière
47 blvd. de l'Hôpital
75634 Paris, Cedex 13, France

Professor Gary Lynch
Department of Psychobiology
University of California, Irvine
Irvine, CA 92650

Professeur Paul Mandel
Centre de Neurochimie
11 rue Humann
67085 Strasbourg, France

Professor Aubrey Manning
Department of Zoology
University of Edinburgh
Edinburgh 9, Scotland

Professor James L. McGaugh
Department of Psychobiology
University of California, Irvine
Irvine, CA 92650

Professor Robert Y. Moore
Department of Neurosciences
School of Medicine
University of California, San Diego
La Jolla, CA 92037

Dr. Phillip G. Nelson
Behavioral Biology Branch
National Institute of Child Health and Human
    Development
Bethesda, MD 20014

Professor John D. Pettigrew
Division of Biology 216–76
California Institute of Technology
Pasadena, CA 91109

Professor David Quartermain
Departments of Neurology and Physiology
New York University School of Medicine
550 1st Avenue
New York, NY 10016

Dr. Geoffrey Raisman
Laboratory of Neurobiology
National Institute for Medical Research
The Ridgeway, Mill Hill
London NW7 1AA, England

Professor Robert A. Rescorla
Department of Psychology
Yale University
New Haven, CT 06510

Professor Donald A. Riley
Department of Psychology
University of California, Berkeley
Berkeley, CA 94720

Professor Steven P. R. Rose
Department of Biology
The Open University
Milton Keynes, United Kingdom

Professor Hugh F. Rowell
Department of Zoology
University of California, Berkeley
Berkeley, CA 94720

Professor Mark R. Rosenzweig
Department of Psychology
University of California, Berkeley
Berkeley, CA 94720

Professor Paul Rozin
Department of Psychology
University of Pennsylvania
Philadelphia, PA 19104

Professor L. T. Rutledge
Department of Physiology
University of Michigan Medical School
Medical Science Building
Ann Arbor, MI 48108

Dr. Arnold B. Scheibel
Dr. Mila Scheibel
Department of Anatomy & Psychiatry
Center for Health Sciences
University of California, Los Angeles
Los Angeles, CA 90024

Dr. Fredrick J. Seil
Department of Neurology
Veterans Administration Hospital
Palo Alto, CA 94304

Dr. J.-L. Signoret
Neurologie et Neuropsychologie
I.N.S.E.R.M. U 84
Hôpital de la Salpêtrière
47 blvd. de l'Hôpital
75634 Paris, Cedex 13, France

Professor Herbert A. Simon
Department of Psychology
Carnegie-Mellon University
Schenley Park
Pittsburgh, PA 15213

Professor Eugene N. Sokolov
Department of Psychology
Moscow State University
Prospect Marxa 18
Moscow, U.S.S.R.

Dr. D. Nico Spinelli
Department of Computer and Information Science
Center for Systems Neuroscience
University of Massachusetts
Amherst, MA 01002

Professor Felix Strumwasser
Division of Biology
California Institute of Technology
Pasadena, CA 91109

Other Participants in the Conference

Dr. Alun Anderson
Department of Zoology
Oxford University
Oxford OX1 3QX, England

Dr. Jacob Beck
Program Director for Psychobiology
National Science Foundation
Washington, D. C. 20550

Professor Seymour Benzer
Division of Biology
California Institute of Technology
Pasadena, CA 91109

Dr. James H. Brown
Program Director, Neurobiology
National Science Foundation
Washington, D. C. 20550

Dr. Jerry Daniels
Division of Biology 216–76
California Institute of Technology
Pasadena, CA 91109

Dr. Sam Deadwyler
Department of Psychobiology
University of California, Irvine
Irvine, CA 92650

Dr. Alben Dunham
Carnegie Corporation
New York, NY

Dr. Pauline M. Field
Department of Human Anatomy
Oxford University
Oxford OX1 3QX, England

Dr. Christopher J. Frederickson
Department of Psychology
Carnegie-Mellon University
Schenley Park
Pittsburgh, PA 15213

Dr. Regina Groshong
Department of Psychology
California State University, Humboldt
Arcata, CA 95521

Dr. H. Thomas James
President
Spencer Foundation

875 N. Michigan Ave.
Chicago, IL 60611

Dr. Kenneth A. Klivington
Program Officer
Alfred P. Sloan Foundation
630 Fifth Ave.
New York, NY 10020

Mr. Andy Kramer
Department of Psychology
University of California, Los Angeles
Los Angeles, CA 90024

Dr. John M. Mays
Science Adviser
National Institute of Education
Washington, D. C. 20208

Dr. Peter Molnar
Department of Psychology
University of Florida
Gainesville, FL 32601

Dr. Morris Moscovitch
Department of Psychology
McGill University
Montreal, Canada

Dr. George J. Mpitsos
Hopkins Marine Station
Pacific Grove, CA 93950

Dr. Keith Murray
Division of Research Grants
National Institutes of Health
Bethesda, MD 20014

Mr. William Quinn
Division of Biology
California Institute of Technology
Pasadena, CA 91109

Dr. Howard Rees
Laboratories for Reproductive Biology
University of North Carolina
Chapel Hill, NC 27514

Professor Larry R. Squire
Department of Psychiatry
University of California, San Diego
La Jolla, CA 92037

Dr. Tom Tomlinson
Assistant Director for Basic Studies
National Institute of Education
Washington, D. C. 20208

Dr. Arthur Wise
Associate Director for Research
National Institute of Education
Washington, D. C. 20208

Name Index

Pages with reference citations are preceded by "cit."

Motta, M., cit., 318
Mountcastle, V. B., cit., 245, 249
Mowrer, O. H., cit., 174, 187, 442
Mpitsos, G. J., cit., 432, 434, 435,
437, 440, 445, 446
Mullan, J., cit., 41, 42
Müller, G. E., 196, 593–594; cit., 200,
561, 583
Mullins, Jr., R. F., cit., 257, 267
Munn, N. L., cit., 150
Murphy, J. M., 213; cit., 212
Murphy, M. R., cit., 571
Murphy, R. A., cit., 366
Murray, M. R., cit., 356, 362, 366,
376, 377, 390
Mushynski, W. E., cit., 263, 264, 312
Muzio, J. N., cit., 231
Myers, R. D., cit., 261
Myers, R. E., 530; cit., 529

Nachmias, J., cit., 112, 137, 139
Nachsohn, I., cit., 15
Nagy, Z. M., cit., 212, 213
Nakai, J., cit., 365, 366, 378
Nakamura, R. K., cit., 57, 58, 60
Nathan, P. W., cit., 20
Nauta, W. J. H., cit., 53, 244, 302, 571
Neale, J. H., cit., 486, 497
Neely, J. E., cit., 551
Negishi, K., cit., 244
Neilson, Jr., D. R., cit., 358, 409
Nelson, M. C., cit., 436, 441, 443, 448
Nelson, P. G., 355–374; cit., 330, 377,
381, 596
Netsky, M. G., cit., 229
Neumann, E., cit., 452
Newell, A., cit., 80, 81, 85, 86, 93
Nicholls, J. G., cit., 420
Nicholson, C., cit., 469
Nicholson, J. L., cit., 256
Nicol, E. C., cit., 378
Nicolson, G. L., cit., 470
Nielson, H. C., cit., 551
Nilsson, N. J., cit., 112, 117, 118
Nirenberg, M., cit., 368, 381, 382, 383
Nissen, C., cit., 382
Njus, D., cit., 473
Nobel, M. E., cit., 212, 220
Noble, E. P., cit., 423, 450
Noell, W. K., cit., 259
Norman, D. A., cit., 79, 86, 87
Norton, A. C., cit., 529
Nottebohm, F., cit., 121, 156
Novitski, E., cit., 441
Nowell, N. W., cit., 259
Nurnberger, J., cit., 443
Nyman, A. J., cit., 261, 262

Oatley, K., 137
Obersteiner, K., cit., 247
O'Brien, J., 272
O'Brien, J. H., cit., 359
O'Connor, N., cit., 15
Offutt, G. C., cit., 440

Ogura, H., cit., 359
Oh, T. H., cit., 367
Oja, S. S., cit., 297
Ojemann, G. A., cit., 24, 30, 51, 72
O'Keefe, J., cit., 576
O'Keefe, O., cit., 124
Okujava, V., cit., 575
Okun, L. M., cit., 357, 378
Olds, J., cit., 124, 125, 129, 200, 202, 203,
359, 445, 576
Olinski, M., cit., 112, 126, 127
Oliver, G. W. O., cit., 447, 449, 450
Oliver, J. M., cit., 471
Oliverio, A., cit., 325
Olson, M. I., cit., 366
Olver, R., cit., 16, 242, 246
Ommaya, A. K., cit., 14, 18
Ontkean, F. K., cit., 357, 378
Opfinger, E., cit., 152
Oplatka, A., cit., 452
Opuda, M. J., cit., 103
Orback, J., cit., 536, 538
Orgel, L. E., cit., 384
Orrego, F., cit., 356
Oscar-Berman, M., cit., 25, 50
O'Shea, M., cit., 465
Oshima, T., cit., 245
O'Steen, W. K., cit., 259
Ott, T., 488; cit., 487, 497
Ottoson, J. O., cit., 567
Overmier, J. B., cit., 186
Overton, D. A., cit., 523, 524

Pagano, R. R., cit., 258, 537
Paivio, A., cit., 70, 88
Pakula, A., cit., 432, 476
Palay, S. L., cit., 334, 337, 344, 345, 570
Palmer, G. C., cit., 341
Palmer, S. M., cit., 366
Pandya, D. N., cit., 129
Pantin, C. F. A., cit., 433
Paolino, R. M., cit., 258, 504, 550, 562
Papert, S., cit., 112, 118, 122–123
Papez, J. W., cit., 23, 51, 571
Papousek, H., 211, 219
Pappas, G. D., cit., 335, 344, 345
Paraskevopoulos, J., cit., 262
Paré, W. P., cit., 216
Parker, M. V., cit., 358
Parkinson, S. R., cit., 99
Parkman, J., cit., 89
Parks, T., cit., 99
Parnas, I., cit., 409, 469
Parnavalas, J. G., cit., 544, 545
Parr, W., cit., 451
Parsons, P. J., cit., 214, 221, 223
Pasik, P., cit., 529
Pasik, T., cit., 529
Patel, J. B., cit., 556, 585
Patten, B. M., cit., 11, 31
Patterson, M. M., cit., 268, 484
Patterson, P. H., cit., 357, 362, 367
Pauling, L., 79
Pavlidis, T., cit., 473

Pavlov, I. P., 165–189, 193, 440, 593;
cit., 409, 433, 439, 441, 475
Peacock, J. H., cit., 357, 362, 363
Pearlman, J. R., cit., 586
Pearson, K. G., cit., 447
Pease, D. C., cit., 246
Peeke, H. V. S., cit., 260, 268, 402, 431,
432, 433, 434, 448, 512, 553
Pelton, E. W., cit., 256
Penfield, W., cit., 22, 24, 41–42, 63, 68,
71, 568
Peper, K., cit., 365
Peretz, B., cit., 415, 432, 433, 434
Perez, R., cit., 112, 141
Perkins, Jr., C. C., cit., 223
Perkins, J. P., cit., 368
Perumal, R., cit., 313
Peters, A., cit., 243, 570
Peters, J., cit., 213
Peterson, E. R., cit., 362, 365, 377, 390,
396
Peterson, G. R., cit., 385
Peterson, L. R., cit., 27, 82, 99
Peterson, M. J., cit., 27, 82
Peterson, R. P., cit., 360, 361, 424, 449
Petit, T. L., cit., 528
Petrinovich, L., cit., 434, 526, 527
Petsche, H., cit., 243, 248
Pettigrew, J. D., 136, 288–289; cit., 134,
201, 255, 336
Pfaff, D. W., cit., 257, 318, 570
Pfaffman, D., cit., 571
Phillips, C. G., cit., 574
Phillips, L., cit., 6, 17, 22, 27, 31, 32, 34,
53
Phillis, J. W., cit., 385
Phoenix, C. H., cit., 257
Piaget, J., cit., 121
Pichichers, M., cit., 366
Pickel, V. M., cit., 344
Piercy, M., cit., 52, 71
Piéron, H., cit., 565
Pilar, G., cit., 420
Pilcher, C. W. T., cit., 306, 451
Pilzecker, A., 593–594; cit., 200, 561, 583
Pinel, J. P. J., cit., 569
Pinneo, J. M., cit., 432, 434, 435, 445
Pinsker, H., cit., 360, 415, 424, 432, 433,
434, 436, 437, 445, 452, 453
Pinsky, C., cit., 385
Pinto-Hamuy, T., cit., 526, 527, 528, 535
Pitres, A., cit., 51
Plaut, S. M., cit., 258
Ploog, D., cit., 118
Pohle, W., cit., 336
Polak, R. L., cit., 385
Pollen, D. A., cit., 112, 136
Polyanskii, V. B., cit., 575
Pomerat, C. M., cit., 365
Poo, M., cit., 471
Porter, K. L., cit., 214
Porter, R., cit., 245
Porter, R. W., cit., 359

Subject Index

Abdominal ganglion, sensitization and, 437

Accessory optic nucleus, visual tasks and, 529

Acetoxycycloheximide
habit strength and, 510
memory and, 490, 494, 497–498, 509
  recovery, 512, 513
norepinephrine and, 514

Acetylcholine
changes with training, 311, 449
excitatory postsynaptic potentials and, 355
membrane voltage and, 470
memory formation and, 502
muscle cell cultures and, 364
neuroblastoma cells and, 368
pacemaker cell and, 477–479
receptors, α-bungarotoxin and, 367–368
sensitivity
  colchicine and, 471
  innervation and, 470

Acetylcholinesterase
cell cultures and, 378, 379, 380
cortical
  enriched environment and, 281, 282, 285
  isolation and, 259, 264
  training and, 269
imprinting and, 304–305, 306
learning and, 449–450
neuroblastoma cells and, 368, 381, 382, 383, 384, 385
synaptic inhibition and, 469

Actinomycin D
circadian rhythm and, 473
denervated muscle and, 470
short-term memory and, 485–486

Action frame, information and, 111

Action potential(s)
of dorsal-root ganglion cells, 362
presynaptic, increased, 335–336
puromycin and, 451
of spinal-cord cells, 362
transmitter receptors and, 469, 470
transmitter release and, 468

Active avoidance. *See* Avoidance

Activity patterns, overcrowding and, 259

Adaptation
fatigue and, 138–139
spatial gratings and, 135–136
species and individual, 321, 323

Adenosine
amnesia and, 486
cyclic AMP and, 356

Adenosine 3′, 5′-monophosphate. *See* Cyclic adenosine monophosphate

Adenosine triphosphatase
neuroblastoma cells and, 383, 384
sodium pump, oubain and, 484

Adenosine triphosphate, cell cultures and, 379

Adenyl cyclase
brain, 325
imprinting and, 304

Adrenal gland
effect of isolation on weight of, 264
effect of overcrowding on weight of, 259

Adrenocorticosteroids. *See* Corticosteroids

Adrenocorticotropic hormone
amino acid incorporation and, 317–318
amygdala lesions and, 537
brain electrical activity and, 318
learning and, 318, 324, 325, 500, 501
memory retention and, 557
release of, 257

Aequorin, calcium and, 468

Affective states. *See* Emotional states

Aflatoxin B1, circadian rhythm and, 473

Afterdischarge, learning and, 114

Aftereffects
figural, 135
relaxation times, 139

Age
brain effects and, 267
complex environment effects and, 262
memory and, 597

Aging
of mammalian cell clones, 384
memory and, 599

Aggression
conditioning of, 153
isolation and, 258, 259
overcrowding and, 259

Agnosia, 41

Alarm calls, habituation to, 149

Alcohol dehydrogenase, cell cultures and, 378, 379

Alcoholism, amnesia and, 22, 23, 50, 51, 52, 54

Alexia
cerebral artery infarction and, 71
nature of, 9

Amino acid
incorporation
  learning and, 269
  stress and, 316–318
pools, levels of, 296
uptake, cyclic AMP and, 304

γ-Aminobutyric acid
changes in, learning and, 449

cultured cells and, 363
glial tumor cells and, 368

2-Aminoisobutyrate uptake, imprinting and, 304

Amnesia
anterograde, characteristics, 7
brain organization and, 9
duration, inhibition of protein synthesis and, 497–501
infantile, 209
  central-nervous-system development and, 227–231
  general neural processes, 225–228
  psychological processes, 222–225
  theories of, 210
motor skills in, 17
perceptual, 565–566
permanence, protein-synthesis inhibition and, 512–514
premorbid, temporal organization of, 18–22
progressive, order of memory function decay, 16
puromycin-induced, reversal of, 318
recovery from, 16
retrograde
  amygdala and, 554–555
  correlates of, 552–553
  factors affecting, 563
  gradients of, 549–552
  temporal characteristics of, 562–564

Amnesic syndromes
basic phenomena, 35
encoding process in, 70–71
fractionation of, 28–30
  consequences and implications, 30–31
introduction to, 5–8
neuropathology of, 22–25
neuropsychology of, 51–53
one or many?, 25–26
psychophysiological interpretations, 53–54
as pure short-term memory, 26–28
synthesis, 35–38
theories, attempts to resolve conflicts among, 33–35
theories about nature of psychological defect, 31
  consolidation block, 31
  encoding defect, 31–32
  retrieval disorder, 32–33

Amphetamine
amnesia and, 514
brain damage and, 524, 527, 531
consolidation and, 584
environmental effects and, 268

Amphetamine (*continued*)
  learning and, 450, 500, 504, 509
  norepinephrine and, 325
Amygdala
  circuit of Papez and, 23
  damage, behavior and, 524–525, 537
  epilepsy and, 41
  olfactory-bulb fibers and, 571, 573, 576
  subseizure electrical stimulation of, 553, 554–555, 556–557, 575, 576
Amyotrophic lateral sclerosis, trauma and, 10
Amytal test, memory storage and, 64
Analysis-by-synthesis, perception and, 111
Anarthria, language function and, 11
Anesthesia
  impaired behavior and, 315–316
  memory and, 18, 25
Animals
  amnesic syndromes, failure to obtain, 15–16, 36, 37
  information storage and memory storage in, 100–105
  trained, breakdown of, 197–198
Anisomycin
  intertrial interval and, 512
  memory formation and, 491–496, 500
  memory recovery and, 513
  norepinephrine synthesis and, 514
  as protein-synthesis inhibitor, 491–492
Annelids
  associative learning in, 150
  conditioning of, 439
  giant fibers of, reflexes and, 402–403
Anomia
  memory traces and, 33–34
  nature of, 9
Anoxia, amnesia and, 22
Anterior commissure, anterior limb, olfactory bulb and, 573
Antibodies
  acetylcholinesterase and, 383
  hippocampal protein, learning and, 300
  nerve growth factor, neuroblastoma cells and, 381
  protein S-100 and, 368
Antimitotic agents, neuron size and, 357
Ants, responses of, 194
Apes, memory capacity of, 14
Aphasia, verbal encoding and, 70
Aplysia
  abdominal ganglion, synaptic input of, 361
  conditioning of, 440, 444–445
    neuronal changes, 446
  egg-laying in, 435
  excitatory postsynaptic potentials in, 419, 437
  habituation in, 432–433, 434
    long-term, 424
  heterosynaptic facilitation in, 133–134
  learned changes, protein-synthesis inhibitors and, 423

learning in, 111
  reflexes of, 404, 412
    habituation and, 407, 415
      long-term sensitization, 409
  sensitization in, 415, 436–437, 438
  synaptic inhibition in, 469
Aplysia californica, circadian rhythm in, 471–473
Appetitive learning
  caudate stimulation and, 553, 564
  medial-reticular-formation stimulation and, 556
Appetitive performance
  environmental complexity and, 261, 262
  isolation and, 258
  overcrowding and, 259
Appetitive reinforcers, Pavlovian conditioning and, 186–187
Appetitive repertoire, learning and, 119–120
Applications of research, ix–xiii, 598–599
Approach behavior, juvenile memory and, 220
Arcuate sulcus lesions, retention deficit and, 534–535
Area inominata, olfactory bulb and, 573, 574
Arousal
  brain damage and, 527, 530
  cortisol and, 502
  drugs and, 524
  footshock and, 567–569
  information storage and, 583, 584, 585, 587–588
  memory recovery and, 514
  metabolite supply and, 304
  subseizure electrical brain stimulation and, 556, 557
Arthropods, conditioning of, 439–443
Asphyxia, memory consolidation and, 200
Association areas, lesions, memory and, 533–536
Associative learning
  cellular theories, 360–362
  cerebellar, 469
  definition, 438
  electrophysiological studies, 359–360
  evolution of, 150
  logical operations and, 149
  nonassociative learning and, 438–439
  paired stimuli and, 181
Astigmatism, visual-system development and, 288
Astrocytes, maturation of, 379
Attention
  selective, 97
  trainability and, 172
Auditory receptors, neutral signal and, 197
Autistic children, operant conditioning of, 199
Automata, theory of, 124

Autoshaping
  conditioning and, 183–184
  elicitation of, 149
Aversion procedure, taste stimulus and, 198
Aversions, age and memory for, 225
Aversive performance, overcrowding and, 259
Avoidance
  active
    amygdala lesions and, 537
    anisomycin and, 494–495
    cycloheximide and, 498
    diethyldithiocarbamate and, 499
    juvenile learning and, 214–215
    memory and, 221
  passive
    age and, 216–219, 221–222, 225
    anisomycin and, 492–493, 495–496
    cycloheximide and, 489–490, 498, 508, 512
    diethyldithiocarbamate and, 499
    pituitary peptides and, 318
    retention, cortical stimulation and, 550
Avoidance learning
  behavioral repertoire and, 152
  colchicine and, 366
  environmental complexity and, 261
  glycoprotein labeling and, 312
  reticular stimulation and, 584
  ribonucleic acid synthesis and, 300–301
  theories of, 186
  types of, 442–443
Avoidance performance, isolation and, 258, 259
Avoidance tasks
  amygdala stimulation and, 555, 556
  cortex stimulation and, 552–553
Avoidance training, effects on biochemical parameters, 300–301
Axon
  branches, training and, 333
  regeneration, 348, 349
  terminals, degeneration of, 345, 349, 350
Axon systems, maturity and direction of flow of, 250
Azaguanine, resistance of neuroblastoma cells to, 383

Babcock sentence, amnesia and, 7
Bait shyness
  anisomycin and, 496–497
  cycloheximide and, 490–491
  Garcia conditioning and, 441–442
Barbiturates
  consolidation and, 584
  state-dependent behavior and, 524
Barbiturate sleeping time, isolation effects, 259

622   SUBJECT INDEX

Learning (continued)
methodological considerations,
159–161
olfactory bulb and, 579
ontogenesis of
complex situations, 215–219
neonatal studies, 210–211
simple tasks, 211–215
performance and, 172
rate
for complex tasks, 215–219
cycloheximide toxicity and, 498
for simple tasks, 211–215
rote, cerebral artery infarction and,
71, 72
sensitization and, 438
"side effects" of, 305
stress-induced amino acid incorporation and, 316–318
studies of, model systems for, 161–163
theoretical approaches, 451–452
types of, 148–150
underlying cellular mechanisms of
biochemical hypothesis, 448–451
circuit-modification hypothesis, 448
reverberation hypothesis, 447–448
unitary nature of, 321–324
use-disuse hypothesis, 329–330
apical dendrites, 332
axon measurements, 333
dendritic spines, 332–333
electrophysiological responses,
330–332
observation limitations, 334
qualitative observations, 333–334
Learning sets, 453
Leech, segmental shortening reaction
in, 404
Lethargy, amygdaloid lesions and, 537
Leucine incorporation
environmental complexity and, 263–
264
learning and, 299
stress and, 316, 317
Leukocytes, colchicine effects, 471
Lidocaine, acetylcholine sensitivity and,
364
Light deprivation
neuronal effects of, 294
visual function and, 258
Limax, Garcia conditioning of, 442
Limbic system
amnesia and, 24, 25, 26
lesions, maze learning and, 531–532,
537–538
maturation of, 227
olfactory bulb and, 579
protein synthesis in, learning and,
299
stimulation, seizures and, 575
Limb innervation, colchicine and, 345
Limulus, lateral inhibition in, 135
Line-spread function, modulation
transfer function and, 135

Lipid synthesis
consequences of, 294–295
learning and, 306
Lithium
memory and, 484, 496
sodium uptake and, 383
Littermates, differences between, 266
Lobotomy
amnesia and, 25
recovery from, 30
Lobular giant movement detector
connections of, 467
input, 465
Locomotor activity, cycloheximide and,
508
Locus ceruleus
iris innervation and, 342
lesions, learning and, 325, 503
Locusts
anterior coxal adductor motoneuron,
firing rate, 410
behavioral hierarchy in, 435
dishabituation of, 418–419
instrumental conditioning of, 443
learning responses of, 405
Long-term memory
amnesia and, 28, 31, 32, 36, 37, 50
central-nervous-system development
and, 225–227
characteristics, 98
components of, 91–92
emergence in rat and man, 225
fixation and retrieval, 84–85
information processing and, 53–54
proactive inhibition and, 100
production-system model of, 93
short-term memory and, 9, 38, 84
slide-file analogy to, 111
word-list recall and, 12
Lysine incorporation
imprinting and, 302, 303–304
training and, 301, 313, 316
visual stimulation and, 296
Lysine vasopressin, avoidance training
and, 318

Macromolecular involvement in learning
inhibition of synthesis, 450–451
synthesis, 448–450
transport, 452
Magnesium
cyclic AMP and, 325
synaptic activity and, 365
Maintained-discrimination task, selective attention and, 101–103
Mammalian cell clones, aging of, 384
Mammals, autoshaping in, 149–150
Mammillary body
amnesia and, 23–24, 51, 52, 54
circuit of Papez and, 23
connections of, 53
maturation of, 227
Mammillothalamic tracts, effect of
damage to, 51, 524

Maple-syrup disease, demyelinization
and, 376
Marr synapse, 134
Mass action, memory and, 57–59, 110
Masturbation, split brain and, 62
Matching-to-sample task, animals and,
101, 103–104
Maturation
information-processing mechanisms,
224–225
motor and motivational, 236–238
neural, 238–240
species-specific behavior, 224
Mauthner cells, occurrence of, 464
Maze learning
amnesia and, 17–18
brain damage and, 531–533, 536
caudate stimulation and, 553
cycloheximide and, 509
environmental complexity and, 260–
261, 262, 267, 268, 284
hippocampus and, 70
by juvenile rats, 212
reticular stimulation and, 584, 587–
588
Medial forebrain bundle, effect of
lesions to, 325
Medial geniculate nucleus, optic-tract
axons and, 341
Melanocyte-stimulating hormone
amino acid incorporation and, 317, 318
memory and, 500
Membrane voltage, acetylcholine and,
470
"Memistors," 323
Memory
amnesia and age of, 21–22
in aneural systems, 163
biogenic amines and, 515–517
brain damage and, 525–540
categories of, 11
consolidation
electrical activity and, 200
time and, 227
early research on, 3–4, 593–596
echoic, 90
emotional state and, 322
equipotentiality and, 59
evolution of, 321–322
formation, RNA synthesis and, 497
intelligence and, 39
James's definition, 4
levels of analysis, 598–599
levels of function in, 16–18
mass action and, 57–59
mechanisms, enriched environment
and, 283–284, 285–286
methodological considerations, 159–
161
model, differential rearing and, 267–
268
model systems in study of, 161–163
modulation, posttrial electrical brain
stimulation and, 552–557

Memory (*continued*)
motivation and, 59–61
multidisciplinary research on, 597–598
nonassociative learning and, 438
nonverbal, right-temporal-lobe
damage and, 29–30
olfactory bulb and, 579
ontogenesis
juvenile studies, 219–222
neonatal studies, 219
perception and, 39–41
processes, unity of, 596–597
protein-synthesis inhibitors and, 488–
497
recently activated, behavior and, 115
recovery of, protein-synthesis inhibition
and, 512–514
research on neural bases, applications
of, 599–600
retrieval of, 195
ribonucleic acid and
inhibitors, 485–487
precursors, 487–488
special, automatic activities and, 246
storage
disruption by subseizure
stimulation, 553–556
facilitation by subseizure
stimulation, 556–557
transfer of, 451
See also Human memory; Long-term
memory; Short-term memory
Memory-scan reaction-time experiment,
101, 104–105
Memory traces, new learning and
activation of, 33–35
Mental retardation
demyelinization and, 376
memory and, 14–15
6-Mercaptopurine, amnesia and, 486
Mesencephalon
habituating units in, 358
rostral, contralateral cortex and, 330–
331
Metabolic rate, paradoxical sleep and,
588
Metacontrast
theories of, 565–566
time and, 565
Methylene blue, staining by, 334
α-Methylmannoside, neurite development and, 378
α-Methyl-*p*-tyrosine, memory and, 500,
516, 517
Metrazol, environmental effects and, 268
Meynert cells, pyramidal-cell dendrites.
and, 245
Mice
active-avoidance task, memory for,
493–495
effects of overcrowding on, 259
isolation syndrome and, 258, 259
jump-pole task, 495
maze reversal, 505–511

passive-avoidance task, 489–490,
492–493
strain comparison, 495
Microglia, reactive neurons and, 544
Microsomes, ribonucleic acid in, 313–314
Microtubules
colchicine and, 366
learning and, 448
neurite outgrowth and, 366
Midtemporal gyrus, memory and stimulation of, 21
Minor hemisphere, face recognition by,
40
Mitochondria
calcium and, 469
depression-prone synapses and, 420
glycoproteins, learning and, 269
ribonucleic acid in, 313–314
Mitral cells, firing, odors and, 574
Mitral valve, innervation after transplant, 343
Modulation transfer function 135, 137,
139
Molluscs, conditioning of, 439. *See also*
specific species
Monkeys
age and delayed responding in, 217
age and visual discrimination in, 215
coding of visual stimuli by, 201
environmental complexity and, 262
juvenile, learning in, 212, 213
memory in, 14
newborn, conditioning of, 211
sensory bias in, 150–151
Monoamine oxidase
cultures and, 377, 378
inhibitors
cell cultures and, 384
memory and, 513–514
performance and, 509
neuroblastoma cells and, 381
synapses and, 469
Monoamines, brain, isolation and, 259
Morphine, cell cultures and, 384–385
Morphological dynamics
in vitro studies, 365–367
in vivo studies, 364–365
Motivation
brain damage and, 522–523
memory and, 59–61, 557
neurobehavioral analysis of, 201–203
Motor activity
brain protein metabolism and, 303,
304, 306
dendrite-bundle development and, 242
environmental effects and, 283
Motor bias, learning and, 151
Motor deficiencies, age-related, 213, 217
Motor memory, development of, 16–17
Motor outputs, neurobehavioral analysis,
203
Motor patterns, specific, development of,
245
Motor skills, amnesia and, 35, 36

Movie cartoons, as memory model, 111
Müllerian mimicry, evolution and, 151
Multiple-memory hypothesis, evidence
against, 98–100
Multiple sclerosis, demyelinization induced by serum from, 376
Muscle
cells, nerve cell synapses and, 366
cultures, nerve explants and, 365–366
denervated, acetylcholine receptors
and, 470
reinnervation, competitive, 361
Myelin
cultured cells and, 362, 363
learning and, 452
Myelinization
age and, 229
of cerebellar explants, 393
of cerebral neocortex explants, 395
stimulation of, 376, 379
time and, 377

α-Naphtholesterases, cell cultures and,
379
Negative discrepancy, multiple stimuli
and, 178
Neocortex
destruction, habits and, 521
lesions
brightness-discrimination tasks,
525–528
mazes and, 531–533
multiple visual-memory systems,
528–530
pattern discrimination, 530–531
synaptosomes, membranes of, 471
See also Cortex
Neonates
learning capacity of, 210–211
memory studies, 219
reflexive behavior, inhibition of, 229–
230
Neostigmine, learning and, 450
Nereid worms
habituation in, 149
withdrawal reflex, 404
Nereis, learning by, 417
Nerve growth factor
dissociated cell cultures and, 378
dorsal-root ganglion cells and, 366
enzyme maintenance and, 378–379
explants and, 376
neuroblastoma cells and, 381
sympathetic ganglion cultures and,
362, 366
Nervous system
adult plasticity of, 336–337
explants, 376–377
hormonal and metabolic effects as "differential experience," 256–258
See also Central nervous system
Network predisposition
ethology and, 118–122
pretheory of, 122–124

Neural circuits, fixed or plastic, 202–203
Neural coding, multiple, 63–65
Neural learning, basic schemes
   perceptron and, 116–118
   without a teacher, 112–116
Neural models, perspective on, 109–112
Neural processes, circuit components, 464
Neural systems, morphological growth
   and increased use of, 334–335
Neurite motility, 366
Neuroanatomy, contributions of, 594–
   595
Neurobehavioral theory, 199–203
Neuroblastoma cells
   clonal cultures, 368, 380–381
     clonal and intraclonal heterogeneity,
      381–382
     differentiation, 381
     metabolic and molecular changes in
      differentiation, 382–384
   drug effects, 384–385
   electrophysiological studies, 368
   hybridization with L cells, 383–384
   muscle innervation by, 470
Neurochemistry, contributions of, 594–
   595
Neuroheuristic programming, active
   subsystems and, 110
Neurological processes and infantile
   amnesia, 225–231
Neuromuscular junctions
   synaptic function analysis and, 355
   vertebrate, depression at, 423
Neurons
   adrenergic, plasticity of, 341–344
   changes in, behavior and, 111
   crustacean, somata of, 423–424
   endogenous firing rate, alteration in,
     409–410
   impulses of, temporal information
     and, 471–473
   labeling of, visual stimulation and, 298
   plasticity of, ontogeny and, 307
   types of, neocortex explants and, 394–
     395
Neuronal models, in vitro, 362–363
Neuropathological approach, advantages
   of, 13
Neuropathology, amnesic syndromes
   and, 22–25
Neuropil synaptic organization,
   alteration of, 344
Neuropsychology, amnesic syndromes
   and, 51–53
Neurotoxin binding, receptor density
   modulation and, 367–368
Neurotransmitters
   environmental complexity and, 264
   lateral hypothalamus and, 201
   memory formation and, 502–505
   See also Transmitters
New learning, amnesia and, 34–35, 36
Nicotine
   avoidance learning and, 259

consolidation and, 584
   memory and, 502
Nissl substance, cell cultures and, 379
N-Nitrosomethylurea, glioma and, 384
Norepinephrine
   cyclic AMP and, 325, 356
   environment and, 264
   glial tumor cells and, 368
   neuroblastoma cells and, 382
   protein-synthesis inhibitors and, 514
   sympathetic ganglion cultures and,
     362
   training and, 514, 516
   unspecific afferents of cortex and, 324
Normetanephrine, neuroblastoma cells
   and, 382
Nucleotides
   changes with training, 311
   metabolism of, 316
Nucleus reticularis thalami, dendritic
   systems, 244–245
Nutrition
   amnesia and, 22
   brain development and, 294

Object discrimination, anisomycin and,
   495, 496–497
OCCAM memory model, 114–116
Octopamine, neuroblastoma and, 368
Octopus, visual system of, 111
Oculomotor defect, brain lesions and, 530
Odor
   affective association with, 323
   mitral-cell firing and, 574, 579
   pheromonelike, behavior and, 571
   See also Scent
Olfaction, mammalian adaptation and,
   570–571
Olfactory bulb
   anatomical features, 573–574
   changes in neuronal activity, 574
   isolated, plasticity in, 577–579
   sensitization and habituation
     experiments, 574–576
   unit activity, plasticity of, 576–577
Olfactory memory, amnesia and, 25
Olfactory nucleus, fibers to olfactory
   bulb, 573
Olfactory system of rodents, 571–574
Oligodendrocytes, differentiation of, 379
Operant conditioning
   classical conditioning and, 149
   reinforcement and, 187
Optic lobe, outputs of, 465
Optic nerve, circadian rhythm and, 471
Oregon junco, song learning by, 156
Orienting response, novel stimuli and,
   475
Orotic acid, incorporation into brain
   RNA, 316
Orthopteran movement-detector system,
   405
Ouabain, short-term memory and, 484
Overcrowding, effects of, 259–260

Overtraining, memory and, 536–537
Owl, habituation to, 149
Oxygen uptake
   in cell cultures, 379
   by neuroblastoma cells, 382

Pacemaker potential, habituation and,
   476–479
Pagurus striatus, learning by, 401–402
Pain response, age and, 224
Paradoxical sleep
   age and, 230–231
   memory consolidation and, 586–589
Parafascicular nucleus, adrenocorti-
   cotropic hormone and, 318
Pargyline
   cycloheximide-induced amnesia and,
     499, 500
   memory recovery and, 513, 517
   norepinephrine and, 504
Parietal lobe
   inferior, memory and, 9
   lesions, perception and, 69
Parietovisceral abdominal ganglion,
   circadian rhythm in, 471–472
Parsimony, learning and, 408–409
Passive avoidance. See Avoidance
Patterns, learning of, 114–115
Pattern discriminations, brain damage
   and, 530–531
Pavlovian conditioning. See Conditioning
Pavlovian relations, instrumental
   learning and, 185–187
Pemoline, as enhancer of learning, 450
Pentylenetetrazol, memory retention
   and, 557
Perception
   brain damage and, 523
   disorders, encoding and, 69
   memory and, 39–41, 111
Perceptive fields, visual cortex and,
   138–140
Perceptron model, 116–118, 126
Performance, brain damage and, 523
Perseveration, frontal-lobe damage and,
   39
Peterson-Peterson paradigm
   amnesia and, 27–28, 29
   nonverbal memory and, 29, 30, 31, 32
   short-term memory impairment and,
     38
Pheniprazine
   cycloheximide-induced amnesia and,
     499, 500
   memory and, 509, 513–514, 515, 517
Phenylethanolamine methyltransferase,
   learning and adrenal levels of, 503
Phenylketonuria, demyelinization and,
   376
Philanthus, learning by, 147
Phobias, illogic of, 120
Phormia
   conditioning of, 441, 446

Senility (*continued*)
  brain dissolution and, 10
Sensitization
  conditioning and, 150, 441
  definition of, 433, 436
  examples of, 436–437
  vs. learning, 438
  olfactory bulb and, 574–576
  repeated stimulus presentation and,
    168
  spinal-cord cultures and, 362
  underlying cellular mechanisms of,
    437–438
Sensory bias, learning and, 150–151
Sensory experience, differential, 258
Sensory inputs, neurobehavioral anal-
    ysis of, 201
Sensory stage, memory and, 9
Septal-area damage, behavior and, 525,
    531–532, 533, 537–538
Septal nuclear complex, innervation of,
    343, 349–350
Septum, subseizure electrical stimulation
    of, 554, 575
Serotonin
  environment and, 264
  memory and, 502–503, 505
  neuroblastoma cells and, 368, 381, 382
  reserpine and, 325
Sexual activity, isolation and, 258
Sexual arousal, imagery and, 62
Sexual behavior, cross-fostering and, 120
Shimbel synapse, modification of, 133
Shock-avoidance training, 188
Short-term memory
  acoustic nature of, 99
  amnesia and, 26–28, 31, 32, 35, 36–37,
    50, 53
  callosal section and, 58–59
  capacity of, 83–84, 85
  characteristics, 98
  physiological basis, 484–485
  production-system model of, 93–94
  right-temporal-lobe damage and, 29
  selective impairment of, 38–39, 70
  semantic encoding and, 99
  slide-box analogy, 111
  structure, 92–94
  visual, 99
  word-list recall and, 12
Shrimp. *See Leander*
Shuttlebox learning
  genetics and, 152
  necortical lesions and, 527
  organism structure and, 196–197
Sickness, reinforcement by, 151
Skill loss, brain damage and, 529
Skinner Box, 195
Sleep
  ontogenesis of, 230–231
  time, environmental complexity and,
    262–263
  See also Paradoxical sleep; Rapid-eye-
    movement sleep

Slide-box metaphor, for internal models,
    110, 111
Snail, associative learning by, 150
Social behavior, cross-fostering and, 120
Social experience, differential, effects of,
    258–260
Sodium
  action potentials and, 362
  channel, tetrodotoxin and, 367
  choline uptake and, 383
  neuroblastoma cells and, 368
  posttetanic augmentation and, 423
Song sparrows, song development in, 118
Sparrows, nonhabituation by, 120
Spatial avoidance, conditioned emotional
    response and, 213–214
Spatial gratings, adaptation and, 135–
    136
Species call, learning of, 155
Sperling paradigm, 82, 83
Spider, memory in, 438
Spinal cat, habituation and sensitization
    in, 358, 574–575
Spinal cord
  cultures of, 362, 366
  use-disuse hypothesis and, 330
Split-brain animals, performance of,
    57–58
Split-brain patients
  encoding process in, 70
  verbal processing in, 12, 13
Spreading depression, memory and, 565
Squirrel, learning by, 155
Stamina, overcrowding and, 259
Startle reflex, number of stimulus
    presentations and, 169
State, electroconvulsive shock
    and, 568–569
State-dependency, brain damage and,
    523–524
Stellate cells, synapses of, 248–249, 265
Stentor, habituation in, 432
Sternberg effect, image encoding and, 62
Stickleback
  habituation of, 149
  operant conditioning of, 149, 153
Stimulation, synaptic ultrastructure and,
    365
Stimulus
  equation for, 137
  external, behavior and, 115
  generalization
    age and, 215
    infantile amnesia and, 223–224, 227
    responses and, 168
  hedonic quality of, 202
  interaction of intrinsic with extrinsic,
    181–183
  intrinsic relations, 180–181
  multiple, conditioned response and,
    175–176
  nature of, conditioning and, 178–179
  onset and duration differences,
    182–183

spatial relations, 179–180
Stimulus-bound behaviors, 201, 202
Stimulus-contingent tasks, age and,
    220–221
Stimulus presentation (noncontingent)
  assessment procedures and outcomes,
    167–168
  latent inhibition and habituation,
    170–172
  sample data, 168–170
Stimulus-response-reinforcement theory,
    failings of, 196–199
Storage deficit, protein-synthesis inhibi-
    tion and, 514–515
Strategy
  changes, behavior and, 94
  encoding process and, 67–68
  free-recall learning and, 98
Stress
  amino acid incorporation and, 316–318
  behavioral responsiveness and, 257
  brain weight and, 267, 283
  isolation and, 258, 264
  metabolite supply and, 304
Striate-area lesions, visual tasks and, 531,
    533
Stroke, memory reconstruction after, 63
Strychnine
  consolidation and, 584, 585
  environmental effects and, 268
Substantia nigra
  subseizure electrical stimulation of,
    553
  visual memory and, 529
Subsystems, isolated or released, 12
Succinate dehydrogenase, cultures and,
    377, 378
Sulfatide synthesis, myelinization and,
    376
Sun-compass reaction, honeybee
    learning and, 154
Superficial cortical response, evocation
    of, 250
Superior cervical ganglion
  axon terminals in, 348–349
  denervation and reinnervation, 349
  explants, synapse formation by, 366
Superior colliculus
  ablation, retinal input and, 340–341
  repetitive stimuli and, 358
  visual tasks and, 529
Suprasylvian gyrus, stimulation of, 330,
    331
Surgery, amnesia and, 22, 24
Symbols, information-processing psychol-
    ogy and, 80, 85
Sympathetic ganglion
  cultures of, 357, 362
  dopamine and, 325
  synaptic function analysis and, 355
Synapses
  alteration of, time and, 273
  altered transmission at, 412
  chemical, differences between, 420